Pathologies

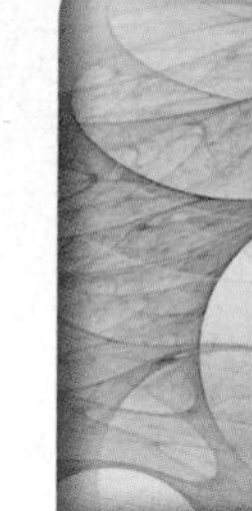

T

U

V

W

A Massage Therapist's Guide to Pathology

FIFTH EDITION

Ruth Werner, LMP, NCTMB

Wolters Kluwer Health | Lippincott Williams & Wilkins

Acquisitions Editor: Kelley Squazzo
Product Manager: Linda G. Francis
Editorial Assistant: Courtney Shell
Design Coordinator: Steven Druding
Manufacturing Coordinator: Margie Orzech
Prepress Vendor: SPi Global

Printed in China

Library of Congress Cataloging-in-Publication Data

Werner, Ruth (Ruth A.)
A massage therapist's guide to pathology / Ruth Werner.
p. ; cm.
Includes bibliographical references and index.
ISBN 978-1-60831-910-7
I. Title.
[DNLM: 1. Massage. 2. Diagnosis, Differential. WB 537]
615.8′22—dc23

2011040201

LWW.com

9 8 7 6 5 4 3 2

CCS0413

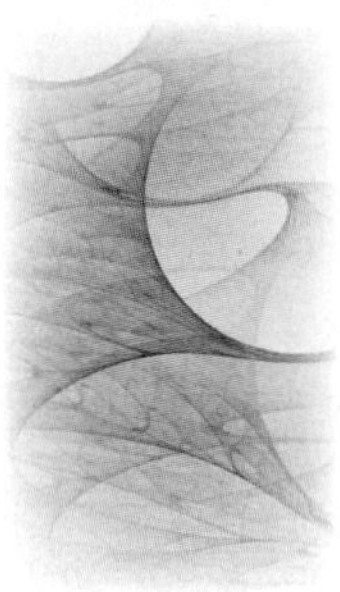

This book is and will forever be dedicated to
the memory of my grandmother, Dora Charak Beckhard,
who probably never got a massage in her life—
but she sure could have used one.

Foreword

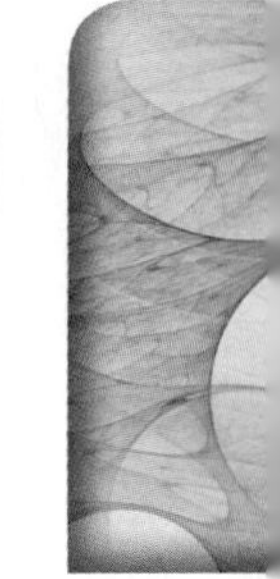

The massage therapy profession is not the same as what it was, even just a few short years ago. Regardless of the work environment where a massage therapist practices, he or she is likely to encounter a wide diversity in clientele who may present with all kinds of different health complications. Consequently, the educational preparation a massage therapist needs is constantly evolving as well.

In the years since this book first appeared on the market, the explosion of accessible information about medical pathologies has been enormous. While there is no question that this increased access to valuable clinical information is a great benefit, there is also a serious challenge for the consumer or student to evaluate high-quality information. The hallmark of a great textbook is one that can both deliver a great quantity of content and help the reader become a discerning evaluator of quality information at the same time. That is no easy task, and with each edition, Ruth Werner has demonstrated an excellent ability to accomplish this challenge.

An example of this improvement in accessibility comes in the new "At a Glance" sections where practitioners can rapidly and easily find concentrated information about special topics of interest. In many cases, the topics presented in these sections are the key questions a practitioner needs immediate information about with a presenting client challenge.

With so many different and exceptional books available on the market today, it can be difficult for the practitioner to determine what should reside in his or her clinical library. Because most clinical books have new editions every few years, there is always the question about what is brought forth in a new edition. However, pathology is one subject where keeping current with the most recent research is a crucial aspect of relevance for the text. Werner's work leading the Massage Therapy Foundation gives her a particular advantage in recognizing the crucial importance of staying current with research findings and implementing them into her writings.

A great example in this text is a new section devoted specifically to conditions affecting fascia. Worldwide interest in the role of fascia in musculoskeletal disorders has blossomed in recent years, particularly as a result of the Fascia Research Congress held every two years. Inclusion of this information in the new edition highlights the necessity of massage practitioners knowing much more about the crucial role played by fascia in many pain complaints.

One of the key challenges of teaching clinical practitioners in every field is helping them move past information they learn in basic training as pure content. In professional practice, the individual is often faced with gray areas that are not answered by simple content knowledge alone. Clinical reasoning and critical thinking skills are crucial to prepare practitioners for the realities they face in clinical practice.

In this edition, discussions of massage are framed as risks and benefits. This is a key issue of importance, as we must teach practitioners that decisions are not simply black-and-white, but evidence must be weighed to make appropriate decisions. Spelling out the use of massage in this fashion with risks and benefits discussed is a great way to encourage the development of these key reasoning skills that are so critical.

When asked to write this foreword, there is another reason that I agreed without hesitation. In the past two decades, I have spent a great deal of effort studying education and how to teach well. There are a handful of educators in our field who clearly stand out above others. From the first time I saw Ruth Werner present, I recognized her as having that great gift that makes an outstanding educator.

Through each edition of her book, I see her infuse that same energy and skill of making it easy, enjoyable, and stimulating to learn about pathology. The ability to take a challenging subject like pathology and make it fascinating for massage therapy students is a clear sign of how skilled and valuable her contributions to our profession have been. This is one book where I'll always want the most recent edition so I can keep inspired and learn as much as possible from what she so generously shares with us all.

Whitney Lowe
Sisters, OR
2011

About the Author

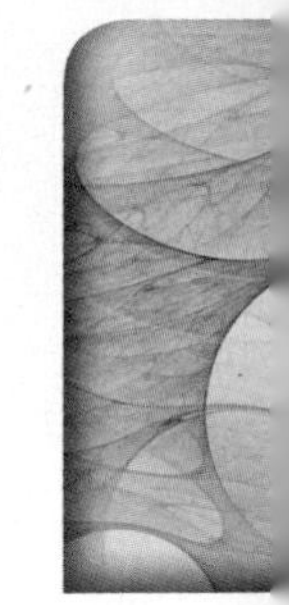

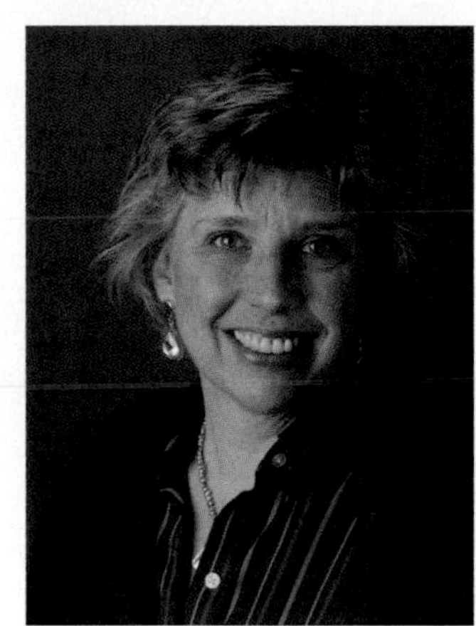

Ruth Werner is a retired massage therapist and lifelong educator with a passionate interest in the role of massage and bodywork for people who struggle with illness. She began teaching while she was still a student of massage and discovered she has a gift for taking complex topics and breaking them down to easily assimilated pieces so that learners can rebuild those ideas in their own framework. Her love of teaching has been a center-point of her career, and in 2005, Ruth was honored with the Jerome Perlinski Council of Schools Teacher of the Year award.

Ruth wrote what became the framework for *A Massage Therapist's Guide to Pathology* as a resource for a massage school in 1993. The first edition of this text was published in 1998. Her second book, *Disease Handbook for Massage Therapists*, was published in 2010.

In addition to keeping *A Massage Therapist's Guide to Pathology* up to date, Ruth is a columnist for *Massage and Bodywork* magazine and is a frequent guest writer in other trade journals.

Her success as a writer has allowed her to devote time and energy to many volunteer efforts. Ruth has served on committees for the American Massage Therapy Association, the National Committee for Therapeutic Massage and Bodywork, the Federation of State Massage Therapy Boards, and the Department of Professional Licensing for the state of Utah. Her most consuming volunteer passion has been to serve first as a Trustee and then as President for the Massage Therapy Foundation: a 501 (c) 3 public charity dedicated to advancing the knowledge and practice of massage therapy by supporting scientific research, education, and community service.

In 2010, Ruth and her family fulfilled a lifelong dream of moving to the Oregon Coast. Now she can see and hear and smell the ocean as she writes.

Preface

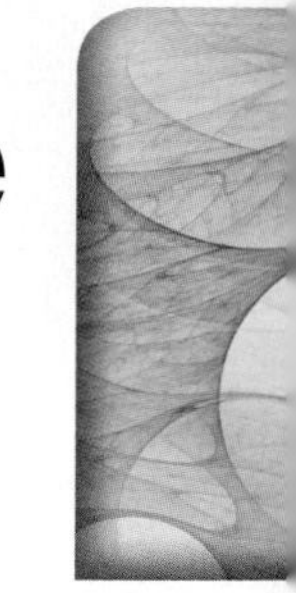

When I began work on the first version of *A Massage Therapist's Guide to Pathology*, I had absolutely no idea of what it would become. For me, it was a labor of love: the chance to explore more about human function and the miracles that occur when injuries heal and sicknesses abate. The fact that it found an unexpectedly eager audience was a huge and happy surprise, and keeping this text at the forefront for pathology education for massage therapists has become my life's joyful calling.

It is always my intent to invite my readers and students into an environment that is friendly without being trivial, clear-cut without being simplistic, and sensitive not only to the struggles that we and our clients may live with but also to the complexities of compassionate and professional decision making in that context.

Ultimately, the study of massage in the context of pathology can be reduced to some basic concepts:

- How does the human body work when it is healthy?
- How does a disease or condition change that process?
- Where does massage or bodywork best enter that dance?

The last question acknowledges that the role of massage therapy for people who live with diseases or disorders simply *cannot* be rubber-stamped to say one condition always indicates massage and another always contraindicates it. The answer to "Is massage safe for this person?" is *always* "It depends." It is the therapist's job to determine what it depends *on*. What are the variables in any given situation? One way to do that is to answer these questions:

- What are the best possible benefits massage can offer this person?
- What are the possible risks?
- How can the therapist use his or her skills to create a session to get the best benefits while avoiding the risks?

Organization of This Text

As in the fourth edition, Chapter 1 is an introduction to basic concepts in pathology, and Chapter 12 focuses only on cancer. Chapters 2 to 11 are dedicated to specific body systems.

Within Chapters 2 to 11, each "Condition" article discusses a condition or set of conditions in an organized and predictable format: *In Brief* boxes provide a thumbnail sketch of the condition under discussion. Then each topic is addressed with the following headings: *Definition, Etiology, Subtypes, Signs and Symptoms*, and *Massage*. All of the articles have been thoroughly updated for this edition.

Changes to This Edition

The book has been reorganized somewhat, as follows:

- You'll find a section on Fascial Disorders in Chapter 3 (Musculoskeletal System Conditions)
- All autoimmune diseases have been moved into Chapter 6 (Lymph and Immune System Conditions)
- Conditions that are rare, or rarely seen in an acute form, have been shortened and moved to Appendix C, Extra Conditions at a Glance. This allows the discussion of more material in the same amount of space as the previous edition.
- A more streamlined presentation of material that is particularly relevant to massage therapy students.

Text Features

- ***Chapter Objectives:*** This study tool at the beginning of the chapter serves as a guide to both students and instructors working with this text.
- ***In Brief boxes:*** Appearing at the beginning of each condition, these boxes provide a "nutshell" version of the article.
- ***New Articles:*** New, fully developed articles have been added, including adhesive capsulitis, Huntington disease, joint replacement surgery, polycystic kidney disease, and several others.
- ***Risks, Benefits, Options Tables:*** This brand-new feature is a highly accessible table appearing at the end of each condition article, in the Massage section. This simple table provides information on potential risks and benefits of massage therapy and bodywork, and a brief look at special options where they are applicable. (A further discussion of modality recommendations is included in the online resources.)
- ***Sidebars***: This popular feature discusses peripheral issues relating to conditions or gives more detailed information.
- ***Compare and Contrast Charts***: These charts lay out aspects of similar conditions side by side, so that readers may better understand where they overlap and where they diverge.
- ***Case Histories:*** These are the stories of people who live with diseases and disorders and are presented to help readers appreciate how these abstract ideas lead to concrete realities.
- ***Notable Cases:*** To help "put a face" on the conditions discussed in this text, this new feature names athletes, political leaders, and other public figures who have been affected by the condition under discussion.
- ***Chapter Review Questions:*** These appear at the end of every chapter. Answers may be found online at http://thePoint.lww.com/Werner5e.
- ***Glossary:*** List of key terms that appear in boldface throughout the text, along with pronunciations and definitions.
- ***Appendixes:***
    - *Appendix A, Medications:* This useful appendix gives directions and precautions for working with clients who are taking medications.

- *Appendix B, Research Literacy, Research Capability:* Appendix B engages students' curiosity with an introduction to reading and understanding the research available on massage therapy, and perhaps even adding to it!
- *Appendix C: Extra Conditions At a Glance:* This new appendix presents 38 conditions that are interesting and pertinent, but rarely seen, at least in an acute state. For instance, most massage therapists will have clients with a history of broken bones but will not be likely to work with an unset fracture; therefore, the discussion of fractures with all their details has been moved into this appendix and shortened. In addition to conditions that were moved from the main chapters, some new conditions are addressed here as well; these include carditis, hyperparathyroidism and hypoparathyroidism, lichen planus, sarcoidosis, and many others.

Helpful Navigation Features

The Pathologies: A full list of all the conditions in this text and their page numbers can be found in the front matter of this book. In addition, every disease covered is listed in the Index at the end of the book.

"Where Can I Find..." boxes: Look for these brightly colored boxes at the beginning of several chapters.

Student Resources

All resources from the previous edition have been fully revised and updated. These, along with our new offerings, may be found at http://thePoint.lww.com/Werner5e:

- **Answers to Chapter Review questions.** Great for test preparation.
- **Animations and film clips.** Pathology animations and film clips, including some from the acclaimed *Acland's DVD Atlas of Human Anatomy.*
- **An audio glossary.**
- **Bibliography.** The full bibliography from the text, with live links to active Web sites.
- **Taking a Client History, with printable forms.** Forms have been generously provided from Diana Thompson's *Hands Heal: Communication, Documentation, and Insurance Billing for Manual Therapists,* Fourth Edition (Lippincott Williams & Wilkins, 2012).
- **Flash Cards.** Students will appreciate these valuable study aids, which are based on the "In Brief" feature that appears throughout the book. Another set of flash cards is based on the Greek and Latin word roots discussed in Chapter 1 of the text.
- **Games.** A wildly popular feature from the previous edition, student activities in the form of a hangman game, crossword puzzle, and quiz show will help to solidify key concepts.
- **Modality recommendation charts.** Charts for each condition with input from subject matter experts give suggestions for massage and bodywork strategies. Modalities include craniosacral therapy, deep tissue massage, lymphatic drainage, polarity, proprioceptive neuromuscular facilitation/muscle energy technique/stretching, reflexology, Shiatsu, Swedish massage, and trigger point therapy.
- **Quiz questions for each chapter**: Test your retention with these multiple choice quizzes!

Instructor Resources

The instructor resources have also been revised and updated. They include the following:

- **Lecture notes for each chapter** that can be adapted and printed for instructor or student use.
- **PowerPoint slides** that are based on lecture notes, with incorporated art and animations.
- **Illustrations** from the fifth edition.
- **Sample syllabi** for 40- and 60-hour pathology courses, along with a curriculum development guide.
- **A full test bank** and test generator software.

Finally…

Finally, my traditional closing words: I invite you to read this with joy. Do more research in what interests you, and share your findings with others. Remember that some of the questions dealt with here will probably never be completely answered. And what we think we know today may be revised or proved wrong tomorrow. Isn't that terrific?

Many thanks and many blessings,

Ruth Werner
Waldport, OR
Summer 2011

User's Guide

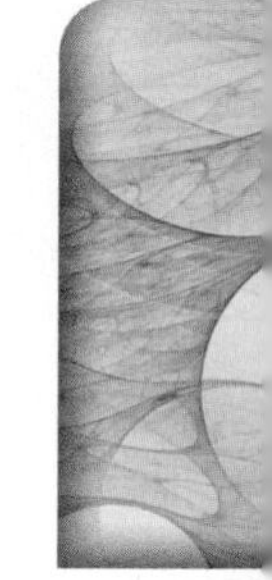

A Massage Therapist's Guide to Pathology gives you the tools to make informed decisions about bodywork for clients who live with a wide variety of diseases and conditions. This user's guide shows how to put the book's features to work for you.

THE PATHOLOGIES

Every condition in the book and its subtypes are listed in alphabetical order with page numbers; this list is in the front matter of the text.

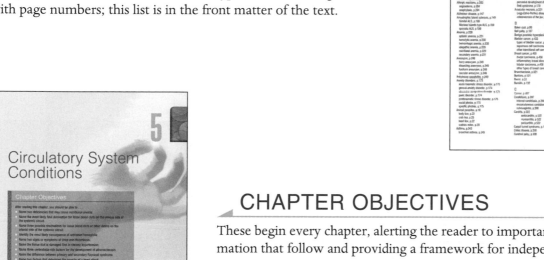

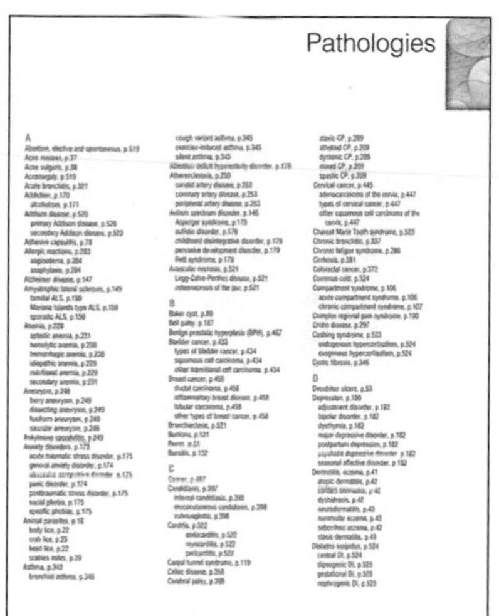

Pathologies

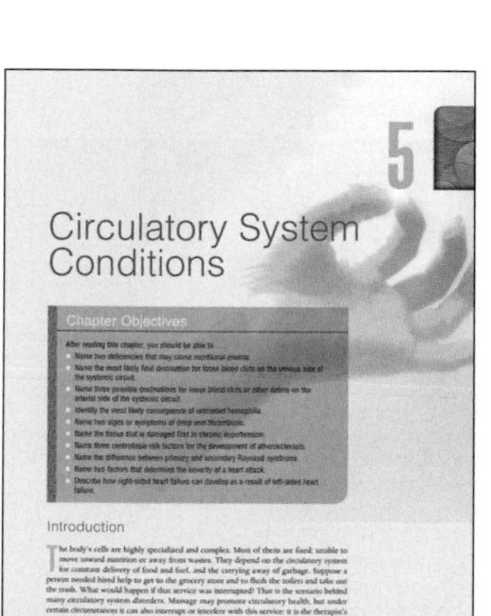

5

Circulatory System Conditions

Chapter Objectives

Introduction

CHAPTER OBJECTIVES

These begin every chapter, alerting the reader to important pieces of information that follow and providing a framework for independent study.

INTRODUCTORY CHAPTER

Chapter 1 introduces key concepts on which the study of pathology is built. Terminology, infectious agents, hygienic methods, and the inflammatory process are discussed here.

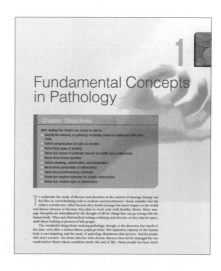

1

Fundamental Concepts in Pathology

Chapter Objectives

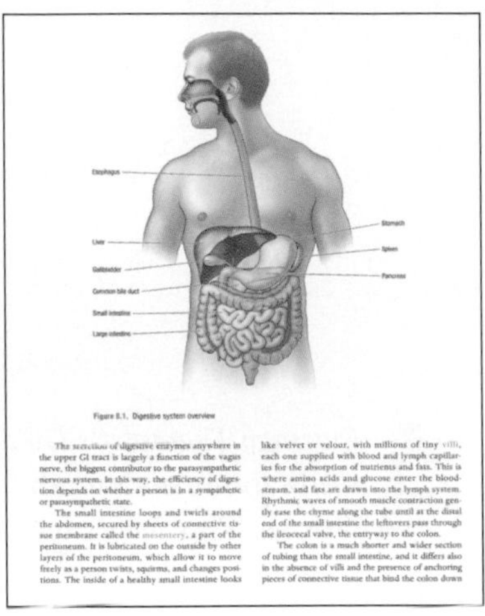

Figure 8.1. Digestive system overview

The secretion of digestive enzymes anywhere in the upper GI tract is largely a function of the vagus nerve, the biggest contributor to the parasympathetic nervous system. In this way, the efficiency of digestion depends on whether a person is in a sympathetic or parasympathetic state.

The small intestine loops and twirls around the abdomen, secured by sheets of connective tissue membrane called the mesentery, a part of the peritoneum. It is lubricated on the outside by other layers of the peritoneum, which allow it to move freely as a person twists, squirms, and changes positions. The inside of a healthy small intestine looks like velvet or velour, with millions of tiny villi, each one supplied with blood and lymph capillaries for the absorption of nutrients and fats. This is where amino acids and glucose enter the bloodstream, and fats are drawn into the lymph system. Rhythmic waves of smooth muscle contraction gently ease the chyme along the tube until at the distal end of the small intestine the leftovers pass through the ileocecal valve, the entryway to the colon.

The colon is a much shorter and wider section of tubing than the small intestine, and it differs also in the absence of villi and the presence of anchoring pieces of connective tissue that bind the colon down

BODY SYSTEM OVERVIEWS

Chapters 2 to 11 open with a brief review of the body system under discussion, with special emphasis on processes that may be interrupted by conditions that change the way we function.

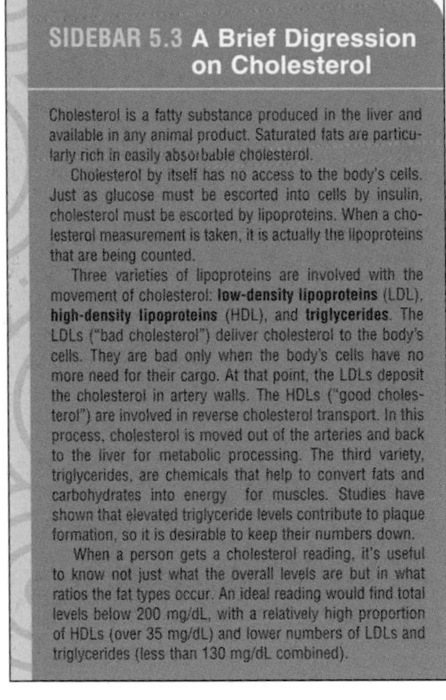
SIDEBAR 5.3 A Brief Digression on Cholesterol

Cholesterol is a fatty substance produced in the liver and available in any animal product. Saturated fats are particularly rich in easily absorbable cholesterol.

Cholesterol by itself has no access to the body's cells. Just as glucose must be escorted into cells by insulin, cholesterol must be escorted by lipoproteins. When a cholesterol measurement is taken, it is actually the lipoproteins that are being counted.

Three varieties of lipoproteins are involved with the movement of cholesterol: **low-density lipoproteins** (LDL), **high-density lipoproteins** (HDL), and **triglycerides**. The LDLs ("bad cholesterol") deliver cholesterol to the body's cells. They are bad only when the body's cells have no more need for their cargo. At that point, the LDLs deposit the cholesterol in artery walls. The HDLs ("good cholesterol") are involved in reverse cholesterol transport. In this process, cholesterol is moved out of the arteries and back to the liver for metabolic processing. The third variety, triglycerides, are chemicals that help to convert fats and carbohydrates into energy for muscles. Studies have shown that elevated triglyceride levels contribute to plaque formation, so it is desirable to keep their numbers down.

When a person gets a cholesterol reading, it's useful to know not just what the overall levels are but in what ratios the fat types occur. An ideal reading would find total levels below 200 mg/dL, with a relatively high proportion of HDLs (over 35 mg/dL) and lower numbers of LDLs and triglycerides (less than 130 mg/dL combined).

SIDEBARS

These present information that is important but peripheral to the core discussion. Disease histories, some statistics, and specific cancer staging protocols are provided in the sidebars.

Anemia in Brief

Pronunciation: ah-NE-me-ah

What is it?

Anemia is a symptom rather than a disease in itself. It indicates a shortage of red blood cells (RBCs), hemoglobin, or both.

How is it recognized?

Symptoms of anemia include pallor, shortness of breath, fatigue, and poor resistance to cold. Other symptoms accompany specific types of anemia.

Massage risks and benefits

Risks: Anemia can sometimes cause neurological damage; this has implications for massage. Any anemia due to bone marrow suppression, inflammation, or premature destruction of RBCs requires that massage be adjusted to meet any limitations set by the underlying pathologies.

Benefits: Massage for idiopathic or nutritional anemia may be safe, but it is unlikely to change the course of this condition.

IN BRIEF BOXES

These give a synopsis of the definition, signs and symptoms, and guidelines for bodywork for each condition discussed. In Brief boxes may be found online, in the form of flash cards, at http://thePoint.lww.com/Werner5e.

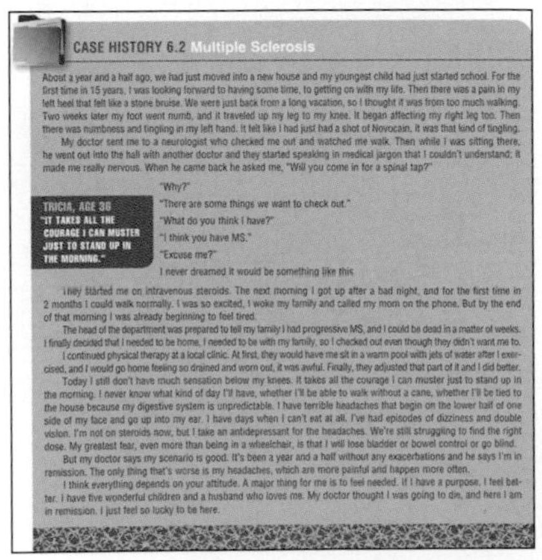
CASE HISTORY 6.2 Multiple Sclerosis

About a year and a half ago, we had just moved into a new house and my youngest child had just started school. For the first time in 15 years, I was looking forward to having some time, to getting on with my life. Then there was a pain in my left heel that felt like a stone bruise. We were just back from a long vacation, so I thought it was from too much walking. Two weeks later my foot went numb, and it traveled up my leg to my knee. It began affecting my right leg too. Then there was numbness and tingling in my left hand. It felt like I had just had a shot of Novocain. It was that kind of tingling.

My doctor sent me to a neurologist who checked me out and watched me walk. Then while I was sitting there, he went out into the hall with another doctor and they started speaking in medical jargon that I couldn't understand; it made me really nervous. When he came back he asked me, "Will you come in for a spinal tap?"

TRICIA, AGE 36
"IT TAKES ALL THE COURAGE I CAN MUSTER JUST TO STAND UP IN THE MORNING."

"Why?"

"There are some things we want to check out."

"What do you think I have?"

"I think you have MS."

"Excuse me?"

I never dreamed it would be something like this.

They started me on intravenous steroids. The next morning I got up after a bad night, and for the first time in 2 months I could walk normally. I was so excited, I woke my family and called my mom on the phone. But by the end of that morning I was already beginning to feel tired.

The head of the department was prepared to tell my family I had progressive MS, and I could be dead in a matter of weeks. I finally decided that I needed to be home. I needed to be with my family, so I checked out even though they didn't want me to.

I continued physical therapy at a local clinic. At first, they would have me sit in a warm pool with jets of water after I exercised, and I would go home feeling so drained and worn out, it was awful. Finally, they adjusted that part of it and I did better.

Today I still don't have much sensation below my knees. It takes all the courage I can muster just to stand up in the morning. I never know what kind of day I'll have, whether I'll be able to walk without a cane, whether I'll be tied to the house because my digestive system is unpredictable. I have terrible headaches that begin on the lower half of one side of my face and go up into my ear. I have days when I can't eat at all. I've had episodes of dizziness and double vision. I'm not on steroids now, but I take an antidepressant for the headaches. We're still struggling to find the right dose. My greatest fear, even more than being in a wheelchair, is that I will lose bladder or bowel control or go blind.

But my doctor says my scenario is good. It's been a year and a half without any exacerbations and he says I'm in remission. The only thing that's worse is my headaches, which are more painful and happen more often.

I think everything depends on your attitude. A major thing for me is to feel needed. If I have a purpose, I feel better. I have five wonderful children and a husband who loves me. My doctor thought I was going to die, and here I am in remission. I just feel so lucky to be here.

CASE HISTORIES

These provide an important voice to the people who live with a variety of diseases and conditions. They offer insight into how some disorders powerfully influence people's lives.

COMPARE AND CONTRAST BOXES

These put key features of closely connected disorders side by side for a point-by-point comparison of similarities and differences.

COMPARE & CONTRAST 2.1 Plantar Warts vs. Calluses

Plantar warts often look like simple calluses: the thick skin that grows on areas of the feet subject to a lot of wear and tear. The problem is that while people may file or snip off their calluses with no ill effects, to do the same with a plantar wart is to risk having that wart virus spread all over the foot and lead to more growths until it becomes difficult to walk.

Massage therapists are in a unique position to observe their clients' feet and notice the subtle differences between plantar warts and callus. They may be able to give clients guidance about getting the right kind of care.

CHARACTERISTICS	PLANTAR WARTS	CALLUS
Location	Anywhere on plantar surface of foot.	Appears in areas of wear and tear, especially back of heels and lateral aspect of feet. Callus usually grows in a similar pattern on both feet.
Appearance	Usually *not* bilateral. May be white, but with darker speckling under thickened skin: this is the capillary supply.	Callus usually grows in a similar pattern on both feet. Thick, white skin.
Sensation	Very hard and unyielding, like stepping on a stone.	No particular sensation.

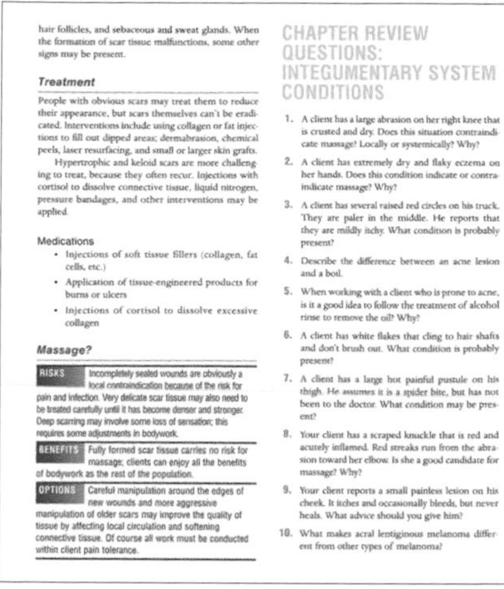

hair follicles, and sebaceous and sweat glands. When the formation of scar tissue malfunctions, some other signs may be present.

Treatment

People with obvious scars may treat them to reduce their appearance, but scars themselves can't be eradicated. Interventions include using collagen or fat injections to fill out dipped areas; dermabrasion, chemical peels, laser resurfacing, and small or larger skin grafts.

Hypertrophic and keloid scars are more challenging to treat, because they often recur. Injections with cortisol to dissolve connective tissue, liquid nitrogen, pressure bandages, and other interventions may be applied.

Medications

- Injections of soft tissue fillers (collagen, fat cells, etc.)
- Application of tissue-engineered products for burns or ulcers
- Injections of cortisol to dissolve excessive collagen

Massage?

RISKS Incompletely sealed wounds are obviously a local contraindication because of the risk for pain and infection. Very delicate scar tissue may also need to be treated carefully until it has become denser and stronger. Deep scarring may involve some loss of sensation; this requires some adjustments in bodywork.

BENEFITS Fully formed scar tissue carries no risk for massage; clients can enjoy all the benefits of bodywork as the rest of the population.

OPTIONS Careful manipulation around the edges of new wounds and more aggressive manipulation of older scars may improve the quality of tissue by affecting local circulation and softening connective tissue. Of course all work must be conducted within client pain tolerance.

CHAPTER REVIEW QUESTIONS: INTEGUMENTARY SYSTEM CONDITIONS

1. A client has a large abrasion on her right knee that is crusted and dry. Does this situation contraindicate massage? Locally or systemically? Why?
2. A client has extremely dry and flaky eczema on her hands. Does this condition indicate or contraindicate massage? Why?
3. A client has several raised red circles on his truck. They are paler in the middle. He reports that they are mildly itchy. What condition is probably present?
4. Describe the difference between an acne lesion and a boil.
5. When working with a client who is prone to acne, is it a good idea to follow the treatment of alcohol rinse to remove the oil? Why?
6. A client has white flakes that cling to hair shafts and don't brush out. What condition is probably present?
7. A client has a large hot painful pustule on his thigh. He assumes it is a spider bite, but has not been to the doctor. What condition may be present?
8. Your client has a scraped knuckle that is red and acutely inflamed. Red streaks run from the abrasion toward her elbow. Is she a good candidate for massage? Why?
9. Your client reports a small painless lesion on his cheek. It itches and occasionally bleeds, but never heals. What advice should you give him?
10. What makes acral lentiginous melanoma different from other types of melanoma?

CHAPTER REVIEW QUESTIONS

These require critical thinking skills and the ability to use information to draw conclusions about the safe practice of bodywork in complicated situations. Answers to the Chapter Review questions are provided at http://thePoint.lww.com/Werner5e.

APPENDICES

This text has three valuable appendices to take readers deeper into pathology studies.

- **Appendix A, Medications:** This appendix addresses the role of bodywork when clients use medications to treat or manage their conditions.
- **Appendix B, Research Literacy, Research Capacity:** This appendix introduces concepts in research literacy so that therapists may become familiar with the skills of reading, interpreting, and possibly even conducting research projects about massage therapy.
- **Appendix C, Extra Conditions at a Glance:** This is a collection of conditions that are interesting and pertinent, but that can be somewhat abbreviated because they are rare or seldom seen in an acute stage.

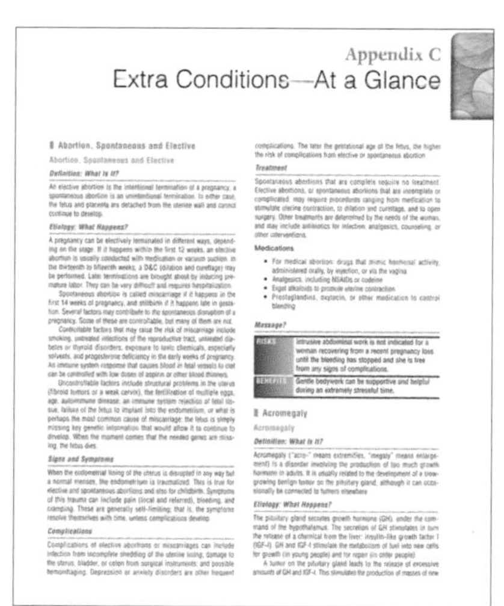

Appendix C

Extra Conditions—At a Glance

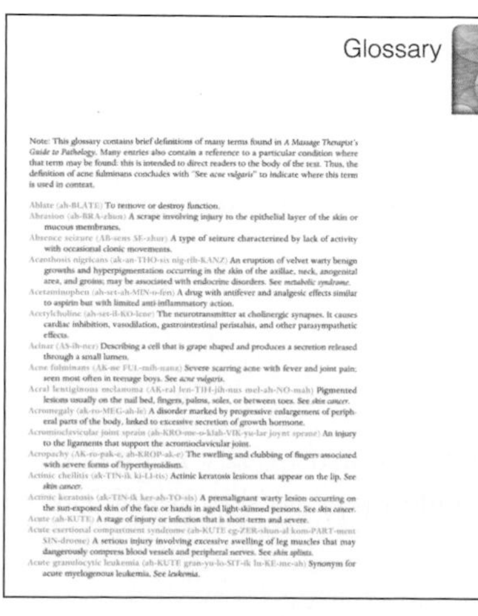

Glossary

GLOSSARY

A full glossary with pronunciations and definitions is provided in the text.

ONLINE RESOURCES

Student Resources:

Several features to support students through learning pathology may be found at http:/ thePoint.lww.com/Werner5e:

- All of the answers to the Chapter Review questions
- Additional practice quiz questions and answers, arranged by chapter
- Animations and video clips to demonstrate several anatomical features or disease processes
- An audio pronunciation guide of glossary terms found in *Stedman's Medical Dictionary for the Health Profession and Nursing*
- Flash cards reinforce key concepts from In Brief boxes and Greek and Latin roots and their English equivalents.
- Games, including crossword puzzles, hangman, and other activities, help build familiarity with important ideas.
- Taking a Client History provides information on how to gather a full picture of each client's health history, with printable intake forms.
- Full bibliography, including the print and electronic resources used to gather information for the text, is listed here to point the way for further research.

Items in the text that refer readers to material on thePoint have this icon 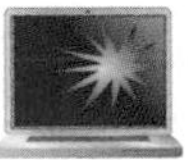

Online Instructor's Resources:

Instructors who adopt this text will be given a password, giving them access to the following helpful resources:

- **Pathology curriculum guidelines.** This document is based on many years of experience. It provides suggestions for how to customize a pathology course to individual needs, including how to choose content, how to use quizzes and examinations, examples of student projects, and much more.
- **Syllabi.** These suggested syllabi for 40- and 60-hour pathology courses have schedules, grading guidelines, and suggested timing for quizzes and examinations.
- **Lecture notes in printable form**. These outlines of the text can be used for teaching notes, student handouts, or both.
- **Lecture notes as PowerPoint slides.** These can project content outlines with images, film clips, and animations embedded in the appropriate places.
- **Images.** All of the art from the text is available in an easily downloadable format.
- **Test bank.** More than 1,000 multiple-choice questions for the new edition have been compiled in a Brownstone test generator. These can be used for quizzes, tests, or homework assignments.

Artwork and Photos

These are rendered in full color throughout the book to help illustrate key points. They provide a valuable resource to help readers recognize a wide range of skin conditions in various stages of severity.

Reviewers

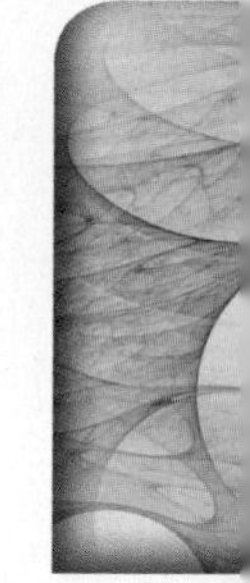

T.J. Ford
East West College
Portland, Oregon

Robert Haase
Haase Myotherapy

Michelle Komm
Pinnacle Career Institute—South Campus
Kansas City, Missouri

Mary McLendon
Mississippi State University
Mississippi State, Mississippi

Kevin Pierce
High Tech Institute, Inc.
Orlando, Florida

Stuart Rice
Bryan College
Gold River, California

David Riedinger
American Institute of Alternative Medicine
Columbus, Ohio

Zefire Skoczen
Renton Technical College
Renton, Washington

Acknowledgments

With every edition of *A Massage Therapist's Guide to Pathology*, the list of people to whom I am grateful grows. A work of this scope can never be done alone, nor should it be. Reader, you hold in your hand the effort of hundreds who have knowingly or unknowingly contributed to the final product. Here is the short list:

- As always, Brian Utting, my first and most influential massage teacher, and Suzanne Carlson, who introduced me to the concept of massage for people who aren't perfectly healthy: Your seeds continue to grow in this project, and I hope they will grow forever.
- Classroom students and continuing education participants: From you I have learned more than I could ever teach. Your generosity informs every aspect of this book, and every reader can be grateful to you.
- Friends and colleagues at Lippincott, Williams & Wilkins: You had the foresight in 1995 to see the potential to leave an important mark on massage education. I am so proud to be part of that legacy.
- The Trustees and Staff and the Massage Therapy Foundation: You show me what it means to "always be learning"—which is my favorite message when I sign books now. The quality of my work has continued to rise mainly because of the inspiration I get from being around people who simply cannot be satisfied with good enough.

And of course, to my ever-evolving family:

Curtis, Nathan, and Lily Anne Rose: You are my heroes. Words fail; love triumphs. All the time, every minute, no matter what.

R. Werner

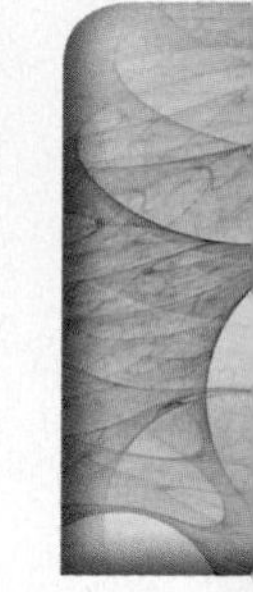

Contents

1

Fundamental Concepts in Pathology

Chapter Objectives

After reading this chapter you should be able to . . .

- Identify the meaning of pathology vocabulary based on Greek and Latin word roots.
- Define *complication* and give an example.
- Name three types of bacteria.
- Name two viruses of particular concern for health care professionals.
- Name three animal parasites.
- Define *cleaning, disinfection*, and *sterilization*.
- Name three components of inflammation.
- Name two proinflammatory chemicals.
- Name two negative outcomes for chronic inflammation.
- Name four cardinal signs of inflammation.

To undertake the study of diseases and disorders in the context of massage therapy can feel like an overwhelming task to students and practitioners. Some consider that the subject is irrelevant, either because they doubt massage has much impact on the health and disease process or because they plan to work only with healthy clients. Many massage therapists are intimidated by the thought of all the things that can go wrong with the human body. They may find medical writing confusing and obscure, or they may be squeamish about looking at pictures of sick people.

The wonderful thing about studying pathology, though, is the discovery that much of the time, even after a serious illness, *people get better.* The reparative capacity of the human body is awe-inspiring, and the study of pathology illuminates that process. And for people who don't recover—for those who live with chronic diseases that can be managed but not eradicated or those whose condition marks the end of life—those people too have much to teach us about living in grace and finding power, pleasure, and fullness from every moment. It is a deep and important privilege for a massage therapist to be invited into that process.

This chapter lays out some of the starting principles for the study of pathology for massage therapists. Being familiar with key concepts will help the reader integrate and mentally organize the rest of the material in this text. This chapter introduces terminology for pathology discussions and looks at common infectious agents, hygienic practices, and the inflammatory process.

Terminology

Many people who are new to the field of massage are surprised to find that the study of anatomy, physiology, and pathology requires learning a new language. It doesn't take much, but a smattering of Greek and Latin not only can help to demystify anatomical terminology but can even make it fun. Knowing that *vermiform appendix* really means *hanging thing that looks like a worm* can add tremendous satisfaction to learning new ways to describe the body.

Much of medical terminology seems steeped in tradition and a desire to confuse people rather than being a tool to understand and celebrate the glories of the human body. Rules about when to use which word elements can seem frustrating and arbitrary. For instance, it can be difficult to work out when to use *syn-*, *sym-*, *con-*, or *com-*, since they all mean the same thing: with. Other patterns are easier to track, since they are linked to the presence or absence of vowels. Thus we say *an*algesic to refer to a painkilling drug but *a*menorrhea to refer to the absence of a menstrual cycle, because *a-* and *an-* mean the same thing: without. Fortunately it is not our job to determine which word roots to use; all we have to do is identify their meaning when we find them.

The list in Table 1.1 includes the Greek and Latin fragments that are most useful in the study of pathology. This is not a comprehensive or exhaustive list, and it omits many of the terms that turn up in beginning anatomy courses. It does include most of the roots for terms that are used in this book, however. Familiarity with these word fragments will make the study of pathology much simpler and even enjoyable.

In addition to Greek and Latin word roots that form the basis for much medical terminology, it is important to define some central ideas. Some terms are used in many pathophysiology discussions, but their meanings are not always consistent. Table 1.2 provides basic definitions for key terms used in this text.

Infectious Agents

Disease-causing organisms are called pathogens. The many thousands of pathogens that can threaten human health have been categorized into five basic types: prions, viruses, bacteria, fungi, and animal parasites. These organisms are the causes of many diseases, some of which are communicable. However, any individual's ability to resist pathogenic invasion may be at least partly determined by other modifiable factors. That is to say, a person who exercises carefully and eats well, who gets plenty of good-quality sleep, and who has a generally positive attitude toward life is often better equipped to fight off the same pathogens that actively threaten someone who is sleep-deprived and stressed out. In other words, while viruses cause colds, other factors may influence immune system activity, which can enhance or interfere with a person's ability to resist getting sick.

Prions

Prions are unique among pathogens: although they are composed of proteins, they contain neither DNA nor RNA. They begin as slightly malformed proteins in neurons that essentially get in the way of normal neuronal activity. For reasons that aren't entirely clear, prions cause infected cells to produce more prions (similarly to the way viruses work). They spread via contaminated blood or transplant tissue, contaminated surgical instruments, or consumption of infected meat products. Prion diseases can also be inherited or the result of spontaneous mutations.

Prions are the causative agents for bovine spongiform encephalopathy (also called mad cow disease), Creutzfeldt-Jakob disease, kuru (a disease that used to be seen among human cannibals), scrapie in sheep and goats, and a few other rare diseases. All prion diseases affect the nervous system, and all are eventually fatal.

TABLE 1.1 Greek and Latin Word Parts

Word Parts	Meaning	Example
a-, an-	Without	Malignant melanoma lesions may show as **a**symmetrical discolorations on the skin.
acro-	Extremity	**Acral** lentiginous melanoma usually begins on the fingers or toes.
adeno-	Glandular	**Adeno**carcinoma is cancer that begins in glands.
-algia	Pain	An an**alge**sic is a painkiller.
angio-	Blood or lymph vessels	**Angio**genesis is the production of new blood vessels.
arthr-	Joint	**Arthro**plasty is surgical implantation of an artificial joint, often to treat osteo**arthr**itis.
brady-	Slow	**Brady**cardia means slow heartbeat.
carcin-	Crab (cancer)	A **carcin**ogen is a cancer-triggering agent.
cardio-	Heart	**Cardio**myopathy refers to damaged heart muscle.
-cele	Swelling, hernia	In spina bifida meningo**cele**, the dura mater and arachnoid protrude through an incompletely closed vertebral arch.
cervi-, cervico-	Neck	**Cervi**cal cancer originates in cells found in the neck of the uterus.
cep-, ceph-	Head, brain	En**ceph**alitis refers to inflammation of the brain.
chole	Bile	**Chole**cyst is another term for gallbladder.
com-, con-	With, together	A **con**centric muscle **con**traction brings the bony attachments closer together.
contra-	Against	A coup-**contre**coup head injury occurs when the brain hits the opposite side of the cranium from the direction of the original blow.
cyst	Hollow organ	Chole**cyst**itis is inflammation of the gallbladder.
demo-	People	**Demo**graphics is recorded information about a specific group of people.
derm-	Skin	**Derm**atophytosis is the condition of having plants (in this case fungi) growing on the skin.
dia-	Through	**Dia**betes mellitus means *sweetness flowing through*, referring to excessive production of urine that is high in sugar.
dys-	Difficulty	**Dys**phagia is difficulty with swallowing or eating.
ecto-, -ectomy	Outside, removal	An append**ectomy** is the removal of the appendix.
-emia	Blood	Septic**emia** is a type of infection of the blood.
endo-	Inside	An **endo**scopy is a test to examine the lining of the gastrointestinal tract.
epi-	Upon	An **epi**demic is a contagious disease that affects a lot of people. (Literally this word means *upon the people*.)
erythr-	Red	**Erythro**poietin is a hormone that stimulates production of red blood cells.

continues

TABLE 1.1 Greek and Latin Word Parts *continued*

Word Parts	Meaning	Example
ex-	Out of	**Ex**ophthalmos is a condition in which the eyes bulge out of their usual position.
-gen	Beginning, producing	An aller**gen** is an allergy-producing substance.
glyco-	Relating to sugar	Hypo**glyc**emia is another term for low blood sugar.
-graphy	Recording, writing	Veno**graphy** is a test to measure blood flow through veins.
hemi-	Half	**Hemi**plegic cerebral palsy affects half of the body.
hemo-	Blood	**Hemo**rrhage means *flowing blood*.
hepat-	Liver	**Hepat**itis is inflammation of the liver.
hydro-	Water	**Hydro**cephalus is a condition involving too much cerebrospinal fluid.
hyper-	Above, too much	**Hyper**uricemia describes having too much uric acid in the blood.
hypo-	Below, too little	**Hypo**tension is another term for low blood pressure.
-itis	Inflammation	Arthr**itis** is inflammation of a joint.
-lepsis	Seizure	Epi**lepsy** is a type of seizure disorder.
leuko-	White	**Leuk**emia is a cancer involving overproduction of white blood cells.
lipo-	Fat	Hyper**lip**idemia describes high levels of fat in the blood.
litho-	Rock	The presence of a kidney stone is nephro**lith**iasis.
-logy	Study	Patho**logy** is the study of disease.
-lysis, -lyso	Destruction	Para**lysis** is the loss of normal function.
mega-	Large	Spleno**mega**ly (enlarged spleen) is a potential complication of mononucleosis.
meno-	Month	**Men**struation is the monthly detachment and expulsion of the uterine lining.
metr-	Mother (uterus)	The endo**metr**ium is the inner lining of the uterus.
micro-	Small	**Micro**graphia (shrinking of handwriting) is a possible symptom of Parkinson disease.
myco-	Fungus	**Myco**sis is any disease caused by a yeast or a fungus.
mye-	Marrow or spinal cord	A **mye**locele is a protrusion of the spinal cord, seen with some types of spina bifida.
myo-	Muscle	Fibro**my**algia describes "fiber muscle pain."
narco-	Stupor	**Narco**lepsy means sleep seizure.
necro-	Death	**Necro**sis is the condition of tissue death.
neo-	New	A **neo**plasm is a new formation; it sometimes refers to a cancerous growth.
nephro-	Kidney	**Neph**ritis is the inflammation of a kidney.
neuro-	Nerve	Peripheral **neuro**pathy is a complication of untreated diabetes mellitus.
-oid	Resembles	The sigm**oid** colon looks like an S.

TABLE 1.1 Greek and Latin Word Parts *continued*

Word Parts	Meaning	Example
-oma	Tumor	A lip**oma** is a benign fatty tumor.
onco-	Tumor	An **onco**logist is a doctor who specializes in cancer.
orchi-	Testes	**Orch**itis is inflammation of the testicles.
-osis	Pathologic condition	Hyperkyph**osis** is the condition of having an accentuated kyphotic curve.
osteo-	Bone	**Osteo**porosis is the condition of developing porous bones.
para-	Alongside, near	The **para**spinal muscles run **para**llel to the spine.
peri-	Around	The **peri**cardium wraps around the heart.
phagia-	Eating	Poly**phagia**, or constant hunger, is a symptom of diabetes mellitus.
-philia	Affinity	Hemo**philia** is a blood clotting disorder.
phleb-	Vein	Thrombo**phleb**itis is inflammation of a vein because of a clot.
phyto-	Plants	Dermato**phyto**sis is another term for fungal infection of the skin.
-plasia	Growth	Hyper**plasia** means too much growth.
-plasm, -plasma	Formed	A wart is a type of neo**plasm**.
patho-	Disease state	A **patho**gen is a disease-causing organism.
physio-	Nature	**Physio**logy is the study of normal life functions.
pseudo-	False	**Pseudo**-gout involves different chemical deposits from those seen with acute gouty arthritis.
psych-	The mind, mental	**Psych**ogenic tremor develops in stressful situations.
ren-	Kidney	The ad**ren**al glands are on top of the kidneys.
-rrhagia, -rrhea	Flowing	Rhino**rrhagia** is a runny nose.
rhino-	Nose	A **rhino**plasty is a nose job.
sarco-	Flesh	Kaposi **sarco**ma is a type of cancer.
sclero-	Hardness, scarring	**Sclero**derma is a disease involving the hardening of the skin.
spondy-	Spine	**Spondy**losis Is osteoarthritis in the spine.
-stasis	Stagnation, standing still	**Stasis** dermatitis is related to poor circulation.
stoma-	An opening; mouth	**Stoma**titis is the development of inflamed lesions at the corners of the mouth.
syn-, sym-	With	The two pubic bones come together at the **sym**physis pubis.
thrombo-	Clot	Deep vein **thrombo**sis is a risk factor for pulmonary embolism.
therm-	Temperature	Hypo**therm**ia is the state of getting too cold.
-trophy, -trophic	Nutrition, growth	Muscular dys**trophy** is a condition in which muscles degenerate.
vaso-	Blood vessel	Raynaud syndrome involves severe **vaso**spasm in the extremities.

TABLE 1.2 Pathology Terms

Term	Definition
Acute	Rapid onset, brief, can be severe
Chronic	Prolonged, long-term, can be low intensity
Complication	A process or event that occurs during the course of a disease that is not an essential part of that disease
Contraindicated	Describing an intervention that may have a negative outcome in a given condition
Demographic	An identified group of people about which information is gathered
Diagnosis	The determination of the nature of a disease, injury, or defect
Endemic	A pattern of disease incidence that is limited to a particular population or area
Epidemic	Widespread outbreak of a contagious disease
Idiopathic	A disease of unknown origin
Incidence	The number of new cases of people falling ill with a specified disease during a specific period within a specific population
Indication	The basis for an intervention that is likely to have a positive outcome in a given condition
Lesion	A pathologic change in tissue
Local	Describing a limited area of the body
Morbidity	A diseased state; the ratio of sick to well people within a population
Mortality	Death rate from a specific disease
Pandemic	A contagious disease affecting the global population
Prevalence	The number of cases of a disease existing in a given population during a specific period or at a particular moment; the proportion of people affected
Prognosis	Expected outcome of a disease or disorder
Sign	An objectively observable indication of a disease or disorder
Stenosis	Abnormal narrowing of any canal or orifice
Subacute	Between acute and chronic; a stage in healing or tissue repair
Symptom	A subjective experience relating to a disease or disorder
Syndrome	A collection of signs and symptoms associated with a specific disease process
Systemic	Describing a whole-body involvement
Trauma	Any physical or mental injury

Viruses

Viruses are packets of DNA or RNA wrapped in a protein coat called a **capsid**. They can't replicate outside of a host; instead, they use the machinery of the cells they target to make more viruses. The infected cell eventually releases many copies of the virus or viral particles called **virions**, which may then invade other nearby cells. Every virus that affects humans has at least one specific target cell, although some viruses have multiple levels of infectious activity. Poliovirus, for example, first invades cells in the gastrointestinal tract and then migrates to motor neurons in the spinal cord.

Outside of a host, many viruses are fragile and disintegrate quickly. Some, however, are extremely stable and can remain infectious for long periods. The most common stable viruses that massage therapists are likely to encounter include herpes simplex and hepatitis B and C. These infections are discussed in detail in Chapters 2 and 8, respectively.

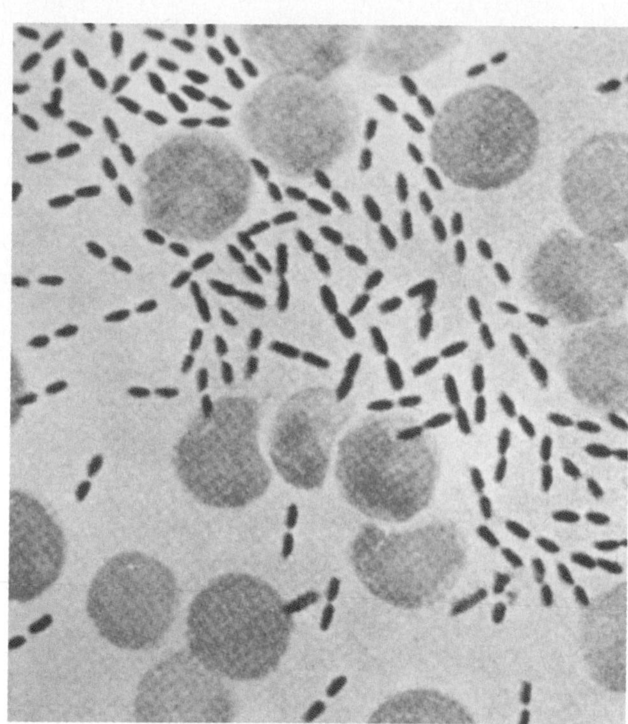

Figure 1.1. Diplococci

Bacteria

Bacteria are single-celled microorganisms that can survive outside of a host. Not all bacteria are pathogenic; some are necessary for good health. But others can cause serious illnesses, either by invading healthy tissues or by releasing enzymes or toxins that destroy healthy cells.

Antibiotics are a group of drugs that either kill bacteria directly or interfere with bacterial replication. Aggressive bacterial infections with a high replication rate often respond to antibiotic therapy better than slow-growing infections. Another feature that helps to determine the virulence of a bacterium is whether it develops a tough waxy coat that protects it from the environment. Coated bacteria, sometimes called **spores**, can survive for extended periods outside a host. Tuberculosis, tetanus, and anthrax are infections caused by bacteria that form resistant spores.

Bacteria come in several basic forms, although some species show an ability to change their shape depending on environmental factors.

- *Cocci* are spherical bacteria that appear in predictable patterns.
    - *Diplococci* are paired cocci. These bacteria are associated with a type of pneumonia (Figure 1.1).
    - *Staphylococci* clump together in groups that resemble bunches of grapes (Figure 1.2). Staph infections of the skin are usually (but not always) local *to* a specific area. Some varieties of staph have become resistant to common antibiotics and can be difficult to treat. One example is methicillin-resistant *Staphylococcus aureus,* or MRSA, which is discussed in the section on staphylococcus infections in Chapter 2.
    - *Streptococci* cling together in chains (Figure 1.3). They tend to cause systemic infections such as

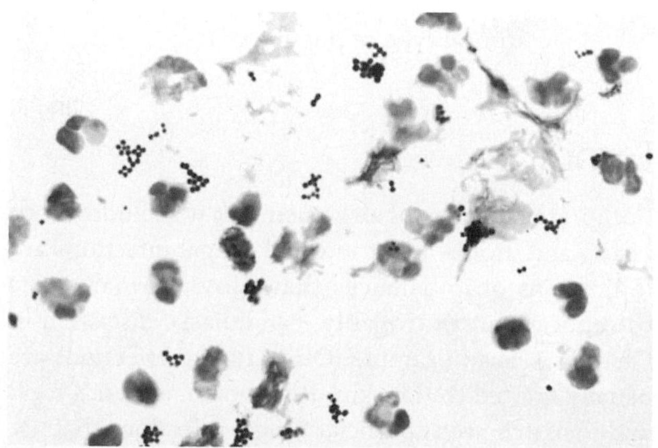

Figure 1.2. Staphylococci

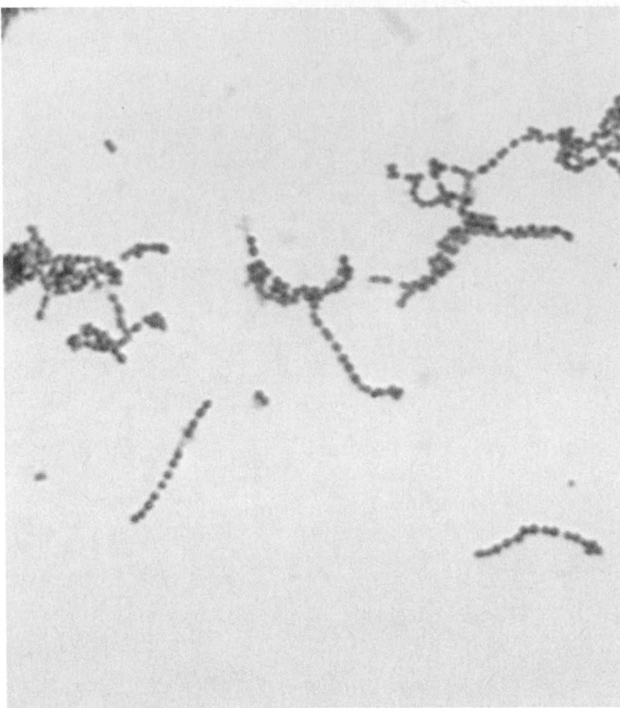
Figure 1.3. Streptococci

strep throat or rheumatic fever. Necrotizing fasciitis, or "flesh-eating bacteria," is often a strep infection, although some other agents have been seen with this as well.

- *Bacilli* are elongated, rod-shaped bacteria. These are the most capable of forming spores.
- *Spirochetes* are spiral bacteria. Technically they are greatly elongated bacilli, with filaments that wind around the cell wall, pulling them into a spiral. Infections caused by spirochetes include syphilis (*Treponema pallidum*) and Lyme disease (*Borrelia burgdorferi*) (Figure 1.4).
- *Mycoplasma* are very tiny microorganisms that cause some sexually transmitted infections and a common type of pneumonia.

Fungi

Fungi are a group of organisms that includes both yeasts and molds. Most internal fungal infections are indications of imbalances that allow normal yeasts to replicate uncontrollably; candidiasis, discussed in Chapter 8, is an example. Other fungal infections are usually limited to the skin. Ringworm, athlete's foot, and jock itch are superficial fungal infections that are discussed in Chapter 2.

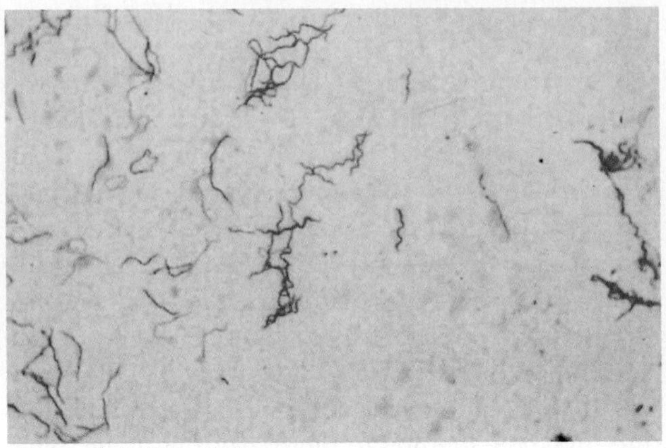
Figure 1.4. Spirochetes

Animal Parasites

Animal parasites can be unicellular or multicellular. The parasites listed here are animals that live on or in a host rather than those that visit one host after another. Animal parasites are annoying in their own right, but they can also function as vectors for other contagious diseases.

- *Protozoa.* These single-celled organisms cause diseases that include giardiasis, malaria, and cryptosporidiosis. The protozoan associated with malaria is vector-borne through mosquitoes, but giardiasis and cryptosporidiosis are transmitted through oral-fecal contamination (Figure 1.5).
- *Helminths and roundworms.* Parasitic worms colonize various places in the body, including the gastrointestinal tract, the liver, and the urinary bladder. Most helminths have been

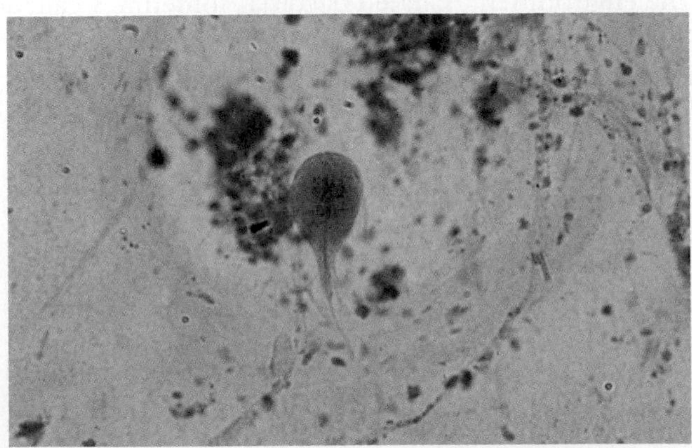
Figure 1.5. Giardia

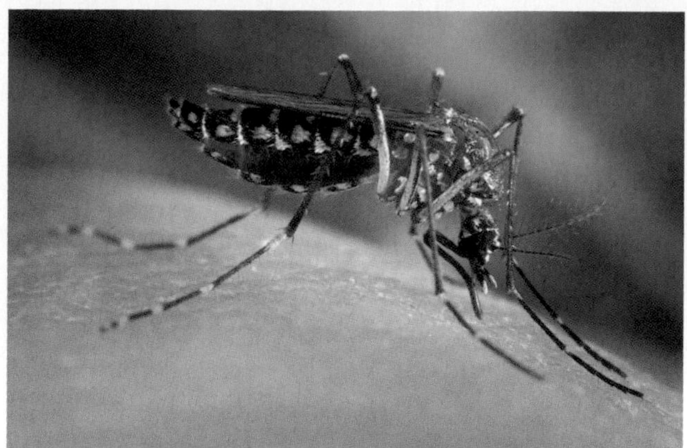

Figure 1.6. Mosquito: vector for West Nile virus

eradicated from the United States, but they are still a significant public health issue in developing countries. Roundworms are still common infestations in the United States and the rest of the world, although they tend to be most prevalent in warm climates. Schistosomiasis, which can cause bladder cancer, and trichinosis are worm-related diseases.

- *Arthropods.* Head lice, crab lice, and the mites that cause scabies are animal parasites that colonize human skin. They are discussed in detail in Chapter 2.
- *Others.* Other animal parasites don't necessarily live on or in a host, but they are worth mentioning because they can spread other pathogens. Mosquitoes (malaria, West Nile virus), ticks (Lyme disease, Rocky Mountain spotted fever), and fleas (bubonic plague) are common disease vectors (Figures 1.6 and 1.7).

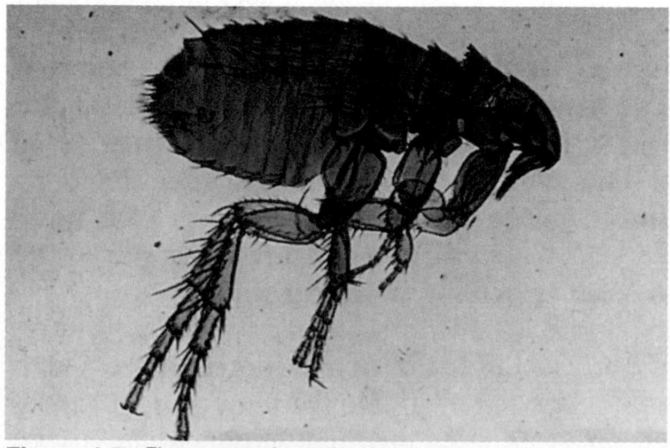

Figure 1.7. Flea: vector for bubonic plague

Hygienic Practices for Massage Therapists

Massage therapists work with a physical intimacy unmatched by practically any other health care profession. How many health professionals, outside of nurses, surgeons, dentists, and dental hygienists, spend an hour or more devoting the total of their concentration and focus, as well as their touch, to the well-being of their clients? This prolonged close contact puts both therapists and clients at risk for sharing pathogens.

The methods for how infectious agents jump the gap from one host to another have been exhaustively studied. The process essentially boils down to three issues: a reservoir or source of the infectious agent, a susceptible new host, and a mode of transport. Possible reservoirs can include other humans or animals or environmental habitats like contaminated computer keyboards or food that harbors potentially dangerous bacteria. The susceptibility of a new host depends on a number of variables, from species to inborn immunity, to variable resistance. Finally the mode of transport can be direct (like blood-to-blood exchange) or indirect through the air with respiratory secretions or from an intermediate object like a doorknob or a light switch. These disease-relaying objects are sometimes called **fomites**.

The hygienic practice guidelines provided here are drawn from recommendations by the Centers for Disease Control and other resources for health care professionals in hospital, dental, and home-care settings. Individual states may also have specific guidelines for massage therapists. These recommendations are probably more elaborate than most massage therapists observe, but bodywork practitioners are conceivably at risk for professional liability if stringent standards of cleanliness and professionalism are not followed.

Definition of Terms

- *Cleaning* is the removal of soil through manual or mechanical means, often in preparation for disinfection or sterilization.
- *Disinfection* is the destruction of pathogenic microorganisms or their toxins by direct exposure to chemical or physical agents. Disinfectants are described as low,

intermediate, and high level. These interventions can kill most pathogens, but bacterial spores may be spared.

- *Sterilization* is destruction of all microorganisms in a given field. It is accomplished with baking, steam under pressure, or chemicals under pressure.
- *Sanitation* is use of measures designed to promote health and prevent disease; it usually refers to creating a clean environment but does not specify the level of cleanliness.
- *Plain soap* is any detergent that contains no antimicrobial products or only small amounts of antimicrobial products to act as preservatives.
- *Antimicrobial soap* is a detergent that contains antimicrobial substances.
- *Alcohol-based hand rub* contains 60% to 95% alcohol (usually ethanol, isopropanol, or both).
- *Universal and standard precautions* are a set of protocols that were introduced in 1987 to create some uniformity in how medical professionals, especially dentists, should limit contact with body fluids in the working environment. Standard precautions were added to universal precautions to include guidelines on how to avoid all potentially harmful body fluids. The following fluids are specifically mentioned in standard precautions as potentially infectious: semen, vaginal secretions, breast milk, cerebrospinal fluid, synovial fluid, pleural fluid, pericardial fluid, amniotic fluid, blood, blood-tinged saliva, and vomit (emesis). Sweat and tears are not described as infectious fluids.

Applications for Massage Therapists

Hand Washing

Healthy skin is composed of several layers of cells that are manufactured deep in the epidermis. As they mature, new cells underneath push older cells toward the surface. By the time they reach the superficial layers of the skin, the cells are dead and they have been filled with keratin to create a tough, waterproof covering. A layer of intercellular lipid anchors the epidermis. This lipid layer, with the stratum corneum, forms an effective barrier between the inside and the outside of the body.

Various types of bacteria colonize the epidermis. Transient bacteria are found in the superficial layers of the skin; these microbes are easily removed with soap and water or other friction. Resident bacteria colonize deeper layers of the skin, and they are more difficult to remove. Fortunately, they also tend to be less aggressive and less likely to cause serious infections.

Hand washing with soap and running water removes new dirt and some transient bacteria, at least temporarily. Depending on the temperature of the water and the nature of the soap, frequent hand washing can also interfere with the function of the lipid layer: hot water and some detergents can reduce intercellular lipids and increase cell proliferation. This can interfere with the uptake of essential fatty acids that help to preserve the impermeability of the skin. In other words, too frequent hand washing with hot water and harsh soap can actually make the skin more vulnerable to infection by compromising the shield.

After extensive research comparing the benefits and risks of frequent hand washing with plain soap and water, antimicrobial soap, and alcohol-based gels, the Centers for Disease Control and Prevention (CDC) has created some recommendations for normal use and for health care workers.[1] It was found that running warm water (not hot water, which raises the risk of skin irritation) plus plain soap for 30 seconds is adequate for most everyday use. This method is also recommended to remove any visible or palpable dirt. It is preferable to dispense soap in liquid form, because bacteria can colonize bar soap.

Using alcohol-based gel or foam according to manufacturers' directions (which means using the amount prescribed and rubbing until the skin is dry) is often faster and more convenient than washing with soap and water, and it is an effective antibacterial and antiviral mechanism, but it does not remove dirt, and it is not effective against spore-forming bacteria. Alcohol-soaked towelettes are specifically not recommended because their alcohol concentration isn't high enough to be effective.

Washing hands with water and antimicrobial soap is effective but carries a higher level of risk of negative reactions in the form of allergies or contact dermatitis than does washing with plain soap. The concern that widespread use of antimicrobial soaps might lead to increasing tolerance among common pathogens appears to be substantiated (some pathogens have increased their resistance), but the changes are extremely minor and not of a scale that presents a challenge.

For people whose skin is very sensitive, it is important to choose a soap with no or minimal dyes or perfumes. These substances raise the risk of developing allergic contact dermatitis, which can compromise the integrity of the skin. In addition, using an emollient that is likewise free of dye or perfume can help support a healthy epidermis and lipid layer while minimizing the risk of an allergic reaction. One benefit of alcohol gels is a relatively low risk of allergic reactions, although skin drying must be counteracted by the use of moisturizing lotion.

Other Hand Care

In addition to keeping hands clean, massage therapists must be vigilant about the risk of open lesions. Hangnails that peel and fray can become portals of entry for serious infections. Hangnails must be kept short and controlled; a good pair of cuticle scissors and appropriate lotion can help with this.

Any other open lesions on the hands must be covered during a massage. This can be done with a simple bandage if it is in a place that doesn't come in direct contact with a client and is changed with each session; a liquid bandage (which can be washed with regular hand washing); or a finger cot, a small latex sheath that must be replaced for every session.

Fingernails must be kept short, of course, and artificial nails should be avoided. Scrapings from the fingernails of health care workers have been cultured to reveal colonies of yeasts and gram-negative bacilli. Imagine getting a massage from someone with long nails, knowing what could be growing under there... how relaxing could that be?

Care of Surfaces and Equipment

In a massage therapy work space, it is a good goal to create an environment where nothing that one client touches directly or indirectly is touched by another client before it is cleaned. This means isolating table linens and other fabrics and cleaning massage furniture, massage tools, lubricant dispensers, and any other items that might come into use during a session.

Fabrics

The fabrics that clients directly contact include linens on the massage table, face cradle covers, bolster and pillow covers, and the therapist's clothing. Any fabric item that a client contacts should be laundered before another client touches it. Similarly, any item that a massage therapist touches during a session with one client should be cleaned or re-covered before it is used again.

Therapists have some choices about their own clothing. Some wear aprons that can be changed with every appointment; this is appropriate as long as the client does not directly contact other articles of clothing. It is also possible to own several uniform shirts that can be changed between sessions. Aprons, uniform shirts, and other clothing items can be laundered with linens.

Guidelines for laundering are not universally agreed upon, but here are some important factors to bear in mind:

- Professional laundering services use water that is 160°F (71.1°C) or above, with a minimum of 25 minutes of agitation to reduce microbial populations.
- Good antimicrobial effect is found with temperatures from 71°F to 77°F (21.6°C to 25°C), if the detergent is strong and used according to manufacturers' directions.
- If bleach is added to the wash, it becomes most active at temperatures above 135°F (62.7°C). Most home hot water heaters heat water to 120°F to 140°F (48.4°C to 60°C), so bleach in the washing machine may not reach its full potential. The recommended amount of bleach is a ratio of 50 to 150 ppm (parts per million).
- Bleached laundry must be thoroughly rinsed to minimize irritation to users.
- Laundry must not be left damp for any significant length of time.
- All laundry should be dried on high heat (160°F, 71.1°C). Ironing adds extra antimicrobial action, but this is probably not a practical suggestion for most massage therapists.
- Clean laundry must be packaged to keep it clean until its next use. It could be wrapped in plastic or stored in a closed, freshly disinfected container.

Therapists who use a professional laundry service will probably rent their sheets from the service. This means the therapist has no control over the quality, texture, color, or newness of the linens. Also, all items except sheets must be laundered by the therapist. This includes towels, face cradle covers, bolster covers, pillow cases, and clothing.

Therapists who do their own laundry should be aware that adding bleach will shorten the life of their fabrics, and of course it is impractical for colored sheets or clothing. Nonchlorine bleach does not have antimicrobial effect. Washing with strong detergent and drying on high heat are sufficient for most situations, however.

Other fabric items include mattress pads, bolsters, pillows, blankets, and heating pad covers. Any of these should be laundered if a client touched it directly, but if the contact was through some other covering (i.e., a mattress pad that is *always* covered by a sheet), then laundering for every session is unnecessary. The exception to this rule is when there are signs of contamination (i.e., bleeding or other fluid seepage) that may penetrate through the protective layer of fabric.

Other Equipment

Massage tables and chairs can be swabbed with disinfectant between clients. This is especially important for face cradles, of course. Therapists may choose which product they prefer, but it should be at least an intermediate-level disinfectant. The CDC recommends a 10% bleach solution for high-touch surfaces; this is inexpensive and easily available. It is important to mix fresh solution frequently, however, as bleach solutions lose potency if they are not used promptly. Bleach-infused wipes can be useful in this application, but it is important to read the labels for best results: some of them require at least 10 minutes of exposure to be effective. Alcohol is specifically not recommended for cleaning surfaces because it evaporates too quickly; it works best with prolonged contact against targeted pathogens.

Massage lubricants must be kept free from the risk of cross-contamination. Lubricants that are solid at room temperature (e.g., beeswax, coconut oil) must be dispensed into individual containers and leftovers discarded so that double-dipping never occurs. Liquid lubricants must be dispensed in bottles that are washed between every session. Bottles should be kept away from possibly contaminated surfaces, such as desktops or the floor.

Hot or cold stones and crystals may be the only massage tools that lend themselves to full sterilization. Depending on their composition, these may be boiled or baked between uses to ensure removal of all pathogens. Items that are not disposable, such as massage tools, vibrators, and hot and cold packs, must have their contacting surfaces disinfected every time they are used.

The Massage Environment

Research indicates that fabrics such as curtains, carpeting, and upholstery are not significant sites of transmission for infectious agents, but they may harbor pet hair or dander that could cause an allergic reaction. For this reason, upholstery and carpets should be vacuumed frequently. Vinyl or leather upholstery can be swabbed with disinfectant. Any carpeting that gets wet can harbor bacteria and fungi; it should be replaced if it isn't completely dry within a few hours. Hard floors can be washed regularly with detergent, but no particular benefit has been found in washing frequently with high-level disinfectants.

Other surfaces that clients and therapists contact should also be cleaned frequently. These include doorknobs, bathroom fixtures, light switch plates, telephones, and coat racks or hooks. If a therapist uses a computer in the office, the keyboard may provide a rich growth medium for pathogens. This can be ameliorated with antiseptic-soaked towelettes or keyboard covers that can be washed in the sink. Also, cash is not called "filthy lucre" for nothing; it is typically handled by numerous dirty hands and is an excellent vector for communicable diseases.

The guidelines suggested here may seem unnecessarily alarmist. However, as more people seek massage, and as new and stronger forms of pathogens develop, it becomes increasingly important for massage therapists in any setting to create the most professional and safest environment possible.

The Inflammatory Process

What Is Inflammation?

Inflammation is a tissue response to damage or the threat of invasion by antigens: bits of nonself. It is typically caused by physical injury (trauma, chemical burn, hypothermia), invasion with foreign bodies (pathogens, splinters, shrapnel), hormonal changes, or autoimmune activity. The inflammatory response is expressed through cellular and vascular functions that are coordinated by chemical mediators.

The purpose of inflammation is to protect the body from pathogenic invasion, to limit the range of contamination, and to prepare damaged tissue for healing. Once an acute inflammatory response has begun, it has only a few possible courses: complete resolution with no significant tissue changes, accumulation of scar tissue, or chronic inflammation, possibly with the formation of cysts and abscesses.

To learn more about inflammation from the author, as well as an animation about the process, visit http://thePoint.lww.com/Werner5e!

Components of Inflammation: Vascular Activity

The vascular component of inflammation comes into play when tissue is damaged by trauma or other factors. For the sake of simplicity, consider a basic laceration or puncture wound as a model, although the same principles hold true for any kind of local injury (Figure 1.8A and B). In the first moments, vasoconstriction occurs. This is easily observable on scratching the skin: a white wheal is followed by a red mark within a few seconds. The vasoconstrictive stage is over within moments for a minor injury, and several minutes for a more serious one.

Vasodilation is the next step in vascular activity. Damaged endothelial cells and mast cells release a host of chemicals that increase the permeability of blood vessel walls, reinforce capillary dilation, attract platelets, and slow blood flow away from the area, limiting the risk of deeper penetration of pathogens.

Vasodilation is short-lived with minor injuries, but it may last for several days with more severe injuries. In some situations the vascular reaction to tissue damage is delayed for several hours; this is the case with sunburns, for instance.

Components of Inflammation: Cellular Activity

Many cells are recruited to manage tissue damage and contamination risk with injury:

- *Endothelial cells.* The endothelial cells of damaged blood vessels release chemicals that activate platelets and allow white blood cells to escape their boundaries. These cells are also sensitive to chemical signals to proliferate: in later stages of healing, endothelial cells build capillaries to supply new tissue growth.

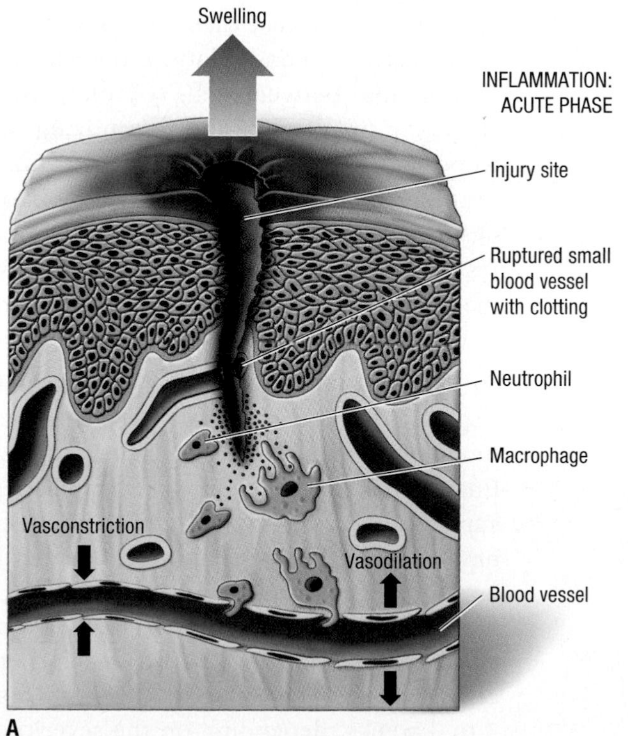

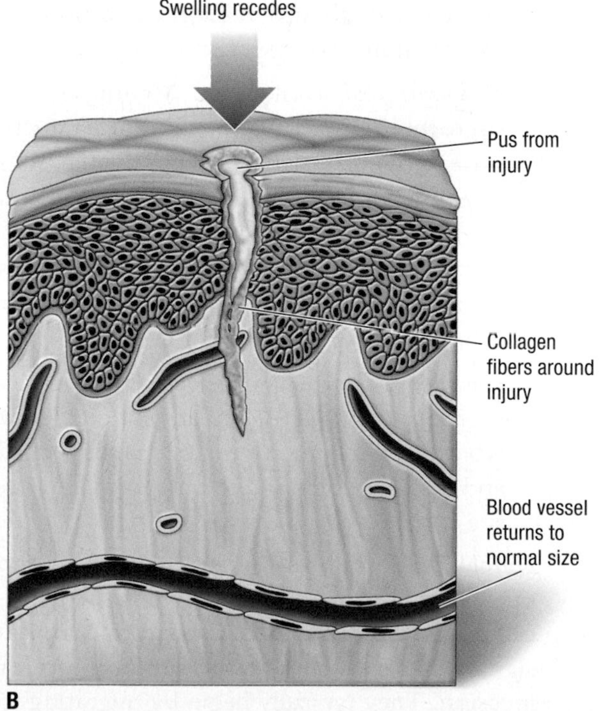

Figure 1.8. Many cellular changes happen with the inflammatory response (**A**) to protect the body from infection and prepare the area for healing (**B**).

- *Platelets.* When platelets are stimulated, they become jagged and sticky, and they release several chemicals that interact with plasma proteins to weave the net of fibrin that forms a blood clot and the scaffolding for future scar tissue.
- *White blood cells.* Several types of white blood cells participate in the inflammatory process. Which types depends on how long the injury has been present and what types of pathogens are involved.
  - *Granulocytes.* **Granulocytes** are the smallest, fastest white blood cells. They are called granulocytes because when they are isolated and stained, they appear to have tiny granules in them. **Neutrophils** are the most common type of granulocyte to be involved in early stages of inflammation. These tiny white blood cells are associated with bacterial infection and musculoskeletal injury. Other granulocytes include **eosinophils** (associated with allergic reactions and parasites) and **basophils** (associated with allergies and histamine release).
  - *Mast cells.* Mast cells are found in tissues most vulnerable to damage: skin, the respiratory tract, and gastrointestinal tract. When they are activated, they release histamine and other chemicals that reinforce and prolong the inflammatory response.
  - *Monocytes and macrophages.* **Monocytes** are large, mobile white blood cells. They are sensitive to chemical signals that call them to sites of injury or potential infection. Monocytes can become permanently fixed **macrophages**. They are typically involved in later stages of inflammation: they help clean up cellular debris to prepare the area for healing.
  - *Lymphocytes.* Some lymphocytes are involved in the resolution of inflammation. They work with macrophages to clean up dead and damaged cells and to help form scar tissue and new blood vessels.
- *Fibroblasts.* Fibroblasts produce collagen and other components of connective tissue extracellular matrix. They also respond to chemical signals that call them to the site of injury or invasion. They typically begin by migrating to local blood clots and may proliferate to create more scar tissue if necessary.

Components of Inflammation: Chemical Mediators

All cells involved in inflammation are coordinated by chemical messages that tell them what to do. Some of these chemicals are suspended in plasma (clotting factors, complement, and a group of chemicals called **kinins** that increase pain sensation and the permeability of capillaries). Platelets, mast cells, and basophils release histamine and serotonin, which also promote vasodilation and capillary permeability. Injured cell membranes release platelet-activating factors and arachidonic acid metabolites that then form prostaglandins and leukotrienes—more inflammatory chemicals. The study of proinflammatory chemicals continues to reveal new secrets about this remarkable and intricate process.

Stages of Healing

The process of healing from injury or infection is extremely complex. It requires the highly coordinated interaction of vascular, cellular, and chemical components to come to a successful resolution. Healing typically happens in three stages.

- *Acute stage.* In this initial inflammatory phase, damaged cells release their chemicals, causing vasoconstriction and dilation, the accumulation of fluid between cells (edema), and the attraction of platelets and fast-moving white blood cells. Tissue exudate begins to form: this can take the shape of the fluid that fills blisters, pus, or other material that indicates immune system activity. Depending on the severity of the injury, the acute stage may last 1 to 3 days or longer.
- *Subacute stage.* Also called the proliferative stage, this is the phase when specific cells accumulate and work to fill in damaged tissue. Endothelial cells grow into new capillaries to supply granulation tissue, the framework for new cells. If the damage affects deeper layers, fibroblasts spin new collagen fibers. At the same time, slower-moving white blood cells begin to clean up dead pathogens and other cellular debris. The subacute stage may last for 2 to 3 weeks, depending on the severity and depth of the injury and the healing capacity of the person who has been injured.

- *Postacute stage.* Also called the maturation stage, this is when new collagen undergoes changes: it is remodeled and reshaped, and it becomes denser and aligns according to force. In other words, if a muscle, tendon, or ligament is injured and accumulates scar tissue, and if that structure is stretched and exercised carefully, those new collagen fibers eventually lie down in alignment with uninjured fibers.

Chronic Inflammation

Occasionally the inflammatory process is not wholly successful. Pathogens or irritants are not removed from the body, the immune system continually attacks some type of tissue, or musculoskeletal structures never regain full function. When this happens, the result is called chronic inflammation. This is different from standard inflammation, involving different types of cells and holding a different prognosis.

When chronic inflammation is connected to an infection or an autoimmune process, several things can happen. Pus that is never reabsorbed is surrounded by a wall of connective tissue: this is a cyst or abscess. It carries a risk of rupture and dangerous infection. Persistent signals to fibroblasts can cause an accumulation of scar tissue that can interfere with organ function, as seen with cirrhosis of the liver. Scar tissue can also block the digestive tract or other passageways; this is called a **stricture**, which can cause stenosis: obstruction of an important passageway. The body sometimes attempts to build new "exit routes" when tubes are otherwise blocked. When these drain into the skin, they are called **sinuses**; when they connect to other hollow organs, they are called **fistulae**. Sinuses and fistulae are possible complications of chronic inflammatory conditions such as ulcerative colitis, Crohn disease, and others.

An unsuccessful inflammatory process can also cause problems in musculoskeletal tissues. Under normal circumstances when a fibrous structure like a muscle, tendon, or ligament is injured, it undergoes a typical inflammatory response. Neutrophils arrive to scout the area for potential invaders; monocytes and fibroblasts follow afterward to clean up the debris and lay down the framework for new collagen fibers. But sometimes the quality of the new collagen is never well established, and the injured structure never satisfactorily heals. While inflammation itself subsides, pain and limitation may continue. This situation, called tendinosis when it affects tendons, is discussed in the section on tendinopathies in Chapter 3.

Finally, when inflammation and the formation of scar tissue are overactive with skin injuries, the resulting lesion can be large and difficult to resolve. This situation is called hypertrophic or keloid scarring and is discussed in the scar tissue section of Chapter 2.

Signs and Symptoms

Every massage therapist should know this litany: the symptoms of inflammation are pain, heat, redness, swelling, and sometimes loss of function. In some cases itching, clotting, and pus formation can be added to the list.

The sources of these symptoms are easy to identify. Vasodilation brings about the redness, heat and swelling by drawing extra blood to an isolated area. Pain and itching can be the result of several factors: edematous pressure, damaged nerve endings, irritating pathogenic toxins, and inflammatory chemicals that increase pain sensation. If the inflammation limits movement, the injured or invaded area loses function. Clotting and pus formation have already been discussed. Not all of these symptoms are present in all cases of inflammation.

Treatment

The typical treatment for inflammation is no surprise; a wide variety of anti-inflammatory drugs have been developed to interfere with the production of proinflammatory chemicals, and decrease pain perception at various steps along the sensory pathways. Several of these medications are discussed in detail in Appendix A. Regardless of their chemical effect on the body, orally administered anti-inflammatories impact massage decisions, because they may hide the results of overtreatment, raising the risk that massage can cause injury. If a client takes anti-inflammatories for a condition that does not contraindicate massage, it is wise to schedule the session when the drug is at its lowest activity. In this way, it is possible to get the most accurate feedback from the client's tissues about the effects of the massage.

Medications

- Over-the-counter anti-inflammatories
- Prescription nonsteroidal anti-inflammatories
- Prescription steroidal anti-inflammatories

Massage?

RISKS	Acute systemic infections like cold or flu contraindicate some types of bodywork because of the risk of communicability to the practitioner, and because the immune system may not keep up with the additional stimulus of rigorous circulatory massage. Acute local skin infections like boils or small lesions locally contraindicate massage because of the risk of communicability, and the possibility of overwhelming the ability of the body to isolate the infectious agents. Inflammation that is not related to infection may be appropriate for various types of bodywork, depending on the stage. Clients who have used anti-inflammatory drugs prior to their massage session may be less sensitive to pressure and consequently vulnerable to overtreatment.
BENEFITS	Lymph drainage techniques can be useful for acute inflammation when no infection is present. Postacute local inflammation may respond well to careful massage, which can help to improve sluggish and congested circulation in the postacute stages of infection and inflammation.

CHAPTER REVIEW QUESTIONS: FUNDAMENTAL CONCEPTS IN PATHOLOGY

1. Define the following terms: sign, symptom, syndrome.
2. What is an epidemic?
3. Name five classes of infectious agents.
4. What is the purpose of universal or standard precautions?
5. What are the risks of repeated hand washing with hot water and harsh soap?
6. What is the recommended handwashing protocol if warm running water and soap are not available?
7. What is the purpose of inflammation?
8. What are three possible outcomes for the inflammatory process?
9. Describe what happens during the postacute, or maturation, phase of inflammation.
10. What adjustments must be made if a client takes anti-inflammatory medication shortly before a massage session?

Reference

1. Centers for Disease Control and Prevention. Guideline for Hand Hygiene in Health-Care Settings: Recommendations of the Healthcare Infection Control Practices Advisory Committee and the HICPAC/SHEA/APIC/IDSA Hand Hygiene Task Force. MMWR 2002;51(No. RR-16). http://www.cdc.gov/mmwr/PDF/rr/rr5116.pdf. Accessed winter 2010.

2

Integumentary System Conditions

Chapter Objectives

After reading this chapter you should be able to...

- Explain why compromised skin contraindicates massage.
- Name three variations on fungal infections of the skin.
- Name what kinds of bacteria are associated with boils.
- Name what kinds of bacteria are associated with cellulitis.
- Identify the causative agent for cold sores.
- Name a feature that distinguishes plantar warts from callus.
- Explain the difference between atopic dermatitis and contact dermatitis.
- Name two dangers associated with widespread burns.
- Identify the ABCDEs of malignant melanoma.
- Name the most dependable sign of nonmelanoma skin cancer.

Introduction: Function and Construction of the Skin

Massage practitioners speak in the language of touch. The messages practitioners give are invitations to a number of different possibilities: to enjoy a state of well-being, to heal and repair what is broken, and to reacquaint a client with his or her own body. All these happen through the skin, a medium equipped like no other tissue in the body to take in information and respond to it, largely on a subconscious level. The goal of massage practitioners is to anticipate these reactions and set the stage for them in a way that is most beneficial to their clients.

Functions of the skin

A student once said that the purpose of skin is to keep our insides from falling out. That's true, but that's not all that skin does; its functions are manifold. Among them are several devices to keep the body healthy and safe, all wrapped up in a tidy 18- to 30-lb package.

Protection

The skin keeps pathogens out of the body, just by being intact, and it discourages their growth on its surface by secreting the acidic substances otherwise needed for keeping hair shafts lubricated. Furthermore, by constantly sloughing off dead cells, it sloughs off potential invaders too.

The skin is the first line of defense against invasion; it is the physical barrier that defines our boundaries. Although it is made of relatively delicate tissue, skin cells quickly and efficiently replace themselves: think of scraping your knuckle on a cheese grater at night, and how the wound is well on its way to healing by the next morning. This capacity for quick replication can sometimes backfire, however, with dangerous results. In addition to fast repair, the skin also offers protection in the abundance of immune system cells located in superficial fascia. When these defense mechanisms become hyperactive, they can cause certain types of rashes and other skin problems.

Homeostasis

The skin protects us from fluid loss, a top homeostatic priority, and one of the most dangerous functions to lose when the skin is damaged. The skin also helps to maintain a constant internal temperature: superficial capillaries dilate or constrict in response to external temperature. Fat in the subcutaneous layer also acts as insulation against cold, and of course the evaporation of sweat is a powerful cooling device when the ambient humidity is low.

Sensory envelope

With as many as 19,000 sensory receptors in every square inch of skin, it's obvious that this is the organ (or tissue, membrane, or system—depending on the source of information) that tells us the most about our environment. Massage therapists must develop the skill of becoming conscious of the subtle information their hands pick up when they touch their clients, and must understand that every sensation on a client's skin causes ripples of reactions all through that person's body.

Absorption and excretion

The skin can be recruited as an organ of absorption and excretion, but only under certain circumstances. The skin does not typically absorb topical substances into the bloodstream unless they are of a particular

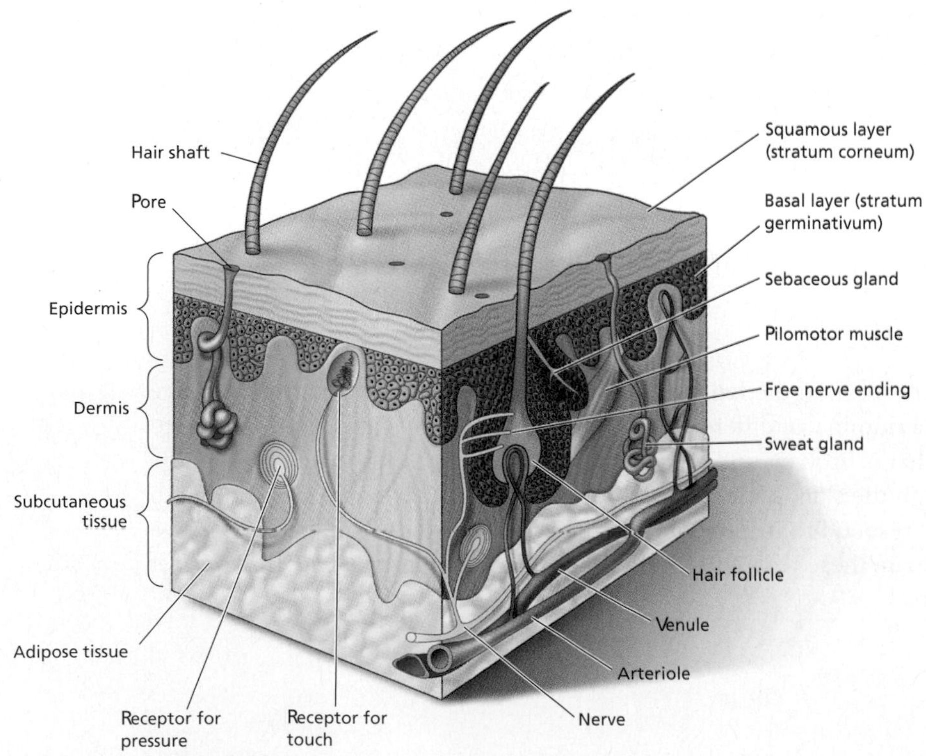

Figure 2.1. Layers of skin

molecular size, or administered with a chemical that allows for transcutaneous absorption; this is the mechanism behind nicotine patches and birth control patches.

The skin can excrete metabolic wastes, but it does so only as a last-ditch option. When the liver, colon, or kidneys are so overwhelmed that they can't process waste products adequately, sweat can carry noxious chemicals out of the body.

Construction of the skin

Skin varies from being very thin (on the lips) to remarkably thick (on the heels). It remodels according to stresses put upon it. **Callus** is an example of this phenomenon: it is simply extra-thick, extra-hard epidermis on places that really take a beating.

The construction of the skin is important, because it has relevance for how disease occurs and how easily it can spread. Three basic layers of tissue define the skin, and within those layers are more layers. The deepest layer has three possible names: the subcutaneous layer, the subdermis, or superficial fascia. It is composed of a loose collagen and elastin framework that holds fat cells and some other structures (Figure 2.1).

The middle layer is the dermis, or "true skin." This is the location of hair follicles, oil and sweat glands, and some nerve endings. The outermost layer of dermis, the basal layer, lies just deep to the epidermis and has the best capillary supply. This is where new skin cells arise. It is also the site of pigment cells or **melanocytes**, which produce melanin to protect people from harmful ultraviolet (UV) rays.

The epidermis is the most superficial layer of skin. It is composed of many layers of cells called keratinocytes that are produced in the basal layer of the dermis. As these cells are pushed toward the surface, they fill with

Integumentary System Conditions

Contagious Skin Disorders

- Animal parasites
  - Head lice
  - Crab lice (pubic lice)
  - Body lice
  - Scabies mites
- Fungal infections of the skin
  - Tinea capitis
  - Tinea corporis
  - Tinea cruris (jock itch)
  - Tinea pedis (athlete's foot)
  - Tinea manuum
  - Onychomycosis
  - Tinea versicolor
- Herpes simplex
  - Oral herpes
  - Genital herpes
  - Herpes whitlow
  - Herpes gladiatorum
  - Herpes sycosis
  - Eczema herpeticum
  - Ocular herpes
- Staphylococcal infections of the skin
  - Boils
  - Folliculitis
  - Methicillin-resistant Staphylococcus aureus
  - Hidradenatis supporitiva
  - Pilonidal cysts
- Streptococcal infections of the skin
  - Cellulitis
  - Erysipelas (St. Anthony's Fire)
  - Necrotizing fasciitis
- Warts
  - Common warts
  - Plantar warts
  - Cystic warts
  - Plane warts
  - Molluscum contagiosum
  - Genital warts
  - Butchers' warts
  - Focal epithelia hyperplasia
  - Epidermoplasia verruciformis

Noncontagious Inflammatory Skin Disorders

- Acne rosacea
- Acne vulgaris
- Dermatitis, eczema
  - Contact dermatitis
  - Atopic dermatitis
  - Seborrheic eczema
  - Dyshydrosis
  - Nummular eczema
  - Stasis dermatitis
  - Neurodermatitis

Neoplastic Skin Disorders

- Seborrheic keratosis
- Skin cancer
  - Basal cell carcinoma
  - Squamous cell carcinoma, actinic carcinoma
  - Malignant melanoma

Skin Injuries

- Burns
- Decubitus ulcers
- Scar tissue
  - Keloid scars
  - Hypertrophic scars
  - Contracture scars

keratin, becoming water resistant and scaly in the process. By the time they reach the surface, they are long dead and are eventually exfoliated to become the major ingredient of household dust. Bacteria colonize these layers of keratinocytes. Transient bacteria, which tend to be more aggressive, are found in the superficial layers. They are removed with friction and running water but are quickly replaced. Resident bacteria, which tend to be less aggressive, colonize deeper layers of the epidermis.

Implications for Massage

Skin conditions have a special relevance for massage therapists because we are in a position to notice lesions and blemishes that clients often don't know are present. This is why it is especially important to be able to recognize most common skin conditions, at least to recommend that clients investigate further with their own doctor. Many skin conditions contraindicate massage, because they might be contagious or they might spread further on the body. But beyond that danger, the one cardinal rule for skin conditions and massage is this: *if the skin in not intact, the client is a walking invitation to infection*. Open skin, broken skin, scabbed skin, oozing skin, or any skin that allows access to the blood vessels inside is a red flag for bodywork practitioners.

Many technical terms describe the ways skin can be injured. Here is a list of common skin lesions:

- Lacerations (rips and tears)
- Incisions (cuts)
- Excoriations (scratches)
- Fissures (cracks)
- Papules (firm raised areas, like pimples)
- Vesicles (blisters)
- Pustules (vesicles filled with pus, like whiteheads)
- Punctures (any kind of hole)
- Avulsions (something has been ripped off, like a finger or an ear)
- Abrasions (scrapes)
- Ulcers (sores with dead tissue that don't go through a normal healing process)

Knowing this vocabulary is important, but it is not as important as knowing that hands-on massage is inappropriate for any situation in which skin is not entirely intact.

For advice from the author about working with contagious skin disorders, view her videos at thePoint.lww.com/Werner5e!

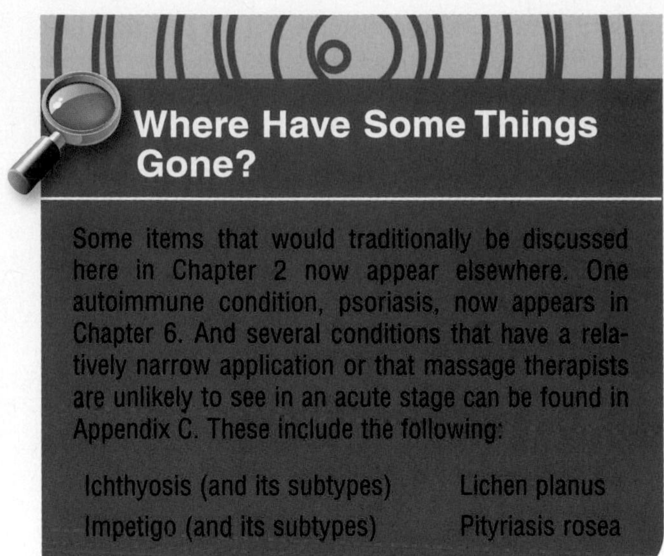

Where Have Some Things Gone?

Some items that would traditionally be discussed here in Chapter 2 now appear elsewhere. One autoimmune condition, psoriasis, now appears in Chapter 6. And several conditions that have a relatively narrow application or that massage therapists are unlikely to see in an acute stage can be found in Appendix C. These include the following:

Ichthyosis (and its subtypes)	Lichen planus
Impetigo (and its subtypes)	Pityriasis rosea

Contagious Skin Disorders

Animal Parasites

Many massage therapists fear parasitic infestations, because bodyworkers are so vulnerable to whatever is crawling around on their clients' skins. But here, as in all things fearful, the best defense is information. This discussion will be limited to animals that live in/on humans or their clothing.

Types of Animal Parasites

Mites

Definition: What Are They?

Tiny mites (*Sarcoptes scabeii*) are arthropods that cause the skin lesions called scabies (Figure 2.2). The females burrow into the epidermis where they feed on damaged skin cells, defecate and urinate, and lay eggs, so the next generation can carry on. The average life cycle of a female mite is 30 to 60 days. As an adult, she lays approximately three eggs per day, although only a small percentage of them hatch. Newly hatched mites migrate to the surface of the skin, where it takes about 14 days for them to achieve maturity.

The mites' waste is highly irritating, causing a delayed itchy allergic reaction in most hosts. If scratching damages the skin, the risk of secondary infection is high.

Animal Parasites in Brief

What are they?
A parasite is any organism that lives by drawing its nourishment from a host. The animal parasites discussed here include mites, head lice, body lice, and crab lice. They live on blood or other materials. They spread primarily through close contact with skin or infested sheets or clothing.

How are they recognized?

- **Mites** are too small to see, but they leave itchy trails or nodules where they burrow under the skin; these lesions are called scabies. Mites prefer warm, moist places, such as the axillae or between fingers.
- **Head lice** are easy to see, but they can hide. A more dependable sign is their eggs: nits are small, rice-shaped flecks that cling strongly to hair shafts.
- **Body lice** look very similar to head lice, but they live primarily in clothing and only visit the host for blood meals.
- **Pubic lice** look like tiny white crabs in pubic and coarse body hair.

All these parasites create a lot of itching through allergic reactions to the toxins they produce.

Massage risks and benefits
Risks: All four parasite infestations are communicable through direct contact. They contraindicate massage until they have been eradicated.
Benefits: Clients who have been treated and have recovered from parasitic infestations can enjoy the same benefits from massage as the rest of the population.

One type of scabies, called crusting or Norwegian scabies, is particularly prevalent among immunocompromised people. It can involve thousands or even millions of mites, and it is highly contagious. The lesions cover large areas and develop dry, flaky scabs, but they tend not to itch.

How Do They Spread?

Mites spread readily through skin-to-skin contact or through contact with something someone else has recently worn or lain on, including massage sheets. Depending on local conditions, mites can live up to 3 days in clothing or bedding.

Signs and Symptoms

Scabies mites are too small to see with the naked eye, so a visual diagnosis is based on the trails they leave behind. Sometimes their burrows are visible; these look like reddish or grayish lines around the areas the mites favor: the groin, axilla, elbows, belt line, or between fingers. Other signs of mite infestation are secondary bacterial infections and the irritated blisters and nodules that arise from allergic reactions to their waste (Figure 2.3). The itching caused by mites has a distinctive unrelenting quality. Where eczema or mosquito bites might itch intermittently and then subside, the itching with mites gets progressively worse.

Scabies lesions can be tricky to diagnose if a parasite isn't isolated and identified. A typical test involves taking a skin scraping to look for mites or their wastes.

Scabies can resemble psoriasis, eczema, and several other skin conditions, so it is important to get an accurate diagnosis. Missing the correct diagnosis increases the risk of further spread and

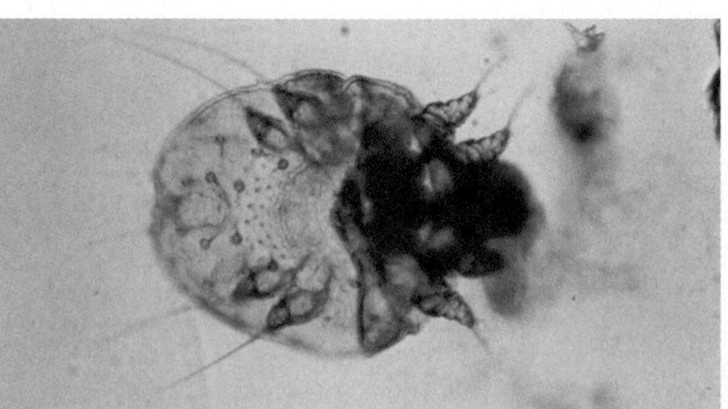

Figure 2.2. Scabies mite (microscopic)

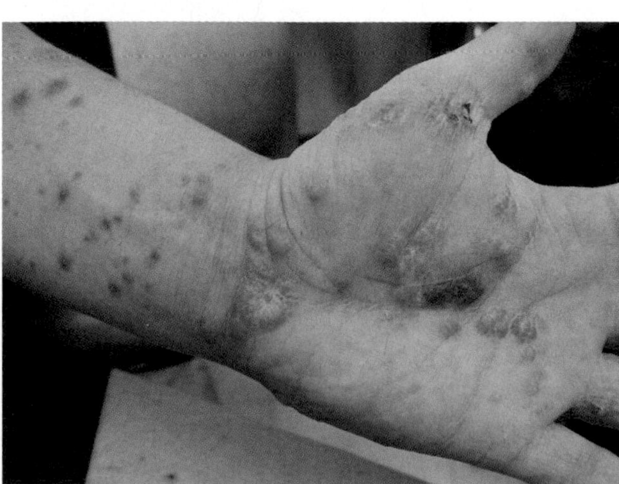

Figure 2.3. Scabies lesions

secondary infection; a false-positive diagnosis means a person may be exposed to potentially toxic material unnecessarily.

Head Lice

Definition: What Are They?

Head lice are wingless insects *(Pediculus humanus capitis)* that live in head hair and suck blood from the scalp. Infestation with lice is sometimes called **pediculosis**. Lice are quite a bit larger than mites and can easily be seen without a microscope (Figure 2.4). Their saliva is very irritating, causing itching and creating the possibility of secondary infection. Lice gestate for 7 to 16 days, depending on ambient temperature. When they hatch, they go through three molts and live an average of 2 to 3 weeks. Their life consists mainly of taking blood meals, mating, and laying eggs.

Historically, head lice and body lice have been vectors of diseases that include typhus, relapsing fever, and trench fever. While no longer considered a health threat in developed countries, these diseases are still spread by lice in refugee camps and other areas where people live in close contact and where good hygiene is difficult to maintain.

How Do They Spread?

Head lice spread most easily through direct contact: human heat allows them to move quickly from scalp to scalp during sports, camping trips, and other close-contact events. When they are separated from a host, they tend to be more sluggish. While head lice don't jump or fly, they can be dislodged to find new hosts with hair dryers, removal of clothing, or rigorous toweling.

Lice can also use hats and scarves to travel from one host to another. They may live in batters' helmets that are shared by Little League teams, hairbrushes that are shared by best friends, and car seats that are shared by carpool buddies. While this is not the most efficient way to spread lice throughout an environment, it is certainly a possible way.

Signs and Symptoms

If a client has lice, the actual insects may or may not be obvious; when they are warm, they move fast and can hide. But they lay eggs called nits that are glued to hair shafts and look like tiny grains of rice (Figure 2.5). (This is the source of the word *nitpicky*.) Newly laid nits are usually found at the base of the hair shaft, mostly behind the ears and along the back of the head. They hatch after about a week on a human host, but nits laid on hairbrushes or clothing may survive up to a month. Dark nits may not yet have hatched, but light-colored nits are usually the empty shells. Nits are a definitive feature for pediculosis; anything else of that size and color (like dandruff or dried hairspray) would brush out easily.

A person with head lice experiences itchiness and the sensation of movement on the scalp. Rigorous scratching can damage the skin and open the door to secondary infection.

Body Lice

Definition: What Are They?

Body lice (*Pediculus humanus corporis*) are closely related to head lice, but they have different living and feeding patterns. Body lice tend not to live directly on their host but in the host's clothing, especially in the

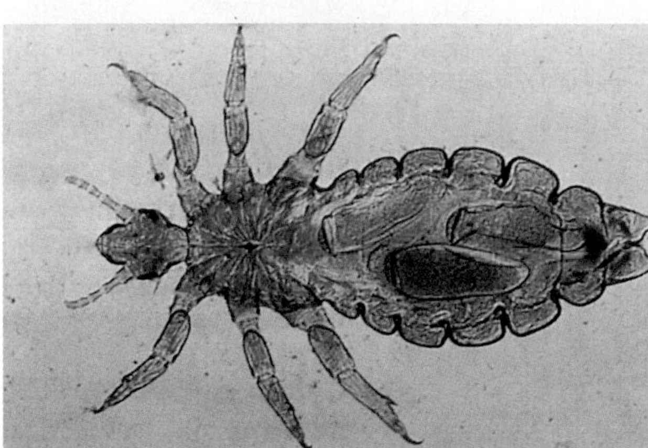

Figure 2.4. Head louse

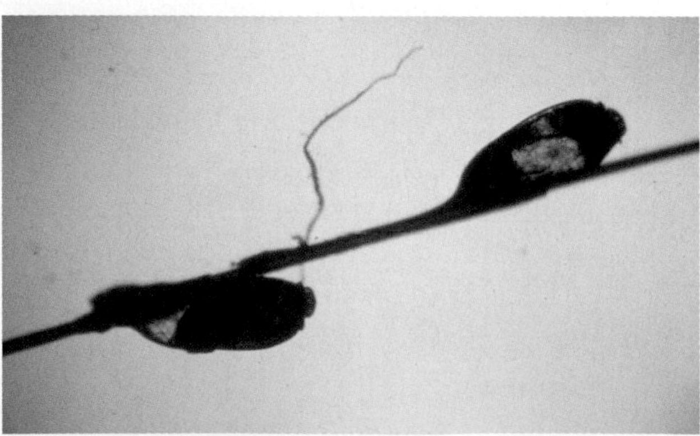

Figure 2.5. Nits attached to a hair shaft

seams. They are a bit bigger than head lice, and they also take blood meals, causing an itchy reaction.

Body lice are fairly rare except among homeless and transient populations who have limited access to laundry facilities and so spend a lot of time in unwashed clothing. Like head lice, body lice are potential vectors of communicable diseases.

How Do They Spread?

Body lice live in clothing, so sharing unwashed clothing is the most efficient way for them to spread from one host to another. They may also crawl from infested clothing to other clothing in a laundry basket in close proximity.

Signs and Symptoms

The primary sign of body lice is an itchy rash that gets worse. The insects seldom live directly on the skin, and they usually lay eggs in clothing, so unless the clothing is examined, a live body louse may not be found.

Pubic Lice

Definition: What Are They?

Pubic lice (*Pthirus pubis*) are tiny insects that look a lot like their nickname, crabs (Figure 2.6). Crabs often infest hair in the groin, but they also live in armpit hair and other coarse body hair (Figure 2.7). They may also be found in mustaches, beards, eyebrows, and eyelashes.

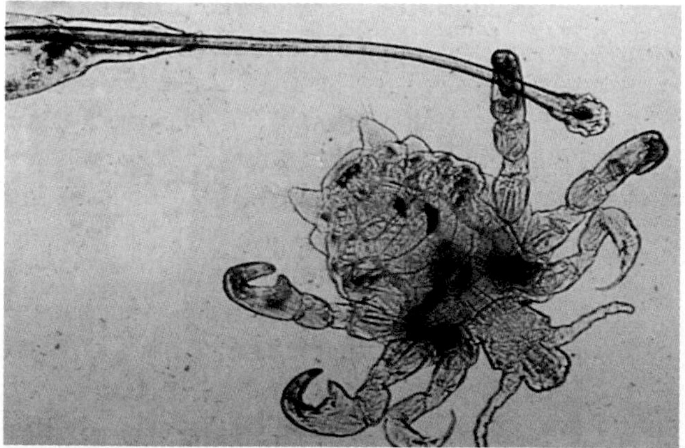
Figure 2.6. Crab louse

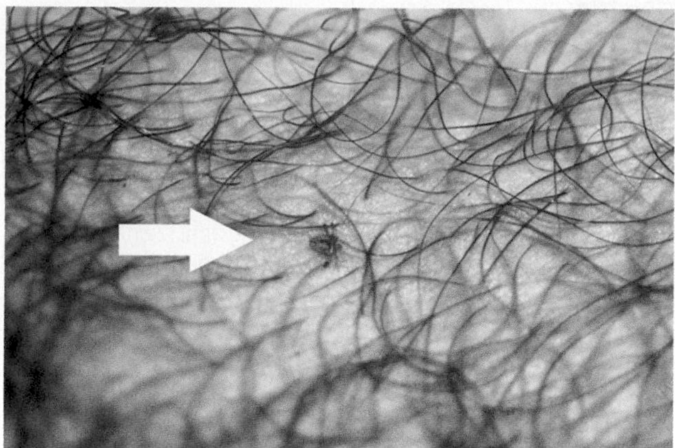
Figure 2.7. Crab louse in body hair (*arrow*)

How Do They Spread?

Pubic lice are usually spread through sexual contact, but infested clothing, linens, or massage sheets can also spread them.

Signs and Symptoms

Pubic lice look like tiny white crabs. Like all of the infestations being discussed, the primary symptom is itching that gets progressively worse without treatment.

Treatment for Animal Parasites

Parasitic infestations carry a powerful social stigma that is negatively (and often inaccurately) associated with poverty and poor hygiene. Anybody can have this problem, and manual therapists are in a position to spread parasites to clients before any symptoms develop, so it is important to be compassionate, nonjudgmental, and well informed.

Of all the infestations discussed here, the easiest to eradicate is body lice: these animals are destroyed with good hygiene and clean clothes. Mites, head lice, and crab lice must be treated with pesticidal cream or shampoo. These substances can be toxic, especially to young children, so they must be used with great care. Head lice can also be treated with less toxic substances, but this must be followed by careful manual removal of adults and nits with a nit comb. Washing or isolating bedding, clothing, upholstery, and soft toys for up to 2 weeks may also be recommended.

Medications

- Topical pesticides include preparations of pyrethrum, malathion, and lindane.

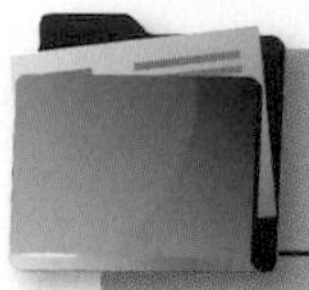

CASE HISTORY 2.1 Scabies, Valerie

Valerie was a massage student. She worked with a variety of people, including fellow students, friends, and her student internship group, people with AIDS.

One day Valerie noted that she had some areas on the outsides of her elbows that were slightly but persistently itchy during the day. They gradually developed red bumps. Ironically, this occurred while Valerie was studying skin conditions in her massage course. "It's natural to convince yourself that you have symptoms of a lot of things. I knew something was going on, and it seemed like it *could* be scabies, but my symptoms were different from anything I'd seen described," she said. The itching was not particularly worse at night and there were no tracks or typical signs of infestation. Even the site of the infestation was unusual: scabies mites usually go for warm, moist, protected areas like skin folds on the *insides* of elbows, but not the outside.

Eventually Valerie went to her general practitioner, who pronounced her condition a "mystery rash" and suggested a corticosteroid cream to limit the itchiness. In a way, Valerie was relieved by this diagnosis. "You never want to think you have scabies," she said. When her husband also developed symptoms, however, he went straight to a dermatologist, who immediately diagnosed scabies and prescribed enough pesticidal soap for both of them.

The cream was applied all over the body up to the chin; evidently mites do not infest the head or face. "That night after I washed off the cream, I was really, really, *really* itchy, and then for 4 or 5 weeks my skin was raw and uncomfortable." The cream itself can cause symptoms that mimic a scabies infestation for weeks at a time. This can lead to scabiosis, in which a person is convinced of the need to medicate for scabies again and again, although the infestation is gone. Scabiosis can become a life-threatening condition if the person repeatedly self-medicates.

Six to eight weeks passed between the onset of Valerie's symptoms and a final diagnosis. During this time, Valerie continued to work on friends and clients and to receive massage from other students. Two other classmates were infested and finally diagnosed. "The first few days [after we knew it was scabies] were full of panic and fear. Within a couple of days of people getting over their fear and paranoia there was a lot of support. People had the attitude that this is just one of the things that can happen when you're a bodyworker."■

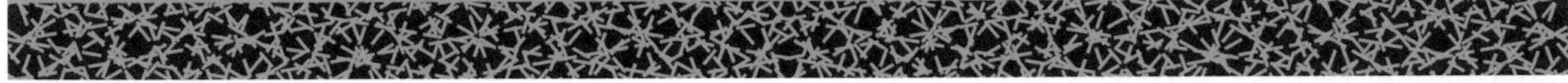

- Oral medications are sometimes prescribed, but they have not been consistently approved by the FDA.
- Antihistamines are used to control itching.
- Antibiotics are prescribed for secondary infection.

Massage?

RISKS Animal parasites are communicable through direct contact. Even though the risk of transmission may be low, the safest choice is to delay massage for a client with an infestation till after treatment is complete.

BENEFITS Any client who has completely treated their condition can enjoy the same benefits of bodywork as the rest of the population.

Fungal Infections

Definition: What Is It?

The nomenclature for superficial fungal infections is dizzying. Fungal infections of human skin, also called **mycoses**, can be caused by several different types of fungi (**dermatophytes**). Dermatophytosis, then, is another term for mycosis. The lesions the infections create are called **tinea**, a Latin word for "gnawing worm": this, and the fact that many lesions look like expanding circles on the skin, is the source for the common and misleading term for these fungal infections, "ringworm."

Etiology: What Happens?

Dermatophytes secrete enzymes that dissolve keratin, which allows them to invade the stratum corneum of

Fungal Infections in Brief

What are they?
Fungal infections of human skin, also called mycoses, are caused by fungi called dermatophytes. The characteristic lesions caused by dermatophytes are called tinea. Several types of dermatophytes cause tinea in different areas; lesions are typically named by location.

How are they recognized?
Most tinea lesions begin as one reddened circular itchy patch. Scratching the lesions spreads the fungi to other parts of the body. As the lesions grow, they tend to clear in the middle and keep a raised scaly red ring around the edges. Athlete's foot, another type of mycosis, produces oozing blisters and cracking between the toes. Fungal infections of toenails or fingernails produce thickened, pitted, discolored nails that may detach.

Massage risks and benefits
Risks: Most fungal infections locally contraindicate massage in all stages.
Benefits: Massage has no particular positive impact on fungal infections, but if the affected areas are very limited, such as only the feet or a small, covered lesion on the body, then massage may be administered elsewhere for general benefit. A client who has fully recovered from a fungal infection can enjoy the same benefits from massage as the rest of the population.

the epidermis. They thrive in warm, moist places like skin folds between toes or around the groin.

Fungal infections are transmitted via touch: either skin to skin or skin to anything that has some fungus on it, like pets, shower floors, or the family hairbrush. It takes anywhere from 4 to 14 days for lesions to appear, and during that time the carrier can spread the fungus, which makes this condition very hard to control.

Several types of dermatophytes may create tinea lesions. Most cases of ringworm are related to colonies of *Trichophyton, Epidermophyton*, or *Microsporum* fungi.

Types of Fungal Infections

- ***Tinea capitis.*** This is a fungal infection of the scalp. It is most common in children before the onset of puberty. It can cause hair loss, and a particularly extreme form can cause an inflammatory response leading to the formation of pus-filled sores called **kerions**. Some of the causative fungi for tinea capitis fluoresce under blacklight: this is a common diagnostic tool for this condition (Figure 2.8).

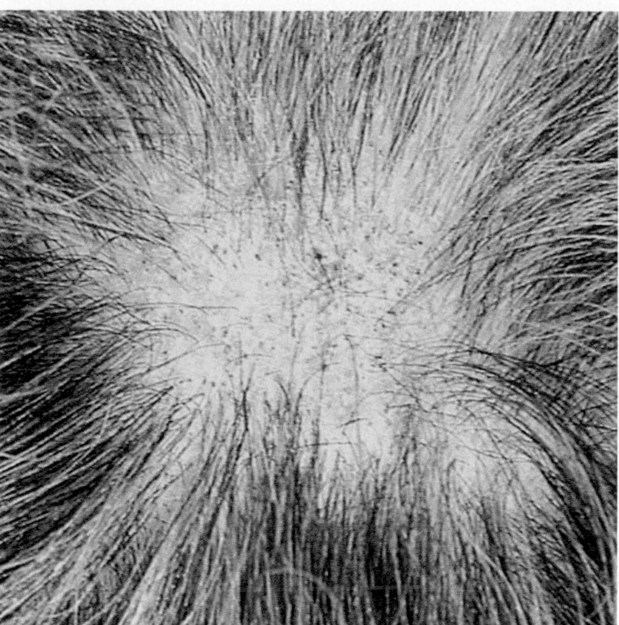

Figure 2.8. Tinea capitis: head ringworm

- ***Tinea corporis.*** This is "body ringworm" that typically develops on the trunk or extremities. It generally begins as one small round, red, scaly, itchy patch of skin on the trunk. Scratching spreads the fungus to other parts of the body, and other lesions appear. They heal from the center first, and they soon take on the appearance of red circles or rings with a scaly edge that may gradually increase in size as the fungus spreads out for new food sources (Figure 2.9).

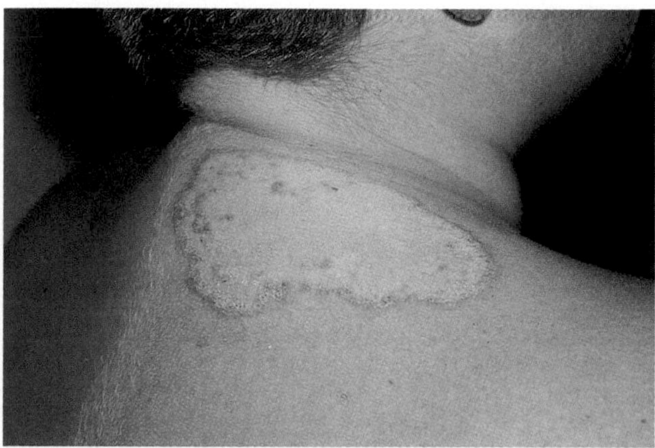

Figure 2.9. Tinea corporis: body ringworm

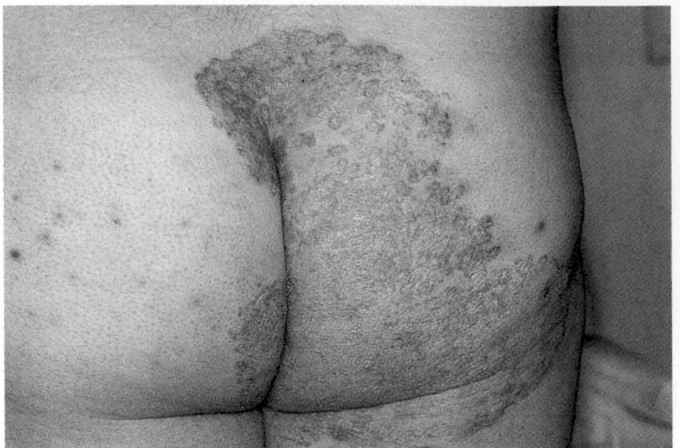
Figure 2.10. Tinea cruris: jock itch

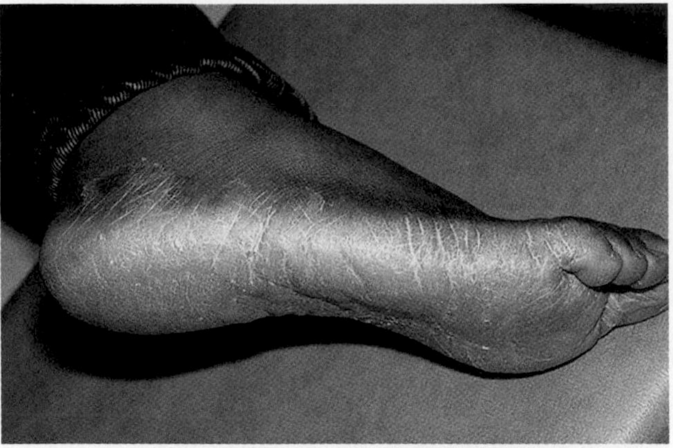
Figure 2.12. Tinea pedis: moccasin distribution

- ***Tinea cruris.*** Also called "jock itch", this is a fungal infection of the groin area. It is much more common in males than females. It is typically associated with damp conditions and tight clothing. It usually spares the penis and scrotum, but may affect the skin around the groin, thighs, and low back (Figure 2.10).
- ***Tinea pedis.*** This is "athlete's foot," but it is not specific to athletes. Tinea pedis is the most common type of fungal infection diagnosed. It is associated with constrictive footwear and moist, humid conditions. It usually starts between the third and fourth digits (Figure 2.11). Athlete's foot burns and itches, and it carries the additional complication of weeping blisters, cracking, peeling skin, and the possibility of a dangerous secondary infection. One variety of athlete's foot fungus presents as dry, scaly, itchy lesions on the heel and sole of the foot. This is called a "moccasin distribution" (Figure 2.12).
- ***Tinea manuum.*** Many people who handle their athlete's foot develop secondary fungal infections on their hands: this is tinea manuum. It resembles tinea corporis (Figure 2.13).
- ***Onychomycosis.*** Also called tinea unguium; this is the result when a fungal infection invades the skin under finger or toenails. It can lead to pitted, eroded, and discolored nails that may eventually detach from the nailbed (Figure 2.14). Destruction of the nail is called **onycholysis**.
- ***Tinea versicolor.*** This fungal infection is unique in that the vast majority of adults have colonies of the causative agent (usually *Malassezia globosa* or *M. furfur*) as part of the normal flora of the skin. In some situations, these normally benign organisms become more aggressive, causing patches of hypo- or hyperpigmented skin that heal within a few months. Because the fungi associated with tinea versicolor are part of most people's naturally occurring skin colonies, tinea versicolor is not considered to be a contagious condition (Figure 2.15).

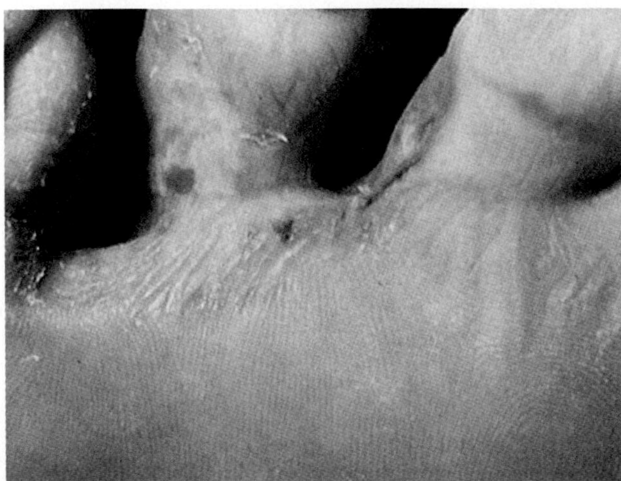
Figure 2.11. Tinea pedis: athlete's foot

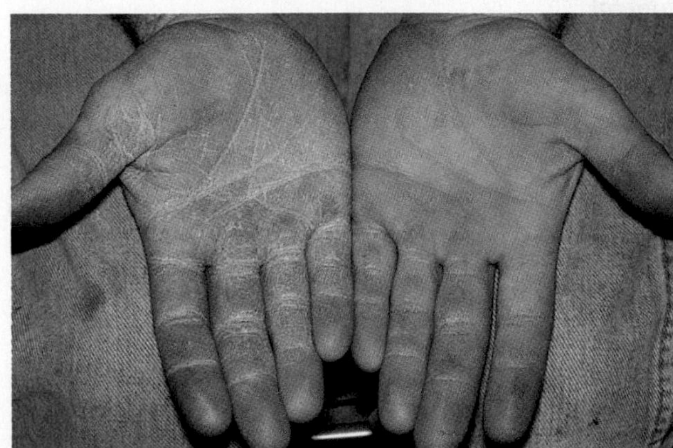
Figure 2.13. Tinea manuum

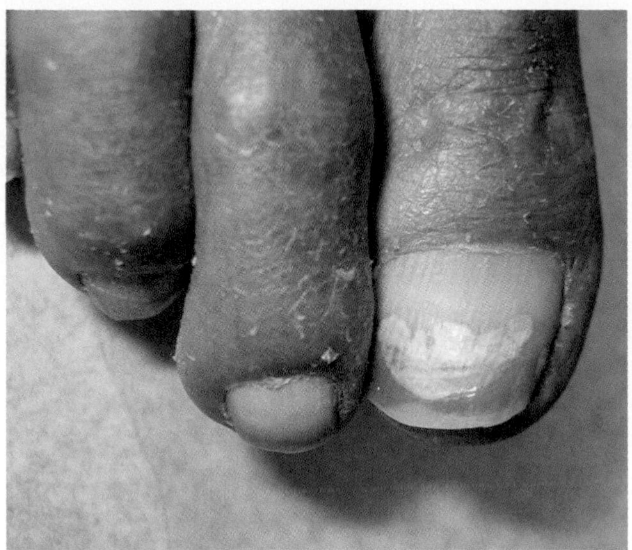

Figure 2.14. Onychomycosis

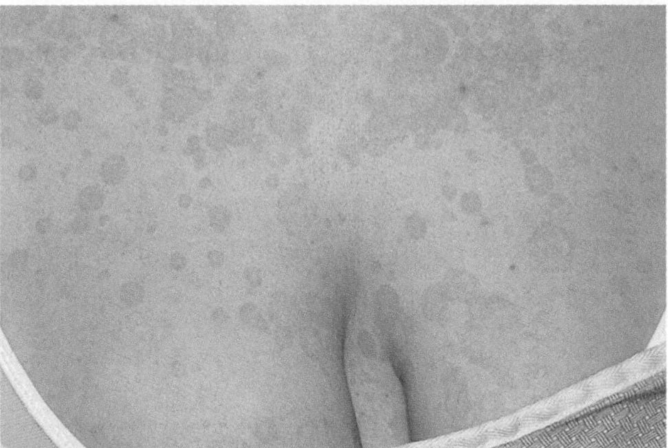

Figure 2.15. Tinea versicolor

Signs and Symptoms

Symptoms of tinea infections vary considerably depending on the causative agent and where they appear. The characteristic "ringworm" lesion is a slowly enlarging reddish scaly circle that is pale in the middle: this shows where the fungi have already taken advantage of the nutrients that are available. Interestingly, mushrooms grow in essentially the same pattern: an enlarging circle around an initial colony.

Subtypes of fungal infections may also involve fluid-filled blisters, ulcerations, or pus-filled sores. It is important to remember that any compromise of the skin creates a risk for secondary bacterial infection.

Treatment

Treatment for any fungal infection typically begins with topical antifungal creams or powders. If these are insufficient, oral antifungal medication may be prescribed. These carry a risk of liver damage though, so patients must be monitored carefully.

Most fungal infections improve when the skin is kept dry. Many patients are advised to avoid tight

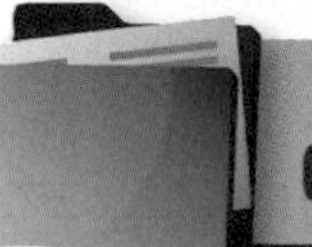

CASE HISTORY 2.2 Ringworm, Delores G.

In June 1994, I was working hard in massage school. I was living in a house where some stray kittens were close by. I wanted to pet them, so I brought them some food. They came out, and I got to pet them while they were eating.

I was sitting down next to them with my knees up. I had shorts on. I was petting them with my left hand, and then I held my legs with the same hand when I was done. I also folded my arms, so my left hand touched my right biceps.

About 9 days later, there were specific round red spots, the size of a half-dollar, on my left calf, and then on my right arm. It wasn't until I remembered petting the kittens that I realized where they came from. About a week after the spots appeared, they started really burning and keeping me awake.

Having ringworm was awful. It turns out that I had massaged only two people between being exposed and being diagnosed, so it didn't spread through the class, but I had to wait until I was cleared up before I could work again. I sat out of practices, which was really depressing, plus it was spreading all over me, from my right arm to my right breast, and on my other calf.

I treated it by showering and then putting tea tree oil and antifungal vaginal cream all over me. I did that for 2 or 3 weeks before it started clearing up. I was all cleared up in about 4 weeks. I waited an extra week just to be sure, so I missed a total of 3 weeks of massage.

When I got ringworm, I was extremely run down from school, which probably made me susceptible. My teacher said it was interesting that my body chose ringworm as the thing that would slow me down, but it worked! ■

clothing that may irritate the skin and exacerbate symptoms. Preventive measures (not sharing towels or clothing; using footwear in public showers, etc.) are important for anyone prone to fungal infections.

Medications

- Topical antifungal applications
- Oral antifungal medications

Massage?

RISKS Tinea infections tend not to be aggressive, but it is important not to promote their spread. Consequently, they at least locally contraindicate bodywork.

BENEFITS If a client has a localized fungal infection that is covered and well controlled, massage on the rest of the body is safe and appropriate.

OPTIONS If a client has athlete's foot but has no open blisters, it may be safe to work on his feet through the sheet. This can minimize the risk of spreading the fungi any further on the foot, or from the client to the therapist.

Herpes Simplex

Herpes Simplex in Brief

Pronunciation: HUR-peze SIM-pleks

What is it?
Herpes simplex is a viral infection resulting in painful blisters on a red base.

How is it recognized?
Herpes outbreaks are often preceded by a prodromic stage: 2 or 3 days of tingling, itching, or pain. Then painful blisters appear, usually around the mouth or genitals. The blisters gradually crust and disappear, usually within 2 weeks.

Massage risks and benefits
Risks: Herpes simplex locally contraindicates massage during the acute stage. Because the virus may also be shed during the prodromic stage, a client who knows he or she may be developing a lesion should be encouraged to reschedule the massage appointment.
Benefits: A client who has no active or prodromic herpes lesions can enjoy the same benefits from massage as the rest of the population.

Definition: What Is It?

Among the several viruses in the herpes family that affect humans, herpes simplex viruses are especially common. Herpes simplex virus type 1 (HSV-1) is typically associated with lesions that appear around the mouth, while herpes simplex virus type 2 (HSV-2) is associated with genital herpes. Exceptions to this rule are increasingly common, however, and because the treatment options for type 1 and type 2 are identical, the distinction between them is less important than it used to be.

Etiology: What Happens?

Oral herpes is transmitted through oral or respiratory secretions. Genital herpes is transmitted through mucous secretions during sexual contact. In either case, the virus spreads most efficiently through direct contact. A person's first outbreak, which usually occurs 2 to 20 days after exposure, is called primary herpes. All subsequent outbreaks are called recurrent herpes.

A primary herpes outbreak may be very severe or almost unnoticeable. Most cases of oral herpes are picked up during early childhood, and the new carrier may never be aware of his or her infection. In extreme cases, the primary infection may be accompanied by fever, swollen glands, and many painful sores that may last 2 to 6 weeks.

One of the distinguishing features of all herpes viruses is that they are never fully expelled from the body. After the primary outbreak, the HSV goes into hiding in the dorsal root ganglia of the spine or the trigeminal nerve. There it waits for an appropriate trigger, which could be a fever, a systemic infection, a sunburn, stress, menstruation, or some other stimulus. When the virus reactivates, a recurrent outbreak occurs, usually at or near the site of the original infection.

Oral herpes lesions are sometimes referred to as "cold sores" or "fever blisters." This reflects the fact that blisters often erupt when the immune system is suppressed and the person is dealing with another infection.

Herpes simplex carries some risk for complications. Secondary bacterial infection is a common problem at herpes lesions. People who are coinfected with HIV and genital herpes have a greater risk of communicating HIV to sexual partners, and people with active genital herpes lesions have an increased risk of contracting HIV from an infected partner. Vaginally delivered newborns of mothers with active genital herpes may develop blindness, pneumonia, or brain damage; this is why women with a history of this condition may be counseled to deliver their children by C-section.

Communicability

While herpes spreads most efficiently through direct skin-to-skin contact, the virus can persist on surfaces from several hours to several days. This means that the face pad used by an infected client can pass the virus to someone else, or the doorknob may now have some virus from when the client touched an itchy blister and then closed the door. Even leaving aside the possibility of spreading an infection to other people, herpes can also spread to other parts of the body: this is called autoinoculation. Touching a cold sore and then touching the eye, for instance, can result in a painful and damaging infection of the cornea or conjunctiva.

It is important to understand that the herpes virus is highly concentrated in the fluid-filled blisters, but it can also be shed from skin that has no visible lesion; this is especially likely during the **prodromic** stage. In other words, the carrier doesn't need to have a visible lesion to spread the virus to other people.

While this sounds very alarming, herpes simplex can only cause a new infection in someone who has never been exposed. Because the vast majority of adults in the United States are positive for herpes simplex virus antibodies, at least for type 1, the risk of triggering a new infection in a client or a therapist is relatively low.

Types of Herpes Simplex

- *Oral herpes* or herpes labialis tends to erupt when immunity is otherwise depressed; during hormonal changes, as in pregnancy or menstruation; after prolonged exposure to sunlight or extreme temperatures; or following any emotional stress. They appear most often on the lips and on the skin around the mouth (Figure 2.16). They may be a lifelong problem.
- *Genital herpes* outbreaks also correspond to depressed immunity and general stress levels, but they typically appear with decreasing frequency until finally they simply never come back. These blisters may appear on the genitals, but they can also be found on the thighs, buttocks, and on the skin over the sacrum (Figure 2.17). People who are immune suppressed tend to have outbreaks over larger areas of the body than others. The lesions are usually quite painful, but if they are inside the vaginal canal, a woman may be unaware of them; this has important implications for communicability. Genital herpes outbreaks are sometimes accompanied by systemic symptoms: fever, muscular aches, swelling in the inguinal lymph nodes, and difficult or painful urination.
- *Herpes whitlow* is an outbreak of lesions around the nail beds of the hands. This condition has

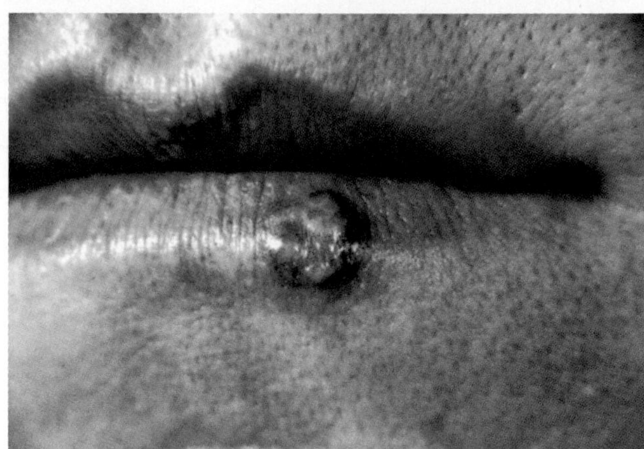

Figure 2.16. Oral herpes

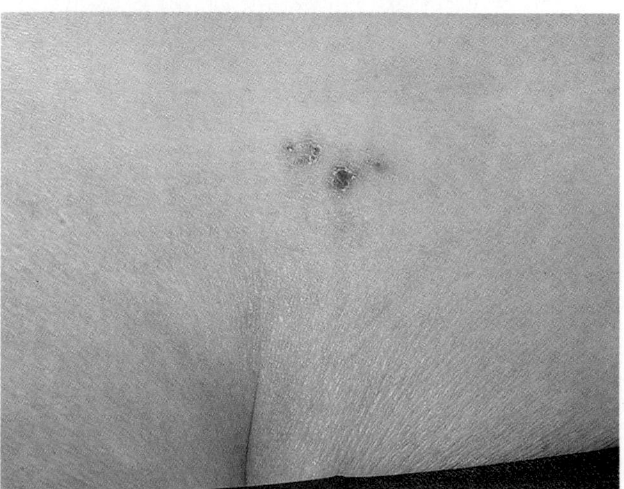

Figure 2.17. Genital herpes

traditionally been associated with children who suck their thumbs, and before the days of consistent glove use by healthcare workers, especially dental hygienists (Figure 2.18). Because massage therapists often work without gloves, they may be at risk for herpes whitlow if clients are shedding virus from any accessible herpes lesion.

- *Herpes gladiatorum* occurs on the trunk and extremities of wrestlers and other athletes who share skin-to-skin contact. In this situation, vesicles often rupture, so the lesions may look more like painful ulcers than blisters on a red base.
- *Herpetic sycosis* is a condition in which multiple herpes lesions develop over the beard area. It is the result of repeated shaving while a lesion is active: this allows the virus to spread into tiny cuts in new areas on the face.
- *Eczema herpeticum* is a condition in which herpes simplex is associated with atopic dermatitis, a type of eczema. It is most common in children and produces a widespread outbreak of herpes lesions.

NOTABLE CASES While many celebrities have been sued for allegedly infecting partners with genital herpes, few have come forward with their own status. Actress Anne Heche is a spokesperson for genital herpes.

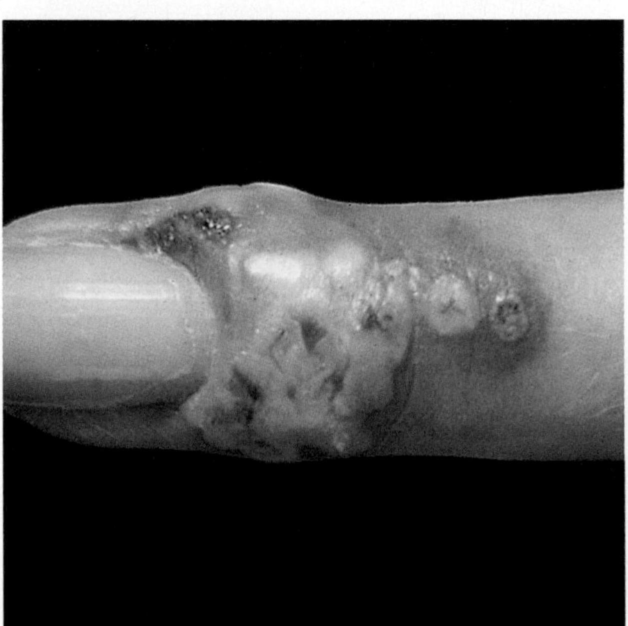

Figure 2.18. Herpes whitlow

- *Ocular herpes* occurs when the virus affects the eyelid, conjunctiva, or cornea of the eye. One outbreak may not cause scarring, but repeated infections can lead to permanent damage.

Signs and Symptoms

Whether type 1 or type 2, herpes simplex usually presents in the same way: the affected area may have some pain or tingling a few days before an outbreak (the prodromic stage); then a blister or cluster of blisters appears on a red base. The blisters erupt and ooze virus-rich liquid all around the area. The blisters scab over after a week or 10 days, ending the most contagious phase of the disease. Altogether the outbreak lasts about 2 to 3 weeks.

Treatment

No treatment fully eradicates herpes simplex from the body, so focus is placed on prevention and reducing the frequency of outbreaks by keeping as healthy as possible.

Medications

- Antiviral medications to shorten the duration of an outbreak
- Topical creams for oral herpes
- Prophylactic medications that reduce the frequency of genital herpes outbreaks

Massage?

RISKS Active herpes locally contraindicates massage, and if a client knows he or she is developing a lesion, it is a courtesy to reschedule a massage appointment.

BENEFITS Massage has no specific benefits for herpes outbreaks, but a client who has no current signs can enjoy the same benefits of bodywork as the rest of the population. Conceivably, the stress-management qualities of massage might reduce the frequency of herpes outbreaks for people who find that stress is a trigger.

OPTIONS Because it is so difficult to resist touching the itchy, burning blisters of herpes simplex, some massage therapists choose not to work with their clients' hands (or to work on the hands through a sheet) while a client has an active outbreak.

SIDEBAR 2.1 When Is a Mouth Sore Not Herpes?

Oral herpes causes the familiar lesions we call fever blisters or cold sores, but not all sores around the mouth are caused by herpes virus.

Angular stomatitis is a condition involving painful irritated cracks around the corners of the mouth. This is often associated with denture wearers, who may drool while they sleep. The accumulation of saliva around the corners of the mouth provides a rich growth medium for the yeast that causes these lesions.

Aphthae, or *"canker sores,"* are lesions inside the mouth, often on the gums and cheeks. These are small, painful ulcers whose cause is unknown. Aphthae may be viral, but they are not contagious.

Staphylococcus Infections of the Skin

Definition: What Are They?

Staphylococcus aureus (named *staphyle,* Greek for grapes, and *aureus* for its yellow color under a microscope), or staph, is a group of bacteria known for colonizing human skin and nasal passages. Staph infections have different names, depending on where they are found or what subtypes of bacteria are present.

Staphylococcus Infections of the Skin in Brief

What are they?
Staphylococcus aureus (staph) is a common group of bacteria that can cause a variety of infections in the body. When they appear on the skin, they usually cause localized infections in the form of boils, folliculitis, or other lesions.

How are they recognized?
Most staph infections form painful, hot, red pustules on the skin. They may occur singly, in groups, or in interconnected clusters.

Massage risks and benefits
Risks: Staph infections involve aggressive and potentially communicable bacteria. They also carry the risk of becoming systemic and life-threatening infections if they are not controlled. Therefore, at least locally they contraindicate massage.
Benefits: Clients who have recovered from staph infections of the skin can enjoy the same benefits from massage as the rest of the population.

Etiology: What Happens?

Staphylococcus bacteria use two mechanisms to cause damage: active invasion of healthy tissue and release of corrosive chemicals that can kill cells. When staph infections occur on the skin, they typically involve painful pus-filled vesicles, occasionally with signs of systemic infection (fever, headache, swollen lymph nodes, malaise).

Most people have colonies of staph bacteria on their skin or in their nasal passages. While these pathogens can be transmitted through person-to-person contact or via contaminated surfaces, they can also be transferred from one area to another. In other words, if a person wipes his nose and then scratches his scabbed knee, the knee injury could develop a new staph infection. Further, once such an infection is established at a site where the skin is damaged, it is possible for the bacteria to travel through the bloodstream to set up infections elsewhere. Pneumonia, bone and joint infections, heart valve damage, and varieties of toxic shock syndrome are all rare but possible complications of superficial staph infections. These are particular risks for people who are already immunocompromised. Staph infections often occur at sebaceous glands or hair shafts that are clogged by dirt, dead skin cells, or other debris, but they can begin wherever the skin has been compromised by a cut, scrape, or friction. An aggressive immune response to this pathogen leads to the classic redness, swelling, pain, and pus formation at the sites of these localized infections.

Types of Staphylococcus Infections

- ***Boils.*** Boils, also called **furuncles**, are local infections of the skin. Boils typically occur one at a time (Figure 2.19). A group of boils connected by channels under the skin is called a **carbuncle**. Boils have much in common with acne, but *S. aureus* is a virulent, aggressive bacterium that actively attacks healthy tissue; this is not true of the pathogen associated with common acne (see Compare & Contrast 2.1).
- ***Methicillin-resistant S. aureus (MRSA).*** MRSA are a group of infection-causing staph bacteria

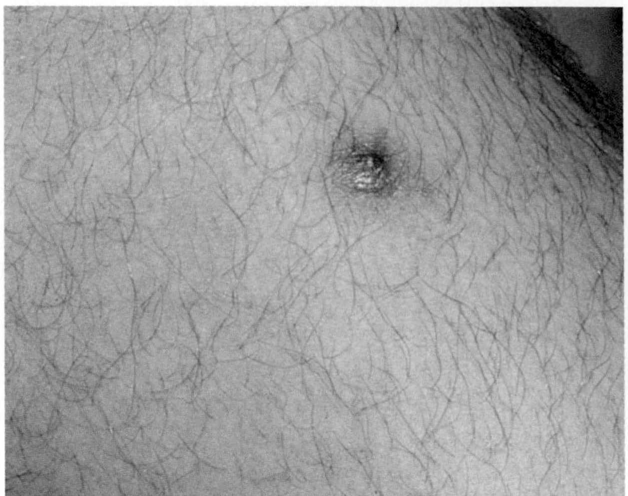

Figure 2.19. Staphylococcus infection: single boil

that have been recognized in hospital settings since the 1950s and have recently been tracked outside of healthcare facilities. Community-acquired MRSA is often associated with athletic facilities and high-density, low-hygiene settings. These skin infections can be spread through indirect contact, like sharing towels or razors. MRSA occurs in several subtypes, but they are all resistant to several antibiotics, including penicillin, methicillin, amoxicillin, and others. MRSA is a particular risk for massage therapists, who must be especially vigilant about hygienic practices with these pathogens.

NOTABLE CASES It is rumored that the original draft of *Das Kapital* was spattered with bloodstains from Karl Marx's lanced boils.

- ***Folliculitis.*** This condition refers to multiple boils in close proximity, usually affecting hair

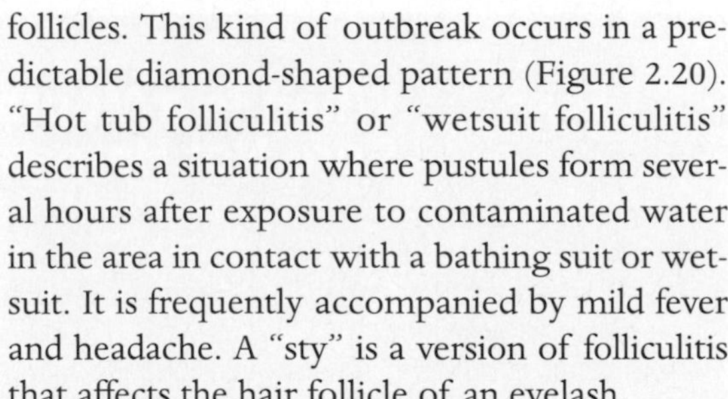

follicles. This kind of outbreak occurs in a predictable diamond-shaped pattern (Figure 2.20). "Hot tub folliculitis" or "wetsuit folliculitis" describes a situation where pustules form several hours after exposure to contaminated water in the area in contact with a bathing suit or wetsuit. It is frequently accompanied by mild fever and headache. A "sty" is a version of folliculitis that affects the hair follicle of an eyelash.
- ***Pilonidal cysts.*** **Pilonidal cysts** describe a large encysted staph infection at the sacrococcygeal region. They are most common among people who have hair growing in the gluteal cleft. These cysts frequently recur and may have to be surgically excised.
- ***Hidradenitis suppurativa.*** This refers to boils that occur where hair follicles and apocrine sweat glands are numerous; the axillae and groin are the most typical locations. **Hidradenitis suppurativa** commonly recurs; it may appear bilaterally and can leave permanent scars (Figure 2.21).

Signs and Symptoms

A staph infection of the skin typically begins as a hard, painful, red or pinkish bump that develops over a day or two. For the next several days, it increases in size, and the center of the abscess fills with pus: bacteria, dead leukocytes, and necrotic tissue. It may grow to the size of a golf ball during this time. Finally, unless it is surgically drained, the boil spontaneously ruptures and resolves. Large infections that penetrate into deep layers of the skin may leave a permanent scar.

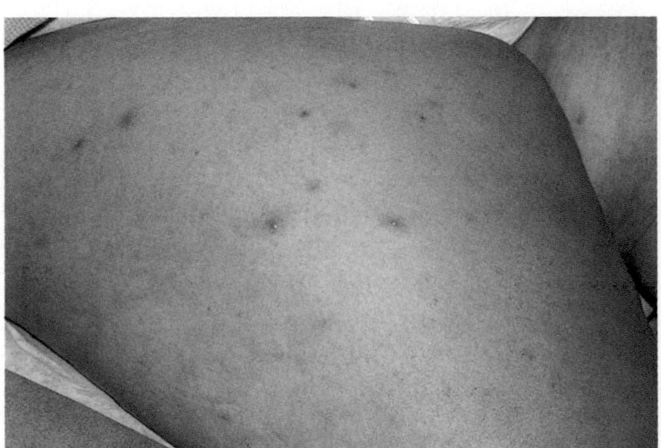

Figure 2.20. Staphylococcus infection: folliculitis

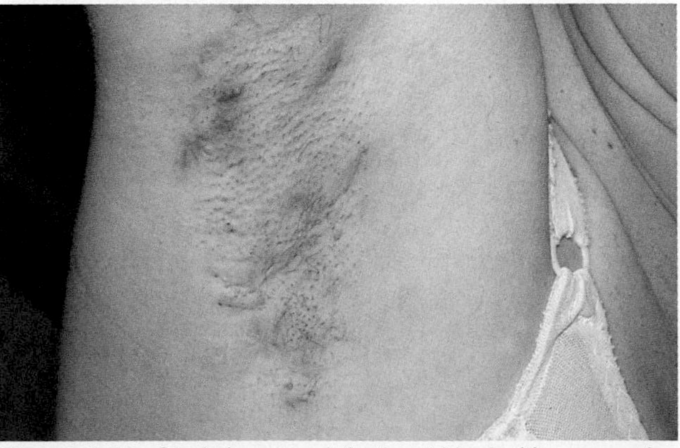

Figure 2.21. Staphylococcus infection: hidradenitis suppurativa

Treatment

Conservative treatment for localized staph infections begins with topical antibiotic ointment and hot compresses. If this is not sufficient, a physician may lance and drain or excise the lesion. Oral antibiotics are sometimes prescribed, but they tend to be slow-acting and have the best effect for people who have a recurring problem.

It is important never to try to squeeze or pop an infection. It could force the infection deeper into tissues or spread the bacteria over the surface of the skin.

Medications

- Topical antibacterial ointment
- Oral antibiotics if necessary

Massage?

RISKS A staph infection involves virulent, hardy bacteria that can spread deeper into the body or from one person to another. If signs of systemic infection (fever, swelling at nearby lymph nodes, discomfort anywhere other than the site of the boil) are present, it is necessary to reschedule the massage.

BENEFITS A client who has recovered from a staphylococcus infection can enjoy the same benefits of massage and bodywork as the rest of the population.

OPTIONS A client who has a well-controlled local infection with no systemic symptoms may receive massage, but not on or near the lesion.

Staphylococcus Infections of the Skin in Brief

What are they?
Streptococci (strep) are a group of bacteria that can cause both local and systemic infections in humans. When these infections start in the skin, they can affect superficial or deep layers, even running along fascial planes into the muscles.

How are they recognized?
Streptococcal infections of the skin are marked by redness and tenderness at the initial site of infection, along with fever, headache, malaise, and other signs of systemic infection.

Massage risks and benefits
Risks: Streptococcal infections involve potentially contagious bacteria that can invade both the lymph and circulatory systems. They systemically contraindicate hands-on bodywork until the infection has been completely resolved.
Benefits: A person who has recovered from a streptococcal infection of the skin can enjoy the same benefits of massage as the rest of the population.

Streptococcus Infections of the Skin

Definition: What Are They?

Streptococcal (strep) infections of the skin usually involve one of the group A class of streptococcus bacteria. These bacteria are also associated with strep throat, impetigo, and toxic shock syndrome.

Etiology: What Happens?

Bacteria, including streptococci, colonize both superficial and deep layers of the skin. Surface pathogens may be temporarily dislodged with washing, but they are quickly replaced. When they gain access through some breach in the defenses, the enzymes they produce can kill healthy cells, causing a very aggressive immune system response.

To cause an infection, streptococcal bacteria must cross the barrier of the skin through some portal of entry. This can be a cut or scratch, athlete's foot, an insect bite, surgery, or some other skin injury. People with stasis dermatitis or unresolved skin ulcers are particularly vulnerable.

A typical streptococcal infection of the skin begins at a skin wound, and may spread to affect a large area. These infections carry a high risk of becoming systemic, even complicating to blood poisoning, so it is important to treat them aggressively.

Types of Streptococcus Infections of the Skin

- ***Cellulitis.*** This is a general streptococcal infection of deep layers of the skin. It is a common complication of simple injuries like a scraped knee or a contaminated blister from athlete's

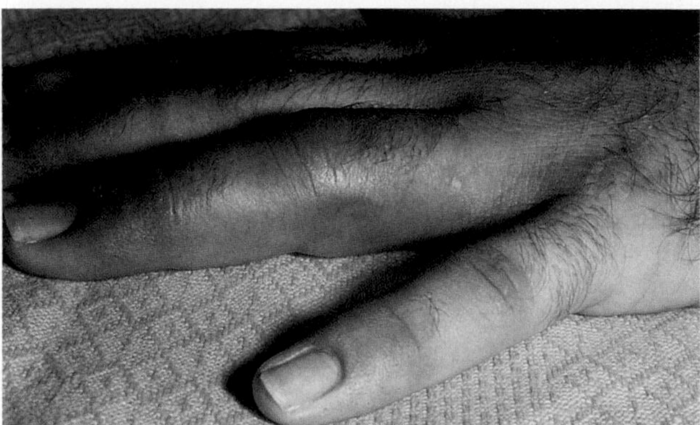

Figure 2.22. Streptococcus infection: cellulitis

foot. Most cases of cellulitis begin on the lower leg; a smaller percentage begin on the face (Figure 2.22).

- ***Necrotizing fasciitis.*** This is "flesh-eating bacteria." In truth, necrotizing fasciitis isn't always a strep infection; it could also be clostridial (as seen with gas gangrene) or it could involve multiple pathogens. The most common cause, however, is group A beta-hemolytic *Streptococcus* bacteria, which excrete powerful toxins that can cause circulatory shock and death. Necrotizing fasciitis moves quickly along fascial planes, and can progress from a minor skin wound to a life-threatening infection in a matter of hours.
- ***Erysipelas (St. Anthony's Fire).*** This describes a streptococcal infection of superficial layers of the skin. Unlike other strep infections, erysipelas shows a sharp margin between involved and uninvolved skin; the red edges are usually very clear (Figure 2.23). The affected area becomes hard, shiny, and red. Blisters may develop, and superficial skin cells may shed. Erysipelas usually has a positive outcome, with no lasting damage unless the patient is especially vulnerable due to age or immune system compromise.

Signs and Symptoms

Sometimes, indications of systemic infection (fever, swollen nodes, headache) precede an obvious skin injury, but signs often begin with a tender, red, swollen area. The wound may develop red streaks running toward the nearest set of lymph nodes. This is also an indicator of lymphangitis: infection of the lymphatic vessels. If the infection starts on the face, a raised, hot, tender, red area may spread across the bridge of the nose and forehead.

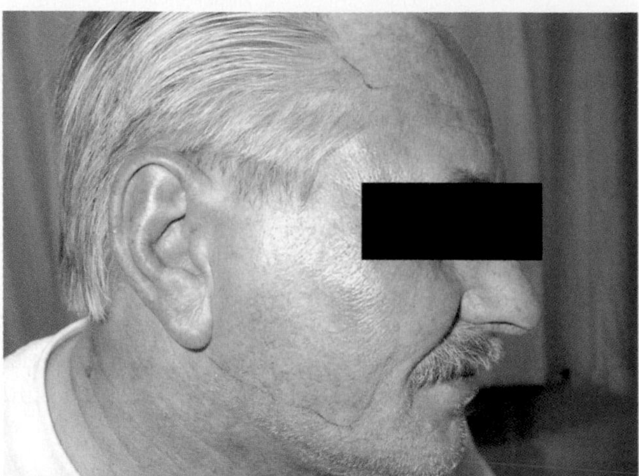

Figure 2.23. Streptococcus infection: erysipelas. Note the clear delineation between involved and uninvolved skin

When the infection has thoroughly engaged the immune system, symptoms include fever, chills, and systemic discomfort. Facial infections are particularly dangerous because of the risk of intracranial spreading through lymphatic capillaries. If strep infections are left untreated, the bacteria may get past the lymph system and enter the circulatory system, leading quickly and perhaps fatally to septicemia, or blood poisoning.

Treatment

Most streptococcus bacteria are sensitive to antibiotics. If the infection is well contained, oral antibiotics are generally recommended. If the infection has penetrated to the lymph or circulatory system, aggressive treatment with intravenous antibiotics is probably called for. Surgical removal of damaged tissue may be part of the treatment for necrotizing fasciitis.

Massage?

RISKS Streptococcal infections of the skin involve tissue damage, a highly contagious bacterial infection, and a risk of blood poisoning. This situation systemically contraindicates massage until all signs of infection have passed.

BENEFITS Clients who have fully recovered from strep infections are good candidates for any kind of bodywork.

Warts

Definition: What Are They?

Warts are small, benign growths caused by varieties of human papillomavirus (HPV) that invade keratinocytes deep in the stratum basale of the skin and some mucous membranes.

Etiology: What Happens?

HPV is a group of over 100 pathogens that have been associated with several types of human warts. These viruses spread when someone with compromised skin directly touches a wart, or through indirect contact, when a new host picks up the virus from a surface or contaminated item. These lesions often develop on areas that take a lot of friction, especially knuckles, knees, and feet. Warts grow extremely slowly, sometimes taking months or years to fully develop.

When a person irritates a wart, or damages skin nearby (like picking at hangnails or biting fingernails near a wart), the virus can spread and more warts may appear. The same caution exists for trying to clip or cut away warts: the blood from these injuries may carry the virus to cause new infections nearby.

Warts in Brief

What are they?
Warts are growths caused by slow-growing viral infections of keratinocytes in the epidermis.

How are they recognized?
The most common warts (verruca vulgaris) look like hard, cauliflower-shaped lumps. They usually occur on the hands or knees. They can affect anyone, but children and teenagers are especially prone to them.

Massage risks and benefits

Risks: Warts locally contraindicate massage. The risk of communicability is low but not zero, and the growths may shed virus in sloughing skin cells and local bleeding.

Benefits: Massage has no direct benefit for warts, but a client with a history of this infection can enjoy the same benefits from bodywork as the rest of the population.

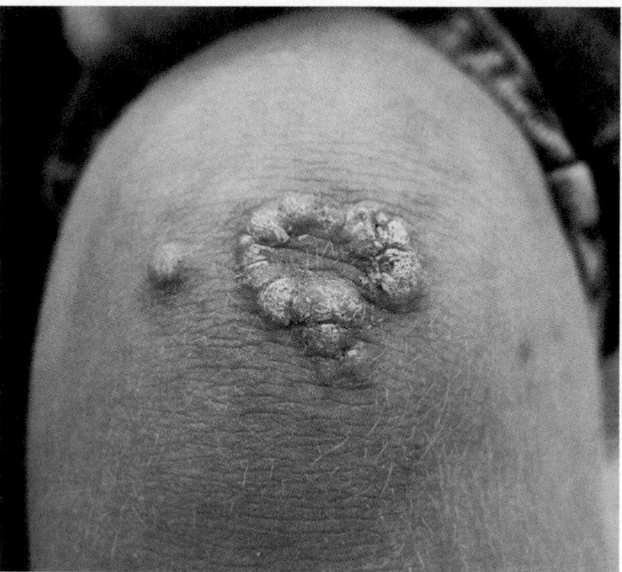

Figure 2.24. Warts on a knee

Types of Warts

- *Common warts* or **verruca vulgaris** typically appear on the hands, knees, and elbows. They are hard flaky nodules that vary in size (Figure 2.24).
- *Plantar warts,* also called **myrmecia**, are warts that grow on the soles of the feet (Figure 2.25). Plantar warts are easy to mistake for callus, but it is important not to try to clip or file them away (see Compare & Contrast 2.1). When several plantar warts grow in the same area, the resulting lesion is called **mosaic warts**.
- *Cystic warts* usually occur on the sole of the foot, but unlike plantar warts, they are smooth and soft. When they are excised, a cheesy substance can be squeezed out. Some experts suggest that

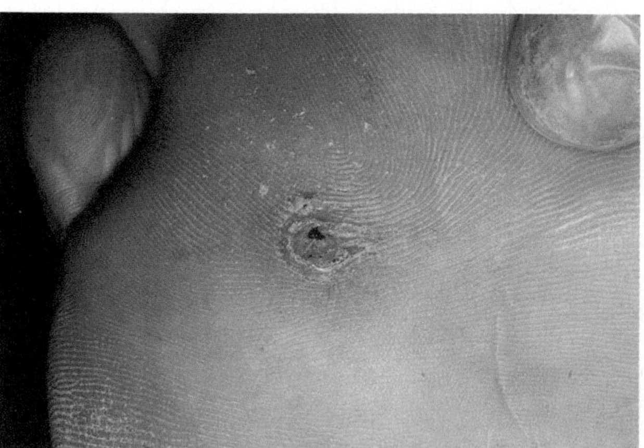

Figure 2.25. Plantar warts

they may involve blocked sweat glands or an attempt to encyst the original viral infection.

- *Plane or flat warts* are small, brown, smooth warts. They can grow a few at a time or with hundreds spread over a large area. They appear most often on the hands, face, and shins. Plane warts may spread during shaving.

NOTABLE CASES Oliver Cromwell demanded that his portraitist portray him, "warts and all." His death mask has clearly discernable warts.

- *Molluscum contagiosum* is usually a children's malady involving small white lumps. The pathogen is not HPV; it is from the pox family of viruses. Molluscum contagiosum in adults can be a sexually transmitted infection.
- *Genital warts* are a sexually transmitted infection caused by several varieties of HPV. Most genital warts come and go with no symptoms, but others may trigger cellular activity leading to cervical cancer, which is discussed elsewhere.
- *Butchers' warts* are associated with meat handling. They look like common warts but are caused by a different variety of HPV.
- *Focal epithelial hyperplasia (Heck disease)* is a form of wart that forms in the mouth, on the lower lip, or on the tongue. It is most common in Native Americans and Aleuts.
- *Epidermodysplasia verruciformis* is a genetic disease involving suppressed immunity and an increased risk of squamous cell carcinoma (SCC).

Signs and Symptoms

Warts come in several different presentations, depending on where they are found and the causative strain of HPV. Sometimes dark spots or "wart seeds" are seen near the base of warts: these are not in fact seeds; they are tiny capillaries that feed the new growths.

Treatment

Treatment options for warts vary from psychosomatic suggestion ("cut a potato into six pieces, then bury each piece in a different place and never tell anyone where you buried them") to low-tech applications of garlic juice or duct tape, to invasive electrocauterization, surgery or lasers. At this point, no single intervention works permanently on all warts, but most people can find relief one way or another.

COMPARE & CONTRAST 2.1 Plantar Warts vs. Calluses

Plantar warts often look like simple calluses: the thick skin that grows on areas of the feet subject to a lot of wear and tear. The problem is that while people may file or snip off their calluses with no ill effects, to do the same with a plantar wart is to risk having that wart virus spread all over the foot and lead to more growths until it becomes difficult to walk.

Massage therapists are in a unique position to observe their clients' feet and notice the subtle differences between plantar warts and callus. They may be able to give clients guidance about getting the right kind of care.

CHARACTERISTICS	PLANTAR WARTS	CALLUS
Location	Anywhere on plantar surface of foot.	Appears in areas of wear and tear, especially back of heels and lateral aspect of feet. Callus usually grows in a similar pattern on both feet.
Appearance	Usually *not* bilateral. May be white, but with darker speckling under thickened skin: this is the capillary supply.	Callus usually grows in a similar pattern on both feet. Thick, white skin.
Sensation	Very hard and unyielding, like stepping on a stone.	No particular sensation.

Wart treatment may be classified as folklore (this would include the potato cure), symptomatic relief that removes the warts but not the virus (including salicylic acid or duct tape application), destructive therapy (using lasers, surgery, or liquid nitrogen), virucidal therapy (using topical or oral antiviral medications), and drugs that interfere with cellular replication.

Medications

- Topical applications of salicylic acid or other irritants
- Antiviral medications (may be topical, injected, or oral)
- Antimitotic therapy (drugs that inhibit cellular replication)

Massage?

RISKS Warts locally contraindicate massage. A massage therapist is unlikely to pick up a new infection, but it is inappropriate to rub on or irritate these growths. Further, warts are often caught and torn around the edges, and if the skin is not intact, the client may be vulnerable to a secondary infection.

BENEFITS Massage probably has no direct impact on warts, but improved immune function in general may be a benefit for someone with a long-term viral infection.

OPTIONS Warts are a local contraindication only, and only for direct and irritating pressure. The affected area can be incorporated into the massage through the sheet.

Noncontagious Inflammatory Skin Disorders

Acne Rosacea

Definition: What Is It?

Acne rosacea is an idiopathic chronic skin condition seen mostly in fair-skinned people between 30 and 60 years of age. It affects the skin of the face, especially the nose and cheeks. It can also affect the conjunctiva and the eyelids. It seldom develops elsewhere on the body.

Acne Rosacea in Brief

Pronunciation: AK-ne ro-SAY-shuh

What is it?
Acne rosacea is a chronic inflammatory condition involving facial skin and eyes.

How is it recognized?
Acne rosacea ranges from mild to severe, starting with occasional flushing and continuing through general inflammation of the face and eyes, the formation of papules and pustules, and finally permanent thickening and distortion of facial skin, especially around the nose.

Massage risks and benefits
Risks: This condition may be exacerbated by local massage, and some clients may be sensitive to some lubricants. For these reasons, the client must be consulted before a massage if the client has acne rosacea.
Benefits: While massage may not have direct benefits for acne rosacea, a client with this condition can enjoy all the general benefits that bodywork has to offer.

Etiology: What Happens?

The pathophysiology of acne rosacea is not well understood. It may be inherited, but no gene has been specifically identified with this condition. Many patients appear to have superficial capillaries that dilate especially easily. Some researchers suggest it may involve an overreaction to normally occurring skin bacteria, including those carried by common mites that colonize hair follicles (*Demodex folliculorum*).

Triggers for rosacea flares are fairly predictable. They may include exposure to sunlight, wind, and cold temperatures; drinking hot liquids or alcohol; eating spicy food; menopause; the use of steroidal anti-inflammatories on the face; and emotional stress.

Signs and Symptoms

Acne rosacea occurs in flare and remission, on a spectrum from mild to severe symptoms. It is often but not always progressive without treatment. While women have rosacea more often than men, men tend to have more severe forms of the disease.

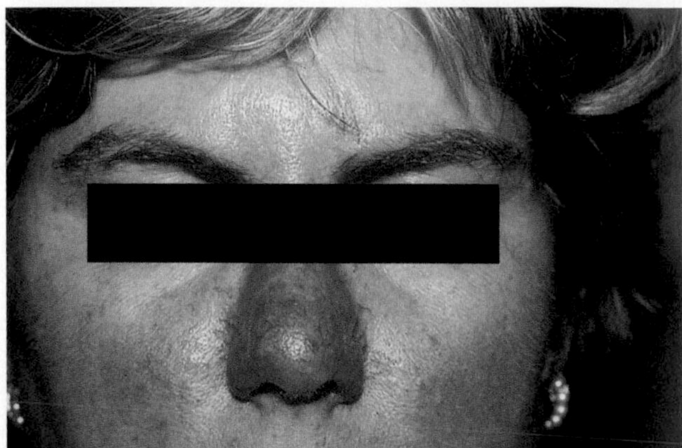
Figure 2.26. Mild acne rosacea

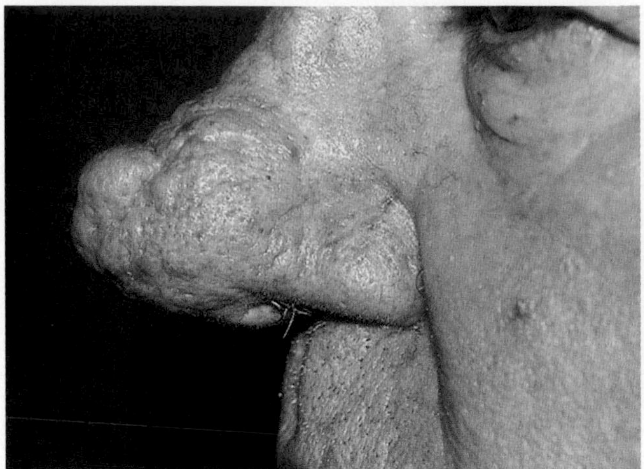
Figure 2.27. Acne rosacea: rhinophyma

At the mild end of the spectrum, a person may experience frequent flushing, with stinging or burning pain (Figure 2.26). **Telangiectasias** are common: these are tiny permanently dilated capillaries on the cheeks and nose. In more severe cases, papules or pustules may develop, but they are not the blackheads or whiteheads seen with acne vulgaris. If the condition affects the eyes, then the conjunctiva and eyelids may become inflamed, and the person may report stinging or the feeling that a foreign body is in the eye. At the most severe end of the spectrum, a person may develop **rhinophyma**: this is permanent distortion and thickening of the skin, usually on the nose (Figure 2.27). In rare cases, similar changes have been seen on the chin and ears.

NOTABLE CASES Comic actor W.C. Fields had rhinophyma, which unfairly contributed to his reputation as an alcoholic. Former President Bill Clinton has rosacea in a milder form.

An important issue for many people with acne rosacea is its effect on self-esteem and public perception. Persons with this disorder may be sensitive to being judged by the appearance of their skin. Furthermore, a traditional but incorrect association between the bulbous nose seen with advanced acne rosacea and alcoholism can lead to social stigmas that are difficult to challenge.

Treatment

Acne rosacea has no permanent cure and so is treated palliatively. In addition to identifying and avoiding triggers, patients may use topical or oral antibiotics. Photodynamic therapy (that combines specialized lights with medication), laser surgery, or dermabrasion may help the appearance of the skin and mask telangiectasias. Plastic surgery may be considered for a person with advanced rhinophyma.

Medications

- Oral antibiotics
- Topical antibiotics
- Topical antimite cream or gel

Massage?

RISKS Acne rosacea may be exacerbated with stimulation of facial skin. Further, some clients may be sensitive to substances in the massage lubricant. It is important to consult with the client about his or her comfort in receiving massage to the face.

BENEFITS Massage from a nonjudgmental therapist may provide welcome relief from the challenges to self-perception that many people with acne rosacea must deal with every day.

Acne Vulgaris

Definition: What Is It?

Acne is a condition in which a person becomes susceptible to small, localized skin lesions. They usually appear on the face, neck, and upper back.

Acne Vulgaris in Brief

Pronunciation: AK-ne vul-GAR-is

What is it?
Acne vulgaris is a condition of sebaceous glands usually found on the face, neck, and upper back. It is closely associated with adolescence, but often persists well into adulthood.

How is it recognized?
Acne looks like raised, inflamed bumps or pustules on the skin, sometimes with white or black tips.

Massage risks and benefits
Risks: Acne locally contraindicates massage because of the risk of infection, causing pain, and exacerbating the symptoms with the application of an oily lubricant.
Benefits: A client with acne can receive massage elsewhere on the body, and enjoy the same benefits from bodywork as the rest of the population.

Etiology: What Happens?

Acne is a multifactoral condition that affects the vast majority of adolescents, although not everyone has it severely. While having some factors in common with boils, acne has a different etiology (see Compare & Contrast 2.2: Acne vs. Boils).

Several issues have been identified in the development of acne:

- Genetic predisposition
- Overactivity of sebaceous glands, with the production of excess keratin that may contribute to blocking ducts
- Androgen production: this begins in puberty, and causes accelerated sebum production among other things
- Colonization with *Propionibacterium acnes*, a bacterium that triggers inflammation
- Some environmental exposures, including hair pomade and some medications (especially steroids, lithium, and some antiepileptic drugs)

Signs and Symptoms

The symptoms of acne are probably familiar to most people (Figure 2.28). It can be locally painful, but it is not usually associated with systemic infection. An exception to this rule is a rare form called acne fulminans: this condition involves fever, joint pain, and general illness.

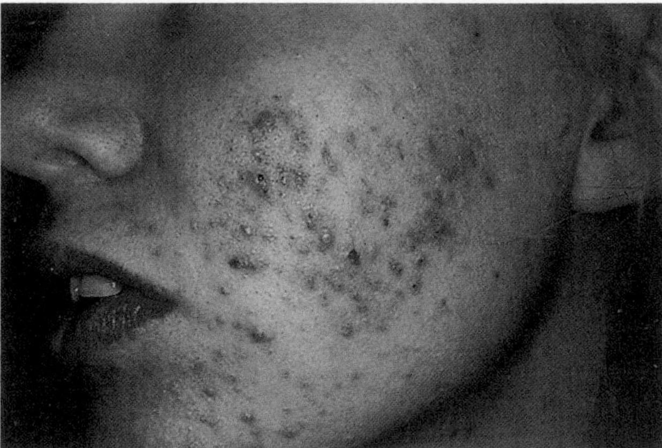
Figure 2.28. Acne vulgaris

Several types of acne lesions have been identified:

- *Pimples* are infections trapped below the surface of the skin; they are raised, red, painful bumps or papules.
- *Cysts* are infections trapped deep in the dermis. They can protrude into the subcutaneous layer and cause permanent scarring. Cysts may or may not be inflamed (Figure 2.29).
- *Open comedones* are also called blackheads. **Comedones** are superficial, and the passage into the hair follicle is open to the air. This allows the trapped sebum to oxidize and turn dark. Blackheads are not, as popular belief would have it, trapped particles of dirt.

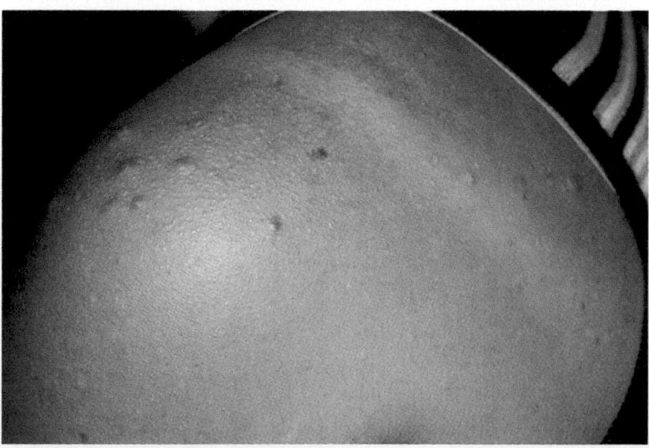
Figure 2.29. Cystic acne

- *Closed comedones* are also called whiteheads, or pustules. They are superficial infections that are covered with a thin layer of epithelium that traps the sebum and pus.

Treatment

For people with acne, the first treatment advice is the most difficult to follow: *don't touch the face*. Touching, scratching, and popping acne lesions does little except to spread the bacteria and create the possibility of permanent scarring.

Dietary interventions currently focus on links between a low glycemic index diet and improvement in acne symptoms (the reduction in insulin is linked to a reduction in androgenic hormones that stimulate sebum production), and a possible connection between increased acne symptoms and the use of hormone-supplemented milk products.

Washing the face twice daily with gentle soap and warm water is generally recommended before trying other interventions. Harsh soaps or scrubbing pads can make this condition much worse. Over-the-counter preparations usually use benzoyl peroxide or other similar substances to limit the activity of *P. acnes*.

Medical interventions usually involve topical or oral antibiotics, often in combination with benzoyl peroxide, which appears to limit drug resistance in *P. acnes*. Low-dose contraceptives may reduce levels of sebum-stimulating hormones. Very extreme acne cases may be treated with a group of drugs called retinoids, which can be used topically or as an oral medication. They are associated with several potentially dangerous side effects, so their use is carefully controlled.

Options for acne-related scars are numerous. They include laser surgery, dermabrasion, and filling pockmarks with fat to smooth out their appearance.

Medications

- Topical antibiotics, especially clindamycin or erythromycin, in combination with benzoyl peroxide
- Oral antibiotics, especially tetracycline, doxycycline, minocycline
- Oral hormones, especially low-dose contraceptives
- Oral or topical retinoids, especially isotretinoin.

COMPARE & CONTRAST 2.2 Acne vs. Boils

Boils and acne have some characteristics in common: they are both bacterial infections that may begin at hair follicles. But boils are far more serious than acne and require different precautions for massage therapists. Here are some differentiating features:

CHARACTERISTICS	BOILS	ACNE
Pattern of appearance	One lesion at a time or a small interconnected group of pustules.	Spread over large areas (face, back, neck)
Virulence	Aggressive bacteria; attack healthy tissue.	Less aggressive bacteria; take advantage of hospitable growth medium.
Symptoms	Extremely painful.	Mildly painful.
Communicability	Can be communicable.	Only with prolonged contact.
Special precautions	Local contraindication; may be systemic contraindication if signs of general infection are present.	Local contraindication; no other precautions necessary.

Massage?

RISKS Active acne lesions locally contraindicate massage. Pimples are infections, and they are associated with a compromised shield: the skin is no longer intact, which means massage can make the infection worse. Further, lesions can be locally painful. And finally, the lubricant can block sebaceous glands, further aggravating an already irritable situation.

BENEFITS Acne can have a devastating effect on self-perception. Massage from a nonjudgmental, welcoming therapist can be a wonderful experience for a person who lives with this disorder.

OPTIONS If a client is concerned about massage lubricant, the best options are to use a water-based lotion instead of oil, or to recommend that the client shower with gentle soap as soon as possible after treatment.

Dermatitis and Eczema

Definition: What Is It?

Dermatitis is an umbrella term meaning skin inflammation, which is stunningly nonspecific. Many of the conditions in this chapter could be called dermatitis, although by convention the term is reserved for disorders that are not infectious. This section focuses on two issues: eczema and contact dermatitis, with some brief discussions of other types of skin inflammation.

Contact dermatitis is a skin inflammation caused by an externally applied irritant or allergen. Eczema is a condition connected to immune dysfunction and hypersensitivity reactions expressed in the skin.

Etiology: What Happens?

Many types of dermatitis are brought about by an overreaction in the immune system to some triggering substance. Hypersensitivity reactions are discussed in detail in the introduction to Chapter 6, but it is useful to look at an abbreviated version here.

The two types of hypersensitivity reactions that create skin symptoms are type I allergic reactions and type IV delayed reactions.

Eczema is a type I reaction. These are systemic immune system responses to nonthreatening stimuli. In this situation, mast cells release vasodilating chemicals, including histamine, and these create an inflammatory response. Eczema is frequently seen alongside allergic sinusitis (hay fever) and asthma. While many young children have signs of eczema, most grow out of it by puberty. For some people, however, this condition persists throughout adulthood.

Allergic contact dermatitis is a type IV delayed reaction, mediated by several immune system agents. Poison oak, poison ivy, and local skin reactions to metals, soaps, dyes, and latex are examples of allergic contact dermatitis. With this type of reaction, symptoms typically develop 12 to 48 hours after exposure.

Both contact dermatitis and eczema can begin a process by which a mildly irritating skin problem becomes a debilitating problem. When a person with dermatitis scratches the mildly itchy lesions, the lesions are stimulated and become itchier. This leads to more scratching, more itchiness, and a vicious circle called the itch-scratch cycle.

Dermatitis and Eczema in Brief

Pronunciation: dur-mah-TY-tis, EK-zeh-muh

What are they?
Dermatitis is an umbrella term for inflammation of the skin. It is usually discussed as a type of eczema or contact dermatitis. Eczema is a noncontagious skin rash brought about by a systemic hypersensitivity reaction. Contact dermatitis is a local reaction on the skin to an irritating or allergenic trigger.

How are they recognized?
Allergic or contact dermatitis presents in various ways, depending on what type of skin reactions are elicited. Exposure to poison oak or poison ivy results in large inflamed wheals; metal allergies tend to be less inflamed and smaller in area.

Eczema may appear as very dry and flaky skin, coin-shaped lesions, yellowish oily patches, or blistered, weepy skin.

Massage risks and benefits
Risks: If the skin is very inflamed or has blisters or other lesions, massage is at least locally contraindicated until the acute stage has passed. If the skin is not itchy and the affected area is highly isolated, as with a metal allergy to a watchband or earrings, massage is only locally contraindicated. It is important to use lotion that will not elicit an allergic reaction for these clients.
Benefits: Massage may not specifically benefit dermatitis or eczema, but as long as it doesn't exacerbate symptoms, clients can enjoy the same benefits from bodywork as the rest of the population.

Persons with dermatitis or eczema are particularly susceptible to secondary infection, because their skin may be delicate and easy to invade. Impetigo, herpes simplex, staphylococcal infections, fungal infections, and warts are common complications of dermatitis and eczema.

Causes of Eczema

Research into the causes of eczema is ongoing, but no single factor has been identified. In addition to a genetic predisposition, contributing factors include two main issues: a deficiency in certain fatty acids that compromises the lipid layer of the stratum corneum, leading to a high risk of damaged skin; and immune dysregulation: an imbalance in the types of T-cells, along with increased proinflammatory chemicals and allergy-related antibodies all contribute to inflammation with capillary dilation, redness, and itching.

Although it seems clear that eczema is connected to a genetically determined immune system dysfunction, flares can be triggered by local irritations such as rough textures, detergents, harsh chemicals, extreme temperatures, and excessive sweating.

Causes of Contact Dermatitis

Contact dermatitis can arise from simple irritation or an allergic reaction. Irritant contact dermatitis is the result of using some substance that could be irritating to anyone. Reliable triggers include prolonged working in water; exposure to harsh cleansers, acids, and alkalis; and ongoing friction. All of these can damage even the healthiest skin, but cessation of the irritation relieves symptoms.

By contrast, allergic contact dermatitis involves an immune response in the skin of the affected person; only people who are allergic have this reaction. Some common triggers include nickel (found in watchbands, snaps, the buttons on jeans, and earrings), preservatives used in lotions, the adhesive used in many medical bandages, some perfumes and dyes, latex, and urushiol: the allergenic substance in the sap of poison ivy (Figures 2.30 and 2.31). Allergic contact dermatitis tends to develop several hours after exposure to the trigger.

Types of Eczema

- *Atopic dermatitis* is the most common variety of eczema. It is usually red, flaky, and dry, occurring in the creases on the sides of the nose and other skin creases, such as knees, elbows, ankles, and hands (Figure 2.32). The skin may thicken and feel rough: this is called **lichenification**.
- *Seborrheic eczema* produces yellowish, oily patches, usually in the skin folds around the nose or on the scalp.
- *Dyshidrosis* produces blisters filled with fluid that appear mostly on hands and feet. It is sometimes described as resembling a

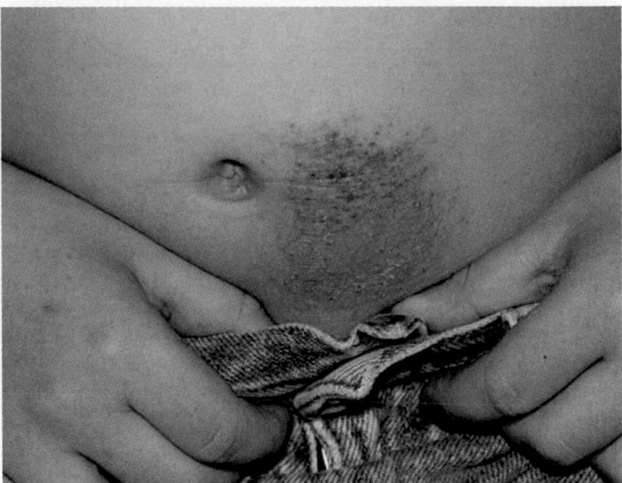

Figure 2.30. Allergic contact dermatitis: nickel in jeans button

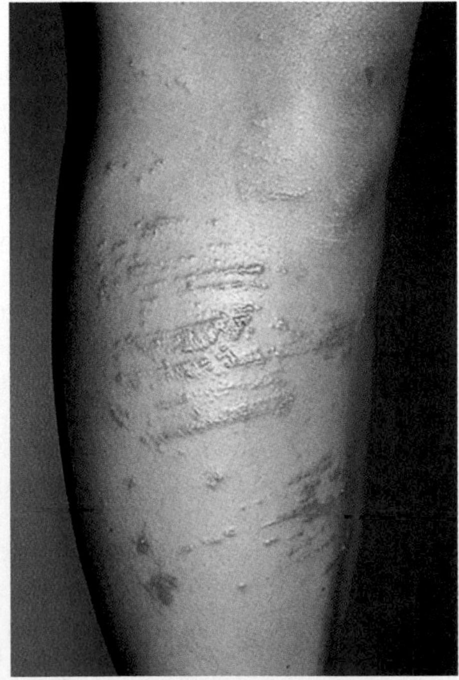

Figure 2.31. Allergic contact dermatitis: poison ivy

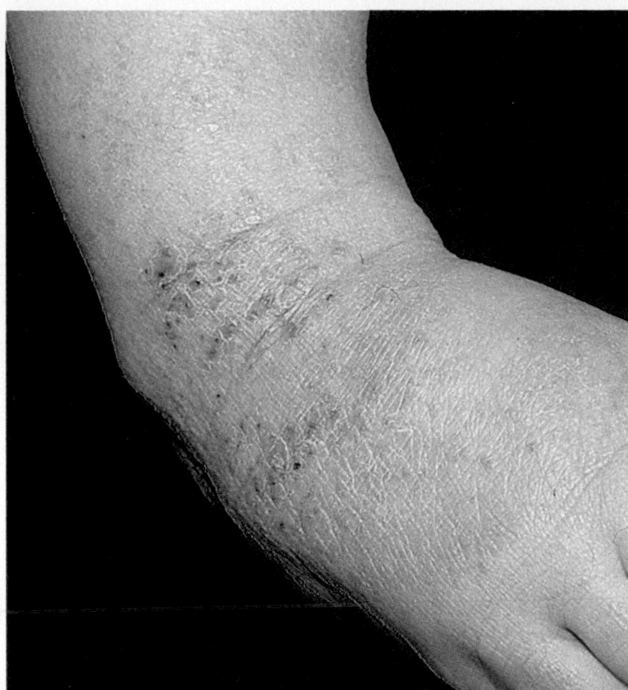

Figure 2.32. Atopic dermatitis

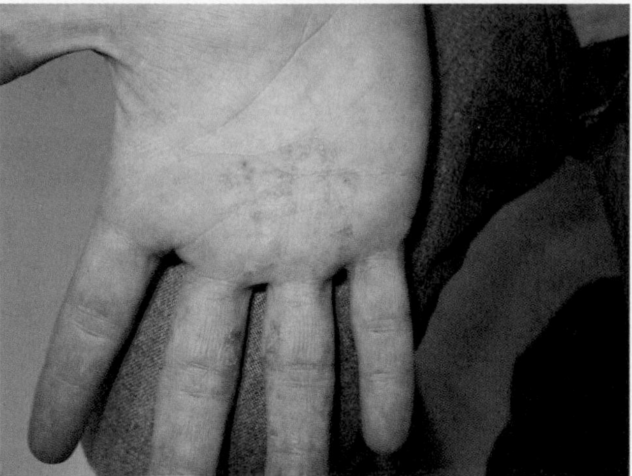

Figure 2.33. Dyshidrosis

combination of fungal infection and a contact allergy (Figure 2.33). It often occurs in response to hot weather or emotional stress.

- *Nummular eczema* appears in small circular lesions, often on the legs and buttocks (Figure 2.34). It can resemble ringworm, and it is often intensely itchy.

Signs and Symptoms of Eczema

Signs and symptoms of eczema vary according to what type is present. Most involve redness, itching, and the risk of secondary infection if the skin is damaged.

Signs and Symptoms of Contact Dermatitis

The symptoms of contact dermatitis vary according to the causative factors. Acute situations are typically locally red, swollen, and itchy or tender, showing exactly where the irritation took place. Long-lasting, low-grade reactions may not show signs of inflammation, although mild itchiness is common.

Other types of dermatitis show specific patterns but are not related to irritation or contact with allergenic substances.

Other Types of Dermatitis

- *Stasis dermatitis* usually appears on the lower legs in association with poor circulation, as seen with diabetes or heart failure. Stasis dermatitis is red or purplish and may occur with small ulcers where the skin has been deprived of nutrition. It often resembles erysipelas, a bacterial infection of the skin.
- *Neurodermatitis* involves a small injury, such as a mosquito bite, that creates an enormous inflammatory response and localized scaly patches of skin.

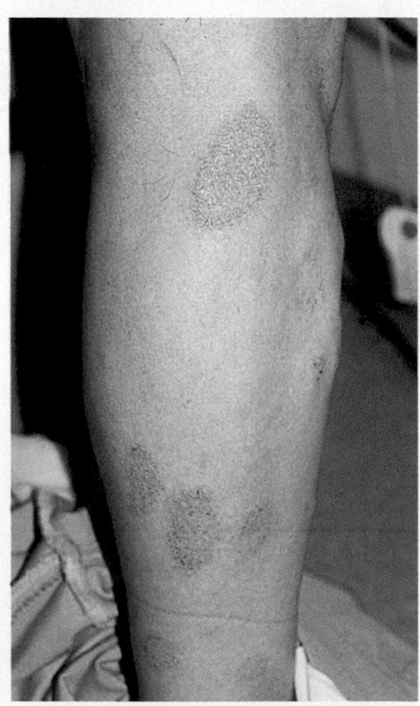

Figure 2.34. Nummular eczema

Treatment

Self-help measures for people with contact dermatitis and eczema begin with trying to identify their triggers, and then avoiding them carefully. Persons with eczema must also try to maintain adequate hydration of the skin, which means finding a moisturizer or emollient that doesn't contain any irritating substances, and applying it while the skin is still wet from bathing. Essential fatty acid supplements that help to strengthen the lipid layer in the skin may also be recommended. Acupuncture appears to decrease the symptoms of acute eczema, as well as the severity of subsequent flares.

Pharmaceutical management of dermatitis and eczema can vary from substances that suppress immune system activity to steroidal anti-inflammatories. Most of these interventions carry a risk of potentially serious side effects that require careful monitoring.

SIDEBAR 2.2 Stress, Allergies, and Cortisol

Stress can ripple through the body in a number of chemical ways. Massage therapists study some of these effects because they too have some influence over what chemicals are being released, and that influence should be informed and intentional.

For people who are prone to allergies, long-term stress creates some special problems. Cortisol is the hormone that is specifically related to long-term stress. When it is secreted over a long time, cortisol can damage the body by systemically weakening the connective tissues. But cortisol has one quality that makes it very, *very* useful: it is a powerful anti-inflammatory agent. When people undergo long-term stress, their cortisol supplies can be depleted. When cortisol is depleted, limited resources are available within the body to quell the inflammatory reaction. And for individuals subject to allergies, this means that they have a difficult time reducing the inflammation from immune system attacks against nonthreatening stimuli such as wheat, pollen, cat dander, and other irritants. If an immune reaction takes the form of a skin rash, it may be called dermatitis or eczema.

This is not to suggest that stress is the only cause of allergies or even the most important one; it's just to point out that long-term stress and cortisol depletion can often make allergies *worse*.

Medications

- Topical immunomodulators
- Topical or oral steroidal anti-inflammatories
- Topical or oral antihistamines

Massage?

RISKS Massage boosts local circulation. If an area is red, warm, and itchy, this could easily exacerbate symptoms of dermatitis or eczema. Further, people prone to these conditions may have an increased risk of having a hypersensitivity reaction to massage lubricants: this must be addressed before beginning a session. Finally, some types of eczema may involve blisters or scratching that damages the skin. These local injuries contraindicate massage because of the risk of secondary infection.

BENEFITS Clients with hypersensitive skin may find that careful massage with a hypoallergenic lubricant is soothing and deeply relaxing. As long as a therapist can find a way to work that does not increase itching or discomfort, the client can enjoy all the benefits that massage has to offer.

Neoplastic Skin Disorders

Seborrheic Keratosis

Definition: What Is It?

Seborrheic keratosis (SK) is a common type of benign skin growth that is most often found with mature adults.

Etiology: What Happens?

The etiology of SK is not well understood. Hyperproliferation of epithelial cells is evident, and a genetic predisposition seems clear, but other factors or triggers have not been identified. Lesions appear most frequently in people over 50 and in areas that have been exposed to sunlight: the chest, back, neck, face, and scalp. It is not seen on palms or soles. SK is not contagious.

SK is not skin cancer, but it can resemble actinic keratosis (AK) (a subtype of squamous cell

Seborrheic Keratosis in Brief

What is it?
Seborrheic keratosis (SK) is a common condition involving single or multiple benign skin growths. It usually affects mature adults.

How is it recognized?
SK can range from very small to the size of a silver dollar. They are typically dark brown or black, but can be lighter. They have a characteristic "pasted on" warty appearance, and usually develop on the trunk, face, or neck.

Massage risks and benefits
Risks: Massage carries no specific risks for SK. The lesions can sometimes be irritated by friction, so they are a local caution if they itch or bleed.
Benefits: Massage has no specific benefits for SK, but can add to the general quality of life of the person who has this condition.

carcinoma) when lesions are relatively new, and malignant melanoma when lesions are advanced. Further, it is possible for malignant cells to develop within the boundaries of SK lesions where they are hard to find; early skin cancer diagnoses may be missed in this way.

SK is usually considered a completely benign condition, but sometimes it has a dramatically rapid onset with multiple lesions. This phenomenon, called the Lesser-Trelat sign, is associated with a risk of other diseases, especially cancer involving the gastrointestinal tract. However, the relationship between SK and internal cancers is unclear.

Signs and Symptoms

SK lesions typically appear one at a time as soft light or dark brown spots on the trunk, face, or scalp. As they mature, they become thicker, and often darker. Eventually, they develop a warty, "pasted on" appearance. They are sometimes described as looking like shiny spots of melted wax, or crusty barnacles adhered to the skin (Figure 2.35).

SK doesn't typically hurt or itch, but when a lesion is irritated by clothing or other sources of friction, it may catch and bleed, opening the door to secondary infection.

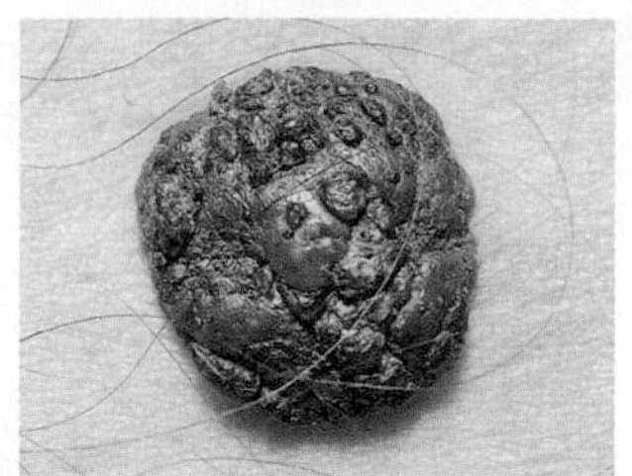

Figure 2.35. Seborrheic keratosis

Treatment

Most of the time, SK isn't treated at all, because the lesions are completely benign and don't usually hurt. Some topical medications may reduce the thickness of the growths. When they are in a location likely to be irritating, it may be worthwhile to remove the growths. This is usually accomplished with cryotherapy, but electrodissection and curettage may be suggested to cauterize and remove the growths surgically.

Medications

- Topical applications to reduce the thickness of SK lesions

Massage?

RISKS Massage carries no risk for seborrheic keratosis (SK) lesions, as long as they aren't irritated or bleeding. These can be considered local contraindications.

BENEFITS Massage has no specific benefits for SK lesions; clients with this disorder can enjoy the same benefits from bodywork as the rest of the population.

Skin Cancer

Definition: What Is It?

Cancer is the uncontrolled replication of cells. Usually, they accumulate into tumors that can invade and damage surrounding tissues. Cells may also leave a primary tumor to travel elsewhere in the body to colonize a new area: this is metastasis.

Cells that are programmed to replace themselves easily (this quality is called lability) are particularly

Skin Cancer in Brief

What is it?
Skin cancer is a group of diseases involving potentially malignant changes in cells of the epidermis. It typically affects keratinocytes (basal cell carcinoma and squamous cell carcinoma) or melanocytes (melanoma).

How is it recognized?
Basal cell and squamous cell carcinomas are often recognized by a giveaway sign: a sore that doesn't heal, or that comes and goes in the same place. These sores can look like almost anything: blisters, pimples, ulcerations, bumps, or abrasions. They are usually painless, but may itch or bleed. Melanoma usually involves a dark lesion that exhibits classic ABCDE signs, but some tumors may be more subtle.

Massage risks and benefits
Risks: Any undiagnosed skin lesions at least locally contraindicate massage until more information is gathered. BCC and SCC have a low metastasis risk, but until the lesions are treated they should be considered local cautions. Decisions about clients with melanoma must be made according to the treatment options they are using.
Benefits: While massage certainly won't cure skin cancer, massage therapists are in a unique position to observe lesions that their clients might not see: many cases of skin cancer have been identified and interrupted in this way.

vulnerable to DNA damage that triggers uncontrolled and disorganized replication. Epithelial cells are highly labile; this explains why cancers of the skin, lungs, breast, prostate, and digestive tract (all epithelial tissues) are the most common cancer diagnoses.

Etiology: What Happens?

Skin cancer begins with a change in epithelial cell function. The trigger for this change is often attributed to UV radiation (especially deep, blistering sunburns) or genetic predisposition, but exposure to other hazards has also been shown to increase the risk of various types of skin cancer. Arsenic, chronic skin inflammation and injury, and the use of immunosuppressant drugs are all associated with an increased risk for skin cancer.

Skin cancer is by far the most commonly diagnosed form of cancer, accounting for about a million diagnoses each year: this is about one-half of all cancer diagnoses in the United States. Most cases are not deadly, however, because the most common forms of skin cancer don't metastasize. People most at risk include those with a long history of sun exposure, those who are fair skinned, those with a personal or family history of skin cancer, and those who are immune-suppressed.

The skin cells that are affected and the results of that change vary with subtypes.

Types of Skin Cancer

Basal Cell Carcinoma

Definition: What Is It?

Basal cell carcinoma (BCC) is by far the most common type of skin cancer, accounting for about 80% of all skin cancer diagnoses. It is a slow-growing tumor of basal cells in the epidermis. It usually appears on the face or head. BCC only rarely metastasizes, but if a tumor is not treated, it may invade and damage healthy tissues, including bones, blood vessels, and nerves.

Signs and Symptoms

BCC has several different presentations. The most common is the nodular form, in which it looks like a small hard lump with rounded pink pearly edges and a soft sunken middle (Figure 2.36). Tiny blood vessels called telangiectasias may be visible. These lesions may itch and bleed easily, but they don't tend to hurt, and they don't heal: the cardinal sign of nonmelanoma skin cancer. Many BCC tumors grow on the face around the nose or orbits (Figures 2.37 and 2.38). Pigmented BCC has darker lesions. Superficial BCC resembles eczema or psoriasis. Micronodular BCC shows multiple well-defined white-yellow lesions. And morpheaform BCC tends to show only subtle scar-like lesions on the skin, while silently and aggressively invading deeper tissues.

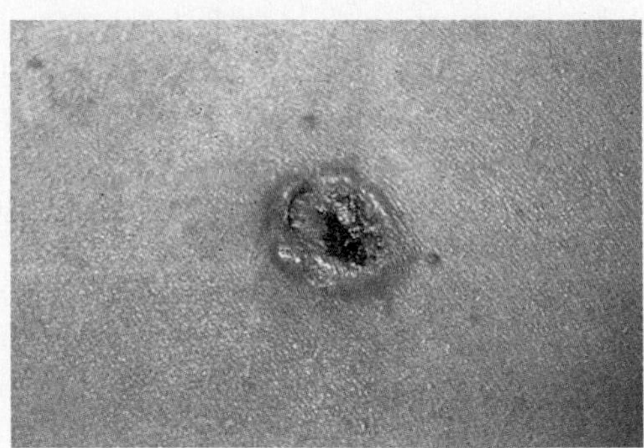

Figure 2.36. Basal cell carcinoma: rodent ulcer

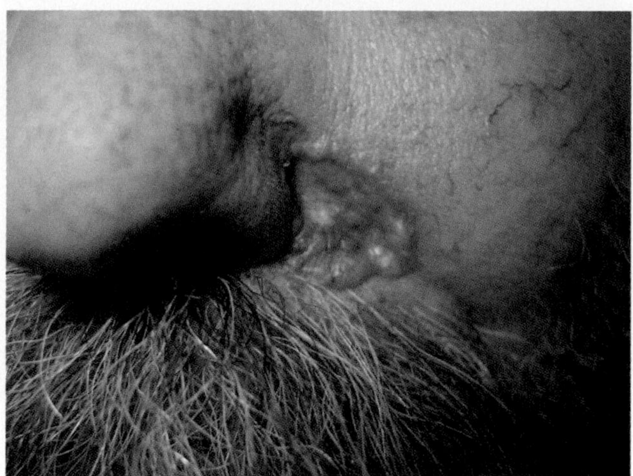
Figure 2.37. Basal cell carcinoma: nose

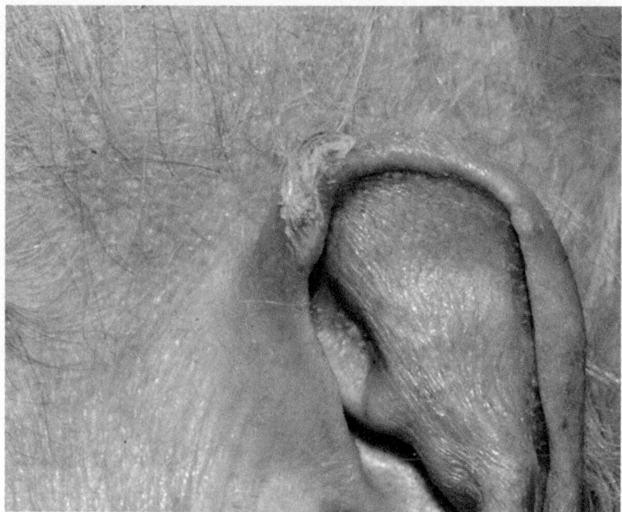
Figure 2.39. Actinic keratosis: ear

Squamous Cell Carcinoma

Definition: What Is It?

SCC is a cancer of skin cells that arises in keratinocytes superficial to the basal layer. It often appears in areas exposed to sunlight, but unlike other skin cancers it also grows in the mouth, affecting the tongue, cheeks, and gums. SCC that grows on the penis or vaginal walls is associated with a history of genital warts.

Exposure to mid-range UV light is the main risk factor for SCC; but this condition can also develop in the presence of long-term skin injury or inflammation like decubitus ulcers, repeating boils, or draining sores.

It is rare but not impossible for SCC to metastasize to other places in the body. For this reason, lesions caught in early stages are typically removed as quickly as possible.

Types of Squamous Cell Carcinoma

- *Actinic keratosis* (AK). Also called solar keratosis; this is often discussed as a precancerous condition that may lead to SCC. However, according to some experts, the cellular changes seen with AK are identical to those seen with invasive SCC. Further, left long enough, most AK lesions do develop aggressive characteristics, and they seldom spontaneously disappear. AK looks like brown or red scaly lesions in sun-exposed areas: forehead, ears, and hands (Figure 2.39).
- *Actinic cheilitis*. This is a form of AK that is found specifically on the lips (Figure 2.40).
- *Leukoplakia*. This form looks like white patches on the tongue and inside the cheek. It is most often associated with tobacco use. It isn't usually dangerous, but in rare cases can become malignant.
- *Bowen disease*. Also called in situ SCC, Bowen disease is similar to AK except that the lesions tend to be larger and browner.

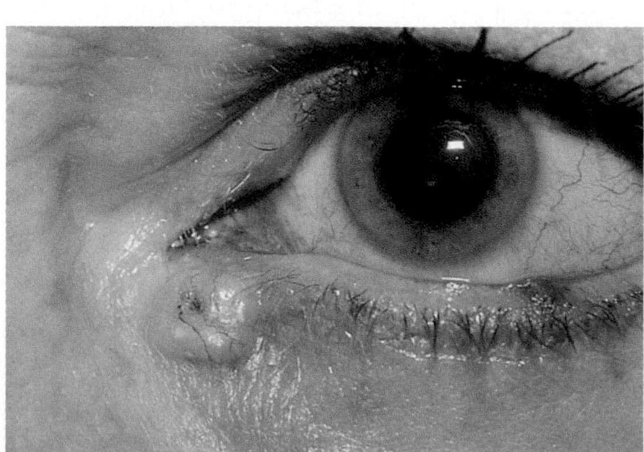
Figure 2.38. Basal cell carcinoma: eye

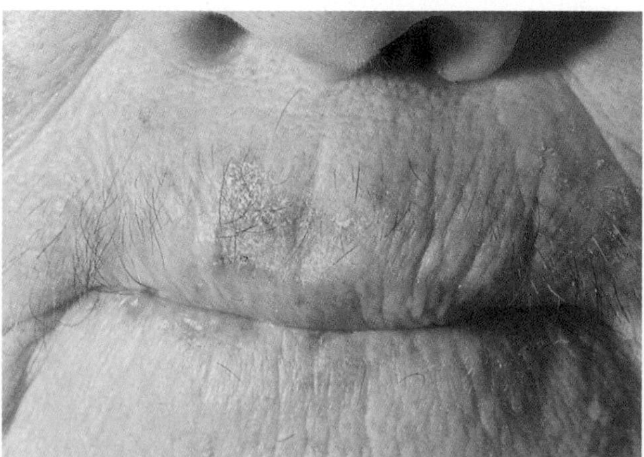
Figure 2.40. Actinic cheilitis: lips

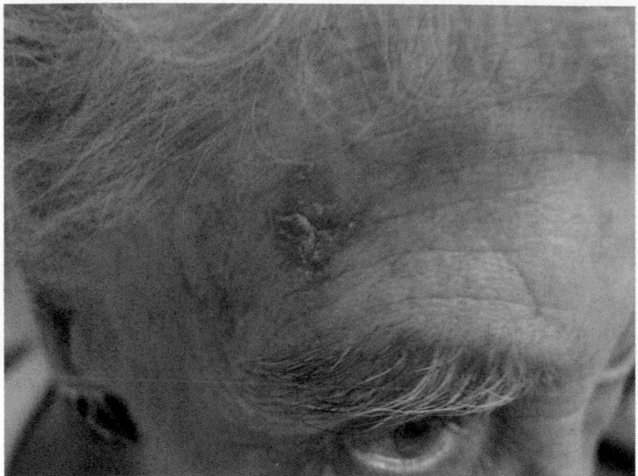
Figure 2.41. Squamous cell carcinoma

Signs and Symptoms of Squamous Cell Carcinoma

SCC lesions often appear on pre-existing injuries, inside the mouth, and in areas with a history of sun damage. They share the typical nonmelanoma skin cancer pattern: they appear as nonpainful sores that may itch or bleed, but don't fully heal. SCC borders are often less distinct than those of BCC (Figure 2.41 and 2.42). Many but not all SCC lesions begin as actinic keratoses.

Melanoma

Definition: What Is It?

Melanocytes are the pigment cells deep in the epidermis that give skin its color. Melanin in skin cells offers some protection from UV radiation, but when melanocytes become overactive and replicate out of control, they can quickly become a life-threatening form of cancer.

Unlike other forms of skin cancer, melanoma metastasizes readily, often leading to tumors in the bones, liver, or central nervous system. It is the leading cause of death by skin cancer. Melanocytes are found in the eye, reproductive and digestive tracts as well as the skin, so while it is rare, melanoma does have the potential to develop in these areas.

Like other forms of cancer, melanoma has a good prognosis if it is found and treated early. An important part of the diagnosis is evaluating how deeply it has penetrated the layers of the skin. Lesions that are less than 0.7 mm deep typically have not yet spread, but lesions that have invaded 4 mm or more are often associated with distant metastasis.

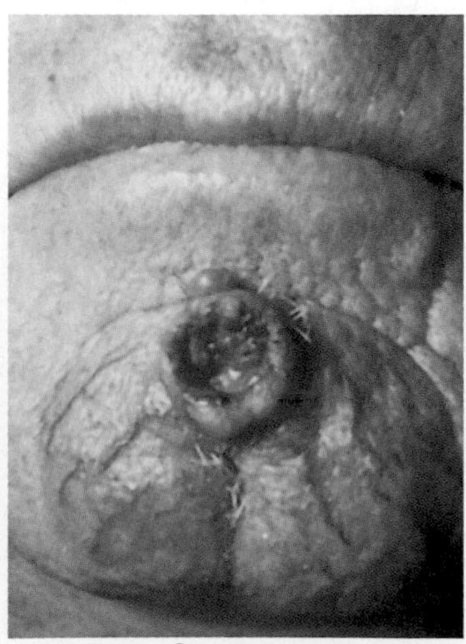
Figure 2.42. Squamous cell carcinoma

SIDEBAR 2.3 Skin Pigmentations

Age and the uneven distribution of melanin in the skin can give rise to several types of skin patches. Because massage therapists work so closely in this context, it is important to be familiar with the most common types of skin markings clients may have.

Moles

Moles, or nevi, are areas where melanocytes replicate, but without threatening to invade surrounding tissues. The melanocytes produce extra melanin, causing symmetrical brown, black, purple, blue, or reddish growths with well-defined borders.

Port-Wine Stains

Port-wine stains are markings that affect blood vessels near the surface of the skin. They are often large, and are usually completely harmless, but may be treated to reduce their appearance.

Freckles

Freckles are simple concentrations of melanin in the skin. They can range from light tan to red, but are always darker than surrounding skin. They are small, but can blend together to form larger shapes. Freckles often darken in response to sun exposure, and fade when protected from UV radiation.

Lentigines

Lentigines (singular is lentigo) are similar to freckles, but they tend to appear on older people and they are much larger than freckles. They are sometimes called "liver spots," although they have nothing to do with liver function.

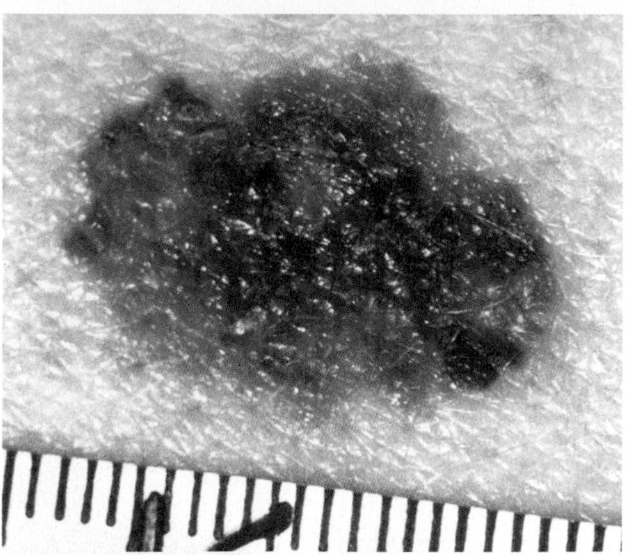
Figure 2.43. Superficial spreading melanoma

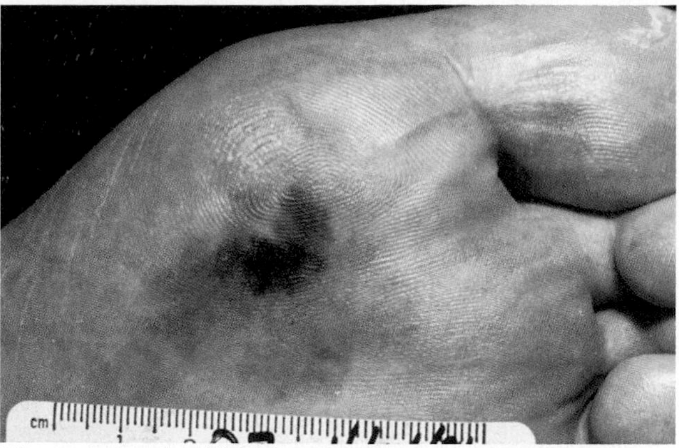
Figure 2.45. Acral lentiginous melanoma

Types of Melanoma

- *Superficial spreading melanoma.* This is the most common variety. It spreads along the surface of the skin before invading deeper tissues. It may be multicolored and slightly elevated (Figure 2.43).
- *Lentigo melanoma.* This also begins as a superficial discoloration, usually in older people. Lesions are often deeply notched, which helps to distinguish them from simple round or oval "age spots" (Figure 2.44).
- *Acral lentiginous melanoma.* This type of skin cancer is as common in people of color as it is in Caucasians. It often begins under the nails or on the palms or soles (Figure 2.45).
- *Nodular melanoma.* This is the most aggressive type of skin cancer. It is significantly elevated from the skin, and it often penetrates deeper into the tissues than other types (Figure 2.46).

Signs and Symptoms

Melanoma often starts from a pre-existing mole that begins to change: it lightens, darkens, thickens, and may become elevated. It may itch or bleed around the edges. The color and texture may change. Many doctors rely on the "ugly duckling" principle: any mole that looks different from others should be examined.

Melanoma doesn't always start as a mole, however, nor does it always begin in places exposed to the sun.

NOTABLE CASES Iconic reggae musician Bob Marley died of acral lentiginous melanoma at age 36. The cancer had metastasized to his lungs and brain. Politician John McCain is a melanoma survivor.

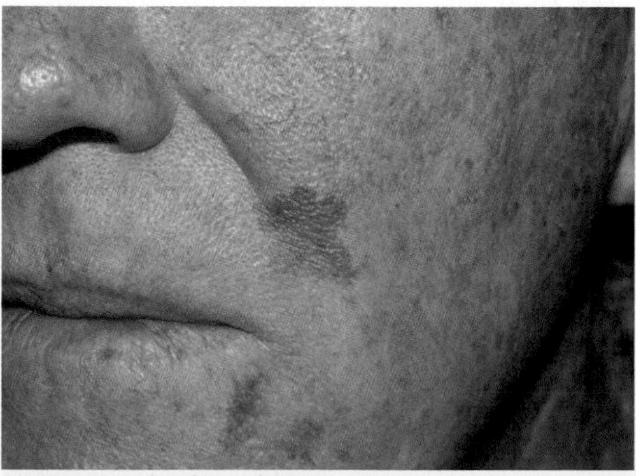
Figure 2.44. Lentigo melanoma

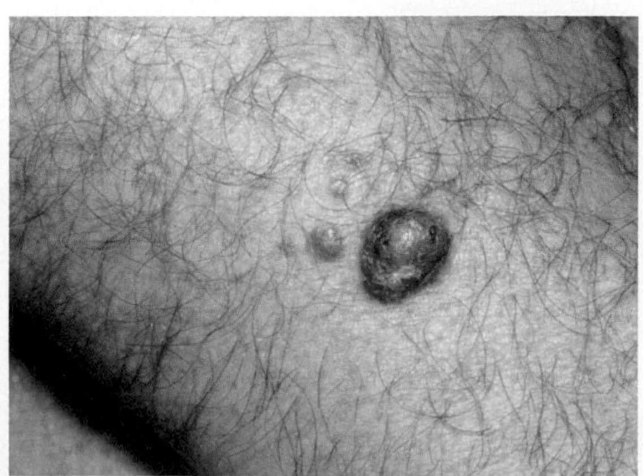
Figure 2.46. Nodular melanoma

Here is the traditional mnemonic to remember key features of melanoma (Figure 2.47):

- A = asymmetrical. Most benign moles are round or oval. Melanomas are irregular in shape.
- B = border. The borders of melanomas are often inconsistent: in some areas, they are clear, and in others on the same lesion, they may be faded or hard to identify.
- C = color. Benign moles are black, brown, or purple. Melanomas tend to be multicolored.
- D = diameter. Melanomas are typically larger than many moles. Any mole greater than 6 mm across should be examined by a dermatologist.

SIDEBAR 2.4 Melanoma Staging

Melanoma staging is a complicated process. It identifies how far the disease has progressed, which allows oncologists to choose treatment options that are most likely to be successful. Staging may be discussed as clinical or pathological:

- Clinical staging is based on a physical exam, imaging tests, and a biopsy of the lesion.
- Pathological staging is based on the biopsy of nearby lymph nodes.

Further, two different ways of describing the depth of lesions have been developed. The Breslow measurement refers strictly to the thickness of the tumor. Alternatively, the Clark level uses the layers of the skin as the primary point of reference. For instance, a Level I tumor only affects the epidermis, while a Level V tumor penetrates into the subcutaneous tissues.

The prognosis for melanoma is consistently worse when the lesion is ulcerated, so this feature is built into the staging protocol: "a" means without ulceration, and "b" means with ulceration.

Tumor	Definition
Tx	Can't be assessed
T0	No evidence of a primary tumor
Tis	In situ: epidermis only
T1a/b	Tumor is <1 mm deep
T2a/b	Tumor is 1.01–2 mm deep
T3a/b	Tumor is 2.01–4 mm deep
T4a/b	Tumor is more than 4 mm deep

N (node) classifications may be qualified by "a" or "b": "a" denotes that all growths are microscopic, while "b" denotes that growths are visible to the naked eye.

Node	Definition
Nx	Can't be assessed
N0	No spread to nodes
N1	Cancer cells are found in 1 node
N2	2–3 nodes are affected, OR the tumor has enlarged with no spread to nodes
N3	4 or more nodes are affected, OR cells are founds in groups of nodes, OR the tumor has spread and affected multiple nodes

Metastasis	Definition
Mx	Can't be assessed
M0	No distant metastasis
M1a	Distant metastases are found in skin and subdermis OR in distant lymph nodes
M1b	Distant metastases are found in lungs
M1c	Distant metastases are found in other organs

Stage	Definition	5-year survival rate (%)
0	Tis, N0, M0	99
IA	T1a, N0, M0	99
IB	T1b or T2a, N0, M0	92
IIA	T2b or T2a, N0, M0	86
IIB	T3b or T4a, N0, M0	68
IIC	T4b, N0, M0	56
IIIA	T1a–4a, N1a, M0	Not available (this is a new classification)
IIIB	T1a/b–4a/b, N1a/b or N2a/b, N3, M0	50–68
IIIC	T any, N any, M0	27–52
IV	T any, N any, M1	18

It is important to remember that skin cancer is usually preventable. The single most important factor in reducing the risk of this disease is to be careful with sun exposure. Experts recommend the following steps:

- Stay out of direct sunlight between 10 A.M. and 4 P.M.
- Cover up with tightly woven clothing
- Cover the ears and back of the neck
- Use sunscreen with a minimum of SPF 15, and reapply after swimming or perspiring
- Use UV-absorbing sunglasses
- Observe these precautions even on cloudy days, because UV radiation penetrates cloud cover

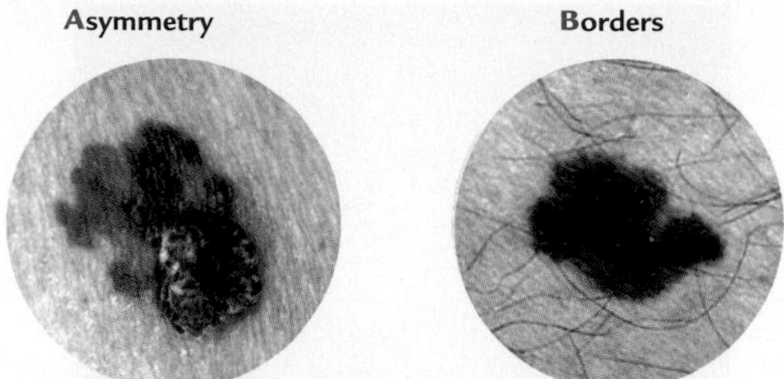

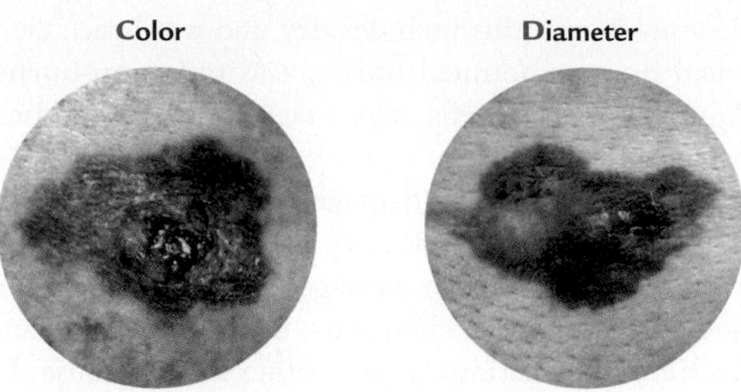

Figure 2.47. ABCDs of malignant melanoma

- E = elevated. The traditional usage refers to the fact that some melanomas, especially the nodular type, are elevated. Another way to use the E in this mnemonic is for "evolving," which refers to the fact that melanomas often change rapidly.

Treatment

Treatment for skin cancer depends on the type and stage at diagnosis.

Typically, options are divided into cryotherapy, surgery, chemotherapy, photodynamic therapy, biological therapy, and radiation.

Medications

- Topical chemotherapy for shallow lesions
- Oral or injected chemotherapy for more invasive cancer
- Medication to cause cancer cells to become sensitive to specific lightwaves, followed by exposure to those lights
- Drugs that mimic cytokines to alter cell activity in and around tumors

Massage?

RISKS The main risk for massage and clients with skin cancer is ignoring an important sign or symptom: a sore that doesn't heal or a suspicious mole or other marking.

BENEFITS Skin cancer is common and, while not usually dangerous in the short run, it requires appropriate and timely care. Massage therapists are in a position to see possible lesions and bring them to their clients' attention. This must be done in a nondiagnostic and nonalarmist way, of course. Clients who have been fully treated for skin cancer can enjoy the same benefits from massage as the rest of the population.

Skin Injuries

Burns

Definition: What Are They?

Many people think about burns in the context of touching a hot iron or brushing a hand across a broiler rack, but the world of burns goes far beyond household appliances. Burns are typically classified as

Burns in Brief

What are they?
Burns are caused by damage to the skin that kills cells. They can be caused by heat, radiation, corrosive chemicals, and electricity.

How are they recognized?
First-degree burns show pain and inflammation of the superficial epidermis: mild sunburns and diaper rash are examples. Second-degree burns involve blistering and damage into deeper layers of the epidermis. Third-degree burns penetrate to the dermis or deeper. They may show white or black charred edges. Later, third-degree burns often result in shrunken, contracted scar tissue that limits movement.

Massage risks and benefits
Risks: All burns locally contraindicate massage while they are acute, because of pain and the risk of secondary infection. (One exception to this rule might be extremely mild sunburns that would benefit from the application of soothing lotion.)
Benefits: People recovering from burns may benefit from the stress-reduction massage offers during a painful process. Healed burns are appropriate for massage as long as sensation is present. Healed third-degree burns often involve itching and restrictive scar tissue, so anything massage can do to ease this is a gift to the client.

thermal burns (this includes dry and wet heat), electrical burns, chemical burns, and radiation burns. Any one of these kills cells, essentially melting their proteins.

In addition to skin damage, burns may also injure other surfaces: the respiratory tract and digestive tract are both vulnerable to damage from overheated air, liquids, or corrosive chemicals. Burns to the face and neck are more serious than to other areas because the resulting inflammation can block breathing passages.

Etiology: What Happens?

The severity of burns is determined by how deep they go, how much surface area they cover, and what part of the body has been affected. Thermal burns occur at temperatures above 115°F (46°C); damage is determined by both temperature and the duration of contact. If a significant amount of skin function is lost, then its functions are compromised: the ability to regulate temperature, control fluid loss, provide a barrier against microbial invasion, and provide sensory information may all be impaired. A burn that affects more than 15% of the skin's surface can put a person at risk for infection, shock, and circulatory collapse.

The severity of chemical burns is based on the pH of the substance, its concentration, duration of contact, and other factors. Because of the way these chemicals act on fat cells, acid burns tend not to penetrate deeply into the skin, but alkali burns, which can effectively melt through the protective fatty layer, can be much more serious.

Types of Burns

- *First-degree (superficial) burns*. These are a mild (but often quite painful) irritation of the superficial epidermis. They are red, but don't involve blisters. Sunburns (Figure 2.48) are a common version of first-degree burns. They usually heal in 2 to 3 days, sometimes with flaking and peeling.
- *Second-degree (partial thickness) burns*. These involve damage into deeper layers of the epidermis. They show redness and instantly appearing blisters. Second-degree burns often leave a permanent scar (Figure 2.49).
- *Third-degree (full thickness) burns*. These penetrate through the epidermis to the dermis or deeper. They destroy not only skin cells but glands, hair shafts, and nerve endings as well. They may present with white or black charred edges (Figure 2.50). If they penetrate into muscle tissue, proteins from the dead cells may accumulate to cause kidney damage. Third-degree burns tend to contract very extremely as they heal, which can cause disfiguring scars and limited mobility of the skin.

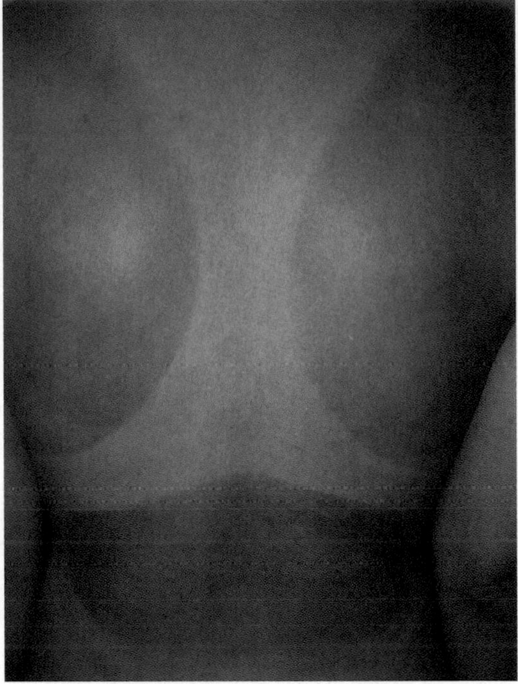

Figure 2.48. First-degree burn

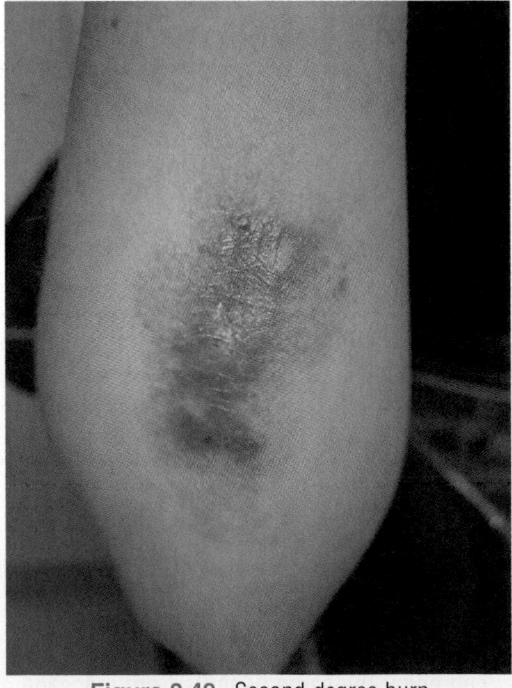

Figure 2.49. Second-degree burn

Signs and Symptoms

The symptoms of burn damage depend on what level of skin has been affected. Details on symptoms by degree of damage are listed with description.

Treatment

First- and second-degree burns are typically treated with soothing lotion. If blistering occurs, antibiotic cream may be recommended to prevent infection. Third-degree burns, however, must be treated with more care to minimize the accumulation of binding scar tissue. This often means wound cleansing and **debridement** (aggressive skin brushing to remove debris), as well as skin grafts and plastic surgery.

Medications

- Antibiotic cream, if necessary
- Analgesics for pain control

Massage?

RISKS Most burns contraindicate massage when they are acute—not just for pain but also for infection risk. The only exception might be very mild sunburn. A client with a history of severe burns might have impaired sensation in those areas: this requires extra care with massage to avoid overtreatment.

BENEFITS A person who is recovering from third-degree burns may have to undergo painful treatments; relaxation massage can help to address the stress that accompanies that challenge. Some evidence also indicates that massage can improve itching, mood, range of motion, and the quality of scar tissue in burn survivors.

Clients who have had burns with no long-term nerve damage can enjoy the same benefits from bodywork as the rest of the population.

OPTIONS Some researchers have developed specific massage protocols for skin rehabilitation. Bodywork practitioners interested in working with these populations can pursue this further at specialized burn treatment centers.

Decubitus Ulcers

Definition: What are they?

Decubitus ulcers, also known as bedsores, pressure sores, and trophic ulcers, are problems massage therapists are most likely to see when working in a hospital, a nursing home, or some other setting with bedridden patients. They stem from inadequate blood flow to the skin that is compressed between bone and another surface.

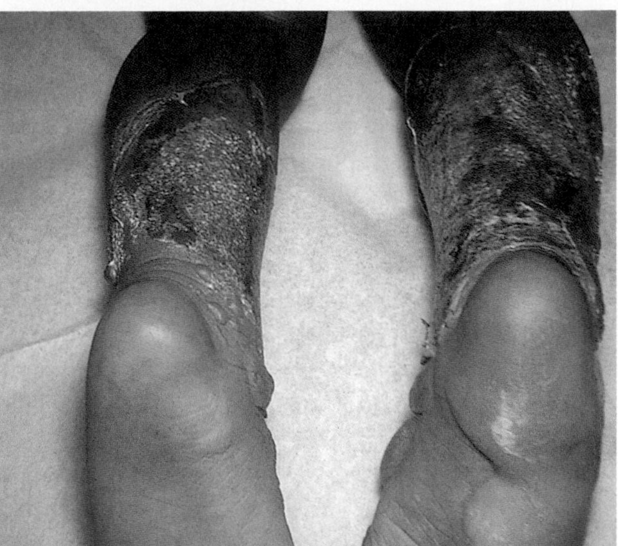

Figure 2.50. Third-degree burn

Etiology: What Happens?

All of the body's cells rely on unobstructed blood flow to deliver oxygen and nutrients, and to carry away wastes.

Decubitus Ulcers in Brief

Pronunciation: de-KYU-bih-tus UL-surz

What are they?
Decubitus ulcers, also called bedsores, are lesions caused by impaired circulation to the skin because of external pressure. This leads to localized cell death and a high risk of secondary infection.

How are they recognized?
Cell damage with bedsores may occur before the skin breaks down: this can be difficult to see until damage is extensive. When ulcers form, they look like open craters in the skin: they don't form a crust, and they may penetrate all the way to the bone.

Massage risks and benefits
Risks: Once tissue damage begins, the risk of infection is so high that decubitus ulcers contraindicate massage.
Benefits: Massage is a tool that prevents bedsores better than treating them. A client with fully healed bedsores can safely receive massage.

If capillaries are compressed between two unyielding surfaces, it doesn't take long for cells to die. This damage can penetrate all the way down to the bone (Figure 2.51). Nearby bacteria may then take advantage of the situation and create a potentially life-threatening secondary infection. Finally, because bedsores involve long-term inflammation, they are also a significant risk factor for developing an aggressive form of SCC.

Decubitus ulcers occur most often in spinal cord injury patients, malnourished people, and older patients who are underweight and immobile. These patients deal with a combination of factors that increase the risk of pressure sores, including impaired pain sensation, poor vasomotor responses in local capillaries, and extremely delicate skin: paradoxically, this means that the shearing and friction forces that occur with positional changes may actually increase the risk of pressure sores. This phenomenon points out how important it is to prevent pressure sores before they happen.

The sacrum, ischial tuberosity, and elbows are the most common sites for decubitus ulcers, but they can develop virtually anywhere that tissue is compressed for more than two hours.

Signs and Symptoms

Stage I of pressure sores shows a marked change in skin temperature (it can become cooler or warmer than the surrounding area). Discoloration may appear to be red, purple, or bluish. Pain and itching accompany these changes. It is difficult to estimate the amount of damage that has accrued at this point: often skin discoloration is the "tip of the iceberg," while extensive tissue loss has developed below.

NOTABLE CASES Spinal cord injury patient Christopher Reeve died from complications related to a pressure sore and subsequent infection.

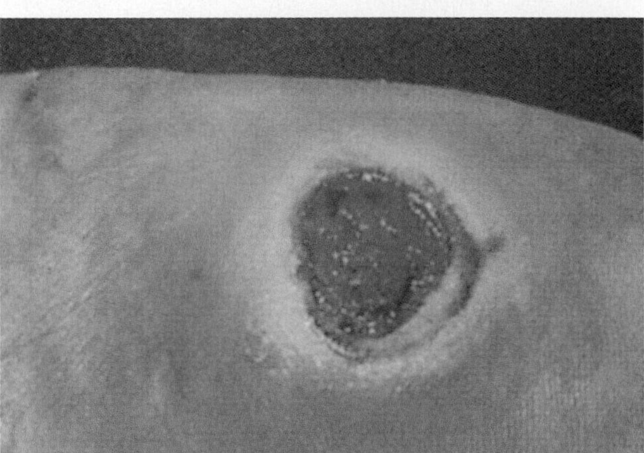

Figure 2.51. Decubitus ulcer

In Stages II through IV, the lesions turn purple, and then necrosis (tissue death) begins. Sores may extend into deep layers of the skin or into fascia, tendons, and down to the bone. Bacteria may invade the damaged tissue, which results in local or systemic infection.

Ulcers differ from other types of sores because poor local circulation prevents a normal healing process. Eventually ulcers can heal, but a permanent dip remains where the dead tissue never grows back.

Treatment

Bedsores are preventable through careful hygiene and frequent bed turning or other postural adjustments. Once they form, however, they are difficult and expensive to treat. Topical antibiotics and special dressings that promote tissue growth may be adequate for some; others may require extensive debridement and surgery to repair. Electrical stimulation may improve local blood flow. Whirlpool baths can support circulation and gentle removal of damaged tissue.

Medications

- Medicated dressings to promote cell growth
- Topical or systemic antibiotics for infection risk

Massage?

RISKS The risk of infection is very high with decubitus ulcers, so any indication that an ulcer has formed or is imminent at least locally contraindicates massage.

BENEFITS Massage may help reduce the risk of pressure sores before they form, but only if the client has good sensation and the skin is resilient enough to accommodate the compression, friction, and shearing forces that even gentle massage may involve. Unfortunately, for many people vulnerable to bedsores, this is not the case.

Scar Tissue

Definition: What is it?

Scar tissue is the development of new cells and extracellular matrix where damage has occurred. An animation about scarring is available at http://thePoint.lww.com/Werner5e.

This discussion is limited to the regenerative capacities of the skin. For information on scar tissue associated with musculoskeletal injuries, see the section on tendinopathies in Chapter 3.

Etiology: What Happens?

The skin, made mostly of relatively delicate epithelial tissue, is our primary barrier against the outside world. Consequently, epidermal cells are genetically programmed to heal fast. Imagine a minor scrape or abrasion: within seconds, clotting mechanisms allow a scab to begin to form. Under the new scab, basal cells detach from the basement membrane and migrate in a single-layered sheet across the wound. When they reach the other side and touch other epithelial cells, a process called **contact inhibition** makes them stop moving.

Back at the original site, stationary basal cells duplicate to build up the ranks of migrating cells. When the whole wound has been covered, the new sheet of basal cells begins dividing to form new strata. Finally, the superficial cells become keratinized, and the scab falls off. Then the wound has healed; the blood supply is protected from the outside world, and the wound is no longer vulnerable to infection. The whole process can take place within 24 hours to several days, depending on the size and location of the injury.

Scar Tissue in Brief

What is it?
Scar tissue is new tissue that grows after an injury, infection, or surgery. It can grow in any kind of tissue, but this discussion is limited to scar tissue that affects any layer of the skin.

How is it recognized?
Deeply scarred skin may lack pigmentation, hair follicles, and sweat glands.

Massage risks and benefits
Risks: Skin that is injured and not yet healed obviously contraindicates massage at least locally, both because of pain and the risk of infection.
Benefits: Skin that is intact but scarred, even if the scar tissue has not fully matured, may benefit from the enhanced local circulation and mobilization provided by careful massage.

If the damage penetrates deeper than the dermis, or if the wound is complicated by any infectious risk, the healing process is more complicated. Fibroblasts migrate to the site, so beneath all that basal cell activity collagen and other extracellular matrices are deposited. Eventually, this delicate granulation tissue may become a dense accumulation of collagenous scar tissue.

Types of Scar Tissue

- *Hypertrophic scars.* These are scars that overflow their boundaries, but don't form permanently enlarged masses. They often appear a month or so after injury, and then stabilize or regress.
- *Keloid scars.* These are the result of overproduction of collagen, leading to a permanently raised mass of collagenous scar tissue. Keloids can be a complication of deep injury, piercing (see Figure 2.52), or surgery.
- *Contracture scars.* Occasionally, a skin injury can cover so much area that as the skin heals, it pulls together in a tight web of connective tissue that may limit the range of motion over joints. This is a potential complication of burns and some surgeries.

Signs and Symptoms

Scar tissue of superficial layers of the skin often leaves no mark after healing is complete. Common permanent scars like striae (stretch marks) and acne scars show where tissue damage that affects layers deeper than the epidermis has occurred. Deeper scars may be marked by discoloration, lack of pigmentation, lack of

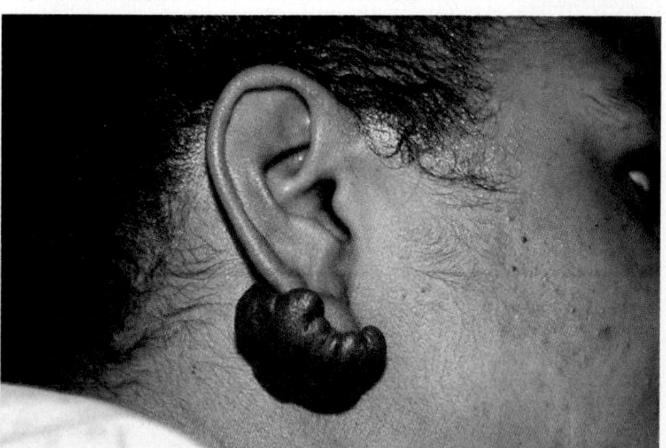

Figure 2.52. Keloid scar

hair follicles, and sebaceous and sweat glands. When the formation of scar tissue malfunctions, some other signs may be present.

Treatment

People with obvious scars may treat them to reduce their appearance, but scars themselves can't be eradicated. Interventions include using collagen or fat injections to fill out dipped areas; dermabrasion, chemical peels, laser resurfacing, and small or larger skin grafts.

Hypertrophic and keloid scars are more challenging to treat, because they often recur. Injections with cortisol to dissolve connective tissue, liquid nitrogen, pressure bandages, and other interventions may be applied.

Medications

- Injections of soft tissue fillers (collagen, fat cells, etc.)
- Application of tissue-engineered products for burns or ulcers
- Injections of cortisol to dissolve excessive collagen

Massage?

RISKS Incompletely sealed wounds are obviously a local contraindication because of the risk for pain and infection. Very delicate scar tissue may also need to be treated carefully until it has become denser and stronger. Deep scarring may involve some loss of sensation; this requires some adjustments in bodywork.

BENEFITS Fully formed scar tissue carries no risk for massage; clients can enjoy all the benefits of bodywork as the rest of the population.

OPTIONS Careful manipulation around the edges of new wounds and more aggressive manipulation of older scars may improve the quality of tissue by affecting local circulation and softening connective tissue. Of course all work must be conducted within client pain tolerance.

CHAPTER REVIEW QUESTIONS: INTEGUMENTARY SYSTEM CONDITIONS

1. A client has a large abrasion on her right knee that is crusted and dry. Does this situation contraindicate massage? Locally or systemically? Why?
2. A client has extremely dry and flaky eczema on her hands. Does this condition indicate or contraindicate massage? Why?
3. A client has several raised red circles on his truck. They are paler in the middle. He reports that they are mildly itchy. What condition is probably present?
4. Describe the difference between an acne lesion and a boil.
5. When working with a client who is prone to acne, is it a good idea to follow the treatment of alcohol rinse to remove the oil? Why?
6. A client has white flakes that cling to hair shafts and don't brush out. What condition is probably present?
7. A client has a large hot painful pustule on his thigh. He assumes it is a spider bite, but has not been to the doctor. What condition may be present?
8. Your client has a scraped knuckle that is red and acutely inflamed. Red streaks run from the abrasion toward her elbow. Is she a good candidate for massage? Why?
9. Your client reports a small painless lesion on his cheek. It itches and occasionally bleeds, but never heals. What advice should you give him?
10. What makes acral lentiginous melanoma different from other types of melanoma?

3

Musculoskeletal System Conditions

Chapter Objectives

After reading this chapter, you should be able to . . .

- Identify the role of dystrophin in muscle function.
- Name three causative factors for muscle spasm.
- Name three factors that can accelerate calcium loss.
- List the three typical stages of adhesive capsulitis.
- Name the difference between strains and sprains.
- Identify the substance that causes damage with gout.
- Identify the causative agent for Lyme disease.
- Explain why knees and hips are vulnerable to osteoarthritis.
- Describe why people with carpal tunnel syndrome may have symptoms proximal to the hand.
- Describe a trigger point "energy crisis."
- Name three structures that may help to pin or trap the structures affected by thoracic outlet syndrome.
- Identify the difference between tendinosis and tendinitis.

This chapter addresses disorders and injuries of muscles, bones, joints, fascia, and associated structures. Together these provide humans with shape, strength, and movement. They are composed almost entirely of the material that provides structure for working cells and permeates every part of the body: connective tissue.

Injury to any of the connective tissue structures (except bone and sometimes cartilage) can be difficult for many medical professionals to identify. Soft tissues don't show well on x-rays, and while magnetic resonance imaging (MRI) can be useful, its ability to locate or identify injury is extremely limited. Ultrasound technology is advancing to the point of being able to see soft tissues in a moving person, but this application is limited to research settings. A thorough clinical examination still yields the most comprehensive information about injury to muscles, tendons, ligaments, and other connective tissues. Massage therapists, with their in-depth understanding of the musculoskeletal system, particularly with the formation of adhesions and scar tissue, are in a unique position to be able to help individuals with these types of injuries.

Bones

Bone Structure

The arrangement of living and nonliving material in bone is elegant and efficient. The collagen matrix on which solid bone is built is arranged as circles within circles. Calcium and phosphorus deposits accumulate on this scaffolding in a similarly circular pattern, leaving holes for blood vessels. In addition, most long bones in the body grow in a slight spiral, much like evergreen tree trunks. The shaft, or **diaphysis**, of long bones is hollow, filled with red marrow in youth and yellow marrow in adulthood. All of these design features give bone remarkable properties: resilience and weight-bearing capacity alongside lightweight construction.

The commands to move rocklike calcium and phosphorus salts around the collagen matrix are carried out by specialized cells. Osteoblasts, or "**b**one **b**uilders," help to lay new deposits, while osteo**cl**asts, or "bone **cl**earers," break them down. These cells are located in the periosteum, around the outside of the bone, the endosteum, which lines the central cavity, and in trabecular or spongy bone.

Osteoblasts and osteoclasts are controlled by hormones. Calcitonin from the thyroid lowers blood calcium by telling osteoblasts to pull calcium out of the blood and deposit it on bone tissue. Parathyroid hormone raises blood calcium by telling the osteoclasts to dismantle calcium deposits and put the valuable mineral back into the bloodstream. There it is available to help with muscle contractions, nerve transmission, blood clotting, and maintenance of the appropriate pH balance in the blood and tissues. Consequently, the density of the bones depends partly on a person's physical activity, and also on whatever other chemical demands the body may make on its calcium banks. This is, in essence, Wolff law: "Every change in the form and the function of a bone, or in its function alone, is followed by certain definite changes in its internal architecture and secondary alterations in its external conformation." In other words, bone is not inert; it is living tissue that remodels according to the stresses that are placed upon it.

Bone Function

The skeleton helps to define our shape, but it has many other functions as well. It provides a bony framework, protection for vulnerable organs, and points of leverage for efficient movement. Red and white blood cells are produced in the red marrow. Bones store calcium, phosphorus, and other minerals for future use, including maintaining a narrow margin of tolerance for acid-base balance in the blood and other tissue fluids. Bones also secrete hormones that help to manage phosphate reabsorption in the kidneys, regulate blood sugar levels by boosting insulin-producing cells, and reduce fat deposition.

Muscles

Muscle Structure

Muscles are composed of specialized threadlike cells called **myofibers** that, with electrical and chemical stimulation, have the power to contract while bearing weight. Myofibers run the full length of the muscle, and each one is encased in a connective tissue envelope, the **endomysium**. Packets of wrapped myofibers are bound in another fascial envelope, creating bundles called **fascicles**. Fascicles are bound together by yet another membrane, the **perimysium** (Figure 3.1). Finally, some large muscle groups are further bound by an external connective tissue membrane (**epimysium**), which blends into the subcutaneous layer of the skin, the superficial fascia (which is—surprise!—another connective tissue membrane).

Muscle Function

Muscles work when a stimulus from a motor neuron crosses the synaptic cleft at the neuromuscular junction. This release of the neurotransmitter **acetylcholine** begins a sequence of events leading to the shortening of myofibers. Muscle contractions are typically classified as **concentric** (pulling the ends toward the center) or **eccentric** (preventing the uncontrolled lengthening of a muscle); or as **isotonic** (keeping the same tone or level of tension) or **isometric** (keeping the same length, while internal tone may change).

When muscles work, they consume fuel and produce both energy (the pulling together of their bony attachments) and wastes. What kinds of wastes are produced depends on how much work is done, how

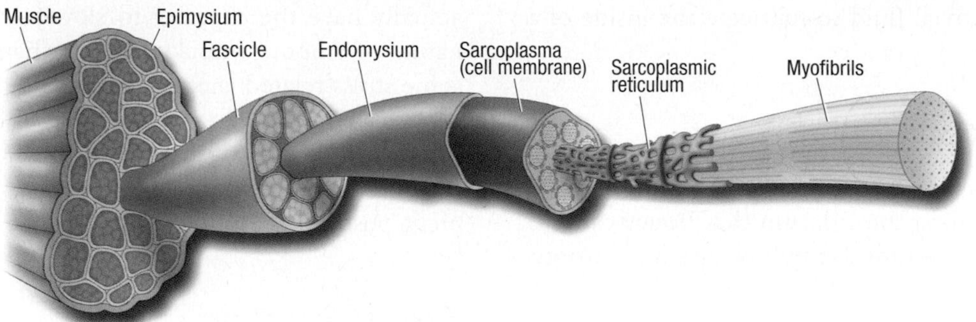

Figure 3.1. Muscles are composed of bundles within bundles, all enveloped by connective tissue membranes

long it takes, and whether adequate oxygen is available during the process. Muscles that work with adequate oxygen supply burn very cleanly: the waste products of aerobic combustion are carbon dioxide and water. But when muscles work without adequate oxygen, a different chemical cascade occurs, which may produce irritants that can contribute to delayed-onset muscle soreness.

The research on massage and muscle soreness has so far borne inconsistent results. The role of lactic acid as an instigator in muscle soreness is no longer generally accepted, so the claim that massage reduces muscle soreness by removing lactic acid and other wastes from the tissues is probably inaccurate. Further, the question of massage and "toxin removal" is far from settled; to date, no research shows evidence of significant changes in toxic excretions after massage. While ample anecdotal evidence has accrued about massage and improved recovery from muscle soreness and overuse, the mechanisms for how this might be accomplished have not been identified.

Joints

Joints are organized into three classes: **synarthroses** ("immovable" joints, such as those between the cranial bones—although even these joints aren't completely immovable), **amphiarthroses** (slightly movable joints, such as those between the bodies of the vertebrae), and **diarthroses** (freely movable joints). Of these classes of joints, the diarthrotic or synovial joints are by far the most vulnerable to injury. For this reason, it is worth a brief review of synovial joints in preparation for a discussion of what happens when they're injured.

Joint Structure

Synovial joints are constructed so that no rough surfaces ever touch, even in joints that bear an enormous amount of weight, such as the knees and ankles (Figure 3.2). Articular cartilage, made of collagen fibers densely arranged around slippery chondroitin sulfate and water, caps the ends of bones where they meet. Maintaining the smoothness of that cartilage is crucial to maintaining the health of the joint. Each synovial joint is equipped with a synovial membrane, which produces synovial fluid, creating a generally slick, eggy environment; synovial means "with egg." As long as the membrane and cartilage stay moist and slick, the joint stays healthy. It takes only a very small

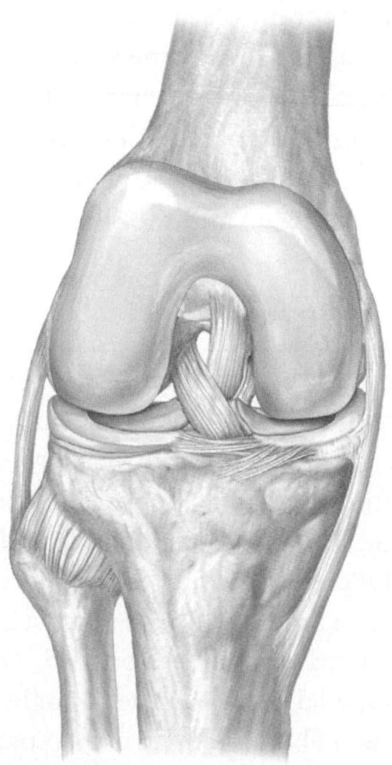

Figure 3.2. Synovial joint

amount of synovial fluid to lubricate the inside of a joint space.

Joint Function

Synovial joints help to produce movement between bones by providing the fulcrum that bones can use for leverage as the muscles pull on them in various directions.

Like most structures, joints are designed to be used regularly. Appropriate movement of the joint capsule stimulates the production of synovial fluid, which circulates through the joint space for the health of all joint components. Lack of movement results in a shortage of synovial fluid; too much movement can damage articular cartilage, or cause the bones to change shape in such a way that smooth surfaces are made rough, thus opening the door to irreversible arthritis. Other factors that can negatively impact joint health include trauma, dehydration, calcium metabolism, nutrition, and autoimmune disease.

Fascia

Until recently fascia was a profoundly understudied tissue. It was the material anatomists removed in order to see the "real" structures: muscles, tendons, ligaments, or organs. It was considered simply to be essentially packing material with little anatomical importance. But recent research into the function and form of fascia has revealed some surprising truths, and much of this information may impact our understanding of how movement and mechanical force is distributed through the body, and how pathologic changes in fascia may affect pain and mobility.

Fascial Structure

Layers of fascia have traditionally been assumed to be essentially passive sheaths made of varying combinations of collagen, elastin, and other reticular fibers. Fascia is often discussed as being superficial or deep; dense or loose. The thickness, density, and elasticity of these layers are determined by the number and type of protein fibers that are present, and in what kind of liquid, gelid, or solid matrix they are suspended. The living cells embedded in fascial sheaths were thought to only produce new protein fibers and matrix material. It turns out that those cells, now sometimes called **myofibroblasts**, actually have the capacity to slowly contract in the nature of smooth muscle cells. Mechanical force and some stress-related chemicals stimulate these contractions, leading to stiffness and rigidity in fascial sheaths. This appears to help distribute the force of muscle contraction across joints and planes to assist with movement, posture, and weight-bearing stress.

Fascial Function

The discovery of contractile cells within connective tissue sheaths changes our understanding of fascial function. Certainly it does the obvious job of separating layers of other tissues, providing lubricated gliding surfaces so that muscles can move easily, and acting as a protective covering to joints and organs. But in addition, it appears to play a role in maintaining long-term postural and movement patterns, especially in its largest form, the lumbodorsal fascia. Fascia is richly supplied with sensory nerves, including the proprioceptors that help determine posture and resting tone. The feedback loops between fascial contraction and efficient skeletal muscular contraction are still being investigated. As this new understanding of fascial function is investigated, common conditions like headaches, low back pain, iliotibial band pain, or even adhesive capsulitis may be found to be at least partly related to fascial hypertonicity and dysfunction.

For more of the author's insights into fascia, view her video at thePoint.lww.com/Werner5e

Other Connective Tissues

Other connective tissue structures are included in the musculoskeletal system and injuries to them are common. Tendons connect muscle to bone, and they are an early line of defense when a joint undergoes traumatic stress. Depending on the force of the trauma, certain ligaments may also sustain injury. The medial and lateral stabilizers outside the joint capsule and the internal stabilizers are generally damaged before the specialized capsular ligament that comprises the joint capsule itself. Bursae, the fluid-filled sacs that cushion areas where two bones might otherwise knock heads or allow tendons to slide over sharp corners, tend to get irritated with repetitive stress. The body grows new bursae anywhere it needs a little extra protection, and these new bursae can also become irritated and painful.

Connective Tissue Problems in General

Every part of the body is supported by connective tissue. It forms the fascial sheaths; it supports blood vessels and the tubes of the digestive tract. It is the framework on which bones grow. Connective tissue provides the scaffolding for the functioning cells of most organs. It gives strength and elasticity to most of the body's membranes. Indeed, connective tissue is such a large proportion of the human body that one way of evaluating a person's general health is by examining the strength, resilience, and power of the connective tissues.

Our three-dimensional connective tissue web links every part of the body to every other part. It demonstrates that, contrary to traditional thinking, the body is not made of a series of interchangeable parts. When a car has a tire that keeps going flat, the owner replaces the tire and the problem is solved. But when a person has an ankle that repeatedly sprains, a back that is so fragile that he can't pick up his child, or headaches that interfere with her day-to-day functioning, the answer isn't just in the ankle, the back, or the neck. It's in the totality of how mental and emotional states ripple into physical experience. It's

Musculoskeletal System Conditions

Muscle Disorders

- Muscular dystrophy
  - Duchenne muscular dystrophy
  - Becker muscular dystrophy
  - Myotonic muscular dystrophy
  - Other forms of muscular dystrophy
    - Facioscapulohumeral; limb-girdle; Emery-Dreifuss; oculopharyngeal
- Spasms, cramps
- Strains

Bone Disorders

- Osteosarcoma
- Osgood-Schlatter disease
- Osteoporosis
- Postural deviations
  - Hyperkyphosis
    - Scheuermann disease
  - Hyperlordosis
  - Scoliosis/rotoscoliosis

Joint Disorders

- Adhesive capsulitis
- Baker cysts
- Gout
- Joint disruptions
  - Dislocations
  - Subluxations
  - Dysplasia
- Joint replacement surgery
- Lyme disease
- Osteoarthritis
- Patellofemoral syndrome
- Spondylolisthesis
  - Congenital spondylolisthesis
  - Isthmic spondylolisthesis
  - Degenerative spondylolisthesis
  - Traumatic spondylolisthesis
- Spondylosis
- Sprains
- Temporomandibular joint dysfunction

Fascial Disorders

- Compartment syndrome
  - Acute compartment syndrome
  - Chronic compartment syndrome
- Dupuytren contracture
  - Plantar fibromatosis
  - Peyronie disease
  - Garrod nodes
- Ganglion cysts
- Hammertoe
- Hernia
  - Direct inguinal hernia
  - Indirect inguinal hernia
  - Epigastric hernia
  - Paraumbilical hernia
  - Umbilical hernia
  - Incisional hernia
  - Hiatal hernia
- Plantar fasciitis
- Pes planus; pes cavus

Neuromuscular Disorders

- Carpal tunnel syndrome
- Disc disease
  - Herniation
    - Bulge
    - Protrusion
    - Extrusion
    - Rupture
  - Degenerative disc disease
  - Internal disc disruption
- Myofascial pain syndrome
- Thoracic outlet syndrome

Other Connective Tissue Disorders

- Bunions
- Bursitis
- Shin splints
  - Medial tibial stress syndrome
  - Periostitis
  - Stress fractures
- Tendinopathies
  - Tendinitis
  - Tendinosis
  - Tenosynovitis
    - De Quervain tenosynovitis
- Whiplash

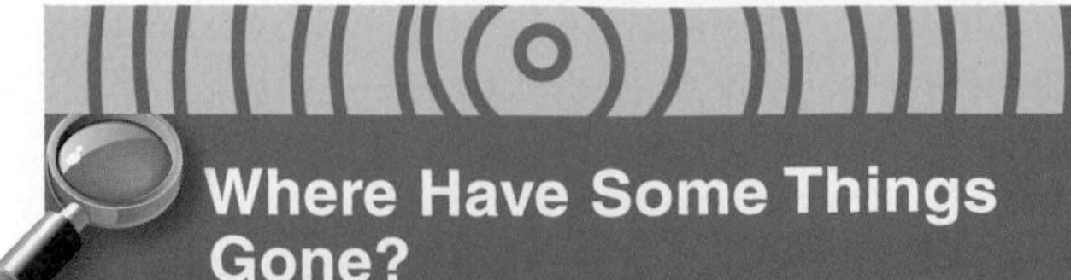

Where Have Some Things Gone?

Some items that would traditionally be discussed in Chapter 3 now appear elsewhere.

Previous editions of *A Massage Therapist's Guide to Pathology* have carried the discussion of fibromyalgia (literally, "fiber-muscle pain") as the first piece in the chapter on musculoskeletal conditions, because its symptoms are mainly **rheumatic**—that is, they involve muscle and joint pain. But the most current research on this common condition reveals that it is primarily a nervous system disorder involving heightened pain sensation, sleep disruption, and several other features concerning neuroendocrine function. Consequently, the discussion of fibromyalgia now appears in Chapter 4.

Three autoimmune conditions—ankylosing spondylitis (AS), rheumatoid arthritis, and scleroderma—now appear in Chapter 6. And several musculoskeletal conditions that have a relatively narrow application or that massage therapists are unlikely to see in an acute stage can be found in Appendix C, Extra Conditions at a Glance. These include the following:

Avascular necrosis	Myasthenia gravis
Ehlers-Danlos syndrome	Osteogenesis imperfecta
Fractures	Osteomalacia
Heterotopic ossification	Osteomyelitis
Marfan syndrome	Paget disease

in how eating habits support or don't support growth and healing. It's in whether a person gets adequate amounts of high-quality sleep. Massage therapists who specialize in helping people with musculoskeletal problems must recognize all these issues when clients have recurring, ongoing, or stubborn injuries that don't follow what is usually considered a normal healing process.

The convenient feature in musculoskeletal problems, as far as massage therapists are concerned, is that most are not related to an infectious agent. A massage therapist can't catch or distribute an epidemic of torn hamstrings. Nor do these injuries usually lead to permanent damage that massage can make worse: massage does not spread bursitis, for instance. But skillful, careful, knowledgeably applied massage administered in the appropriate stage of healing can help many musculoskeletal conditions to improve. Sometimes that improvement is just a temporary cessation of pain (which is a fine purpose in itself), but often this work can bring about the lasting changes that make structural massage an important factor in the healing process.

Muscle Disorders

Muscular Dystrophy

Definition: What is It?

Muscular dystrophy (MD) is a group of several closely related diseases characterized by genetic anomalies that lead to the degeneration and wasting away of muscle tissue. It usually begins in skeletal muscles of the extremities, but ultimately it can affect the breathing muscles and the heart.

Muscular Dystrophy in Brief

Pronunciation: MUS-kyu-lar DIS-tro-fe

What is it?
Muscular dystrophy (MD) is a group of related inherited disorders characterized by degeneration and wasting of muscle tissue.

How is it recognized?
Different varieties of MD affect different areas of skeletal muscles. The age of onset, initial symptoms, and long-term prognosis depend on what kind of genetic problem is present.

Massage risks and benefits
Risks: Patients with MD may be fragile, and any bodywork must fit within their capacity to adapt. Late stages may involve respiratory or cardiac weakness, which must be accommodated.
Benefits: Because it doesn't affect sensation, it is safe for MD patients to receive massage. Bodywork as part of a healthcare strategy may help to delay contractures and preserve function as long as possible.

The two most common varieties of MD are X-linked inherited diseases. This means the affected gene is carried by the mother, but passed on only to her sons. Other types of MD are autosomal dominant or recessive; they may affect females as often as males (see Sidebar 3.1).

Etiology: What Happens?

Normal muscles convert fat or glycogen into fuel to do their work of pulling bony attachments together. They do this with the assistance of a protein called dystrophin, which is produced in muscle cells, just under the sarcolemma. The most common versions of MD involve a genetic mutation that either prevents the production of dystrophin altogether, or allows its production only at inadequate levels. Other forms of MD involve low production of other vital proteins.

In the absence of dystrophin or other key chemicals to help convert nutrients into energy, muscle cells atrophy and die, to be replaced by fat and connective tissue. Antagonists to affected muscles have no resistance, and eventually their connective tissue shrinks, pulling bony attachments closer together in a permanent contracture.

MD may also affect the heart and breathing muscles, making patients vulnerable to cardiac and respiratory weakness.

Types of Muscular Dystrophy

- *Duchenne muscular dystrophy*. This X-linked genetic anomaly is the most common and most severe variety of the disease. Boys with this condition cannot produce any dystrophin at all.
- *Becker muscular dystrophy*. This is a less common and less severe form of MD that also affects only boys. In this version, some dystrophin is produced, but not enough for normal function.
- *Myotonic muscular dystrophy*. This is the most common form of adult-onset MD. Its primary symptom is myotonia: stiffness or spasm following muscular contraction. Myotonic MD is a progressive disorder that affects many systems. It can cause cataracts, gastrointestinal dysfunction, and heart problems.
- *Other varieties of muscular dystrophy*:
  - Congenital MD includes several rare varieties that are diagnosed at birth or in early infancy.
  - Facioscapulohumeral dystrophy primarily affects the muscles of the face, shoulder, and upper arm.
  - Limb girdle dystrophy begins in the shoulders, upper arms, and pelvic area.

SIDEBAR 3.1 What's in Your Genes?

Genes are part of the building blocks of human cells. They are arranged along pairs of chromosomes, and each parent contributes one side of the pair. Some diseases are caused by anomalies in genetic structure. While these anomalies can be inherited from one or both parents, they can also occur with no family history as spontaneous mutations. Breakthroughs in the study of molecular genetics have revealed the specific anomalies responsible for various forms of muscular dystrophy, as well as other inherited disorders such as sickle cell disease, Marfan syndrome, hemophilia, and osteogenesis imperfecta.

Inherited diseases have three variations: they can be autosomal dominant, autosomal recessive, or X-linked disorders.

- **Autosomal dominant** inheritance means that one parent has a defective gene and the other does not. Each child has a 50% chance of inheriting the defective but dominant gene, which causes the disease. Males and females are at equal risk for autosomal dominant inheritance.
- **Autosomal recessive** inheritance means that each parent carries one defective gene, but it produces no symptoms. Each child has a 25% chance of inheriting both defective genes and developing the associated disease. Alternatively, each child has a 50% chance of inheriting only one gene and becoming a carrier for the next generation.
- **X-linked** inheritance means that a woman carries a defective gene on one X chromosome. Each of her sons has a 50% chance of inheriting the faulty gene from her. Each of her daughters has a 50% chance of carrying the faulty gene to her sons. It is rare for females to be severely affected by X-linked diseases. Women who carry these genetic defects are at increased risk for developing some but not all of the characteristics of the genetic disease. Men who have X-linked mutations may pass the genes onto their daughters, who may become carriers, but no sons are directly affected.

- Emery-Dreifuss MD shows contractures of the Achilles tendon, elbow, and spine.
- Oculopharyngeal MD affects the eyes and pharynx muscles first.

Signs and Symptoms

Signs and symptoms of MD vary according to type, but the two most common varieties, Duchenne and Becker, are very similar in presentation: symptoms often begin during toddlerhood, when a little boy begins to have trouble walking or climbing stairs. He may complain of leg pain. He develops a waddling gait with an accentuated lumbar curve to compensate for the weakness in his legs. Eventually he may not put his whole foot down at all; instead, he walks on tiptoes. His calves may seem to become disproportionately large in a condition called **pseudohypertrophy**; in actuality, the muscle mass is being replaced with fat and connective tissue.

MD can progress to affect the spine, joints, the heart, and the lungs. Many patients die at a young age of cardiac or respiratory failure.

Duchenne MD is usually diagnosed between 3 and 5 years of age, and an affected child will probably be in a wheelchair by his twelfth birthday. Its progression is fairly dependable, and the best life expectancy is typically mid-20s.

Becker MD has a similar progression, but it is usually diagnosed later and has a less severe impact. The outlook may be a great deal brighter, depending on how much dystrophin individual patients may produce.

MD is occasionally but not always accompanied by mental disability. Other conditions that accompany these diseases include contractures and severe postural deviations that develop as the skeletal muscles tighten and pull on the spine and rib cage. Severe scoliosis can in turn restrict lung capacity, which raises the risk for both cardiac impairment and respiratory infection.

Treatment

Because this is a genetic disorder, no treatment to reverse or cure MD exists. Some interventions work to prolong the use of muscles and limbs, including massage and physical therapy. Surgery is sometimes recommended to release tight tendons or to straighten a distorted spine. Gene therapies are in development, but nothing so far has improved the function or outlook for MD patients.

Outside of these interventions, a child with MD is aided to be as comfortable and as functional as possible. This usually means learning to use leg braces, a standing walker, and ultimately a wheelchair.

Medications

- Corticosteroids appear to slow progression of muscle loss in Duchenne MD
- Anticonvulsants or muscle relaxants for myotonic MD
- NSAIDs for pain
- Tricyclic antidepressants for pain and depression

Massage?

RISKS A person with MD may have general fragility, in the area of muscle contractures. Advanced cases of serious forms of MD may involve heart or respiratory weakness; any bodywork must allow for this fragility. Further, the drug regimen used may alter massage choices; steroids and muscle relaxants have specific cautions for bodywork.

BENEFITS Massage and physical therapy may be recommended to preserve function, ease pain, and slow the process of contractures in muscles that are antagonistic to those weakened by the disease. Because sensation is intact with MD, massage is safe as long as systemic weaknesses are recognized and respected.

Spasms, Cramps

Definition: What is It?

A spasm or cramp is an involuntary contraction of a voluntary muscle. The difference between spasms and cramps is somewhat arbitrary; cramps are strong, painful, usually short-lived spasms. One could say that chronically tight, painful paraspinals are in spasm, while a gastrocnemius with a charley horse is a cramp. The severity of these episodes depends on how much of the muscle is involved. Spasms and cramps can be distinguished from muscle twitching or **fasciculations** by the scale of the tissues involved: twitching

Spasms, Cramps in Brief

What are they?
Spasms and cramps are involuntary contractions of skeletal muscle. Spasms are considered to be low-grade, long-lasting contractions, while cramps are short-lived, very acute contractions.

How are they recognized?
Cramps are extremely painful, with visible shortening of muscle fibers. Long-term spasms are painful and may cause inefficient movement but may not have acute symptoms.

Massage risks and benefits
Risks: Muscles in acute, painful contraction do not invite rigorous massage on the belly; this may be more irritating or even damaging than not. Some underlying pathologies may cause muscle cramping; these must be ruled out or accommodated if this is a frequent event.
Benefits: Stretching along with massage at attachment sites of contracting muscles are often effective strategies for reducing tone. Muscles that have been in involuntary contraction respond well to massage, which can reduce residual pain and improve local circulation.

is typically a painless momentary contraction of a small number of superficial muscle fibers; spasms and cramps can be painful and involve whole muscles or muscle groups.

The terms "spasms" and "cramps" are sometimes used in reference to visceral muscle too (i.e., spastic constipation), but this discussion is restricted to the involuntary contraction of skeletal, or so-called voluntary muscle.

Etiology: What Happens?

Muscles involuntarily contract for many reasons. Some of the most common situations are addressed here.

- *Nutrition.* Calcium and magnesium deficiencies, in addition to causing problems later in life, can make one prone to cramping, especially in the feet. Other important substances for efficient muscle contraction include water, glucose, and sodium. If any of these is in short supply, muscles can't work to their best potential.
- *Ischemia.* When a muscle, or part of a muscle, is suddenly or gradually deprived of oxygen, it can't function properly. Rather than becoming loose and weak, it becomes tighter and tighter. Often this is a gradual process, but sometimes it is a sudden and violent reaction to oxygen shortage.

  Anything that impedes blood flow into the affected areas can cause a local oxygen shortage, but chronic contraction is a common offender. Consider a typical tight, painful iliocostalis, one of the paraspinal muscles that holds the back erect. Here is a muscle that is typically chronically overworked. The fibers are shortened and thickened with the effort of keeping the spine upright, and this makes it harder for the supplying capillaries to deliver oxygen. Consequently, the iliocostalis draws up even tighter. This further inhibits the influx of oxygen, starting a vicious circle of ischemia causing spasm, causing pain, which leads to spasm, and so on. Furthermore, muscles that are forced to work without oxygen accumulate the chemical byproducts of anaerobic combustion, which may inhibit efficiency and increase pain and irritation. The whole picture is complicated by the fact that as postural habits develop, the brain comes to interpret these sensations as being normal. Proprioceptors eventually reinforce the patterns that cause the problem. This situation can persist without any real relief until the circle of ischemia-spasm-pain is interrupted (Figure 3.3).

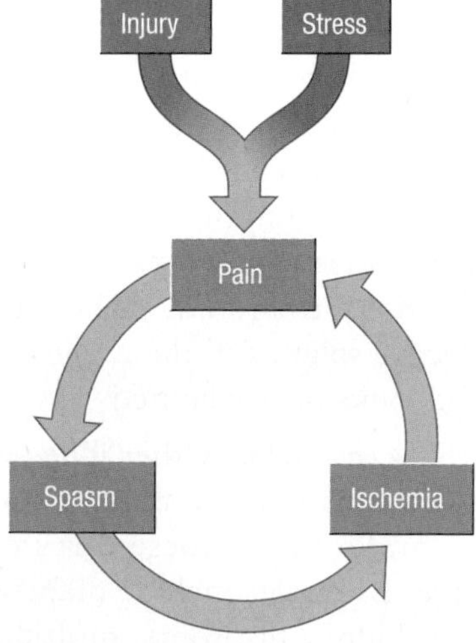

Figure 3.3. Pain-spasm-ischemia cycle

3 Musculoskeletal System Conditions

Pregnancy can be another cause of ischemic cramping. As the fetus lies on the femoral artery (just where it splits off from the abdominal branch), it can interfere with blood flow into the leg, prompting a violent contraction of the calf muscles. This is a classic example of an acute cramp, or charley horse. Other kinds of circulatory interruptions or nervous system problems can cause cramps too, so in a decision about whether massage is appropriate, it's important that no unrecognized pathology is creating an oxygen deficiency.

- *Exercise-associated muscle cramping*. Athletes often report problems with muscles cramping at or near the end of vigorous work. Dehydration, electrolyte imbalance, and hyperthermia may all be contributing factors, but these cramps may be primarily due to a neurological abnormality that overexcites muscle spindles (the proprioceptors involved in tightening) while inhibiting the activity of **Golgi tendon organs** (the proprioceptors that allow muscles to let go). The target muscles usually cross two joints, and they cramp when they are contracted from a shortened position. Stretching the muscles and manipulating the tendons limit these cramps, but they tend to recur if the athlete is inadequately warmed up or stretched out before beginning to exercise.
- *Splinting*. This is a reflexive reaction against injury. Consider an acute whiplash: the supraspinous and intertransverse ligaments have been severely wrenched, and the body senses a potentially dangerous instability in the cervical spine. The postural neck muscles contract in response; as far as they're concerned, they are keeping the head from falling off. This kind of spasm is an important protective mechanism, because it prevents movements that could cause further injury. The muscles create an effective splint, and the range of motion of affected joints is very limited.
- *Underlying conditions*. Other illnesses or conditions can contribute to muscle cramping and spasm, and some of these carry cautions for massage. Examples include diabetes mellitus, anemia, kidney disorders, multiple sclerosis, peripheral neuropathy, dystonia, or local nerve compression.

Treatment

Massage is a much-used strategy to manage long-term, low-grade muscle spasms. Muscle cramps and spasm may also be treated with heat or ice, or local applications of ointments that create hot and cold sensations to alter local blood flow. Ongoing mild but painful situations may be treated with analgesics, but muscle relaxants are usually reserved for very extreme situations.

Medications

- Analgesics for pain management
- Muscle relaxants for severe spasm, often in conjunction with trauma

Massage?

RISKS Muscles that are chronically tight or cramping may not respond well to direct and aggressive bodywork delivered to the muscle bellies.

Underlying conditions or pathologies that contribute to involuntary contractions must be addressed if cramping is a frequent occurrence.

A client taking painkillers or muscle relaxants for muscle spasm will not be able to give accurate feedback to the massage therapist about pain or stretching limitations.

When muscles are splinting a new injury, it is important to respect this protective mechanism until the acute stage has passed.

BENEFITS Cramping muscles can respond well to bodywork that is not at the muscle belly, and muscles that have been in spasm or cramp benefit from the circulatory turnover that massage can provide.

When a spasm that splints an injured area has outlived its usefulness, massage can help to reestablish efficient movement, but this is best done incrementally to avoid the risk of reinjury.

OPTIONS Acute muscle cramps can often be relieved through stretching and massage to their attachment sites. After the cramp releases and pain is resolved, rigorous massage is safe and useful for local circulatory turnover.

Strains

Definition: What Are They?

Strains are injuries to muscle fibers involving the tearing of myofibers and production of scar tissue. They

Strains in Brief

What are they?
Strains are injuries to muscles involving torn fibers.

How are they recognized?
Pain, stiffness, and occasionally palpable heat and swelling are all signs of muscle strain. Pain may be exacerbated by passive stretching or resisted contraction of the affected muscle.

Massage risks and benefits
Risks: Rigorous massage to an acute muscle injury may exacerbate inflammation and tissue damage.
Benefits: Massage after the acute stage of inflammation has passed can powerfully influence the production of useful scar tissue, reduce adhesions and edema, and reestablish range of motion.

are sometimes difficult to distinguish from tendon injuries, which are discussed in the section on tendinopathies later in the chapter.

Etiology: What Happens?

Muscle strains and other soft tissue injuries may arise from specific trauma, but they often develop in the context of chronic, cumulative overuse patterns with no specific onset.

When a muscle is injured, myofibers are torn, the inflammatory process begins, and fibroblasts flood the area with collagen to knit the injury back together. The accumulation of scar tissue within contractile tissue is a normal process, but it has some potentially important implications:

- *Impaired contractility*. Scar tissue can impede the efficiency of uninjured muscle fibers. When the muscle cells try to contract, they bear the weight not only of their bony attachments but also of the fibers that are disabled by the mass of collagen that binds them up. This increases the load on uninjured fibers and raises the chance of repeated injury, more scar tissue, and further weakening of the muscle.
- *Adhesions*. Collagen that is manufactured around an injury isn't laid down in perfect alignment with the muscle fibers; instead, it is deposited quickly but in haphazard form. Randomly arranged collagen fibers tend to bind up different layers of tissue that are designed to be separate: these are adhesions. Adhesions can occur wherever layers of connective tissue come in contact with each other. They may occur within the muscle, as is frequently seen with the paraspinals, or between muscles, when muscle sheaths stick to other muscle sheaths. Hamstrings are a common place for this phenomenon. Wherever they occur, adhesions limit mobility and increase the chance of injury (Figure 3.4).

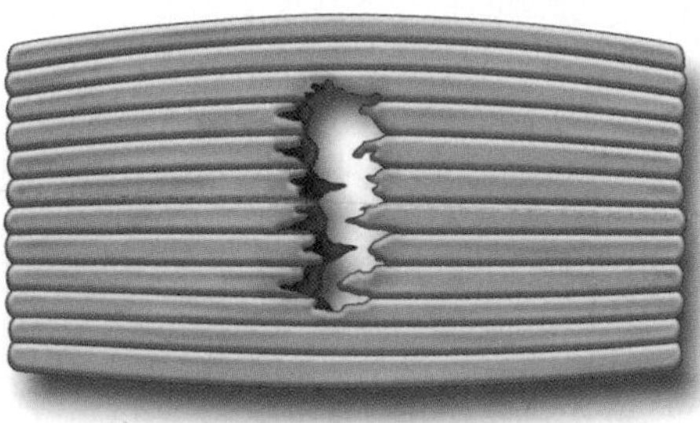

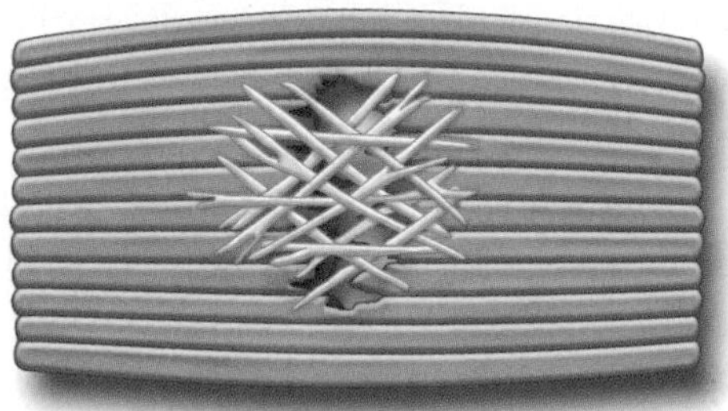

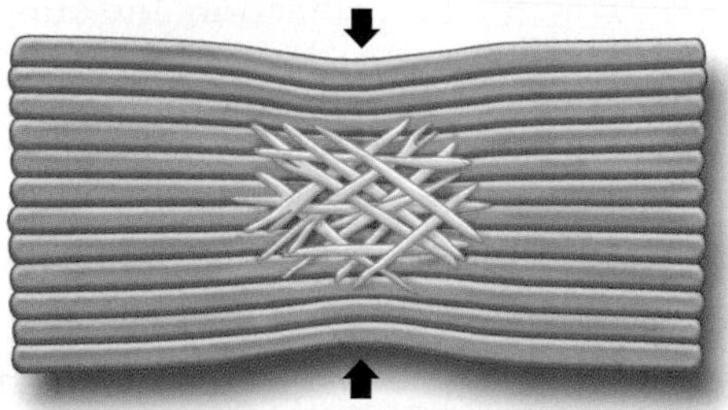

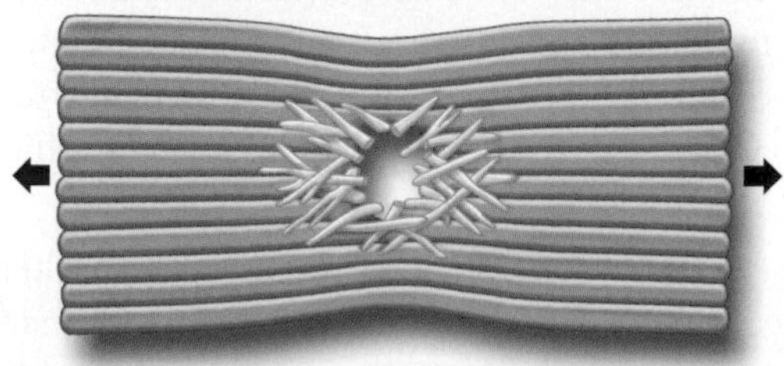

Figure 3.4. Strains and sprains: the injury-reinjury cycle

Signs and Symptoms

Symptoms of muscle strain include mild or intense local pain, stiffness, and pain on resisted movement or passive stretching. Unless it is a very bad tear, no palpable heat or swelling is usually present.

Strains are graded by severity. First-degree strains are mildly painful but don't seriously impede function, while third-degree strains involve ruptured muscles and possibly the avulsion of bony attachment sites.

Treatment

It is now generally recognized that early intervention in the healing process for injured muscles significantly improves the prognosis for full recovery. Although individual specialists approach musculoskeletal injuries with different tactics, several of their priorities are predictable:

- *Get an accurate diagnosis.* Evaluating muscular injuries requires a thorough patient history and a skilled clinical examination. Other diagnostic procedures (e.g., radiographs, bone scans, CT, and MRI) may be recommended as well.
- *Control inflammation.* Inflammation is a valuable process, but it can outlive its usefulness and end up causing more harm than good. Inflammation can often be controlled by RICE (rest, ice, compression, elevation), but some physicians now use the PRICES protocol, which adds protection and support to the list.
- *Rehabilitate damaged tissues.* This part of the treatment involves exercises that add incremental amounts of weight-bearing stress to the injured muscle to help the scar tissue realign with the original fibers and to gradually increase strength and fitness. This may be the most vulnerable time in the process, as athletes who are eager to resume training may try to go too fast and get injured again, and others may neglect the need to exercise and allow scar tissue to accumulate to inefficient levels.
- *Prevent further injury.* Most chronic muscle injuries are related to controllable factors that can be adjusted to help prevent future problems. These include dealing with muscle imbalances that make one area weaker while another may be tighter, improving technique in specific sports, making sure that equipment is appropriate and in good repair, adjusting training schedules so that changes are incorporated slowly, taping or bracing vulnerable areas, and being careful about good warm-up and cool-down procedures.

Medications

- NSAIDs for pain and inflammation

Massage?

RISKS Vigorous deep massage to a new or acute injury may exacerbate inflammation and tissue damage.

BENEFITS Carefully performed massage at the appropriate stage of healing can be an important contributor to the recovery from a simple muscle injury, turning a potentially painful and long-lasting injury into a relatively trivial event with a successful outcome.

OPTIONS In acute strains, lymphatic drainage or other work to limit edema is appropriate. Later, crossfiber and linear friction along with passive stretching and carefully calibrated exercises can help the new scar tissue to align in the best possible formation for efficient contractions and range of motion.

Bone Disorders

Osteosarcoma

Definition: What is It?

Osteosarcoma is a relatively rare form of cancer that originates in bone tissue. It is most common in adolescents and young adults. This distinguishes it from metastatic carcinoma, which is the development of secondary tumors in bone tissue: these usually arise from cancer of the breast, prostate, or lung and are usually found in people aged 50 years and older.

Osteosarcoma in Brief

What is it?
Osteosarcoma is a type of cancer that originates in bone tissue.

How is it recognized?
Osteosarcoma is often silent until damage is extensive. Deep aching pain with activity is the key sign, along with palpable enlargement of the affected bone or bones.

Massage risks and benefits
Risks: Because the earliest signs of osteosarcoma mimic orthopedic injury, it is possible that a person could delay an important diagnosis by pursuing bodywork instead of medical treatment. The threat of damaged bones with the possibility of fractures is another risk for these clients.
Benefits: Massage has many benefits for clients undergoing cancer treatment, including reducing stress, improving sleep, and mitigating some of the side effects of treatment. This should always be done as part of a healthcare team.

A client who has fully recovered from osteosarcoma can enjoy the same benefits from massage and bodywork as the rest of the population.

Etiology: What Happens?

Cancer is the development of cells that replicate in a hyperactive and disorganized way. It most commonly affects cells that naturally grow fast, which is why epithelial cancers are more common than any other kind. Bone cancer, or osteosarcoma, is relatively rare because bone tends not to grow quickly—except in children and young adults: these are the people most vulnerable to osteosarcoma.

It is important to differentiate between osteosarcoma and metastatic carcinoma. Osteosarcoma begins in bone cells, whereas metastatic carcinoma is the result of cancer that begins elsewhere (see Sidebar 3.2).

Osteosarcoma has three main subtypes: osteoblastic, chondroblastic, and fibroblastic. These refer to the originating cells. It typically grows as one major tumor at a time, and it is most commonly found near the growth plates of the long bones: the femur, the proximal tibia, and the proximal humerus are the most common locations (Figure 3.5). Tumors can originate in either trabecular or cortical bone tissue. Left untreated this cancer can destroy the bone and metastasize to other tissues: the lungs are the most frequent site.

No specific risk factors have been identified for osteosarcoma, other than childhood exposure to radiation and genetic predisposition.

SIDEBAR 3.2 Staging Metastatic Carcinoma

Metastatic carcinoma is a term to describe the development of cancerous tumors that have migrated and colonized new tissues: the original tumor is somewhere else. Bone tissue is a frequent site of metastatic carcinoma, but this is not bone cancer: it is breast, liver, or lung cancer that has metastasized to the bone. Metastatic carcinoma of the bone is far more common than bone cancer, and it is usually seen in mature patients, while bone cancer usually affects adolescents and young adults.

Until fairly recently osteosarcoma had no formal staging system, so treatment strategies were haphazard at best. In 1980, a staging system was developed that is now the standard. It is known as the Enneking system, or the Musculoskeletal Tumor Society system. In this system, tumors are graded by the aggressiveness of their cells, and also by whether the growths are contained within a compartment or not. In this situation, "compartment" means within the boundaries of a bone, an intra-articular space, or a fascially enclosed space.

Stage	Grade	Compartment status
I-A	Low-grade tumor	Intracompartmental
I-B	Low-grade tumor	Extracompartmental
II-A	High-grade tumor	Intracompartmental
II-B	High-grade tumor	Extracompartmental
III-A	Any signs of metastasis	Intracompartmental
III-B	Any signs of metastasis	Extracompartmental

Signs and Symptoms

Like many types of cancer, osteosarcoma tends to be silent until it is well established. The earliest symptoms include pain with activity, which progresses to pain at rest. Because this usually

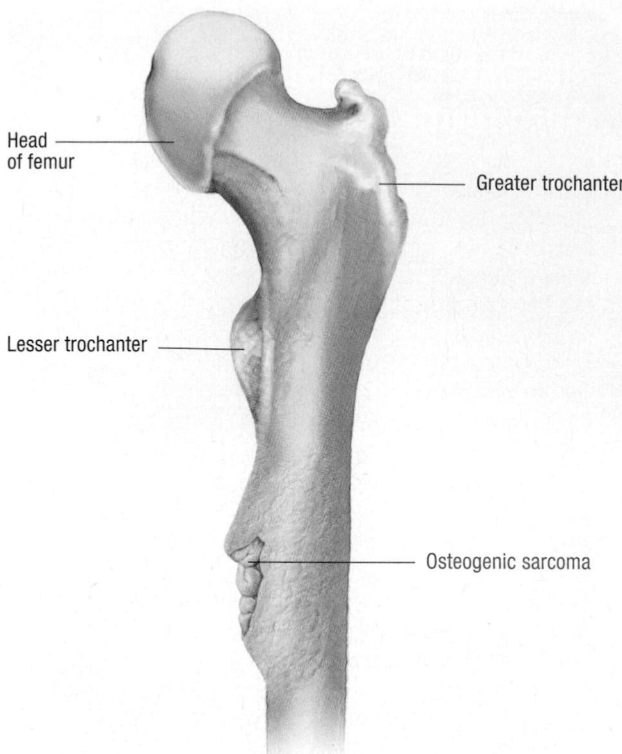

Figure 3.5. Osteosarcoma

happens in an adolescent or young adult, it is easy to mistake these warning signs for growing pains or soft tissue injuries. A palpable mass develops on the affected bone, and left untreated, respiratory symptoms eventually indicate metastasis to the lungs.

Treatment

Osteosarcoma is typically treated with orthopedic surgery to biopsy the growth, to remove it with clean margins, and to support the remaining bone, sparing the limb if possible. Because the vast majority of osteosarcoma patients experience a relapse without further treatment, chemotherapy is a standard follow-up strategy.

Medications

- Chemotherapeutic drugs to minimize the risk of further cancer development
- Drugs to help manage the symptoms of chemotherapy

Massage?

RISKS The symptoms of osteosarcoma can look like growing pains or simple soft tissue injury. This may lead patients to seek massage rather than medical treatment, which can delay an important diagnosis. Once the cancer has been identified, care must be taken around the damaged bone, because fractures are a possibility. And of course any massage or bodywork strategy must accommodate for the challenges of cancer treatment which in this situation involves surgery and chemotherapy at least.

BENEFITS Massage offers many benefits to cancer patients, including improving mood, lessening anxiety and depression, promoting good quality sleep, and decreasing the negative side effects of cancer treatments. All this must be done in coordination with the rest of the healthcare team, of course.

A client who has fully recovered from osteosarcoma can enjoy the same benefits of bodywork as the rest of the population.

Osgood-Schlatter Disease

Definition: What is It?

Osgood-Schlatter disease (OSD) is irritation and inflammation at the site of the quadriceps attachment on the tibia. It can also be called tibial tuberosity apophysitis. It occurs when the quadriceps muscles are vigorously used in combination with rapid growth of the leg bones, typically during an adolescent growth spurt in athletic children.

Etiology: What Happens?

When children enter their teens, they begin a time of rapid bone growth, especially in their femurs and tibias: the bones that determine how tall they will be. The quadriceps group attaches at the tibial tuberosity, a bony landmark that doesn't fully calcify until late in adolescence. This structural weak spot is vulnerable to constant, repeated forceful contractions of the quadriceps that can lead to inflammation and injury.

With acute inflammation of the quadriceps attachment, the tendon can pull away from the bone, causing multiple tiny fractures and enlargement of the

Osgood-Schlatter Disease in Brief

Pronunciation: OZ-good SHLAH-ter dih-ZEZE

What is it?
Osgood-Schlatter disease (OSD) is the result of chronic or traumatic irritation at the insertion of the quadriceps tendon in combination with adolescent growth spurts.

How is it recognized?
When OSD is acute, the tibial tuberosity is hot, swollen, and painful. The tibia may grow a large permanent protuberance at the site of the quadriceps attachment.

Massage risks and benefits
Risks: An acute flare-up of OSD locally contraindicates circulatory massage, which could exacerbate pain and inflammation.
Benefits: Techniques for reducing lymphatic congestion and work elsewhere on the body are certainly appropriate. A client with a history of OSD but no current inflammation at the knee may benefit from the pain relief and balance in quadriceps muscle tone that massage can supply.

tibial tuberosity. In extreme cases, an **avulsion** can form: this is a separation of a part of the bone. It is common for OSD patients to develop a large, permanent bump at the tibial tuberosity; this is where the bone adapts to the constant pull of the quadriceps insertion. OSD is usually unilateral, but some athletes develop inflammation at both knees.

The severity of OSD varies greatly from one person to the next; one person may have to be careful warming up before playing soccer, while another athlete may have to quit the team altogether. It is generally a self-limiting condition, which means that when the connective tissue growth catches up with the bone growth, the pain and irritation subside even though a bone spur remains. Most cases subside when the tibia fully ossifies, late in adolescence.

Signs and Symptoms

OSD is easy to identify because the people susceptible to it are such a well-defined group: athletic teens. In acute stages of OSD, the knee is hot, swollen, and painful just distal to the patella at the tibial tuberosity. Any activity that stresses or stretches the quadriceps aggravates symptoms.

When OSD is not acute, pain and inflammation are resolved, but the characteristic bump of the remodeled tibia may be permanent (Figure 3.6). A person who had OSD as a child may never be comfortable kneeling because of tibial distortion.

Treatment

Treatment for OSD focuses on reducing pain and limiting damage to the tibia. Mild cases can be managed by carefully warming up and stretching the quadriceps and hamstrings before exercise, and icing them afterward. Nonsteroidal anti-inflammatories may be suggested to help with pain and inflammation. A strap worn below the patella may ease pain during play, and kneepads can help if activities require kneeling.

Severe cases may require that the athlete suspend activity until the pain and inflammation have been gone for several weeks. In the meantime, the knee may be supported with a brace or cast. This period is followed by rehabilitative exercise to strengthen the muscles and reduce the chance of a recurrence when the athlete becomes active again.

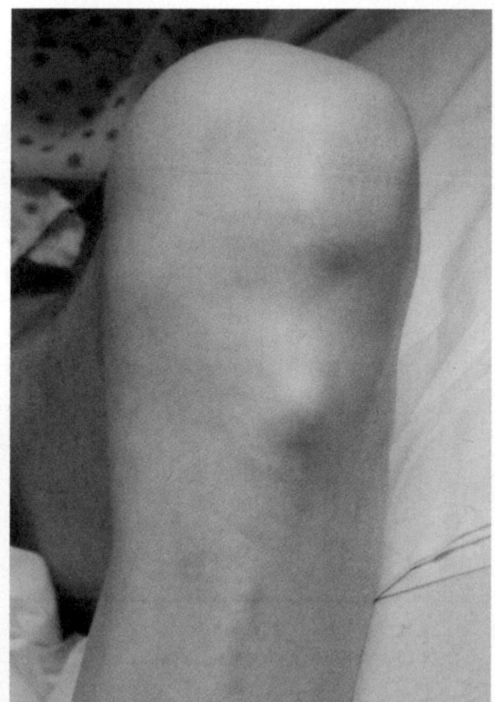

Figure 3.6. OSD: a non-tender enlargement of the tibial tuberosity

In rare cases, the knee may need surgery to remove bits of the tibia that were pulled off and suspended in the tibial tendon.

Medications

- NSAIDs for pain and inflammation

Massage?

RISKS Some types of massage may exacerbate pain and inflammation during acute flares of OSD.

BENEFITS Lymphatic work may help resolve acute inflammation. In nonflared cases, massage may ease pain, improve flexibility, and reduce tension in the quadriceps.

Osteoporosis

Definition: What is It?

Osteoporosis literally means "porous bones." In this condition, calcium is pulled off the bones faster than it is replaced, leaving them thin, brittle, and prone to injury. It affects about 10 million Americans, but many more may have a preosteoporotic condition called **osteopenia**. Women with osteoporosis significantly outnumber men, for a variety of reasons. This condition is usually diagnosed in people over 60, but it is closely tied to events, habits, and activities of earlier years.

> **Osteoporosis in Brief**
>
> Pronunciation: os-te-o-por-O-sis
>
> **What is it?**
> Osteoporosis is loss of bone mass and density brought about by endocrine imbalances, poor metabolism of calcium, nutritional, and other influences.
>
> **How is it recognized?**
> Osteoporosis in the early stages is virtually silent. In later stages, compression or spontaneous fractures of the vertebrae, ribs, wrists, or hips may occur. Hyperkyphosis brought about by compression fractures of the thoracic vertebrae is a frequent indicator of osteoporosis.
>
> **Massage risks and benefits**
> ***Risks:*** Acute fractures or risk of fracture contraindicates rigorous massage.
> ***Benefits:*** Massage is unlikely to change the course of osteoporosis, but done carefully it can ease pain and improve the quality of life for people who live with this common and painful condition.

Etiology: What Happens?

Bones are composed of hard mineral deposits (mostly calcium phosphate) formed on a scaffolding of collagen fibers. The volume of mineral deposits determines bone density. People normally accumulate most of their bone density by about age 20, but small gains are made until around age 30 to 35. After that point, density is either maintained at a stable level or withdrawals are made from this "calcium bank." The turnover of mineral deposits happens constantly, but this activity occurs in trabecular bone at a higher rate than in cortical bone. Osteoporosis develops when calcium is withdrawn from bone tissue faster than it is deposited.

Risk factors for osteoporosis are typically described as controllable or noncontrollable. Noncontrollable factors include gender (women are more at risk because of childbearing and breastfeeding, as well as having smaller bones to begin with), age, body size (smaller people are more at risk than larger ones), ethnicity (whites and Asians have this more often than other races), and family history. Controllable factors include hormone levels, a history of anorexia, levels of calcium and vitamin D, medications, sedentary lifestyle, diet, and cigarette and alcohol use.

Logically, high calcium consumption should lead to high bone density, and high bone density should be linked to a low risk of osteoporosis and bone fractures. However, many factors beyond calcium consumption influence bone health, including the accessibility of other vitamins and minerals, exercise habits, pH balance in the blood (especially as it is influenced by meat-based proteins), other diseases, medications, and even emotional state. The factors that help to determine a person's risk for osteoporosis boil down to issues around calcium absorption, calcium loss, and bone density maintenance.

- *Calcium absorption.* Calcium requires an acidic environment in the stomach to be absorbed into the bloodstream. If calcium enters the body in a form that impedes its contact with hydrochloric acid (for instance, in dairy products), the body has only limited access to this mineral. Similarly, if natural secretions of hydrochloric acid are reduced, as in older adults, it becomes harder to absorb whatever calcium is consumed.

Some vitamins influence how the body uses calcium. Vitamin D controls absorption and retention of this important mineral. The body synthesizes vitamin D in response to direct sunlight (it takes about 15 minutes of exposure per day, depending on latitude), but vitamin D can also be easily supplemented. Vitamin K, found in many dark, leafy greens, also supports calcium absorption. Preformed vitamin A, however, can increase the risk of fractures if it is consumed in high quantities.

- *Calcium loss*. Calcium is constantly lost in sweat and urine. Some substances, specifically meat-based proteins, cause higher levels of calcium to be excreted in urine. So a person who takes in ample amounts of dietary calcium but who also eats a lot of meat tends to lose a lot of calcium.

  Several other factors can lead to calcium loss. High caffeine consumption (more than three or four cups of coffee or servings of caffeinated soda per day) has been seen to have a negative impact. Other factors include medications (chemotherapeutic agents, corticosteroids, some diuretics, anticonvulsant drugs); hyperthyroidism; heavy alcohol use; smoking; inflammatory bowel disease (Crohn disease, ulcerative colitis); a history of eating disorders; and endocrine disorders, including Cushing syndrome, low testosterone, and low estrogen.
- *Bone density maintenance*. The shape and density of bones are determined by the activity of osteoclasts and osteoblasts. These cells work to remodel bones according to the commands of calcitonin, parathyroid hormone, estrogen, and progesterone. If hormones tell the osteoclasts to work faster than the osteoblasts, bone density declines. Bone cells are most active in **trabecular** bone, which is found in **epiphyses** of long bones and vertebral bodies. The loss of key struts of calcium deposits in these areas can cause bones to collapse.

  Bones are not the only part of the body that needs calcium. Calcium is consumed in nearly every chemical reaction that results in muscle contraction and nerve transmission, and it is essential to blood clotting and nerve transmission. It also works as a buffer to help maintain the proper pH balance. The body has a strict prioritizing system for these important functions: chemical reactions that promote moment-to-moment survival are more important than maintaining the density of the vertebrae or femoral neck.

NOTABLE CASES Many celebrities have shared their osteoporosis experiences with the public, including actress Sally Field and comedienne Joan Rivers. Several influential men have had this condition as well, including Pope John Paul II, Winston Churchill, Clarence Darrow, and very possibly Benjamin Franklin.

When a person develops osteoporosis, it is usually because the balancing act between calcium absorption, calcium loss, and bone density maintenance is upset, and the calcium stored in the bones is pulled off faster than it is replaced. The bones, especially in the spine and femur, become progressively less dense, leaving the person vulnerable to the primary

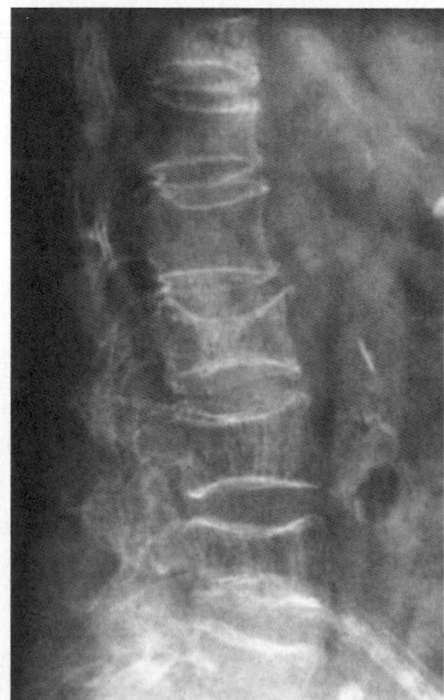

Figure 3.7. Demonstrable bone loss at vertebral bodies with osteoporosis

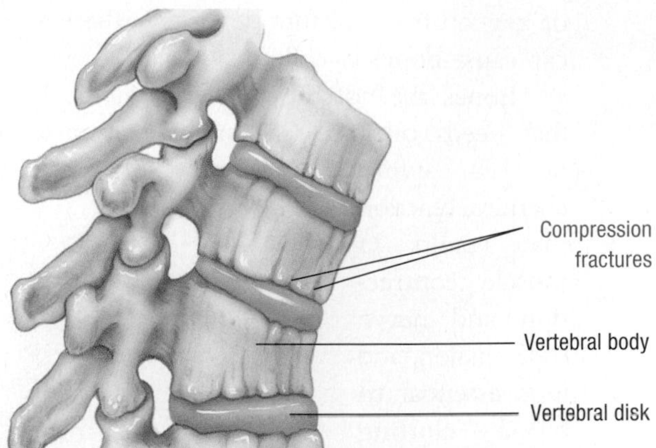

Figure 3.8. Vertebral bodies with compression fractures

complications of this disease: spinal or hip fractures (Figures 3.7 to 3.9).

Signs and Symptoms

Osteoporosis has no symptoms in its early stages. People who are at particularly high risk may undergo testing to try to identify it early, but it is often missed until complications, specifically fractures, develop.

Symptoms of osteoporosis center on pathologically weak bones. Thinned or collapsed vertebrae lead to a loss of height and the characteristic rounded "widow's hump" of hyperkyphosis. Chronic or acute back pain appears in this stage as the vertebrae continue to degenerate.

Complications

People with osteoporosis are prone to fractures with little or no cause; these are called spontaneous or pathological fractures. Hips (usually the femoral neck rather than the ilium), vertebrae, and wrists are particularly vulnerable to breakage. Brittle ribs are often associated with corticosteroid use. And since in advanced age, people are naturally low on both living **osteocytes** and growth hormone to support the healing process, it is difficult to recover from any injury of this severity. Most people who break a hip never return to prefracture levels of activity.

Treatment

Once osteoporosis has been recognized, a number of treatment options are available to keep it from getting worse. Pharmaceutical interventions include hormone replacement therapy to influence estrogen or calcitonin, **bisphosphonates, SERMs** (selective estrogen receptor modules), and some others. None of these interventions is harmless, however, and osteoporosis patients must weigh risks and benefits of these medications carefully.

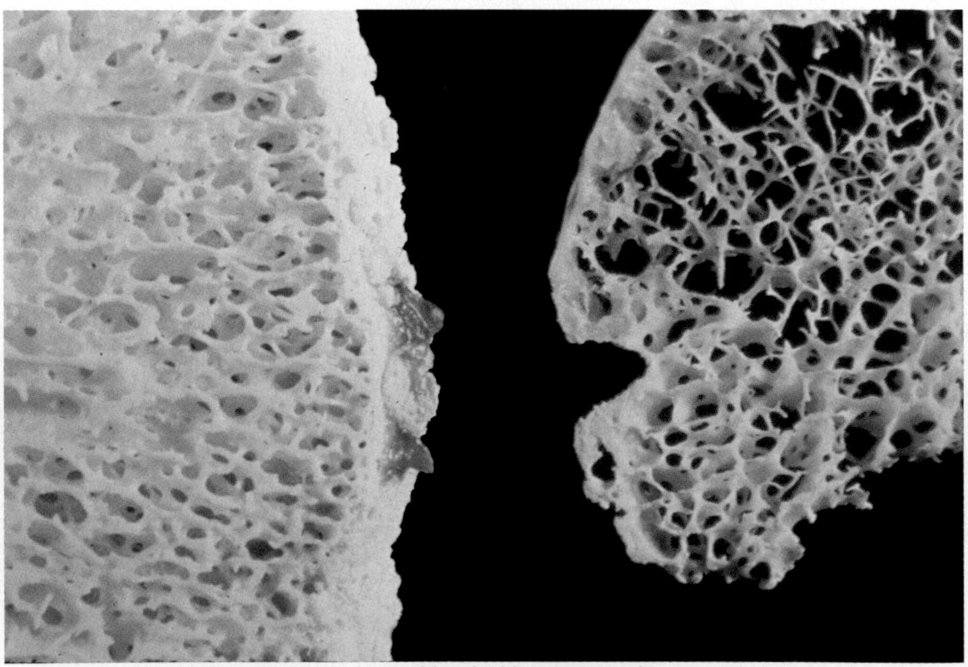
Figure 3.9. Loss of bone density in femoral head with osteoporosis

Exercise is almost always a part of the osteoporosis treatment strategy. Since bone remodels according to the stresses placed on it, weight-bearing stress ensures that maintaining healthy mass is a high priority. Diet also plays an important part in dealing with osteoporosis. Specific vitamins and other substances may improve calcium uptake, even for postmenopausal women, but that subject is outside the scope of this book.

Medications

- Vitamin and mineral supplements, including calcium, vitamin D, and others
- Hormone replacement therapy (including calcitonin) for slowed bone loss
- SERMs for slowed bone loss
- Bisphosphonates for slowed bone loss
- Parathyroid hormone for accelerated bone growth
- **RANK ligand inhibitors** to interfere with osteoclast formation

Prevention

It is possible to prevent osteoporosis, feasible to slow it down or halt it, but difficult to reverse it. The causes of this disease are many and varied, but they center on one main theme: the time to build up calcium reserves is in youth and early adulthood. The skeleton grows in height until about age 20, but it continues to accumulate density until about age 30. After that point, it either stays stable or progressively demineralizes. Four main steps have been recommended to achieve and maintain optimal bone density and avoid osteoporosis:

- *Get dietary calcium from absorbable sources.* Dairy products are abundant and convenient, but not the most efficient source for all people. Other recommended calcium sources include beans and greens: legumes and most green leafy vegetables. (Spinach and chard, while rich in calcium and other nutrients, also have substances that limit calcium absorption.) Calcium supplements vary in absorbability; calcium carbonate, calcium phosphate, and calcium citrate are generally recognized to have good accessibility.
- *Exercise.* Weight-bearing stress makes it necessary for the body to maintain healthy bone density.
- *Get vitamin D.* The RDA for vitamin D is 200 units, or 5 μg/day. This can be ingested in supplement form or naturally synthesized by exposure to sunlight.
- *Avoid substances and behaviors that pull calcium off bones.* These include excessive salt, animal-based proteins, caffeine, alcohol, and tobacco exposure.

Massage?

RISKS The primary risk for a person with osteoporosis who receives massage is that a fracture may occur because of undue pressure or problematic positioning on the table. It is important also to remember that elderly clients are unlikely to have only one pathology: this is a population that may have several problems in addition to osteoporosis that may influence bodywork choices.

BENEFITS Massage won't reverse osteoporosis, but it can be a powerful modality to help with pain and limited movement. Any work that respects a client's fragility while working for pain relief is welcome.

OPTIONS Clients with osteoporosis may need imaginative bolstering to create a setting in which it is safe to receive massage. Pillows, bolsters, rolled up towels, or other tools may be needed to firmly "nest" them into the table for maximum comfort.

Postural Deviations

Definition: What Are They?

Although it is tempting to think about the spine like a ship's mast, a column, or a tent pole held erect by muscular tension, it is actually much stronger than any of those. The curves in the cervical, thoracic, and lumbar regions give the spine many times the resistance it would have if it were straight. Sometimes these natural curves are overdeveloped though, which reduces resiliency and strength rather than enhancing it. Hyperkyphosis (humpback),

Postural Deviations in Brief

What are they?
Postural deviations are overdeveloped thoracic or lumbar curves (hyperkyphosis and hyperlordosis, respectively), or a lateral curve, possibly with a twist, in the spine (scoliosis, rotoscoliosis).

How are they recognized?
Extreme curvatures are easily visible, although radiography is used to pinpoint exactly where the problems begin and end.

Massage risks and benefits

Risks: Extreme postural deviations are sometimes connected to serious underlying diseases that influence the growth patterns of bone and soft tissues. Severe compression of the rib cage may lead to respiratory or cardiac impairment, along with a risk of pneumonia and rib fragility.

Benefits: As long as underlying factors are addressed and bodywork is well tolerated, massage may have a powerfully positive effect on postural deviations, helping to balance soft tissue stress and improve alignment, efficiency of posture, and ease of movement.

hyperlordosis (swayback), and scoliosis (S, C, or reverse-C curve) and rotoscoliosis (scoliosis with a twist) are the specific postural deviations addressed here (Figure 3.10).

Etiology: What Happens?

Postural deviations occur when the spine's normal curvature is overexaggerated, or moves out of normal planes. Mild forms may not cause any visible signs or impairment in function, but more severe cases can interfere with pain-free posture, movement, and overall function.

The causes of most postural deviations are not fully understood, so the term "**idiopathic**" is often applied. As researchers continue to explore this problem, we may find that some situations are tied to several factors, including bone density, environmental exposures, genetic predisposition, and other postural compensations, especially at the cranium and sacrum.

Postural deviations may be discussed as functional or structural problems. In the early stages, it may be that soft tissues pull the spine out of alignment: a functional problem. Functional deviations

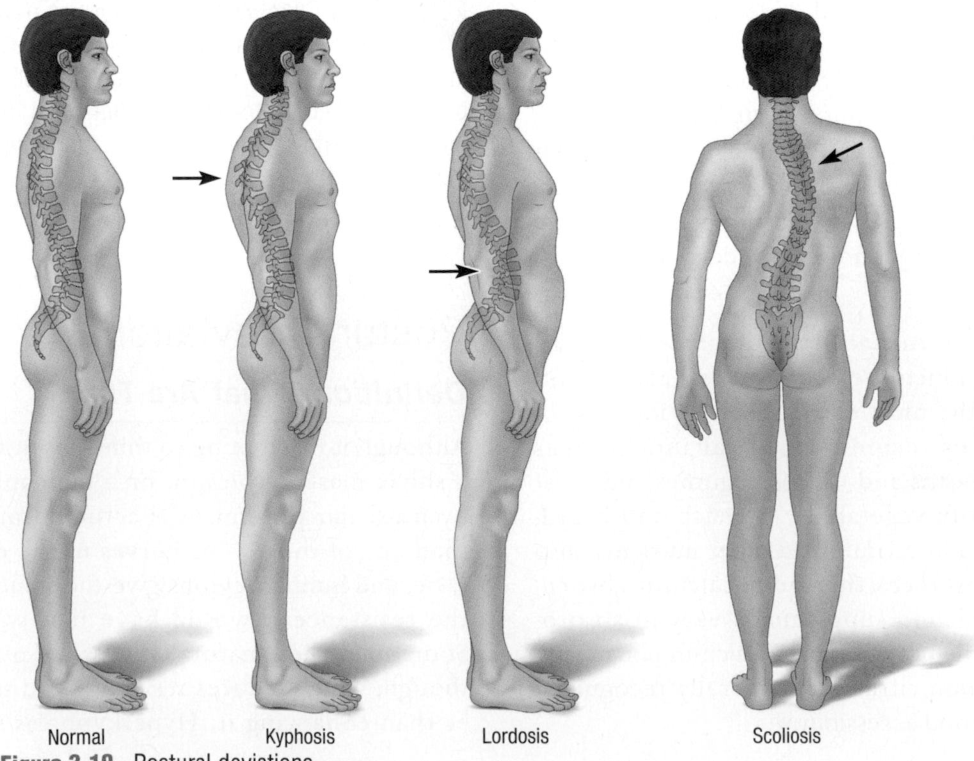

Figure 3.10. Postural deviations

are often identified if observable curves disappear or are significantly reduced when the patient goes into trunk flexion or side flexion. The condition is most treatable at this point: muscles, tendons, and ligaments can be exercised, stretched, and manipulated into new holding and movement patterns.

Functional deviations can also be brought about by problems elsewhere in the body: unequal leg length, for instance, or a sacrum that isn't level. These are correctable, but if the soft tissues are left untreated and the bones are constantly pulled in one direction or another, they eventually change shape to adapt to those stressors. Vertebral bodies and discs adopt a wedge shape, and the facet joints may become distorted. At this point, the condition becomes a structural deviation, which is much harder to reverse. And some structural deviations are related to underlying conditions that affect how bones grow. These create soft tissue pain and dysfunction, but they are not caused by it.

Most cases of postural deviations are idiopathic, that is, of unknown origin. However, a small percentage of structural problems in the spine can be related to congenital or neuromuscular problems such as cerebral palsy, polio, muscular dystrophy, osteogenesis imperfecta, or spina bifida.

Types of Postural Deviations

- **Hyperkyphosis.** Hyperkyphosis is an overdeveloped thoracic curve. In young people, it is very often a result of muscular imbalance. In older people, it may be due to muscular imbalance, but it can also be a complication of osteoporosis or ankylosing spondylitis. A kyphotic curve of 20 to 40 degrees is considered normal. Surgical intervention isn't usually suggested for anything under a 75-degree curvature.
    - **Scheuermann disease.** This is a type of hyperkyphosis that mostly affects young men. It involves uneven growth of the vertebrae, and can create an extreme "hunchback" appearance. It is corrected with bracing, physical therapy, or surgery.
- **Hyperlordosis.** Hyperlordosis is an overdeveloped lumbar curve. The architecture and musculature of the low back makes it particularly vulnerable to this kind of imbalance. Hyperlordosis can often be much improved by exercise and physical therapy (including massage). Although not dangerous in itself, hyperlordosis can lead to serious low back pain.
- **Scoliosis, rotoscoliosis.** Scoliosis is a problem for approximately 1% to 2% of teenagers. It progresses in girls much more frequently than boys, and almost always involves a bend to the right. If it appears with a spinal rotation, the term rotoscoliosis is appropriate. This condition usually appears during the rapid-growth years of late childhood and early adolescence. Complications include nerve irritation as misshapen bones press on nerve roots, spondylosis, and serious heart and lung problems arising from a severely restricted rib cage.

Signs and Symptoms

Postural deviations range from being quite subtle to being painfully obvious. A visual examination can yield information about hyperkyphosis and hyperlordosis, and even mild scoliosis may be visible with a forward-bending test. Patients often report muscular tension and sometimes nerve impairment along with chronic ache and loss of range of motion. If the condition is very advanced, movement of the ribs may be impaired, leaving the patient vulnerable to cardiac and respiratory problems and lung infections.

Treatment

Most postural deviations that are not related to underlying conditions are treated (if at all) with chiropractic or osteopathic manipulation, physical therapy, and exercise protocols. Bracing for external support may be recommended. When a deviation goes beyond a predetermined boundary, surgical intervention involving implants or bony fusions may be recommended. This is not always a permanent solution; however, many patients require follow-up procedures later in life.

NOTABLE CASES Actress Elizabeth Taylor had scoliosis that she credited with restricting her to a wheelchair.

Massage?

RISKS Some postural deviations are the result of serious underlying conditions. These must be identified and accommodated as part of a massage therapy strategy. Of special note: hyperkyphosis may be related to osteoporosis and extremely brittle bones.

Outside of these cautions, massage has few risks for a person with postural deviations that do not interfere with lung or cardiac function.

BENEFITS Carefully performed massage that targets the complicated tangle of soft tissue stresses on the spine can be tremendously useful in addressing many postural deviations.

OPTIONS The muscular component in most postural deviations presents a circular puzzle that must be explored by a massage therapist and client looking for long-term change. Addressing chronically lengthened as well as shortened muscles, adding hydrotherapy components, and being rigorous about tracking progress will help move toward the goal of pain-free posture and efficient movement. Many therapists and clients find the best results when bodywork is combined with movement training to learn new habits that preserve best function.

Adhesive Capsulitis in Brief

What is it?
Adhesive capsulitis, also known as frozen shoulder, is an idiopathic condition in which the connective tissues of the glenohumeral joint capsule and surrounding areas become progressively inflamed, painful, and thickened, which radically limits the range of motion.

How is it recognized?
Adhesive capsulitis has a predictable pattern of slowly progressive pain and loss of both active and passive range of motion, followed by a period of stability, which then usually fully or mostly resolves. The whole process can take between several months and two to three years.

Massage risks and benefits
Risks: When this condition is acute and worsening, massage may exacerbate pain and inflammation. Also, patients may use mild to very strong analgesics to manage this process, which can mean that bodywork must be done with extra care.
Benefits: During the phases when pain and inflammation are less extreme, massage and other manual therapies may be used in addition to other interventions to help restore freedom of movement and shorten recovery time.

Joint Disorders

Adhesive Capsulitis

Definition: What is It?

Adhesive capsulitis, or "frozen shoulder," is a poorly understood condition in which the connective tissues that surround the glenohumeral joint become first inflamed, and then thickened and restrictive. This process typically takes several months to fully develop, then it is stable for several months, and then for most patients it eventually spontaneously resolves, and most or all of the lost range of motion is restored.

Adhesive capsulitis is most common in people in their 50s and 60s. Women are slightly more likely to have it than men. People with diabetes, hyperthyroidism, or pathologically high triglycerides appear to be most susceptible. It is also more common among people who have had recent shoulder injuries, chest or breast surgery, or who have been immobilized for other reasons.

Etiology: What Happens?

The etiology of adhesive capsulitis is not at all clear. Some experts suggest that it always begins with an adhesion between the anterior part of the glenohumeral capsule to the head of the humerus; others propose that it begins in extracapsular tissues like local ligaments and the subacromial bursae, and the thickening that happens in the joint capsule is a secondary development.

An anomaly in the quality of collagen fibers in the area is similar to that seen with Dupuytren contracture, although the prognosis for frozen shoulder is much better than for other connective tissue contractures. The fact that it is significantly more common in people with high triglycerides, diabetes, and hyperthyroidism suggests that it may be connected to disorders involving problems with tiny blood vessels, leading to extra inflammation and the excessive production of connective tissue fibers. Finally, the excessive pain signals that are recorded with this condition suggest some similarities to complex regional pain syndrome, a condition that involves a self-sustaining pain feedback loop between the central nervous system and peripheral tissues.

Signs and Symptoms

A typical presentation of adhesive capsulitis involves a person in her 50s or 60s who experiences pain in one shoulder, especially at night. Often, no precipitating event or factor is ever identified. The pain is slowly progressive, and the shoulder gradually loses its range of motion: this is sometimes called the "freezing" phase. As the pain progresses and intensifies to become constant and acute, the shoulder becomes increasingly stiff. Over a period of several months, a person with adhesive capsulitis can lose up to 85% of normal joint mobility.

Eventually the progression stabilizes, and for several months the shoulder is extremely stiff, but no longer acutely painful. This is the "frozen" phase. Both active and passive motion is severely limited, especially in external rotation, abduction, and flexion.

Finally, for reasons that are still a mystery, the whole process reverses: pain is relieved, and full or nearly full range of motion is restored; this is the "thawing" phase. The whole cycle from beginning to end can take anywhere from nine months to three years.

It is unusual for adhesive capsulitis to occur in both shoulders at one time, but many people who have it on one side may develop it on the other side later in life.

Treatment

Treatments for adhesive capsulitis are recommended depending on the stage of progression to manage pain and to restore mobility as much as possible. Research shows that while some interventions may increase range of motion and decrease pain in the short term, no single treatment is consistently better in the long term than simply letting this condition run its course from "freezing" to "frozen" to "thawing."

Analgesics ranging from aspirin to narcotics may be recommended in the early stages, as this condition is extremely painful.

Injections of painkillers with corticosteroids are often used in the "freezing" or "frozen" stage, with and without physical therapy. If they are successfully administered, injections serve the double purpose of introducing anti-inflammatories into the affected area, and mechanically stretching and distending the joint capsule. If these are unsatisfactory, some physicians recommend surgery to loosen the joint capsule. Other options include joint manipulation under anesthesia, or a nerve block to temporarily deaden the subscapular nerve.

Medications

- Analgesics, including NSAIDs and stronger drugs
- Corticosteroid injections to manage inflammation

Massage?

RISKS Especially in the first "freezing" phase, adhesive capsulitis may be acutely painful and involve active inflammation. Direct and intense bodywork on and around the shoulder capsule at this time may only exacerbate symptoms. Furthermore, patients with adhesive capsulitis in its most painful presentation may be prescribed painkillers that mask important information. It is important that massage therapists don't overtreat this condition while symptoms are temporarily quelled.

BENEFITS Manual therapies get generally good results with this condition, as long as care is taken not to exacerbate pain or inflammation. Physical therapy, exercise, and good self-care are often part of the successful treatment plan as well.

OPTIONS Careful and specific work around the shoulder girdle with active participation from the client may be effective to help restore range of motion. It is important to work in a way that doesn't exacerbate inflammation, which may set the client back.

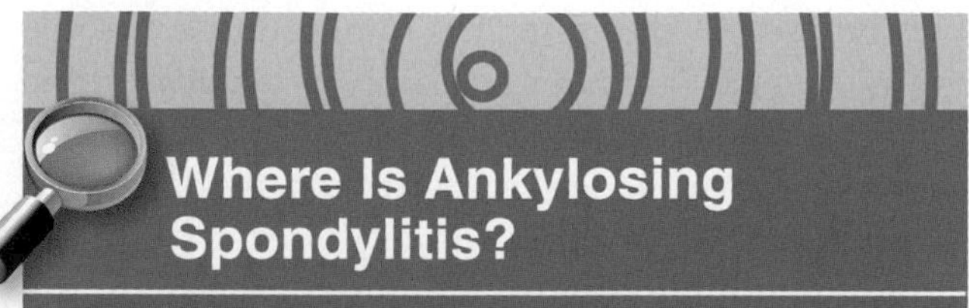

Where Is Ankylosing Spondylitis?

Ankylosing spondylitis (AS) is an autoimmune disorder in which the immune system mistakenly attacks facet joints in the spine, along with other tissues. This leads to inflammation and progressive fusions in vertebrae. AS now appears with several other autoimmune disease discussions in Chapter 6.

Baker Cysts

Definition: What Are They?

Baker cysts are synovial cysts found in the popliteal fossa, usually on the medial side. They are also called popliteal cysts.

Etiology: What Happens?

Baker cysts form when the joint capsule at the knee develops a pouch at the posterior aspect. They usually protrude into a small gap between the medial head of the gastrocnemius and the tendon of the semimembranosus (Figure 3.11). Some experts theorize that Baker cysts are a protective mechanism to prevent too much fluid accumulation at the knee in the context of chronic inflammation: a one-way valve directs the flow of excess fluid into many cysts, and prevents it from returning to the joint capsule.

Baker cysts in adults are almost always connected to other joint problems: osteoarthritis, rheumatoid arthritis (RA), lupus, or knee injuries, including cruciate ligament tears or meniscus tears.

Baker cysts are not usually dangerous, but a cyst can become big enough to impair blood flow through the lesser saphenous vein in the back of the leg. If that is the case, the patient is at risk for thrombophlebitis or deep vein thrombosis (DVT). Other complications include the risk of rupture (which creates symptoms that resemble DVT), bleeding into the joint, infection, or posterior compartment syndrome (blockage of fluid flow from the posterior compartment of the lower leg).

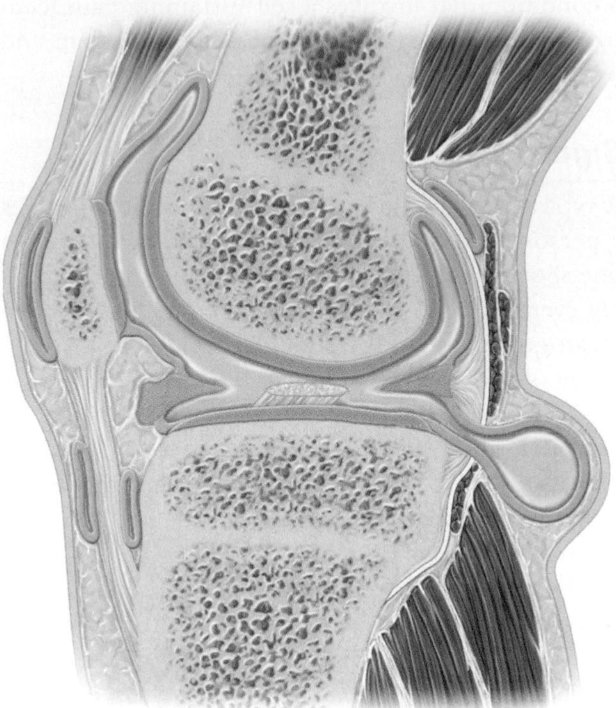

Figure 3.11. Baker cyst

Baker Cysts in Brief

What are they?
Baker cysts are synovial cysts, usually found on the posterior aspect of the knee. They are often connected to the synovial capsule of the knee.

How are they recognized?
Baker cysts are palpable deep to the superficial fascia in the popliteal fossa. They may cause pain on knee extension or a feeling of tightness in flexion.

Massage risks and benefits
Risks: Deep work in the popliteal fossa is generally not recommended, regardless, but the presence of a cyst that could rupture makes it even more important to avoid intrusive pressure in this area. In addition, Baker cysts may be large enough to interfere with blood return from the leg. This raises the risk of thrombosis, which must be cleared before bodywork is safe.
Benefits: While large Baker cysts locally contraindicate massage, bodywork elsewhere is safe. A client who has fully recovered from Baker cyst can enjoy the same benefits from massage as the rest of the population.

Signs and Symptoms

Baker cysts themselves are generally asymptomatic, but the affected knee often has pain from the underlying cause of inflammation. The cysts usually extend into the medial side of the popliteal fossa and may protrude down the leg, deep to the gastrocnemius. Patients with Baker cysts often report a feeling of tightness or fullness when the knee is in flexion and mild pain on extension. Large cysts may create visually asymmetrical legs (see Figure 3.12).

Treatment

Most Baker cysts are first treated with ice and nonsteroidal anti-inflammatories in the hopes that they

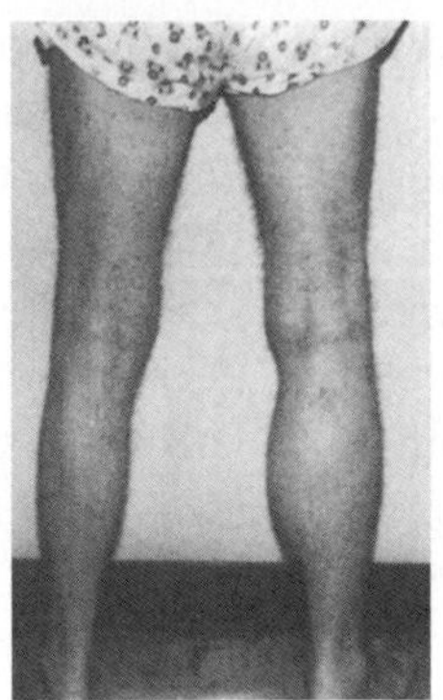

Figure 3.12. Baker cyst: note the disparity in size between two calves

will resolve spontaneously. If this is unsuccessful, they may be aspirated, followed by cortisone shots to resolve joint inflammation. This is often an impermanent solution, however, as they easily recur until the underlying joint disruption has been resolved, often through surgery.

Medications

- NSAIDs for pain and inflammation control

Massage?

RISKS Baker cysts present a local contraindication for massage, with the caution that if signs of thrombosis are present, then medical intervention is called for.

BENEFITS Massage away from the affected area is safe and appropriate. Clients who have successfully treated their Baker cyst can enjoy the same benefits from massage as the rest of the population.

Gout

Definition: What is It?

Gout is one of the oldest diseases in recorded medical history; treatment recommendations that are still in use date back to 580 A.D. Gout is a type of inflammatory arthritis that is relatively common in men between 40 and 50 years old, and women who are postmenopausal. Its incidence appears to be increasing as baby boomers with long histories of problematic eating and drinking habits enter maturity.

Gout in Brief

What is it?
Gout is an inflammatory arthritis caused by deposits of monosodium urate (uric acid) in and around joints, especially in the feet.

How is it recognized?
Acute gout causes joints to become red, hot, swollen, shiny, and extremely painful. It usually has a sudden onset.

Massage risks and benefits
Risks: Acute gout locally contraindicates massage simply because of pain, inflammation, and the risk of exacerbating damage. It may also systemically contraindicate all but the most gentle types of bodywork: this is a severe and acute condition that suggests serious metabolic problems that must be addressed.
Benefits: Joints with a history of multiple gout episodes may be permanent sites of caution, depending on how much damage might have accrued. A client with a history of successfully treated gout but no current symptoms can enjoy all the benefits of massage everywhere else on his or her body.

Etiology: What Happens?

Uric acid is a naturally occurring byproduct of digestion. Foods and liquids that are high in a substance called purine are particularly potent sources of uric acid. Under normal circumstances, uric acid is extracted from the blood by the kidneys. Having higher than normal levels of uric acid in the blood is called hyperuricemia: this is a predisposing factor for gout.

Hyperuricemia may develop for a couple of reasons. If the kidneys function normally but a person has a high protein and alcohol intake, they can't keep up with demand. Alternatively, the uric acid load may be normal but the kidneys are somehow impaired. This may be an inherited weakness, or related to other problems like diabetes or lead poisoning. And of course a person can have low-functioning kidneys with a high protein and alcohol intake: this is gout, waiting to happen.

NOTABLE CASES Gout has been known as the disease of kings, associated with rich diet and decadent living. This is witnessed by a list of some famous gout patients: Alexander the Great, Henry VIII of England, Charles V of Spain and his son Philip II, Dr. Samuel Johnson, Wolfgang von Goethe, and Benjamin Franklin.

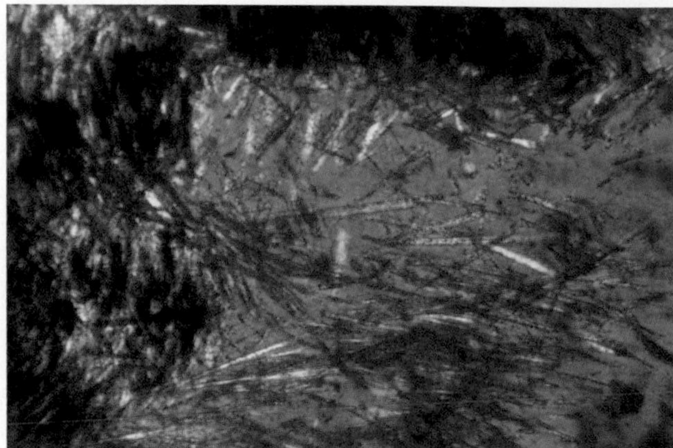

Figure 3.13. Gout: crystals erode joint capsules

The transition from hyperuricemia to an acute gouty attack is often precipitated by some specific event: binge eating or drinking, surgery, sudden weight loss, or a systemic infection. When uric acid consolidates, it forms sharp, needlelike crystals that accumulate in and around the joint capsule, grinding on and irritating synovial membranes, bursae, tendons, and other tissues (Figure 3.13). The crystals attract neutrophils, and these white blood cells initiate an exaggerated inflammatory response. This can happen in a short period: typically a person goes to bed feeling fine, and wakes in the night with a foot that is red, throbbing, and painful; this is called **podagra** (Figure 3.14).

The joint between the first metatarsal and proximal phalanx of the great toe may be the most frequent site for uric acid crystal accumulation because of gravity, but it may also have to do with the lower temperature found in extremities that aids in the crystallization process.

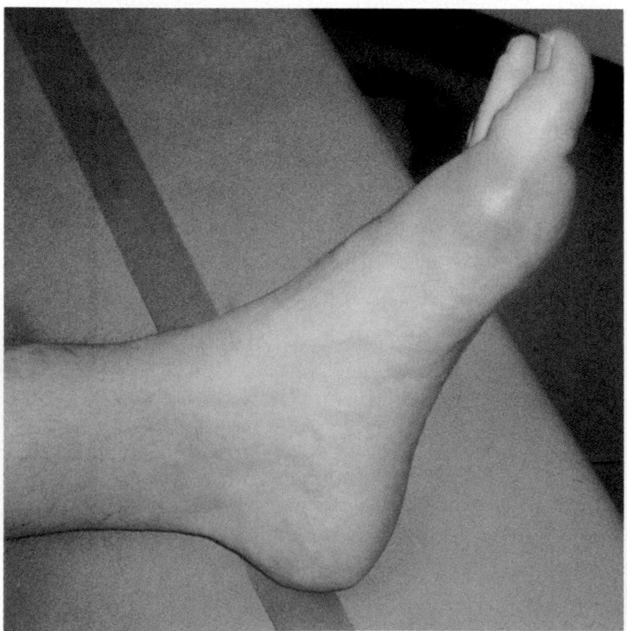

Figure 3.14. Gout: inflammation at the medial metatarsal-phalangeal joint (podagra)

In later stages of the disease, deposits of sodium urate called **tophi** may develop inside and around joints. These tophi erode the joint structures, leading to a complete loss of function. Tophi also grow along tendons and in subcutaneous tissues.

Hyperuricemia is clearly connected to gout, but the cause and effect link is not always consistent. Many people have hyperuricemia without ever having gout. Conversely, some people with gout show normal or even below-normal levels of uric acid in the blood. Experts theorize that under normal circumstances, the uric acid crystals are coated with serum proteins. When gout is triggered, the crystals are uncoated, and can directly interact with local cells to stimulate pain and inflammation.

Sometimes a person has just one attack of gout and then is never bothered by it again. If a second attack occurs, it comes several years later. The third attack happens after a shorter interval, and the fourth one, shorter still. Each event resolves itself in a few days or weeks. After 10 to 20 years, a patient may end up with almost constant acute attacks of this disease, but often by that time the associated problems of this condition may make toe pain the least of his worries.

Signs and Symptoms

Acute gouty arthritis has some very predictable patterns. It has a sudden onset and almost always happens in the feet first, especially at the joints of the great toe. Cumulative damage creates a characteristic punched-out pattern of bony erosion. Gout may also appear elsewhere on the foot, or in other body areas.

An acute gouty joint shows all of the signs of extreme inflammation. The joint may swell so much that the skin is hot, red, dry, shiny, and exquisitely painful. This phase of inflammation is often accompanied by a moderate fever (up to 101°F, or 38.3°C) and chills.

Complications

The complications of gout are related to having too much uric acid in the bloodstream, which indicates that kidneys are not functioning at adequate levels. Uric acid crystals may also cause kidney stones, which can contribute to renal failure. Impaired kidneys can't process fluid adequately. This stresses the rest of the circulatory system, causing high blood pressure, the end result of which can be atherosclerosis or stroke. All these problems—hyperuricemia, kidney insufficiency, gout, high blood pressure, and cardiovascular disease—are closely related.

Treatment

It is important to get a reliable diagnosis to treat gout successfully. A condition called pseudogout has similar symptoms, but because it involves different chemicals, it requires different treatment options (see Compare & Contrast 3.1).

A standard medical approach to gout has three prongs: pain relief (with analgesics other than aspirin, which inhibits uric acid excretion), anti-inflammatory drugs, and finally, drugs that modify metabolism and uric acid management. Preventive measures include increasing fluid intake (other than caffeine or alcohol, which act as diuretics), losing weight, and limiting purine-rich foods.

Medications

- NSAIDs, but not aspirin, for pain and inflammation
- Steroids (oral or injected) for inflammation
- Colchicine to treat or help prevent attacks
- Metabolic drugs (allopurinol, probenecid) to alter uric acid formation and excretion

Massage?

RISKS Acutely inflamed gouty joints at least locally contraindicate massage. This situation often involves fever and general malaise, which contraindicates all but the gentlest bodywork systemically.

Any joints that have had multiple gout attacks may be permanently distorted and vulnerable to irritation with pressure or movement: these are local cautions even when the acute stage has passed.

Some massage therapists talk about "grinding out uric acid crystals" in the feet. For a person with a history of gout, work of this pressure and intent is not appropriate.

A client who complains of pain and shows extreme inflammation around a joint should consult a doctor before applying ice: if it is gout, ice will promote the crystallization of uric acid.

BENEFITS When gout is not acute and is successfully treated, patients can enjoy the same benefits from massage as the rest of the population.

COMPARE & CONTRAST 3.1 Gout vs. Pseudogout

Gout is a variety of arthritis brought about by the accumulation of uric acid (monosodium urate) crystals in and around joint capsules, especially in the feet. Calcium pyrophosphate dihydrate deposition (CPDD), or pseudogout, has a very similar presentation, but since it doesn't involve uric acid or hyperuricemia, it requires a different treatment plan. Massage therapists are not required to be able to tell the difference between gout and pseudogout, but we can certainly counsel our clients to explore options if the treatment they receive doesn't seem to meet their needs.

CHARACTERISTICS	GOUT	CPDD (PSEUDOGOUT)
Prevalence	100:100,000	Unknown
Primary symptom	Exquisitely painful inflammation, usually around great toe, instep, or heel. May affect other joints as well.	Exquisitely painful inflammation, usually at knee or wrist
Implications for massage	Most patients have hyperuricemia, a risk of kidney stones, other urinary system challenges that may in turn impact the circulatory system.	CPDD is idiopathic, and may or may not be related to underlying problems. Clients must be screened for contributing factors, but none may be present.

Joint Disruptions

Definition: What Are They?

Dislocations and associated joint disruptions describe situations where the articulating bones of a joint are not in correct relationship. In a full dislocation, the surfaces have no contact and the joint cannot be used. In a **subluxation**, the surfaces have partial contact; the joint may be functional but limited in range of motion. **Dysplasia** of a joint involves bony deformation that prevents a normal articulation. This happens most frequently at the hip.

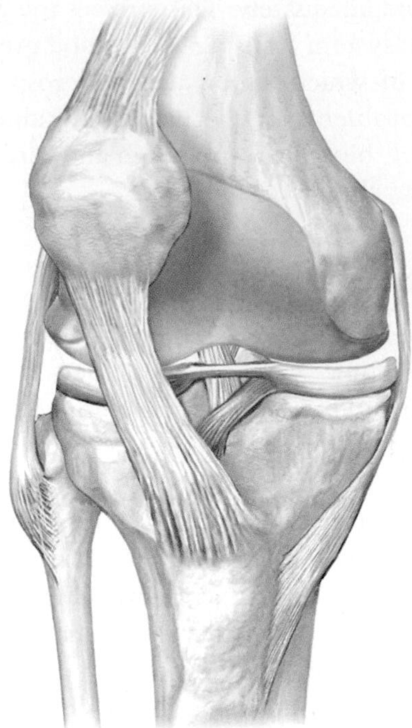

Figure 3.15. Joint disruption: dislocated patella

Etiology: What Happens?

Synovial joints are composed of two or more bones with articulating cartilage, a synovial membrane, a ligamentous capsule, and varying types and amounts of supporting fascia, ligaments, tendons, and muscles. When the bones in a joint are not in their optimal relationship, joint function is impaired. This can happen because of specific trauma, because of a congenital problem with the shape of the bones, or it can be a slowly progressive chronic problem of instability without full dislocation.

Joint Disruptions in Brief

What are they?
Joint disruptions include any situation that interferes with the proper alignment between bones in a joint. A dislocation means that the articulating bones within a joint capsule are separated. A subluxation involves bones that are incompletely dislocated: the joint can function, but has limited range of motion. Hip dysplasia involves abnormalities in the shape of the acetabulum or femoral head that prevents a fully functioning hip joint.

What do they look like?
Traumatic joint disruptions are obvious and painful, with swelling, loss of function, and obvious displacement of the bones. Chronic subluxations and dysplasia can be more subtle.

Massage risks and benefits

Risks: Massage at the site of an acute situation may exacerbate symptoms and inappropriate joint manipulations may lead to a dislocation or subluxation episode.

Benefits: Massage for subacute dislocations or subluxations may be appropriate and helpful if the compromised range of motion is respected. Massage elsewhere on the body is safe, and may help to address some of the compensation patterns that develop with chronic musculoskeletal problems.

Types of Dislocations and Joint Disruptions

- **Dislocation.** The articulating bones are no longer touching; the shared surfaces have become disconnected, usually because of trauma. Dislocations are common for the shoulder, the fingers (especially the metacarpal-phalangeal joints), and the patella, although they can certainly occur elsewhere (Figures 3.15 and 3.16). A joint with a history of dislocation that is

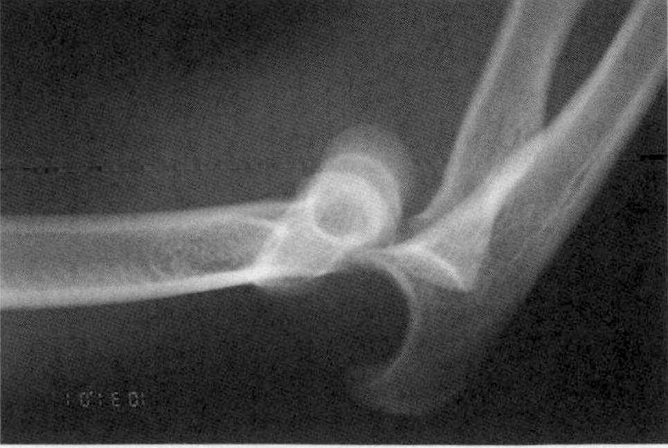

Figure 3.16. Joint disruption: dislocated elbow

not surgically corrected is at increased risk for spontaneous dislocation in the future.

- **Subluxation.** Bones are out of best alignment, but the joint capsule is intact. The joint is functional, but lacks a full range of motion. Joints that commonly subluxate include the intervertebral facet joints, the patellofemoral joint, and the radial head (this is sometimes called "nursemaid's elbow" from dangling a child by his or her forearm).
- **Dysplasia.** A congenital anomaly, dysplasia involves the formation of an abnormal acetabulum or femoral head. This can often be detected in early infancy, but if it causes no symptoms (usually this means it occurs bilaterally), it may require no treatment. Ultimately, a person with hip dysplasia is at very much increased risk for both subluxation and dislocation of the affected hip.

Signs and Symptoms

Joint disruptions can create various signs and symptoms, depending on the cause. Acute traumatic situations are obvious, with pain, swelling, and very often damage to other nearby tissues that may include bleeding, bone fractures, torn or irritated nerves, and damaged ligaments, muscles, and tendons (Figure 3.17).

Subluxations can be related to trauma, but more often they involve low-level pain that is chronic and progressive. When they occur at the vertebrae, some experts suggest that they can put mechanical pressure on nerve roots, leading to referred pain and other symptoms in the extremities and viscera.

Hip dysplasia may be silent and undetected, or it may lead to uneven limb length and significant problems with walking in childhood.

Complications

A person with a history of dislocations may have permanently compromised ligaments, which can contribute to joint instability and an increased risk for both subluxation and osteoarthritis. In addition, the muscles that cross the affected joints may become hypertonic in an attempt to stabilize the nearby structures. This can lead to pain, trigger points, and limited range of motion.

Treatment

Treatment for joint disruptions depends on the cause. Traumatic situations that involve other tissue damage may call for surgery. Closed injuries and small-scale subluxations may be reducible through manipulation and traction of the affected joint. Chronic and congenital situations may be treated with splints, braces, physical therapy and exercise to strengthen the muscles surrounding the compromised structures.

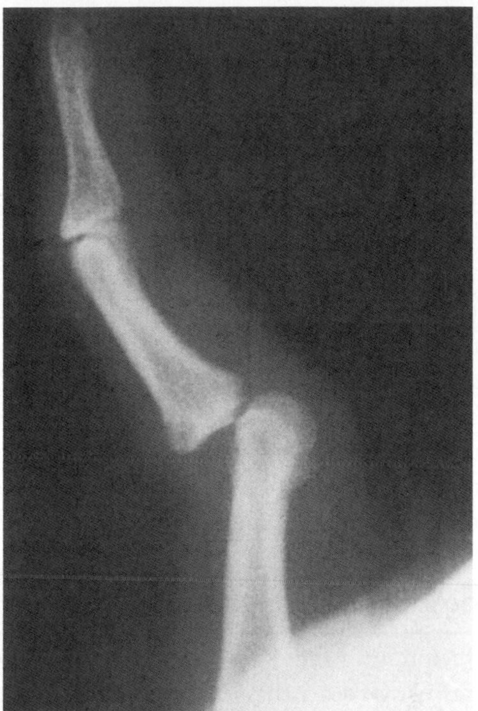

Figure 3.17. Joint disruption: soft tissue damage

Medications

- NSAIDs to manage pain and inflammation for acute situations

Massage?

RISKS Acute traumatic joint disruptions obviously contraindicate massage at least locally. For subacute or chronic problems, the practitioner must respect limitations in range of motion.

BENEFITS Massage to the adjoining soft tissues around a weak or unstable joint may be helpful not only to manage pain but also to improve muscle and connective tissue function.

OPTIONS Very specific protocols for work around the knee, hip, and shoulder may be applied specifically to these joints, with positioning adjustments to prevent spontaneous dislocations or subluxations. Additionally, any work that augments the goals of a physical therapy protocol may be helpful.

Joint Replacement Surgery

Definition: What is It?

Joint replacement surgery, also called **arthroplasty**, is a procedure designed to repair articulating surfaces within a synovial joint. The goal is to have pain-free (or pain-reduced) movement, although the range of motion may be permanently limited. Arthroplasty is not a condition in itself, but it is a common surgery; it carries some long-term consequences that may inform bodywork choices.

Between 700,000 and 800,000 joint replacement surgeries are conducted in this country each year. The vast majority are for knees and hips, but shoulder replacements are becoming more common.

Etiology: What Happens?

The precipitating factor for most joint replacement surgeries is osteoarthritis, or "wear-and-tear" arthritis. Rheumatoid arthritis, avascular necrosis, or serious trauma (sometimes related to osteoporosis) may also contribute to reasons for an arthroplasty. In any case, this surgery is only conducted when all other options, including exercise, braces, anti-inflammatory medication, cortisone injections, and less invasive surgeries are no longer adequate interventions. The x-rays of a good candidate for joint replacement surgery typically show a loss of space in the joint cavity, bony remodeling, bone spurs, and the possibility of debris inside the joint cavity.

In a joint replacement surgery, the contacting bony surfaces are replaced by artificial components called **prostheses**. Historically, these have been made of various materials ranging from ceramic to titanium, but today, they are most likely to include a highly polished ball made of cobalt chrome on one surface and a polyethylene cup or socket on the other. The average lifespan of a weight-bearing joint prosthesis is ten to fifteen years, at which time the components are likely to be worn down or loosened, and in need of another replacement.

Joint Replacement Surgery in Brief

What is it?
Joint replacement surgery is a surgical procedure to replace one or more articulating surfaces in a synovial joint. This surgery may be performed because of osteoarthritis, trauma, or other causes of permanent joint damage.

How is it recognized?
A joint replacement patient has scars at the surgical site, and may have a permanently restricted range of motion.

Massage risks and benefits
Risks: Postsurgical acute inflammation requires specific adjustments in massage goals and pressure. Massage therapy that involves stretching may put the patient at risk for joint failure, even if the surgery was many years earlier.
Benefits: Massage therapy has been shown to help reduce postsurgical pain and inflammation. It can improve the quality of scar tissue, allowing for better freedom of movement. These benefits may allow the arthroplasty patient to resume healthy levels of activity sooner than otherwise might be expected. For people with older surgeries and no long-standing problems, massage that doesn't challenge their range of motion has the same benefits as for the rest of the population.

Types of Joint Replacements

- *Shoulders.* Arthroplasty of the glenohumeral joint is a relatively new surgical procedure, but it is becoming increasingly common. This is done when the joint is no longer competent: trauma, ongoing damage to the rotator cuff, or bone spurs have made the head of the humerus and the glenoid fossa incompatible in shape. Shoulder joint repairs can take two forms. The most common version replaces the ball of the humerus and the cup of the glenoid. Some patients are candidates for a "reverse" shoulder replacement, in which a ball is attached to the scapula, and the head of the humerus is replaced with a shallow cup, thus reversing the typical relationship between the bones.
- *Hips.* Hip joints are frequently replaced, either as a consequence of arthritis that wears away at this huge weight-bearing joint or as a result of femoral trauma. This situation, which combines femoral repair with joint resurfacing, is frequently associated with osteoporosis or other problems that make the femoral neck vulnerable to fracture (Figure 3.18).
- *Knees.* Knees are unique in that they combine a large range of motion with strict limitation in direction—that is, they flex and extend only (unless the knee is bent, in which position it can slightly rotate). Consequently, knees are vulnerable to shearing forces that can damage their stabilizing ligaments and put the internal cartilage at risk for permanent damage. Small repairs

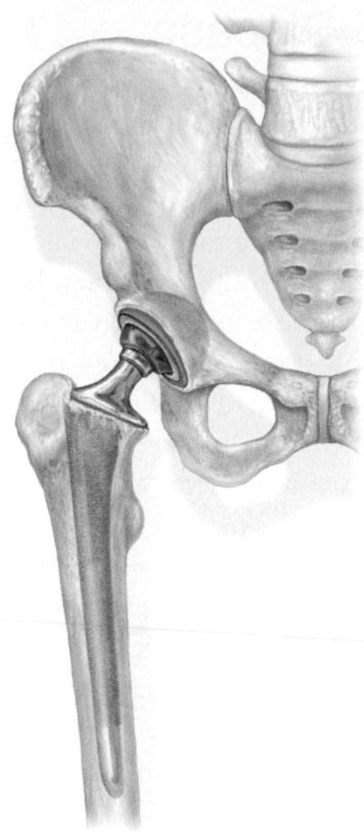

Figure 3.18. Joint replacement surgery: hip prosthesis

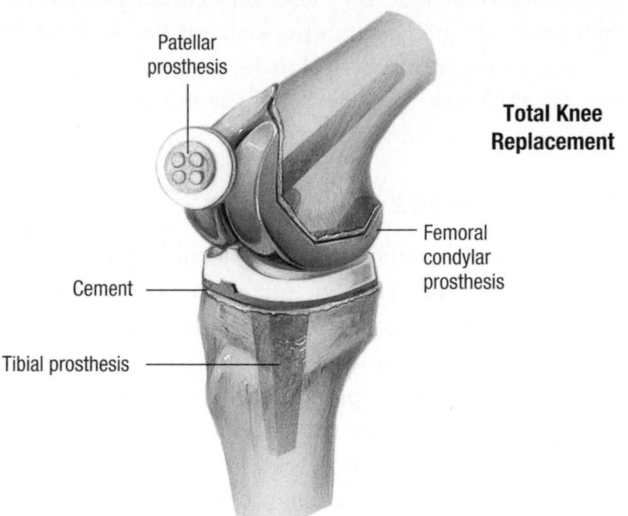

Figure 3.19. Knee prosthesis

to the menisci can be made with arthroscopic surgery, but eventually the joint may be reduced to "bone-on-bone" contact. Knee joint replacements can sometimes involve resurfacing only one part of the joint, or they can involve replacing the ends of the tibia, femur, and the contacting surface of the patella. Cruciate ligaments may be replaced with polyethylene posts to help stabilize the new mechanism (Figure 3.19).

- *Other joints*. Arthroplasty can be conducted on ankles, various carpal-metacarpal and interphalangeal joints, the saddle joint of the thumb, and the temporomandibular joint (TMJ).

Several variables influence exactly how a joint replacement surgery is conducted. Older and less active patients may have their prostheses simply glued to their existing bone: this allows for a speedier recovery, but carries a risk of loosening and poor adherence between the bone and the implant. Younger or more active patients are better candidates for implants that have tiny pores where new bone tissue can grow to blend with the synthetic material. This is a lengthier process, but the long-term strength of the joint tends to be much better.

The surgical approach through the soft tissues is another important variable in the predication for how quickly or successfully a joint replacement surgery will heal. Longitudinal approaches are less damaging to the muscles, but they may require a much longer incision than a lateral approach. The angle at which the socket is implanted and the size of the prosthesis are other important factors. Women obviously have differently sized and angled joints than men, but these differences have only recently been recognized by manufacturers of prostheses, which are now available in a range of sizes.

Signs and Symptoms

The symptoms that lead to a joint replacement are typically related to osteoarthritis or some other form of joint inflammation and damage. Most people report a deep ache that is made worse with movement, although it often progresses to the point of being painful all the time.

A person who has had an arthroplastic surgery has a significant scar at the surgical site. The only other dependable sign is a loss of normal range of motion. People with reconstructed hips, knees, or shoulders are limited in the degree and direction of movement that is safe for their prostheses. Going beyond a safe range puts the implants at risk for loosening, which then requires surgical correction. It is preferable to avoid this because each successive surgery has a lower success rate, and leads to a more limited range of motion.

Treatment

Joint replacement surgery is a major undertaking, involving general anesthesia, anywhere from two to four hours of surgery, and a 3- to 5-day hospital stay. Postsurgical treatment includes immediate mobilization (often starting on the same day as the surgery), pain medication, and because DVT is a common and dangerous complication, compression stockings and anticoagulant drugs.

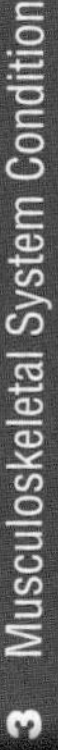

Knee surgery patients may also use a continuous passive motion machine that keeps the knee moving even when the patient is at rest. Physical therapy typically begins on the day after surgery, and may be recommended for several weeks following the procedure.

Complications

The possible complications that accompany any surgery are daunting. They include a reaction to anesthesia; arrhythmia; and the consequences of blood clots, including DVT, pulmonary embolism, and circulatory shock. Hospital-borne pathogens may lead to an infection in the joint, urinary tract infection, or pneumonia.

Complications related specifically to arthroplasty also include inadvertent fracture of the articulating bones, excessive scarring, and a loss of range of motion that is far beyond what was expected. Later complications can arise relating to a poorly seated prosthesis, or failure to bond correctly with bone tissue.

Medications

- Analgesics for pain control
- Anticoagulants for blood clot limitation
- Antibiotics (if infection develops)

Massage?

RISKS New joint replacements carry specific risks in relation to surgical complications. Older joint replacements must be carefully maneuvered to avoid stressing the joint and putting it at risk for loosening or failure. Always check with the client for limitations in range of motion.

BENEFITS Evidence suggests that massage can improve the symptoms of some kinds of arthritis, which may delay the need for a joint replacement surgery: a definite benefit.

Massage can also reduce postsurgical pain and inflammation, and it can improve the quality of scar tissue for better mobility. For clients with older surgeries and no other complications, massage that respects their limited range of motion has the same benefits as it does for the rest of the population.

OPTIONS It is important to determine why a client had a joint replacement surgery. Usually the reason is osteoarthritis, which means more than one joint may be affected. Look for postural compensation patterns that may cause pain and interfere with the most pain-free and efficient function possible.

Lyme Disease

Definition: What is It?

Lyme disease is an infection with a spirochetal bacterium called *Borrelia burgdorferi*. This pathogen spreads by the bite of two species of ticks: deer ticks (*Ixodes scapularis*) and Western black-legged ticks (*I. pacificus*). These ticks are very small, especially in the nymph stage, when they most frequently affect humans. This can make it difficult to find them on the skin. An unfed deer tick nymph is slightly larger than the period at the end of this sentence (Figure 3.20).

Lyme disease has been reported in most states, but the highest concentrations are in the Northeast and mid-Atlantic states, the upper Midwest, and northwestern California. Persons most at risk are those who work or play outside in grassy or wooded areas; the ticks don't thrive in sunny or arid environments.

Etiology: What Happens?

Deer ticks and Western black-legged tick live about 2 years. The life phase when they find human hosts is usually their second spring or summer when they

Lyme Disease in Brief

What is it?
Lyme disease is a bacterial infection spread by the bites of certain species of ticks. The immune response to the bacteria causes inflammation of large joints along with neurological and cardiovascular symptoms.

How is it recognized?
The hallmark early symptom of Lyme disease is a circular bull's-eye rash at the site of the tick bite. The skin is red, itchy, and hot but not usually raised. The rash may be accompanied by fever, fatigue, and joint pain. Later symptoms may include acute intermittent inflammation of one or more large joints, numbness, poor coordination, Bell palsy, and an irregular heartbeat.

Massage risks and benefits
Risks: When inflammation due to Lyme disease is acute, any bodywork must be noninvasive and gentle.
Benefits: During subacute phases, massage may be appropriate to maintain joint function and relieve pain.

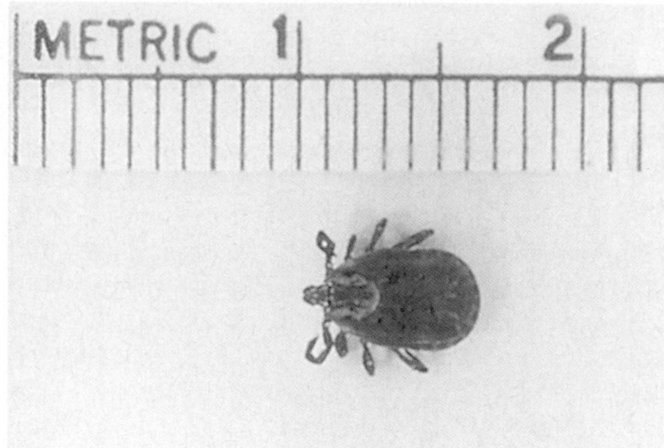

Figure 3.20. Deer tick: vector for Lyme disease

climb onto grass or bush stems and wait for a warm-blooded host to brush close by.

Ticks pick up the spiral bacterium *B. burgdorferi* from the blood of their animal hosts, especially mice. If an infected tick subsequently bites a human, that bacterium may be transmitted to the human host. It is the bacterial invasion, not the tick bite, that causes the damage seen with Lyme disease. The bacteria enter the bloodstream with the tick's saliva, and from there can access joints and other tissues.

B. burgdorferi is a slow-growing bacterium. This creates several problems, including a delayed immune response and difficulties in getting accurate blood tests. So far three subspecies of the bacterium have been found, and up to 100 different strains of the infection are active in the United States. Further, *B. Burgdorferi* is not the only tickborne infection found in the United States; see Sidebar 3.3 for more on tickborne infections.

Sidebar 3.3 Is It Just Lyme Disease?

Lyme disease is caused by tickborne bacteria that infect joints and cause debilitating arthritis. Some Lyme disease patients live with pain and progressive inflammation for years, in spite of antibiotics that should provide relief. It turns out that some of these patients may have more than Lyme disease alone: deer ticks can carry two other pathogens that affect humans:

- **Ehrlichiosis** is a tickborne bacterial infection that can easily coexist with Lyme disease. Consequences of **ehrlichiosis** infection include low white blood cell and platelet counts. This infection can be cleared with antibiotics from the tetracycline family, but this is a different class of antibiotics from that usually used for Lyme disease alone. Ehrlichiosis is less common than Lyme disease, so some patients may live with this infection for a long time before it is discovered.
- **Babesiosis** is a parasite similar to the protozoan that causes malaria. It can also coexist with Lyme disease. **Babesiosis** can cause anemia and an enlarged spleen, as well as other serious problems, especially for immunosuppressed people. Babesiosis responds well to quinine *if* it is identified as an infection separate from Lyme disease.

To complicate matters further, two other tickborne illnesses may also be confused with Lyme disease:

- **Southern tick-associated rash illness (STARI)** is a condition endemic to southeast and south central states. It is spread by the Lone Star tick, which carries the spirochete *B. lonestari*. **STARI** also causes a bull's-eye rash and is treatable with antibiotics.
- **Rocky Mountain spotted fever (RMSF)** is an infection with the bacterium *Rickettsia rickettsii*, spread by hard ticks all over the United States. Early symptoms include fever, headache, muscle pain, and malaise, followed by a spotty rash (as opposed to a bull's-eye rash). Although RMSF is treatable with antibiotics, it is a potentially life-threatening infection that can affect blood and blood vessels all over the body, leading to serious long-term consequences.

Signs and Symptoms

Lyme disease moves in stages, with signs and symptoms particular to each.

- *Early localized disease.* This is the first stage of a Lyme disease infection. Ticks are slow feeders, so it may take several days for the bacteria to enter the body and some days after that for symptoms to appear. Early symptoms generally appear 7 to 30 days after an initial tick bite. They include a circular red rash (a bull's-eye rash) that is hot and itchy but not raised from the skin (Figure 3.21), accompanied by high fever, fatigue, night sweats, headache, stiff neck, and swollen lymph nodes. If no rash appears (as in more than 50% of cases), these early symptoms may be mistaken for flu, mononucleosis, or meningitis.
- *Early disseminated disease.* This is the second stage, during which the infected person develops systemic symptoms of infection with *B. burgdorferi*. These include cardiovascular symptoms (especially irregular

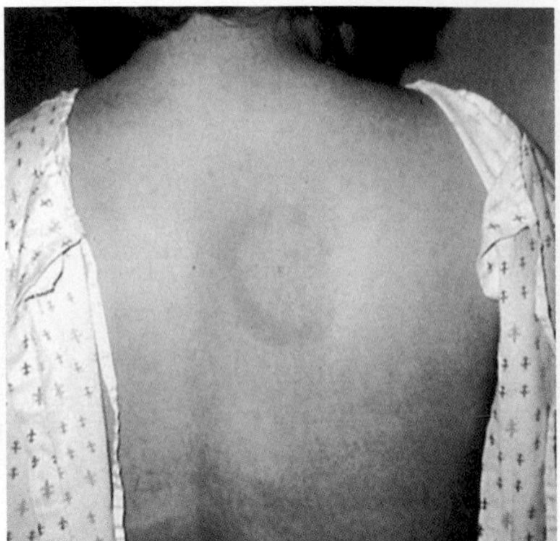

Figure 3.21. Lyme disease: bull's-eye rash

heartbeat and dizziness), neurological symptoms (chronic headaches, cranial nerve palsy that resembles Bell palsy, numbness, tingling, forgetfulness, and poor coordination), along with more general problems, including debilitating fatigue.

- *Late disease.* This is the final outcome of a Lyme disease infection. It is associated with extreme inflammation of one or more large joints. The knees are the most commonly affected area, but elbows and shoulders are often inflamed as well. Most patients don't have the infection in more than three joints at a time. The inflammation can be extreme enough to damage the joint permanently, especially if it is untreated.

NOTABLE CASES Authors Amy Tan (*Joy Luck Club*), Rebecca Wells (*Divine Secrets of the Ya-Ya Sisterhood*), and Alice Walker (*The Color Purple*) have all struggled with Lyme disease. Singer Darryl Hall (Hall and Oates) has also been diagnosed with it.

The tendency for Lyme disease to affect joints is what classifies it as an arthritic condition. In fact, the first cases of Lyme disease ever identified were among a group of children who were all initially misdiagnosed with juvenile rheumatoid arthritis (see Sidebar 3.4).

Most people with Lyme disease have symptoms for several weeks or months, and then they subside. A small number develop a chronic condition, which can progressively get worse. It is unclear whether these patients have a continuing chronic infection or develop an autoimmune response that is originally triggered by the bacterial infection.

SIDEBAR 3.4 History of Lyme Disease

Although Lyme disease was only definitively identified and named in 1982, it has probably been present for much longer.

In the early 20th century, doctors made note of target-shaped red rashes, which were named **erythema migrans**. People who developed these rashes seemed to have a high incidence of arthritis, but if they were treated with penicillin, their chances of developing arthritis were significantly lessened.

Then in 1974, a group of children in Lyme, Connecticut, were diagnosed with juvenile rheumatoid arthritis. Parents were skeptical about such a high concentration of a disease that was not understood to be in any way communicable. This led to intensive research, during which a scientist named Burgdorfer isolated the spirochete now called *B. burgdorferi.* He found it in highest concentrations in the midgut of deer ticks. It lives here until ticks feed on a host, when it may exit the tick to invade new territory.

Treatment

Accurate diagnosis of Lyme disease is an ongoing challenge, as both false-positive and false-negative blood tests are common. Further, without the signature bull's-eye rash as an indicator, the signs of Lyme disease can resemble several common chronic conditions. Doctors in endemic areas are encouraged to consider Lyme disease when investigating conditions like fibromyalgia, chronic fatigue syndrome, and multiple chemical sensitivity syndrome.

B. burgdorferi is sensitive to antibiotics, so the outlook for someone who is accurately diagnosed with Lyme disease in the early stages is often hopeful. The type and duration of antibiotic treatment for Lyme disease is a topic of much debate, as some patients seem to require different treatment regimens than others.

The best protection against Lyme disease is protection from disease-bearing ticks. This means wearing long sleeves and long pants when working or playing in areas where tick infestation is high. Tucking pants into socks or boots may make it harder for ticks to gain access to skin. Wearing light-colored clothing is recommended, to make it easier to find and remove ticks. Using insect repellants can also reduce the risk of tick bites.

Examining the skin after being in a high-risk area is another important preventive measure. Ticks prefer to occupy warm, protected areas such as the groin, axilla, backs of knees, and insides of elbows. If a tick is found, it should be carefully removed with tweezers to keep the mouth parts intact, and then the person should report being bitten and take the tick to the doctor. If the tick is found and removed within 24 hours, the risk of infection is very low.

Medications

- Antibiotics for infection control

Massage?

RISKS The arthritic phase of Lyme disease involves intermittently severe and painful inflammation of joints; this contraindicates massage, at least locally. Lyme disease can also affect the nervous and circulatory systems, and because treatment can take a long time to take effect, it is especially important for massage therapists to operate as part of a client's healthcare team.

BENEFITS As long as sensation is present and inflammation is not acute, a person with Lyme disease may enjoy the relaxation, relief from anxiety, and general sense of well-being that massage can offer.

OPTIONS Massage therapists who live and work in areas where Lyme disease is especially common should be aware of what deer ticks and Western black-legged ticks look like, so that if they find these parasites during a session, they can counsel clients to receive appropriate medical care.

Osteoarthritis

Definition: What is It?

Also called degenerative joint disease, osteoarthritis (the most common form of arthritis) is a condition in which synovial joints, especially weight-bearing joints, lose healthy cartilage. This condition is distinguished from other types of arthritis by being directly related to age and wear and tear of the joint structures. The etiology of osteoarthritis is restricted to synovial joints. Arthritis at the spine has some important differences, and is discussed in the section titled Spondylosis.

Osteoarthritis in Brief

Pronunciation: os-te-o-arth-RY-tis

What is it?
Osteoarthritis is joint inflammation brought about by wear and tear causing cumulative damage to articular cartilage.

How is it recognized?
Affected joints are stiff, painful, and occasionally palpably inflamed. Bony deformation may be easily visible or palpable. Osteoarthritis most often affects knees, hips, and distal joints of the fingers.

Massage risks and benefits
Risks: Acutely inflamed arthritis (which isn't typical) at least locally contraindicates massage that may promote local fluid flow and exacerbate inflammation.
Benefits: Full body and specific massage for painful joints can reduce stiffness and pain, and improve the quality of life for people with osteoarthritis, even though it is unlikely to contribute to any internal joint repair process.

Etiology: What Happens?

Joints, especially knees and hips, put up with tremendous weight-bearing stress and repetitive movements; their design is a marvel of efficiency and durability. But the environment inside a joint capsule is precarious; any imbalance can have cumulative destructive impact. This can take the shape of excessive stress on a healthy joint or normal stress on a joint that has already been compromised. Once the process of arthritis has begun, it may be possible to stop it, but capacity for regeneration and repair is limited at best (Figure 3.22).

Osteoarthritis is now understood to be a process of degeneration that may begin with the cartilage, but it progresses to affect the synovium and the connecting bones. Hyaline or articular cartilage is constructed of a relatively small number of living **chondrocytes** that produce collagen (mostly type II fibers), along with **proteoglycans**: large negatively charged molecules that attract water. The cells, protein fibers, and molecules of fluid are arranged in slightly different patterns, depending on whether they are superficial, intermediate, or attached directly to the chondral surface of the articulating bone. These

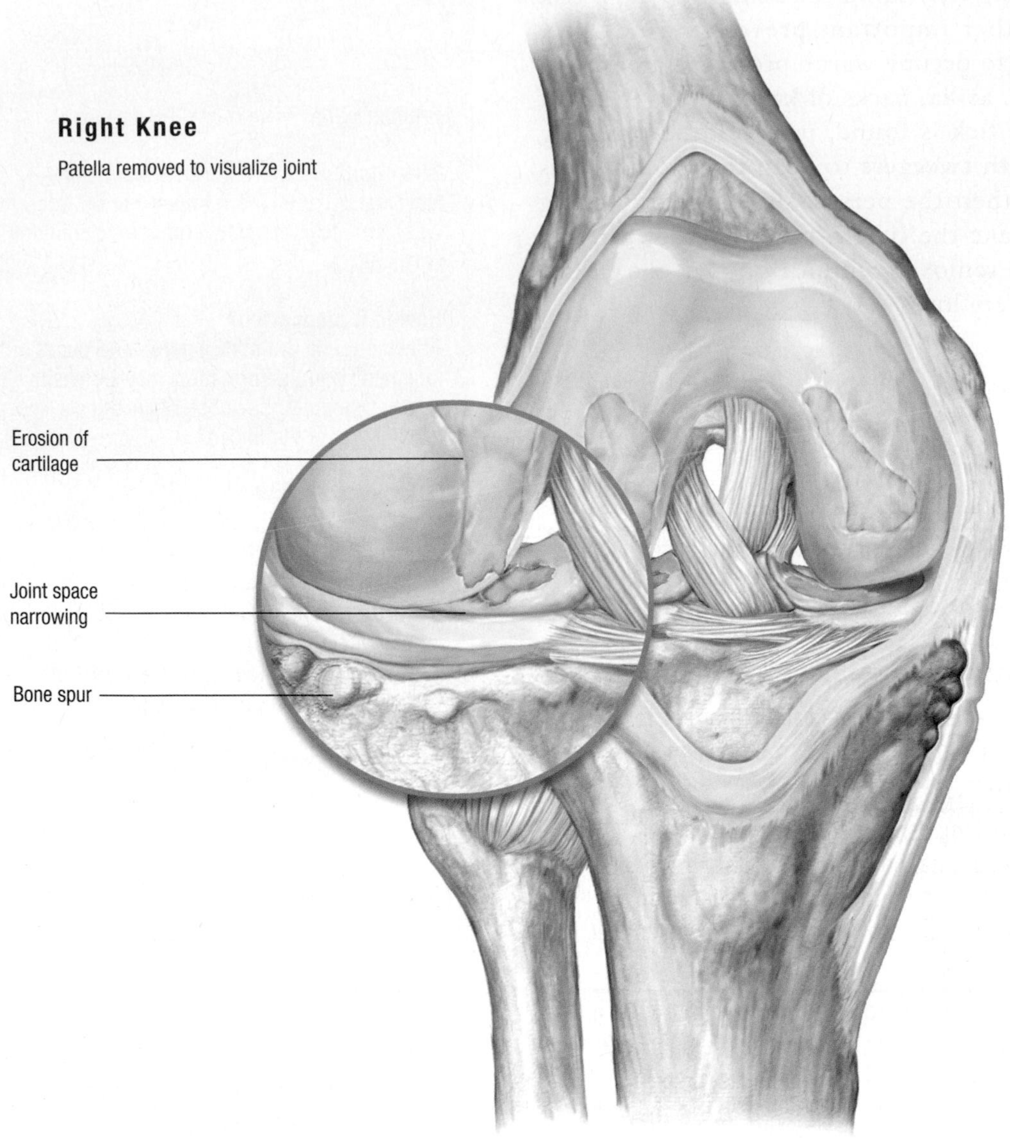

Figure 3.22. Osteoarthritis

varying zones give cartilage the ability to resist both shearing and compressive forces.

Chondrocytes remain active all through life, constantly replacing and rebuilding the cartilage surface, but they don't actively proliferate, and they don't migrate to damaged areas. Further, chondrocytes become less active with age. When cartilage degenerates, chondrocytes make less fluid and collagen, and the structure degrades. The process is accelerated by the production of local proinflammatory chemicals that also inhibit normal chondrocyte activity. Local irritation can also trigger the synovial lining to become inflamed and to produce other chemicals that damage the cartilage. Ultimately, the breakdown of cartilage stimulates osteocytes in the epiphyses of the affected bones to become more active: the condyle of the bone may become enlarged, **osteophytes** (bone spurs) may develop, and in some cases cyst-like cavities develop under the cartilage of the affected bone.

Many changes may trigger joint degeneration. Age alone changes the quality of articular cartilage, making it drier and more prone to injury. Being overweight adds stress to knees and hips, and some evidence now points to a biochemical link between adipocytes (fat cells) and cartilage degeneration. If the ligaments that surround the joints are chronically lax, the joint can become unstable, raising the risk of arthritis; this can be a long-term problem with joints that have been dislocated. A history of trauma or surgery (to remove pieces of the meniscus, for instance) is another predisposing factor. Repetitive pounding stress, such as running or jumping with inadequate support, can also open the door to problems. Hormonal imbalances and nutritional deficiencies, including dehydration, inadequate calcium metabolism, and foods that trigger inflammatory responses, may compromise the health of joint structures.

Some features of osteoarthritis overlap with those of an etiologically different disease, rheumatoid arthritis (RA). The discussion of RA appears in Chapter 6, but a chart comparing the two conditions can be found in this chapter: see Compare & Contrast 3.2.

Signs and Symptoms

The symptoms of osteoarthritis are related to irritation of the joint structures. This condition is seldom hot, painful, or visibly swollen. More often, it lingers in a chronic stage in which the joints have ongoing deep pain and stiffness, especially when they are not warmed up or when they have been overused. Many osteoarthritis patients report that a change in weather triggers symptoms: this may be a reflection of ambient air pressure and its effect on joint capsules. Osteoarthritis can be crippling when it occurs at the

COMPARE & CONTRAST 3.2 Osteoarthritis vs. Rheumatoid Arthritis

Of the 100 conditions that cause painful inflammation of joints, the two most commonly recognized are osteoarthritis and rheumatoid arthritis (RA). Osteoarthritis is a wear-and-tear disorder that could possibly be exacerbated by over-enthusiastic bodywork but can't be spread through the body. RA is an autoimmune disorder, and it can progressively affect more joints.

The following is a brief list of the most common patterns seen with osteoarthritis compared with RA.

CHARACTERISTICS	OSTEOARTHRITIS	RHEUMATOID ARTHRITIS
Prevalence	Radiographs show bony deformation in 33%–90% of people over 65.	Up to 1.5% of the population.
Demographics	Most common in people over 40. Men and women affected equally.	Women affected two to three times as often as men; men more likely to have systemic symptoms. May affect children.
Pain patterns	Spine, knees, hips most frequently affected. Distal finger joints, saddle joint (trapezium, first metacarpal) also at risk.	Proximal joints in hands and feet, ankles, wrists usually affected. Extreme distortion of joint capsules can cause joints to be visibly misshapen. Pain appears in flare and remission stages.
Other symptoms	None	In early stages and acute episodes, fever, malaise, lack of appetite, muscle pain may be present.
Implications for massage	Can be useful to maintain range of motion and relieve pain in muscles that cross over affected joints, as long as inflammation is not acute.	Can be useful for joint function during remission.

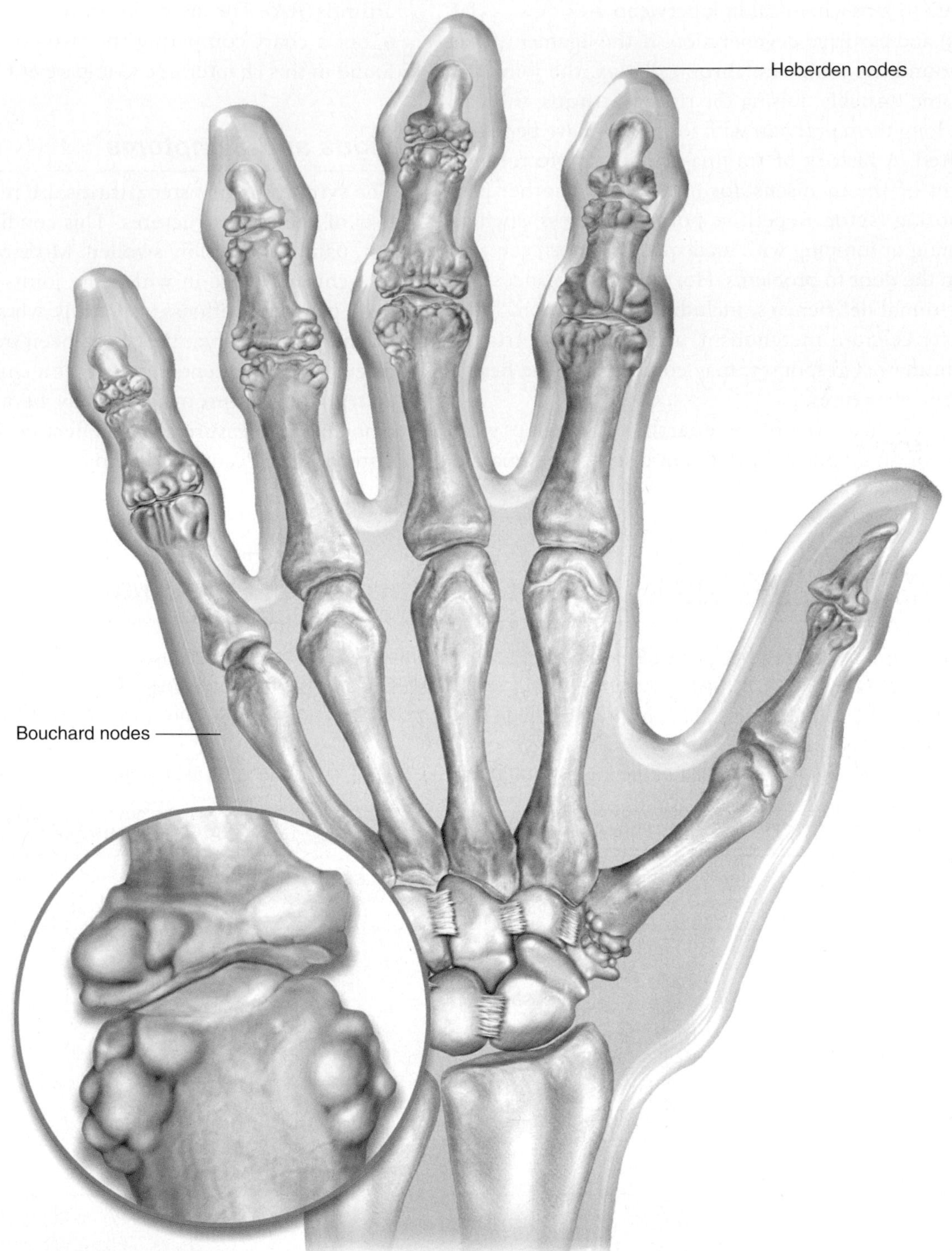

Figure 3.23. Osteoarthritis at the hand

hip or knee, because the pain and limitation are badly exacerbated by walking.

When osteoarthritis develops in the fingers, characteristic thickening of the phalangeal epiphyses is present. Bulges at the distal interphalangeal joints (DIPs) are called **Heberden nodes**. When they appear at the proximal interphalangeal joints (PIPs), they are called **Bouchard nodes** (Figure 3.23).

Treatment

The goals of treatment for osteoarthritis are to reduce pain and inflammation and to limit or reverse the damage to the joint structures. These are accomplished in a number of different ways, depending on how advanced the condition is.

NSAIDs may be recommended for pain control, but many patients find that the risk of negative side effects outweigh their benefits. Topical applications of **counterirritant** ointments can be helpful. Exercise can address multiple goals by helping to maintain a healthy range of motion, increasing stamina, promoting weight loss, and improving the strength of muscles surrounding the affected joints. Nutritional supplements are sometimes recommended, including **glucosamine** and **chondroitin sulfate**. The research on their effectiveness is mixed and they do carry some risks of negative interactions with other substances, so they should be used with the advice of a primary care provider.

Arthroscopic procedures include injections of corticosteroids to reduce inflammation (this can be done only a few times a year), injection of substances to improve joint viscosity, aspiration of excess joint fluid, and joint **lavage** and **debridement** work to remove loose bits of cartilage (these are sometimes called "joint mice") and to smooth articulating surfaces.

Joint replacement surgery is addressed elsewhere in this chapter.

Medications

- NSAIDs, including Cox-2 inhibitors, for pain control
- Injected steroidal anti-inflammatories

Massage?

RISKS Acute inflammation contraindicates massage that promotes local circulation, but this is rare in osteoarthritis. As long as bodywork is well tolerated, it carries few risks for osteoarthritis patients.

BENEFITS Carefully performed massage, including general work that does not specifically focus on affected joints, has been seen to reduce pain and stiffness, and to improve function in osteoarthritis patients.

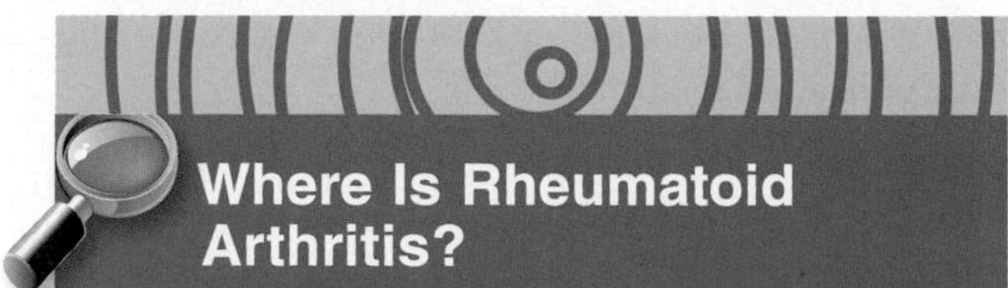

Where Is Rheumatoid Arthritis?

Rheumatoid arthritis is an autoimmune disorder in which the immune system mistakenly attacks structures in and around synovial joints, leading to inflammation and deformity. It now appears with several other autoimmune disease discussions in Chapter 6.

Patellofemoral Syndrome

Definition: What is It?

Patellofemoral syndrome (PFS) is a condition in which the patellar cartilage becomes irritated as it contacts the femoral cartilage. This situation can be a precursor of osteoarthritis.

PFS is almost always associated with overloading or overuse of the patellofemoral joint, although it may be precipitated by a specific injury or trauma. The term PFS used to be considered synonymous to **chondromalacia patellae**. The term chondromalacia is now reserved for fraying and chipping of the patellar cartilage, often because of a genetic weakness in the cartilage, rather than as an overuse problem. More current synonyms for PFS include jumper's knee,

Patellofemoral Syndrome in Brief

Pronunciation: pah-tel-o-FEM-or-al sin-drome

What is it?
Patellofemoral syndrome (PFS) is an overuse disorder that can lead to damage of the patellar cartilage.

How is it recognized?
PFS causes pain at the knee, stiffness after immobility, and discomfort in walking down stairs.

Massage risks and benefits
Risks: Massage carries no particular risks for PFS.
Benefits: If damage has already occurred to the patellar cartilage, massage is unlikely to reverse that process. However, both general and specific massage can help deal with discomfort and muscular tension that may develop when the knee is stiff and painful.

movie-goer's knee, anterior knee pain syndrome, and over utilization syndrome.

Etiology: What Happens?

When the knee is bent, whether or not it is bearing weight, the femur and the patella press together. Furthermore, the range of motion for the patella is broader than most people understand. This bone moves superiorly and inferiorly, but it can also move medially and laterally, and it can rotate or tip in any direction. If pressure is not evenly distributed across the back of the patella, disruptions to the patellar cartilage can occur. While this condition can be stopped or even reversed if it is caught early, long-term irritation can ultimately lead to permanent cartilage damage and osteoarthritis at the knee.

Two main issues have been identified as contributors to PFS: overuse or overloading, and poor alignment.

Overuse can be a result of percussive activities, especially with twisting and jumping. Overloading of the joint can occur even without repetitive percussive activity if the person is overweight.

Inefficient alignment at the knee can take many forms. Poor footwear or running on uneven surfaces can change how force moves up the leg into the knee. Flat feet, jammed arches, or problems in how the foot hits the ground can do the same thing. Unequal development of the medial and lateral quadriceps muscles is frequently identified; PFS almost always involves a lateral pull on the patella. Muscular imbalances between the quadriceps, hamstrings, and iliotibial band are factors. An exaggerated **Q-angle** is sometimes suggested as a factor in PFS, but this has not been reliably demonstrated as a factor.

Signs and Symptoms

Symptoms of PFS include pain that is usually felt on the anterior aspect of the knee, stiffness after long immobility, difficulty walking down stairs, and a characteristic crackling, grinding noise on movement called **crepitus**.

One of the issues that makes this condition challenging is that it can be difficult to distinguish from—and frequently occurs concurrently with—another condition: patellar tendinosis. This is significant because while PFS is largely unaffected by massage, patellar tendinosis may respond well, with a virtually pain-free resolution. Consequently, it is important to have a clear idea of what a client really has. One clue that is sometimes useful is that patellar tendinosis often hurts going up stairs (resisted extension of the leg) while PFS may hurt more going down stairs (the weight of the femur pushing on the patella).

Treatment

The best treatment options for PFS involve finding strategies to slow or stop the progression, while not becoming sedentary in the process. Running and jumping types of exercise may need to be replaced with swimming or cycling. Physical therapy often includes exercises to strengthen and balance tension in the muscles that cross the knee and that influence knee alignment. The quadriceps, hamstrings, tensor fascia latae, and deep lateral rotators are often addressed in the challenge to improve alignment and stop the progression of damage that PFS can cause.

Other interventions include ice, nonsteroidal anti-inflammatories for pain management, orthotics to improve alignment in the feet, and improved footwear. Some orthopedists recommend the use of a knee brace or sleeve to stabilize the patella, or special taping of the knee for the same purpose. If noninvasive options aren't sufficient, surgery might be recommended. This may be in the form of arthroscopy to smooth out the articular cartilage, or a procedure called a "lateral release" that detaches a portion of the lateral stabilizing ligaments from the patella.

Medications

- NSAIDs for pain management

Massage?

RISKS Massage carries no particular risk for a person with patellofemoral syndrome (PFS), but direct downward pressure on the patella may be irritating.

BENEFITS Bodywork aimed specifically at the knee, but also systemically, can help to address the tension, stiffness, and chronic low-grade pain that many people with PFS experience.

OPTIONS A good strategy might focus on equalizing tension on either side of the patella, and retraining the knee extensors to track the patella appropriately over the joint.

Spondylolisthesis

Definition: What Is It?

Spondylolisthesis is a condition in which a structural problem in the lumbar spine allows one or more vertebral bodies to slip anteriorly. This can involve tiny or large bone fractures, and put pressure on nerve roots at the intertransverse foramina, or on the spinal cord itself in the spinal canal. For more information on spine-related vocabulary, see sidebar 3.5.

Etiology: What Happens?

The facet joints in healthy lumbar vertebrae occur on an essentially coronal plane. The superior facets of one lumbar vertebra contact the front sides of the inferior facets of its upstairs neighbor; this prevents the higher bone from sliding forward.

A structural weak spot in lumbar vertebrae can be found at the **pars interarticularis**, which forms the bridge between the lamina and the pedicle. Sometimes the pars is underdeveloped, and tiny microfractures allow for the anterior portion of the vertebra to shift forward. Alternatively, if the orientation of the facets is on a sagittal plane, or if the pars interarticularis has to accommodate for extreme shearing forces, the bone may fracture, allowing the vertebral body to slide forward (Figure 3.24).

SIDEBAR 3.5 "Spondylo-" Tongue Twisters

The terminology used in the discussion of arthritis and stenosis in the spine can be puzzling. Here is a brief look at some of the most confusing terms:

- ***Spondylosis***. A general term for any degenerative condition of the vertebrae. This comes from the Greek root *spondylo-*, for *vertebra*.
- ***Spondylolysis.*** A specific defect in vertebrae, usually in the lumbar spine, that impairs the weight-bearing capacity of the bone. The word roots are *spondylo-* and *lysis, or loosening.*
- ***Spondylolisthesis***. An anterior displacement of the body of a lumbar vertebra onto its inferior vertebra or onto the sacrum. This is a combination of *spondylo-* and *olisthesis*, Greek for *slipping and falling.*

All three of these conditions can contribute to stenosis, or a narrowing of the spinal canal that may involve nerve pressure.

Spondylolisthesis in Brief

What is it?
Spondylolisthesis is a condition in which structural anomalies or injuries allow one or more lumbar vertebral bodies to slide forward.

How is it recognized?
Leading symptoms of spondylolisthesis include low back pain and spasm, tight hamstrings, radiating pain into the buttocks and thighs, and the possibility of some weakness in the affected dermatomes.

Massage risks and benefits
Risks: The main risk for a client with spondylolisthesis is that lying on a table in a mild state of low back extension may temporarily exacerbate low back pain. This is easily addressed with careful bolstering. Very extreme cases may indicate surgery, in which case massage is best left for the recovery period.
Benefits: Many people with spondylolisthesis experience chronic low back pain, paraspinal muscle spasm, and tight hamstrings. All these issues may be successfully managed with massage. Bodywork is unlikely to reverse this problem, but it can address many of its worst effects.

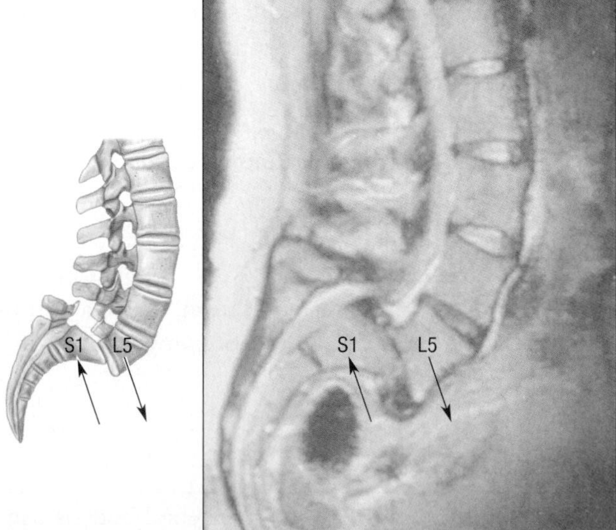

Figure 3.24. Spondylolisthesis

3 Musculoskeletal System Conditions

Tiny microfractures of the pars interarticularis can have several outcomes. They can essentially heal with a false joint that allows permanent hypermobility; they can grow a bony bridge that lengthens the vertebral arch; or the fibrous bands that extend between the edges of the injury may never fully calcify.

When it occurs in adolescents and young adults, spondylolisthesis is often associated with activities that involve repetitive twisting and back extension. Gymnasts, wrestlers, rowers, weightlifters, tennis players, and football players have a particularly high risk.

Types of Spondylolisthesis

- *Congenital spondylolisthesis*. This occurs when a person is born with facets that are oriented on a sagittal rather than coronal plane in the lumbar vertebrae. This may never cause a problem unless physical activity challenges the integrity of the facet joints.
- *Isthmic spondylolisthesis*. This involves a structural weakness at the pars interarticularis. While it may not create symptoms during childhood, adolescent growth spurts combined with athletic activities often create multiple microfractures of the bone, along with pain and loss of range of motion.
- *Degenerative spondylolisthesis*. This type is most common in women and men over 40 years old. Unlike other forms, it may not involve any damage to the vertebral arch. Instead, it may begin with arthritis at the facet joints along with disc thinning that allows supporting ligaments to slacken and destabilize the lumbar joints. Then the joint capsule stretches as the bone is shifted forward.
- *Traumatic spondylolisthesis* is a rare situation where an accident or trauma damages the pars interarticularis.
- *Pathologic spondylolisthesis*. This occurs as a complication of some other event. It could involve tumors from metastatic cancer, an infection in the bone or joint capsule, or complications of a previous spinal surgery.

Signs and Symptoms

Anterior slippage of the lumbar vertebral body is usually described by degree of severity:

Grade 1	1%–25% slippage
Grade 2	26%–50% slippage
Grade 3	51%–75% slippage
Grade 4	76%–100% slippage
Grade 5	100% or more slippage

Signs and symptoms of spondylolisthesis generally correspond to the severity of the vertebral displacement. Grade 1 or 2 slippages are by far the most common, and they are associated with central low back pain, tight hamstrings, spasm of the lumbar paraspinal muscles, and in some cases pain that radiates into the buttocks and thighs.

More severe cases may demonstrate a palpable shelf in the lumbar spine when the patient flexes the trunk. Nerve compression is more likely in this situation, which may result in pain, numbness, or weakness along the affected dermatomes. Rarely, the damage to the spine may result in pressure directly on the spinal cord, which leads to an emergency situation called **cauda equina syndrome**. This can cause permanent loss of bladder and bowel control as well as other complications, so it is important to deal with this as quickly as possible.

One problem with degenerative spondylolisthesis is that it often has a slow onset, and it affects a population (people over 40 years old) who may be at risk for other conditions that create a s imilar picture. The radiating pain and numbness that sometimes is seen with spondylolisthesis can easily be confused with symptoms of peripheral artery disease or peripheral neuropathy, and vice versa. These symptoms must be explored in order to be sure of their origin.

Treatment

The majority of spondylolisthesis cases can be treated with mild pain relievers, exercise to strengthen the abdominal muscles, and massage to ease back pain and hamstring tightness. Very severe cases involve a completely disrupted vertebral arch and may indicate surgery for correction and stabilization.

Medications

- Nonsteroidal anti-inflammatory drugs for pain management

Massage?

RISKS When a client's back is acutely painful, massage therapists must be careful not to exacerbate pain or inflammation. Any instability in the low back must be addressed with careful positioning. If symptoms include areas of numbness or reduced sensation, that needs to be pursued with a neurologist.

BENEFITS The chronic low back pain, paraspinal spasm, and tightness in the hamstrings that many spondylolisthesis patients experience can all be addressed with massage. Bodywork won't correct structural problems with the vertebrae, but it can be an effective way to deal with the symptoms.

OPTIONS Hyperextension of the back can be addressed by using bolsters under the abdomen and ankles when the client is prone, and under the knees when the client is supine.

Spondylosis in Brief

What is it?
Spondylosis is a form of degenerative arthritis that occurs in the spine.

How is it recognized?
Spondylosis is identifiable by radiography, which shows a characteristic thickening of the affected vertebral bodies, facets, and ligamentum flava. Symptoms are present only if pressure is exerted on nerve roots, causing pain, numbness, paresthesia, and specific muscle weakness. Otherwise, the only sign of spondylosis may be slow, progressive loss of range of motion in the spine.

Massage risks and benefits
Risks: Spondylosis can cause nerve impingement that is exacerbated by certain positions; clients with this condition must be positioned carefully to reduce the risk of nerve pressure.
Benefits: Massage is unlikely to reverse spondylosis, but it can be a strategy to address pain, stiffness, and general quality of life.

Spondylosis

Definition: What is It?

Spondylosis is a form of degenerative arthritis, involving age-related changes of the vertebrae, discs, joints, and ligaments of the spine.

Etiology: What Happens?

The section on osteoarthritis describes in some detail the changes that happen when damage occurs at synovial joints. Spondylosis has some features in common with osteoarthritis, but some important differences distinguish the two conditions.

The connections between the vertebral bodies and the intervertebral discs are not synovial joints, but they are vulnerable to some of the same problems that freely movable joints can develop. It can be a useful analogy to think of the vertebral bodies as articulating bones, the tough annulus fibrosus as a capsular ligament, and the softer gelatinous nucleus pulposus as the synovial fluid inside a joint. As the spine ages, especially if the connecting ligaments are lax or if the vertebrae are out of optimal alignment, shearing and compressive stresses can affect the joint. The disc thins and bone spurs may develop around the vertebral body or on the facet joints (Figures 3.25 and 3.26).

Spinal ostoephytes usually appear on the anterior or lateral aspects of the vertebral bodies but occasionally grow on the facets or in a place to put pressure on the nerve roots or spinal cord. Back and neck pain with spondylosis happens only when the growths put mechanical pressure on nerve roots or the spinal cord, and this occurs only when the foramen is significantly less than its normal size. This narrowing of the nerve space is called spinal stenosis.

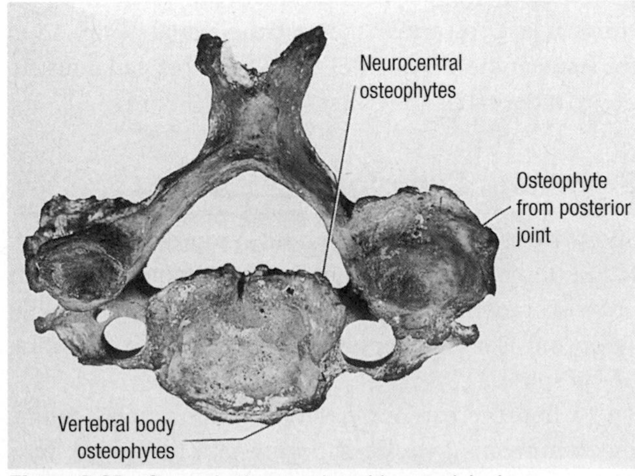

Figure 3.25. Osteophytic growths with spondylosis

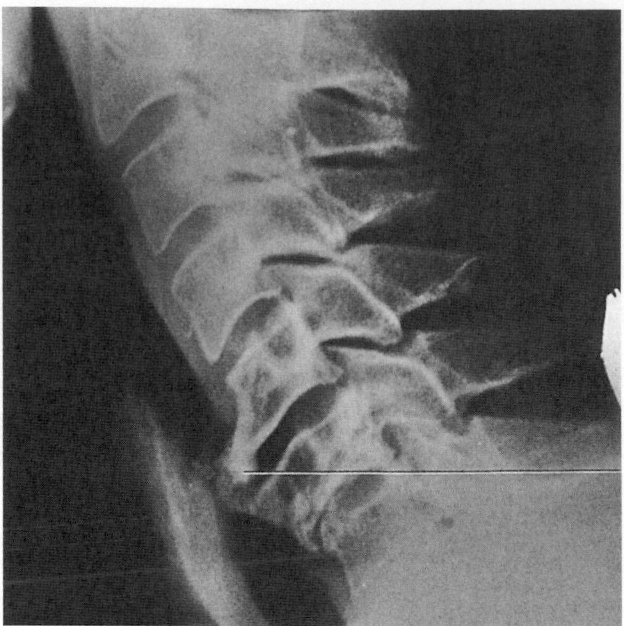

Figure 3.26. Fusion of vertebral bodies with spondylosis

In addition to excessive calcium deposits on vertebrae, advanced age may contribute to the ossification of the long vertical ligaments that stabilize the spine. The anterior longitudinal ligament runs on the anterior aspect of the vertebral bodies. **Diffuse idiopathic skeletal hyperostosis** is a common condition involving calcium deposits along this structure. This may be a major contributor to the gradual painless loss of range of motion that is frequently reported with spondylosis. The posterior longitudinal ligament runs along the posterior aspect of the vertebral bodies (on the anterior side of the spinal canal). Ossification may occur here as well; this carries a higher risk of spinal cord pressure. Finally, the **ligamentum flavum**, which runs on the posterior aspect of the spinal canal, often thickens and even buckles with age; this can contribute to stenosis that impinges the spinal cord.

Signs and Symptoms

Spondylosis often has no painful symptoms whatever. If the bony changes do not press on nerve roots but grow somewhere that impedes movement, the main symptom is slow, painless, but irreversible stiffening of the spine.

When the osteophytes do press on nerve roots, the symptoms include shooting pain, tingling, pins and needles, numbness, and muscle weakness only in muscles supplied by the affected nerve. If the pressure is on the spinal cord, symptoms are bilateral and may include loss of bladder or bowel control.

One distinguishing feature of nerve pressure from osteophytes is that the pain is absolutely consistent; if the bone spurs are in a place to create pain when a person is in a certain position or posture, then that pain is predictable and tends to get worse over time instead of better.

Complications

Spondylosis is a slowly progressing condition that mostly affects middle-aged and elderly people. Usually it is not dangerous, but it can have some serious complications.

- *Spreading problems in the spine.* This is not a progressive disease that travels through the blood or lymph, but if two vertebrae become fused through bony remodeling, that puts much more stress on the joints above and below the fusion to provide mobility. Those joints can become unstable, develop arthritis, and undergo the same bony remodeling that created the first problem. Alternatively, the stress of hypermobility may cause disc problems. Disc disease can be both a predisposing factor and a complication of spondylosis.
- *Nerve pain.* This is the consequence of having osteophytes grow where they can put pressure on nerve roots in the foramina.
- *Secondary spasm.* This accompanies nerve pain. Muscle spasm may be confined to the paraspinals, where it exacerbates the problem by compressing the affected joints, or it may follow the path of referred pain. Muscles may also work to protect the spine from movement that would otherwise be excruciatingly painful.
- *Blood vessel pressure.* Osteophytes in the neck sometimes press on the vertebral arteries as they go up the transverse foramina. If the head is turned or extended in a certain position, the patient may feel dizzy or have headaches or double vision from impaired blood flow into the head.
- *Spinal cord pressure.* This is an extremely serious complication of spondylosis in the neck. Osteophytes may grow in a location to put pressure not on the nerve roots but in the spinal cord itself, a condition called **cervical spondylitic myelopathy**. This is felt as progressive

weakening down the body, possible loss of bladder and bowel control, and even eventual paralysis.

Treatment

Treatment for spondylosis depends on which complications are present. Anti-inflammatories and pain control are the usual first recourse. Movement, bracing, and exercise can limit progression once the damage has begun. Massage, acupuncture, and hydrotherapy are often recommended before more intrusive steps are tried.

If noninvasive measures are insufficient, local injections of steroids can provide temporary relief. A variety of surgeries can create more space for nerve roots or the spinal cord. These often involve spinal fusions, however, and they work best for younger patients who have not been having arthritic symptoms for a long time or in more than one joint.

Medications

- NSAIDs for pain control
- Narcotic or opioid drugs (Vicodin, Percocet) for pain control if NSAIDs are not sufficient
- Muscle relaxants for spasm
- Antiseizure drugs for paresthesia
- Injected steroidal anti-inflammatories

Massage?

RISKS The main risk for clients with spondylosis is that careless positioning may allow bone spurs to put pressure on nerves. Also, muscles that surround affected areas may be hypertonic for good reason: they could be protecting the spine from movement that may be painful.

BENEFITS Massage can help reduce pain and stiffness, and improve the general quality of life for clients with spondylosis—as long as general cautions for frailty and positioning are observed.

Sprains

Definition: What Are They?

Sprains are tears to ligaments, the fibrous connective tissue strapping tape that links bone to bone throughout the body.

Sprains in Brief

What are they?
Sprains are injured ligaments. Injuries can range in severity from a few traumatized fibers to a complete rupture.

How are they recognized?
In the acute stage pain, redness, heat, swelling, and loss of joint function are evident. Later these symptoms are less extreme, although perhaps not entirely absent. Passive stretching of the affected ligament is painful until all inflammation has subsided.

Massage risks and benefits
Risks: Acutely inflamed sprains locally contraindicate intrusive work until the inflammation has subsided, but lymphatic work to decrease edema may be safe and appropriate. Sprains can sometimes mask symptoms of minor fractures; if symptoms are not significantly relieved within a few days, this possibility should be pursued with a medical professional.
Benefits: Damaged ligaments that are not acutely inflamed respond well to specific massage along with passive stretching and full use within pain tolerance.

Etiology: What Happens?

The traditional image of ligament tissue has been that it is composed mostly of linearly arranged collagen fibers, invested with a few fibroblasts, with the function of linking bone to bone. Research has revealed that ligaments are highly invested with sensory neurons, many of which are proprioceptors that help to control the function of nearby muscles. This understanding has created new strategies in dealing with ligament injuries and the accompanying muscle adaptations that they inevitably involve.

Dense fibrous structures like ligaments are injured when some of their fibers are stretched or ripped. The severity of the injury depends on what percentage of the fibers is affected. First-degree injuries involve just a few fibers, second-degree injuries are much worse, and third-degree injuries are ruptures: the entire structure has been ripped through (Figure 3.27).

Injury to ligaments triggers the rapid production of new collagen fibers. These are laid down in a haphazard mass early in the healing process. Then the perfect combination of movement, stretching, and weight-bearing stress in the maturation phase of recovery helps to reorient the fibers in alignment with

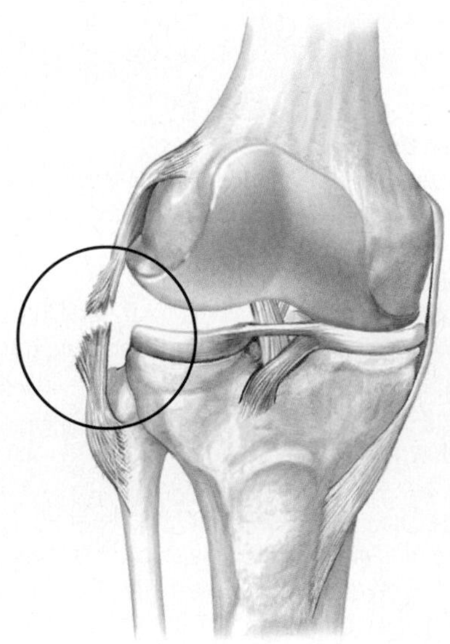

Figure 3.27. Third degree sprain: ligament rupture

the uninjured structure. If this happens in the best possible way, the new scar tissue seamlessly blends with the uninjured portions of the ligament. But if a new injury is immobilized and kept from movement, the scar tissue may become dense and contracted, pulling on all the healthy fibers nearby and significantly hampering the weight-bearing capacity of the ligament. This situation can involve chronic, low-grade inflammation that slowly degrades the whole structure.

A few things distinguish sprains from strains and tendon injuries, which are discussed in other sections.

- *Ligament structure*. The dense linear arrangement of collagen fibers in ligaments affords little stretch and almost no rebound. Further, the mechanics of ligament construction makes them vulnerable to injury under special circumstances: a sudden snap with no warming up, or a prolonged but extreme stretch after activity can injure fibers. If a ligament becomes loose, it cannot stabilize the joint as well as it did before the injury. This ligament laxity contributes to chronic injury-reinjury situations and is a factor to the risk of osteoarthritis.
- *Severity*. Sprains are more serious than strains and tendinosis. Because tendons and muscles tend to be more elastic and less densely arranged than ligaments, they stretch before a ligament does. Furthermore, ligaments don't have the same rich blood supply as muscles, and they are denser than tendons. Consequently, they don't have the same access to circulation, which makes them heal slower than muscles or tendons.
- *Swelling*. With a few exceptions, acute sprains swell much more than muscle strains or tendinosis; this is one way to differentiate between injuries. Swelling is a protective measure that recruits the body's healing resources and limits movement, which prevents further injury. Ligaments are often contiguous with the joint capsules of the joints they cross over, so an injury to them may signal the joint to swell too. Ligaments that are not attached to joint capsules swell much less than those that are.

Signs and Symptoms

Acute sprains show the usual signs of inflammation: pain, heat, redness, and swelling, along with loss of function because rapid swelling splints the unstable joint and makes it extremely painful to move. Inflamed ligaments are especially painful with passive stretches of the structure.

An acute sprain may mask the symptoms of a bone fracture, especially in the foot. This is important to clarify because the treatment and activity recommendations for sprains and fractures are very different.

In the subacute stage, signs of inflammation may still be present, but the joint begins to regain function. The physiological processes are no longer geared toward blood clotting and damage control; they have shifted toward clearing out debris and rebuilding torn fibers.

The amount of time that passes between acute and subacute stages varies with the severity of the injury, but 24 to 48 hours are typical. However, some injuries waver back and forth between acute and subacute, especially in response to overuse or intrusive massage.

Sprains can happen at almost any synovial joint, but the anterior talofibular ligament of the ankle is the most commonly sprained ligament in the body. Ligaments overlying the sacroiliac joint are also very commonly injured, as are various ligaments around the knees and fingers.

Treatment

At one time, the recommendation for treating a sprain suggested soaking it in hot water and casting it to immobilize it during healing. Clearly, this was counterproductive: heat increases edema and the accumulation of scar tissue, while immobilization prevents the new fibers from aligning with the rest of the structure.

These days RICE therapy (rest, ice, compression, elevation) is considered the norm, with an emphasis on moving the joint within range of pain tolerance as soon as possible. The potential benefits are clear: ice keeps edema at bay, limiting further tissue damage from ischemia. Compression does the same. Elevation also encourages lymph flow out of an already congested area. Orthopedic specialists sometimes recommend adding protection in the form of taping or a brace, and modalities that may include ultrasound, exercise, and proprioceptive training to reduce the risk of a recurrence of injury.

Medications

- NSAIDs for pain and inflammation

Massage?

RISKS Massage other than lymphatic work is not appropriate in the area of an acute sprain. Sprains that are not significantly better within a few days may be complicated by a bone fracture; this must be pursued with another medical professional.

BENEFITS Massage can be extremely helpful for subacute or mature sprains. It can address poor-quality scar tissue and muscle holding around affected joints for improved local nutrition and efficiency of movement.

OPTIONS Specific work on affected ligaments is appropriate in subacute or postacute situations: with-fiber and crossfiber friction may be used, along with any variety of pin-and-stretch techniques that may work to improve mobility and work with proprioceptive affect on muscles.

Temporomandibular Joint Disorder

Definition: What is It?

TMJ disorder is an umbrella term that can refer to a multitude of common problems in and around the jaw. This collection of signs and symptoms is usually associated with malocclusion (a dysfunctional bite), **bruxism** (teeth grinding), and loose ligaments surrounding the jaw. These issues can lead to excessive movement between the temporal and mandible, damage to the internal cartilage, and possible dislocation of the joint. TMJ disorder is sometimes referred to as TMD: **t**emporo**m**andibular joint **d**isorder. TMJ disorders occur mostly in people between 30 and 50 years old, and women diagnosed with this disorder outnumber men about 4:1.

Temporomandibular Joint Disorder in Brief

What is it?
Temporomandibular joint (TMJ) disorder describes any problem that causes pain and loss of function at the TMJ.

How is it recognized?
Symptoms of TMJ disorder include pain in the head, neck, shoulder, ear, and/or mouth; clicking or locking in the jaw; and loss of range of motion of the jaw.

Massage risks and benefits
Risks: TMJ disorders can be difficult to diagnose, and they can resemble several other problems that require different treatment options; massage therapists working with clients who have long-lasting symptoms need to be careful about getting an accurate diagnosis.
Benefits: Massage can be useful for a client with TMJ disorder at any stage, but especially if the intervention occurs before permanent bone or cartilage damage develops.

Etiology: What Happens?

The temporomandibular joint is like none other in the body. Far from being a simple hinge joint, the TMJ allows the mandible to move up, down, forward, back, and side to side. The jaw is unusually mobile, as the joint capsule actually stretches with the position of the mouth (Figure 3.28). A fibrocartilage disc cushions the temporal bone as it contacts the condyle of the mandible, but this disc is sometimes pulled awry or injured, which can lead to problems in the joint (see video online). Furthermore, the muscles that work together to control jaw movement during chewing and speech are particularly prone to developing trigger points, which can refer

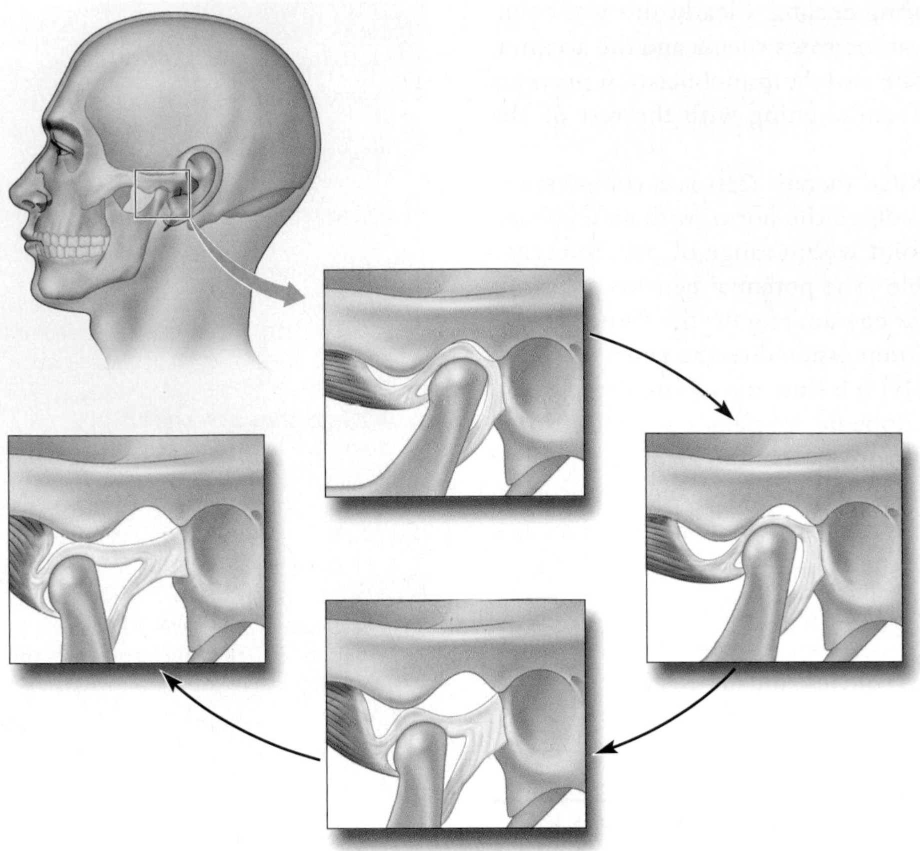

Figure 3.28. The TMJ allows great mobility as the jaw protracts

pain into the jaw, the face, over the head, and into the neck. The tension in the muscles of mastication (the masseter, the medial and lateral pterygoids, and the temporalis among others) can be both a symptom and trigger of TMJ disorders.

TMJ disorders are often categorized as three issues, but overlap can occur between these factors:

- *Myofascial pain*. Trigger points in the jaw muscles can refer pain to the face, head, and neck.
- *Internal derangement*. The cartilaginous disc or other structures may be abnormal or damaged.
- *Osteoarthritis*. Progressive wear and tear at the jaw can lead to permanent remodeling of the joint (Figure 3.29).

TMJ problems are often circular—that is, the factors that cause TMJ disorders can also be the symptoms. In this way, tight muscles can lead to pain and tissue damage, which can lead to arthritis at the jaw, which reinforces muscle tightening. Rheumatoid arthritis occasionally occurs here, but osteoarthritis is a far more frequent contributor to TMJ problems. Other factors include misalignment of the bite and congenital malformations of the bones.

When the highly specialized joints at the jaw undergo chronic misalignment, trauma, or muscle tension, a person may find it difficult to open or close

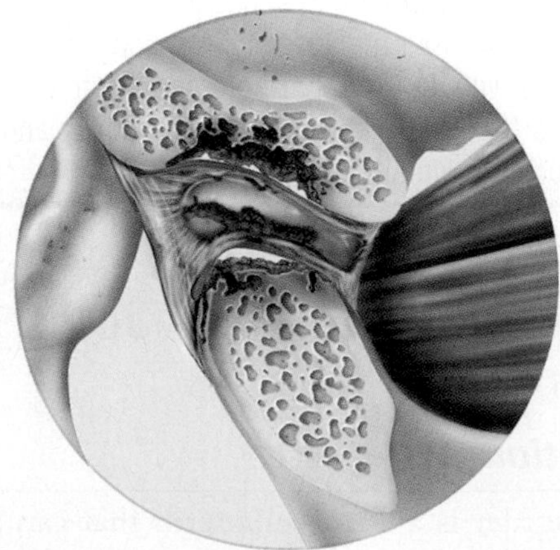

Figure 3.29. TMJ disorder: damage to the disc and articulating bones

the mouth without pain. Chewing and swallowing become problematic, and pain in the jaw can reverberate systemically throughout the body.

Signs and Symptoms

The signs and symptoms of TMJ disorders are as follows:

- *Jaw, neck, and shoulder pain.* This can be from deterioration of bony structures inside the capsule (arthritis), or it can be local and referred pain generated by tight, trigger point–laden muscles.
- *Limited range of motion.* Deformation or displacement of the cartilage inside the joint can make it difficult or impossible to open the mouth all the way, or to move through a normal range of protraction, retraction, and side-to-side action.
- *Popping, clicking in the jaw.* This is usually attributed to having the disc or bone out of alignment, which interferes in jaw opening.
- *Locking of the joint.* Again, this is a result of having the fibrocartilage disc interfere with normal joint movement.
- *Grinding teeth (bruxism).* Like many issues with this disorder, this symptom is also a possible cause of the problem. Chronically shortened jaw elevators contribute to clenching and grinding of teeth, especially during sleep, when the joint should be as relaxed as possible.
- *Ear pain.* Because of the location of the joint, pressure may be exerted directly on the eustachian tubes. Symptoms in this case include a feeling of stuffiness in the ears, and loss of hearing or tinnitus.
- *Headaches.* These can also be related to the enormous pressure translated through the teeth to the cranium, to trigger points of muscles in spasm, and to cervical subluxation.
- *Chronic misalignment of cervical vertebrae.* This is probably a result of the muscular hypertonicity that is generated by this problem. As pain refers from the jaw to the neck and shoulders, the muscles there tighten up and pull asymmetrically on the neck bones. No matter how often the neck is adjusted or how brilliantly the neck muscles are massaged, this pain-spasm cycle is unlikely to resolve until the jaw situation is addressed.

Treatment

Several other injuries have similarities with TMJ disorder, and part of successful treatment is ruling these out. A short list includes **Ernest syndrome** (a sprain of a nearby ligament); trigeminal neuralgia, occipital neuralgia, and osteomyelitis, perhaps from an infected tooth.

Once a conclusive diagnosis is made, treatment options are typically divided into nonsurgical and surgical options. Nonsurgical options include applying heat or cold to painful areas, physical therapy, ultrasound and massage for jaw muscles, anti-inflammatories, and local anesthetics. Special splints that reduce bone-to-bone pressure may be prescribed. **Proliferant** injections to tighten the ligaments that surround the jaw may also be effective. If these noninvasive techniques are successful, the TMJ disorder may be averted before permanent bony distortion or cartilage damage inside the joint occurs.

NOTABLE CASES A punch to the jaw radically affected actor Burt Reynolds' quality of life. Wracked by pain, he didn't work for 3 years. He lost about 50 lb because he couldn't eat solid foods. A long, slow recovery brought him out of this disability, but he was severely affected by this injury.

If these are not satisfactory, surgeries for TMJ disorder range from an outpatient procedure in which scar tissue and adhesions are cleared out or dissolved with injections into the joint, to arthroscopic surgery to manipulate the cartilage, to full prosthetic joint replacement.

Medications

- NSAIDs for pain and inflammation
- Steroidal anti-inflammatories, including injections into the joint
- Tricyclic antidepressants for pain, stress
- Muscle relaxants
- Botulinum toxin injections to temporarily paralyze jaw-clenching muscles (this has not been approved by the FDA, but some specialists use it)

Massage?

RISKS Not all jaw pain is caused by TMJ disorder, and it is important to have an accurate diagnosis for the best outcome. Some of the disorders that mimic TMJ disorder contraindicate massage in certain circumstances.

BENEFITS Massage can help reduce muscle tone, resolve trigger points, and improve client awareness of bruxism and other habits, all of which can improve the outlook for a person with TMJ disorder.

OPTIONS Intraoral massage to the pterygoid muscles can be a successful part of TMJ disorder treatment, especially combined with specific work to address other jaw and neck muscles.

Fascial Disorders

Compartment Syndrome

Definition: What Is It?

Compartment syndrome is a condition in which an injury or repetitive stress creates pressure inside a tight fascial compartment that can lead to the starvation and death of muscle and nerve cells.

Etiology: What Happens?

Two forces operate to maintain fluid balance within tight fascial compartments, especially in the lower leg: tissue pressure (which is partly determined by the rate and volume of incoming fluid) and **perfusion pressure** (which describes the ratio of blood in the arteries compared to that in the veins within an enclosed space). When tissue pressure rises above perfusion pressure, then fluid enters the capsule, but the usual delivery system to move it out is compromised. The result is a vicious circle: fluid pours into the area, but cannot leave because exit routes are compressed; starving and damaged cells release proinflammatory chemicals that boost capillary permeability, and attract and retain more fluid (Figure 3.30). Eventually permanent damage may occur, including the death of muscle and nerve cells, and toxic levels of cellular debris in the bloodstream that could lead to renal failure and death.

Compartment Syndrome in Brief

What is it?
Compartment syndrome is a situation in which a fascial compartment is under so much pressure that oxygen and nutrients can no longer reach cells. It can be acute, which is a medical emergency, or chronic and less severe. It usually happens in the lower leg, but can occur in any fascially contained space.

How is it recognized?
Acute compartment syndrome usually follows a trauma (a crushing injury, arterial damage, a long bone fracture). It is extremely painful, especially when tissues are passively stretched, and patients often report a tight, full feeling.

Chronic compartment syndrome is typically connected to a specific repetitive athletic activity. Cramping, pain, weakness, and numbness are all possible symptoms. Exercise makes it worse, but symptoms subside when the activity is suspended.

Massage risks and benefits
Risks: Any modality that manipulates soft tissues during an acute phase of compartment syndrome may make a bad situation worse by drawing more fluid to an area that is already impacted.
Benefits: Massage and stretching (or both simultaneously) may help to delay the onset of pain with chronic compartment syndrome. Massage may also be an effective preventive measure for athletes at risk for this condition.

Types of Compartment Syndrome

Compartment syndrome usually affects one of the four fascial compartments of the lower leg, but it has been seen in other areas, including compartments of the foot, hand, forearm, buttocks, and abdomen. A special variant on the phenomenon of fluid-compressed nerves is seen in the lateral thigh with a condition called **meralgia parasthetica**: this version is usually related to weight gain, tight-fitting clothing, or seatbelt injury.

- *Acute compartment syndrome*. This describes a sudden onset of massive swelling within an enclosed space. It is usually due to a crushing injury, a closed long bone fracture, or a penetrating injury that damages an artery (a gunshot or stab wound, for instance). Burns and venomous bites or stings can trigger this reaction, and it can also happen if arterial circulation is

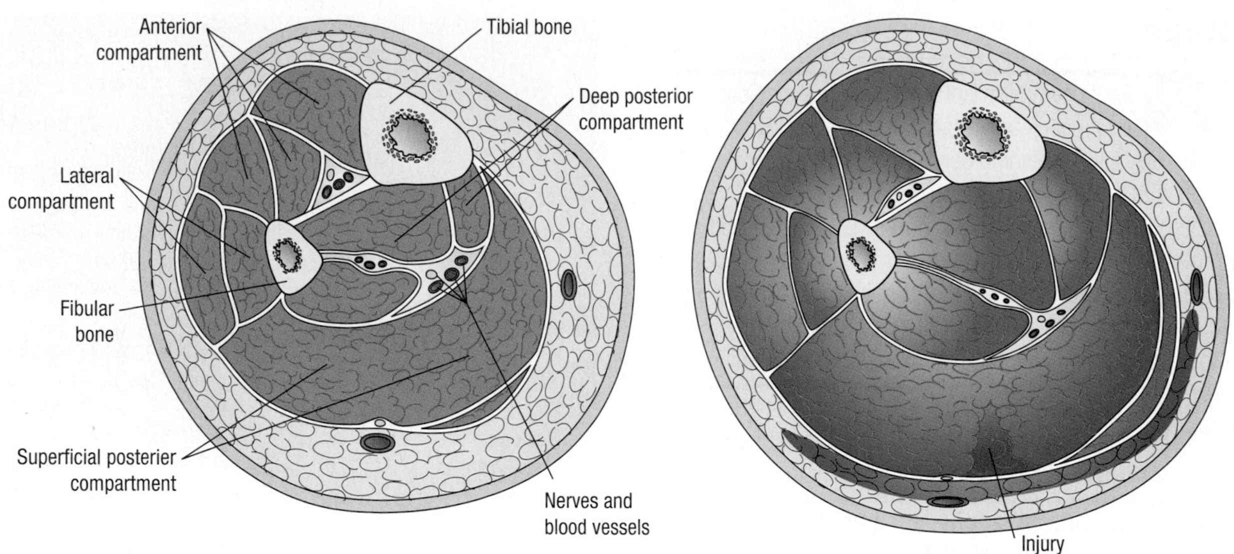

Figure 3.30. Compartment syndrome: injury-related inflammation compresses soft tissues and may lead to serious damage

compressed and then suddenly restored: this is an occasional complication of surgery.

- *Chronic compartment syndrome.* This is a much less serious condition that is usually related to repetitive athletic activity. Also called exertional compartment syndrome, this describes a situation in which the increased circulation and normal muscle expansion that happens with exercise overwhelms the body's capacity to maintain proper fluid pressures within a fascial capsule. Chronic compartment syndrome may often be considered when an athlete complains of shin splint symptoms.

Signs and Symptoms

Acute compartment syndrome is usually related to some clear trauma, but in rare cases, it can arise from intense exercise, or even from no discernable cause. It involves pain that is out of proportion to the extent of the injury; this is often described as "tight" or "burning" pain. Passive stretching of the tissues is especially painful. The area is hot and hard to the touch.

Chronic compartment syndrome is almost always a response to a repetitive athletic activity, and the symptoms may include pain, cramping, weakness, numbness, and changes in gait. Symptoms develop during exercise, and subside when activity stops. However, many people report that this condition is progressive: it takes less and less exercise to elicit symptoms, and pain lingers for longer and longer afterwards.

Treatment

Compartment syndrome of any kind is typically diagnosed with an instrument called a **tonometer**: this uses a needle to penetrate targeted muscles and measure internal pressure. In acute cases, this is self-evident, but for chronic compartment syndrome, measures are taken at rest and immediately after exercise. If that pressure is reliably higher than 30 to 45 mm Hg, intervention is suggested, usually in the form of a **fasciotomy**: a surgical split of the affected fascial sheath to relieve internal pressure. Hyperbaric oxygen and drugs to support kidney health may also be recommended. Acute compartment syndrome is so extreme that if surgery is not performed within a few hours of the trauma, the patient may experience permanent loss of function, amputation, or potentially life-threatening kidney damage from debris released by dying muscle cells.

A person with chronic compartment syndrome may also consider surgical release of the fascial sheath, but obviously this is not a medical emergency. Before reaching this point, patients are usually counseled to try orthotics or improving footwear, to stretch carefully, to warm up and cool down appropriately around exercise, to use massage (which has been shown to delay the onset of symptoms but not to affect the pressure within internal compartments), and to add more variety to the exercise they do.

Medications

- For chronic compartment syndrome: anti-inflammatories to manage swelling and pain

Massage?

RISKS Acute compartment syndrome is a medical emergency and must be treated quickly to avoid potentially life-threatening complications. Any client presenting with these signs needs to be referred out immediately. Chronic compartment syndrome may respond well to massage when it is not active or irritated, but when the client is in pain, manipulating affected tissues with anything but the lightest touch is likely simply to interfere with the body's ability to compensate for increasing compartmental pressure.

BENEFITS Chronic compartment syndrome in the lower leg may respond well to massage as a strategy to prevent or delay the onset of pain.

OPTIONS In acute situations, it is important to secure medical care as soon as possible.

Because the fascial compartments in the lower leg are so dense and inelastic, and because the normal range of motion at the tibiotalar joint prevents extensive stretching, massage with a "pin and pump" approach to the anterior and posterior lower leg muscles can be a powerful way to engage those muscles in preparation for activity, or as a postexercise protocol.

If the leg is in a flared-up stage of chronic compartment syndrome, lymph drainage modalities may be useful to help move fluid appropriately through the area.

Dupuytren Contracture

Definition: What is It?

This condition, also called palmar fasciitis, is an idiopathic thickening and shrinking of the palmar fascia that limits the movement of the fingers. Usually, the ring and little fingers are most severely affected, although the index and middle fingers may also be bent.

NOTABLE CASES Some of the best-known people affected by Dupuytren contracture include US President Ronald Reagan, British Prime Minister Margaret Thatcher, playwright Samuel Beckett, and actors Bill Nighy and David McCallum

Dupuytren contracture is most common among middle-aged white men of Northern European descent. Statistically, it is seen most often along with physical labor that involves vibration, smoking, alcohol use, and type I and type II diabetes.

Etiology: What Happens?

It is unclear exactly what begins the fascial changes seen with Dupuytren contracture. Local ischemia appears to trigger a sequence of events leading to the production of free radicals, which then stimulate the proliferation of myofibroblasts. These cells produce type III collagen (normal palmar fascia is composed mainly of type I collagen), and the myofibroblasts both contract, and form crosslinks with the collagen fibers. As the condition progresses, the collagen thickens and toughens, leaving tight, thick bands of connective tissue that interfere with the use of the hand.

Flexion of the fingers is normal for patients with Dupuytren contracture, but they cannot extend their fingers normally (Figure 3.31). When the extension is limited by 30 degrees or more, patients are considered to be candidates for corrective surgery. People with the most severe presentations are sometimes also

Dupuytren Contracture in Brief

Pronunciation: du-pwe-TRON kon-TRAK-chur

What is it?
Dupuytren contracture is an idiopathic shrinking and thickening of the fascia on the palm of the hand.

How is it recognized?
This is a painless condition that usually affects the ring and little fingers, pulling them into permanent flexion.

Massage risks and benefits
Risks: Massage has no particular risks for Dupuytren contracture as long as it is performed within limits for pain tolerance.
Benefits: Massage may be useful to slow the progression of this disease, or to help with the development of healthy and functional scar tissue post surgery.

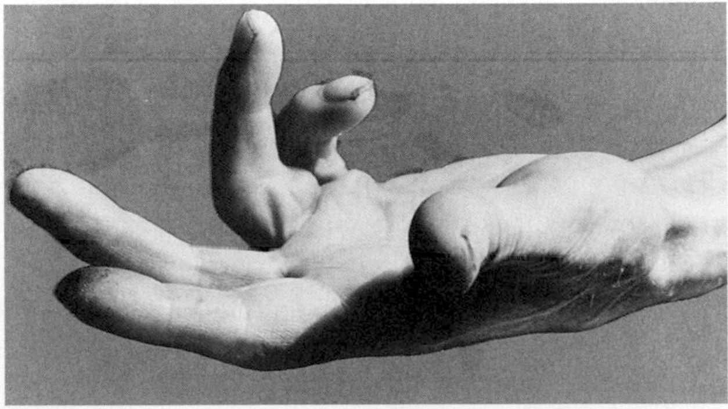

Figure 3.31. Dupuytren contracture

susceptible to other fascial restrictions elsewhere in the body, as discussed below.

Types of Dupuytren Contracture

- *Plantar fibromatosis* (Ledderhose disease). This is essentially the same as Dupuytren contracture, but it develops on the plantar aspect of the foot.
- *Peyronie disease*. This is a condition in which scar tissue develops under the skin of the shaft of the penis.
- *Knuckle pads* (Garrod nodes). These are deposits of connective tissue at the interphalangeal joints of the hands.

Signs and Symptoms

The typical pattern of Dupuytren contracture is that a middle-aged man develops a mildly tender or painless bump just proximal to his ring finger on the palmar aspect of the hand. Over months or years, the nodule extends into a cord in his palm and out to the PIP joint. The little finger might develop a cord as well. The fingers are slowly drawn toward the palm, and they can't be straightened out. Dupuytren contracture is bilateral in almost half of cases, although one side is usually more extremely affected than the other.

This condition may be mildly painful in early stages, but then often becomes painless. It is usually slowly progressive, although some people have a relatively fast onset. Some people have only the growth of tough, fibrous bumps on their hands, while others end up with severely bent, strangulated, unusable fingers. If the constriction to nerve and blood supply is very severe, the affected fingers may be amputated.

Treatment

If Dupuytren contracture is treated before too much atrophy occurs, corticosteroid injections can be effective to limit progression. Injections of **collagenase**, an enzyme that dissolves collagen, is another option, and release of the cord by way of tiny punctures (**needle aponeurotomy**) is a procedure with little risk of complications.

Surgical intervention is generally not recommended until fingers become bent and too stiff to move. At that point, the surgery involves making several zig-zag cuts in the palm to release the fascia, followed by skin grafts, physical therapy, and massage to limit the growth of scar tissue. Even when surgery is successful, Dupuytren contracture recurs in about one-third of cases.

Medications

- Corticosteroid injection at the site of connective tissue overgrowth
- Enzyme injection at the site of connective tissue overgrowth

Massage?

RISKS If nerves have been damaged, sensation could be impaired in the hand, and this requires special care. Steroid injections may alter the strength of the fascia, which may require adjustments in the intensity of treatment. Otherwise, massage within a client's pain tolerance has no specific contraindications for Dupuytren contracture.

BENEFITS As long as sensation is intact, massage may be helpful in slowing the progression of Dupuytren contracture, or in supporting the growth of healthy functional scar tissue after surgery.

Ganglion Cysts

Definition: What Are They?

Ganglion cysts are small connective tissue pouches filled with fluid that grow on joint capsules or tendinous sheaths. They usually appear on the wrist, the hand, or the top of the foot, but they have been found elsewhere as well. Ganglion cysts are found in women about three times more often than men.

Etiology: What Happens?

A ganglion cyst is essentially a connective tissue pouch filled with a viscous fluid. Cysts may have a single chamber, but many have multiple lobes that are connected by tiny channels. Experts suggest that they are related to a chronic degeneration of fascia, leading to proliferation of collagen and other substances.

Ganglion cysts are not inherently dangerous, but they can grow in places that interfere with function. This can lead to pain and a loss of range of motion,

Ganglion Cysts in Brief

Pronunciation: GANG-le-on sists

What are they?
Ganglion cysts are small fluid-filled sacs that are attached to tendinous sheaths or joint capsules.

How are they recognized?
Ganglion cysts form small bumps that usually appear on the hand, wrist, or ankle. They are not usually painful, unless they are in a place to be irritated by frequent activities.

Massage risks and benefits
Risks: Friction or pressure directly on a cyst may be irritating; these growths locally contraindicate specific massage.
Benefits: Massage has no specific effect on ganglion cysts; clients with this condition can enjoy the same benefits from bodywork as the rest of the population.

among other problems. They usually grow on the wrist (Figure 3.32), hand, or foot, but have been found in many other locations.

One type of ganglion cyst is called a mucous cyst. This grows on the distal interphalangeal joint, usually of older people with osteoarthritis at the same joints. Mucous cysts can damage the joint capsule or distort the growth of the fingernail.

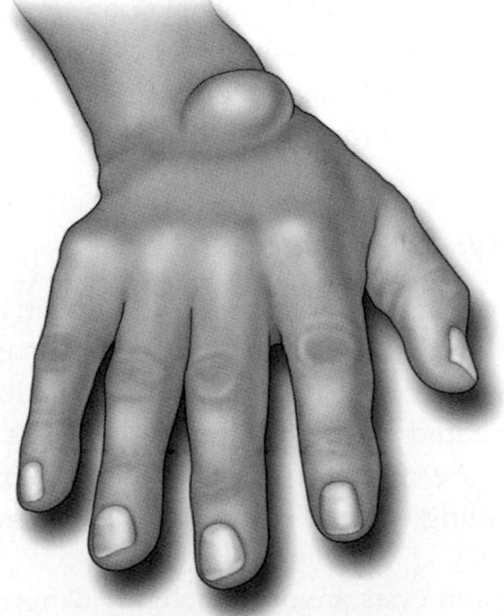

Figure 3.32. Ganglion cyst

Signs and Symptoms

Ganglion cysts may be too small to notice, or they may grow nearly to the size of a tennis ball, obstructing joint function and interfering with normal range of motion. They may have a gradual or sudden onset. Most ganglion cysts are not painful, except when they grow in places where they can be easily irritated, such as on the fingers and around the wrists. This can put them in a state of chronic irritation, and it can be difficult for them to subside spontaneously.

Treatment

Generally, the treatment for ganglion cysts is to leave them alone: they often resolve without interference. They may be aspirated to relieve internal pressure, but they often grow back. The traditional home remedy for ganglion cysts used to be to smash them with a Bible. Patients are not advised to use this option, however, as smashing a ganglion cyst with a book or any other heavy object can obviously cause a lot of other soft tissue damage.

Cysts may be excised through open surgery or arthroscopy if they are big enough to be a significant problem. If they grow back, they are usually not as large as the original cyst.

Massage?

RISKS While massage is unlikely to rupture a cyst, deep specific work in the area may be irritating. Of course, undiagnosed bumps need to be evaluated by a primary provider.

BENEFITS Bodywork is not likely to improve a client's ganglion cyst, but massage elsewhere is safe and appropriate: these clients can enjoy the same benefits from massage as the rest of the population.

Hammertoe

Definition: What is It?

Hammertoe is a foot deformity that affects the lateral toes. The second toe is most commonly affected, especially when this digit is longer than the great toe. In this situation, the muscles and tendons that cross the foot joints become permanently shortened. The result is hyperextension at the metacarpal-phalangeal

Hammertoe in Brief

What is it?
Hammertoe is a type of foot deformity that affects the lateral toes.

How is it recognized?
Hammertoe involves a characteristic contracture that puts the proximal interphalangeal joint into flexion, and both the metatarsal-phalangeal and the distal interphalangeal joints into hyperextension. It can be passively flexible, or completely rigid.

Massage risks and benefits
Risks: This condition can involve acute and painful inflammation; any massage or manipulation that exacerbates this should be avoided.
Benefits: If the condition is treated while tissues are still soft and malleable, and other environmental factors are changed, massage with stretching and support could help to slow the progression of a hammertoe situation. Massage may also help with postural or gait distortions.

joint and distal interphalangeal joint, and flexion at the proximal interphalangeal joint, (Figure 3.33).

Closely related deformities include claw-toe (with flexion at both interphalangeal joints), mallet toe (with flexion only at the DIP), and curly toe (with flexion at all interphalangeal joints).

Etiology: What Happens?

Hammertoe and other toe problems are multifactoral conditions. They are seen most often in people with second toes that are longer than the great toe, and they occur frequently along with bunions and pes cavus. The main contributing factor is usually footwear that causes the second toe to curl over, but other issues include the use of high heels that force pressure onto the long second toe, trauma, underlying disease (diabetes, rheumatoid arthritis, and osteoarthritis are sometimes seen with hammertoe), and a genetic predisposition for this condition to develop, as seen with Charcot-Marie Tooth syndrome.

Hammertoe is a progressive condition. It generally starts with an involuntary contracture as the normal balance between toe flexors and extensors is lost, but the tissues are soft and malleable. It gradually becomes rigid as the connective tissues thicken and shrink around the contracted muscles.

Signs and Symptoms

The primary signs of hammertoe and other toe problems include a visible deformity, involuntary contraction of the foot muscles, and pain where the toe is irritated by friction. This often results in corns or callus on the dorsal aspect of the toe joints, where they rub against shoes. Left untreated, this can lead to open sores and the risk of infection.

Hammertoe in its early stages can be flexible, but it becomes progressively more rigid over time.

Treatment

Changing footwear, using pads to treat corns and callus, orthotics, and using tape or splints to straighten toes are the first recommendations for a person with hammertoe. Some specialists may suggest steroid injections for inflammation and to address connective tissue thickness. If these are insufficient, surgery may be recommended. Surgeries vary according to whether the tissues are soft or rigid, but most involve opening and correcting the involved joints. If a bunion is present, this can be corrected at the same time.

Medications

- Nonsteroidal anti-inflammatory drugs to manage pain and inflammation
- Corticosteroid injection

Massage?

RISKS If a client's foot is hot and inflamed, this is obviously a local caution for any but the lightest touch. Otherwise as long as sensation is intact and work is not painful, hammertoe has no specific contraindications for massage.

BENEFITS If a client's hammertoe is rigid, massage may have little immediate or local impact. However, if this situation is still passively malleable, massage may work along with taping, splints, or other devices and stretching to help restore balance between the musculotendinous forces in the foot.

OPTIONS A client with hammertoe in any form is likely to compensate for a loss of foot strength in both posture and gait. Massage can certainly address these issues to reduce pain and improve efficiency of movement.

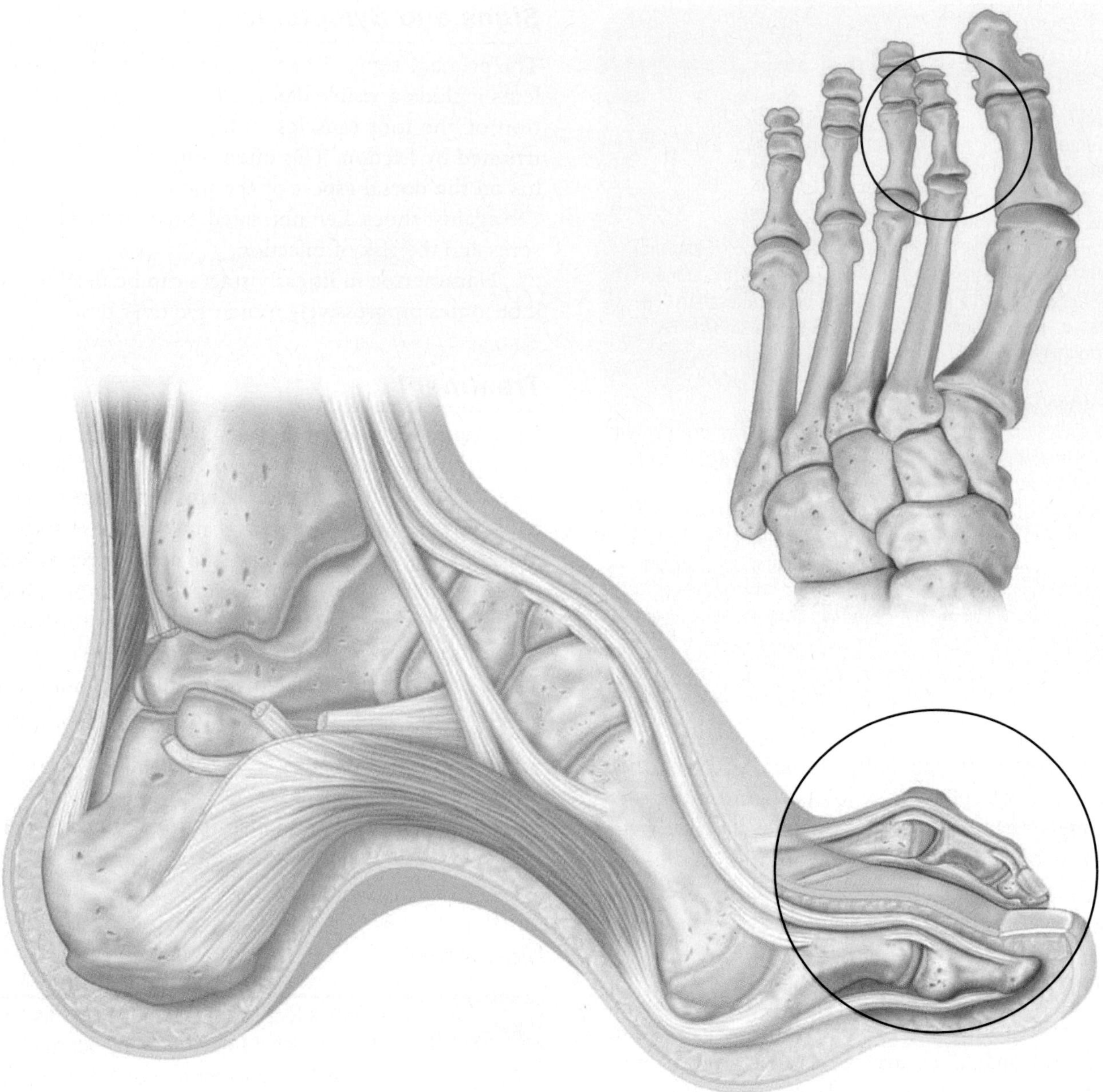

Figure 3.33. Hammertoe

Hernia

Definition: What Is It?

Hernia means "hole." A variety of hernias can occur in the body: muscles may herniate through fascial walls; vertebral discs may herniate; the brain may even herniate through the cranium. This discussion focuses on abdominal hernias: holes or weak spots in the abdominal wall or diaphragm, through which contents may protrude or become trapped.

Hernias are common: about 5 million are diagnosed each year in this country. Men have abdominal hernias much more frequently than women.

Etiology: What Happens?

Abdominal hernias can be classified as fascial disorders because they involve weakness in the connective tissues that are meant to form strong containers. When the fascia is stressed through mechanical forces or

Hernia in Brief

Pronunciation: HUR-ne-a

What is it?
A hernia is a hole or rip through which structures may protrude.

How is it recognized?
Abdominal hernias usually involve bulging and mild to severe pain, depending on whether a portion of the small intestine is trapped. Hiatal hernias show heartburn or other signs of gastroesophageal reflux disorder.

Massage risks and benefits
Risks: An untreated hernia locally contraindicates massage: it is a situation that requires a different kind of intervention.
Benefits: A client whose hernia has been successfully treated can enjoy the same benefits from bodywork as the rest of the population.

congenital flaws, a hole forms and the abdominal contents (usually loops of small intestine) can be forced through.

Many hernias are reducible, which means that the contents can be put back where they belong without surgery. But they may progressively get worse, bulging more often, while a bigger hole develops. Therefore, once a hernia has been identified, surgery to tighten up or close the hole is recommended sooner rather than later. Where a hernia develops and what it feels like depend mainly on gender and what forces push the abdominal contents against their walls. A hernia that cannot be reduced is said to be **incarcerated**, and the entrapped structures are at high risk for strangulation and infection.

Types of Hernia

- **Direct inguinal hernia.** This is a hole in the abdominal wall at the inguinal ring. This opening for the spermatic cord to enter the abdomen is a weak spot. A sudden change in internal abdominal pressure, like coughing, sneezing, or heavy lifting (especially with simultaneous twisting) may force a section of small intestine right through this weak spot (Figure 3.34).
- **Indirect inguinal hernia.** In this situation, structures protrude into the inguinal canal and, in men, down into the scrotum.
- **Epigastric hernia.** This is a bulge superior to the umbilicus. The linea alba splits, and a portion of the omentum pushes through. The symptoms, besides a visible lump above the navel, may include a feeling of tenderness or heaviness in the area, but seldom extreme pain. This hernia happens with women and men, but it is more common in men.
- **Paraumbilical hernia.** This is another split of the linea alba, this time right at the navel. It is sometimes a complication of childbirth. This type of hernia is almost exclusive to women.
- **Umbilical hernia.** This occurs at the **umbilicus**, and it is a common condition in newborn babies. It usually closes without intervention by age 2. In adults, umbilical hernias may occur with obesity, ascites, or as a result of multiple pregnancies.
- **Incisional hernia.** This is a fairly common surgical complication in which scar tissue at an incision site breaks down.
- **Hiatal hernia.** This is an enlargement of the diaphragmatic hiatus, the opening in the dome of the diaphragm where the esophagus and other structures pass from the thorax to the abdomen. When this opening is enlarged, the stomach can protrude up into the thoracic cavity (Figure 3.35). Hiatal hernias are a major contributor to gastroesophageal reflux disorder (GERD).
- **Other hernias.** These are rare. Femoral hernias involve a bulge inferior to the inguinal ligament into the femoral canal. **Obturator hernia** is a bulge of pelvic contents into the obturator foramen. **Spigelian hernia** is a bulge at the lateral aspect of the rectus abdominus.

Signs and Symptoms

Signs and symptoms of hernias depend on the location and size of the opening. Sharp or mild pain, a feeling of fullness, and a palpable bulge are common indicators. Hiatal hernias are recognized by the signs of GERD, along with shortness of breath as the stomach protrudes between the lungs.

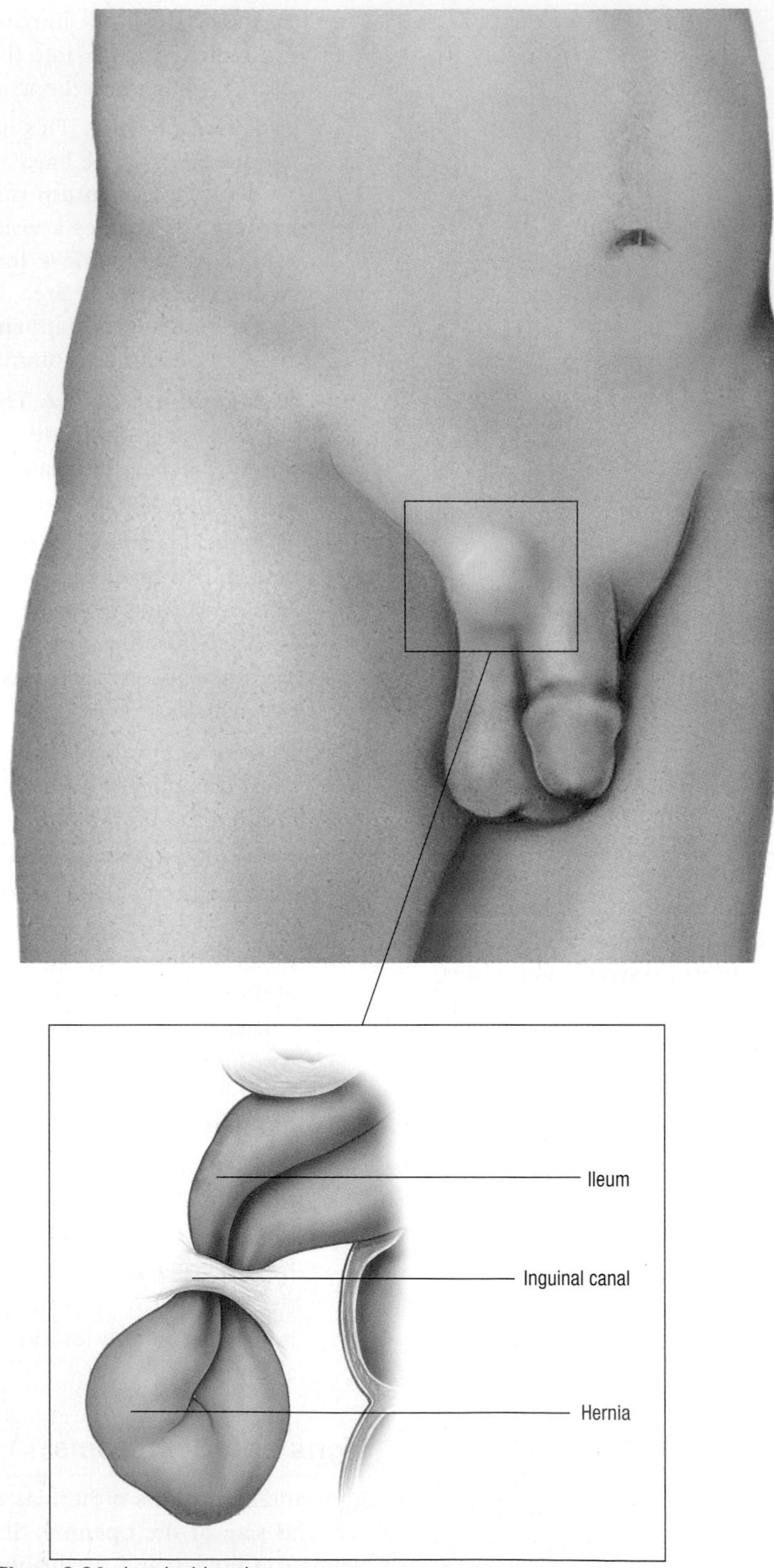

Figure 3.34. Inguinal hernia

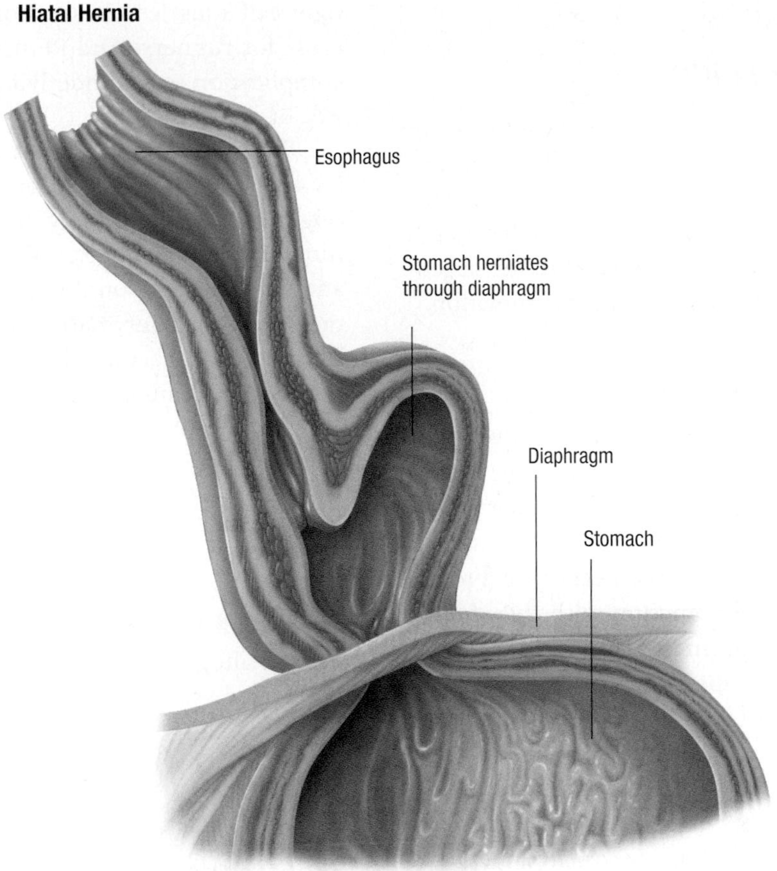

Figure 3.35. Hiatal hernia: the stomach protrudes through the diaphragm

The seriousness of a hernia is determined by how big it is. Paradoxically, the bigger the hernia, the safer it is, at least for the short term. Small holes can be more dangerous: structures can become trapped and strangulated. Signs of this complication range from discomfort and vomiting to an area becoming red, enlarged, and excruciatingly painful.

Treatment

Surgery is frequently recommended even for mild hernias because they tend to get worse as time goes on, and a small repair has lower risks than a large one. The standard surgical technique entails inserting a small piece of mesh at the site of the tear. This helps to distribute the force of abdominal pressure more evenly than stitches or staples alone, reducing the risk of a recurrence. This procedure can be conducted as open or laparoscopic surgery.

A variety of surgeries to repair hiatal hernias have been developed.

If a person doesn't need immediate surgery, a special corset or truss may be recommended to prevent sudden changes in abdominal pressure, but these days trusses are considered only temporary measures, not a solution to the problem.

Medications

- Antibiotics if strangulation of internal structures occurs
- Medications to manage acid reflux for hiatal hernias

Massage?

RISKS Untreated hernias are local contraindications for specific massage, because the fascial wall is already compromised: any extra pressure or stretching would not be helpful.

BENEFITS Gentle massage around the edges of postoperative scars may be helpful in scar tissue organization. Clients who have successfully treated a hernia in the past can enjoy all the benefits of bodywork as the rest of the population.

Plantar Fasciitis

Definition: What is It?

Plantar fasciitis (PF) is a common condition involving pain at the plantar fascia, which stretches from the calcaneus to the proximal phalanges on the plantar surface of the foot. While the suffix "-itis" implies that this is an inflammatory condition, PF is related to the degeneration of collagen more than to acute inflammation.

Etiology: What Happens?

The plantar fascia is a tough band of connective tissue that supports the medial longitudinal arch of the foot. It is thickest in the middle of the band and thinner on the medial and lateral aspects. It is vulnerable to damage through anatomic and repetitive biomechanical forces.

PF often occurs in conjunction with the growth of bone spurs on the calcaneus. While these spurs were once assumed to be the source of heel pain, that assumption is no longer taken for granted.

Excessive running, especially in worn down shoes, is a contributor to PF. Being overweight can predispose some people to PF, as can sudden changes in activity levels. Unequal leg length, flat or pronated feet, and jammed arches are associated with this problem. Very tight calf muscles are also contributing factors, especially for runners. And PF may occur as a secondary complication to an underlying disorder such as gout, RA, or diabetes.

When the plantar fascia is overused or stressed, its fibers tend to fray or become disorganized (Figure 3.36). The quality of the tissue degrades, and function is gradually lost. Despite its name, PF is not an inflammatory condition, but rather the degeneration of the collagen matrix of the plantar aponeurosis. The absence of acute inflammation has some implications for determining the best treatment options, so it is an important point to consider.

Plantar Fasciitis in Brief

Pronunciation: PLAN-tar fah-she-Y-tis

What is it?
Plantar fasciitis (PF) is a condition caused by repeated microscopic injury to the plantar fascia of the foot.

How is it recognized?
PF is acutely painful after prolonged immobility. Then the pain recedes when the foot is warmed up, but comes back with extended use. It feels sharp and bruise like, usually at the anterior calcaneus.

Massage risks and benefits
Risks: If the plantar fascia is acute inflamed (which is unlikely), local deep massage should be delayed. Massage to the plantar fascia for a client who has recently had a cortisone injection may increase the risk of rupture.
Benefits: Massage can help release tension in deep calf muscles that put strain on the plantar fascia; it can also help to affect the quality of scar tissue at the site of the injury.

Signs and Symptoms

PF follows a distinctive pattern that makes it easy to identify: it is acutely painful for the first few steps after a period of immobility. Then the pain subsides or disappears altogether, but becomes a problem again with prolonged standing, walking, or running. A sharp bruised feeling either just anterior to the calcaneus on the plantar surface or deep in the arch of the foot often marks this disorder.

Treatment

The most important thing to do for PF is to manage the tensions that cause the plantar fascia to be irritated after periods of immobility, especially first thing in the

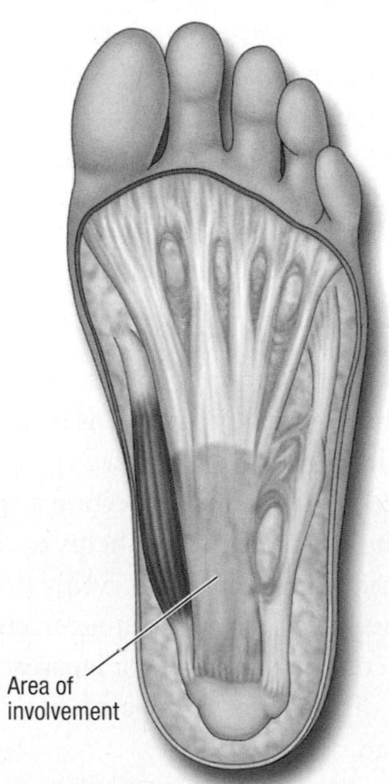

Figure 3.36. Plantar fasciitis

morning. Warming and massaging the foot and lower leg before getting out of bed can make the tissue more flexible. Shoe inserts or heel cups can keep the foot from going into deep dorsiflexion. Some experts suggest that heel cups in particular are better targeted at heel fat pad degeneration rather than PF. Another device that many patients find helpful is a night splint that holds the foot in a slightly dorsiflexed position. This allows the plantar fascia fibers to knit in a way that won't be stressed and irritated so easily.

Ice, stretching, and deep massage to the calf muscles and at the site of the irritation are frequently prescribed for PF. Corticosteroid injections are sometimes given if other interventions are unsuccessful, but steroids damage the fat pads on the heels and may weaken the collagen fibers and increase the risk of plantar fascia rupture, so they are used only sparingly. **Extracorporeal shockwave lithotripsy**, similar to that used to break up kidney stones, is used with some success for PF. As a last-ditch option, surgery may be performed to divide sections of the plantar fascia.

No single treatment is universally effective; each patient must experiment with the treatments that meet his or her own needs. Most people eventually find relief, but it may take 6 to 18 months before all symptoms are resolved.

Medications

- NSAIDs for pain management
- Cortisone injection for anti-inflammatory and collagen-dissolving effect

Massage?

RISKS If a client has used cortisone injections to treat his PF, massage at the site should be avoided until the tissues have stabilized. When acute inflammation (which is probably rare) is present, massage should be locally avoided in order to not exacerbate symptoms. Otherwise, massage for PF is safe and appropriate.

BENEFITS Massage is often suggested both to decrease tension in nearby muscles and to have an organizing influence on collagen fibers within the plantar fascia itself.

OPTIONS A bodywork focus not only on the affected foot but also on the deep calf muscles that control foot alignment is often recommended.

Pes Planus, Pes Cavus

Definition: What Are They?

Pes planus ("flat feet") is the technical term for feet that lack the medial arch between the calcaneus and the great toe, the lateral arch between the calcaneus and the little toe, and the transverse arch that stretches across the ball of the foot.

Pes cavus ("caved feet") is the term for feet with jammed arches, or a hyperaccentuated arch that does not flatten out with each step, but instead stays high and immobile.

Etiology: What Happens?

The feet are architecturally complex. Each one has 26 bones, 33 joints, and more than 100 muscles, tendons, and ligaments to mediate our relation to gravity when we stand. Imbalance at the forefoot, midfoot, or hindfoot can lead to problems in how weight is distributed over the whole surface and how the stress of weight-bearing is translated to the rest of the body.

Pes planus and pes cavus may develop for several reasons. A congenital problem in the shape of the foot bones or the strength of the foot ligaments

Pes Planus, Pes Cavus in Brief

Pronunciation: pes PLANE-us, pes KAV-us

What are they?
These are the technical terms for flat feet or jammed arches.

How are they recognized?
In pes planus, the feet lack arches. Eversion of the ankle, sometimes referred to as pronation, may also be present. Persons with pes cavus have extremely high arches that don't flatten with weight bearing.

Massage risks and benefits
Risks: Massage carries little risk for a client with pes planus or cavus, unless the foot problems are brought about by an underlying condition that requires some adjustment with bodywork.
Benefits: In some cases, the health of intrinsic foot muscles and ligaments can be improved through bodywork, especially if it is combined with increased awareness of posture and movement patterns. If the ligaments are lax through genetic or other problems, then massage may not correct the situation, but it could work with other factors to reduce pain and improve function.

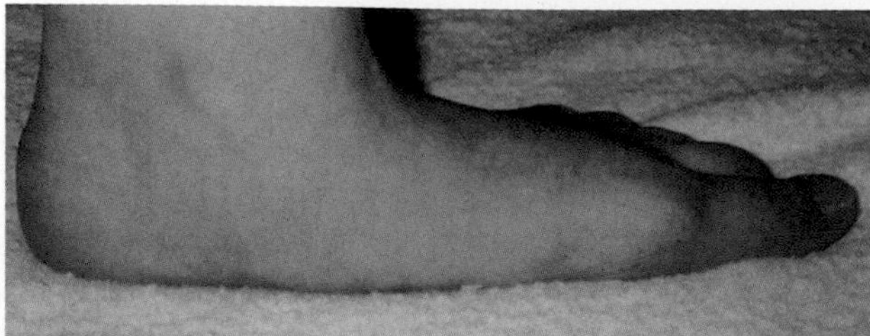
Figure 3.37. Pes planus

is one cause. Foot trauma and malunion fractures of the calcaneus or talus may alter the shape of the foot. Problems may also arise from the ongoing battle between the deep flexors and everters, combined with poorly functioning ligaments and footwear that offers little or no support (Figure 3.37).

Pes planus in particular has been studied in relation to a problematic tibialis posterior tendon. This leads to hypertonicity and imbalanced pulling, especially at the peroneus muscles on the lateral aspect of the foot. A failure of ligaments that support the arches of the feet contributes to symptoms. Ultimately, while the medial arch is flattened, the foot veers laterally, exerting excessive pull on the medial deltoid ligament

Pes cavus, when it is serious enough to interfere with function, is often examined as a complication of an underlying or preexisting disorder. Malunion fractures and compartment syndrome are often considered. Neuromuscular disorders, such as Charcot-Marie-Tooth syndrome, MD, polio, or cerebral palsy, may contribute to jammed arches. When pes cavus has a sudden onset and is bilateral (i.e., not related to a specific trauma), a neurological cause is investigated: it could be related to a tumor or other problem in the central nervous system leading to spasticity in lower leg muscles.

Whatever the source of distortion, if the foot bones lack spring and mobility, shock absorption is lost (Figure 3.38). Each time the foot hits the ground, thousands of pounds of downward pressure that should be softly distributed through the tarsal bones, reverberates through the rest of the skeleton. In this way, flat feet or jammed arches can lead to arthritis in the feet, plantar fasciitis, neuromas, and then knee problems, hip problems, back pain, even headaches, and TMJ disorders. Furthermore, foot problems can be especially dangerous for people with poor peripheral circulation, because chronic friction and irritation at isolated spots can lead to sores on the feet.

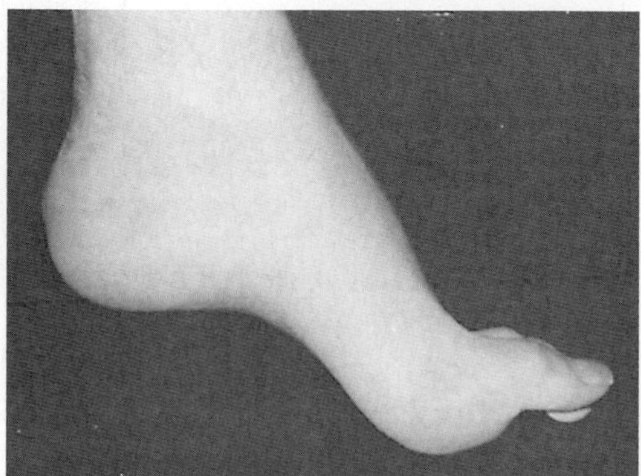
Figure 3.38. Pes cavus: arched foot

Signs and Symptoms

Pes planus signs may be subtle until complications develop. Pain, a visible lack of an arch while standing, and a laterally deviated heel are typical indicators. Pes cavus tends to be more severe and dramatic, especially when it is related to an underlying neuromuscular condition. Along with a rigid arch, patients experience lateral foot pain, extensive callus, and ankle instability.

Treatment

A person who is aware that the alignment of his or her feet is a problem may be recommended to switch to highly supportive shoes. Physical therapy to rebalance the peroneus longus and tibialis posterior muscles may be suggested. Orthotics or braces to improve foot alignment can help with pain and dysfunction. Rarely, surgery may be performed to repair injured tendons that can contribute to flat feet, to reshape foot bones, or to fuse foot joints for reduced pain and improved stability.

When pes cavus is related to an underlying condition and function could be restored by surgically releasing tight tissues, this may be considered a viable choice.

Massage?

RISKS Pes cavus is often connected to an underlying disorder that may require modifications in bodywork. Outside of this caution, massage has little risk for a person with flat feet or jammed arches.

BENEFITS Deep specific massage to the feet and muscles of the lower legs may improve the local environment to the extent that secondary symptoms are decreased and function improves.

Neuromuscular Disorders

Carpal Tunnel Syndrome

Definition: What is It?

Carpal tunnel syndrome (CTS) is a set of signs and symptoms brought about by entrapment of the median nerve between the carpal bones of the wrist and the transverse carpal ligament that holds down the flexor tendons (Figure 3.39; see video online at http://thePoint.lww.com/Werner5e). The median nerve supplies the thumb, forefinger, middle finger, and half of the ring finger (Figure 3.40). If it is caught, pinched, or squeezed in any way, it creates symptoms in the part of the hand the nerve supplies.

CTS is the most common peripheral nerve compression syndrome. It is an occupational hazard for massage practitioners and anyone else who performs repetitive movements for several hours every day, including people who work with keyboards, string musicians, bakers, assembly line workers, and checkout clerks. Women with CTS outnumber men; this may be because their carpal tunnels are smaller to begin with, so less irritation may lead to symptoms.

Carpal Tunnel Syndrome in Brief

What is it?
Carpal tunnel syndrome (CTS) is irritation of the median nerve as it passes under the transverse carpal ligament into the wrist.

How is it recognized?
CTS can cause pain, tingling, numbness, and weakness in the part of the hand supplied by the median nerve. Complications or related problems can also create pain in the proximal wrist or forearm.

Massage risks and benefits
Risks: Any work that elicits symptoms must be modified to avoid irritation to the median nerve.
Benefits: Depending on underlying factors, CTS may respond well to massage that helps create more space for the median nerve to function.

Etiology: What Happens?

The source of the pain associated with CTS is debatable. While some experts claim that pressure directly on the nerve causes pain, others suggest that pressure impedes blood flow to the nerve, and that is the source of the problem.

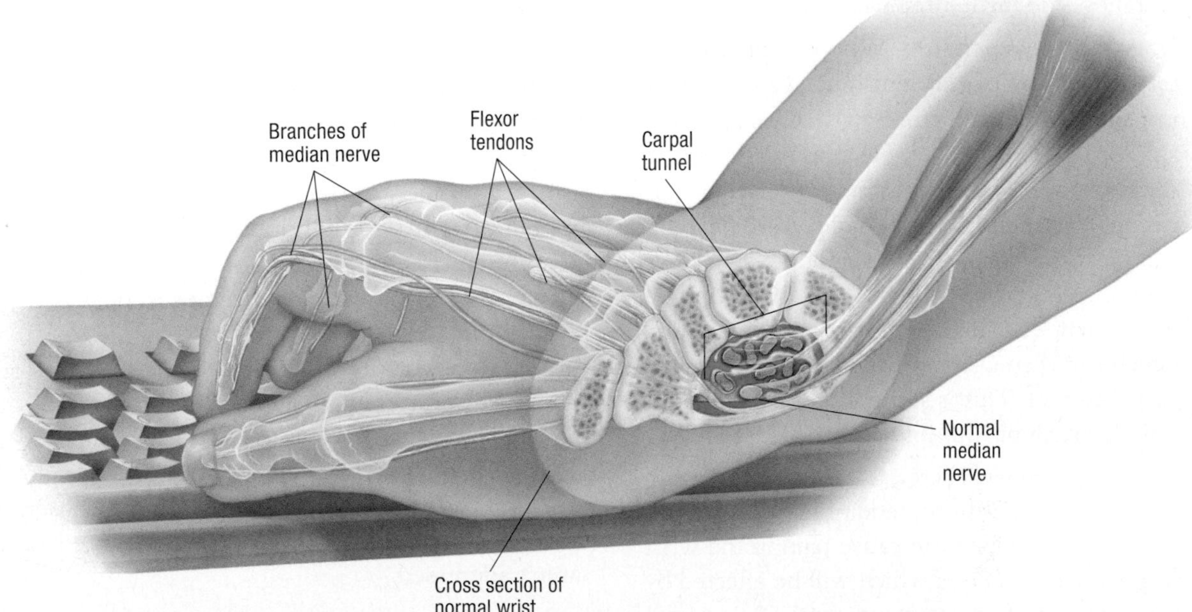

Figure 3.39. Carpal tunnel syndrome is often caused by repetitive motion, such as typing on a keyboard

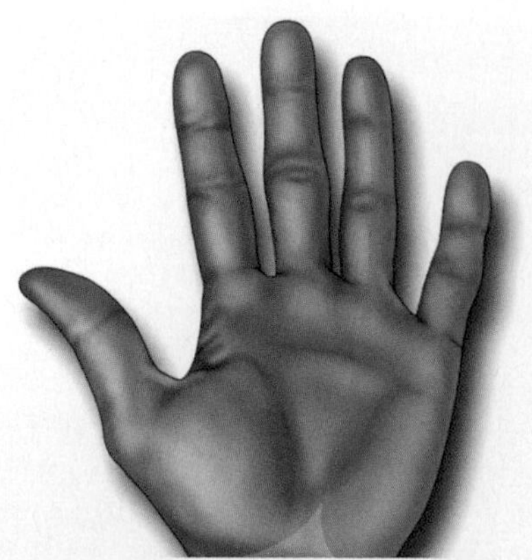

Figure 3.40. Carpal tunnel syndrome affects the thumb, index finger, middle finger, and half of the ring finger

Whether the damage is to the nerve itself or to its blood supply, irritation within the carpal tunnel may arise from several sources. To develop a treatment strategy (and to assess the appropriateness of massage), the aggravating factors must be determined. These factors include edema, subluxation of a carpal bone, or what is probably the most common situation: fibrotic buildup of connective tissues in the wrist due to repetitive use.

What makes CTS especially challenging to identify and treat, however, is that many things can mimic or contribute to nerve pain in the hand, and these must also be addressed for successful outcomes. The possibilities include but are not limited to the following:

- *Neck injury*. Herniated discs and irritated neck ligaments refer pain distally. The worse the irritation, the further the pain refers.
- *General nerve impairment*. When a nerve is irritated, the flow of nutrients and wastes can be impaired along its entire length. This puts it at risk for irritation at multiple sites in addition to the wrist, all of which must be addressed for successful treatment (see video clip). Cervical disruption, disc pressure, thoracic outlet syndrome (TOS), or entrapment or elongation elsewhere in the arm can all irritate the median nerve, which can then also become compressed at the carpal tunnel. This is sometimes referred to as **double crush** or **multiple crush syndrome**.
- *Other wrist injuries*. These can include osteoarthritis, rheumatoid arthritis, tendinitis, and ligament sprains, all of which can cause pain in the wrist and hand and none of which will be affected by any of the standard treatments for CTS.

CTS can also be a symptom or consequence of several other systemic diseases. Diabetes mellitus, hypothyroidism, lymphedema associated with cancer staging, acromegaly, rheumatoid arthritis, and gout can all involve pressure at the carpal tunnel.

Signs and Symptoms

Depending on the source and severity of the problem, CTS can manifest as tingling; pins and needles; burning, shooting pains; intermittent numbness; and weakness as innervation to the hand muscles is interrupted. The thenar pad may flatten out as the thumb muscles atrophy. It is often worse at night, when people may sleep on their arm, or turn their wrist into awkward positions. It can be painful enough to wake someone out of a deep sleep. If pressure is taken off the nerve promptly, symptoms tend to disappear. But the worst-case scenario is permanent damage to the median nerve, resulting in loss of muscle function and sensation in the hand.

The median nerve supplies the lateral aspect of the hand with sensation and motor function. About 90% of the fibers in the median nerve are sensory and 10% are motor. This means that motor problems (weakness or atrophy) may indicate more significant nerve damage than is seen with sensory problems alone.

Treatment

Treatment for CTS often begins with a wrist splint. The goal is to keep the carpal tunnel in a neutral position (in which it is as spacious as possible) and to require less work from the supportive tissues. Anti-inflammatories may be recommended or prescribed. Corticosteroid injections into the wrist may also be recommended to reduce inflammation and dissolve excess connective tissue. Exercises to stretch and mobilize tight wrist tendons may be recommended. Acupuncture, chiropractic, or yoga may be suggested as other noninvasive strategies to deal with CTS symptoms.

If no other intervention is successful, CTS treatment culminates in surgery. The transverse carpal ligament is split, and some of the accumulated connective tissue is scraped away. This may be done as an open or endoscopic procedure. Surgery isn't entirely successful, however, if other sites of nerve irritation aren't addressed.

Medications

- NSAIDs for pain and inflammation
- Injected steroids for connective tissue dissolution and anti-inflammatory action
- Injected lidocaine for pain relief

Massage?

RISKS Any work that creates CTS symptoms should be modified immediately. Otherwise, CTS is only a local caution that may be appropriate for careful work that doesn't cause pain.

BENEFITS Massage that doesn't exacerbate symptoms has been shown to contribute to improvement in strength, function, and symptoms for CTS patients.

OPTIONS Specific work within pain tolerance on the hand, wrist, forearm, and shoulder of a person with CTS may have some success at decompressing the median nerve.

Disc Disease

Disc Disease in Brief

What is it?
Disc disease refers to any situation in which the intervertebral disc is damaged in such a way that it puts pressure on nerve roots, the cauda equine, or the spinal cord.

How is it recognized?
Symptoms of nerve pressure include local and radicular pain, specific muscle weakness, paresthesia, and numbness.

Massage risks and benefits
Risks: Many problems can cause nerve pain that looks similar to disc disease. Before bodywork can be conducted safely, it is important to have as clear a diagnosis as possible. Acutely inflamed discs may do best with gentle work that doesn't irritate surrounding muscles or other tissues. Muscle splinting around a weakened area must be treated with great care because reducing tone prematurely may aggravate symptoms. Any type of positioning that exacerbates symptoms should be avoided, of course.
Benefits: A person with a damaged disc may derive great benefit from careful bodywork that focuses on decompressing the spine, reducing the muscle splinting (when the area is stable), and addressing compensatory postural patterns that often accompany nerve pain.

Definition: What is It?

Disc disease is an umbrella term referring to a collection of problems in which the nucleus pulposus and/or the annulus fibrosus of an intervertebral disc extends beyond its normal borders. Pain is present if the disc presses on the spinal cord or spinal nerve roots. If the bulge or crack doesn't happen to interfere with nerve tissue, no symptoms may be present at all.

Etiology: What Happens?

A typical intervertebral disc is a complex package. It has an outer wrapping of very tough, hard material called the annulus fibrosus. This wraps around a soft, gelatinous center called the nucleus pulposus. Ideally, the nucleus should be roughly spherical, with the harder annulus layers forming flat surfaces above, below, and around the ball. This combination of textures gives the disc the ability to resist both compressive and shearing forces (Figure 3.41, also see video clip).

The annulus fibrosus is an arrangement of concentric circles of collagen fibers. These fibers are arranged in such a way that the tighter they're pulled, the stronger they become. On the other hand, the closer the vertebrae are, the looser (and weaker) the annulus is. This has great implications for the nucleus pulposus, which relies on a tight, solid exterior wall for support.

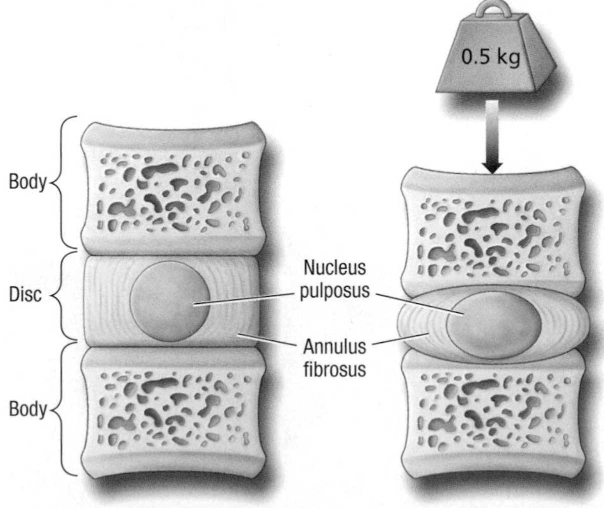

Figure 3.41. Intervertebral discs increase the weight-bearing capacity of the spine

Most people's nucleus pulposus becomes thinner and dry with age. This means more stress is placed on the annulus to bear weight and absorb shock, so the annulus has an increased risk for cracks or fissures. The whole degeneration of the disc then adds stress to the connecting vertebrae; osteophytes frequently develop on the lip of the vertebral bodies or around the facet joints. In this way disc disease is closely aligned to spondylosis.

Causes of disc injury may vary according to the general resiliency and age of the connective tissues of the person involved. For some people, it takes a major trauma such as a car accident or a bad fall to damage a disc. But some people with weak, loose intervertebral ligaments have a risk of disc damage from ordinary everyday activity. The classic scenario for this kind of disc damage is an incident that involves simultaneous lifting and twisting:

- A person bends over to pick up something heavy. Trunk flexion flattens the anterior portion of the nucleus and opens up a posterior space, while stretching the posterior fibers of the annulus, making them taut and strong.
- The person jerks into an erect posture, possibly twisting at the same time, while carrying a heavy load. Suddenly coming into extension, especially while carrying something heavy, quickly redistributes the nucleus and shoots it into that posterior space with great force. The posterior annulus fibers are now at their weakest, most lax position.
- The nucleus presses against the weakest part of the posterior annulus, and breaks through, putting pressure on nerve roots. Or the force of the motion, combined with the brittleness of the annulus, causes the annulus to crack and put pressure on nerve tissue. The chemical substance of the nucleus pulposus creates a very extreme inflammatory response that can be a major contributor to the nerve pain that accompanies these injuries.

The kind of lifting-and-twisting injury described here usually affects the discs below L4 and L5. Cervical disc lesions can occur with sports injuries, whiplash, and similar trauma, usually at the disc below C5 or C6. Thoracic injuries are possible but rarer, since the ribs make the thoracic spine much more stable than its cervical and lumbar counterparts. Discs that cause pain usually bulge posterolaterally, because that is the path of least resistance in the tight space they inhabit, but they can also go to the left or right side (Figures 3.42 and 3.43).

Most injured discs are temporarily painful but don't lead to permanent or serious problems. The most serious complication of a disc injury is the threat of pressure exerted directly posteriorly. In the neck, this means the spinal cord is compressed; in the lumbar spine, it is called **cauda equina syndrome**

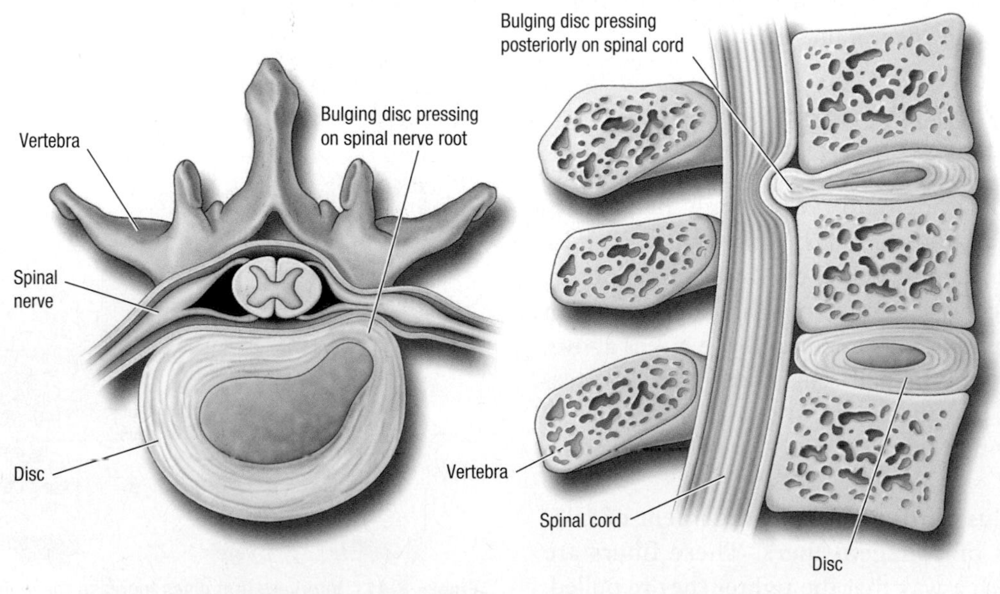

Figure 3.42. Herniated nucleus pulposus

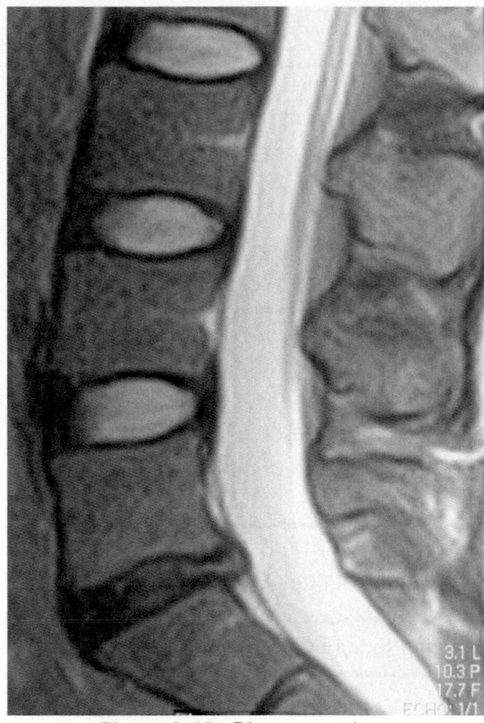

Figure 3.43. Disc protrusion

because the disc material presses on the extensions of spinal nerves between T1 and S5 called the cauda equine (video clip available at http://thePoint.lww.com/Werner5e). Direct spinal cord compression leads to some specific signs, including hyperactive reflexes; bilateral pain, paresthesia, or numbness in a "saddle" distribution; and the loss of bladder or bowel control. Any of these problems can become permanent, or paralysis can develop, if pressure is not resolved quickly.

Types of Disc Problems

It is useful to be able to recognize the terminology for disc problems that may turn up in a diagnosis. Disc problems are generally discussed as three major issues:

- *Herniated disc*. The nucleus pulposus extends beyond the margin of the vertebral body. These injuries are most common in young adults. The nucleus may be damaged in these ways:
  - *Bulge*. The entire disc protrudes symmetrically beyond the normal boundaries of the vertebral body.
  - *Protrusion*. The nucleus pulposus extends out of the annulus at a specific location. If it protrudes posterolaterally (the most common version), it may press on nerve roots. If it protrudes straight back, it may press on the spinal cord or cauda equina.
  - *Extrusion*. A small piece of the nucleus protrudes, with a narrow connection back to the body of the nucleus. In some cases, the protrusion can separate from the nucleus altogether; this is called a sequestration.
  - *Rupture*. The nucleus pulposus bursts and leaks its entire contents into the surrounding area.
- *Degenerative disc disease*. This refers to small, cumulative tears of the annulus, along with decreased disc height and dehydration of the nucleus. Eventually, the annulus may press against a nerve root or the spinal cord.
- *Internal disc disruption*. This condition is often related to trauma in addition to degenerative disc disease. In this case, the nucleus protrudes through the annulus but stays within the boundaries of the whole disc.

Signs and Symptoms

Symptoms associated with disc disease arise from pressure on nerve tissue or from an extreme inflammatory response that occurs when the nucleus pulposus leaks. Nerve pressure can come and go as the patient's position and alignment shift, and so once the initial inflammation subsides, pain may be intermittent.

- *Local and radicular pain*. pain that radiates along the dermatome of the affected nerve root. Pain is often described as shooting, burning, or electrical. When pain originates from a lumbar disc injury, it may cause pain through the buttocks and down the back of the leg: this is often called sciatica, although other professionals use that term to mean irritation of the sciatic nerve elsewhere than at the spinal roots.
- *Specific muscle weakness*. weakness or even atrophy in the muscles that are affected by irritated nerves. (This is different from general muscle weakness that can arise from overall deconditioning.)
- *Paresthesia*. "pin and needles" in the affected dermatome.
- *Reduced sensation*. This can also be a sign of ligament damage instead of or in addition to disc damage.

- *Numbness*. Total numbness is one distinguishing factor between disc problems and ligament injuries.

Treatment

The most successful treatment outcomes for disc injuries depend on an accurate diagnosis. Red flags that must be ruled out include the possibility of cancer, infection, spinal fracture and, in the cervical spine, problems with the structure or function of the vertebral artery. One situation that mimics a disc problem but is actually much less serious is a ligament sprain: irritated spinal ligaments running between spinous or transverse processes can refer pain along the same dermatomes as the nearby discs. Ligament injuries do not cause total numbness or specific muscle weakness, however, and they respond well to specific types of massage.

The main goal of disc disease treatment is to create a situation where pressure on nerve roots is removed. Chiropractors and osteopaths work to correct bony alignment and to create a maximum of space for the nucleus to retreat back to its normal boundaries. Medical doctors recommend short-term bed rest or traction, followed by movement within tolerance, for the same reason. Physical therapy and education on correct posture and body mechanics are often recommended to people recovering from disc problems.

If noninvasive strategies are insufficient, a variety of other options exist. Injections of cortisone to deinflame the area are sometimes used. Injected **papain** (derived from papaya enzymes) may be used to dissolve some of the disc material. Surgery to remove the disc (discectomy), with or without spinal fusion of the connecting vertebrae is also possible.

Medications

- NSAIDs for pain and inflammation control
- Short-term narcotic analgesics if necessary
- Antiseizure drugs or tricyclic antidepressants for nerve pain
- Steroidal anti-inflammatories, including injected cortisone, for inflammation control
- Injected papain to help dissolve displaced proteins
- Injected lidocaine to myofascial trigger points causing pain around injured discs
- Muscle relaxants

Massage?

RISKS Disc problems can be complex and difficult to pin down; these are situations where massage therapists can benefit most by working as part of a healthcare team. Acute inflammation and/or muscle splinting to guard an unstable area call for bodywork that respects these processes rather than interfering with them.

BENEFITS Massage for low back pain in general is often successful. Bodywork with the intent to create space for a disc to retreat and to reduce muscle spasm and inflammation (after the acute stage has passed) may be especially useful for clients with disc problems.

OPTIONS People with disc problems may have difficulties with any position that puts their back into hyperextension. Bolsters or body cushions may be needed to avoid aggravating symptoms.

Myofascial Pain Syndrome

Definition: What Is It?

Myofascial pain syndrome (MPS) is a condition that is identified when a person develops many trigger points: pain-generating spots in muscles that are palpable as knots or taut bands. It affects men and women about equally.

Etiology: What Happens?

Myofascial trigger points probably develop as a multifactoral process. Traditionally, it was thought that they began as microscopic injuries to individual muscle fiber, and that these fibers descend into a pain-spasm-ischemia cycle. This may be the situation with some trigger points, but many trigger points are more closely related to problems with the synapse between the motor neuron and the motor end plate of the myofiber: this makes MPS primarily a neuromuscular condition.

The main issue in a trigger point is a sustained, involuntary contraction of an isolated group of **sarcomeres** (the overlapping units of myofibrils that create the striations associated with skeletal muscles). If this occurs close to the neuromuscular junction, it is called a central trigger point. Contractions that develop close to the tenoperiosteal junction may also involve

Myofascial Pain Syndrome in Brief

MY-o-fash-al pane SIN-drome

What is it?
Myofascial pain syndrome (MPS) is a collection of signs and symptoms associated with the development of myofascial trigger points in muscles.

How is it recognized?
MPS is recognized mainly by the trigger points that arise in predictable locations in affected muscles. Active trigger points create hard painful knots or taut bands; the pain may refer to distant locations. Latent trigger points may not generate pain unless they are irritated.

Massage risks and benefits
Risks: The only risk massage has for clients with MPS is that overtreatment could leave them sore. This condition involves pain-sensitizing chemicals that must be addressed in addition to reducing tone at and around trigger points.
Benefits: MPS indicates massage, which can interrupt the cycles that promote painful trigger points and help to mitigate the causes of pain and soreness that accompany these phenomena.

folded and dehydrated collagen fibers; these are called attachment trigger points.

When a microscopic contraction pulls on the rest of the myofiber, it creates a taut band. This gives rise to two simultaneous problems: an increased need for fuel, and a decreased supply of blood due to local ischemia. This situation is sometimes called an ATP energy crisis. Chemicals that increase sensitivity and pain are released, including prostaglandins, bradykinin, serotonin, substance P, and others: this helps to generate and reinforce pain sensation. In response to pain, more of the muscle attempts to tighten, causing more secretion of acetylcholine (ACh). Poor local circulation limits the availability of ACh-neutralizing enzymes, it keeps irritating chemicals present, and it inhibits the movement of calcium back into channels in the cell membrane. The consequence: a tiny, involuntary, but prolonged and painful contraction of one part of a muscle cell (Figure 3.44).

Prolonged immersion in pain-causing chemicals carries a toll for local sensory neurons. Some research suggests that the neurons become locally demyelinated, which may contribute to the unique referred pain pattern seen with trigger points.

Trigger points that are not frequently irritated may become latent: they are not painful, and they do not refer pain. But latent trigger points are associated with restricted range of motion and muscle weakness. Further, very little stimulus can turn a latent trigger point into an active one, which is locally and distantly painful even when the muscle is at rest.

Satellite points are trigger points that form as secondary issue to primary trigger points. They may develop in areas where referred pain is perceived, in areas where muscle fibers are overloaded because of compensation patterns to protect a primary trigger point, in the antagonists to muscles with active trigger points, or in muscles that are referred pain areas for the heart or other organs.

Signs and Symptoms

Trigger points have some qualities that make them unique among muscle disorders.

- *Taut bands or nodules.* Trigger points can be palpated in muscle tissue as taut, hypertonic bands of fibers within a mass of muscle that is less tight (Figure 3.45) or as small nodules that dissipate under static or pulsing manual pressure. A muscle flicker, or twitch response, is often seen when a trigger point is palpated.
- *Predictable trigger point map.* Each skeletal muscle in the body has an area or group of areas where trigger points are most likely to form. These areas have been extensively mapped.
- *Referred pain pattern.* Active trigger points are always locally painful under digital pressure, but they often refer pain to other areas in the body as well. Their referred pain patterns are consistent from person to person (Figure 3.46).
- *Regional pain.* MPS is seldom a whole-body dysfunction. More often, trigger points flare up in specific regions, often around the neck and shoulders. Jaw muscles are notorious for developing trigger points, which refer pain all over the face and head. This variety of MPS is often discussed in the context of TMJ disorders.

Other symptoms of MPS are less predictable than trigger point development. Sleep disorders occur occasionally but not consistently. Depression and anxiety are also possible, especially when a person has little success in getting an accurate diagnosis and effective treatment. These make MPS resemble

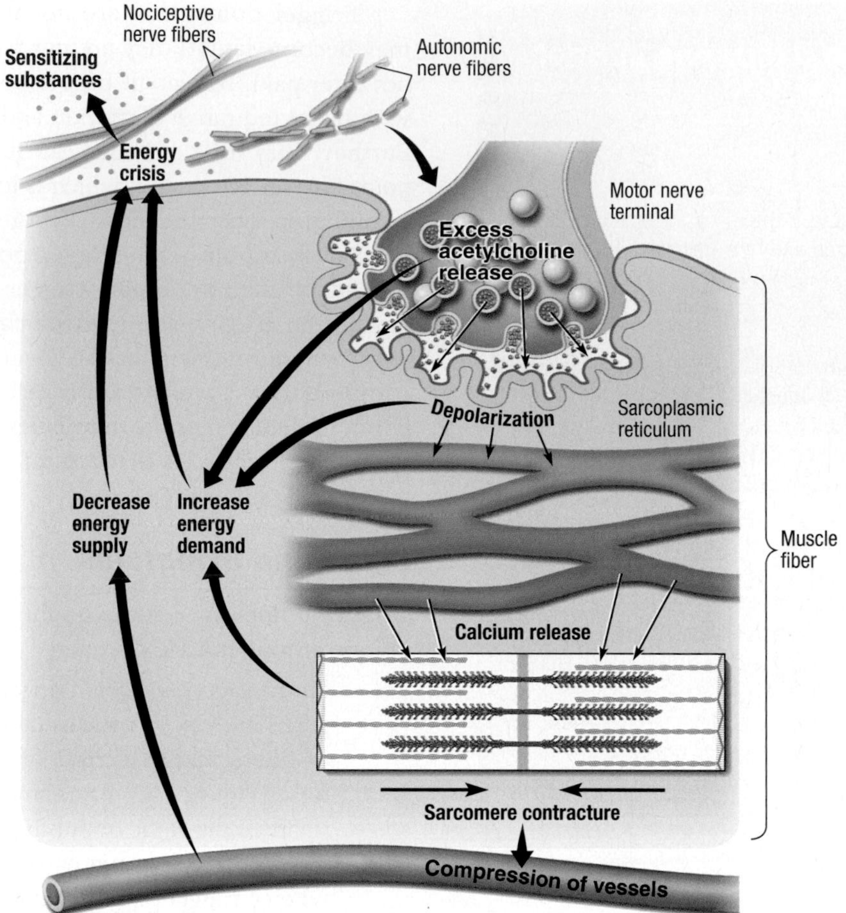

Figure 3.44. Trigger point energy crisis

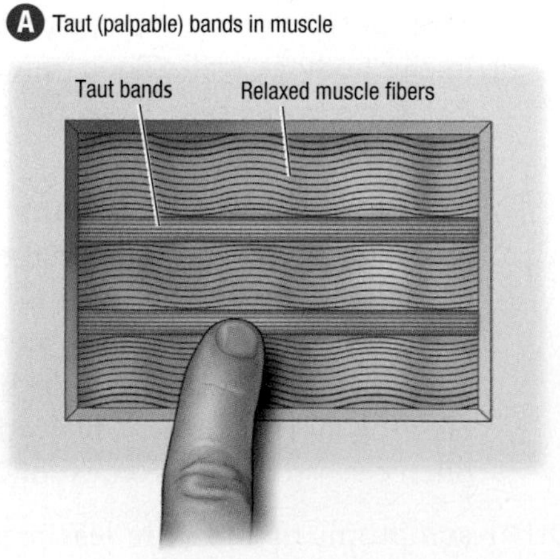

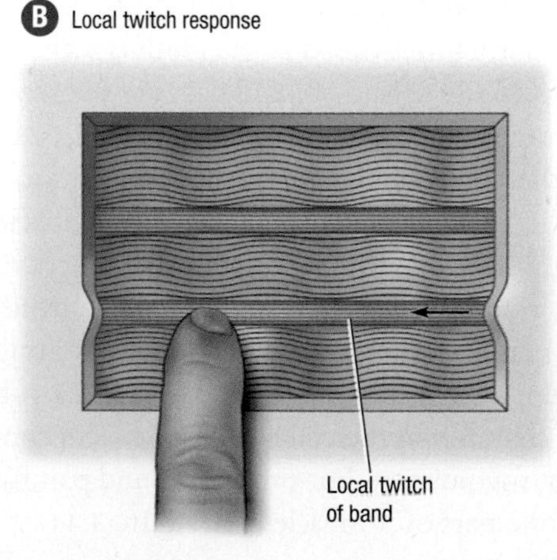

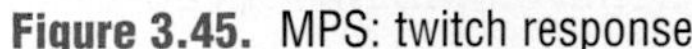
Figure 3.45. MPS: twitch response

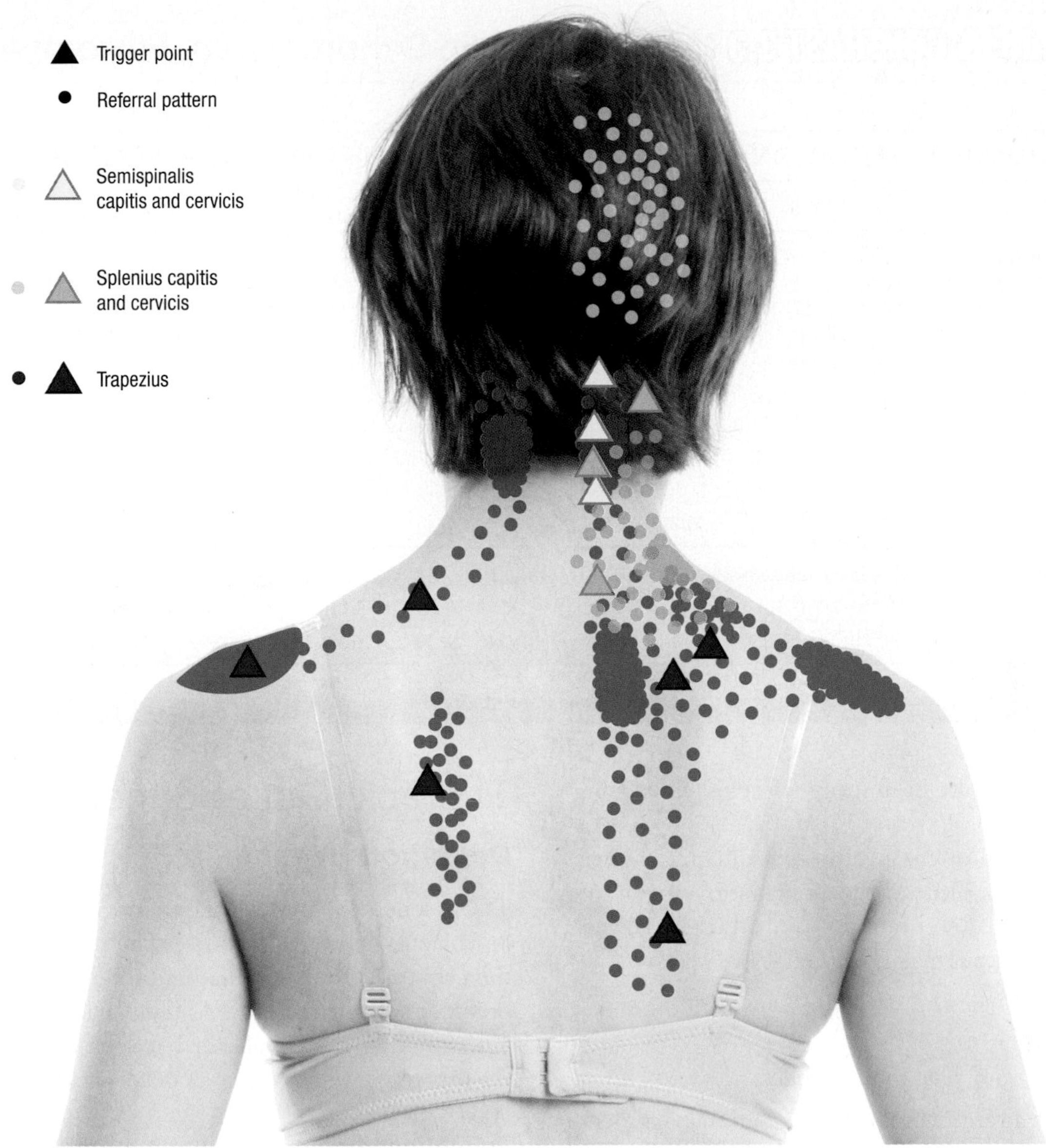

Figure 3.46. Trigger points refer pain

another chronic pain syndrome, fibromyalgia. The fibromyalgia discussion appears in Chapter 4. It is important to distinguish between the two conditions, however, because their treatment protocols, especially for bodywork, are different (see Compare & Contrast 3.3).

Treatment

The top priority for MPS treatment is to eradicate both active and latent trigger points. This is accomplished in a number of ways, including the use of vapocoolant spray, local injections of anesthetics, dry needling, and acupuncture. Injections of botulinum toxin have been explored to block ACh release at the neuromuscular junction. All of these approaches work to interrupt the pain-spasm cycle or the ATP energy crisis, allowing the tight fibers to relax while the muscle is stretched.

Manual therapies in several forms have been seen to have success in the resolution of trigger points. Prolonged ischemic pressure has been the traditional strategy, but approaches to trigger points typically find that pulsing pressure that follows the taut band

COMPARE & CONTRAST 3.3 Myofascial Pain Syndrome vs. Fibromyalgia

CHARACTERISTICS	MYOFASCIAL PAIN SYNDROME	FIBROMYALGIA SYNDROME
Prevalence	Unknown.	Up to 3% of U.S. population.
Demographics	Women and men equally affected.	85% women.
Prognosis	Can be a short-term problem that is permanently resolved.	Life-long problem; can be managed, but may never be eradicated.
Distinguishing symptom	Trigger points: predictable spots in individual muscles, areas of hypertonicity. May be nodular or appear as a taut band that generates a twitch response. Manual pressure on active trigger point elicits pain locally, and also in predictable patterns of referral.	Tender points: predictable areas; light pressure yields intense, diffuse pain. Tender points are often hypotonic, and are not always in muscle tissue.
Implications for massage	Responds well to massage; rhythmic pressure can interrupt pain-spasm cycle to eradicate trigger points.	Massage can help, but manual pressure exacerbates tender points.

of the muscle may be even more effective while being far less painful.

Because MPS often develops out of chronic overuse or poor ergonomics, the patient's movement and work habits are often examined and adjusted, so that perpetuating factors may be eliminated.

Medications

- NSAIDs for pain management
- Tricyclic antidepressants for pain management
- Injected anesthetics or botulinum toxin

Massage?

RISKS A person with many active trigger points not only experiences chronic pain but may also be easy to overtreat because of an abundance of pain-sensitizing chemicals in the tissues. Massage can help to resolve trigger points, but it must also address the residual "clean up" that must follow.

BENEFITS Careful massage can be effective to resolve MPS, by addressing the pain-spasm cycle and the ATP energy crisis that occurs where trigger points develop. Various subspecialties of bodywork have been developed to address these issues, and evidence shows both efficacy and safety for their application.

Thoracic Outlet Syndrome

Definition: What Is It?

TOS is a neurovascular entrapment. The nerves of the brachial plexus or the blood vessels running to or from the arm (or some combination thereof) are impinged or impaired at one or more of three places: between the anterior and medial scalenes; between the clavicle and the first rib, or under the coracoid process (Figure 3.47).

Etiology: What Happens?

The brachial plexus, the network of nerves that supplies the arm with sensation and motor control, consists of spinal nerves C5 to T1. These nerves travel from intervertebral foramina through the anterior and medial scalenes, between the clavicle and the first rib, under the pectoralis minor, and around the humerus. If some part of the plexus is somehow compressed along the way, symptoms develop along the distance of that nerve. The nerve roots C8 and T1, both of which contribute to the ulnar and median nerves, are most at risk for compression with TOS.

Pinched nerves are only one aspect of TOS. This is a neurovascular entrapment, and the vessels at risk are the subclavian vein and the axillary artery, which is a distal portion of the subclavian artery. These vessels

Thoracic Outlet Syndrome in Brief

Pronunciation: thor-AS-ik OUT-let SIN-drome

What is it?
Thoracic outlet syndrome (TOS) is a collection of signs and symptoms brought about by occlusion of nerve and blood supply to the arm.

How is it recognized?
Depending on what structures are compressed, TOS shows shooting pains, weakness, numbness, and paresthesia (pins and needles) along with a feeling of fullness and possible discoloration of the affected hand and arm from impaired circulation.

Massage risks and benefits
Risks: Care must be taken not to exacerbate pressure on delicate structures, either with massage or with positioning on the table. Outside of this limitation, massage has no specific risks for clients with TOS.
Benefits: Massage that works to create space for unimpeded blood and nerve impulse flow can have a profound positive impact on TOS. If the problem arises from structural anomalies, massage may not make much difference beyond temporary symptomatic relief. Muscular imbalances must be addressed from multiple dimensions and directions to achieve lasting change.

can be mechanically obstructed when muscles in small spaces get too tight.

TOS is discussed in many ways in medical literature: It is labeled as "neurological TOS" if it involves only nerve compression (the most common presentation). It is called "vascular TOS" if it involves only blood vessels. Often it is called "disputed TOS," because while the patient may have severe symptoms, the exact point of nerve or vascular impression may not be identified.

TOS can be caused by anything that impinges brachial plexus nerves or blood vessels, anywhere from the anterior neck to the anterior chest. Although postural habits and bony growth patterns can make a person susceptible to TOS, it often seems to be precipitated by a specific traumatic event: a hyperextension injury, or a repetitive stress situation similar to the factors seen with CTS.

The most common contributing factors to TOS include the following:

- *Muscle imbalance.* The anterior and medial scalenes and the pectoralis minor are the muscles most immediately involved with TOS. These tight muscles tend to become shrunken and fibrotic, while their antagonists (rhomboids, trapezius, neck extensors) become weak. This leads to a characteristic stooped or caved-in posture that significantly raises the risk of TOS.
- *Connective tissue bands.* Many people with TOS symptoms are found to have excessive connective tissue accumulation around the attachments of the scalenes. This material can put mechanical pressure on nerves and blood vessels. Whether the connective tissue bands are a congenital problem or a result of long-term postural habit is debatable.
- *Cervical ribs.* In about 1% of the population, the transverse processes of the cervical vertebrae grow longer than normal, extending into the soft tissues of the neck. They are usually unilateral, and C7 is the vertebra that grows them most frequently.

Although TOS is diagnosed only when the impingement occurs at the scalenes, costoclavicular space, or under the coracoid, other factors can contribute to identical symptoms. To treat this condition successfully, it is important to find out exactly where that interference is happening. Some possibilities include misalignment at the cervical vertebrae; spondylosis; rib misalignment; injuries to the wrist, elbow, or shoulder (including CTS); or nerve entrapment in the arm that causes the whole nerve to become inflamed. In rare cases, serious nonorthopedic conditions can create symptoms that look like TOC. Lung tumors in the apex of the lung, aneurysm, thrombus, or nerve damage from surgery can all lead to the collapse of the shoulder girdle and pressure on delicate structures.

Signs and Symptoms

Symptoms of TOS include all signs of nerve irritation: shooting pains, numbness and similar sensations, weakness, tingling, and pins and needles. Spinal nerves C8 and T1 are affected most often; these contribute to the ulnar nerve. Vascular symptoms include a feeling of fullness when blood return from a vein is blocked, or cold and weakness when blood flow to the axillary artery is impaired. In rare cases, a throbbing lump above the clavicle may be palpated. A difference in color or temperature of the affected arm may also be noticeable. Neurologic and vascular symptoms tend to be worst at night, when the patient lifts the affected arm over the head, or when the person is tired from other activities.

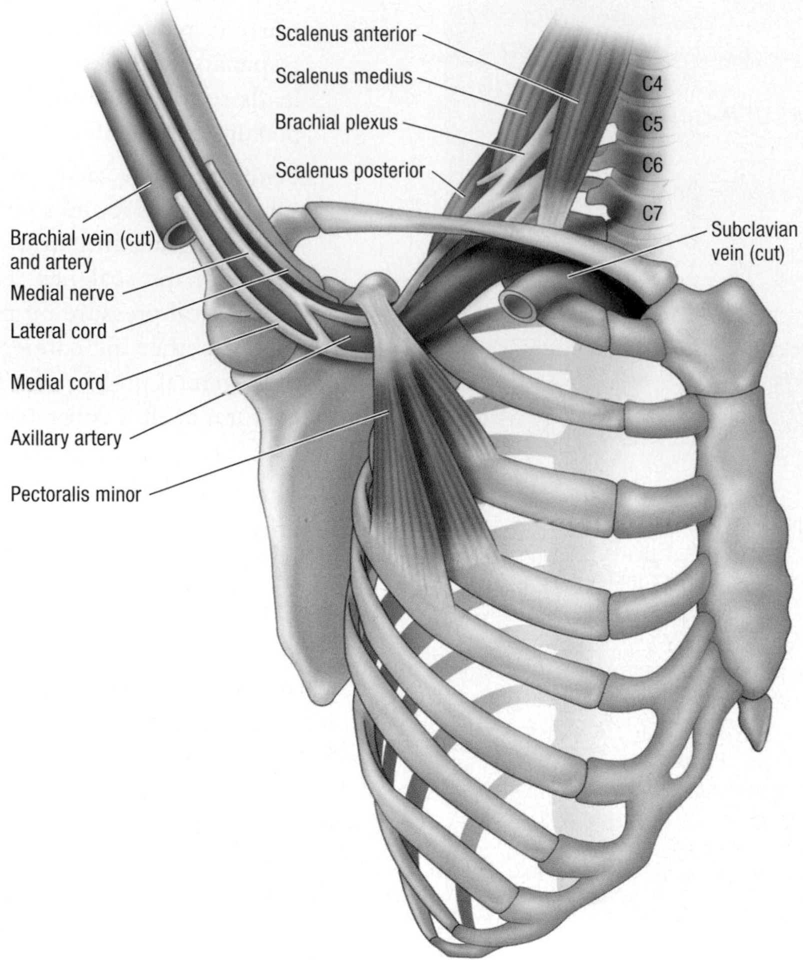

Figure 3.47. Thoracic outlet syndrome

Treatment

TOS is typically treated conservatively. Analgesics, gentle physical therapy, and stretching are the first lines of strategy. If these don't work, surgery to correct a bony anomaly or to remove connective tissue bands may be suggested. If the obstruction is found to interfere with blood flow, treatment may be more aggressive to avoid the risk of embolism.

Medications

- NSAIDs for pain
- Opioids if NSAIDs are not sufficient
- Antiseizure drugs (including Gabapentin or Clonzepam) for intractable nerve pain
- Antidepressants for nerve pain
- Anticoagulants with vascular compression to reduce the risk of thromboembolism

Massage?

RISKS Some forms of thoracic outlet syndrome (TOS) are related to anatomical anomalies, and massage will not resolve this situation. Careful positioning and sensitive work is important to avoid exacerbating impingement of delicate nerves or blood vessels. Therapists must be aware of what drugs the client may be using to make appropriate adjustments.

BENEFITS Massage along with postural and movement education can drastically improve TOS for a person with due to muscular imbalances. Even in cases where the impingement is not muscular, massage may be able to lessen the pressure on inflamed nerves in the arms, leading to improved function.

OPTIONS Focus on the shoulder girdle, the scalenes, and the postural muscles of the neck is key to unlocking the postural pattern that contributes to this condition.

SIDEBAR 3.6 Thoracic Outlet Syndrome Tests

Several tests for TOS have been developed that are available for massage therapists to use, although a client with positive tests must still be diagnosed by a primary care provider.

One of the most dependable tests for TOS is the **EAST** (elevated arm stress test). The client is seated, and his or her arms are abducted to 90 degrees. The elbows are flexed and hands point toward the ceiling. The client opens and closes the fists for 3 minutes. Most people with TOS are unable to complete this task before their symptoms interfere.

In the **Wright hyperabduction test**, the arm points to the ceiling, and the head is turned toward the affected side. If this exacerbates symptoms or reduces the strength of the pulse of the affected side, impingement to the axillary artery and lower brachial plexus nerves is suspected.

For **Adson's test** the head is extended and rotated toward the affected side. The client takes a deep breath, and the radial pulse on the affected side diminishes or even completely disappears.

TOS that is due to muscle atrophy may show best when a client lies on his affected side and the pulse is diminished by axillary artery compression.

Other Connective Tissue Disorders

Bunions

Definition: What Are They?

Bunions are also known as hallux valgus, which means "laterally deviated big toe." The first phalanx of the great toe is distorted toward the lateral aspect of the foot. The joint capsule stretches, a bursa grows at the irritated site, and callus grows over the protrusion. A smaller version of the same problem sometimes appears at the base of the little toe; this is called "tailor's bunion" or "bunionette."

Women have bunions about 10 times more often than men. High-heeled, narrow-toed shoes are factors, but a genetic weakness in the toe joints may predispose some people to bunions regardless of footwear.

Etiology: What Happens?

Several factors can contribute to the misalignment between the first metatarsal and the proximal phalanx of the great toe. Feet with exaggerated arches, or even with no arches, can force pressure onto the targeted spot. Muscle imbalances within the foot and the lower leg can influence how force is distributed through the joint. Further, the shape of the head of the first metatarsal determines the stability of the metatarsophalangeal joint: the rounder the head, the less stable the joint and the more prone it is to valgus stress.

Any of these issues, in combination with footwear that squeezes the toes or forces weight onto the medial aspect of the foot (i.e., high-heeled, narrow-toed shoes or cowboy boots), can open the door to the painful distortion that bunions involve.

Pressure at the metacarpophalangeal joint can cause erosion and irritation, but the acute pain of bunions is also often related to local friction bursitis. Ultimately, if this misaligned weight-bearing joint is not corrected or supported in a way that limits erosion of the joint structures, the bunion patient can also develop bone spurs and arthritis, which can make it prohibitively painful to walk.

Signs and Symptoms

Bunions look like a large lump on the medial side of the metatarsophalangeal joint of the great toe. If the bunion

Bunions in Brief

Pronunciation: BUN-yunz

What are they?
A bunion is a protrusion at the metatarsophalangeal joint of the great toe that occurs when the toe is laterally deviated.

How are they recognized?
Bunions are recognizable by the large bump on the medial aspect of the foot. When they are inflamed, they are red, hot, and painful.

Massage risks and benefits
Risks: Bunions locally contraindicate deep specific massage, which may exacerbate inflammation and pain.
Benefits: Lymphatic work to reduce local inflammation may help with some bunion pain, and work elsewhere on the foot and with other gait compensation patterns may be helpful for a client with this painful condition.

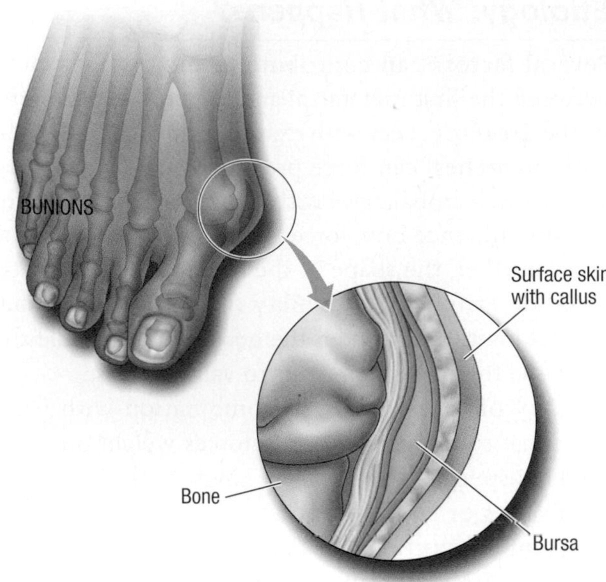

Figure 3.48. Bunion

is not irritated, a simple protrusion, often covered with a thick layer of callus, is obvious (Figure 3.48). If the bursa is inflamed, the area is red, hot, and extremely painful.

Treatment

The highest priority in treating a bunion is to remove whatever irritants contribute to the problem. This may mean switching footgear or even cutting holes in shoes to make room for the protrusion. Other noninvasive strategies include massage and exercise: range-of-motion stretches, gentle traction, and friction around (not on) the affected area are recommended to limit pain and slow progression, but these interventions do not necessarily realign the toe.

Elevating the heel to an appropriate height can relieve some pain, and a corticosteroid injection can reduce inflammation. But if damage has developed inside the joint and if the bunion is painful enough to limit the patient's activity, surgery may be recommended. A variety of surgeries have been developed to remove the bunion, reshape the foot bones, or fuse the joint. The success rates are determined by how badly the foot was distorted and whether joints other than the metatarsophalangeal joint were involved.

Medications

- NSAIDs for pain and inflammation management
- Injected cortisol for inflammation

Massage?

RISKS Acutely inflamed bunions locally contraindicate deep, specific massage, which may exacerbate swelling and pain.

BENEFITS Massage won't reverse a bunion, but it can certainly improve the quality of life for a person with this painful condition.

OPTIONS Focus on intrinsic foot muscles and other postural and gait compensation patterns that arise when walking is painful may improve efficiency of movement and reduce overall pain.

Bursitis

Definition: What is It?

Bursae are small closed sacs made of connective tissue. They are lined with synovial membrane and filled with synovial fluid. Bursitis is inflammation of the bursae. When these fluid-filled sacs are irritated, internal cells proliferate and generate excess fluid, which causes pain and limits mobility.

Bursitis in Brief

What is it?
A bursa is a fluid-filled sac that acts as a protective cushion, eases the movement of tendons and ligaments moving over bones, and cushions points of contact between bones. Bursitis is the inflammation of a bursa.

How is it recognized?
Acute bursitis is painful and is aggravated by both passive and active motion. Muscles surrounding the affected joint often severely limit range of motion. It may be hot or edematous if the bursa is superficial.

Massage risks and benefits
Risks: Acute bursitis locally contraindicates any massage that is deep or specific. Bursitis due to infection contraindicates massage until the infection has been treated and eradicated.
Benefits: Lymphatic work to reduce local inflammation may help with some bursa pain, but doesn't address the root of the problem. Massage elsewhere on the body during an acute phase and directly to the muscles around the affected joint (within pain limits) in a subacute phase is appropriate.

The human body has about 160 bursae, but new ones can be generated in areas that need protection. Most bursae are very small, but the ones that protect the knee, shoulder, and hip can be quite large.

Bursitis comes in all shapes and forms, some of which have descriptive names, like *housemaid's knee* and *student's elbow,* which occurs on the point of the olecranon. *Weaver's bottom* is bursitis on the ischial tuberosity. Bursitis at the greater trochanter is a common variety, as is bursitis at the insertion of the iliopsoas on the lesser trochanter and at the calcaneus. Subacromial bursitis (Figure 3.49) is probably the most common presentation.

Etiology: What Happens?

Imagine stretching a rubber band over the sharp edge of a table. Now imagine moving it back and forth for several minutes. In a short time, the rubber band frays and then breaks. But if you put tiny water balloon between the rubber band and the edge of the table, the rubber band has freedom to move without the friction from the table: the water balloon protects it from damage. Bursae are the water balloons; they serve to ease the movement of tendons (rubber bands) over bony angles (table edge) (see Figure 3.50). Bursae also cushion the bones where they would otherwise bang against each other. Bursae pad people's sharpest corners: they are on elbows, knees, heels, and ischial tuberosities and between layers of fascia. Some bursae are present at birth, but others grow in response to wear and tear.

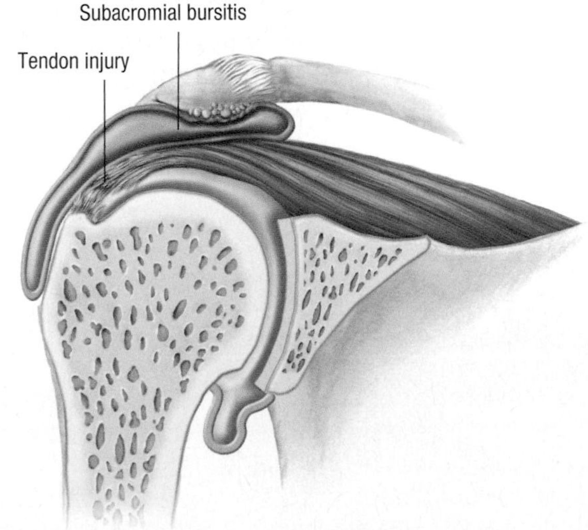

Figure 3.49. Subacromial bursitis

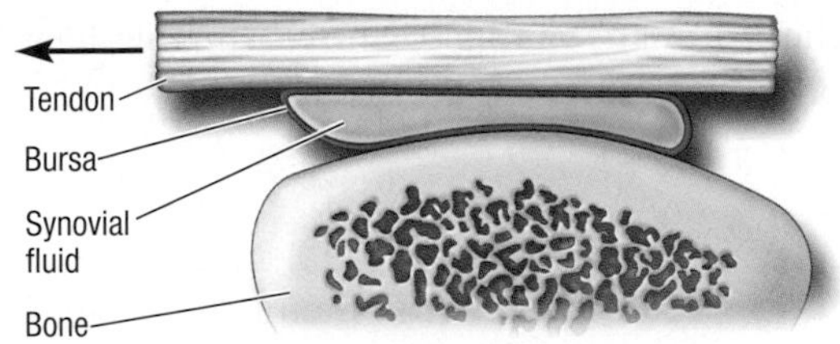

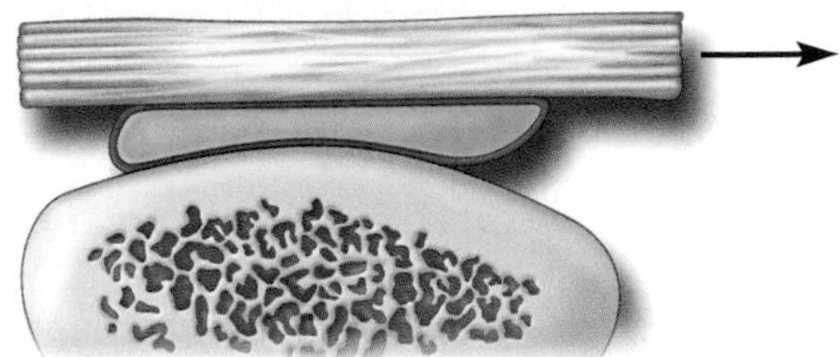

Figure 3.50. Bursae allow tendons to move freely over bony prominences

Without bursae to protect them, many tendons would fray and rupture in short order. Some bones that are not meant to touch would touch, and with great force. Sharp corners like elbows or bunions would have no protection.

Repetitive stress is the most common bursitis trigger. Chronic irritation leads to changes in the synovial lining: the walls of the bursa thicken, and the inflammatory process stimulates a massive production of fluid. Nearby muscles contract to splint the perceived injury, drastically limiting the range of motion of the affected joint. Sometimes the muscles actually aggravate and prolong an episode of bursitis by compressing the joint and the bursa at the same time.

Bursitis often occurs in concert with other inflammatory conditions. It tends to accompany general area inflammation, so if a person has a tendon injury, bursitis is often present as well. It also attends gout, rheumatoid arthritis, and tuberculosis.

The most common sites of bursitis are at the subacromial bursae, several of the 11 bursae around the knees, at the greater trochanter, and at the ischial tuberosities. Bursae can also be inflamed through a local infection, usually with *Staphylococcus aureus*. This happens most often with superficial bursae, especially at the elbow and the knee.

Signs and Symptoms

The symptoms of bursitis include pain on passive and active movement, along with extremely limited range of motion because of muscular splinting. Superficial bursitis may also show palpable heat and swelling.

Treatment

Treatment strategies for bursitis include oral anti-inflammatories, hot or cold packs, aspiration of excess fluid, and corticosteroid injections.

Medications

- NSAIDs for pain and inflammation management
- Injected cortisone for inflammation

Massage?

RISKS Acute bursitis can be exacerbated if deep specific massage is applied to the irritated area. Any infection must be resolved before bodywork is applied as well.

BENEFITS Massage that respects the limitations of acute inflammation is safe for clients with bursitis. Clients who have a history of bursitis can enjoy the same benefits of bodywork as the rest of the population.

OPTIONS Careful work to muscles that cross the affected joint may help to restore a normal range of motion, decompress the area, and reduce some of the bursal irritation.

Shin Splints

Definition: What Are They?

Shin splints is a term referring to a variety of lower leg problems. **Medial tibial stress syndrome** is the injury most commonly associated with shin splints, but closely related problems include **periostitis** and stress fractures. Chronic or acute compartment syndrome can be related injuries, but they are discussed elsewhere.

Etiology: What Happens?

Several features make the lower leg susceptible to certain injuries. One of them is the fact that the lower leg muscles have long attachments. Their endomysial sheaths blend directly into the deep crural fascia, and the periosteum and interosseous ligament of the tibia and fibula. This means any irritation of these muscles and fascia easily translates into irritation of the attaching periosteum.

Another key to lower leg function is the shock-absorbing capacity of the feet. Feet are designed to spread out and rebound with each step. If the foot has inadequate shock absorption—because of flat feet or jammed arches (pes planus or pes cavus, respectively), worn-out shoes, hard surfaces, or any combination thereof—the tibia and the muscles in the lower

Shin Splints in Brief

What are they?
The term "shin splints" refers to a collection of lower leg injuries, including muscle injuries, periostitis, hairline fractures, and other problems. They are usually brought about by overuse and/or misalignment at the ankle.

How are they recognized?
Pain along the tibia may be superficial or deep, mild, or severe. The pattern of pain differs with the specific structures that are injured.

Massage risks and benefits
Risks: Some shin splint situations may contraindicate massage until more information is gathered, or the acute stage has passed. Compartment syndromes (discussed elsewhere) can be a serious complication, and bone fractures need different treatment options and healing times than other injuries.
Benefits: Massage therapy can be helpful to treat uncomplicated muscle injuries around the tibia, and it can also be a useful strategy to augment training and reduce the risk of injury to the lower leg muscular and fascial structures.

Where Is Scleroderma?

Scleroderma is an autoimmune disorder in which the immune system mistakenly attacks the lining of small blood vessels, leading to the abnormal production of collagen in the skin and other tissues. It now appears with several other autoimmune disease discussions in Chapter 6.

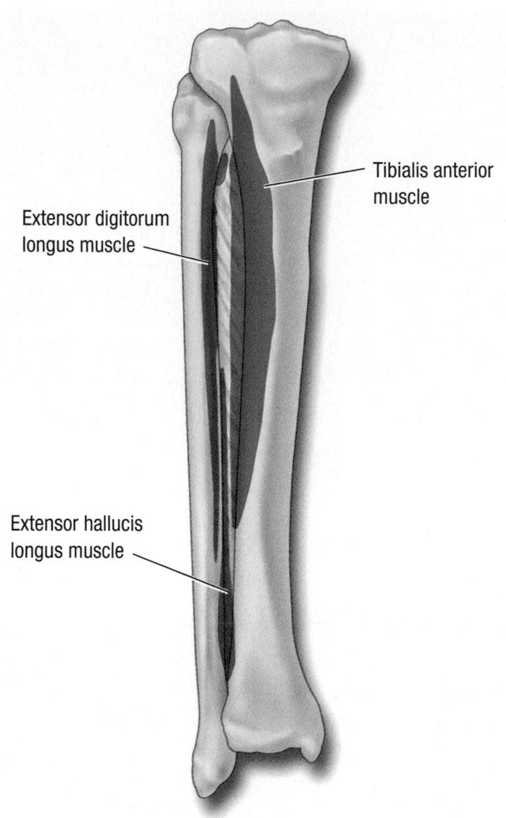

Figure 3.51. Shin splints: anterior leg muscles blend into the tibial periosteum

leg, especially the soleus, tibialis anterior, and tibialis posterior, absorb a disproportionate amount of the shock. They are not designed for this job, and ongoing stress may cause the periosteum to become irritated, the bone to crack, and the muscles to fray and become inflamed.

Shin splints often develop when a training routine is suddenly changed, or in relation to worn-out footwear or running consistently on hard surfaces. Running all uphill or all downhill can also be triggers.

Compartment syndrome, a situation in which swelling within the tough fascial compartments of the lower leg dangerously impedes function, is a possible complication of shin splints. This condition is discussed elsewhere.

Types of Shin Splints

- *Medial tibial stress syndrome*. This may be the most common presentation of shin splints. It involves muscular injury on the medial side of the tibia, specifically to the soleus and tibialis anterior. It is typically painful at the distal third segment of the medial tibia.
- *Tibialis anterior, tibialis posterior injury*. The pain associated with these injuries may be familiar to many people. The ache often runs most of the length of the tibia on the lateral side (for tibialis anterior) or deep in the back of the calf (for tibialis posterior).
- *Periostitis*. This inflammation of the periosteum may develop with damage to the soleus, the anterior tibialis, or posterior tibialis muscles. That seamless connection of membranes begins to rip apart, and the fibers of the muscles pull away from the bone.
- *Stress fractures*. These hairline fractures of the tibia can be extremely painful, and they don't heal unless activity is suspended. They are frequently the result of "running through the pain." Stress fractures of the tibia often don't show up well on radiographs: they are best diagnosed by bone scan, which looks for areas of increased circulatory activity.

Signs and Symptoms

Pain from shin splints can be mild or severe, and the location varies according to which of the structures has been damaged. It gets worse with whatever actions the affected muscles do: dorsiflexion, inversion, or plantarflexion. Simple muscle injuries are rarely visibly or palpably inflamed. If the anterior lower leg is red, hot, and puffy, a more severe injury than muscle damage may be present.

Treatment

The typical approach to mild shin splints is to reduce activity, and to alternate applications of heat and cold to the affected area. Changing footwear and analyzing inefficient movement or training patterns are helpful. Patients may be counseled to replace their normal activity with nonpercussive exercise while their legs recover. If pain is intense or long lasting, further evaluation for stress fractures or compartment syndrome may be necessary.

Medications

- NSAIDs for pain and inflammation control

Massage?

RISKS Any palpably hot or inflamed situation in the lower leg musculature requires medical attention before massage is appropriate. If a case of shin splints seems particularly long lasting, evaluation for a stress fracture is important: a massage therapist may be in a position to give good advice in this instance.

BENEFITS Mild muscle injury or periosteum irritation can respond well to massage, which may allow the client to return to pain-free activity sooner than otherwise.

OPTIONS Pin-and-stretch techniques that focus on the accessible shin muscles can target structures that are otherwise difficult to stretch and mobilize.

Tendinopathies in Brief

Pronunciation: ten-dih-NOP-ath-ez

What are they?
Tendinopathies are injuries or damage to tendons and their fascial sheaths. While it is possible for these injuries to involve acute inflammation (as indicated in the traditional terms tendinitis or tenosynovitis), most long-term tendon injuries are related to collagen degeneration rather than inflammation. The term for this condition is tendinosis.

How are they recognized?
Pain and loss of range of motion are often present with tendinopathies. Pain is exacerbated by resisted exercise of the damaged muscle-tendon unit. Damage to the tenosynovial sheath may also create pain, resistance to movement, and **crepitus**: a grinding texture as the tendon moves through its fascial covering.

Massage risks and benefits
Risks: Tendinopathies with true inflammation are rare, but when they occur, bodywork is best delayed until the acute phase is complete. An exception to this is lymphatic work, which may help to limit some of the negative aspects of swelling.
Benefits: Most tendinopathies indicate massage, which aims to help improve the quality and function of the affected connective tissues.

Tendinopathies

Definition: What Are They?

Tendinopathies is an umbrella term that covers injury and damage to tendons and tenosynovial sheaths. These conditions can include acute tears and ruptures but are most often related to chronic degeneration due to injury, repetitive use, age, nutrition, and other factors.

Etiology: What Happens?

When tendons are injured, a number of changes in the tissue occur. Acute injuries involve inflammatory cells (various types of white blood cells), edema, and pain; the correct term in this situation is tendinitis. But most tendinopathies do not involve acute inflammation. Rather, they are conditions in which the collagen degenerates and the tendon loses its weight-bearing capacity. This situation is more correctly termed tendinosis, or pathologic condition of the tendon.

Tendons are made mostly of type I collagen fibers suspended in liquid ground substance. A small number of elastin fibers are woven into the structure to lend some limited stretch and rebound, but the bulk of the tissues are dense, linearly arranged collagen fibers. Healthy tendons look hard, shiny, and white. By contrast, tendons with chronic degeneration look dull, gray or brown, and soft.

The causes for the chronic degenerative processes of tendinosis can be discussed as a combination of intrinsic and extrinsic factors. Intrinsic factors include direct or shearing forces transferred through the tendon, overuse without recovery time, poor flexibility, underlying disease, or a history of corticosteroid injection. Extrinsic factors can include training errors of athletes, problems with equipment, or a fall or blow that damages the tendon from the outside.

Tendinopathies occur most often at the rotator cuff and biceps tendon, medial and lateral epicondyles of the humerus, around the patella, at the distal attachment of the iliotibial band, and at the Achilles tendon.

Types of Tendinopathies

- *Tendinitis*. This is a new injury that leads to the classic signs of inflammation: pain, heat, redness, and swelling.

- *Tendinosis*. In this condition of long-term degeneration, microscopy shows more liquid ground substance than in a healthy tendon, and the collagen fibers are disrupted and discontinuous. Fibroblasts are active, and new blood vessels are present also. The collagen fibers are predominantly type III fibers, which are thinner and weaker than the normal type I fibers of healthy tendons (Figure 3.52).
- *Tenosynovitis*. In this condition, irritation develops where tendons slide through their synovial sheaths. It happens most often at the wrist and flexor aspect of the fingers, and is often characterized by a gritty sensation called crepitus during movement (Figure 3.53).
  - *DeQuervain tenosynovitis*. This is tenosynovitis specifically of the abductor and extensor pollicis tendons. It is often acutely inflamed, and may be related to a systemic bacterial infection.

Signs and Symptoms

The symptoms of tendinopathies are very similar to those of muscle strains, though they may be more intense. The acute stage may show some heat and swelling, depending on which tendons are affected. Most tendon swelling is not visible or palpable with a few exceptions: the Achilles tendon and the posterior tibialis tendon at the medial ankle may swell significantly with injury. In all stages of tendinosis, stiffness and pain are present, especially with resistive movements and in stretching.

Tenosynovitis has an added feature of resistance as the affected tendon moves through its sheath. This can show as crepitus (a grinding sensation), and as a loss of smooth motion: fingers with this condition are easy to flex, but difficult to extend; this gives rise to a layman's term for this: "trigger finger."

Treatment

The quality of the healing of a damaged tendon or sheath depends largely on what happens with the production of new collagen fibers. Because inflammation turns out not to be a significant issue in most long-lasting tendon injuries, the use of anti-inflammatories and steroid injections is being reconsidered.

A combination of rest, ice, stretching, and carefully gauged exercise turns out to be the most

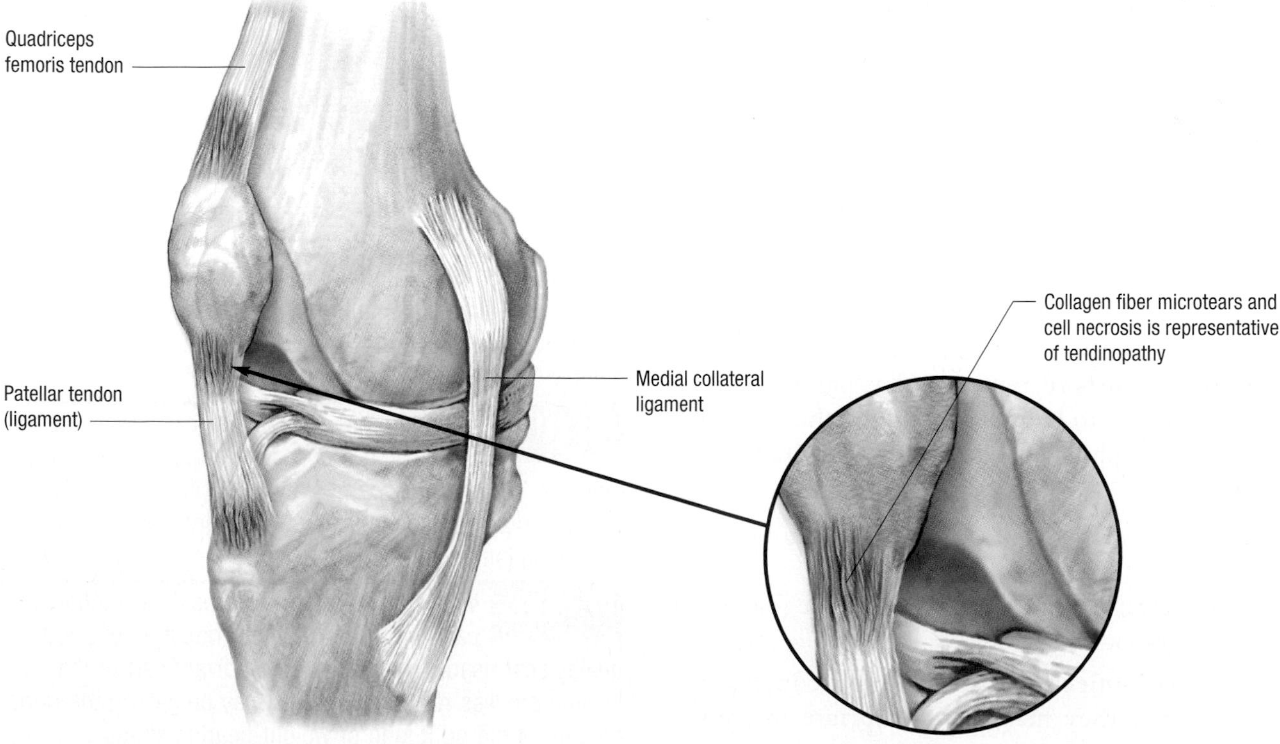

Figure 3.52. Tendinopathy

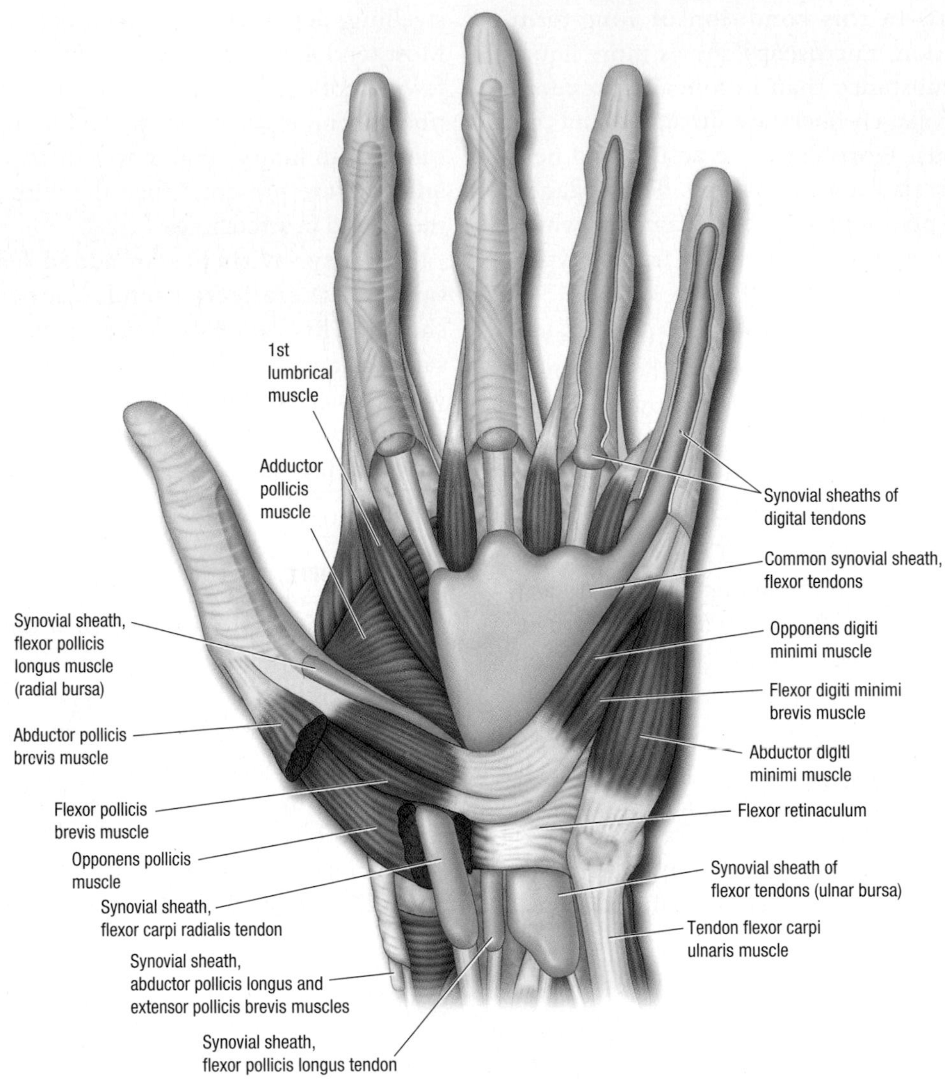

Figure 3.53. Tenosynovitis: synovial sheaths should allow tendons to slide easily over each other

effective treatment options for these injuries. Ultrasound or extracorporeal shock wave therapy also get good results, especially in combination with exercise. Eccentric contractions appear to be particularly useful to rebuild a damaged tendon. Some orthopedists recommend that patients wear a splint or brace to help bear some of the force of a damaged tendon, especially with DeQuervain tenosynovitis.

Medications

- NSAIDs for pain (but usually not for anti-inflammatory action)
- Steroid injections (this is now controversial but they may be appropriate in some circumstances)

Massage?

RISKS Acute injuries locally contraindicate deep massage until the inflammation has begun to resolve, but lymphatic work during this phase may be helpful.

BENEFITS Various types of massage can contribute to the healing process for chronically irritated tendons. Whether that comes about because of impact on circulation or the mechanical impact of movement and stretching isn't clear, however.

OPTIONS With-fiber friction and crossfiber friction can help promote the production of good-quality scar tissue, but the most important part of the healing process for these injuries may be getting the right amount of the right kind of weight-bearing stress.

Whiplash

Definition: What is It?

Whiplash, or cervical acceleration-deceleration (CAD), is a broad term used to refer to a mixture of injuries, including sprains, strains, and joint trauma. Bone fractures, herniated discs, nerve damage, and concussion are commonly seen along with these soft tissue injuries and so are often addressed simultaneously. Whiplash injuries are usually, but not always, associated with motor vehicle accidents (MVAs) in which the head whips backward and then forward in rapid succession (Figure 3.54).

Etiology: What Happens?

The nature of damage incurred by whiplash accidents depends on many variables. In MVAs, some of the most important factors are the direction of impact, the speed with which the vehicles were moving, the relative weight of the vehicles involved, whether the individual was wearing a seatbelt, the position of the individual's head, and whether the person was aware of the impending impact and had time to brace. Analysis of rear-impact accidents shows that as the momentum of the car seat forces the thorax forward, the head initially stays stable. About 100 milliseconds later, the head is propelled into flexion. The momentum of this movement is magnified by the leverage of the neck.

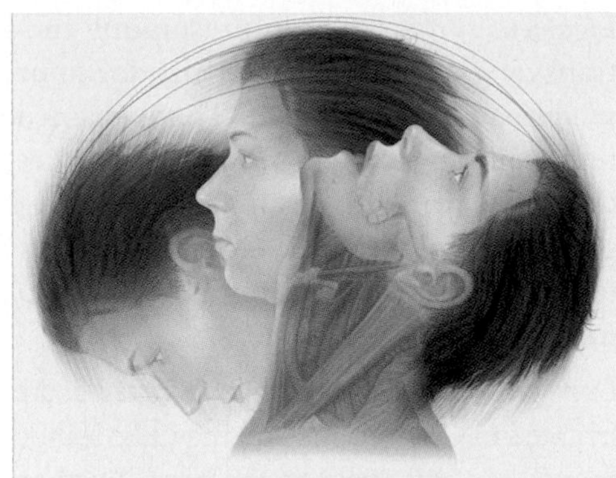

Figure 3.54. Cervical acceleration and deceleration: whiplash

Whiplash in Brief

What is it?
Whiplash is a collective term referring to a collection of soft tissue injuries that may occur with cervical acceleration followed by deceleration. These injuries include sprained ligaments, strained muscles, damaged joint capsules, and TMJ problems. Although whiplash technically refers to soft tissue injury, damage to other structures, including vertebrae, discs, and nerve tissue, frequently occurs at the same time.

How is it recognized?
Symptoms of whiplash vary according to the nature of the injuries. Posttrauma pain at the neck and referring into the shoulders and arms, along with chronic headaches, are the most frequent indicators.

Massage risks and benefits
Risks: Acute injuries, along with those that have not been fully diagnosed, contraindicate any but the gentlest bodywork. The risks of exacerbating inflammation or of disrupting unstable bones or joints are important to respect.
Benefits: Postacute and mature whiplash injuries can benefit from massage that focuses on restoring healthy muscle tone and movement patterns, along with improving the quality of any connective tissue scarring that may have occurred.

While MVAs account for the majority of diagnosed whiplash cases, it is important to remember that other injuries can create the same scenario. Sports injuries and falls can involve a similar injury process, especially when a collision affects the neck and head.

Accidents of this nature put the cervical muscles (especially the sternocleidomastoid, scalenes, and splenius cervicis) at risk for strains. Supraspinous and intertransverse spinal ligaments are frequently sprained. Two internal structures, the anterior and posterior longitudinal ligaments, may also be traumatized. Other damage may affect the capsules of the facet joints; the esophagus and larynx; intervertebral discs; vertebrae, which may subluxate or fracture; the TMJ; spinal nerve roots; the spinal cord, which may be compressed or stretched; and the brain, which is vulnerable to concussion.

Signs and Symptoms

A lot of crossover exists between whiplash-related injuries and subsequent complications; both are discussed here. Basic signs and symptoms include head and neck pain, which may radiate into the trunk or arms; loss of range of motion; and **paresthesia**. One of the curious aspects of whiplash is that it is common for symptoms to be delayed for days, weeks, and occasionally months before coming to full intensity. This phenomenon is not well understood.

- *Ligament sprains.* The supraspinous and intertransverse ligaments are at risk for injury in a whiplash type of accident. These ligaments can refer pain up over the head, into the chest, and down the arms: this can be difficult to distinguish from nerve pain. Ligament sprains often take a long time to heal, and they tend to accumulate excessive scar tissue.
- *Damaged facet joint capsules.* Joint capsules are often irritated in CAD events and they, like spinous ligaments, can refer pain to the head. Furthermore, these joint capsules are richly equipped with **nociceptors** that may intensify pain messages sent to the spinal cord. They also have proprioceptors that can send confusing messages to the brain, leading to dizziness or disorientation.
- *Subluxated cervical vertebrae.* Vertebrae may be displaced to the front, back, or side or rotated one way or another. In some very extreme cases, fractures may occur. Left untreated or incompletely treated, misaligned vertebrae with lax ligaments and lack of structural support may develop spondylosis.
- *Damaged discs.* This is not inevitable, but it may happen that the force of trauma causes the annulus fibrosus of the discs to crack, allowing the nucleus pulposus to bulge or herniate.
- *Spasm.* When a neck injury is acute, the paraspinals and other neck muscles go into spasm to splint the stretched neck ligaments. But this reaction has a tendency to outlive its usefulness. Spasm of neck muscles significantly limits its range of motion.
- *Trigger points.* Traumatized muscles often develop trigger points: local tight areas that refer pain, often into the head, causing chronic headaches. This is one form of myofascial pain syndrome.
- *Neurological symptoms.* These can include dizziness, blurred vision, abnormal smell or taste, tinnitus (ringing in the ears), or loss of hearing. These signs indicate cranial trauma: the brain has been bruised and may have some internal bleeding. This is usually the result of a specific blow, but postconcussion syndrome can also happen without direct impact.

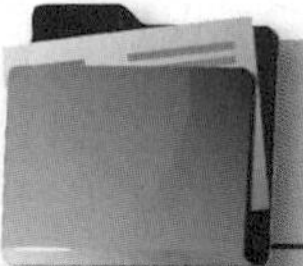

CASE HISTORY 3.1 Whiplash

A massage therapist met with a first-time client approximately 1 year after the client was in a car accident. The client was still in considerable pain. He was diagnosed with whiplash and was seeking massage under prescription from his doctor.

The therapist worked slowly and carefully, and was encouraged by the client to go deeper into his neck muscles, all the way down to the transverse processes of the neck vertebrae. He felt better after the massage; his muscles were looser, and he had an improved range of motion.

Several hours later, the client sneezed. The force of the motion wrenched his neck and reinjured the tissues, so that he was in greater pain, more spasm, and had much less range of motion than he had before his massage. He returned for another session, but it was ineffective at reducing his pain and dysfunction. He never sought massage again.

What is the moral here? It is utterly unclear whether the first massage put the client at risk for reinjuring himself just by sneezing. The therapist followed all the rules of good sense, worked with a doctor's recommendation, and let the client guide her into how much pressure felt comfortable. Yet it is necessary to entertain the possibility that the massage somehow did put the client at risk, even though the therapist was well informed and made what seemed to be the right decisions. No two people go through the same kind of healing process, and no two people respond to massage the same way. Massage therapists must weigh the benefits and risks of their work on a case-by-case basis. It is impossible to rely only on books and rules to make decisions about whether to give massage.■

- *TMJ disorders*. Direct impact of the jaw can damage the TMJ, but it is possible that the joint can be traumatized simply through the rapid acceleration and deceleration that accompany whiplash injuries. This is sometimes called "jawlash."
- *Headaches*. These arise for a variety of reasons, including, but not limited to, referred pain and trigger points from spasms in the neck, sprained ligaments that refer pain up over the head, irritated facet joint capsules, cranial bones that may be out of alignment, stress and its autonomic action on blood flow, muscle tightness in the neck and head, TMJ problems, and concussion.

Treatment

Neck collars are used for acute whiplash patients to take the stress off their wrenched ligaments and to try to reduce muscle spasm. But the sooner the injured structures are put back to use, the less scar tissue accumulates. Therefore, collars are strictly for short-term use, as this kind of immobilization can create more long-term problems than benefits.

Other treatment recommendations for whiplash patients include heat, ice, electrical stimulation, massage, myofascial release, traction, and stretching and strengthening programs.

Medical intervention typically focuses on pain relievers, anti-inflammatories, and muscle relaxants. These substances can change the quality of the tissues and sensory responses, so massage therapists should be aware when clients use them.

Medications

- NSAIDs for inflammation and pain control
- Narcotic analgesics for pain control
- Tricyclic antidepressants for sleep aid, pain control, and sedation
- Muscle relaxants for pain and spasm
- Injected steroids for inflammation
- Injected analgesics for pain
- Injected botulinum toxin into cervical trigger points for pain
- Oral steroids for inflammation

Massage?

RISKS The risk of exacerbating inflammation or inappropriately disrupting damaged tissues with vigorous massage during the acute phase of whiplash is important to respect. Further, because damage can affect the vertebrae, central nervous system, and structures in the anterior neck, it is important for a client with a recent neck trauma to be fully evaluated by a primary care provider before using bodywork as a treatment strategy.

BENEFITS In the subacute and postacute phases of whiplash recovery, massage can be an excellent strategy to deal with pain, proprioception, muscle tone, movement patterns, and dysfunctional scar tissue. Massage in combination with bony manipulation can be an especially powerful combination.

CHAPTER REVIEW QUESTIONS: MUSCULOSKELETAL CONDITIONS

1. What kind of muscle spasm serves an important function in healing?
2. What part of the bone is affected most severely by osteoporosis? What implications does this have for complications?
3. Describe the difference between functional and structural postural deviations.
4. What is a synonym for adhesive capsulitis?
5. Your client has a subluxated vertebra. Can you work with him? Why or why not?
6. Your client had a hip replacement surgery last year. What accommodations can you expect to make for her?
7. Your client has been diagnosed with Lyme disease. What extra hygienic measures do you need to take to prevent contracting this infection?

8. Where do massage therapists often get osteoarthritis?
9. What is a common feature of spondylosis that distinguishes it from other types of arthritis?
10. Your client has a three-week-old ankle sprain. It is still painful but not palpably hot or swollen. What benefits might massage offer this person?
11. Describe why bruxism is both a cause and a symptom of TMJ disorder.
12. What does hernia mean? Name three kinds of abdominal hernias.
13. Describe how pes planus can lead to headaches.
14. Your client has electrical pain and weakness in the hand, especially at the thumb and first three fingers. What condition is probably present?
15. With the understanding that carpal tunnel syndrome is often a part of a multiple crush phenomenon, list at least two other places where the median nerve might be irritated or obstructed.
16. Your client has been diagnosed with degenerative disc disease at L4. Name three symptoms he is likely to report.
17. Your client has excruciating pain at the base of the great toe. The skin is red, shiny, hot, and throbbing. What condition is probably present?
18. Your client has excruciating pain at the base of the great toe. The skin is thick and callused, and a large bump protrudes medially. What condition is probably present?
19. What condition is associated with the accumulation of trigger points?
20. Your client was in a motor vehicle accident 2 days ago, and has been diagnosed with whiplash. Name three possible associated injuries that contraindicate massage in the acute phase.

4

Nervous System Conditions

Chapter Objectives

After reading this chapter, you should be able to...

- Name a feature that Alzheimer disease and amyotrophic lateral sclerosis have in common.
- Name a caution for massage for clients with peripheral neuropathy.
- Name the causative agent of shingles, and another common infection caused by the same pathogen.
- Name three types of depression.
- Name three types of anxiety disorders.
- Name the most subtle type of autism spectrum disorder.
- Name two types of stroke, and explain how they differ.
- Name the nerve involved in Bell palsy.
- Name three complications of spinal cord injury.
- Name the differences between fibromyalgia syndrome tender points and myofascial pain trigger points.
- Name a trigger for tension-type headaches and migraine headaches.
- Name three major cautions for massage in the context of nervous system disorders.

By the time most massage therapists finish their core education, they probably know more about the nervous system than they ever suspected existed, and they may still feel like rank amateurs on the subject. That feeling is common to most people who study this topic: it is a complex system about which we are still learning, so detailed information changes often. Fortunately, only a passing familiarity with the structure and function of this system is needed to make educated decisions about massage and many nervous system disorders.

Many of the conditions considered here affect the peripheral nerves rather than the central nervous system (CNS), so this introductory discussion focuses mainly on the structure and function of the parts of the nervous system massage therapists can touch—which, not coincidentally, are also the parts of the system that are most vulnerable to injury.

Function and Structure

Nerves are bundles of individual neurons: fibrous cells capable of transmitting electrical impulses from one place to another. At their most basic level, the function of neurons is to transmit information from the body to the brain (sensation) and responses from the brain to the body (motor control). Interconnecting neurons in the brain also provide the potential for consciousness, learning, creativity, memory, and other fascinating abilities, but they are beyond the scope of this book.

Peripheral nerves are composed of bundles of long filaments (neurons) that run from the spinal cord to the area in the body to which they supply sensation or motor control. Each neuron is a single living cell. Some of them are tiny, but the neurons that signal when we stub our toe run from the toe up the leg, through the buttocks, into the spine, and up to the spinal cord, terminating around T_{12} to L_1. Each of these cells is several feet long.

Neurons have three parts: the **dendrite** (which carries impulses toward the cell body), the cell body with a nucleus, and the **axon** (which carries impulses away from the cell body). Sensory neurons therefore have exceptionally long dendrites to carry information from the periphery toward the cell body in the dorsal root ganglia; they have short little axons to continue carrying their impulses into the spinal cord. Motor neurons have tiny dendrites and cell bodies inside the spinal cord, and very long axons to carry messages out to their terminating sites in the muscles and glands.

Neurons connect via **synapses**. Motor and sensory neurons sometimes use combinations of central or association neurons to pass messages. When a stimulus enters the spinal cord via a sensory neuron, the message can cross the synapse to multiple neurons. Some carry it up to the brain to be consciously processed, but others immediately exit the spinal cord through a motor neuron that allows an even faster response to the stimulus. This loop is called a **reflex arc** (Figure 4.1).

Most neurons in the peripheral and central nervous systems have a waxy insulating coating called **myelin**. This layer of material speeds conduction along

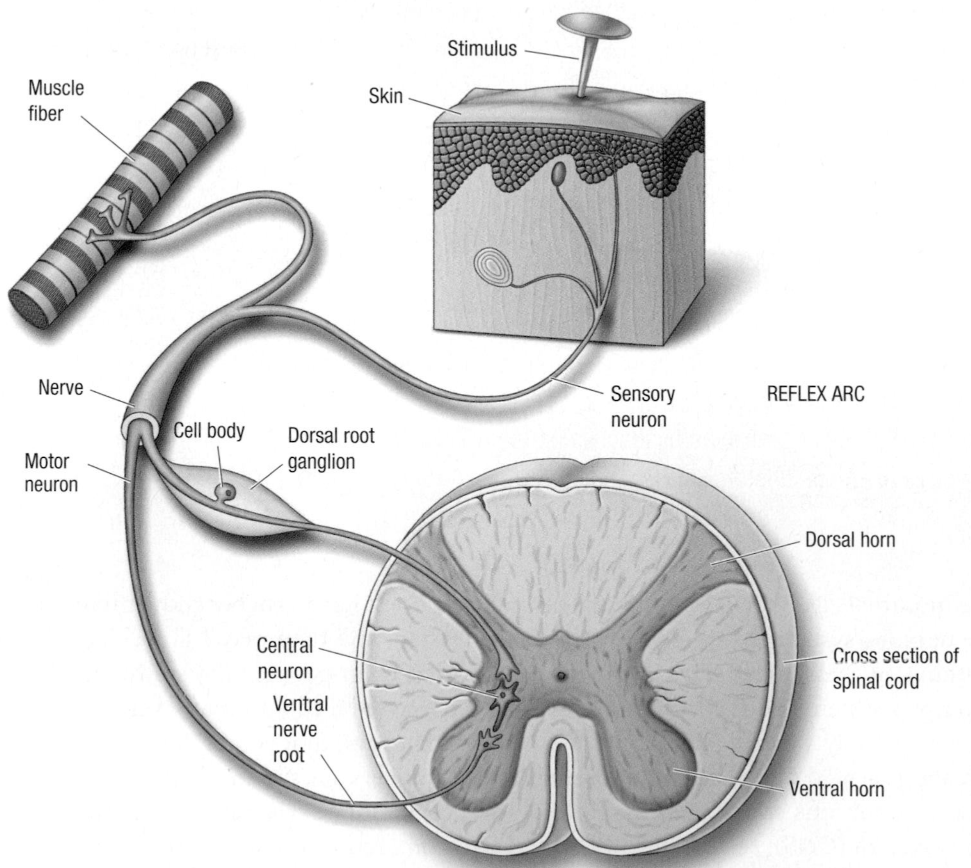

Figure 4.1. The reflex arc: connecting sensation to motor response

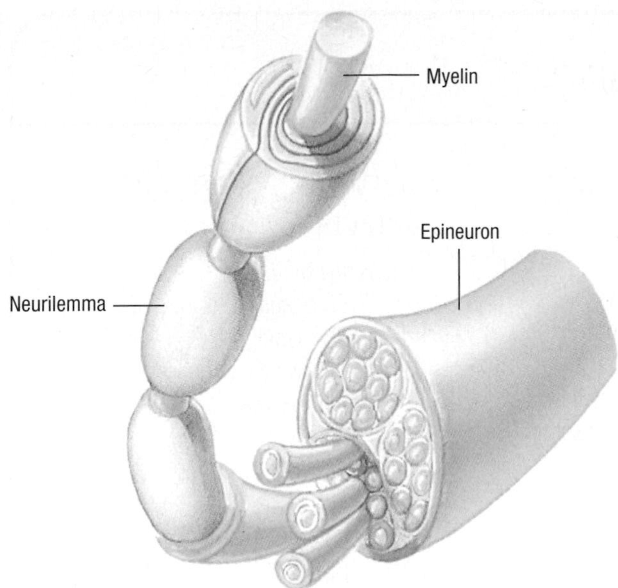

Figure 4.2. Nerve coverings: myelin, neurilemma, connective tissue epineuron.

the fiber and also prevents the electrical impulses from jumping from one fiber to another. In the peripheral nervous system, neurons have another protective feature in **neurilemma**, an outside covering of fibers that can help to regenerate damaged tissue (Figure 4.2).

It is a convenient analogy to think about nerves as bundles of electrical wires. The similarities are obvious: here are thousands of filaments carrying electrical impulses, each one wrapped by an insulating layer of myelin, and they are bundled together in packages. The analogy stops, however, when one considers the effect of external pressure on nerve fiber transmission. Nerves function with a combination of electrical and fluid flow; this flow may be severely limited by external pressure. Consider the implications of that pressure on a femoral nerve that is hugged by a psoas in spasm, or the brachial plexus nerves running through a tangled maze of scalenes and pectoralis minor muscles: the obstruction of fluid flow in living nerve tissue interferes with function, and leads to many problems.

General Neurological Problems

Most of the nervous system disorders that massage can mechanically affect involve some kind of pinching or distortion of peripheral nerves as they wend their way from the spinal cord to their destination in the body. Peripheral nerve damage often has a good prognosis because of the regenerative properties provided by the neurilemma.

Other neurological problems involve the central nervous system (CNS), which have very limited ability to regenerate, and which massage obviously cannot directly access. But even when the spinal cord has been injured, overlapping patterns of innervation created by the **plexi** often allow at least partial function of what would otherwise be a totally useless limb. This remarkable advantage begins to explain the benefits of the complicated interweaving patterns of spinal nerves that supply the extremities. The best plan, when faced with a client who has sustained CNS damage, is to address the symptoms of these disorders as well as possible, looking for sensation where it is present, and to create as hospitable an internal environment as possible.

Various kinds of CNS damage often leads to the progressive loss of motor function. This has traditionally been viewed as an inevitable consequence of CNS injury, but this idea may prove to be a myth. It has been found in many cases that loss of motor function may be an issue of proprioceptive adaptation more than true nerve loss. In other words, a stroke or traumatic brain injury survivor may lose some strength in an arm or a leg, and the compensatory movement patterns allow for further degeneration of affected muscle fibers. Massage, stretching, and careful exercise may help make it possible to interrupt and even reverse this type of progressive loss.

Organic and mechanical problems with the central and peripheral nervous systems are one class of neurological problems, which massage therapists encounter. Psychiatric disorders, which can also be classified as

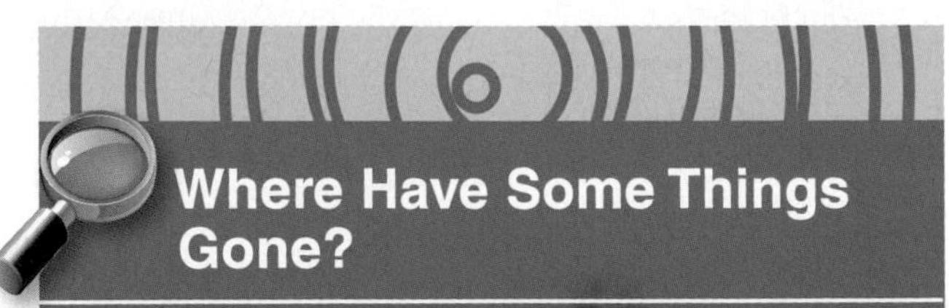

Where Have Some Things Gone?

Some items that would traditionally be discussed in Chapter 4 now appear elsewhere. Multiple sclerosis, an autoimmune disorder, now appears in Chapter 6. And several conditions that affect the nervous system but that have a relatively narrow application, or that massage therapists are unlikely to see in an acute stage, can now be found in Appendix C, **Extra Conditions At A Glance.** These include the following:

Acromegaly	Guillain-Barre syndrome	Multiple system atrophy
Charcot-Marie-Tooth syndrome	Myasthenia gravis	

Nervous System Conditions

Chronic degenerative disorders

- Alzheimer disease
- Amyotrophic lateral sclerosis:
  - Sporadic
  - Familial
  - Mariana Islands type
- Huntington disease
- Peripheral neuropathy

Movement disorders

- Dystonia
  - Focal
    - Spasmodic torticollis
    - Vocal dysphonia
    - Oromandibular dystonia
    - Blepharospasm
    - Writer's cramp
  - Segmental
    - Meige syndrome
    - Multifocal dystonia
    - Hemidystonia
    - Generalized dystonia
- Parkinson disease
- Tremor

Infectious disorders

- Encephalitis
  - Viral encephalitis
    - Primary
    - Secondary
  - Other types of encephalitis
- Herpes zoster
  - Chickenpox
  - Shingles
  - Postherpetic neuralgia
  - Ramsey-Hunt syndrome
  - Sine herpete
- Meningitis
  - Bacterial meningitis
  - Viral meningitis
- Polio, postpolio syndrome

Psychiatric disorders

- Addiction
  - Alcoholism
- Anxiety disorders
  - General anxiety disorder
  - Panic disorder
  - Acute traumatic stress disorder
  - Posttraumatic stress disorder
  - Social phobia
  - Specific phobias
- Attention deficit hyperactivily disorder
- Autism spectrum disorders
  - Autistic disorder
  - Asperger syndrome
  - Pervasive development disorder
  - Rett syndrome
  - Childhood disintegrative disorder
- Depression
  - Major depressive disorder
  - Psychotic depressive disorder
  - Adjustment disorder
  - Dysthymia
  - Bipolar disease
  - Seasonal affective disorder
  - Postpartum depression
- Eating disorders
  - Anorexia
  - Bulimia
  - Binge eating disorder

Nervous system injuries

- Bell palsy
- Complex regional pain syndrome
- Spinal cord injury
- Stroke
  - Ischemic stroke
    - Transient ischemic attack
    - Cryptogenic stroke
  - Hemorrhagic stroke
- Traumatic brain injury
- Trigeminal neuralgia

Nervous system birth defects

- Spina bifida
  - SB occulta
  - SB meningocele
  - SB myelomeningocele
- Cerebral palsy
  - Spastic CP
  - Athetoid CP
  - Ataxic CP
  - Dystonic CP
  - Mixed CP

Other nervous system conditions

- Fibromyalgia
- Headaches
  - Tension type
  - Migraine
  - Cluster
  - Rebound
- Ménière disease
- Seizure disorders
  - Epilepsy
- Sleep disorders
  - Insomnia
  - Obstructive sleep apnea
  - Central sleep apnea
  - Restless leg syndrome
  - Narcolepsy
  - Circadian rhythm disruption
- Vestibular balance disorders
  - Benign paroxysmal positional vertigo
  - Labyrinthitis
  - Acute vestibular neuronitis
  - Perilymph fistula

neurological problems, are another matter altogether. Many people have a bewildering array of mental or psychological qualities that set them apart from what is labeled "normal." Some of these people seek massage as a way to deal with some of the difficulties that their conditions create. This is often a good impulse; touch is an integral part of physical and psychological health. Research on massage and mood disorders shows a strong and reliable positive effect. In fact, it could be said that touch is an important link between physical and psychological health (Sidebar 4.1).

Major Cautions for Massage Therapists

In the context of nervous system problems and massage, a few cautions emerge as common themes:

- *Numbness*. When a client can't feel part of his or her body, it is inappropriate to try to change the quality of those tissues. It is fine to include the numb area as a part of the incorporating aspect of massage, but extra care must be taken not to damage tissues where the client has no sensation.
- *Verbal communication*. Some types of nervous system problems make it difficult or impossible for clients to communicate verbally. While massage can still be safe and supportive, it is especially important for therapists to be sensitive to nonverbal cues about comfort and pain from these clients.
- *Medications*. Clients who take medication to help manage their mood or other mental states may find that massage is especially helpful—so much so that they want to change or stop taking their medication altogether. While this sounds like wonderful progress, it must only be done with the guidance of the prescribing physician.

SIDEBAR 4.1 The Stress Response System

The stress response system is the link between the CNS and the endocrine system that allows humans to respond to both short-term and long-term stressors. It is controlled by the hypothalamic-pituitary-adrenal axis, the communication loop between the hypothalamus, the pituitary gland, and the adrenal glands. A healthy stress response system allows immediate reactions that are appropriately gauged to the circumstances: big reactions to big threats, small reactions to small threats. And when the stress response system works well, the chemical changes it brings about are transitory and quickly neutralized once the threat has passed.

Some people have a stress response system that doesn't work well. The chemical messages issued first from the hypothalamus, then by the pituitary gland, are slow to leave the brain and reach the adrenals. This takes longer to have an effect on the body, decreasing the ability to respond quickly to threat. But the stress reaction, once it takes hold, is tenacious, and after-effects linger much longer than for someone who has a healthy stress response system. Furthermore, people who have a sluggish stress response system also tend to have more stress responses with less threatening stimuli. This is a person who fumes in a long checkout line, who frets in heavy traffic, and who blows up when the kids leave their bikes in the driveway. This is someone who may have a sluggish but overactive stress response, and this person has a high propensity to develop several diseases, including depression and anxiety disorders.

What determines the health of the stress response system? Studies with animals reveal one reliable predictor for a sluggish stress response: lack of tactile stimulation, or touch. Understimulated animals have consistently slower, longer lasting, and more frequent stress responses than animals that were regularly petted and fondled. Consider what this means for the average undertouched person in our society: low-functioning but long-lasting stress reactions that occur with unnecessary and unhealthy frequency.

A solid body of evidence supports the use of massage for several psychiatric conditions, including depression and some types of anxiety. The mechanism for how massage helps in these situations isn't yet clear, but it seems possible that welcomed, educated touch can be an important link between physical experience and psychiatric health.

Chronic Degenerative Disorders

Alzheimer Disease

Definition: What Is It?

Alzheimer disease (AD) is a progressive degenerative disorder of the brain causing memory loss, personality changes, and eventually death.

The incidence of AD is strongly tied to age. While about 10% of people over 65 have it, about 50% of those over 85 have been diagnosed with it. It affects more women than men, but that may be more tied to life expectancy than to a gender-based predisposition.

Alzheimer Disease in Brief

Pronunciation: ALZ-hy-mur dih-ZEZE

What is it?
Alzheimer disease (AD) is a degenerative disorder of the brain involving shrinkage and death of neural tissue.

How is it recognized?
AD is difficult to definitively diagnose in a living person, but signs and symptoms include progressive memory loss, deterioration of language and cognitive skills, disorientation, and lack of ability to care for oneself.

Massage risks and benefits
Risks: AD patients may become disoriented, and some have difficulty with verbal communication. A therapist in this setting must be sensitive to nonverbal signals. Further, because this is often a disease of elderly people, other conditions that require bodywork accommodations may also be present.
Benefits: Massage has been seen to have much to offer AD patients: they tend to be calmer, better oriented, and less combative when bodywork is part of their care strategy.

Etiology: What Happens?

AD is named after a German doctor, Alois Alzheimer, who first documented the trademark lesions in the brain seen with this disorder in 1906. He performed an autopsy on a female patient who died in a mental institution in her mid-50s, and he noticed two specific changes in her brain tissue: plaques and tangles. These observations have become the primary postmortem diagnostic features of this disease, and they have become the focus of the leading edge of research today.

- *Plaques*. Sticky deposits of a naturally occurring cellular protein called **beta amyloid** have been noted on neural cells of people with AD. Beta amyloid is produced by many cells in the body, and it occurs in various lengths and qualities, depending on where it is found. In the brain it seems to be particularly sticky. When it accumulates in sufficient amounts, the deposits stimulate an inflammatory response in the brain that kills off not only the cells affected by the plaques but nearby unaffected cells as well.
- *Neurofibrillary tangles*. Another Alzheimer-related protein is called **tau**. This substance helps to physically support long fibers in the CNS, so they can connect at synapses. When tau proteins in AD patients degenerate, the long fibers collapse and become twisted and tangled together. Eventually the cells, which are incapable of transmitting messages to each other, shrink and die. The brain of a person with AD shows predictable patterns of atrophy, with deeper **sulci** (Figure 4.3), a smaller hippocampus, and larger ventricles than the brains of people without AD.

The presence of beta amyloid plaques and tau-related tangles means that fewer brain cells function at normal levels. With the loss of neural tissue, levels of neurotransmitters in the brains of AD patients become pathologically low. This makes it difficult for the functioning nerve cells that remain to communicate with each other. Further, the **hippocampus** (the part of the brain that processes and stores new information and knowledge) shrinks and loses function. Consequently, the AD patient loses access to memories and loses the ability to process new information.

Plaques and tangles were the first features associated with AD. Other contributing factors include

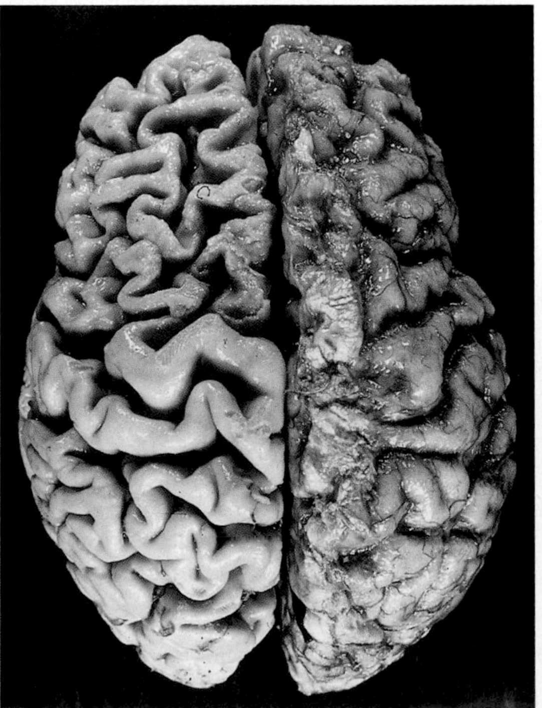

Figure 4.3. Visible atrophy associated with (AD)

genetics, chronic inflammation, a history of head injury, exposure to environmental toxins, high cholesterol levels, low estrogen levels (in women), the presence of cardiovascular disease and diabetes, and many other variables. These discoveries reveal many new possibilities for treatment and prevention of this disease.

While the exact causes of AD remain a mystery, it seems clear that some choices influence the chance of developing this disease. Regular physical activity, a healthy diet, frequent interactions with others, and a habit of lifelong learning are factors that appear to lessen the risk of developing this disease.

Signs and Symptoms

The degeneration associated with AD can occur across a wide spectrum over many years. Although each individual's experience of this disease is unique, a loose staging system has been developed:

- *Mild cognitive impairment (MCI).* This situation occurs in many older people, and may be simply age-related memory loss. However, a higher percentage of people with MCI go on to develop AD than those without MCI.
- *Mild Alzheimer disease.* In this stage, the affected person may easily get lost, have trouble with handling money, take longer to do basic tasks, and undergo some personality changes.
- *Moderate Alzheimer disease.* At this stage, memory loss and confusion are major problems. The patient may fail to recognize family and friends. Hallucinations, paranoia, and delusions are all possible.
- *Severe Alzheimer disease.* At this stage, verbal communication has been lost and the patient is completely reliant on others for all care. The swallow reflex is impaired, leading to a high risk of aspiration and subsequent pneumonia. Alternatively, the end of life may come as progressive organ shut down.

Treatment

Because AD is a complex condition that is not fully understood, no single treatment can address all the symptoms, and no intervention either prevents or reverses this disease. Treatment strategies focus on slowing the process, and dealing with the other conditions that frequently occur alongside, especially depression and anxiety.

Medications

- Cholinesterase inhibitors for memory improvement
- Antidepressants
- Antianxiety medication
- NSAIDs (excluding aspirin and acetaminophen) to limit inflammatory responses to plaques

Massage?

RISKS Elderly clients with Alzheimer disease (AD) may have a collection of other long-term diseases that require adaptations in bodywork: it is important to be fully informed about a client's health profile. Further, AD patients may be not able to communicate verbally, and they may become disoriented and confused. For this reason, it is especially important for massage therapists working in this setting to be sensitive to nonverbal signals about their client's sense of safety and well-being.

BENEFITS Although bodywork doesn't slow or reverse AD, it does improve the quality of life for patients in that they become less disruptive, show a better sense of orientation, and have more positive interactions in nursing home settings.

Amyotrophic Lateral Sclerosis

Definition: What Is It?

Also known as Lou Gehrig disease in the United States and motor neurone disease in Great Britain, amyotrophic lateral sclerosis (ALS) is a progressive and fatal condition that destroys motor neurons in the central and peripheral nervous systems, leading to the atrophy of voluntary muscles. The cells most at risk are the large motor neurons in the lateral aspects of the spinal cord. These are replaced by fibrous **astrocytes**, which make the spinal cord hard and scar like. "Amyotrophic" refers to muscle atrophy, "lateral" refers to the parts of the spinal cord that are affected, and "sclerosis" refers to the hardening of the spinal cord tissue.

Etiology: What Happens?

The cause or causes of ALS are unknown. When the disease develops, motor neurons in the central and

Amyotrophic Lateral Sclerosis in Brief

Pronunciation: am-e-o-TRO-fik LAT-er-al skler-O-sis

What is it?
Amyotrophic lateral sclerosis (ALS) is a progressive disease characterized by degeneration of upper and lower motor neurons and consequent atrophy of voluntary muscles.

How is it recognized?
Symptoms of ALS include weakness, fatigue, and muscle spasms. It appears most frequently in patients between 40 and 70 years old.

Massage risks and benefits
Risks: Some patients experience painful spasms with certain stimuli, and any massage must be designed to minimize this response. Patients with advanced ALS become frail and vulnerable to secondary infection. They may use devices to help with eating and breathing. All of these require adjustments in bodywork.
Benefits: Because patients with ALS have full sensation, massage that respects frailty, medical equipment, and other risks can be safe and welcome. Massage may help to maintain muscle function and mobility, and to delay the atrophy that is part of this disease.

peripheral nervous system die. Many ALS patients also have tissue damage in parts of the frontal lobe that are involved in the planning and execution of movement. This damage may also lead to some cognitive changes, which can contribute to some of the emotional aspects of this disease.

Surviving neurons in the peripheral system grow new axon branches to supply deprived muscle fibers, which increases the size of each motor unit. When those neurons ultimately fail, progressive and irreversible atrophy of voluntary muscle occurs (Figure 4.4). About one-third of the motor neurons that supply a muscle must be destroyed before atrophy becomes noticeable.

Several possible contributing factors for ALS have been identified, including genetic predisposition, oxidative injury, mitochondrial dysfunction, premature cell death, glial cell pathology, and glutamate excitotoxicity. Glutamate is a neurotransmitter that, for reasons that are not clear, is not neutralized or reabsorbed by presynaptic neurons, and it eventually damages and even kills the motor neuron it is meant to stimulate.

SIDEBAR 4.2 Dementing Diseases

Alzheimer disease (AD) is one of several conditions that can cause dementia and memory loss. Some conditions involve permanent brain damage, whereas others may be only temporary problem, if they are treated appropriately. Causes of permanent memory loss other than AD include the following:

- *Vascular dementia* is caused by a narrowing of the arteries to the brain, usually associated with advanced cardiovascular disease.
- *Stroke and transient ischemic attack (TIA)* cause brain tissue to die because of an interruption in blood supply.
- *Parkinson disease (PD)* involves the degeneration of certain motor centers in the brain, but it also often involves dementia.
- *Lewy body dementia* is the result of protein deposits (**Lewy bodies**) similar to the beta amyloid plaques that lead to dementia. This disease has features in common with both Alzheimer and PD.
- *Huntington disease* (*HD*) is another progressive degenerative central nervous system disease. It is characterized by destruction of nerve cells and resulting changes in personality and intellect. HD is a genetic disorder.
- *Creutzfeld-Jakob disease* is a type of dementia that can affect young and middle-aged people as well as the elderly. It is the human variant of **bovine spongiform encephalopathy** (mad cow disease).

Other conditions can cause memory loss that is recoverable. Naturally, it is important to consider these possibilities before concluding that a patient has irreversible AD. Some examples include high blood pressure, depression, diabetes, hypothyroidism, side effects of medication, and vitamin B_{12} deficiency.

Types of Amyotrophic Lateral Sclerosis

- *Sporadic ALS*. This is the most common type, accounting for 90% to 95% of all cases in the United States.
- *Familial ALS*. This form shows a genetic link for ALS. It accounts for about 5% to 15% of all cases in the United States, and is characterized by an earlier onset than the sporadic variety of ALS.
- *Mariana Islands type*. This is endemic to a specific population in the Western Pacific Islands,

especially Guam. It may be related to food sources that are limited to that region.

Signs and Symptoms

Symptoms of ALS are sometimes classified by whether the disease affects spinal nerves or cranial nerves, and whether the symptoms demonstrate damage to upper motor neurons or lower motor neurons. (Upper motor neurons are entirely within the brain and the descending tracts of the spinal cord, and lower motor neurons begin in the ventral horn of the spinal cord and go to voluntary muscles throughout the body.)

About 75% of ALS cases are diagnosed as the spinal variation, with early symptoms in the arms or legs. Difficulty with fine motor skills in the hands (writing, buttoning a shirt) may be the first sign of a problem. When early symptoms occur in the legs, frequent tripping or stumbling may be the first indication of the disease. Both sides may be affected, but one side is typically worse than the other. Fatigue, cramping, stiffness, and weakness move proximally up the limb and eventually affect the voluntary trunk muscles that control breathing.

About 25% of ALS cases first present as difficulties with speech, swallowing, or motor control of the tongue. This is the **bulbar** form, and it is often more serious, with a faster progression, than the spinal form of the disease. Bulbar ALS is also associated with extreme and rapid mood swings, or "emotional incontinence."

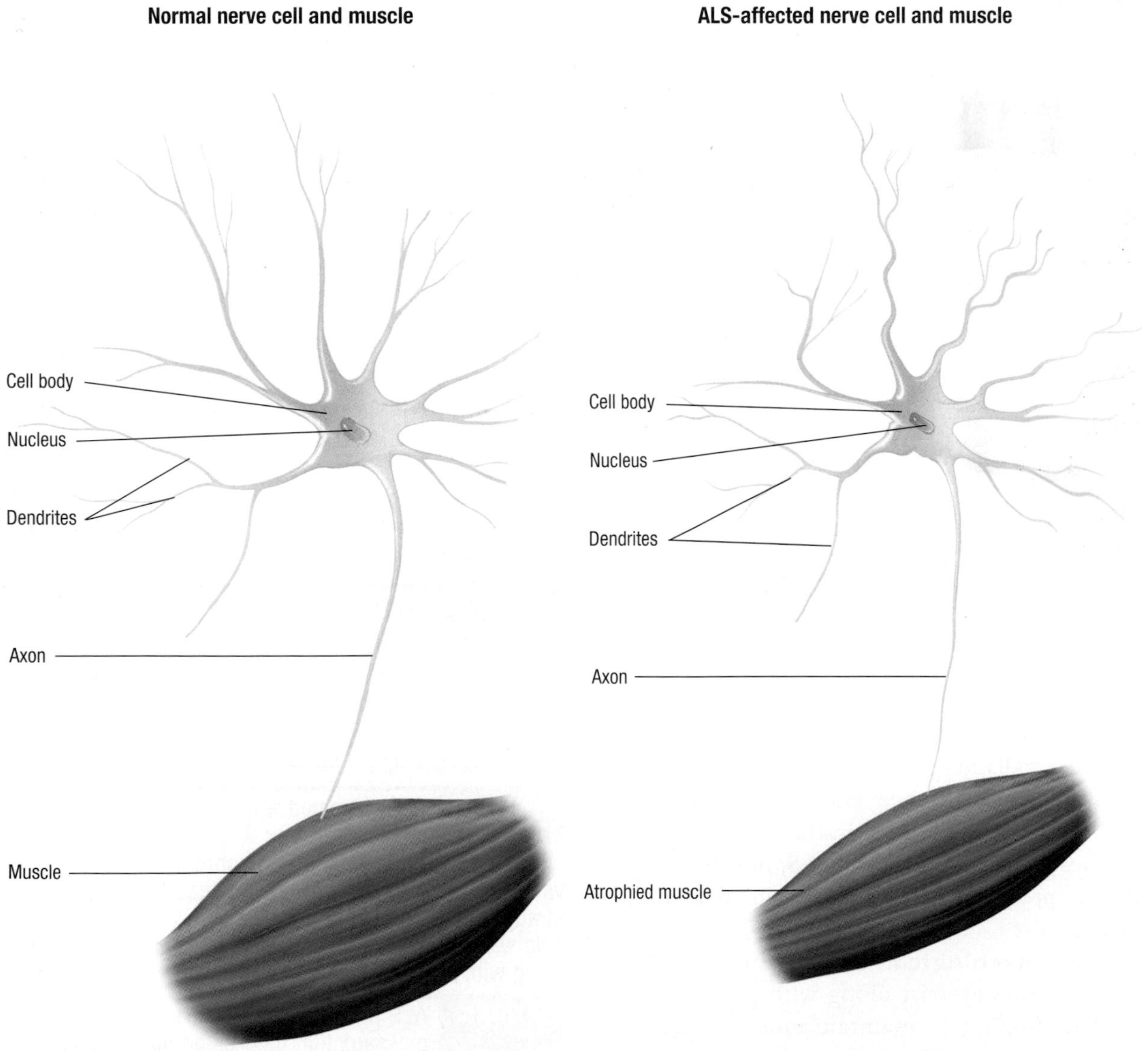

Normal nerve cell and muscle

ALS-affected nerve cell and muscle

Figure 4.4. Nerve damage with ALS

Upper motor neuron problems manifest as progressive **spasticity**, exaggerated reflexes (including the gag reflex), and a positive **Babinski sign** (the great toe goes into extension rather than flexion when the plantar surface of the foot is stimulated). Lower motor neurons are involved when weakness, atrophy, muscle cramps, and **fasciculations** (uncontrolled twitching) are present. Both upper and lower motor neurons are damaged in ALS.

NOTABLE CASES First baseman "Iron Horse" Lou Gehrig was a successful baseball player until he was diagnosed with amyotrophic lateral sclerosis (ALS) after he began dropping catches and tripping over his own feet. In his 1939 farewell speech, he famously declared, "Today I am the luckiest man on the face of the earth." He died 2 years later.

Physicist and author of *A Brief History of Time* Stephen Hawking is one of the longest living and most famous ALS patients. He has had this condition for many years, and has built a rich career while being essentially paralyzed by this disease.

The massage therapy community lost a great friend and resource when Nina McIntosh, author of *The Educated Heart* died of ALS in 2010. She is greatly missed. This section is for you, Nina.

The nerve damage seen with this disease affects motor neurons only; sensory neurons are left intact. This can be a painful process, however, with wracking muscle spasms, constipation, and the gradual collapse of the body as gravity puts demands on muscles that have no power to respond.

Treatment

Drug treatment for ALS is designed to deal with general fatigue, muscle spasms, and secondary infections. In addition, some drugs can limit the amount of glutamate in the CNS, so motor nerves function for a longer period. Interventions that limit saliva production (low-dose radiation or Botulinum toxin injections to the salivary glands) can help with swallowing problems and lower the risk of aspiration-related pneumonia. These are not a cure for ALS, but they may significantly prolong the lives of people affected by this disease.

Nonpharmacological treatment for ALS includes moderate exercise along with physical and occupational therapy to maintain muscle strength for as long as possible. Heat and whirlpools are used to control muscle spasms, and speech therapy helps with difficulties in swallowing and speech. Assistive devices such as leg braces, arm braces, wheelchairs, voice aids, and computers can improve a patient's ability to function. A healthy diet is critical for as long as patients can eat easily. In advanced cases, swallowing may be so difficult that the insertion of a stomach tube (gastrostomy) may be recommended. Breathing support can help with both lung function and fatigue. Psychological therapy for ALS patients and their families to deal with anxiety and depression is an important part of the treatment plan.

Treatment options for ALS can delay the inevitable, but once diagnosed, this disease, which has no known cure, usually results in death within 2 to 10 years. Most ALS patients die of pneumonia or **cachexia** (extreme weight loss). Some ALS patients, however, have survived for decades, and it is unclear why.

Medications

- Riluzole to reduce neuron damage due to glutamate toxicity
- Muscle relaxants for spasm and spasticity
- Antidepressants for depression
- Anxiolytics for anxiety
- Dextromethorphan and quinidine to ameliorate involuntary emotional responses seen with bulbar type ALS

Massage?

RISKS Many amyotrophic lateral sclerosis (ALS) patients struggle with painful cramping, and any massage must be designed to minimize that symptom. Patients with advanced ALS become very frail and vulnerable to secondary infection, so bodywork must be careful about those risks.

BENEFITS ALS is treated with heat, exercise, and physical therapy. Any bodywork that fits within these parameters is also appropriate, especially when delivered as part of a coordinated healthcare strategy. Massage has been used with some success to help with the pain of muscle spasms, and the stress of living with a fatal disease.

OPTIONS ALS patients can find special value in massage that focuses on pain and strong breathing.

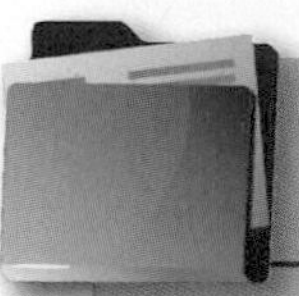

CASE HISTORY 4.1 Amyotrophic Lateral Sclerosis

Six months after he married the love of his life and built her a home, Eric was diagnosed with amyotrophic lateral sclerosis (ALS). Rather than succumb to sadness, the couple decided to go to Paris for a vacation and try to conceive a child. Nine months later, a baby girl joined the household.

For the past 2 years, I have treated Eric for 90 minutes in his home every week. Before he lost control of his facial muscles, I could understand his slurred speech; he sounded like a poststroke patient or a fellow hammered with too many whiskeys. Now all he can do is grunt and point, so he communicates with the aid of a small computer keyboard through which a stilted robotic male voice "speaks" as he types. He can no longer walk, and he moves about his huge home with a fancy battery-operated wheelchair.

In these 2 years, he has changed from being a hearty, muscular chiseled strong man to a man who leans on one side of my body as he takes slow, uneven steps from his wheelchair to the massage table.

Eric says that without the weekly massage sessions, his medication level would be much higher, he would have more muscular spasms, and the pain in his shoulder would be unbearable.

Approaching a body with ALS is more than a little tricky. Spasms occur without warning; the beginning of slow, even, medium-pressure effleurage while applying lotion to a lower extremity can result in a board-hard leg that extends as if levitating off the table of its own accord. All I can do is place my hand on the leg and slowly coax it back down to the table. Arms that used to open wide to hug those around him would contract against his body were it not for the slow, sometimes painful range-of-motion exercises we perform on all arm joints each week. Every bit of therapy takes twice as long as working on a "normal" body: if he's not stretched, he contracts; if I go too fast, he spasms; communication is cumbersome; and causing pain, though unintended, is always a possibility.

The end of life for an ALS patient is often related to diaphragm function. It can slow down to the point that the decreased lung capacity invites pneumonia, which is the ultimate threat to any sedentary human. For this reason, aggressive (though careful) resisted breathing exercises are part of every session. This means I have to get up on the table and place my hands just at his tenth rib, trying not to dislodge his feeding tube or the dressing around his diaphragmatic monitor. Then I encourage him to push against me with his breath while I'm wobbling all over and trying hard not to fall off the table. This brings on a lot of laughter—therapeutic in itself for someone with limited lung capacity. I hover above him while he laughs and tries to take a deep breath. I watch as he deems himself victorious if he can take at least one deep inhale and exhale; it's enough to bring a strong woman to tears. The victory is minuscule to most of us, but this effort could help extend his life.

Presently, there is no cure for this frustrating and frightening disease. But massage therapy can make a profound difference in the patient's pain and in the progression of muscular contractions. Every case is different, but the intelligent and dedicated therapist can adapt her skills to these very special patients and help make the damnable progression of ALS more tolerable as it is accompanied by loving touch.■

—Charlotte Versagi

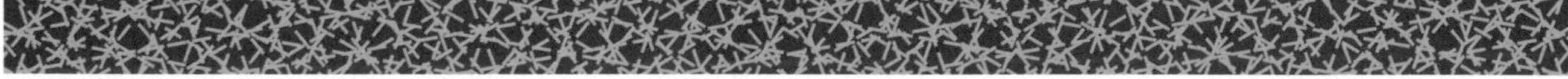

Huntington Disease

Definition: What Is It?

Huntington disease (HD) is a progressive degenerative disease of the CNS that is ultimately terminal. It is brought about by an autosomal dominant genetic mutation. This means that only one gene must be present for the disease to manifest; it can be passed to children by both mothers and fathers; and every child of a parent with the HD gene has a 50% chance of having the gene—and therefore developing the disease—as well.

Today HD has been diagnosed in about 30,000 Americans, but about 250,000 people are at risk for carrying the HD gene.

Etiology: What Happens?

Symptoms of what was probably HD have been in medical records since the Middle Ages, but it wasn't

Huntington Disease in Brief

What is it?
Huntington disease (HD) is a genetic disorder that leads to the destruction of certain neurons in the brain. It is progressive and terminal.

How is it recognized?
Signs and symptoms of HD vary by individual, but they involve dysfunction of motor control, emotional instability, and impaired cognitive processing.

Massage risks and benefits
Risks: A client with HD is facing a terminal condition with both physical and mental degeneration. As the disease progresses, a person's orientation may become challenged, so being touched or manipulated may be perceived as threatening. Also people with advanced Huntington disease may become quite frail with a risk for pneumonia and other infections. Finally, the twitching and writhing that distinguishes this disease arise from signals deep inside the brain. While massage may help the client to relax, it probably won't fundamentally change the progression of this condition.
Benefits: HD patients are counseled to stay strong and active as long as possible. If massage can support these efforts, then their physical degeneration may be delayed, and the risk of injury from clumsiness or falling may be somewhat lessened.

until 1872 that a British doctor named George Huntington put together a comprehensive list of signs and symptoms of this genetic disorder. Since then it has been known as dancing mania, hereditary chorea, Huntington chorea, and finally HD.

This disorder is the result of a genetic mutation that alters the behavior of certain neurons in the brain leading to cell death and irreversible and progressive loss of brain function. Intensive research has revealed that the mutation occurs when a gene has an abnormal number of repeating base pairs in a section of the DNA molecule. HD symptoms are most likely to develop when the repeating "stutter" of abnormal base pairs is over 40. The more repeating pairs that are present, the earlier symptoms tend to develop. Each successive generation of HD patients shows an increasing number of repeating pairs, especially among males: children who inherit the HD gene from their father are more likely to develop symptoms earlier than those who inherit the gene from their mother.

NOTABLE CASES Iconic American activist and folk singer Woody Guthrie ("This Land is Your Land," "This Train is Bound for Glory") may be the most familiar face of Huntington disease. For many years, it was assumed that Guthrie was an alcoholic or schizophrenic; he was not appropriately diagnosed until 1954, and he died in 1967—a month before his son Arlo released his own signature album, "Alice's Restaurant."

It is unclear exactly how these mutated genes lead to HD symptoms. Theories include the secretion of an abnormal protein that damages neurons, mitochondrial dysfunction, the presence of oxygen-free radicals, and a disruption in how the brain accumulates cholesterol. Understanding the process will create better treatment options in the future, but regardless of the mechanism, predictable patterns of neuron damage are demonstrable. Degeneration of neurons stimulates astrocytes (glial cells that surround neurons) to multiply, which can further interfere with neuron function. Damage appears to concentrate in certain areas of the basal ganglia that have to do with organizing motor control. Sections of the frontal lobes and cerebral cortex are also vulnerable to damage, and many HD patients have abnormally large ventricles: the hollow areas inside the brain where cerebrospinal fluid circulates. When key neurons in the brain die, they not only lose their own function, but the neurotransmitters they would have secreted are also in short supply; this imbalance may account for some HD symptoms.

Ultimately, every person who carries the HD gene will develop the disease, and the disease is progressive, degenerative, and terminal, usually from pneumonia, complications of an injury, or suicide. New tests that identify the HD gene early are available, but they don't predict the time of onset or life expectancy. Children of a parent with HD are now faced with the difficult decision of finding out whether they are positive for the gene, and whether to risk passing that gene along to their own children.

Signs and Symptoms

A person's age at the onset of HD symptoms has been recorded as young as 3 years old, and as old as 80, but most patients report the beginning of symptoms between ages 35 and 50. Typically, the younger a person is when symptoms develop, the more rapid the progression of the disease is likely to be.

Early signs and symptoms vary widely from one patient to another, but all of them can be categorized into three main types: changes in motor function; changes in emotional stability; and changes in cognition.

- **Motor function**. Some HD patients begin their symptoms with mild clumsiness and occasional loss of balance. Twitching, tics, and dystonia may start at the extremities and face, but may progress to involve the whole body. "Chorea" (from the Greek root word for dance, as in choreography) refers to the involuntary writhing, twisting movements of the face, trunk, and arms many HD patients experience.

  When HD occurs in children, they may experience muscular rigidity, slow movement, tremors, and seizures.

  Advanced HD patients have extreme balance and coordination problems, and the risk of falls can be extremely threatening. Loss of facial coordination can make swallowing and speaking prohibitively difficult.

- **Emotional stability**. Personality changes are sometimes the first sign of HD onset. These can include rapid and very extreme mood swings, irritability, apathy, hostility, and extreme depression.

  Depression is a common complication of HD, as it is of many progressive and terminal diseases. Unfortunately, depression and suicidal ideation are common side effects of some HD medications, making this aspect of the disease particularly difficult to manage.

- **Cognition**. Most HD patients experience significant cognitive decline as their disease progresses. Unlike the dementia seen with AD, HD dementia is centered on attention, learning, judgment, and decision making rather than on language and memory loss.

Treatment

As a genetic mutation, HD is not treatable at this time. Drug therapies are aimed at controlling the worst symptoms and complications. Outside of drugs, HD is treated with psychiatric counseling, speech therapy, occupational therapy, and physical therapy designed to preserve maximum motor functioning for as long as possible.

Genetic counseling is available both for children of HD-positive parents and for HD patients who are considering being a parent themselves.

Medications

- Tetrabenezine to treat chorea symptoms; it raises the risk of depression, however, which is already a risk for HD patients
- Antipsychotic medications (haloperidol) for delusion and psychosis
- Tranquilizers (clonazepam) for anxiety and paranoia
- Antidepressants (fluoxetine, sertraline, nortriptyline)

Massage?

RISKS A client with Huntington disease (HD) may experience any combination of motor problems, emotional volatility, and cognitive decline. If that person becomes disoriented and confused during a session, massage may feel unwelcomed at best, and actively threatening at worst: this situation obviously contraindicates any bodywork that the client does not desire.

Clients in an advanced state may be physically frail and vulnerable to infection; any bodywork must be gauged by their ability to adapt.

BENEFITS Because HD affects motor control and may lead to a high risk of falls and other injuries, many patients are counseled to exercise and stay physically fit for as long as possible. Massage may be a helpful part of this strategy. Also any symptoms that are aggravated by stress may be at least mitigated by massage, as long as it is welcomed.

OPTIONS HD can involve involuntary muscle contractions, including twitching, tics, and jerking. Depending on how any individual receives the stimulus of massage, it may be safer and more comfortable to work with a massage chair than on a table.

Peripheral Neuropathy

Definition: What Is It?

Peripheral neuropathy (PN) is usually not a disease in itself, but a symptom or a complication of other underlying conditions. Peripheral nerves, either singly or in groups, are damaged through lack of circulation, chemical imbalance, trauma, or other factors.

Etiology: What Happens?

PN can affect one nerve at a time (**mononeuropathy**) or multiple nerves (**polyneuropathy**). It is typically

Peripheral Neuropathy in Brief

Pronunciation: per-IF-er-al nur-OP-ath-e

What is it?
Peripheral neuropathy (PN) is damage to peripheral nerves, often as a result of some other underlying condition or exposure to pathogens or toxic substances.

How is it recognized?
Symptoms include burning or tingling pain that begins distally and moves proximally, cramping or twitching, hyperesthesia, or autonomic dysfunction, which could include problems with digestion, heart rate, breathing, or other issues.

Massage risks and benefits
Risks: PN contraindicates specific massage when it involves numbness that could interfere with a client's ability to give accurate feedback. Alternatively, pain or increased sensitivity may make massage difficult to receive. Finally, when PN is the result of an underlying disorder that contraindicates massage, this must be addressed before bodywork is safe.
Benefits: If massage improves symptoms rather than exacerbating them, and if underlying conditions allow for bodywork, a client with PN may derive benefit from soothing touch.

classified by whether it affects sensation, voluntary muscle control, or autonomic function.

PN is occasionally related to a genetic anomaly, but it is usually a consequence of some other injury, infection, or systemic disease; this is called acquired PN. Some common causes of acquired PN include the following:

- *Injury*. Carpal tunnel syndrome, thoracic outlet syndrome, Bell palsy, disc disease, and trigeminal neuralgia are all examples of PN related to acute or chronic injury.
- *Infection*. Herpes simplex, herpes zoster (shingles), HIV/AIDS, Lyme disease, hepatitis, syphilis, and Hansen disease (leprosy) can all cause damage and irritation to peripheral nerves.
- *Systemic disease*. Diabetes (type 1 or type 2), renal failure, vitamin B_{12} deficiency, cancer, and other tumors can all contribute to nerve damage, as can some autoimmune diseases, including lupus, Sjögren syndrome, sarcoidosis, and Guillain-Barré syndrome.
- *Toxic exposure*. Chronic alcoholism, sniffing glue, some medications, exposure to heavy metals (especially lead and mercury), solvents, and other environmental contaminants can damage peripheral nerves.

Signs and Symptoms

Most cases of PN begin subtly and slowly, and symptoms depend on what combinations of sensory, motor, and autonomic nerves are damaged. Injury to sensory neurons produces burning pain or tingling in the hands and feet, which gradually spreads proximally into the limbs and finally the trunk. Extreme sensitivity to touch (**hyperalgesia** or **allodynia**) can follow, but this may eventually be replaced by reduced sensation (people feel like they are always wearing socks or gloves, even when they're not), or numbness. Numbness is problematic because if a person can't feel something—a toe, for instance—he or she can't tell if it's been injured or infected. Secondary infections and ulcers are common complications of numbness with any disease.

Damage to motor nerves can lead to twitching, cramps, and eventually atrophy of the affected muscles.

Damage to autonomic nerves is often the most serious; this can interfere with digestion, maintaining heart and respiratory rates, sweating, blood pressure, and control of the bladder or bowel.

Treatment

Treatment for PN depends entirely on the underlying pathology that is causing the nerve damage: controlling the primary disease can help to control associated nerve pain. Topical ointments with lidocaine or **capsaicin** sometimes offer some relief. Other therapies include **TENS units** (transcutaneous electrical nerve stimulation that interrupts pain transmission), biofeedback, acupuncture, relaxation techniques, and massage to improve circulation in the affected extremities.

The good news is that if PN is interrupted before damage affects cell bodies, the peripheral nerves may be able to regenerate.

Medications

- Analgesics for pain control
- Anti-inflammatories, especially for autoimmune disease

- Immunoglobulins to suppress immune system response
- Antiseizure drugs
- Tricyclic antidepressants

Massage?

RISKS Undiagnosed pain, tingling, or numbness needs to be evaluated by a primary care provider before massage can be known to be safe. Numbness and reduced sensation can interfere with a client's ability to know when pressure is sufficient. Other clients with peripheral neuropathy (PN) may experience that any touch is irritating, so massage may have to be adjusted or even delayed until the contributing factors to PN have been addressed.

BENEFITS Massage, through soothing touch, relief of general stress, or improvements in local circulation, may improve the quality of life for a person with PN, but this can only be determined on a case-by-case basis.

Dystonia

Definition: What Is It?

Dystonia is a common condition that involves repetitive, involuntary, sometimes sustained contractions of skeletal muscles. Symptoms often reach a peak and then stabilize or subside in intensity, but they may recur. Dystonia can occur without an identifiable cause, due to a genetic anomaly, or as a secondary symptom of an underlying disorder or drug reaction.

Dystonia is found among all ages and races, but women are affected more often than men.

Etiology: What Happens?

Like other movement disorders, dystonia appears to be linked to problems with the basal ganglia. It involves an inability to process certain neurotransmitters, including **dopamine**, **GABA** (gamma-amino butyric acid, an inhibitory neurotransmitter), **serotonin**, and **acetylcholine**. The result is prolonged bursts of electrical activity in the affected muscles. This distinguishes it from other movement disorders such as Parkinson disease or tremor, which result in rhythmic, oscillating shaking in one plane of movement.

Dystonia in Brief

What is it?
Dystonia is a movement disorder resulting in repetitive, predictable, but involuntary muscle contractions.

How is it recognized?
The primary symptom of dystonia is repetitive involuntary muscle contractions, especially during stress or in relation to specific tasks. Some forms involve only the head or face, the vocal cords, or one limb, but other forms are progressive or involve the whole body. The contractions themselves are not always painful, but they can lead to painful tissue changes including arthritis, muscle strains, and contractures.

Massage risks and benefits
Risks: Some of the drugs used to treat dystonia may have implications for massage, so therapists should be aware of how clients with dystonia treat their condition.
Benefits: This condition doesn't affect sensation, so any bodywork that is comfortable to receive is safe. Some dystonia patients may seek massage to help with fatigue and to reduce stress.

Causes of dystonia vary. Genetic predisposition, underlying neurological disorders, and reactions to medications are the most frequent triggers.

Dystonia can be classified by age of onset (childhood, adolescent, or adult) or by cause (primary, secondary, or dystonia-plus syndromes). Most often, however, dystonia is described by what part or how much of the body is affected.

NOTABLE CASES National Public Radio talk show host Diane Rehm is affected by vocal dysphonia. Other influential people who have had dystonia include late actress Katharine Hepburn, Supreme Court Justice Sandra Day O'Connor, the late Senator Robert Byrd, and Founding Father Samuel Adams.

Types of Dystonia

- *Focal dystonia*. These conditions affect specific muscles or muscle groups.
    - *Spasmodic torticollis*. This is the most common form of dystonia. Also called **cervical dystonia**, it involves unilateral involuntary contractions of neck rotators, usually the sternocleidomastoid. For other types of torticollis, see Sidebar 4.3.

SIDEBAR 4.3 Other Types of Torticollis

Spasmodic torticollis is classified as a type of dystonia, a movement disorder that starts in the CNS. Other forms of torticollis are related to musculoskeletal problems, which of course have very different implications for massage.

- *Congenital torticollis.* A genetic anomaly results in the development of only one sternocleidomastoid muscle. Because so many other muscles can rotate and flex the head, this problem may be dealt with through physical therapy.
- *Infant torticollis.* In the late stages of pregnancy, the fetus may lie with the head twisted to one side. This can create a shortened or weakened sternocleidomastoid and cranial bone distortion. This condition is usually successfully treated with exercise and a special helmet designed to reshape the cranial bones.
- *Wryneck.* This is a simple stiff neck, often caused by irritation of the intertransverse ligament at C7. A cervical misalignment may also create the problem, which will not be relieved until both the muscles and the bony alignment have been addressed. Trigger points and spasm in the splenius cervicis are other possible causes. Short-lived cases of wryneck may be brought about by sleeping in a bad position or some other event or trauma that might cause irritation in the neck muscles.

Torticollis can, on rare occasions, be the earliest presenting sign of a more serious condition. In some documented cases, it was the first symptom of bone cancer in the spine (the tumor may affect the motor and/or sensory neurons), bone infection, and even a bad infection of the adenoids.

- *Vocal dysphonia.* This affects the vocal cords, leading to difficulty with speech, and a shaky, hoarse, or whispery quality to the voice.
- *Oromandibular dystonia.* This affects the face and lower jaw muscles. It can lead to problems with eating and swallowing.
- *Blepharospasm.* This leads to repetitive, forceful blinking, and squinting of the eyes. It can be severe enough to cause functional blindness, even though the eyes themselves are not affected.
- *Meige syndrome.* This is a combination of blepharospasm and oromandibular dystonia.
- *Writer's cramp.* This is a condition in which the dominant hand develops painful cramps during activity.
- *Multifocal dystonia.* This affects disconnected parts of the body, the left leg, and the face, for instance.
- *Hemidystonia.* This affects the left or right side of the body. It is an occasional repercussion of stroke.
- *Generalized dystonia.* This is the most severe form of this disorder. It usually starts in the leg and progresses to affect the whole body.

Signs and Symptoms

Signs and symptoms of dystonia are related to what type is present and at what age symptoms began. People who develop this disorder in childhood tend to have it in more severe forms than those who develop dystonia in maturity.

The primary symptom is involuntary contraction of an area. Contractions may be quick or sustained, and they often involve multiplane movement and twisting. Episodes tend to be exacerbated by stress or fatigue. Contractions are often related to specific tasks and disappear when other tasks that use the same muscles are substituted: walking backward instead of forward, for instance. Many dystonia patients develop a habit of repeatedly touching the affected area, which serves to reduce local contractions. This pattern is called **geste antagoniste**.

Dystonic contractions may not be painful, but they can lead to painful consequences. Headaches can result from spasmodic torticollis or facial contractions. Muscle irritation and arthritis may develop in areas where contractions are continually sustained. Eventually, the muscle fibers may shrink and the connective tissue sheaths around them thicken into a permanent contracture. Another complication is the functional blindness that occurs when blepharospasm interferes with normal eyelid contractions.

Treatment

Treatment options for dystonia work to modulate motor function in the affected muscles. Physical therapy and gentle stretching are often recommended. Oral or injected medications can affect neurotransmitter secretion or uptake. Injections of botulinum toxin can block the acetylcholine receptors in the affected muscles. A device can be implanted in the brain to help regulate motor function (deep brain stimulation). If no other interventions are satisfactory, surgery can disrupt portions of the basal ganglia or interrupt nerve transmission to the muscle or in the spinal cord.

Medications

- Benzodiazepines to limit messages to motor neurons
- Baclofen to reduce spasticity and spasm
- Anticholinergic medications to block acetylcholine activity
- Injected botulinum toxin to locally affect acetylcholine uptake

Massage?

RISKS Some of the treatment interventions for dystonia may impact choices for massage. When a client uses a drug that makes muscles less responsive, the therapist must accommodate by limiting the intensity of the pressure or the extent of any passive stretching that is part of the session.

BENEFITS Dystonia is exacerbated by fatigue and stress, so patients may seek massage as a coping mechanism.

Parkinson Disease

Definition: What Is It?

Parkinson disease (PD), first discussed by the British physician James Parkinson in 1817 as the "shaking palsy," is a movement disorder involving the progressive degeneration of nerve tissue, and a reduction in neurotransmitter production in the CNS.

It affects about 1.5 million people in the United States, mostly over age 60. Men with PD outnumber women by about 3 to 2.

Etiology: What Happens?

The basal ganglia are small pockets of gray matter deep in the brain that work with several other structures to provide learned reflexes, motor control, and coordination: smooth movement that is balanced between prime movers and their antagonists.

Healthy basal ganglia cells are supplied with a vital neurotransmitter, dopamine, by cells in a nearby structure, the substantia nigra (aka "black stuff"). In PD, the substantia nigra cells die off, depriving the basal ganglia cells of dopamine. Without dopamine, the basal ganglia cells cannot do their job, so coordination and controlled movement degenerates.

It is not clear why the substantia nigra degenerates in most PD cases. Environmental agents may be found to be one cause; risk factors for PD include exposure to some pesticides, herbicides, fertilizers, and other industrial chemicals. The presence of Lewy bodies in the basal ganglia cells and other areas may predict PD, but these deposits are associated with other disorders as well. In some families, a genetic connection is clear, and specific sites of genetic abnormality have been located.

The term parkinsonism refers to conditions that display Parkinson-like symptoms but differing etiologies. Some of these cases can be traced to specific issues, including certain drugs, repeated head trauma (pugilistic parkinsonism affects boxers), and neurovascular disease.

Parkinson Disease in Brief

What is it?
Parkinson disease (PD) is a degenerative disease of some dopamine-producing cells in the brain. Dopamine helps the basal ganglia to maintain balance, posture, and coordination.

How is it recognized?
Early symptoms of PD include general stiffness and fatigue; resting tremor of the hand, foot, or head; and slowed movement. Later symptoms include muscle rigidity, poor balance, a shuffling gait, a masklike appearance to the face, and a monotone voice.

Massage risks and benefits
Risks: PD patients can have problems moving on and off the table. Attendance during these transitions may be important for their safety. Also, because PD is most common among elderly clients, other conditions that influence choices for bodywork may also be present.
Benefits: PD patients may experience great benefit from massage, as it can help with muscle spasm, fatigue, and the quality of sleep.

Signs and Symptoms

Symptoms of PD can be divided into primary and secondary problems. Primary symptoms arise from the disease itself, while secondary symptoms are the result of primary symptoms.

Primary Symptoms

- *Nonspecific achiness, weakness, and fatigue.* PD has a slow onset and is most common in elderly people, so these early symptoms are often missed.
- *Resting tremor.* This phenomenon is present in most PD patients and is often one of the first noticeable symptoms. A rhythmic shaking or pill-rolling action of the hand is often seen. Tremor may also affect the foot, head, and neck. This tremor is most noticeable when the patient is at rest, but not sleeping. It often disappears entirely when the patient is engaged in some other activity. This distinguishes it from essential tremor, which is discussed elsewhere.
- *Bradykinesia.* This is difficulty in initiating or sustaining movement. It can take a long time to begin a voluntary movement of the arm or leg, movement may be halting and interrupted midstream. PD patients with bradykinesia sometimes report feeling rooted to the floor when they can visualize moving a leg, but it doesn't happen without sustained effort.
- *Rigidity.* Because of changes in motor function, flexor muscles become chronically tight. This can give rise to a characteristically stooped posture, as the trunk flexors contract more strongly than the paraspinals. This is particularly obvious when PD accompanies osteoporosis, as it often does in elderly patients. Rigidity also makes it difficult to bend or straighten arms and legs and can cause a particular masklike appearance as the facial muscles lose flexibility and ease of movement (Figure 4.5). Rigidity also accounts for a reduced rate of blinking, increased drooling, and difficulty with eating, swallowing, and digestion: painful constipation is a frequent result.
- *Poor postural reflexes.* Disruption in the activity of basal ganglia cells results in uncoordinated movement and poor balance. PD patients are particularly susceptible to falling.

NOTABLE CASES Perhaps the most recognized spokesperson for Parkinson disease (PD) at present is actor Michael J. Fox who was diagnosed at age 41 with this disease. Other well-known PD patients include "The Man in Black" Johnny Cash, Heavyweight boxing champion Mohammed Ali (who has pugilistic parkinsonism), and Pope John Paul II.

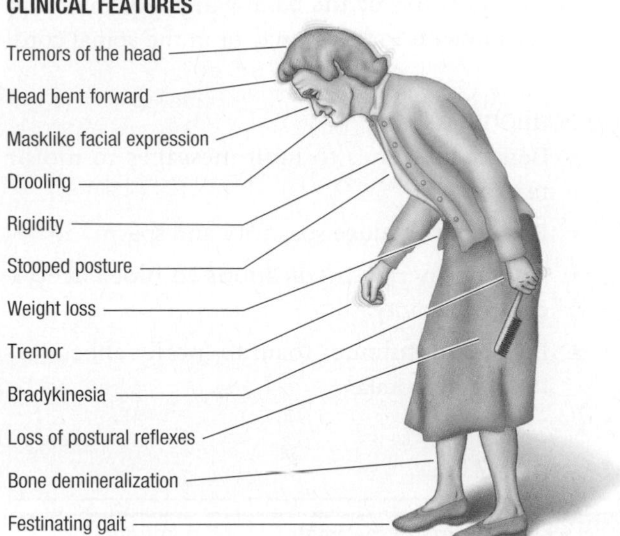

Figure 4.5. Clinical features of Parkinson disease.

Secondary Symptoms

- *Shuffling gait.* Difficulty in bending arms and legs makes walking a special challenge. Often the ability to swing the arm is noticeably diminished on one side. The patient takes small steps and may then have to stumble forward to avoid falling. This chasing after the center of gravity is called a **festinating gait**.
- *Changes in speech and eating.* PD causes progressive rigidity of the muscles in the larynx that control vocalization. The speech gradually becomes monotone and expressionless. Muscular changes in the mouth and throat also create problems with swallowing and drooling, particularly while lying down.
- *Changes in handwriting.* The loss of coordination in fine motor muscles changes the ability of a PD patient to write by hand. **Micrographia**, or progressively shrinking, cramped handwriting, is one of the later symptoms of this disease.
- *Sleep disorders.* PD patients are subject to a variety of sleep disorders, from a complete reversal of normal sleeping schedules to extra-active REM sleep, to chronic sleeplessness.
- *Depression.* The progressive nature of PD makes anxiety and depression a very predictable part of the disease process. Depression can also be related to insomnia, or it can be a side effect of medication. Sometimes the symptoms

of depression can outweigh the symptoms of the disease, and treatment for depression can lessen PD symptoms as well.

- *Mental degeneration.* Advanced PD patients may have memory loss and deterioration of cognition, but these can also be side effects of PD drugs.

Treatment

Pharmacologic treatment for PD patients is a complicated subject. Doctors must balance the benefits of early intervention to slow the progression of this disease with the many unacceptable side effects that accompany long-term drug use. Choosing which drugs to prescribe, in which sequence, and in which combinations, is an ongoing challenge.

Because PD is related to a lack of dopamine in the basal ganglia, the most common strategy is to supplement a synthetic form of this neurotransmitter. **Levodopa** (L-dopa) can cross the blood-brain barrier, especially with a companion drug called **carbidopa**, but it tends to have a lot of negative side effects, and many patients develop resistance, so it is a temporary solution.

Other drug therapies include substances that slow the metabolism of dopamine, so that whatever is available stays for a longer time, and substances that stimulate dopamine receptors in the basal ganglia, so that uptake of the neurotransmitter happens more easily. Anticholinergic agents work to limit muscle contraction. None of these is a permanent solution, however, and all of them carry risks of serious side effects. Doctors working with PD patients must monitor their medications carefully and make frequent adjustments.

Physical, speech, and occupational therapies are often employed to maintain the health and general functioning levels of PD patients for as long as possible. Psychotherapy and support groups are recommended to cope with the effects of depression.

Some PD patients find that deep brain stimulation (an electrode activates the thalamus by way of a magnet implanted under the skin) can help to control tremors. Other neurosurgery options have worked to modulate motor dysfunction at other locations in the brain. These interventions are typically employed only when other options have failed.

Medications

- Levadopa, carbidopa to cross the blood-brain barrier and supplement dopamine in the brain
- Catechol *O*-methyltransferase inhibitors (COMT inhibitors) to prolong the effects of levadopa and carbidopa therapy
- Monamine oxidase-B inhibitors to protect damaged neurons, act as antioxidants
- Anticholinergics to block acetylcholine and manage muscle rigidity

Massage?

RISKS Many Parkinson disease (PD) patients have difficulty getting on or off a table, and may need assistance to do so. Because this is usually a disease of the elderly, other disorders may be present along with PD, so these must also be addressed for the safety of massage.

BENEFITS Massage can help with many aspects of PD, including sleep quality, muscle rigidity, anxiety, and depression. Because it is an option with little risk of negative side effects, massage is one of the most frequently used complementary therapies by PD patients.

OPTIONS Some massage therapists report that they see the best benefits for their clients with PD when massage sessions are short but frequent, as opposed to longer and less frequent.

Tremor

Definition: What Is It?

The term tremor refers to involuntary movements, which can be a freestanding disorder, or a symptom of a number of different types of CNS problems. The key characteristics of tremor disorders are that the movements are rhythmic oscillations of antagonistic muscle groups, and the movement occurs in a fixed plane: this distinguishes tremor from dystonia, which may involve involuntary movement in any plane. Tremors vary by velocity, body parts involved, and amplitude.

Etiology: What Happens?

Tremors can occur in a variety of ways. Most situations appear to be related to dysfunction in the links between the brainstem, the cerebellum, and the thalamus.

Tremors affect the hands, face, and head more often than other areas. They are sometimes

Tremor In Brief

What is it?
Tremor is rhythmic, involuntary muscle movement. It can be a primary disorder (unrelated to other problems), or it can be a symptom of other neurological diseases.

How is it recognized?
Tremor is identified through rhythmic, predictable, but uncontrolled fine or gross motor movements.

Massage risks and benefits
Risks: The main risk for massage in this context is that tremor could be a symptom of some underlying condition that contraindicates massage.
Benefits: Massage may or may not have impact on tremor, but as long as contraindicating conditions have been addressed, it can certainly add to the quality of life for a client with this condition.

classified by whether they are physiologic or pathologic. Physiologic tremors are exacerbated by stress, fear, or underlying problems like alcohol withdrawal, hypoglycemia, hyperthyroidism, or drug reactions. Pathologic tremors are either idiopathic or caused by some other condition.

Types of Pathologic Tremor

- *Essential tremor.* This is an idiopathic chronic tremor that is not secondary to any other pathology. Up to 10 million people in the United States have essential tremor. This condition is slowly progressive, but not usually debilitating. Onset can occur as early as adolescence, but essential tremor most often shows up at about 45 years of age. It can be an inherited disorder.
- *Secondary tremor.* This is a situation where tremor develops as a part of some other CNS disorder. PD, multiple system atrophy, and HD all list tremor among their symptoms.

Signs and Symptoms

Tremors are generally classified as resting tremor, action tremor, or psychogenic tremor.

- *Resting tremor.* Oscillations occur when the person is at rest, but not during sleep.
- *Action tremor.* This has three subtypes:
  - *Postural tremor.* Oscillations occur when the patient attempts to hold a limb against gravity, that is, holding an arm out in front of him.
  - *Isometric tremor.* Shaking occurs with isometric contractions, that is, squeezing the examiner's fingers.
  - *Intention tremor.* This is worst when the patient attempts to use his hands for fine or complex tasks.
- *Psychogenic tremor.* This is present in everyone, but is usually so subtle it is unnoticeable. When it becomes pronounced, it is often stress-related and disappears when the person is distracted.

Treatment

Several medications can help control tremor symptoms. Surgical interventions may be used if the tremor is debilitating and unresponsive to medication; these include implanting a deep brain stimulation device or creating interruptions at the thalamus or globus pallidus.

Medication

- Beta blockers appear to inhibit receptors in muscle spindles
- Tranquilizers, including benzodiazepines or phenobarbitals to inhibit muscle function
- Antiseizure medications
- Botulinum toxin (specifically for muscles of the face or head)
- Controlled doses of alcohol

Massage?

RISKS Tremor can occur as part of serious underlying disorders. These must be identified before massage can safely proceed. Some clients may find that the physical challenges of getting on or off a massage table or chair may make them feel unstable. In these situations, it is important to be in attendance during transition times.

BENEFITS A client with essential tremor that is exacerbated by stress may find that his or her symptoms are lessened with massage.

Infectious Disorders

Encephalitis

Definition: What Is It?

Encephalitis is an infection of the brain, usually caused by any of a variety of viruses. It frequently occurs along with inflammation of the spinal cord (myelitis) and/or inflammation of the meninges (meningitis). While some strains of infection-causing pathogens used to be found only in certain geographical areas, the ease of world-wide travel has made the phenomenon of **endemic** infections less limiting than they used to be (Sidebar 4.4).

Etiology: What Happens?

Most cases of encephalitis are viral, although they can be related to bacterial infections or fungi. Viral infections can be primary (a direct attack on the nervous system) or secondary (a complication of viral infection elsewhere in the body).

Encephalitis infections affect the **parenchyma** (working areas) of the brain and sometimes the meninges and spinal cord. Inflammation is an inevitable result. Infections are often mild and do not always lead to long-lasting damage, but occasionally, and especially if the patient is very young or very old, encephalitis infections cause permanent neurological damage, cognitive changes, stroke, seizures, paralysis, or even death.

Encephalitis in Brief

Pronunciation: en-sef-uh-LY-tis

What is it?
Encephalitis is inflammation of the brain. It is usually brought about by a viral infection, but other pathogens can cause it as well.

How is it recognized?
Signs and symptoms of encephalitis include fever, headache, confusion, and personality and memory changes. In rare cases, encephalitis causes permanent neurological damage or even death.

Massage risks and benefits
Risks: Acute encephalitis, like most acute infections, contraindicates massage. If an infection has been very severe, then some complications may require adaptation in a bodywork session.
Benefits: A client who has fully recovered from encephalitis with no long-lasting damage can enjoy the same benefits from massage as the rest of the population.

SIDEBAR 4.4 West Nile Encephalitis: Watching a Virus Take Hold

In August 1999, six residents of Queens, New York, checked into local hospitals with high fever in combination with debilitating headaches. Five of them also developed alarming neurological symptoms: weakness, paralysis, and even coma.

Initial tests suggested an outbreak of Saint Louis encephalitis, a mosquito-borne viral infection. But patients showed a different pattern from that usually seen with St. Louis encephalitis; several of them were much sicker than medical professionals expected to see. Within days several more people in the area were reporting similar symptoms.

At the same time, a few miles away from the epicenter, birds in the Bronx Zoo were dying at a startling rate. Crows all over the city were dying, too. Horses in nearby suburbs were falling to a mysterious brain fever.

It took some time, but epidemiologists finally put the phenomena together and realized that the viruses attacking humans were the same as those attacking the birds and horses. It was firmly established that the infectious agent was one never before seen in the United States: West Nile encephalitis virus was being transmitted from horses and birds to humans by common mosquitoes.

By the time the first frost killed the mosquito population, 56 confirmed cases were identified among humans, with 7 deaths. The people who died of encephalitis were all over 68 years of age.

It has never been firmly established exactly how the West Nile virus got to New York. One of the patients had been to Africa the previous June and might have been infected then, or it is possible that one of the birds in the Bronx Zoo carried the virus into the United States. Aggressive mosquito abatement programs limited the spread of the disease for that season, but studies of both mosquitoes and birds indicate that the virus has now expanded over much of the continent.

The virus continues to be watched closely, but mortality rates are now generally low. This suggests that most people now have been exposed and developed resistance to the virus. It is still important to be vigilant about this infection, which can be life threatening, but the initially aggressive phase appears to be over.

Types of Encephalitis

- *Viral encephalitis*
  - *Primary:* these can be **enteroviruses** (by way of the gastrointestinal tract) or **arboviruses** (vector-borne, usually by way of a mosquito).
  - *Secondary:* these are infections that spread from elsewhere in the body. Herpes simplex, herpes zoster, mumps, and measles are all viral infections that can later attack the CNS.
- Other types of encephalitis: these can include bacterial, fungal, or protozoan infections, but they are in the minority of encephalitis diagnoses in the United States.

Signs and Symptoms

Symptoms of encephalitis can range from so mild that they are never identified, to extremely severe. How the disease presents depends on the pathogen and the age and general health of the patient. Infants, the elderly, and immunosuppressed people are most vulnerable to the very extreme forms of the disease, while others only rarely have any lasting damage from the inflammation.

The mild end of the symptomatic scale includes a sudden onset of fever with headaches, drowsiness, irritability, and disordered thought processes. In severe cases, drowsiness can progress to stupor and then coma. The patient may also have double vision, confused sensation, impaired speech or hearing, convulsions, and partial or full paralysis. Changes in personality, intellect, and memory may develop, depending on which parts of the brain are affected.

NOTABLE CASES In 2000, actor Liza Minnelli experienced a severe bout of viral encephalitis that was originally mistaken for a stroke.

Treatment

Viral encephalitis is treated with antiviral medications, along with steroids to limit inflammation, sedatives to moderate convulsions, and "supportive therapy," which is to say, rest, good nutrition, and adequate hydration.

Medications

- NSAIDs, especially acetaminophen, for fever and headache relief (mild cases only)
- Antiviral medication to interrupt viral replication
- Anti-inflammatories, including steroids, to limit inflammation in the CNS
- Antiseizure drugs
- Sedatives

Massage?

RISKS A client with an acute infection of any kind needs to reschedule a massage appointment, but if along with fever he or she has headache, confusion, and changes in speech, sensation or motor control, it is important to seek immediate medical attention.

BENEFITS A client who has fully recovered from an encephalitis infection can enjoy the same benefits from massage as the rest of the population.

Herpes Zoster

Definition: What Is It?

Varicella zoster virus (VZV) is an infection of the nervous system. In this case, the targeted tissues are the dendrites at the end of sensory neurons, which leads to painful, fluid-filled blisters on all of the nerve endings of a specific dermatome.

Chickenpox is usually the first interaction people have with this virus, but subsequent outbreaks are called *shingles*. This comes from the Latin *cingulum*, which means girdle or belt. This describes the typical distribution of blisters around the chest or abdomen along a dermatomal line.

Etiology: What Happens?

VZV is a virus in the herpes family that attacks sensory nerve cell endings, leading to painful, itchy blisters on the skin. Most people's first exposure to this pathogen is through a childhood bout of chickenpox. Like other herpes viruses, VZV is never fully expelled from the body. Instead, it goes dormant, in this case in the dorsal root ganglia (the meeting point for all the sensory neurons in each dermatome) or the geniculate ganglion of the trigeminal nerve. Later in life, when circulating antibodies are low, the virus may reactivate, this time as shingles.

Herpes Zoster in Brief

Pronunciation: HUR-peze ZOS-ter

What is it?
Herpes zoster is an infection of sensory neurons with varicella zoster virus (VZV). This virus causes chickenpox, but can have other presentations as well.

How is it recognized?
Itchy, painful blisters on a red base are the signature mark of a herpes zoster infection. In chickenpox, these can appear all over the body; in shingles they appear along the affected dermatome.

Massage risks and benefits
Risks: This is an extremely painful condition, and the blisters carry live virus, although most massage therapists have probably already been exposed. Both of these features are good reasons to postpone a massage until after the blisters have healed.
Benefits: Some clients with postherpetic neuralgia may find that massage is soothing (although others may not). Clients who have fully recovered from shingles can enjoy the same benefits from bodywork as the rest of the population.

VZV is initially spread through mucous secretions. Triggers for later reactivations can be difficult to pin down. Contributing factors include stress, old age, and impaired immunity because of other diseases. Shingles is notorious for accompanying HIV, Hodgkin lymphoma, advanced tuberculosis, pneumonia, chemotherapy, or as a result of having had an initial infection before 18 months of age. Shingles occasionally occurs after severe trauma or as a drug reaction.

Although the fluid in zoster blisters carries live virus, among adults it isn't particularly contagious because most people are exposed to chickenpox in childhood and have protection. This does not hold true, however, for a person who comes in contact with shingles while his or her own immune system is depressed, or who has never been exposed to the virus in the first place. In this case, an adult may get either shingles or chickenpox, but shingles is more likely.

Complications of VZV include the risk of secondary bacterial infection of the blisters, and damage to the eye when the trigeminal nerve is affected. A poorly understood phenomenon of pain outlasting blisters by several months or years is a frequent complication of shingles; this is called postherpetic neuralgia, and is described below.

Types of Herpes Zoster

- *Chickenpox*. This is the first infection with VZV that most people experience, although with the development of a vaccine for this condition, this may become rare (Sidebar 4.5). Chickenpox involves itchy blisters on a red base, but unlike shingles, they are spread all over the body.
- *Shingles*. This is a resurgence of VZV, usually later in life. It involves the outbreak of painful blisters along the dermatome that is colonized by virus from an earlier infection.
- *Postherpetic neuralgia*. In this situation, the pain generated by the shingles outlives the blisters by a minimum of 3 months, and may persist for years. The risk for developing postherpetic neuralgia (PHN) rises significantly with age: 60% of 60-year-old patients with shingles develop PHN, while 75% of 70-year-old patients have this complication.

SIDEBAR 4.5 Vaccines for Chickenpox and Shingles

A chickenpox vaccine for young children was licensed in the United States in 1995. Many schools now require or strongly recommend that children entering kindergarten be vaccinated against this infection. While this protects children from an uncomfortable time (and a small but significant risk of dangerous complications), perhaps the greater incentive is for their parents, who would otherwise have to miss a week of work to stay home with a sick child.

But two unexpected consequences came out of this vaccination campaign. One is that the chickenpox vaccine wears off within several years, leaving vaccinated children vulnerable to breakout infections with the virus, although these tend to be less severe than typical infections. Another consequence is that adults now seldom spend time with children who have chickenpox. Without this additional exposure, the incidence of shingles among older adults has gone up.

This has led to the development of an adult booster vaccine for varicella zoster that can prevent the outbreak of shingles and its painful complication, postherpetic neuralgia.

- *Zoster sine herpete*. Occasionally, a person can have a reactivation of VZV with all the pain sensation, but with no visible lesions. This condition is called zoster sine herpete ("sine" means "without", so this means "zoster without herpes lesions"). It can be easily misdiagnosed as a herniated disc, a heart attack, or multiple other painful but invisible conditions.
- *Ramsey-Hunt syndrome*. The trigeminal nerve is the main sensory nerve for the face. When this is the target for herpes zoster, eye damage, hearing loss, and temporary or permanent facial paralysis resembling Bell palsy can occur.

Signs and Symptoms

Pain and itching are the primary symptoms of a zoster infection. In chickenpox, an outbreak can take several days to resolve, but in shingles, pain is present for 1 to 3 days before the blisters break out, and for the 2 to 3 weeks in which blisters develop, erupt, and scab over. Pain is often present for months even after the lesions have healed and the skin is intact again.

Chickenpox blisters can be all over the body, and some people report blisters inside the mouth and down the digestive tract as well. Shingles blisters may grow along the entire dermatome of the host dorsal root ganglion, but more often they appear along an isolated stretch. It is nearly always a unilateral attack (Figure 4.6). Sensory nerves that supply the trunk and buttocks are the most frequently affected, although the trigeminal nerve may also be attacked.

Treatment

Herpes zoster is treated mainly palliatively. Cool baths and soothing lotion are recommended for chickenpox. More aggressive intervention may be required for shingles and postherpetic neuralgia.

Medications

- NSAIDs for pain and inflammation (note: *not* aspirin for children)
- Steroidal anti-inflammatories for inflammation
- Antiviral medications to shorten the outbreak
- For postherpetic neuralgia:
  - Opioid analgesics
  - Tricyclic antidepressants
  - Antiseizure medication
  - Topical lidocaine or capsaicin patches

Massage?

RISKS A client with an active case of chickenpox or shingles is unlikely to seek massage, simply because touch is uncomfortable. Cautions for this condition center around both the client's pain and the risk of spreading infection, although most people have been exposed to varicella zoster virus by adulthood, so that risk is relatively low. Clients with PHN may want to avoid touch, but that is unpredictable; others may find careful touch to be soothing.

BENEFITS Any client who has fully recovered from shingles or chickenpox can enjoy the same benefits from massage as the rest of the population. Clients with PHN may seek the soothing qualities that massage can offer.

Meningitis

Definition: What Is It?

Meningitis is inflammation of the **meninges** that surround the brain and spinal cord. The pia mater is the layer most affected. Most infections are found within three groups: children under 5 years old, young adults living in dormitories or close quarters, and elderly people. It is most threatening for the very young and very old.

Meningitis in Brief

Pronunciation: men-in-JY-tis

What is it?
Meningitis is an infection of the meninges, specifically the pia mater.

How is it recognized?
Symptoms of acute meningitis include very high fever, rash, photophobia, headache, and stiff neck. Symptoms are not always consistent; however, they may appear in different combinations for different people.

Massage risks and benefits
Risks: Meningitis is a communicable inflammatory disease with serious potential outcomes. It contraindicates massage while it is acute.
Benefits: Clients who have completely recovered from meningitis can enjoy the same benefits from massage as the rest of the population.

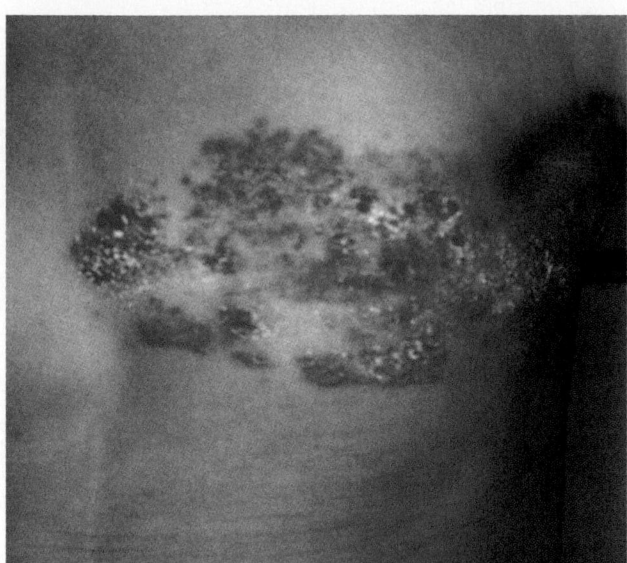

Figure 4.6. Shingles

Etiology: What Happens?

Meningitis is usually caused by bacterial or viral infection. Fungi and amoebae can also cause it, but this is relatively rare in the United States. It is important to find the causative factor, because the severity and treatment options vary according to the pathogen.

When a pathogen enters the CNS, it causes a number of changes that can be very dangerous. Infection in the cerebrospinal fluid increases the permeability of the blood-brain barrier. This in turn leads to cerebral edema and invites an influx of toxic waste products that would otherwise be filtered out. Intracranial pressure can damage cranial nerves (CN VIII is especially at risk, and damage here can lead to permanent hearing loss or deafness), obstructive **hydrocephalus** (which limits the normal circulation of cerebrospinal fluid within the brain and spinal cord), and inflammation of internal blood vessels with a high risk of blood clots and ischemic damage to brain cells: a type of stroke. Ultimately, the body's autoregulating centers are damaged, and the person dies of diffuse brain injury.

The pathogens that cause meningitis can infect other tissues as well. Most people with pneumococcal infections of the CNS concurrently have pneumonia, for instance. And bacterial infections of the blood can lead to the distinctive reddish purple rash associated with meningitis, along with a risk of blood clotting in capillaries, which opens the door to gangrene in the extremities.

Bacterial meningitis can be contagious. Its mode of transmission is much like the common cold: an infected person sneezes or coughs and then touches some surface, such as a doorknob or light switch. An uninfected person touches the surface, and then touches his or her eye or mouth. Meningitis brought about by the intestinal **enterovirus** family can also be spread by oral-fecal contact, which is an issue when it occurs in young children or in day care settings.

Some parts of the world are subject to epidemics of meningitis. The meningeal belt of sub-Saharan Africa has seasonal outbreaks of the severe bacterial version of this disease.

Types of Meningitis

- *Bacterial meningitis.* This infection is usually due to an invasion of *Streptococcus pneumoniae* (also called pneumococcus) or *Neisseria meningitides* (also called meningococcus). Bacterial meningitis tends to be more severe than the viral infection, and the risk of long-term CNS damage, specifically hearing loss or loss of mental function, is much higher. It does respond to antibiotics if the correct ones are administered early in the disease process.
- *Viral meningitis.* The viruses that can cause meningitis are many and varied, including a number of enteroviruses (usually associated with intestinal infections), herpes, HIV, coxsackievirus, and others. Viral meningitis tends to be less severe than bacterial meningitis and seldom causes permanent damage.

Signs and Symptoms

The symptoms of an acute meningitis infection include a rapid onset of high fever and chills, a deep red or purple rash, extreme headache, irritability, aversion to bright light, and a stiff rigid neck—this is because any stretch or pull of the meninges is acutely painful. Confusion, drowsiness, slurred speech, nausea, delirium, and convulsions may accompany severe infections.

Incubation between exposure to a disease-causing organism and the development of symptoms can be anywhere from several hours for bacterial infections to 3 weeks for viral ones. Symptoms typically peak and then taper off over a period of 2 to 3 weeks.

Treatment

The most common forms of bacterial meningitis can be prevented with the *Haemophilus influenzae* type B (HiB) vaccine. Vaccines for viral types can be obtained, but are recommended only for people traveling to areas where the infections are endemic.

Once an infection has developed, if the pathogen is identified as a bacterium, large doses of antibiotics are administered immediately to forestall the possibility of CNS damage. Steroids may also be prescribed to limit inflammation in the brain. Viral meningitis is generally treated with supportive therapy consisting of rest, fluids, and good nutrition while the patient's immune system fights back.

Medications

- Oral and/or intravenous antibiotics for bacterial infection
- Antiviral medication for viral infection
- Steroidal anti-inflammatories for inflammation control
- Antiseizure medications if necessary

Massage?

RISKS Meningitis is inflammatory, potentially communicable, and has the possibility of creating very severe damage. It contraindicates massage while it is acute.

BENEFITS Clients who have fully recovered from meningitis can enjoy the same benefits from bodywork as the rest of the population.

Polio, Postpolio Syndrome

Definition: What Are They?

Poliomyelitis, or infantile paralysis, as it used to be known, is a viral infection. The poliovirus targets intestinal mucosa first, and motor nerve cells in the anterior horn of the spinal cord later. Polio is becoming a rare disease, especially in developed countries (see Sidebar 4.6), but many survivors are still alive.

Postpolio syndrome (PPS) is a progressive muscular weakness that develops 10 to 40 years after an initial infection with the poliovirus. Anywhere from 25% to 60% of polio survivors eventually develop PPS.

Etiology: What Happens?

Wild poliovirus occurs in three subtypes. It can be spread through aerosol droplets, but the most efficient mechanism is oral-fecal contamination. It usually enters the body through the mouth in contaminated water, and sets up an infection in the intestine. New virus is concentrated and released in fecal matter, possibly to contaminate water elsewhere.

For over 99% of people exposed to the poliovirus, nothing else happens. But in a small portion of people, the virus travels into the spinal cord, where it targets and destroys motor nerve cells in the anterior horn. This impedes messages leaving the spinal cord, which in turn leads to rapid deterioration and atrophy of muscles and motor paralysis.

The paralysis caused by polio is motor only; sensation is still present. And because the motor nerves overlap muscle groups in the extremities, some muscle fibers may still function, even though many motor neurons may have been damaged. In other words, consider the dermatomes for the quadriceps. Even if all of the impulses to the motor neurons in L_2 have been eliminated, L_3 supplies other motor neurons to the same muscle group (Figure 4.7). Furthermore, nerve cells that survive the initial attack can grow new terminal axons to enervate muscle cells that were otherwise cut off. This increases the size of each motor unit, and puts

Polio, Postpolio Syndrome in Brief

What are they?
Polio is a viral infection, first of the intestines and then, for about 1% of exposed people, the anterior horn cells of the spinal cord. Postpolio syndrome (PPS) is a group of signs and symptoms among polio survivors, particularly those who had significant loss of function in the acute stage of the disease.

How are they recognized?
The destruction of motor neurons leads to degeneration, atrophy, and finally paralysis of skeletal muscles in polio patients. Later in life, polio patients may develop a sudden onset of fatigue, achiness, and weakness. Breathing and sleeping difficulties may also occur.

Massage risks and benefits
Risks: As long as an infection is not acute, massage is safe for polio patients, because sensation is not affected.
Benefits: Massage has been used for polio and PPS patients to help with strength, muscle tone, and fatigue.

SIDEBAR 4.6 Polio: It's Almost Extinct

In 1988, the Global Poliomyelitis Eradication Initiative combined efforts by the World Health Organization (WHO), UNICEF, Rotary International, and the Centers for Disease Control in the largest public health effort for the eradication of a disease. As a result of this initiative, the last new case of wild poliovirus in the Western Hemisphere was diagnosed in Peru in August 1991. The western Pacific region was certified polio free in October 2000. The last reported case in Europe was in 1998.

Countries with little or no incidence of polio infection are still vulnerable to invasion with the virus, especially along borders with countries where the virus is still active. Therefore, it is recommended that even "safe" countries maintain their vaccination schedules until the globe is free of the poliovirus.

excessive demand on the cell body of the enlarged motor neuron to supply the fiber with nutrition. In the long run, these motor neurons may wear out, leading to muscle weakness and possible atrophy: this is PPS.

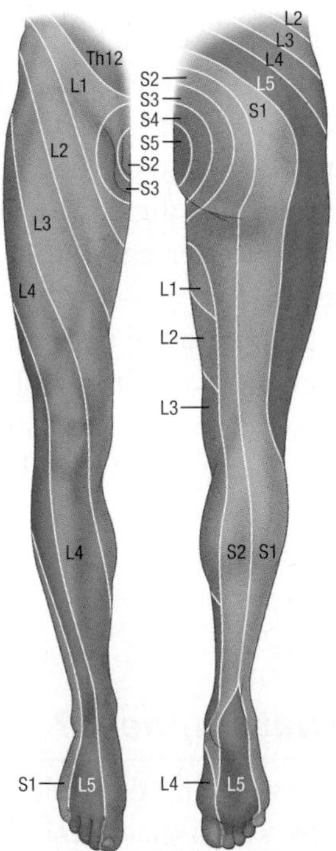

Figure 4.7. Dermatome patterns in the leg muscles allow multiple nerves to supply muscle groups; if one nerve root is damaged, the muscle group is still usable

Polio is rarely seen now because two inexpensive, stable, easy-to-administer vaccines have enabled eradication efforts in most countries. It is important to note, however, that the Sabin vaccine, which is given orally, introduces weakened viruses into the digestive system, where they stimulate the production of polio antibodies. The virus is concentrated in the feces, and people who handle the diapers of recently vaccinated infants need to be aware of this. Immunosuppressed persons should avoid contact with infants who are undergoing this treatment.

Signs and Symptoms

A new infection of polio is unlikely to occur in this country, but PPS is common among childhood polio survivors. This is marked by a sudden and sometimes extreme onset of fatigue, pain, and weakness. Spinal changes including the onset of spondylosis and postural deviations are common. Many patients report a decreased tolerance for cold. Breathing difficulties, sleep disturbances, and trouble swallowing may also develop. These symptoms usually begin 10 to 40 years after the original infection. They tend to run in cycles in which function is progressively lost, followed by periods of stability and then more loss of function.

NOTABLE CASES The list of well-known people who have had polio is long and diverse. It includes musicians Joni Mitchell and Neil Young; actors Donald Sutherland, Alan Alda, and Mia Farrow; science fiction novelist Arthur C. Clarke; professional golfer Jack Nicklaus; artist Frida Kahlo, and President Franklin Delano Roosevelt.

Treatment

Moist heat applications, physical therapy, and massage have been used to treat polio survivors once the initial infection has subsided. Together, hydrotherapy and massage can help to keep functioning muscle fibers healthy and well nourished.

PPS is treated by reducing muscular and neurological stress: adjusted braces, changing activity levels, and exercise programs that encourage the use of muscles not supplied by the damaged nerves are often suggested. People with PPS need to avoid excessive use of affected muscles, since exercise to these compromised tissues can cause permanent damage to the working fibers.

Massage?

RISKS Because polio is a motor paralysis with full sensation, the only caution for massage is that it should not take place during acute infection, and this is unlikely to happen if the therapist practices in a developed country.

BENEFITS Postpolio syndrome indicates massage that may help improve the efficiency of weakened muscles, improve sleep, reduce fatigue, and add to the quality of life for these patients.

Psychiatric Disorders

Addiction

Definition: What Is It?

Addiction is a complex topic. While definitions of chemical use, abuse, and dependency are relatively clear, the whole issue is clouded by the legal status of the substance in question. For instance, a person may become addicted to caffeine or to cocaine, but caffeine is not generally considered an addiction problem, while cocaine certainly is. Alcoholism is a form of addiction that, because of its prevalence in the culture and the profound effects it has on virtually every system of the body, is discussed as a subset of addiction in this article.

The issue of addiction falls into three categories: use, abuse, and dependency.

- *Use.* If a person ingests a substance specifically to change mood or physical experience, it is substance use.
- *Abuse.* Abuse is the use of a substance in a way that is potentially harmful to the user or to other people. It is further identified when substance use leads to impairment or distress, and when within a 12-month period at least one of the following facts is true: the user finds that he or she cannot fulfill obligations to work, family, or school; recurrent use puts the user in dangerous situations; the user has legal problems in relation to substance use; or the user has social or interpersonal problems in relation to substance use.
- *Dependency.* The line between use, abuse, and addiction is sometimes blurry, and it is not always connected to length of time or amount of substance ingested. Dependency occurs when three or more of the following are true: the user develops increasing tolerance for the substance; the user has withdrawal symptoms when access to the substance is interrupted; increasing amounts of the substance are used; the user cannot voluntarily limit use; the user devotes significant time to using or recovering from use; the user replaces other activities with substance use; or the user continues to abuse the substance even when fully aware of the dangers involved.

Addiction in Brief

What is it?
Substance abuse is the use of substances in ways or in dosages that result in damage to the user and people close to the user. It can involve the use of both legal and illegal substances. Addiction develops when the user becomes dependent on the substance to achieve a desired state of experience, or to avoid withdrawal symptoms.

How is it recognized?
Specific symptoms of addiction are partly determined by what substances are being consumed. Generally speaking, they include a craving for the substance in question, an inability to voluntarily limit use, unpleasant or dangerous withdrawal symptoms, and increasing tolerance of the substance's effects.

Massage risks and benefits
Risks: Long-term substance abusers may accrue multiple physical problems that can influence whether massage is a good choice. Clients who are intoxicated at the time of a massage need to reschedule.
Benefits: Because it can offer many benefits without the complications of using chemical tranquilizers, massage can be a helpful part of the detoxification period of addiction treatment. Clients who are in long-term recovery can enjoy the same benefits from massage as the rest of the population.

Etiology: What Happens?

The process of developing dependency on a particular substance depends on the chemical makeup of that product and the susceptibility of the user. Some drugs work in the CNS by slowing the rate at which neurotransmitters are reabsorbed at key synapses. This can lead to changes in the numbers of neurotransmitter receptors, which is then perceived as an increased need for the drug. This is the process seen with nicotine exposure, and it is why smoking is one of the most difficult addictions to overcome. Other disruptions in neural pathways and neurotransmitter relationships have been noted as well, and brain studies have revealed that some people are predisposed for addiction even without a history of exposure.

Alcohol and sedatives such as tranquilizers and barbiturates work by depressing CNS arousal. While alcohol is technically a depressant, the loss of inhibitions felt by the drinker can give the impression that it is a stimulant. Some people have a genetic susceptibility to alcohol addiction, but many alcoholics develop the disease over many months or years of repeated use that finally and permanently changes the chemistry in the brain.

Once a person becomes dependent on a substance, two things happen: it takes more and more to achieve the desired affects, and to stop using the substance can create physical responses that are daunting to contemplate. Addiction is defined in two categories: psychological and physical. Psychological addiction is dependency on the pleasurable or satisfying sensations that some substance provides—in other words, the addict loves the feeling the drug gives. Physical addiction is a dependency arising from the need to avoid withdrawal symptoms, which can include general physical pain, hallucinations, nausea, vomiting, seizures, and in extreme cases, death.

Risk Factors

Several risk factors contribute to a person's susceptibility to addiction.

- *Genetic predisposition.* The rate of drug abuse and alcoholism is demonstrably greater in the families of other addicts than in the general population. This is partly an environmental and availability issue, but studies have shown that even children who are not raised with their chemically dependent parents have a higher than normal incidence of addiction.
- *Other mental illness.* Depression and/or anxiety disorders raise the risk of a person becoming a substance abuser, as he or she may attempt to self-medicate to cope with problems.
- *Environmental factors.* These include availability of the substance in question, peer pressure, low self-esteem, a history of physical or sexual abuse, being a child in the household of a substance abuser, and other stressors that may make drug use look like a reasonable choice.
- *Type of drug being used.* Some drugs are simply more addictive than others, but most substances can cause dependency if they are used consistently enough.
- *Age.* The younger a person is at the beginning of use of an addictive substance, the more likely he or she is to develop a long-term dependency on it.
- *Medical reasons.* A patient's need for medication sometimes outlives the problem that required the initial prescription. Addictions to painkillers and sleeping pills are examples of this phenomenon.

Complications

Complications of drug addiction can range from paranoid delusions to coma or even death. Some of the worst effects of drug use are not limited to the users, however. People close to substance abusers are also at risk. Drug-related violent crime, car accidents, industrial accidents, impaired judgment leading to the spread of sexually transmitted infections, and high rates of domestic violence and child abuse are other complications of chemical dependency that affect many people beyond the user.

The complications of alcoholism can be progressive and insidious, and its use affects virtually every system of the body. Here is a brief synopsis:

The digestive system. Alcohol irritates the stomach lining, and high levels of consumption are responsible for a specific type of gastritis. It is also very rapidly absorbed through the gastric mucosa into the portal system. The portal vein dumps the alcohol directly into the liver, where it enters the rest of the bloodstream. The effects of alcohol are felt until the liver has finished neutralizing it.

People who have preexisting gastrointestinal problems are especially vulnerable to the worst effects of alcohol. It is implicated in the development of cancer in the upper gastrointestinal tract, especially in the esophagus, pharynx, larynx, and mouth. Alcoholism can cause ulcers, internal hemorrhaging, pancreatitis, and cirrhosis.

The cardiovascular system. Alcohol use decreases the force of cardiac contractions and can lead to irregular heartbeat or arrhythmia. Alcohol is also toxic to myocardial tissue and can lead to alcoholic cardiomyopathy. Alcohol tends to agglutinate red blood cells, making them stick together. This leads to the possibility of thrombi, not only in the brain but in the coronary arteries as well. Alcohol use can also have the opposite effect: liver damage can lead to reduced clotting factors and poor vitamin K synthesis, which may result in uncontrollable bleeding.

Moderate alcohol consumption may actually help prevent cardiovascular disease by increasing high-density lipoprotein levels (the "good" cholesterol) in the blood.

The nervous system. Memory loss frequently occurs for biochemical reasons as well as from agglutinated red blood cells blocking cerebral capillaries, causing brain cells to starve to death. Even some social drinkers sustain measurable brain damage from repeated agglutination. In the short term, alcohol slows reflexes, slurs speech, impairs judgment, and compromises motor control. In the long term, the same effects can happen on a permanent basis, often due to a thiamine deficiency. This is also known as Wernicke-Korsakoff syndrome. In advanced stages of cirrhosis, the blood accumulates levels of metabolic wastes that can cause brain damage.

NOTABLE CASES The list of famous people who have battled addiction is too long to explore. Rather than lingering on the many creative souls lost to the complications of alcoholism and drug abuse, in this context, it is more fitting to wonder what works of art we might have enjoyed if their lives had not been shortened by this disease.

The immune system. Prolonged alcohol use severely impedes resistance, especially to respiratory infections. Alcoholics are especially vulnerable to pneumonia.

The reproductive system. Alcoholism can cause reduced sex drive, erectile dysfunction, menstrual irregularities, and infertility. Babies of alcoholic women are susceptible to **fetal alcohol syndrome**, the most common type of environmentally caused mental disability in the United States.

Alcoholic families. Children raised in homes with one or more alcoholic adults have an increased risk of becoming substance abusers themselves. Their chances of developing depression, anxiety disorders, and phobias are higher than in the general population. And their health costs are higher than those of other children, and many children in foster care settings are from alcoholic homes.

Other complications. Alcohol is frequently a factor in traffic injuries, drownings, falls, burns, and unintentional shootings.

Signs and Symptoms

Symptoms of chemical dependency vary according to the substance, but main features are consistent:

- The person feels a persistent craving for the substance.
- The person goes to great lengths, including actions that could be illegal, to ensure that the substance is always available.
- The person cannot voluntarily control use of the substance.
- The person develops an increasing tolerance to the effects of the substance and so must consume more to achieve the same results; the substance is necessary for the person to feel "normal."
- The person puts himself or herself and others at risk for harm while under the influence.
- Cessation of use creates unpleasant, alarming, and even physically dangerous withdrawal symptoms.

In addition to these signs, the addict or alcoholic may devote a significant amount of time to using and then recovering from substance use. He or she may neglect responsibilities to family, job, friends, and other relationships while distracted by substance use. And finally, the addict often denies that substance use seriously impedes or endangers his or her life: "I'm not dead yet, so obviously, I'm okay."

Treatment

The first and most important step in treating any kind of addiction is for the addict to accept that a problem exists. Once a person has reached that point, many treatment programs have good success rates, although the recurrence rate is high until a person reaches about 5 years of sobriety. Treatment goals for addiction are threefold: abstinence, rehabilitation, and prevention of relapses.

Most programs begin with detoxification, during which the drugs are expelled from the body. This may be ameliorated with sedatives, tranquilizers, or less potent versions of the drug in question until all chemical remnants have been processed out of the body.

The time this takes varies according to the substance in question.

Detoxification is followed by rehabilitation, during which the patient is taught about the effects of chemical use and trained in avoidance behaviors to provide some tools to handle the temptation to fall back into old habits.

Aftercare has been shown to be the most important part of treatment for chemical dependency. This sets up the patient with a support system that will carry him or her throughout a lifetime choice of abstinence.

Some medications can help to suppress the craving for alcohol or can cause violent physical illness when alcohol is consumed, but this doesn't eradicate the effects of alcohol. The potential for relapse into substance abuse lasts indefinitely, so this is a condition that is treated most successfully with long-term coping skills rather than short-term patches.

Medications

- Benzodiazepines in low doses to mitigate the stress of withdrawal symptoms
- Neurotransmitter receptor blockers to lessen the "reward" response in the brain and reduce craving for alcohol or narcotics
- Disulfiram to create negative physical responses (nausea, vomiting, headache) to alcohol use

Massage?

RISKS A client with a history of drug or alcohol abuse is at high risk for secondary health problems, including liver damage, bacterial infections, HIV/AIDS, hepatitis, and heart problems. All of these require adjustments in bodywork choices.

BENEFITS Some rehabilitation facilities employ massage therapists to help ameliorate withdrawal symptoms, speed detoxification, and reduce the need for tranquilizers and other drugs.

Clients who are in long-term recovery and good health can enjoy the same benefits from bodywork as the rest of the population.

OPTIONS Current alcohol or other drug use at the time of an appointment contraindicates massage, mainly because of the risk of overtaxing a liver that is already occupied. This guideline can be a judgment call, based on the level of intoxication (one glass of wine is different from a fifth of vodka), the setting of the massage session, the behavior of the client, and the boundaries set by the therapist.

Anxiety Disorders

Definition: What Is It?

Anxiety disorders are a collection of distinct psychiatric disorders that have to do with irrational fears and extensive efforts to avoid or control them. These conditions often overlap, so a person can meet the diagnostic criteria for multiple conditions. Anxiety disorders range in severity from mild to completely debilitating.

Etiology: What Happens?

"*Am I safe*?" At this moment, every person who is alive and awake is asking this question at some level of consciousness. The answer for people with anxiety disorders is "*Probably not*." This interpretation of environmental signals is reflected in emotional and physical experiences that can be completely debilitating. Contributing factors include genetic vulnerability, a history of traumatic events, and situations or

Anxiety Disorders in Brief

What are they?
Anxiety disorders are a group of conditions that involve exaggerated, irrational fears and attempts to control those fears. Some anxiety disorders come and go; some are chronic progressive problems; others reach a peak and then recede or remain stable.

How is it recognized?
While triggers for individual cases may vary, many anxiety disorders involve sympathetic reactions including fast heart rate, sweating, dizziness, faintness, and nausea. In addition, feelings of impending death, a sense of physical detachment, unwelcome or frightening thoughts, and other reactions are possible.

Massage risks and benefits
Risks: The main risk for bodywork in the context of anxiety disorders is that a client may not feel safe, or touch may not be welcomed. This can arise at any time, so it is important for practitioners to be very sensitive to verbal and nonverbal signals about how massage is being received.
Benefits: As long as a client feels safe and touch is welcomed, massage can help clients with anxiety disorder feel less anxious and more secure and capable of dealing with everyday challenges.

circumstances that trigger a stress response that is out of proportion to the actual threat.

To aid in the investigation of these conditions, careful distinctions have been drawn between the terms arousal, fear, and anxiety. *Arousal* is preparation for the possibility of a stressful event. It is directly linked to a perceived trigger or stressor (the deer that might dart across the darkened highway; the tsunami warnings on the TV). *Fear* occurs when the possibility of a stressful event is confirmed. The deer is in front of you; the waves are rising quickly. *Anxiety*, by contrast, is a state of prolonged heightened arousal or fear, but with no discernible immediate or significant threat: no deer, no tsunami, but all the physical and emotional reactions that accompany the feeling of impending disaster.

NOTABLE CASES Many historical figures left records of their struggles with anxiety disorders, although they were never officially diagnosed. Abraham Lincoln, Sir Isaac Newton, Emily Dickenson, and John Steinbeck may be among the most influential figures to show signs of problems ranging from social phobia to general anxiety disorder to disabling agoraphobia.

Anxiety disorders take a huge toll on a person's ability to complete school or hold a job. Consequently, a disproportionately high percentage of people with anxiety disorders never earn a high school diploma and are in the lowest end of socioeconomic ranking. Furthermore, complications of anxiety disorders include an increased risk for substance abuse, sleep disorders, eating disorders, cardiovascular disease, and depression (with an increased danger for suicidal thoughts or behaviors).

Two major issues are consistent with anxiety disorders: problems with the limbic system and the hypothalamic-pituitary-adrenal (HPA) axis, and neurotransmitter imbalances.

- *The limbic system and the HPA axis*. The **limbic system** is a part of the brain that is responsible for determining a person's sense of safety in any given moment. It does this through two regulatory centers, the **amygdala** and the **hippocampus**. When a person experiences a threatening stimulus, these structures work together to recognize the threat and translate this information to the **hypothalamus** (mediator of sympathetic or parasympathetic reactions), which uses links with the pituitary and adrenal glands to establish a stress response: this is the **HPA axis**. In perfect health, the HPA axis produces electrical and chemical signals that allow a person to respond appropriately to a stressor. But when the HPA axis is overactive, it can lead to the release of excessive amounts of glucocorticoids (of which cortisol is the dominant hormone) from the adrenal glands. Excessive levels of glucocorticoids in the blood can damage several processes. They can weaken connective tissue, suppress immune system responses, and—most pertinent to a discussion of psychiatric disorders—they can shrink the hippocampus. One line of thought about anxiety disorders links the atrophy of the hippocampus (by up to 20% in some circumstances) to difficulties with connecting stimuli to appropriate responses.
- *Neurotransmitters*. The neurotransmitters that are most frequently disturbed in anxiety disorders include norepinephrine (chemically related to adrenaline), GABA, serotonin, corticotrophin-releasing factor, and some others. These are so tightly interdependent that disruption in one of these chemicals tends to cause disruptions in all of them.

Types of Anxiety Disorders

- *General anxiety disorder (GAD)*. GAD consists of chronic, exaggerated, consuming worry, and the constant anticipation of disaster. It does not cause the person to avoid stressful situations, but he or she lives in a constant state of anxiety that makes it difficult to accomplish many tasks. It appears earlier and develops more slowly than other anxiety disorders.

  GAD is diagnosed when at least three of the following symptoms persist for 6 months or longer: restlessness or a feeling of being on edge, easy fatigability, poor concentration, irritability, muscle tension, and sleeping problems.
- *Panic disorder*. Panic disorder is characterized by the sudden onset (often with no identifiable trigger) of very extreme sympathetic symptoms: a pounding heart, chest pain, sweatiness, dizziness, faintness, and alternating flushing and chilling. Hyperventilation causes numbness and tingling in the lips and extremities. A feeling of being smothered, of impending doom, and the nearness of death usually lasts for about 10 minutes but may persist for many hours.

A person can have a panic attack without having panic disorder. But when episodes repeat, especially if they are associated with a certain place or situation, panic disorder is diagnosed.

Panic disorder is complicated by worrying about having another attack: fear of fear. When it causes a person to avoid situations in which panic attacks have happened before or may happen in the future, it can cause another anxiety disorder, **agoraphobia**, or fear of open places. Gradually, a person's perceived safety zone shrinks to the point where he or she becomes reluctant to leave the immediate environment. About one-third of panic disorder patients develop agoraphobia.

Panic disorder is one of the most successfully treated of all anxiety disorders, but treatment is most successful if it is initiated before the onset of agoraphobia.

- *Posttraumatic stress disorder (PTSD)*. Traditionally, associated with soldiers returning from the horrors of war, PTSD has also been known as "shell shock."

  PTSD is characterized by visceral memories of a specific ordeal, such as combat, physical or sexual abuse, rape, assault, torture, natural disaster, terrorist attack, or any other life-threatening event. Sometimes a patient was a witness to an attack or threat to someone else. Memories of the event are relived in nightmares and waking flashbacks. The patient often becomes withdrawn, irritable, and occasionally aggressive as these memories intrude more and more frequently into his life. Startle reflexes tend to be exaggerated, and hypervigilance is common. **Dissociation,** the detachment of the mind from physical or emotional experiences, is a hallmark of PTSD. Some patients find that their symptoms subside with time and eventually no longer affect them, but others find that without treatment this is a lifelong problem.

  Symptoms of PTSD usually appear within 3 months of the triggering event, but some patients aren't affected until many months or years later; this is called delayed-onset PTSD.
- *Acute traumatic stress disorder*. Acute traumatic stress disorder has much in common with PTSD, but it is characterized by development of symptoms within 1 month of a triggering event.
- *Obsessive-compulsive disorder (OCD)*. OCD is a combination of intrusive, uncontrollable, unwelcome thoughts (obsessions), and highly developed rituals designed to try to quell or control those thoughts (compulsions). Unlike many other anxiety disorders, OCD can come and go throughout a lifetime and is not always progressive.

  Some of the most common obsessions of OCD patients include fear of contamination by dirt, germs, or sexual activity; fear of violence or catastrophic accidents; fear of committing violent or sexual acts; and fears surrounding disorder or asymmetry. The rituals used to battle these fears include repeated hand washing (often to the point of damaging the skin); refusing to touch other people or contaminated surfaces; repeatedly checking locks, stoves, irons, or other appliances; counting telephone poles; carefully and symmetrically arranging clothes, food, or other items; and persistently repeating words, phrases, or prayers. While many people occasionally engage in some of these behaviors, OCD patients often devote hours every day to the rituals that are designed to keep them safe.
- *Phobias, Social and Specific*

  Social phobia. Also called social anxiety disorder, social phobia is characterized by intense, irrational fears of being judged negatively by others or of being publicly embarrassed. It can involve specific situations, such as speaking or performing in public, or it can involve any social setting at all. Physical symptoms include blushing, sweating, trembling, and nausea, but many social phobia patients display no outward signs of their disorder. While many people feel shy or nervous among strangers, patients with social phobia are significantly distressed and even disabled by their fear, which can interfere with work, school, or relationships.

  Specific phobias. A specific phobia is an intense, irrational fear of something that poses little or no real danger. Some common phobias include fear of animals (including larger animals such as dogs, cats, or birds but also insects and spiders); closed-in places (claustrophobia), open spaces (agoraphobia), heights (acrophobia), flying, elevators, and blood. Untreated phobias can severely restrict a person's ability to hold a certain kind of job, live in a certain kind of building, or perform mundane tasks, such as grocery shopping. Persons with this disorder often respond better to controlled desensitization and relaxation techniques than they do to medication.

Signs and Symptoms

Signs and symptoms of anxiety disorders vary according to type. While they usually involve irrational fears and inappropriate sympathetic nervous system responses, they present differently by variety and patient. Brief descriptions of their signs and symptoms are included in the descriptions.

Treatment

Most anxiety disorders are treated with a combination of medication and psychotherapy. Some varieties respond better to psychotherapy and the development of coping skills alone, while others also require chemical intervention to reestablish neurotransmitter balance in the CNS. Most patients with anxiety disorders can find some combination of therapies that successfully treat their problem—if they seek treatment. Sadly, many patients are inadequately treated or never seek treatment at all.

Psychotherapeutic techniques used for anxiety disorders vary from supported resistance to compulsive behaviors for OCD patients, to controlled exposure to frightening stimuli for people with specific phobias, to various forms of behavioral-cognitive therapies to help patients learn ways to address and often overcome the irrational fears that limit their lives.

Other interventions have been shown to improve the quality of life for anxiety disorder patients, including relaxation techniques, meditation, yoga, acupuncture, and massage.

Medications to treat anxiety disorders fall into three classes: antidepressants, antianxiety drugs, and beta blockers.

Medications

- Benzodiazepines for sedative effect (these carry a high risk for dependence)
- Buspirone for sedative effect
- Antidepressants, including selective serotonin reuptake inhibitors (SSRIs), tricyclics, and monoamine oxidase (MAO) inhibitors
- Beta blockers to control symptoms of panic disorder

Massage?

RISKS Some anxiety disorder patients have a history of physical or sexual abuse; this can create problematic reactions to touch. It is vital that these clients feel safe and in control within a massage environment.

BENEFITS Massage has been documented to help clients with anxiety disorder feel calmer and more able to cope with the everyday stresses that life offers. The mechanism for this benefit is not well understood, however. It could be any combination of parasympathetic response, support of a healthy hypothalamic-pituitary-adrenal axis through welcomed touch, and the results inherent in a supportive therapeutic relationship between the client and therapist.

OPTIONS It is vital to be flexible to meet the needs of clients with anxiety disorders. Adjustments like working through clothing, with another person in the room, or with the office door open may help them to feel safer. It is also important to remember that progress is not a smooth curve, and clients' needs may fluctuate from one session to the next.

Attention Deficit Hyperactivity Disorder in Brief

Definition: What Is It?

Attention deficit hyperactivity disorder (ADHD) is a neurobiochemical disorder resulting in difficulties with attention, movement, and impulse control. It has been recognized in children since the early 1900s, but was not discussed in medical literature as an issue for adults until 1976.

An argument can be made that the ADHD label is a misnomer. In this condition, a person pays attention to matters that are peripheral to a central task, and may not be able to filter what is important from what is trivial in any moment. This is not attention deficit; rather, it is too much attention to too many things.

Etiology: What Happens?

ADHD is a neurochemically mediated disorder. It has been traced to problems with dopamine production,

Attention Deficit Hyperactivity Disorder in Brief

What is it?
Attention deficit hyperactivity disorder (ADHD) is a neurobiochemical imbalance in the brain resulting in problems with focus, impulse control, and motor activity. It occurs among children and adults.

How is it recognized?
ADHD is marked by the behavior changes it brings about: inattention, inappropriate impulsivity, and when hyperactivity is present, difficulty with controlling movement. The diagnosis of ADHD depends on the observations of people close to the patient, along with ruling out other possible causes for the symptoms.

Massage risks and benefits
Risks: Massage has no particular risks for clients with ADHD, except that some people have limited tolerance for spending a long time on the table.
Benefits: As long as the client is comfortable, massage provides the benefit of an opportunity for a quiet, focused, nonjudgmental physical experience.

transportation, and reabsorption, and with noradrenaline disruption in the frontal cortex, basal ganglia and cerebellum: areas in the brain that have to do with decision making and movement.

While the causes of ADHD are still unclear, some contributing factors have been identified. Genetic predisposition is certainly an issue; many ADHD patients have a first-degree relative with the same disorder. Altered brain function is observable, as motor control and planning centers in the brain are affected by disturbed chemical levels. And maternal behaviors (smoking and alcohol consumption) and exposure to toxins (lead, **dioxins**, and **PCBs**) have been seen to increase the risk of ADHD in children.

Signs and Symptoms

Three specific patterns of behavior indicate ADHD: inattentiveness, hyperactivity, and impulsivity. A person with ADHD may only be inattentive or have a combination of these features, but behaviors are consistent in multiple settings, for instance, at school or work, at home, and in social situations.

Signs of inattention include becoming easily distracted by irrelevant sights and sounds; failing to pay attention to details and making careless mistakes; having difficulty with following instructions carefully and completely; and losing or forgetting things such as toys, or pencils, books, and tools needed for a task.

Some signs of hyperactivity and impulsivity include feeling restless, fidgeting with hands or feet, or squirming; running, climbing, or leaving a seat when sitting or quiet behavior is expected; blurting out answers before hearing the whole question; and having difficulty waiting for others to complete a task.

NOTABLE CASES Olympic swimming champion Michael Phelps was diagnosed with attention deficit hyperactivity disorder (ADHD) at age 8, and was able to turn his "hyperfocus" to a gold medal–winning goal. It is not surprising that people with ADHD are known as class clowns; other celebrities diagnosed with this condition include actors Jim Carrey and Will Smith.

Treatment

Diagnosis and treatment of ADHD in children and adults is complicated by the fact that several disorders commonly occur along with it, including sleep disorders, oppositional defiant disorder, depression, and anxiety disorders.

At this moment, the most common treatment for ADHD is psychostimulants, usually from classes of drugs called methylphenidates or dextroamphetamines. These drugs work by stimulating areas in the brain where activity is diminished. Another option is a norepinephrine reuptake inhibitor; this is not a stimulant; instead, it works to keep norepinephrine available in some synapses for a longer period.

Research suggests that ADHD responds best to medication, but that when medication is coupled with family counseling or parental training, the average required dosage is smaller for children who are treated with medication alone. In adults, an expanded version of counseling called metacognitive therapy has been found to be effective.

Side effects of ADHD medications are a concern, especially if the patient is a young child. They can include appetite suppression, increased blood pressure and heart rate, sleep problems, and sometimes the development of facial or vocal tics. These signs indicate that a medication is poorly tolerated or the dosage needs to be adjusted. Some ADHD medications cannot be combined with some asthma medications.

Other approaches for ADHD include the use of nutritional supplements and adjusting the diet to avoid sugar, caffeine, and other stimulants.

Untreated or undertreated ADHD carries the risk of several serious consequences. Children with this disorder have difficulty with self-esteem, maintaining relationships, and performing well with schoolwork or other jobs. Later in life, untreated or unsuccessfully treated ADHD patients have a higher-than-average rate of automobile accidents, and an elevated risk of developing substance abuse or other addictive behaviors (i.e., gambling, shopping, engaging in sexual encounters) in attempts to self-medicate to manage their disease.

Medications

- Psychostimulants
  - Methylphenidate
  - Dextroamphetamine
- Norepinephrine reuptake inhibitors
- Antidepressants

Massage?

RISKS Massage holds no risks for children or adults with attention deficit hyperactivity disorder (ADHD), except that some people are uncomfortable being asked to be still for as long as a typical massage may take.

BENEFITS Bodywork has been seen to improve anger control, sleep quality, classroom behavior, mood, and interpersonal relationships in people diagnosed with ADHD.

OPTIONS While some clients with ADHD love the stimulation of a rigorous, fast-paced sports massage type of bodywork, others prefer the chance to achieve the stillness found with subtler energy techniques.

Autism Spectrum Disorders

Definition: What Are They?

Autism spectrum disorders (ASD) are a group of disorders characterized by problems with connecting emotionally with other people, including parents and family members, communication difficulties, specific and predictable movement patterns, and sensory problems. ASD begins in early childhood. It is usually diagnosable by age 3, although many children with ASD aren't identified until they start kindergarten.

Autism Spectrum Disorders in Brief

Pronunciation: AW-tizm SPEK-trum dis-OR-derz

What are they?
Autism spectrum disorders (ASD) are a group of conditions that present in early childhood, involving problems with communication, socialization, and movement behaviors.

How are they recognized?
ASD can range from mild to severe. Symptoms can involve language development, difficulties in connecting emotionally to other people, tactile hypersensitivity and hyposensitivity, repetitive and restrictive movement patterns, and several other issues, depending on the type and severity of the individual disorder.

Massage risks and benefits
Risks: While massage has no specific physical risks for ASD patients, many of these patients do not spontaneously welcome touch.
Benefits: If a bodywork practitioner can create a relationship and a working strategy so that a client with autism can accept and welcome touch, massage can be a valuable way to connect other people to this client's life.

Etiology: What Happens?

The difference in CNS function between people with ASD and people without it is the subject of intense study. Abnormalities are present within various neural systems linking the brainstem, limbic system, basal ganglia, cerebellum, corpus callosum, and cerebral cortex of people with ASD, but no predictable pattern is present for all patients.

The most easily distinguishable factor behind some cases of ASD is a genetic anomaly. **Fragile X syndrome** is a condition in which a pinch appears in the X chromosome; this is the most common form of inherited mental disability, and is found in many ASD patients. **Tuberous sclerosis**, another genetic anomaly, involves the growth of benign tumors in the CNS and other vital organs. Children with tuberous sclerosis have a higher chance of also being autistic. Siblings of children with ASD have a much greater chance of having ASD than the general public (and the chance for identical twins is much higher still) clearly pointing to a genetic factor, although the specific mutations are not always identifiable.

Other theories for the development of ASD include mitochondrial dysfunction within neurons; early exposure to some virus that stimulates an autoimmune response; exposure to mercury, lead, or other heavy metals; and allergies.

Types of Autism Spectrum Disorders

- *Autistic disorder*. This may also be called "severe autism" to distinguish it from the milder form. It is characterized by the three basic traits associated with ASD: impairment in communication skills; poor social interactions; and restricted, repetitive patterns of movement.
- *Asperger syndrome*. This is a mild form of ASD involving difficulties with socializing, but language skills and mental development are often normal or above normal. Some people classify Asperger syndrome as an entity distinct from mild autism, but not all experts agree on this. Many people with Asperger syndrome develop a consuming interest in some subject that completely engages them.
- *Pervasive developmental disorder, not otherwise specified*. This is a condition in which the child exhibits several ASD signs, but doesn't meet the diagnostic criteria for any other label.
- *Rett syndrome*. This is a genetic disorder that typically results in severe symptoms. Almost all diagnoses are in girls, because affected boys are usually lost through miscarriage. Where this was once considered a rare and extreme form of ASD, genetic testing now allows the identification of milder cases of Rett syndrome.
- *Childhood disintegrative disorder*. This is a rare condition, occurring mostly in boys. It has a later onset than other forms of ASD: around age 3 or 4. It is characterized by a dramatic and sudden loss of vocabulary, motor, and communication skills.

Signs and Symptoms

Signs and symptoms of ASD vary according to what type is present. Three major issues are present for most types: deficits in verbal and nonverbal communication, problems with social interaction, and repetitive behaviors or movements. These occur in varying combinations and severity for each person. In addition, many ASD patients show unusual reactions to some sensory stimuli: they often seem to be impervious to cold or pain, while some sounds and textures, even soft ones, appear to be unbearable.

One common theme that many people with ASD share is the phenomenon of being locked within their own perspective. The recognition that other people also have consciousness is slow to come and difficult to integrate. People with ASD don't automatically register nonverbal signs such as facial expressions or body language, and it is difficult to interpret the emotional tone behind speech. "Come here" to a child with ASD means the same thing whether it's offered with a kiss and a cookie, or with a frown and a punishment in store. Consequently, the people in these children's lives, including parents and family members, can appear to be completely unpredictable and therefore to be avoided.

NOTABLE CASES Perhaps the most notable spokesperson for autism spectrum disorder is Temple Grandin, a writer and animal behavior consultant who invented a "hug machine" to help calm hypersensitive people.

ASD frequently occurs with other conditions. About 25% of ASD patients also have seizures, and most have some level of cognitive disability. By contrast, of ASD patients with an IQ of 35 or above, many show signs of savant characteristics, that is, extremely highly developed skills with some narrow set of interests, such as numbers, music, reading, or other talents.

Early indicators of ASD include a lack of babbling, pointing, or smiling at 12 months; no word use at 16 months; no word linkage at 24 months; no response to the child's name; and observable regression in language and social skills. Other signs include little or no eye contact, no imaginative play with toys, obsessive lining up of objects, extreme attachment to one object, and the appearance of a hearing deficiency. Many children show restricted, repetitive behaviors, such as hand wringing, rocking, or other movements, especially when they are tense or upset.

Treatment

ASD is treated according to type and the individual characteristics of the child. Experts agree that children with ASD do best in highly structured, specialized programs that reinforce positive behaviors and work to reduce negative ones.

Applied behavioral analysis is an intensive one-on-one intervention that occurs for many hours every week. Children who undergo this kind of therapy, especially in early years (preschool is preferable) often have significant improvement in function. Sensory integration therapy uses touch, pressure, vibration, massage, and lots of play equipment to help patients better organize their sense of touch.

Many ASD patients also have symptoms of other disorders, especially ADHD, obsessive compulsive disorder, and depression. Treating these can improve the possibility that other ASD interventions are successful.

Some parents find that dietary adjustments help their children. Avoiding gluten and casein (a protein found in dairy products) reduces symptoms for some, but not all, ASD patients. Supplementing vitamin B_6 with magnesium has similar results: some patients benefit, and others have no response.

In addition to these interventions, medication may be prescribed to help manage seizures, anxiety, and depression, but no medication addresses the issue of autism itself.

Medications

- Antipsychotics to manage anger, irritation, aggressive, or self-destructive behaviors
- Antidepressants, especially SSRIs for depression and anxiety
- Psychostimulants for ADHD symptoms
- Antiseizure drugs for seizures

Massage?

RISKS The most important caution for working with clients who have autism spectrum disorder (ASD) is that the sensation of touch is not always welcome. Therapists may have to be patient and imaginative to create an environment where the best outcomes can occur.

BENEFITS If the ASD patient is comfortable receiving touch, massage can have a profound impact on a person's ability to connect with the world in a positive way.

Depression

Definition: What Is It?

Depression is a group of disorders that involve negative changes in emotional state. One of the best descriptions of this disease is "a genetic-neurochemical disorder requiring a strong environmental trigger whose characteristic manifestation is an inability to appreciate sunsets."[1]

In other words, depression is a CNS disorder involving a genetic predisposition, chemical changes, and a significant triggering event that results in a person losing the ability to enjoy life. Depression is more than a temporary spell of the blues; it can be a long-lasting, self-propagating, and ultimately a debilitating—even life-threatening—disease.

Depression in Brief

Pronunciation: de-PRESH-un

What is it?
Depression is an umbrella term covering a number of mood disorders that can result in persistent feelings of sadness, guilt, and/or hopelessness.

How is it recognized?
Symptoms vary according to the type of depression and the individual, but they usually include a sad mood, loss of enjoyment derived from usual hobbies and activities, and some combination of disappointment with oneself, hopelessness, irritability, a change in sleeping habits, and thoughts of suicide.

Massage risks and benefits
Risks: Massage has no particular risks for clients with depression, unless the client decides to stop taking medication: this is something that must be done with medical supervision.
Benefits: Massage has been shown to be very beneficial for people with depression, although the mechanism isn't understood.

Etiology: What Happens?

The pathophysiology of depression is not well understood. Several distinctive features have been noted in the brain and endocrine system of depressive individuals, but whether these features cause the problem or are caused by the problem is still a mystery. The most significant and consistent distinguishing feature of depression is a neurotransmitter imbalance, especially with serotonin, norepinephrine, and dopamine: these may be in short supply, or receptor sites for them may not function well. Either way, the drugs most often prescribed for depression work to increase the accessibility of these important chemicals.

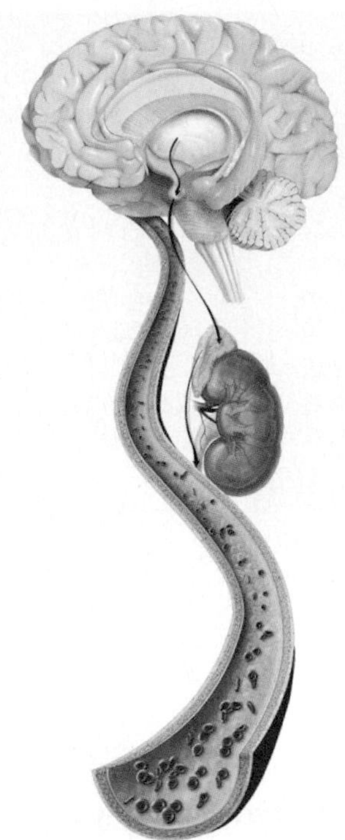

Figure 4.8. HPA axis

The HPA axis is another factor in depression and chemical imbalances. The HPA axis describes the tight connection between the CNS and the endocrine system: the pituitary gland, under the control of the hypothalamus, controls the adrenal glands by way of corticotrophin-releasing hormone (Figure 4.8). Depressive people tend to secrete excessive amounts of corticotrophin-releasing hormone, meaning that they create stress responses to minimal stimuli, and those responses tend to have a longer lasting effect on the body.

Many factors contribute to depressive episodes. Some of them are controllable, but many are not. Whether or not someone develops depression depends on personal chemistry, genetics, emotional and environmental triggers, and unique personality qualities and problem-solving tendencies. Other psychiatric conditions commonly overlap with depression, especially PTSD and obsessive compulsive disorder. In addition, chronic illness increases the risk for this disorder. This is easy to understand, as chronic pain, or the prospect of sliding into inevitable disability naturally deprives a person of a sense of hopefulness or investment in life. Often the symptoms of depression outweigh the symptoms of the chronic illness: if the depression can be resolved, coping skills for the illness may also improve.

Several other problems can contribute to depression, but these are often much more easily controlled than the ones so far discussed. Hypothyroidism, smoking, alcohol, drug use, or side effects of medication can all create depressive symptoms. Also, certain nutritional deficiencies, notably vitamin B_{12} and folate, can contribute to depressive symptoms.

Complications

The most obvious and serious complication of depression is suicide. About 30,000 people successfully commit suicide each year in the United States, and up to 200,000 suicide attempts are recorded. It is estimated that half of those attempts are related to depressive episodes. Although men have depression about half as often as women, they are four times more likely to successfully commit suicide.

NOTABLE CASES Artist Vincent Van Gogh probably lived with bipolar disease, as well as gonorrhea, absinthe addiction, and possible poisoning from the paints he was using. In one manic period of 2 months, he produced 90 spectacular paintings, none of which found a buyer in his lifetime. He died at age 37 of a self-inflicted gunshot wound.
Sophie's Choice author William Styron was a depression patient whose eloquence is haunting. This comes from his memoir, *Darkness Visible*: "Mysteriously and in ways that are totally remote from normal experience, the gray drizzle of horror induced by depression takes on the quality of physical pain… it is entirely natural that the victim begins to think ceaselessly of oblivion." He did eventually recover to become a vocal advocate for mental health issues. He died of pneumonia at age 81 in 2006.

In addition to suicide risk, a history of depression is now found to be a risk factor for several other conditions, notably stroke, heart attack, and other forms of cardiovascular disease. Further, the severity of the preexisting depression can be a predictor for how well a person recovers from a stroke or heart attack. Although the cause-and-effect relationships between depression and cardiovascular disease have not been fully identified, an obvious connection can be made between depression and the physical manifestations of long-term stress.

Finally, depression frequently accompanies other long-term diseases. The symptoms of depression can make the consequences of other conditions worse (e.g., pain sensation is amplified, sleep is disrupted), and people who are depressed are not likely to take good care of themselves by eating well, taking medication according to prescription, and staying in contact with supportive friends and loved ones.

Types of Depression

Experts recognize several etiologically distinct types of depression.

- *Major depressive disorder.* This is classic debilitating clinical depression. It is recognized when very severe symptoms persist for periods longer than 2 weeks. Left untreated, episodes of major depression may last anywhere from 6 to 18 months and on average recur anywhere from four to six times over a lifetime. Each successive episode can be triggered by a less important event: in other words, the person becomes increasingly vulnerable. Ultimately, someone who doesn't seek treatment for a major depressive disorder can expect to spend many years feeling hopeless, helpless, and worthless.
- *Psychotic depression.* This is major depressive disorder with **psychosis**: that is, hallucinations (a distortion of perception with a powerful sense of reality) and/or delusions (beliefs that are not changed by reason or contradictory evidence).
- *Adjustment disorder.* This is depression related to a specific event that triggers an emotional response, but the symptoms significantly outlast what might be considered a normal recovery or grieving period.
- *Dysthymia.* This is a less extreme version of depression, with fewer symptoms in less extreme forms, but it can last for years at a time. Someone who has dysthymia can function but won't ever feel normal or at his or her best. Dysthymia can occur simultaneously with major depressive disorder, in a condition called **double depression**.
- *Bipolar disorder.* This is also called manic depression. It is marked by mood swings on a continuum from major depression to mania (Sidebar 4.7). Mania is defined by heightened energy, elation, irritability, racing thoughts, increased sex drive, decreased inhibitions, and unrealistic or grandiose notions that lead to decisions made with extremely poor judgment. Someone in a manic state might undertake a huge new project, spontaneously quit a job, buy a car, or make some other major life change without realizing the long-term implications—which will of course be waiting when the manic episode subsides.

SIDEBAR 4.7 Arc of Mood States

Depression is sometimes discussed in the context of a continuum of moods. Bipolar disorder in particular refers to swings from one place on the scale to another, and the extremity of mood determines the subtype of bipolar disorder that is diagnosed.

The descriptors for moods along this continuum are these:

- Severe depression (as seen with major depressive disorder)
- Moderate depression
- Mild low mood (as seen with dysthymia)
- Balanced mood (no pathology is present)
- Hypomania
- Severe mania (as seen with the most extreme version of bipolar disorder)

- *Seasonal affective disorder.* This is depression related to the absence of sunlight. Its incidence goes up according to distance from the equator. It is thought to be related to low levels of melatonin, a neurotransmitter stimulated by exposure to sunlight. It is most prevalent during December, January, and February.
- *Postpartum depression.* This is the depression that affects new mothers, usually developing within the first few months after giving birth. It is related to several factors, including vast hormonal shifts, a sense of inadequate social support, and biologic vulnerability: women with a history of other types of depression, especially bipolar disorder, are at increased risk. A woman with postpartum depression has all of the symptoms of major depression, along with the deep-rooted fear of having harm come to or of actually doing harm to her baby. A different condition, called **postpartum psychosis**, involves hallucinations or delusions that may put the mother or her children in danger.

Signs and Symptoms

The signs and symptoms of depression depend partly on what type is present. The two leading symptoms include a persistent sad or empty feeling and experiencing less enjoyment from usual activities and hobbies. Other common symptoms include a deep sense of guilt or disappointment with oneself, a feeling of hopelessness—that things will never get better—irritability, and a change in sleeping habits: the person either sleeps very little or sleeps much more than usual.

Additional signs and symptoms can include a decreasing ability to concentrate, weight changes (the person either eats much more than usual or loses all interest in food), a loss of energy, a feeling of helplessness, persistent physical pain that is unresponsive to treatment (especially headaches, backache, and digestive discomfort), and suicidal thoughts, plans, or attempts. A person is typically diagnosed with depression when five or more of these symptoms are present in a new pattern for a minimum of 2 weeks.

Treatment

Most types of depression are treatable, although finding the right combination of therapies can be time consuming, frustrating, and expensive. Several different classes of antidepressant medications have been developed, each with advantages and disadvantages, and new medications are in development all the time.

The success of a person's treatment for depression depends largely on patience, as many medications can take several weeks to achieve their full potential. It is important to try to treat depression fully, because when people find relief but have lingering symptoms, they are at high risk for recurrent episodes.

Medications used for major depressive disorder usually fall into one of four categories: **SSRIs** (selective serotonin reuptake inhibitors, including Prozac and Zoloft), **SNRIs** (serotonin norepinephrine reuptake inhibitors, including Effexor and Cymbalta), **MAOIs** (monoamine oxidase inhibitors, including Nardil), and **tricyclic antidepressants** (TCAs, including Elavil). All of these classes of medication aim to make neurotransmitters more easily accessible in the mood-determining areas of the brain.

Antidepressants work by making targeted neurotransmitters more available in brain synapses, often by inhibiting the reuptake of those chemicals. They are effective for most people, but they have two major disadvantages: they take several weeks to establish any noticeable mood changes, and they tend to produce unpleasant side effects during that initial adjustment period. Side effects usually include dry mouth, dizziness, constipation, skin rashes, sleepiness or sleeplessness, sexual dysfunction, and restlessness. Side effects generally subside within 4 to 6 weeks, which is about when the benefits of the medication begin to be felt.

Lithium is used specifically with bipolar depression. Rather than altering levels of neurotransmitter reuptake or recycling, lithium works simply to smooth out mood swings. It can be toxic and is associated with several complications, so several alternatives to lithium for bipolar disease have been developed.

Psychologists and psychiatrists may also employ various types of talk therapy to help patients improve coping skills and reduce both the effects and the recurrence of depressive episodes. Some evidence suggests that talk therapy along with medication leads to more successful outcomes. Three major approaches have been found to be most useful, depending on the personality and needs of the affected individual. **Cognitive-behavioral therapy** focuses on the patient's skills at managing life and making beneficial choices. **Interpersonal therapy** focuses on how relationships color a person's life for better or worse. And **psychodynamic therapy** looks at how unresolved inner conflicts can affect the way a person makes choices and lives with those choices.

Other therapies for depression include:

- *Light therapy*. Persons living with seasonal affective disorder may not need medication or talk therapy; they need sunlight. Exposure to broad-spectrum lights can help to reduce symptoms.
- *Electroconvulsive therapy*. Some major depressive disorder patients don't respond to medication, and they are at high risk for suicide. Electroconvulsive, or shock, therapy may be the best choice for these patients. It is not entirely clear why it works, but it can be a highly effective intervention for people who don't get relief from other options.
- *St. John's wort*. This herbal extract has received a lot of attention as a mood enhancer without the side effects that other antidepressants carry. While some studies indicate that it can be effective for mild dysthymia, it has been shown to be ineffective as a treatment for major depressive disorder. St. John's wort has some risks; if a person takes medication to control HIV or any cytotoxic drugs (to reduce the risk of organ

rejection, for instance), St. John's wort has been seen to make these medications less effective.

- *Others*. A number of other interventions for depression continue to be explored, including vagus nerve stimulation, SAM-e (S-adenosyl-methionine), omega-3 fish oil, 5-hydroxytryptophan (a supplement that provides the building blocks for serotonin), and others.

Acupuncture, massage, and exercise have also been seen to be helpful to manage depression symptoms.

Medications

- Antidepressants, including SSRIs, SNRIs, TCAs, and MAOIs
  - Note: MAOIs carry a high risk of dangerous interactions with other drugs, but new application strategies minimize that danger.
- Mood stabilizers, including lithium and lithium analogues for bipolar disorder
- Antiseizure drugs as mood stabilizers for bipolar disorder
- Antianxiety medication if needed for postpartum depression and others

Massage?

RISKS No specific physical risks exist for a person with depression who wants to receive massage. It is important to bear in mind, however, that massage may be so well received that the client may want to reduce or completely abandon his or her medications. It is vital that this does not happen without the oversight of the prescribing physician.

BENEFITS Although the mechanisms for how it works are not understood, massage has a powerful positive influence on mood, anxiety, and the perceived ability to deal with the stressors of daily life. Depression of any kind indicates massage.

Eating Disorders

Eating Disorders in Brief

What are they?
Eating disorders are a group of problems consisting of compulsions about food and weight gain or loss. Anorexia, bulimia, and binge eating are distinct problems, although they frequently overlap.

How are they recognized?
Signs and symptoms of anorexia and bulimia may be hard to recognize in early stages, since these behaviors are often done in private. Long-term consequences include esophageal and colon damage, tooth damage, electrolyte imbalance, arrhythmia, low cardiac stroke volume, hormonal disturbance, osteoporosis, and many other problems. Binge eating is recognizable by eating habits in combination with significant weight gain, sometimes in a short period of time.

Massage risks and benefits
Risks: A person with a severe eating disorder may have several complications that influence massage choices. Dangerous arrhythmia, osteoporosis, and other conditions require adaptation from massage therapists.
Benefits: Massage can be a wonderful option for people with eating disorders, if they welcome the touch and attention. It is an opportunity to feel their bodies in a positive way, which can be an unusual experience for them.

Definition: What Are They?

Eating disorders are a variety of unhealthy eating habits that become difficult or even impossible to reverse. Eating disorders often arise in response to emotional or physical stressors. They may begin as a short-term coping mechanism, but they can become a serious long-term impairment to health. The disorders discussed here include anorexia, bulimia nervosa, and binge eating disorder.

Most anorexia and bulimia patients are young women, although men can also have these problems. Demographics on binge eating disorder are difficult to gather, but given the fact that about two-thirds of the adults in the United States are overweight, and 60 million adults are classified as obese (with a body mass index of 30 or above), it is reasonable to suggest that many people in this country have a dysfunctional relationship with food.

Etiology: What Happens?

The personality profiles of anorexia and bulimia patients point toward young women with high expectations of themselves. They are often eager-to-please overachievers who do well in school and may be involved in athletics that emphasize thinness or strength-to-weight ratios: dancing or gymnastics among girls, for instance, and wrestling for young men.

Anorexia and bulimia tend to center on control among a population that often feels powerless: adolescent girls in a culture that bombards them with impossible standards to live up to. A young woman may not be able to control how people treat her, but she can at least control what goes into her mouth. For many, that feels like a major victory, at least in the short run.

In addition, some neurotransmitter levels appear to be different among eating disorder patients compared to the general population. Whether this is a cause or a result of anorexia and bulimia is debatable, but it does open the door to some treatment options.

When a person begins to pathologically limit her diet in order to stay thin, ultimately it doesn't matter whether it's because of a neurotransmitter imbalance or because she's desperate to get on the gymnastics team. Her choices eventually change the way her body functions. If this persists for long enough, she may reach the point at which it's impossible for her digestive system to work properly: she can lose the ability to break down nutrients, absorb nutrition, or process waste. Anorexia and bulimia can be terminal illnesses.

The phenomenon of overeating can also be a control issue, but it is also a complex mixture of other physical and psychological factors, many of which are not well understood. It has significance for massage therapists for several reasons, but touch and protection are perhaps the most immediately pertinent.

The experience of welcomed touch is a basic human need, and its presence or absence has an impact on overall health. In our culture, nonsexual touch between adults is almost exclusively limited to greeting and leave taking, sports and violence, and personal care, that is, health care or aesthetician services. Consequently, if a person doesn't get touch on the outside, she can at least get touch on the inside: the sensation of eating past the point of satiation can be perceived as an internal "hug." Eating for comfort can become a vicious circle, as our culture places a high premium on physical attractiveness (i.e., being slender), which means that overweight people may have a harder time making and keeping supportive touch-rich relationships. This can drive them to the short-term comfort measure of overeating more frequently. Massage therapists are in a position to provide nurturing, restorative, educated, and nonjudgmental touch to a population of people who may have little or no other access to this important sensory nourishment.

Weight gain creates a physical barrier between a person and the world. This protective device may be a person's conscious or subconscious attempt to distance herself from experiences she wants to avoid. It is common to see overeating and weight gain, for instance, in people who are subject to physical, verbal, or sexual abuse. Survivors may use overeating as a strategy to discourage their abusers. Many survivors of touch abuse are binge eaters. Many survivors also eventually explore massage as a way to experience touch that is positive and nurturing. Massage therapists who work with this population must be very aware of how closely these clients' emotional state may be reflected in their physical state.

> **NOTABLE CASES** Many public figures have battled eating disorders, some of them unsuccessfully. Princess Diana of Wales struggled with bulimia related to the stress of her public position. Singer Karen Carpenter died of complications due to anorexia at age 32. Supermodels Isabella Caro and Ana Carolina Reston both lost their battles with anorexia. Olympic hopeful gymnast Christy Henrich died of multiple organ failure at age 22, which opened the possibility for many gymnasts to share their struggles with anorexia and bulimia.

The complications associated with eating disorders can be divided into mental/emotional issues and physical issues. Many eating disorder patients struggle with depression, irritability, sleep disorders, and anxiety disorders, especially OCD.

Physical complications can include a slow heart rate (**bradycardia**), low blood pressure, and arrhythmia. Changes in hormone secretion with **amenorrhea** can cause early-onset menopause, with **osteopenia** or even osteoporosis—exactly at a time when young adults should be adding to their total bone mass instead of losing it. Overuse of laxatives can cause colon dysfunction, and self-induced vomiting can lead to tooth damage, esophageal erosion and scarring, and dangerously imbalanced electrolytes. Eventually a person who regularly induces vomiting may find it difficult to keep food down, even if she wants to.

Binge eaters are at risk for cardiovascular disease, osteoarthritis, type 2 diabetes, gallbladder disease, and other physical problems associated with being overweight if their eating habits are never modified. However, these patients do not accrue the same life-threatening chemical imbalances that anorexic or bulimic patients do. If eating behaviors are changed, binge eaters may sustain few if any long-term problems.

Types of Eating Disorders

- *Anorexia nervosa*. This is a situation in which a person drastically limits his or her caloric intake. It is essentially self-starvation. It may be restrictive, in which a person simply doesn't take in enough calories to sustain her or purge type, in which calorie intake may be adequate for sustenance, but it is negated by compensatory activities, including vomiting; use of laxatives, diuretics, and/or enemas, and excessive exercise.
- *Bulimia nervosa*. Bulimia translates literally to "ox hunger." This is a disorder in which a person may appear to eat normally in public, but then in private binges on "forbidden" or self-indulgent foods. This behavior then leads to compensatory activity including self-induced vomiting, laxative use, or excessive exercise. It is also important to note that many patients fluctuate between anorexic and bulimic behaviors.
- *Binge eating*. This describes a situation where a person engages in overeating that is accompanied by a distressing sense of loss of control. Because this is not followed by excessive exercise, fasting, or purging, binge eaters tend to gain a lot of weight. If the behavior is related to a specific trauma or emotional problem, this can take place over a relatively short time.

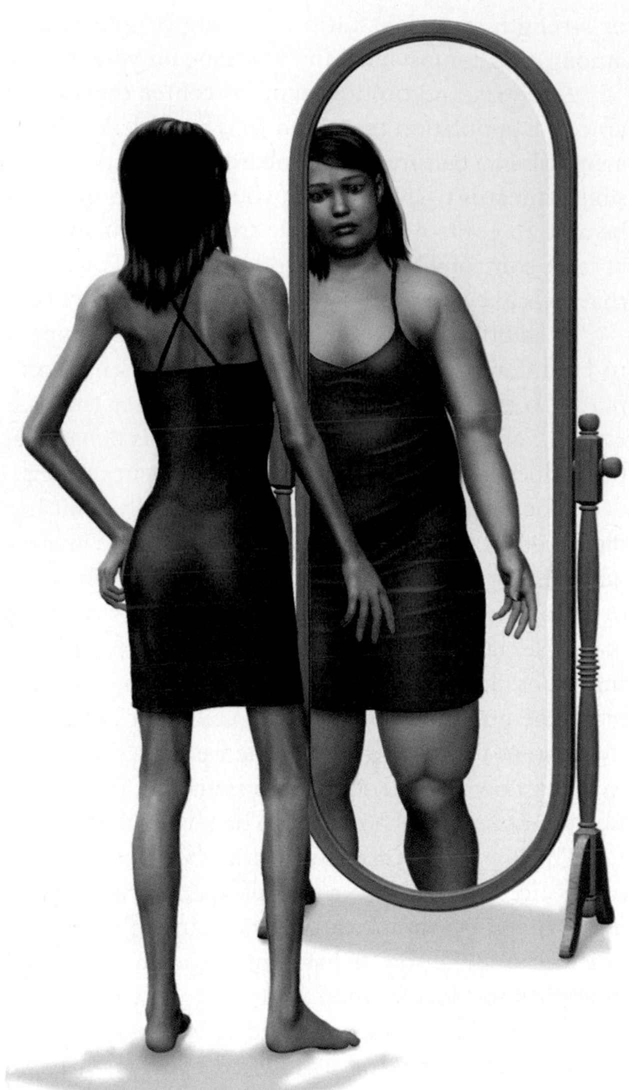

Figure 4.9. Anorexia: distorted body image

Signs and Symptoms

Signs and symptoms of eating disorders obviously depend on which type is present. Diagnostic criteria for anorexia include intense fear of gaining weight, distorted self-perception (Figure 4.9), and a loss of the menstrual cycle. Advanced anorexics, in addition to being extraordinarily thin, sometimes develop lanugo: fine, downy hair usually seen only in early infancy. This grows all over the body, possibly as an effort to compensate for the absence of any insulating fat in the superficial fascia.

Bulimia patients experience recurrent episodes of binge eating coupled with damaging compensatory behaviors that include self-induced vomiting, laxative use, and excessive exercise.

Binge eating disorder is characterized by bouts of uncontrollable eating that occur at least twice a week for 6 months or more. These episodes are marked by a sense of powerlessness and significant distress.

Treatment

Treatment for eating disorders is most successful when the emphasis is less on gaining or losing weight than on resolving the issues that led to the behaviors in the first place. While it is important to stabilize weight and support patients with healthy eating habits, these interventions are generally unsuccessful until the patient's psychological and emotional issues have been addressed. If a patient has progressed to the point where they are at risk for very serious complications or death, then treatment may begin in a hospital setting.

Research revealing neurotransmitter imbalances in the brain of many eating disorder patients has opened the door to medications that may help. Medication with individual or group psychotherapy support often leads to successful outcomes for all types of eating disorders.

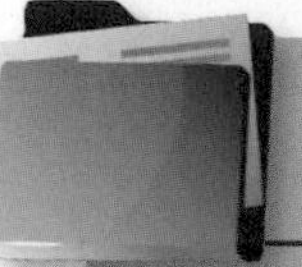

CASE HISTORY 4.2 Eating Disorders

I think my eating problems began when I was around 12 years old. I was an only child and a gymnast, working hard in my program. All my coaches wanted muscle, muscle, muscle—no flab. At that time I got in the mindset that the more I worked out, the more muscle I'd have, so I started skipping meals to have more body-building time. Having muscles and doing my routines perfectly were the only things on my mind.

I went on a pretty much just rice diet. Rice doesn't have any fat but lots of carbs to burn for energy. I'd have a bowl of rice and some water, which would make me feel really full. I think because of that my stomach shrank; just eating regular foods became really hard. Since I was always by myself, my parents didn't realize my problem. I always wore baggy clothes because I was constantly cold, and if I wore something tighter, my mother would say I looked fat; but in truth I was barely 5 ft tall and about 70 or 75 lb.

When I was 15 my grandfather, who had been the center of my life, died. I went into a deep depression. I had already lost gymnastics because of an injury. So I'd just go to school, go home, go to sleep, get up for a little bit to eat, and go back to sleep to do it all over again. When I slept, I had terrible dreams, and I heard voices when I was awake. I started to lose a lot of hair and have irregular menstrual cycles.

JESSICA, AGE 19: "Food was the one thing I thought I could control completely."

At this time and up until I turned 18, I felt like my parents controlled everything: what I wore, who I spent time with, where I was, every minute of the day. Food was one thing I thought I could control completely. Sometimes I'd get up in the middle of the night and eat and eat like I was about to die. I would feel awful later, but I would never make myself throw up. I saw a movie on bulimia once and saw how much damage it caused, so instead I would not eat for a day or two after I binged. I still do that sometimes, but not as severely as I used to.

Now I'm in massage school. I eat about two and a half meals a day. I was kind of surprised that getting massage was so easy for me. I did have some fears about lying supine on the table, but I'm over it. I have chronic back pain, and I enjoy deep massage.

I know I was lucky. I was able to control my eating before it got so bad that I needed to be admitted to the hospital. My whole sense of who I am and what makes me feel good is different now. I still really like getting compliments. If I hear, "You look great," or "That shirt looks good on you," then I feel like I can eat a chicken sandwich or a bowl of ice cream without feeling guilty later. But for the most part, for stuff like the grades I get in school or what courses I take, no one decides what I need now. I am my own person, and I am in control of my life once again. It feels really good. ■

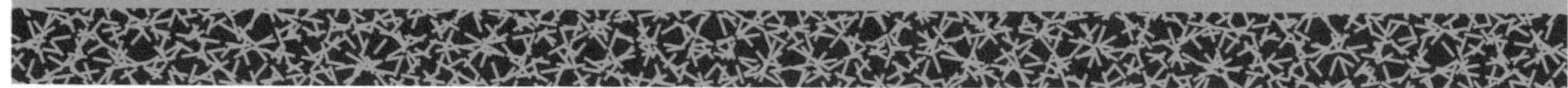

Medications

- Antidepressants, especially SSRIs
- Mood stabilizers, including antiseizure drugs

Massage?

RISKS Anorexia and bulimia can lead to changes in body function that affects the gastrointestinal tract, the cardiovascular system, and bone density. A frail client requires accommodation for bodywork to respect these challenges.

BENEFITS Clients who struggle with eating disorders tend to have a distorted and strongly negative perception of their physical being. Massage can be a powerful way to experience their bodies as safe, strong, and healthy. Some studies indicate lower anxiety ratings and improved body image for eating disorder patients who receive massage.

Nervous System Injuries

Bell Palsy

Definition: What Is It?

Bell palsy is the result of damage to or impairment of CN VII, the facial nerve. This nerve is composed almost entirely of motor neurons and is responsible for providing facial expression, blinking the eyes, and providing some taste sensation (Figure 4.10). It travels a complicated route from its origins to the face and exits the cranium through a small foramen just behind the earlobe.

This is a fairly common condition, especially among people who are pregnant, those with diabetes, or those who are immunocompromised.

Bell Palsy in Brief

What is it?
Bell palsy is flaccid paralysis of one side of the face caused by inflammation or damage to CN VII, the facial nerve.

How is it recognized?
Symptoms of Bell palsy include a sudden onset of weakness in the muscles of the affected side of the face. Ear pain, headaches, hypersensitivity to sound, and drooling may also occur.

Massage risks and benefits
Risks: It is important to identify the cause of cranial nerve damage if possible, since some factors that contribute to Bell palsy may contraindicate massage. Otherwise, because sensation is intact so the client can give accurate feedback, massage has no specific risks for this condition.
Benefits: Massage may help to keep facial muscles flexible and nourished during the period of nerve repair that follows an episode of Bell palsy.

Etiology: What Happens?

Bell palsy is a type of peripheral neuritis, that is, inflammation of a peripheral nerve. The facial nerve (CN VII) begins in the brain and passes through several narrow spaces before emerging to supply the tongue with some taste sensation, and the muscles of the face with motor control. When the nerve is inflamed in a tight passageway, it sustains damage that affects both sensory and motor function.

Several possible factors may contribute to Bell palsy, but most cases are linked to the herpes simplex virus. This pathogen, which lies dormant in the nervous system, stimulates the production of antibodies when it reactivates. This elicits an inflammatory response against the facial nerve. Other causative agents for Bell palsy can include Lyme disease, Epstein-Barr virus, and cytomegalovirus.

Bell palsy can range from mild to severe. A mild case may cause damage only to the myelin sheath, but a more serious episode can damage the facial

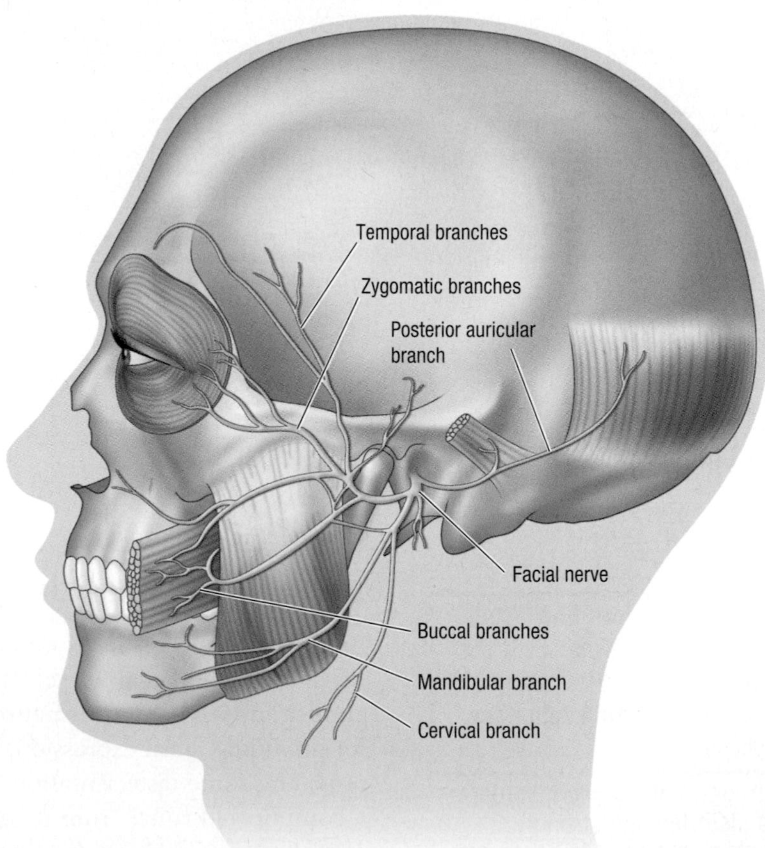

Figure 4.10. The facial nerve

nerve fibers. Since CN VII provides motor control for muscles of facial expression and the platysma, damage results in weakness or total paralysis of the face on the affected side. Fortunately, the facial nerve has the potential to regenerate, so the prognosis for Bell palsy is generally very good: about 85% of people who have it regain full or nearly full function within a few months.

One serious complication of Bell palsy can develop if the lubrication and cleaning of the eyeball provided by blinking is impaired. Another rare complication occurs when the facial nerve forges some new and inappropriate connections as it heals. The result may be unpredictable muscle activity in the face (**synkinesis**) or secretion of excessive tears during salivation.

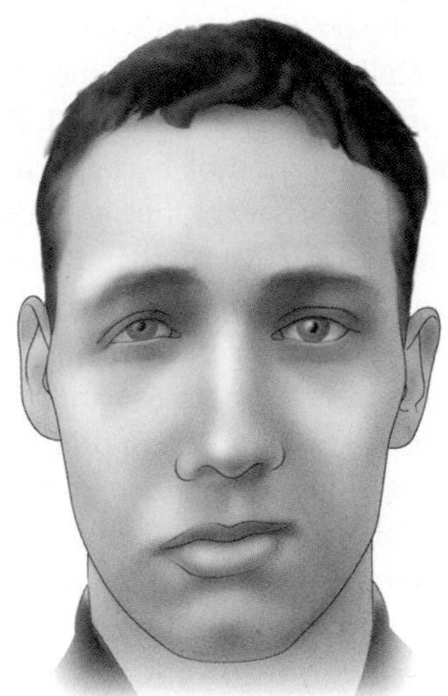

Figure 4.11. Bell palsy

Signs and Symptoms

Symptoms of Bell palsy are brought about by loss of nerve supply to the muscles on one side of the face. Classic signs include a sudden onset (often overnight) of flaccid paralysis of the muscles of the upper and lower face (Figure 4.11). It is difficult to eat, drink, and close the eye of the affected side. Production of saliva may be increased or decreased, and taste may be distorted. Sometimes the ear on the affected side becomes hypersensitive, because a muscle connected to the eardrum (the **stapedius**) is paralyzed; this is called **hyperacusis**. The affected side may have pain, but it is more likely to be in the form of headaches or an ache behind the ear than electrical nerve pain. This is motor, not sensory, paralysis (except for some taste buds that may be affected), so sensation throughout the face stays intact.

Treatment

Treatment for Bell palsy depends on the causative agent, which means it is important to have an accurate

CASE HISTORY 4.3

JIM S: "No dimple for a year!"

When I think about what may have precipitated my bout with Bell palsy, I remember one of the most stressful years of my life. I had recently moved to the Pacific Northwest and had to go back to school to receive Washington State licensure as a massage practitioner. I was working three jobs and going to school. I had also spent some days plunging into the cold water of a tributary of the Breitenbush River. I was overcooked!

When the paralysis started, I thought it was a temporary effect of some bodywork I had received. I was told to take Advil and ice my neck. I was given massage to help with the pain. But nobody recognized the seriousness of the symptoms. Within a day I had full-on Bell palsy complete with hyperacusis (abnormal acuteness of hearing), full facial muscle paralysis, an eyelid that would not blink (with the inherent rolling of the eye up and out of danger when the lid would normally blink), and a distorted soapy beer taste on the affected side of my tongue.

Because I neglected to see a neurologist for over a week, my facial nerve degenerated, and it took almost a year for nearly full function to resume. I couldn't use my dimple for a year! I'm adamant about people seeing a neurologist immediately these days when I hear of a case of Bell palsy.

The whole experience was generally frustrating because there's a lot of poor information out there, but it was a great emotional process; when you've used your face for a calling card all your life and suddenly it's not available to you anymore, you have to really deal with what's underneath. ■

diagnosis. Facial paralysis can also be related to multiple sclerosis, Guillain-Barré syndrome, sarcoidosis, or tumors on or around CN VII or CN VIII. Ramsay-Hunt syndrome is a complication of herpes zoster (shingles) that can affect the facial nerve, but it tends to be much more painful and longer lasting than Bell palsy.

Bell palsy treatment is usually conservative because most cases are self-limiting, that is, they resolve without interference. Steroids and antiviral medications are the typical prescription, although their use is somewhat controversial because most patients heal regardless of medication. Patients are counseled to tape the affected eye closed at night, and to use drops and protect it from drying and dust during the day. Massage is often recommended to stretch and mobilize facial muscles until the nerve repairs itself.

Medications

- Steroidal anti-inflammatories to manage nerve inflammation
- Acyclovir or other antiviral medications to shorten the duration of attack
- NSAIDs for pain relief

Massage?

RISKS If the underlying cause of facial paralysis doesn't contraindicate massage, then massage has no specific risks for Bell palsy.

BENEFITS Massage keeps the facial muscles elastic and the local circulation strong. This sets the stage for a more complete recovery when nerve supply is eventually restored.

Complex Regional Pain Syndrome

Definition: What Is It?

Complex regional pain syndrome (CRPS) is a collection of signs and symptoms including long-lasting pain and changes to the skin, muscles, joints, nerves, and blood vessels of the affected areas. CRPS 1 is the most current label for what used to be called reflex sympathetic dystrophy syndrome (RSDS); this is abnormal pain and other signs related to soft tissue or other injuries, usually to a distal portion of the arm or leg. CRPS 2 (formerly known as causalgia) is pain related to a nerve injury that again outlives a normal process and often exceeds the boundaries of the affected nerve (Sidebar 4.8). CRPS is a progressive disorder that can be completely debilitating.

Complex Regional Pain Syndrome in Brief

What is it?
Complex regional pain syndrome (CRPS) is a chronic, progressive condition in which an initial trauma, usually to the distal part of the arm or leg, causes pain that is more severe and longer lasting than is reasonable to expect. The pain can become a severe and self-sustaining phenomenon that is a lifelong problem.

How is it recognized?
CRPS is identified primarily by pain that outlasts a normal healing period for a trauma or injury. Other signs include changes in the quality of the skin around the area, muscle weakness, joint stiffness, and atrophy.

Massage risks and benefits
Risks: Touch of any kind at the initial site of injury is often unbearable for CRPS patients, so this presents at least a local caution. These clients are likely to use very powerful analgesics and medical devices, and this must also inform decisions about bodywork.
Benefits: If any touch anywhere on the body can be received without pain, this is a wonderful gift for patients with CRPS. Massage may also be employed with physical therapy to maintain mobility and slow atrophy, as long as it is welcomed.

Etiology: What Happens?

When a person receives a stimulus, a sensory neuron carries that information to the spinal cord. That efferent neuron has a synapse with ascending sensory neurons that carry the stimulus to the brain where it is interpreted, but it also communicates with motor neurons in the spinal cord to elicit a faster response: this is the reflex arc in a nutshell.

If the stimulus is something soothing (a smooth, confident effleurage stroke, for instance), the result is a relaxation response in the tissues. But if the stimulus is threatening or painful, the brain-mediated response is a sympathetic reaction.

In CRPS, an initial trauma (often to a hand or foot, but anywhere on the body can be affected)

SIDEBAR 4.8 Pain by Any Other Name...

In October 1864, a group of doctors compared their observations of Civil War soldiers recovering from gunshot wounds. Their comments were remarkably astute, and they provide a vivid picture of the experience of the condition eventually termed causalgia, from the Greek *kausis* (burning) and *algia* (pain).

> "In our early experience of nerve wounds, we met with a small number of men were suffering from a pain which they described as 'burning' or as 'mustard red-hot' or as 'red-hot file rasping the skin'... Its intensity varies from the most trivial burning to a state of torture, which can hardly be credited, but which reacts on the whole economy, until the general health is seriously affected..."[2]

Over the years, this condition, now called complex regional pain syndrome (CRPS), has been known by many names. Sympathetic maintained pain syndrome is another term, along with shoulder-hand syndrome and Sudeck atrophy. Causalgia itself is now considered to refer to pain related to any peripheral nerve injury (CRPS 2), while reflex sympathetic dystrophy syndrome refers to pain that begins in the extremities (CRPS 1).

begins a pain sensation that is mediated by the sympathetic nervous system. This disorder is often associated with high-velocity trauma such as bullet or shrapnel wounds, but it has also been seen with minor strains and sprains, as a postsurgical complication, with fractures, at injection sites, following strokes, as a consequence of disc disease, and sometimes with no identified causative trauma at all.

Regardless of the trigger, pain creates a sympathetic response, which reinforces pain sensation. In addition, pain sensors in the affected area become increasingly sensitive. In other words, the pain becomes a self-fulfilling prophecy: a person hurts, which causes stress, which makes the pain worse, and the healing processes that should interrupt this sequence are unable to overcome the power of the vicious circle.

Eventually the physiologic changes that occur when a specific part of the body is stuck in a sympathetic loop cause their own damage, which may eventually be irreversible: circulation affects the skin, the bones become thin, joints may fuse. This pain cycle also has the potential to spread proximally on the affected limb, to the contralateral limb, and elsewhere.

Signs and Symptoms

Signs and symptoms of CRPS vary widely, but three major issues are usually present: One is burning pain around the site of initial injury. Another is autonomic dysfunction that shows as changes in skin temperature and texture, edema, hair and nail growth, and changes in local blood supply that can lead to bone density loss. The third is motor dysfunction that begins as weakness and spasms in local muscles along with joint stiffness but may progress to contracture and atrophy of muscle, bone, and joint structures. In any case, **hyperalgesia** (excessive pain sensation) and **allodynia** (pain reaction to touch) are dependable symptoms.

CRPS has been broken into three loosely defined stages. Not all experts agree on the sequence of progression, as this disorder is experienced differently by every person who has it, but they can be a useful organizing principle to understand the process of the problem.

- *Stage I.* These signs and symptoms are prevalent during the first 1 to 3 months of pain. They include severe burning pain at the site of the injury; muscle spasm; reduced range of motion, excessive hair and nail growth if the injury is on a hand or foot; and shiny, hot, red, sweaty skin (Figure 4.12). Stage I is sometimes called the acute stage.
- *Stage II.* This is characterized by changes in the growth pattern of the affected tissues. The swelling spreads proximally from the initial site, the hair stops growing, and the nails become brittle and easily cracked. Skin that was red in stage I takes on a bluish cast in stage II. In this intensely painful stage, the muscles

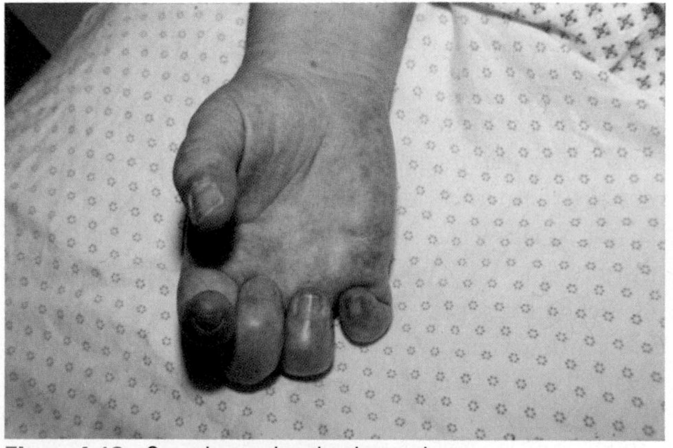

Figure 4.12. Complex regional pain syndrome

begin to atrophy from underuse, and the nearby joints may thicken and become stiffer. Stage II usually lasts 3 to 6 months. It is also called the dystrophic stage.

- *Stage III*. At this point, irreversible changes to the affected structures have occurred. The bones are thin and brittle, the joints are immobile, and the muscles tighten into permanent contracture. The condition may spread proximally up the limb, to the contralateral limb, or anywhere else in the body, including internal organs. At this point, the pain sensation is a self-sustaining phenomenon, and not responsive to most treatments. This is known as the atrophic stage.

Treatment

Treatment for CRPS is a challenging process. Evidence suggests that the best outcomes occur when treatment is instituted early, but it can be difficult to distinguish this condition in early stages. Physical and occupational therapy are recommended to preserve function and prevent or delay atrophy of the affected areas; this is problematic for many people who are in significant pain that is exacerbated by movement or exercise. Other noninvasive therapies include hydrotherapy (within tolerance), biofeedback training, topical analgesics, and **TENS units** to block some pain perception.

Psychotherapeutic intervention is useful, as the pain and disability involved with this condition can lead to extreme forms of depression, anxiety, and sleep disorders, and these complications can make CRPS symptoms worse.

Chemical nerve blocks are often used to block nerve transmission at the sympathetic ganglia near the spinal cord and other locations. These are often useful, but they are temporary and cannot be used indefinitely.

Intrathecal pumps that deliver painkilling medications directly into the spinal cord allow patients to manage their own pain. These bypass the blood-brain barrier to allow the same results with smaller doses of drugs.

Some patients undergo a full sympathectomy, that is, their sympathetic motor neurons are surgically severed. While it has been effective for some, others find that this extreme intervention is also temporary and has many serious side effects.

Pharmocologic approaches to CRPS run the gamut from NSAIDs to antidepressants to muscle relaxants. Because this is such a painful condition, doctors and their patients tend to be willing to experiment with many options, although many of these are strictly experimental at this point. A short list of medications for CRPS includes the following.

Medications

- NSAIDs for early-stage CRPS to control pain and inflammation
- Oral analgesics, including opioids, narcotics, and ketamine for pain control; although these drugs carry many risks and potential side effects, they can be useful for CRPS
- Antidepressants, especially tricyclics, for pain relief and improved sleep
- Antiseizure drugs for pain control

Massage?

RISKS CRPS locally contraindicates massage because touch is so painful. It is important to know what treatment options clients with CRPS use, because some medications or medical devices may require adaptation with bodywork.

BENEFITS If massage can be offered in a way that doesn't exacerbate symptoms, it could be a wonderful addition to the quality of life of someone who lives with this extremely challenging condition.

Spinal Cord Injury

Definition: What Is It?

The definition of spinal cord injury (SCI) is self-evident: this is damage to nerve tissue in the spinal canal. How that damage is reflected in the body depends on where and how much of the tissue has been affected.

Traumatic SCI falls into one of five categories: In **concussion**, tissue is jarred and irritated but not structurally damaged. In **contusion**, bleeding in the spinal cord damages tissue. In **compression**, a damaged disc, a bone spur, or a tumor puts mechanical pressure on the cord. In **laceration**, the spinal cord is partially cut, as with a gunshot wound. In **transection**, the spinal cord is severed.

Spinal Cord Injury in Brief

What is it?
A spinal cord injury (SCI) describes a situation in which some or all of the fibers in the spinal cord have been damaged, usually by trauma, but occasionally by other problems such as tumors or bony growths in the spinal canal.

How is it recognized?
The signs and symptoms of SCI vary with the nature of the injury. Loss of motor function follows destruction of motor neurons, but that paralysis may be flaccid or spastic, depending on the location of nerve damage. Loss of sensation follows the destruction of sensory pathways. If the injury is not complete, some motor or sensory function remains in the affected tissues.

Massage risks and benefits
Risks: SCI patients are vulnerable to infections and other complications that may contraindicate massage. Numbness contraindicates any bodywork that aims to substantively change the quality or elasticity of tissues; without pain sensation the client can't give informed feedback about comfort or safety. Care must be taken not to trigger painful spasms, and therapists much watch for signs of autonomic dysreflexia.
Benefits: Massage can be a powerful way to weave together functioning and nonfunctioning parts of the body for a person with permanent nerve damage, as long as care is taken in areas with limited sensation. If sensation is present and other contraindicating factors are addressed, massage to unaffected areas can be as rigorous as the client prefers.

An injury that affects the lower abdomen and legs but leaves the chest and arms intact is called **paraplegia**. An injury that affects the body from the neck down is called **tetraplegia** or **quadriplegia**. For more terminology in the context of CNS injuries, see Sidebar 4.9.

About 250,000 people in the United States live with an SCI, and males outnumber females by about 4:1.

Etiology: What Happens?

A primary injury to the spinal cord is usually a crushing blow (Figure 4.13), but the cord can also be injured through direct compression exerted by tumors, bone spurs, or cysts. Gunshot wounds may lacerate the cord. Spinal cords are rarely completely transected; when they are, the mortality rate is very high.

SIDEBAR 4.9 Nerve Damage Terminology

Nerve damage can manifest in several ways. Familiarity with some of the vocabulary of nervous system damage can make it much easier to "talk shop" with clients and doctors dealing with these problems.

- *Paresthesia* is any abnormal sensation, particularly the tingling, burning, and prickling feelings associated with pins-and-needles sensation.
- *Hyperkinesia* is excessive muscular activity.
- *Hypokinesia* is diminished or slowed movement.
- *Hypertonia* is a general term for extreme tension, or tone, in the muscles.
- *Hypotonia* is an abnormally low level of muscle tone, as seen with flaccid paralysis.
- *Spasticity* is a type of hypertonia in which the stretch reflex is overactive. The flexors want to flex, but the extensors don't want to give way. Finally, the extensors are stretched too far, and they release altogether. This phenomenon is called the clasp-knife effect.
- *Paralysis* is loss of any function controlled by the nervous system. The word comes from the Greek for loosening.
- *Paresis* is partial or incomplete paralysis.
- *Flaccid paralysis* is typically a sign of peripheral nerve damage. It accompanies conditions such as Bell palsy. Flaccid paralysis occurs with muscles in a state of hypotonicity.
- *Spastic paralysis* is the result of central nervous system (CNS) damage. It combines aspects of hypertonia, hypokinesia, and dysreflexia. It is never resolved, which distinguishes it from mere spasm. These are types of spastic paralysis:
  - *Hemiplegia* means the left or right side (or hemisphere) of the body is affected. This is the variation that most often accompanies stroke.
  - *Paraplegia* means the bottom half of the body or some part of it has been affected. These patients still have at least partial use of their arms and hands.
  - *Diplegia* is symmetrical paralysis of upper or lower extremities resulting from injuries to the cerebrum.
  - *Tetraplegia*, or *quadriplegia*, means that the body has been affected from the neck down. Tetraplegics can eat, breathe, talk, and move their head because these functions are controlled by the cranial nerves, which are usually protected from injury.

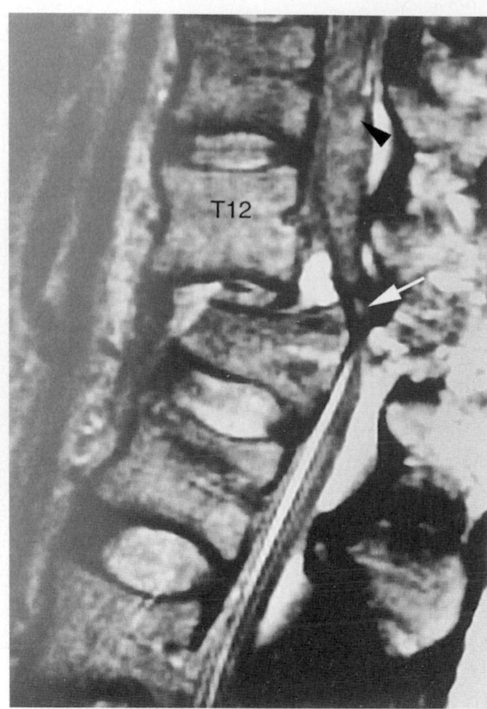

Figure 4.13. Spinal cord injury

A newly injured spinal cord goes through an initial period called spinal cord shock. During this time, the cord swells, and many body functions are severely impaired: blood pressure is dangerously low, the heart beats slowly, peripheral blood vessels dilate, and the patient is susceptible to hypothermia. In this acute phase of injury, the affected muscles may be hypotonic. Then when the inflammatory process begins to subside, the muscles supplied by damaged axons begin to tighten, and their reflexes become hyperreactive. Spasticity along with **dysreflexia** is a hallmark of SCI. If muscles stay flaccid and reflexes are dull or nonexistent, the damage is probably to the nerve roots or peripheral nerves, rather than to the spinal cord itself. Depending on the nature of the accident, it is perfectly possible to sustain injury to both the spinal cord and the nerve roots, especially in the **cauda equina** (see video clip, online at http://thePoint.lww.com/Werner5e).

A person's ultimate level of function after sustaining an SCI is related to how much tissue damage accrues. A significant portion of the damage to delicate CNS tissue is incurred not by the trauma, but by posttraumatic reactions that damage tissue adjacent to the injury site. This understanding opens the possibility for treatments that provide a much improved prognosis for SCI survivors.

Some of the most serious posttraumatic reactions include these:

- Excessive bleeding in and around the spinal cord; this can also contribute to circulatory shock, dangerously low blood pressure, and slowed heart rate.
- Free radical activity that destroys cell membranes.
- The secretion of excessive glutamate, an excitatory neurotransmitter in the spinal cord can damage motor neurons; this is called **excitotoxicity**.
- Immune system activity with inflammatory cytokines that contribute to cell damage and the accumulation of scar tissue in the spinal cord.
- Accelerated apoptosis, or cell death. This process seems to affect the oligodendricytes in particular: these are glial cells that form myelin in the CNS. When they degenerate, CNS cells are stripped of the covering that would otherwise speed transmission and provide electrical insulation from other fibers.

Complications

Spinal cord injuries can lead to many serious long-term complications. An SCI patient must invest a lot of time and energy in working to prevent, manage, or recover from these secondary problems:

- *Respiratory infection.* When the chest can't fully expand and contract and the cough reflex is limited (as is often seen with injuries higher than T_{12}), it is difficult to expel pathogens from the body.
- *Deep vein thrombosis, pulmonary embolism.* The formation of blood clots in the venous system is a high risk for new SCI patients, and the risk decreases only slightly with the passage of time.
- *Urinary tract infection.* SCI patients who must use a catheter to urinate are at high risk for contamination and infection of the urinary tract. Left untended, the risk of these infections invading the kidneys is significant.
- *Decubitus ulcers.* Also known as bedsores or pressure sores, these can arise anywhere circulation is limited by mechanical compression of the skin. Because these wounds don't heal quickly or easily, they are highly susceptible to infection, which can easily complicate to **septicemia**.

- *Heterotopic ossification*. This is the formation of calcium deposits in soft tissues. It typically occurs around the hips or knees, where it can be acutely painful. It can be corrected only with surgery.
- *Autonomic dysreflexia*. Damage to the spinal cord above T_6 raises the risk of developing **autonomic dysreflexia**, in which a minor stimulus (e.g., a full bladder or bowel, a ridge of cloth caught under the skin, and menstrual cramps) creates an uncontrollable sympathetic reaction. It causes a pounding headache, increased heart rate, flushing, sweating, and other symptoms, including dangerously high blood pressure. Autonomic dysreflexia can be a medical emergency.
- *Cardiovascular disease*. Suddenly changing from an active life to confinement in a wheelchair means a significant reduction in physical activity for most SCI patients. The risk of developing hypertension, atherosclerosis, and other cardiovascular problems is high for this sedentary population.
- *Numbness*. Most SCI patients have some numbness or reduction in sensation, depending on which part of the spinal cord has been damaged. The absence of pain is dangerous, because it allows damage to occur without warning. Small cuts or abrasions can become infected, and an SCI patient may never know.
- *Pain*. Many SCI patients have various kinds of pain along with numbness and lack of sensation. Some chronic pain is generated in the nerve tissue, but refers to the damaged limbs. Nerve root pressure may refer pain along the associated dermatome. Pain may be generated by the development of calcium deposits. Also, pain may be related to musculoskeletal injury, as a person must learn to use the arms and shoulders in new ways to propel the wheelchair and get into and out of it.
- *Spasticity, contractures*. As the muscles supplied by damaged motor axons begin to tighten, an SCI patient progressively loses range of motion. Chronically tight muscle fibers eventually atrophy, to be replaced by thick, tough layers of connective tissue; this is called a **contracture**. If any sensory or motor function is left in the limb, temporary episodes of **spasticity** may also be a problem. These may be caused by any kind of stimulus; the reflexes of active muscle fibers in SCI patients are very extreme and sensitive.

Signs and Symptoms

The motor and sensory impairment caused by SCI is determined by what parts of the cord are damaged and at what levels. The higher the damage, the more of the body is affected. Injuries to the anterior cord affect motor function, while damage to the posterior aspect affects the senses of touch, proprioception, and vibration. Damage to the lateral parts of the cord interrupts sensations of pain and temperature. Most SCIs involve damage to multiple areas.

NOTABLE CASES When "Superman" Christopher Reeve fell off his horse in 1995, the world of spinal cord injury treatment and prognosis changed radically. Having such a high-profile and charismatic advocate brought attention, funding, and research to this field. Mr. Reeve died in 2004 from cardiac arrest, a sequence of septicemia from an infected decubitus ulcer.

Mark Beck, the author of *Theory and Practice of Therapeutic Massage*—one of the first contemporary textbooks for the massage therapy profession—had a catastrophic skiing accident at age 42: "I caught a tip, flew down the hill and landed on my head." He shattered the lamina of C_6 and it dislocated anteriorly over C_7, crushing the spinal cord. Over 20 years later, he is thriving as a quadriplegic, still writing, teaching, and deeply involved in the industry. He credits regular bodywork with range-of-motion exercises, skin brushing, lymphatic work below the injury level, and clinical massage where sensation is present, for his longevity.

Treatment

If something presses directly on the spinal cord or cauda equina, emergency surgery to remove it is indicated. The other very important early intervention with these traumas is to limit secondary reactions that may damage uninjured tissue, so powerful anti-inflammatories and other medications are usually administered as quickly as possible.

Some later treatments for SCI include procedures to implant electrodes that can help with movement, or transplantation of tendons for improved strength. Another line of treatment focuses on spinal reflexes for walking and other movements. Even when the patient needs extensive help, going through the motions on a treadmill or stationary bike improves motor function, exercises functioning muscles, and benefits the cardiovascular system. Furthermore, these interventions appear to improve reflexes in general, which leads to a better overall prognosis.

SCI survivors must learn new skills to live as fully as possible. Physical and occupational therapists specialize in helping these patients gain the skills they need to function; mental/emotional therapists are also essential, especially for those who are adapting to their paralysis as a new way of life.

Medications

- For recent spinal cord injuries:
  - Steroidal anti-inflammatories
  - Anticoagulants (usually heparin) to control blood clot risk
- For long-term SCI patients:
  - Anticoagulants (usually heparin) to control blood clot risk
  - Fast-acting antihypertensives for autonomic dysreflexia
  - Antibiotics for respiratory and urinary tract infections
  - Muscle relaxants for spasm and spasticity
  - Botox injections for spasm and spasticity
  - NSAIDs for pain
  - Opioids for pain
  - Antiseizure drugs for pain

Massage?

RISKS Massage carries many potential risks for spinal cord injury (SCI) patients, including numbness that interferes with accurate feedback and a host of possibly life-threatening complications. Still, as long as these are addressed, massage can be safely administered in this context.

BENEFITS It is hard to overstate the benefit of nontask-related touch for a person who lives with a medically complicated condition. Massage may help maintain function for SCI patients, but it is also a powerful positive physical experience for people who live with a great challenge. Some research suggests that SCI patients use massage more than any other alternative healthcare modality, and report that it is consistently helpful for dealing with pain.

OPTIONS In addition to working for pain relief, focus on proprioceptors and muscle tone may forestall muscle tightness due to habit rather than central nervous system damage; this may allow an SCI patient to maintain a level of dexterity and postural strength that would not otherwise be achievable.

Stroke

Definition: What Is It?

Stroke, also called brain attack or cerebrovascular accident (CVA), is damage to brain cells due to oxygen deprivation brought about by thrombosis (a clot forms onsite), embolism (a clot travels from elsewhere), or hemorrhage (internal bleeding). It is the single most common type of CNS disorder. It is the third leading cause of death in the United States, coming in behind heart disease and cancer. It is the leading cause of adult disability.

About 700,000 people have a stroke each year in this country. Of them, 500,000 will have their first attack, while 200,000 will have a repeat stroke. About 160,000 Americans die of stroke each year. About 5 million stroke survivors are alive in this country today.

Etiology: What Happens?

Oxygen deprivation in the cranium kills brain cells, leading to dysfunction in the rest of the body. The

Stroke in Brief

What is it?
A stroke is damage to brain tissue caused either by a blockage in blood flow or by an internal hemorrhage.

How is it recognized?
The symptoms of stroke include paralysis, weakness, and/or numbness on one side; blurry or diminished vision on one side with asymmetrically dilated pupils; dizziness and confusion; difficulty in speaking or understanding simple sentences; sudden extreme headache; and possibly loss of consciousness.

Massage risks and benefits
Risks: A person who survives a stroke is at increased risk for a repeat episode and may have other cardiovascular conditions, so a massage therapist needs to make appropriate adjustments for both the client's resiliency and medications. Massage in the carotid area for a client with any risk of carotid artery disease is a particular caution.
Benefits: Massage for someone who is rehabilitating from a stroke can be very supportive and useful. It can be employed along with physical and occupational therapy to promote healthy muscle tone and to preserve function in affected tissues.

oxygen shortage can come about either because of a blockage, which is a variety of ischemic stroke, or because of bleeding, in which case it is a hemorrhagic stroke (see Animation at http://thePoint.lww.com/Werner5e).

The amount of damage a stroke causes is determined primarily by the location and number of neurons that are damaged by oxygen deprivation. Secondary responses to tissue damage have also been seen to contribute heavily to stroke damage. Inflammatory reactions, free radical activity, and other factors can cause tissue damage that far exceeds the oxygen deprivation brought about by the stroke itself. The injured area around the site of the stroke is called the **ischemic penumbra**. Interrupting the cascade of secondary responses with appropriate treatment can limit the extent of this area.

Motor damage from strokes can result in partial or full paralysis of one side of the body; this is called **hemiparesis** for weakness or **hemiplegia** for complete loss of function. The side of the body is opposite to the side of the brain affected by the stroke. **Aphasia** (loss of language), **dysarthria** (slurred speech), memory loss, and mild or severe personality changes may also occur. Sensory damage may result in permanent numbness and/or vision loss. Depression is another complication that is frequently seen after stroke; this condition has a complex intersection with stroke that is discussed in Sidebar 4.10.

SIDEBAR 4.10 Depression → Stroke → Depression...

The relation between stroke and depression is fascinating and complicated. It is well established that depression is an independent risk factor for stroke, but the mechanism is not well understood. One theory suggests that a low serotonin level changes the function of platelets and increases inflammation. This is also an issue for heart attack and atherosclerosis. Interestingly, while cognitive-behavioral (talk) therapy is effective to relieve the symptoms of depression, it does not reduce the risk of other vascular problems—but antidepressants that improve the uptake of serotonin have been seen to reduce the risk of future vascular problems, especially heart attack.

Massage therapists should be interested in this phenomenon, since one of the most consistently measured effects of massage is a rise in serotonin. Wouldn't it be interesting if massage and bodywork had an influence on the risk of depression-related stroke?

Many stroke survivors develop depression after their incident; this is called poststroke depression. This number is not separated from the people who had depression before their stroke, however. Depression tends to make all stroke treatments less effective and significantly affects the prognosis for recovery.

Risk Factors

Although a person can have a genetic predisposition toward a CVA, many of the factors that contribute to stroke are well within the reach of personal control.

Risk Factors That can be Controlled

- *High blood pressure*. Untreated hypertension is the biggest single contributing factor to the risk of stroke.
- *Smoking*. Nicotine constricts blood vessels and raises blood pressure.
- *Atherosclerosis, high cholesterol*. These conditions also contribute to high blood pressure and raise the risk of emboli.
- *C-reactive protein*. This substance is present with long-term low-grade inflammation. A high C-reactive protein level is a dependable predictor for both ischemic stroke and atherosclerosis.
- *Atrial fibrillation*. Left untreated, this condition can help to form the emboli responsible for some ischemic embolic strokes.
- *High alcohol consumption*. This is generally considered to be more than 2 drinks per day.
- *Drug use*. Cocaine, crack, and marijuana have all been seen to increase stroke risk.
- *Obesity and sedentary lifestyle*.
- *Diabetes*. Untreated, this condition can contribute to high blood pressure and atherosclerosis. Poorly treated diabetes triples the risk of stroke.
- *High-estrogen birth control pills*. These pose a risk especially when taken by a person who smokes.
- *Hormone replacement therapy*. Some women who supplement estrogen and progesterone

as a way to manage symptoms of menopause have a significantly increased risk of stroke.

- *Depression.* Depression has been seen to be a predictive factor for stroke: one-third of stroke patients are diagnosed for depression before their CVA.
- *Overall stress.*

Risk Factors That Cannot be Controlled

- *Age.* Three-quarters of stroke patients are over 65 years of age. The risk of stroke doubles each decade after 55.
- *Gender.* About 25% more men than women have strokes, but strokes kill more women than men.
- *Race.* African Americans have a higher incidence of hypertension than whites. They are about twice as likely to have a stroke as whites, and they are almost twice as likely to die of it.
- *Family history.* Having a family history of stroke and cardiovascular disease can be a predisposing factor. Structurally weak blood vessels can be an inherited problem.
- *Previous stroke.* Having one stroke usually predisposes a person to having another. Predisposition is not predestination, however; by taking control over whatever factors are within reach, a person can take big steps toward reducing the chances that he or she will have another stroke.

Types of Stroke

- *Ischemic stroke.* This is the most common version of CVA. The ischemia can be caused by cerebral thrombosis (a blood clot or blockage forms inside a vessel in the brain) or embolism (a clot forms somewhere else and travels to the brain to create a blockage) (Figure 4.14).

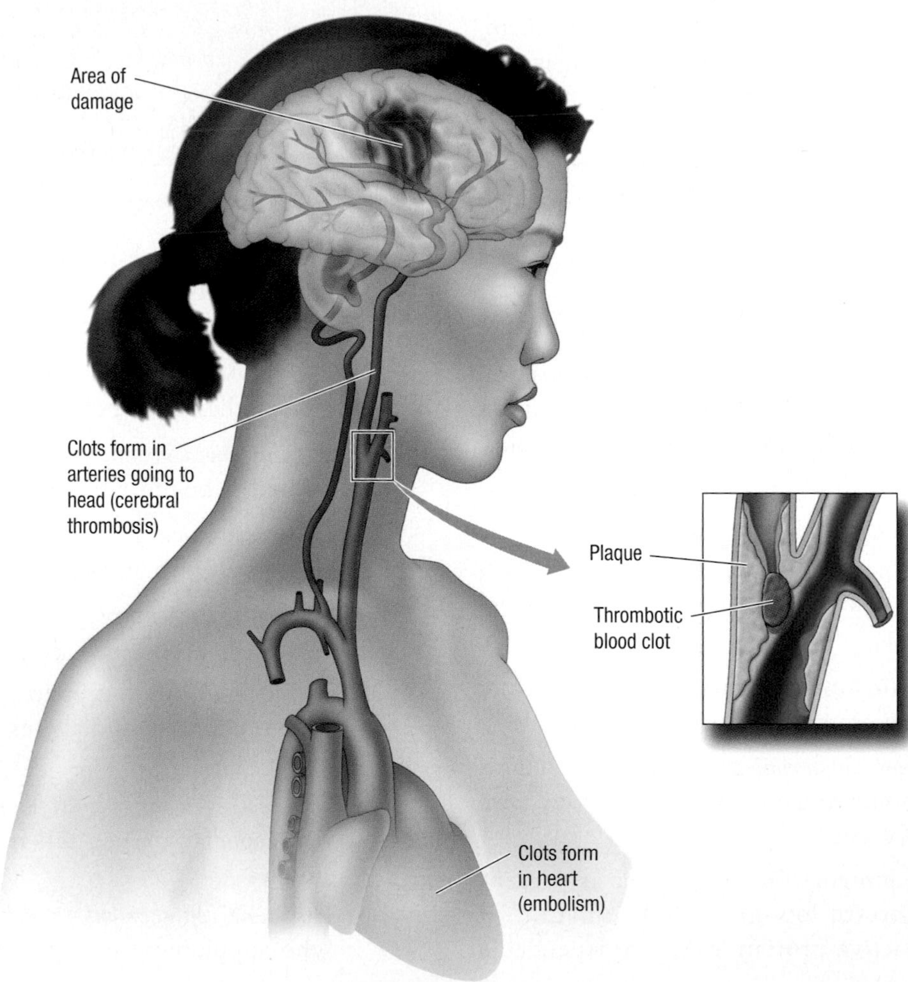

Figure 4.14. Ischemic stroke

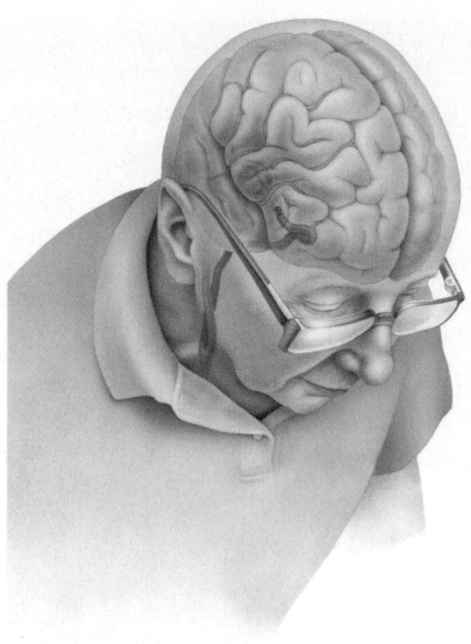

Figure 4.15. TIA: a tiny clot is trapped but quickly dissolves

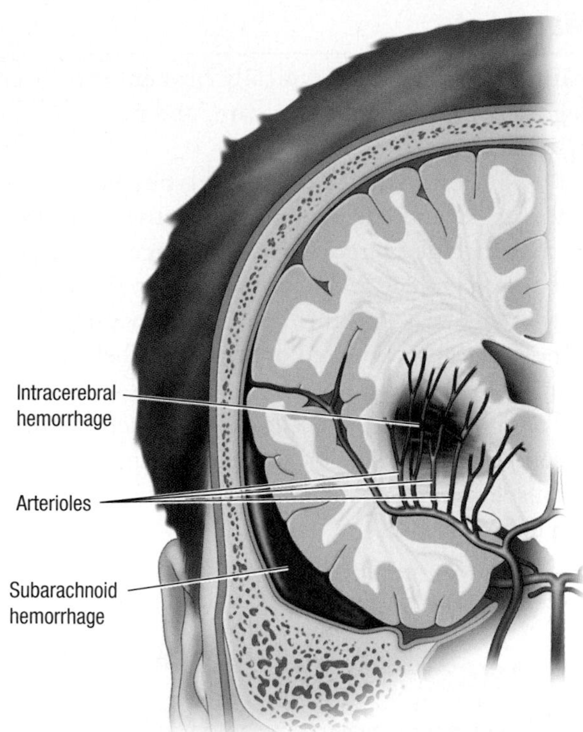

Figure 4.16. Hemorrhagic stroke

Emboli that cause strokes may originate in the carotid artery, or in the chambers of the heart, especially if valves are damaged or the heartbeat is unsteady so blood can pool and thicken (see Animation Insert: at http://thePoint.lww.com/Werner5e).

- *Transient ischemic attack (TIA).* Also called a "ministroke"; this occurs when the blockage is due to a small clot that melts within a few hours. Damage may be mild, but cumulative: a person may have many TIAs, and they can serve as a warning signal for the risk of a more serious event: a full stroke or heart attack. Someone who has had many TIAs may also appear to have dementia (Figure 4.15).
- *Cryptogenic stroke.* This is a CVA with no known cause. It may be connected to a **patent foramen ovale**, an abnormal opening in the septum of the heart that allows blood (including clots) from the pulmonary circuit to cross over into the systemic circuit, where it can get to the brain. This is especially likely when a stroke occurs in a person younger than 55 years of age.

- *Hemorrhagic stroke.* These account for about 20% of all strokes. They can involve bleeding deep inside the brain (intracerebral hemorrhage), or on the surface of the brain (subarachnoid hemorrhage) (Figure 4.16). These strokes are often associated with aneurysms, which may be a result of genetic anomaly, chronic hypertension, bleeding disorders, head trauma, or a malformation of blood vessels called **arteriovenous malformation** (AVM).

Signs and Symptoms

It is important to be able to recognize the signs of stroke; the sooner treatment is administered, the less damage will occur. The signs of someone having a stroke are these:

- Sudden onset of unilateral weakness, numbness, or paralysis on the face, arm, leg, or any combination of the three.
- Suddenly blurred or decreased vision in one or both eyes; asymmetrical dilation of pupils.
- Difficulty in speaking or understanding simple sentences; confusion.
- Sudden onset of dizziness, clumsiness, vertigo.
- Sudden extreme headache.
- Possible loss of consciousness.

Treatment

Treatment for stroke is typically broken into three categories: prevention, acute care, and postacute or long-term care.

Prevention includes identifying people at high risk for stroke and encouraging preventive measures. This may include exercise and diet changes, antiplatelet or anticoagulant drugs, or surgery on the carotid artery (Sidebar 4.11). Intracranial aneurysms may also be surgically corrected or reinforced before they rupture.

The treatment of choice for acute ischemic stroke is thrombolytic medication to melt existing clots, but this must be administered within the first few hours of onset to be effective.

If the CVA was from a hemorrhage on the other hand, thrombolysis could be dangerous or even deadly. Hemorrhagic strokes are treated by working to relieve pressure in the brain.

Once it is clear how much function was lost during a stroke, postacute care begins. The patient must relearn how to do basic tasks, including walking, speaking, eating, and self-care. At one time, the main focus with physical and occupational therapy was to teach the patient how to manage self-care with the unaffected side of the body. However, studies of nerve activity show unexpected potential for new growth if motor use demands it. This phenomenon is called **neuroplasticity** (see Sidebar 4.12). The finding that the brain grows in response to use and movement has led to rehabilitation programs that focus on strengthening the function of the weakened side of the body, with much better results.

SIDEBAR 4.12 Neuroplasticity

Neuroplasticity refers to the potential for neurons to grow and adapt after damage or injury. Contrary to traditional belief, it has been found that nerve cells in the central nervous system (CNS) have the capacity to change under the right circumstances. This can happen in several ways: they may sprout new axon terminals to establish new synapses; redundant nerve pathways may be recruited post injury; or latent nerve pathways may become newly viable.

One of the most exciting aspects of this discovery is that some brain chemicals appear to promote neuroplasticity. Introduced at the key moments in CNS injury, they may significantly improve the prognosis for a stroke, traumatic brain injury, or spinal cord injury patient. Using neuroprotective drugs in the context of CNS injury is a new field that is still undergoing testing, but it may become the industry standard.

SIDEBAR 4.11 Carotid Artery Disease: Nowhere to Go but Up

The discussion of atherosclerosis points out that because of chronically high blood pressure, both the aorta and coronary arteries are particularly prone to the development of atherosclerotic plaque. The carotid arteries, which emerge from the aortic arch, are similarly vulnerable. Although they are farther from the heart, blood pressure in the arteries that supply the head is ordinarily high to ensure adequate blood flow to the brain. This puts the carotid arteries at risk for the same endothelial damage and plaque development seen with the aorta and the coronary arteries; this is called carotid artery disease.

The problem with carotid artery disease is that if any fragment of plaque or blood clot should break free, it has only one direction to go: straight up into the brain. When this happens in very tiny increments, it is called transient ischemic attack, or TIA. But the presence of carotid artery disease significantly raises the risk of a major stroke—so much so that identifying this disorder often leads to aggressive treatment, in the shape of carotid **endarterectomy:** the artery is surgically opened, cleaned out, and closed up again.

Massage therapists working with clients who know they have carotid artery disease must stay away from the neck, especially the anterior triangle, which is bordered by the sternocleidomastoid muscle, which runs superficially over the carotid arteries.

Medications

- Thrombolytics for ischemic stroke to dissolve blood clots
- Anticoagulants and antiplatelet drugs for ischemic stroke to limit the formation of new clots
- Insulin for blood glucose management (high blood glucose is associated with poor outcome for stroke patients)
- Antihypertensive medications to control blood pressure

Massage?

RISKS The main risks for stroke patients who want to receive massage concern the possibility of another cardiovascular compromise and the threat of another cerebrovascular accident. If these concerns are addressed, careful massage can be helpful and appropriate. The drugs these patients take and the complications to which they are vulnerable also require adaptation for bodywork.

BENEFITS Much of the lost function for stroke patients is related to changes that happen outside the central nervous system: consistent tightness and lack of use allow any functioning muscle fibers finally to degenerate. Massage and other therapies that challenge this process through gentle stretching, exercises, and building awareness can help to minimize unnecessary loss of function.

Traumatic Brain Injury

Definition: What Is It?

TBI is an insult to the brain, not brought about by congenital or degenerative conditions, that leads to altered states of consciousness, cognitive impairment, and disruption of physical, emotional, and behavioral function.

TBI is usually due to external force: a direct blow, a rapid acceleration/deceleration incident, or a bomb blast in a war zone. Motor vehicle accidents, gunshot wounds, war injuries, falls, sports injuries, and physical violence are leading causes. They occur most often among children under age 4, adults aged 15 to 25, or those over 75.

Etiology: What Happens?

Several classifications for head injuries have been created to try to organize the vast number of ways the brain, although encased in a protective casing, can be injured. Head injuries are sometimes distinguished as primary or secondary issues. Primary injuries are related to the mechanical force that causes damage. Secondary injuries are the consequences or complications of primary injuries.

Primary injuries include these:

- *Skull fracture* occurs when the bones around the skull are broken, usually by a direct blow.

Traumatic Brain Injury in Brief

What is it?
Traumatic brain injury (TBI) is brain damage brought about by trauma rather than by a congenital condition or chronic degenerative disease.

How is it recognized?
Symptoms of TBI vary according to the location and severity of the injury. Long-term effects range from mild cognitive impairment (MCI), learning problems, and motor control difficulties, to varying types of coma or persistent vegetative state.

Massage risks and benefits
Risks: People with TBI may experience numbness, spasticity, and psychiatric disturbance. Any of these may require adaptation of bodywork.
Benefits: Many TBI patients undergo intensive physical, occupational, and speech therapy to preserve or recover motor function. Carefully administered massage is also appropriate, as long as it is incorporated into the patient's healthcare plan.

Surprisingly, the prognosis for an open head injury is often better than for a closed head injury, because the risk of damage from too much pressure is less.

- *Penetrating injury* is usually due to a gunshot wound, but may also be from a knife or other object. Penetrating injuries are the leading cause of death among TBI patients.
- *Concussion* is any temporary loss of brain function. **Concussion** is the most common type of TBI. When it occurs in an athlete, it is essential that the tissues heal completely before the athlete returns to play. If he has another head injury too soon, he can develop **second impact syndrome**, a much more serious condition than a simple concussion.
- *Contusion* is bruising inside the cranium. When a **contusion** happens at the point of impact and also where the brain hits the opposite wall, it is a **coup-contrecoup** injury.
- *Diffuse axonal injury* is internal tearing or shearing of nerve tissue throughout the brain. It is often related to acceleration/deceleration

accidents, as seen with whiplash or shaken baby syndrome.

Secondary injuries include these:

- *Anoxic brain injury* is complete lack of oxygen in the brain. It can be brought about by airway obstruction or sudden apnea.
- *Hypoxic brain injury* is an inadequate supply of oxygen, often associated with ischemic stroke, edema, or toxic exposure, especially carbon monoxide poisoning.
- *Hemorrhage* is bleeding inside the brain, often associated with ruptured aneurysms.
- *Hematoma* is development of a large amount of coagulated blood, either pressing outside or within the brain.
- *Intracranial pressure* is a secondary inflammatory response that can follow any or all of the causes of TBI. The swelling of brain tissue and action of free radicals against healthy tissue may ultimately be responsible for more damage than the original source of the trauma.

Preventive measures to guard against the risk of TBI are self-evident but worth repeating. Most TBIs happen as a transport injury, that is, in an event involving cars, motorcycles, bicycles, scooters, skates, or skateboards. Driving only while alert and sober, using a seat belt, and wearing a helmet can reduce the risk and severity of these accidents. Other preventive measures include making sure the home is safe for young children and elderly people to reduce the risk of falls, and ensuring the appropriate storage of firearms.

NOTABLE CASES Professional American football players are, not surprisingly, particularly prone to TBI. The seriousness of complications related to multiple head injuries has led to rules that now dictate some limitations in how soon an injured athlete can return to play.

Signs and Symptoms

Signs and symptoms of a TBI vary according to what areas of the brain are affected and how severe the injury is. Trauma to the frontal lobes is most common and may result in language and motor dysfunction; trauma to structures close to the brainstem is more likely to lead to massive loss of autonomic function.

Symptoms of an acute TBI include leakage of cerebrospinal fluid from the ears or nose; dilated or asymmetrical pupils; visual disturbances; dizziness and confusion; apnea or slowed breathing; nausea and vomiting; slow pulse and low blood pressure; loss of bowel and bladder control; possible seizures, paralysis, numbness, lethargy, or loss of consciousness. In infants, chronic crying, lethargy, or unusual sleep patterns are cause for concern. Symptoms may occur immediately or grow in severity over a course of days or even weeks.

Long-term consequences of TBI include mild to severe cognitive dysfunction, especially with memory and learning skills. Movement disorders may range from hypertonicity to spasticity. Seizures are a frequent complication. Permanent changes in behavioral and emotional function are also common; many TBI survivors are emotionally volatile and may develop new patterns of aggressiveness and hostility. Severe cases of TBI (usually ones that affect the brainstem) may lead to stupor, coma, locked-in syndrome, persistent vegetative state, or brain death.

Treatment

TBI is treated with surgery to remove pressure on the brain if necessary, followed by intensive physical, recreational, occupational, and speech therapy to preserve or recover function. The prognosis with children is generally best, since their brains seem to be most capable of establishing new pathways to relearn skills. Nonetheless, our understanding of how to take advantage of the brain's ability to grow (neuroplasticity) grows daily, and continues to brighten the outlook even for mature TBI survivors.

Medications

- Antiseizure medication
- Antidepressants
- Antipsychotic medications
- NSAIDs to manage pain
- Muscle relaxants for spasm and spasticity
- Cholinesterase inhibitors for memory improvement

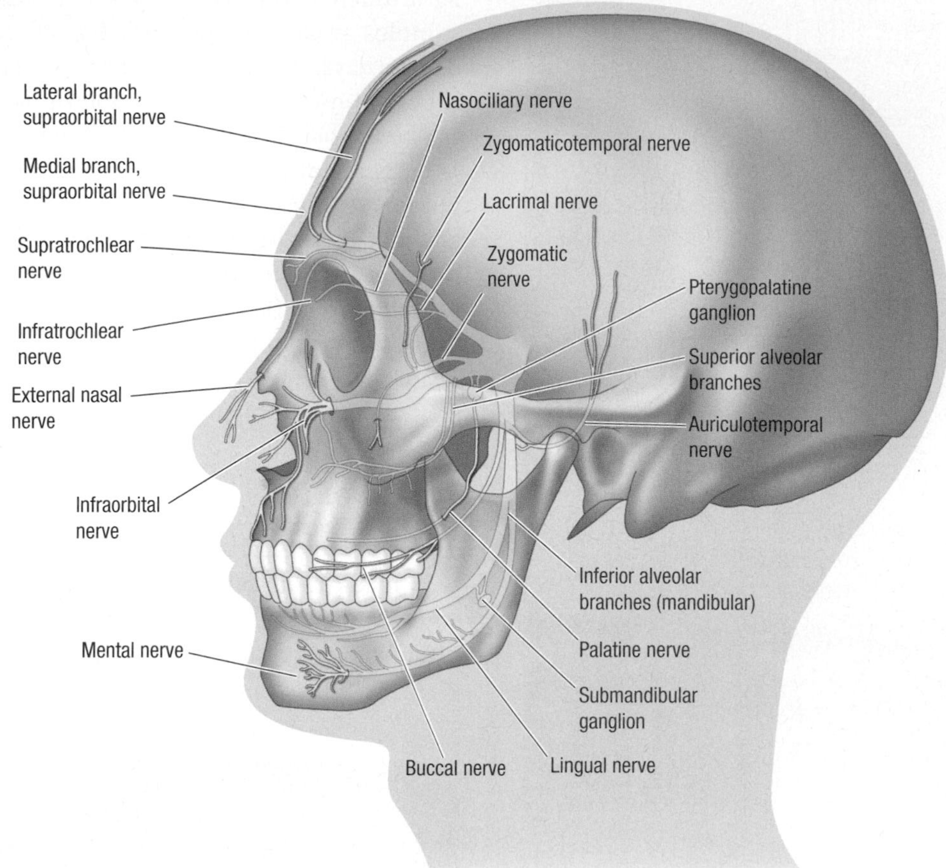

Figure 4.17. Trigeminal nerve

Massage?

RISKS Traumatic brain injury is a complicated, serious problem, and a massage therapist working with a client who has this condition is best doing so as part of an integrated healthcare team. If a client has numbness or is noncommunicative, massage or other stroking techniques may be performed to help preserve the health of the tissues and prevent some complications, but this must be performed with caution, since the client cannot give feedback.

BENEFITS If sensation is present and the client is able to communicate clearly about comfort, massage can be an important part of a rehabilitation strategy to maintain healthy muscles and connective tissues.

OPTIONS As with other central nervous system injuries, massage or bodywork that focuses on proprioception and muscle tone may be especially helpful to maintain strength and flexibility in affected areas.

Trigeminal Neuralgia

Definition: What Is It?

TN is neuro-algia ("nerve pain") along one or more of the three branches of Cranial Nerve V, the trigeminal nerve (Figure 4.17). It is also called tic douloureux, which is French for painful spasm or unhappy twitch.

Etiology: What Happens?

TN is usually classified as primary or secondary. In either case, the trigeminal nerve is irritated, and the result is brief, repeating episodes of sharp, electrical, burning, or stabbing pain on one side of the face.

The typical presentation of primary TN is usually related to a blood vessel that wraps around or irritates the trigeminal nerve where it emerges from the pons at the base of the brain. This vessel may essentially wear away the myelin covering on some of the fibers, which allows the nerve to misfire. Autopsies of people

Trigeminal Neuralgia in Brief

Pronunciation: try-JEM-ih-nul nur-AL-je-ah

What is it?
Trigeminal neuralgia (TN) is a condition involving sharp electrical or stabbing pain along one or more branches of the trigeminal nerve (CN V), usually in the lower face and jaw.

How is it recognized?
The pain of TN is very sharp and severe. Patients report stabbing, electrical, or burning sensations that occur in brief episodes, but that repeat with or without identifiable triggers. A tic is often present as well.

Massage risks and benefits
Risks: TN contraindicates massage to the face unless the client can guide the therapist into what feels safe and comfortable. Clients may not be comfortable lying face down if the face cradle of the table elicits symptoms.
Benefits: Massage elsewhere to the body, especially to the neck and shoulders, may offer great relief to TN patients.

with TN are not always consistent about this, however, and many people have this structural anomaly with no painful symptoms. Ultimately, the source of the pain may be a combination of factors.

Secondary TN is due to some other problem, which could include tumors, bone spurs, recent infection, complications of dental surgery, or multiple sclerosis.

Signs and Symptoms

Some people call the pain of TN among the worst in the world. It's often described as a sharp, electrical, stabbing, or burning sensation. These episodes may last for 10 seconds to 2 minutes, or several jabs may occur in rapid succession. A muscle tic or grimace goes along with the nerve pain.

In the most common form of TN, episodes take the form of sharp blasts of pain on one side of the face in response to some mild trigger. A rarer version involves a constant ache or burning sensation that may be interrupted by bolts of electrical stabbing or burning pain.

Episodes of trigeminal nerve pain can be triggered by speaking, chewing, swallowing, sitting in a draft, a light touch to the wrong spot, and sometimes by no stimulus at all. Episodes may happen several times a day for days, weeks, or months and then suddenly disappear—only to begin again months or years later. TN can be a debilitating lifelong condition if it is not treated.

TN is not painful during sleep, nor does it cause numbness, muscle weakness, or hearing loss. It is usually unilateral, and the right side is affected about five times more often than the left. All these factors help to differentiate TN from other conditions that might cause similar symptoms, including migraine or cluster headaches, Ramsay-Hunt syndrome, stroke, or other cranial nerve problems (Sidebar 4.13).

Treatment

The conventional medical approach to TN starts with medication, but typical analgesics are ineffective. Antiseizure drugs that inhibit nerve conduction are often successful in the short run, but many patients

SIDEBAR 4.13 Other Cranial Nerve Disorders

Any damage or irritation to a cranial nerve may lead to symptoms in the face. Trigeminal neuralgia (TN) and Bell palsy are two of the most common disorders that may cause facial symptoms. But a few other cranial nerve disorders can create confusion, so they are listed here:

- *Postherpetic neuralgia* is a complication of herpes zoster. It may occur wherever the shingles blisters appeared but can outlast the visible lesions by several weeks or months. When the herpes infection affects the optic nerve, postherpetic neuralgia can create extremely painful facial symptoms.
- *Glossopharyngeal neuralgia* is etiologically identical to vascular compression on the trigeminal nerve, but this condition affects CN IX, which supplies sensation to the back of the throat.
- *Atypical face pain* is a condition similar to TN and in some cases may be a predecessor to it. It is characterized by pain that is less severe than TN, but it tends to involve continuous rather than intermittent pain. The pain may go up over the back of the head and into the scalp, and it may involve the occipital as well as the trigeminal nerve.
- *Hemifacial spasm* creates a painless tic that is related to blood vessel compression of the facial nerve rather than the trigeminal nerve.

don't tolerate them well, or they experience "breakthrough pain" that requires a change in dosage or a combination of drugs. Muscle relaxants and tricyclic antidepressants may also be prescribed.

Several other interventions have been developed to treat TN. These usually involve the controlled destruction of part of the nerve with lasers, radiation, a heated probe, or injected chemicals. These options often provide some relief, with the understanding that the patient may have permanent numbness and some facial muscle weakness as a result. Microvascular surgery to relieve pressure on the trigeminal nerve is the most invasive procedure. It entails unwrapping the strangulating blood vessel from around the trigeminal nerve. This process leaves sensation intact and has the longest lasting success, but it carries more risks of complication than other approaches.

Medications

- Antiseizure medications for pain control
- Muscle relaxants
- Tricyclic antidepressants

Massage?

RISKS Trigeminal neuralgia (TN) contraindicates any bodywork that might elicit symptoms, which means that touching the face or head is probably off-limits unless the client can guide the therapist into work that is soothing instead of irritating. Further, the pressure of a face cradle may trigger symptoms, so prone work may not be possible.

BENEFITS A person with TN often has musculoskeletal consequences that can be successfully addressed by massage. Tension in the neck and shoulders is predictable, as people chronically guard against the possibility of an episode.

Nervous System Birth Defects

Spina Bifida

Spina Bifida in Brief

Pronunciation: SPY-nah BIF-ih-dah

What is it?
Spina bifida is a neural tube defect resulting in an incompletely formed vertebral arch, damage to the meninges and/or spinal cord, and a high risk of distal paralysis and infection.

How is it recognized?
Spina bifida occulta can be completely silent and detected only through incidental tests. Cystic spina bifida can be detected through prenatal testing, but the most obvious sign is a protrusion, sometimes covered by skin, of a cyst containing layers of the meninges, cerebrospinal fluid, and usually the spinal cord as well.

Massage risks and benefits
Risks: Spina bifida patients live with numbness, paralysis, and accompanying complications. Any bodywork must be carefully gauged to clients ability to adapt and give informed feedback about pressure.
Benefits: Infants with cystic spina bifida go through multiple surgeries followed by rigorous physical therapy to establish and maintain the best function possible, especially in the trunk and legs. Massage can be helpful in this context as well.

Definition: What Is It?

Spina bifida (literally, "cleft spine") is a neural tube defect in which the vertebral arch fails to close completely over the spinal cord. Sometimes this defect is so subtle that it is found only through incidental radiography or MRI, but in other cases it can be so severe that the spinal canal is open and the baby may not survive the birth.

Etiology: What Happens?

Several types of neural tube defects may occur between day 14 and day 28 after conception (Sidebar 4.14). At this time, the woman may not know she is pregnant, and the fetus is about the size of a grain of rice, but the cells that eventually differentiate into connective, muscle, and epithelial tissue at various levels of the spinal cord are in place. If something interrupts their development, spina bifida may occur.

The main risk factors for spina bifida include genetic predisposition, environmental exposure, and a deficiency of folic acid at conception and in the earliest weeks of fetal development. Because this condition

NOTABLE CASES Musician Hank Williams Sr. had spina bifida occulta, which probably contributed to a lifelong struggle with back pain leading to alcohol and drug abuse problems. World-renowned athlete and motivational speaker Jean Driscoll is a wheelchair rider who has won eight championships in the Women's Wheelchair division of the Boston Marathon.

may be determined before a woman knows she is pregnant, it is especially important for women who want to have children to be sure they are getting enough folic acid in their diet.

Spina bifida is a complex disorder with several possible complications. Meningitis is a threat if the CNS is exposed. **Hydrocephalus** affects about 85% of children with diagnosed spina bifida. The insertion of a shunt that drains cerebrospinal fluid down the neck and into the abdominal cavity prevents hydrocephalus from damaging the brain. Hydrocephalus is sometimes related to **Chiari II formation**: a defect in which the brain protrudes into the spinal canal, blocking off the flow of cerebrospinal fluid. While most children with spina bifida have normal intelligence, some have mild to severe learning disabilities that may make it difficult to function in a mainstream classroom. Many spina bifida patients develop a very severe latex hypersensitivity, possibly from having multiple intrusive surgeries and other medical procedures. This allergy may create a dangerous anaphylactic reaction later in life.

Other common complications include **tethered cord** (the spinal cord doesn't slide freely within the spinal canal), decubitus ulcers, bowel and bladder problems with a high risk of renal failure, obesity, and severe muscle imbalances that can lead to severe scoliosis.

SIDEBAR 4.14 Other Neural Tube Defects

The neural tube is composed of fetal cells that fold in on themselves during the earliest days of development. Under normal circumstances, the tube is complete and closed by day 28, when the fetus is about the size of a grain of rice.

Sometimes those cells, which are the starting material of the vertebrae, skull, spinal cord, spinal nerves, and brain, deform. Spina bifida occulta, meningocele, and myelomeningocele describe problems with the spinal cord, but the brain can also be affected. Some neural tube defects that can occur apart from or along with spina bifida include the following:

- *Encephalocele.* In this condition, the bones of the skull don't develop properly. A cyst protrudes from the head, containing cerebrospinal fluid and possibly brain tissue as well.
- *Anencephaly.* In this condition, the brain forms incompletely or doesn't form at all. These babies tend to be stillborn or die soon after birth.
- *Arnold-Chiari malformation.* This is a rare disorder except in the presence of myelomeningocele, with which it is relatively common. In this situation, the brainstem and some of the cerebellum protrude into the spinal canal in the neck. This leads to hydrocephalus, difficulties with swallowing and breathing, and impaired coordination of the arms.

Types of Spina Bifida

- *Spina bifida occulta (SBO).* In this situation, the vertebral arch, usually in a lumbar vertebra, does not completely fuse, but no signs or symptoms are obvious. A person with SBO may never be aware of the condition unless a low back radiograph is taken for another reason. Some people with SBO have a small dimple, birthmark, or tuft of hair on the spine at the location of the abnormality, but they have no dysfunction because of it. While SBO is usually inconsequential, it can be serious. Two or more vertebrae may be affected, and the person may develop a tethered spinal cord. This can manifest as problems in the feet (especially pes cavus) and problems with bladder and bowel control. These often arise during puberty, when the child goes through a growth spurt that stretches the spinal cord.
- *Spina bifida meningocele.* This is the rarest type of cystic spina bifida. Only the dura mater and arachnoid layers of the meninges press through at the site of the vertebral cleft, forming a cyst that is visible at birth. It is easily reparable with surgery and generally has few or no long-term consequences for the baby.
- *Spina bifida myelomeningocele.* This is the most common and most severe version of cystic spina bifida, accounting for about 94% of diagnosed cases. In this case, the spinal cord or extensions of the cauda equina protrude along with the meninges through several incompletely formed vertebral arches. Occasionally, the skin doesn't cover the protrusion, raising a

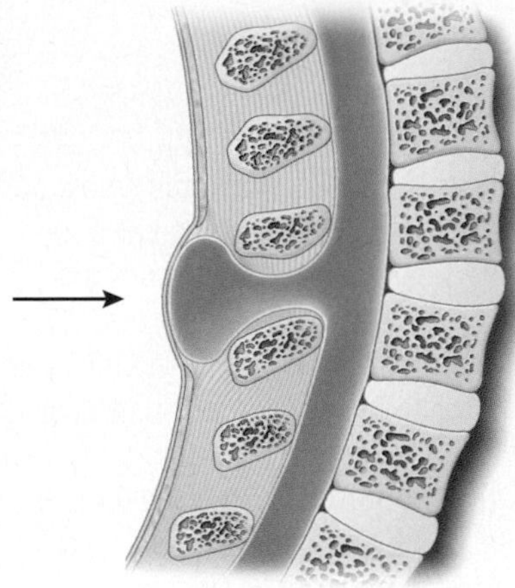

Figure 4.18. Spina bifida occulta. The vertebral arch is incompletely fused; no external sac is present

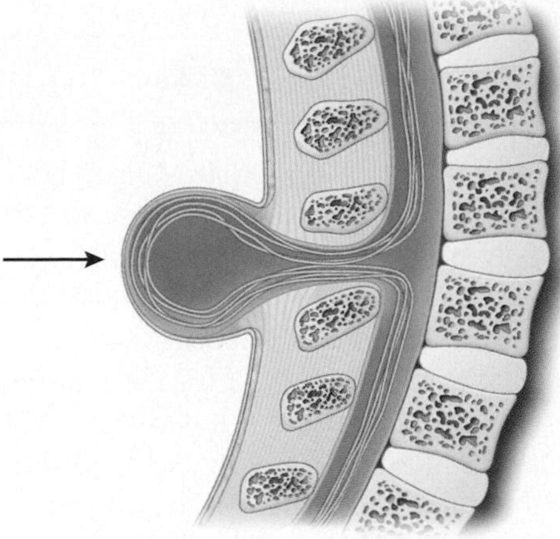

Figure 4.20. Spina bifida myelomeningocele. An external sac contains the meninges and cerebrospinal fluid, peripheral nerves, and spinal cord tissue

serious risk of CNS infection if no immediate intervention takes place.

Signs and Symptoms

SBO is not obvious at birth, although it sometimes causes a birthmark, patch of hair, or a dimple at the site of the abnormality. Cystic spina bifida is obvious, because a sac containing meninges and/or spinal cord material protrudes on the back of the newborn infant. It usually occurs in the lumbar spine, and the sac is often red and raw looking (Figures 4.18 to 4.20).

The severity of cystic spina bifida is determined by the location and size of the cyst: nerve function below the cyst is severely impaired or absent. Most cases present in the thoracic or lumbar spine.

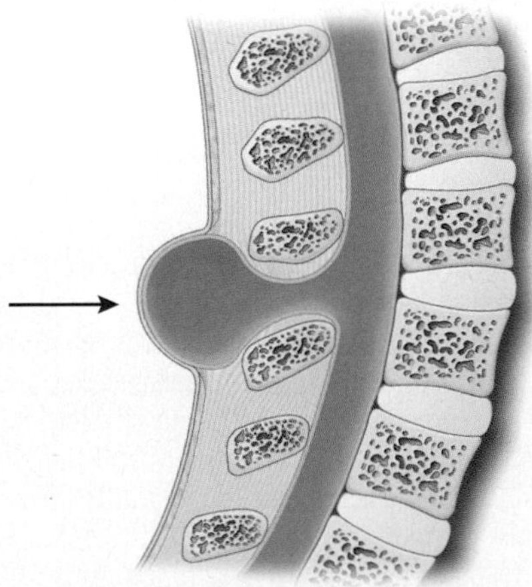

Figure 4.19. Spina bifida meningocele. An external sac contains the meninges and cerebrospinal fluid

Treatment

A baby born with cystic spina bifida needs surgery within a few days to reduce the cyst and preserve as much spinal cord function as possible. Afterward, even tiny babies are supported with rigorous physical therapy and exercises to maintain function in the leg muscles as much as possible. As children mature and their functional level becomes clear, they may be taught to use crutches, braces, wheelchairs, or other equipment as necessary.

Many spina bifida patients undergo multiple surgeries, not only to reduce the protruding cyst but also to correct a tethered cord, to deal with the complications of hydrocephalus, and to address complications brought about by severe scoliosis.

Medications

- Anticholinergic drugs to help with bladder function
- Alpha-adrenergic drugs to help with bladder function
- Tricyclic antidepressants

Massage?

RISKS The risks related to massage for people with spina bifida revolve around paralysis, numbness, and complications like decubitus ulcers or scoliosis.

BENEFITS As long as risks are addressed, massage can be helpful and supportive for spina bifida patients.

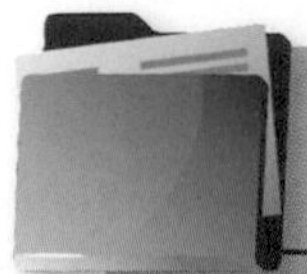

CASE HISTORY 4.4 Spina Bifida

With an effortless motion, he pulled himself onto the table. He grasped his lifeless legs and twisted his whole body until he was lying prone. To gaze on his body was to grasp two opposing realities at once. His legs, clad in a loose-fitting pair of sweatpants, were shriveled and limp. Even his hips and buttocks were hollowed out and gaunt after years of frustrated growth and nearly useless service to the greater whole.

Yet beginning with his lower back and especially with the lower border of his rib cage, a transformation of epic proportions occurred. The sides of his torso tapered out dramatically to accommodate his thickly muscled back. Indeed, his entire upper body resembled that of a professional bodybuilder. Thus, while the lower half of his body revealed a life of disease, death, and despair, his upper body reflected a life filled with drive, determination, ambition, and hope.

At the end of the session, when my client had gotten off my table, dressed, and left the building, I reflected on the meaning of wholeness. It dawned on me that wholeness is not a disease-free condition, at least in this life, in this reality.

Instead, wholeness is a realized and used connection between the human will and a greater purpose, a greater goal. This athlete thrives because his sights are set on goals that diminish the significance of his lower body and magnify the significance of his upper body, including, especially, his mind. Similarly, I thrive when my sights are set on goals that are adorned in truth and immersed in love—on my best days and even on my worst days. ■

—Jan Fields, observations on the 2002 Paralympic Games

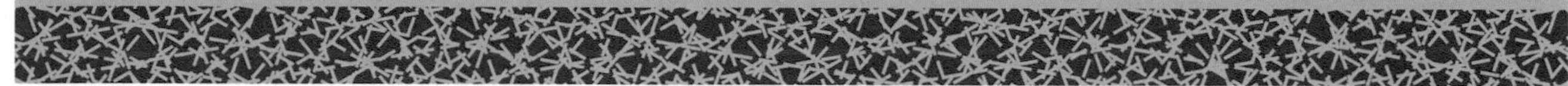

Cerebral Palsy

Definition: What Is It?

Cerebral palsy (CP) is a collective term for many possible injuries to the brain during gestational development, birth, and early infancy. Several types of CP have been identified, each involving damage to different parts of the brain at different moments in development.

In spite of improved prenatal care, the incidence of CP in the United States has remained unchanged for several decades, and in some areas has even gone up. This may be related to the fact that more premature babies are surviving than ever before, and they are especially vulnerable to these problems. Other high-risk populations are hard to identify, but statistics are highest among children of mothers who smoke, who live in poverty, who don't receive prenatal care, and who have previously had preterm babies.

Etiology: What Happens?

CP is the result of brain damage, usually to motor areas of the brain, specifically the basal ganglia and the cerebrum. Intracranial hemorrhage, damage to the white matter around the ventricles, and toxicity due

Cerebral Palsy in Brief

Pronunciation: ser-E-bral (or SER-eh-brul) PAWL-ze

What is it?
Cerebral palsy (CP) is an umbrella term used to refer to a variety of CNS injuries that may occur prenatally, at birth, or in early infancy. These injuries usually result in motor impairment, but they may also lead to sensory and cognitive problems as well.

How is it recognized?
CP is usually diagnosed early in infancy, when voluntary motor skills typically begin to develop. CP patients may have hypertonic or hypotonic muscles, suppressed or extreme reflexes, and poor coordination, and they may show random involuntary movement.

Massage risks and benefits
Risks: The main risks for CP patients receiving massage are seizures, numbness, and difficulties with communication. In this situation, the therapist must take extra care not to overchallenge damaged tissues, and to be sensitive to nonverbal signals about comfort.
Benefits: As long as sensation is intact and the client can communicate, massage can be helpful for people with CP as a strategy to manage pain and stress, to maintain elasticity, and to improve motor function.

to extreme infantile jaundice are leading factors in CP. Causes of CP can fall into three groups, according to when they occur.

- *Prenatal causes*. Many cases of CP can be traced to maternal illness during pregnancy. Contributing factors include infection with rubella or toxoplasmosis, hyperthyroidism, diabetes, Rh sensitization (the mother essentially has an allergic reaction to the blood type of her unborn child), toxic exposure, or abdominal trauma. Pregnancy-induced hypertension and infection of the placental membrane can also increase the risk of CP. Other prenatal causes involve random mutations of genes that affect brain growth.
- *Birth trauma*. CP can result if the child undergoes **anoxia** or **asphyxia** (lack of air from a mechanical blockage) during birth. Respiratory distress and head trauma (often from a difficult presentation or the use of forceps in delivery) may also increase the risk of brain damage.
- *Acquired CP*. This is CP that develops in early infancy. Causes include very extreme jaundice that can lead to brain damage and deafness, head trauma (often from car accidents or child abuse), infection with meningitis or encephalitis, brain hemorrhages, or neoplasms in the brain that may lead to brain damage.

Regardless of the cause of the brain damage, a child with CP has some impairment of function. The problem may be subtle, or it may be completely debilitating both physically and mentally: it all depends on what part and how much of the brain has been affected.

Complications of CP include several other serious challenges. Seizures, hearing loss, and **strabismus** (eyes that don't focus on the same axis) are common. Digestive difficulties, including gastroesophageal reflux disease, poor gastrointestinal motility, and urinary incontinence, are common, as are low bone density and heart disease. CP is also associated with excessive drooling and a high risk of cavities.

Although it doesn't always involve cognitive problems, many CP patients have some level of mental disability, and fully cognizant patients may have challenges in communicating clearly. Many CP patients have seizure disorders, which can require very powerful medication to control.

The muscles of CP patients can become so chronically tight that they are replaced with tight, restrictive contractures. Contractures can pull on the skeleton so constantly and so powerfully that the patient is at risk for developing osteoarthritis, hip dislocation, or extreme scoliosis that can make it painful to sit or stand and difficult to breathe.

NOTABLE CASES Irish author, painter, and poet Christy Brown had cerebral palsy. He was the subject of the award-winning film *My Left Foot*, which chronicled his life from infancy, when it was assumed he was hopelessly disabled, through the discovery that he could write and draw with his toes, to his recognition as a leading artist in his country.

Perhaps the most pervasive and least studied complication of CP is the pain that these children and adults must deal with on a daily basis. The disorder itself can be painful as it twists the body into stressful postures and positions, but the treatments, from frequent surgeries, to aggressive rehabilitation exercises, can also be severely painful.

While CP is discussed as the types described below, it may also be classified by what part of the body is affected. These terms are consistent with those used for other CNS disorders: hemiplegic CP means the left or right side is affected; diplegic CP means either the arms or the legs are affected; and quadriplegic CP means all the extremities are affected to some extent.

Types of Cerebral Palsy

- *Spastic CP*. This is the most common form of the condition. In some areas, muscle tone is so high that the tight muscle's antagonists have completely let go. This is called the **clasp-knife effect**.
- *Athetoid CP*. This involves very weak muscles and frequent involuntary writhing movements of the extremities, face, and mouth.
- *Ataxic CP*. This is a rare variety of the disorder, involving chronic shaking, intention tremors, and very poor balance.
- *Dystonic CP*. This involves slow, involuntary twisting movements of the trunk and extremities.
- *Mixed CP*. This is a combination of the forms, and it affects many CP patients.

Signs and Symptoms

Signs and symptoms of CP vary according to the location and extent of brain injury. They typically develop between age of 6 months and early toddlerhood. Some of the most common features of CP include hypotonicity, hypertonicity, problems with walking, poor coordination and voluntary muscle control, unusually weak muscles, random movements, and early hearing and/or vision problems.

Adults with CP tend to age faster than others; it takes much more energy and effort to move for someone with CP than for someone without. Simple activities are more draining, and adult patients tend to be prone to fatigue, exhaustion, and overuse syndromes.

Treatment

The CNS damage that occurs with CP is incurable and irreversible. CP is therefore managed, rather than treated, by providing skills and equipment to live as fully and functionally as possible. For some CP patients, this means braces, crutches, or orthotics; for others, it means intensive occupational, physical, and speech therapy for many years. Computers have become an important tool for many patients with CP; these appliances can improve communication and open many new opportunities for this population.

Speech therapy helps with communication and safe swallowing. Intensive physical and occupational therapy, often combined with massage, is used to maintain and improve muscle function and elasticity.

Medication for CP is prescribed to help manage seizures and to reduce muscle spasm. Botox injections can limit excessive salivation and involuntary muscle contractions for several months at a time. Some surgical interventions have been developed to correct hip dislocations, to lengthen contracted muscles, to realign vertebrae that have become distorted by scoliosis, to sever some motor neurons to the legs, and to alter nerve pathways in the brain to reduce the severity of tremors.

Medications

- Oral or injected muscle relaxants for spasticity
- Injected Botox to reduce spasticity
- Injected antispasmodic medication to reduce spasticity
- Antiseizure medications for seizures and chronic pain
- Bisphosphonates for improved bone density

Massage?

RISKS Some people with cerebral palsy (CP) may not be able to verbally communicate easily; massage therapists must be sensitive to nonverbal signals from these clients. In addition, any numbness contraindicates intrusive massage that may overchallenge the tissues, and care must be taken not to trigger seizures, if that is part of a client's symptomatic profile.

BENEFITS Massage can be a wonderful addition to the healthcare strategy of a person with CP: it can be used to help with pain and stress, digestive function, and muscle tension.

OPTIONS Bodywork that focuses on muscle tone and proprioception can be especially useful for clients with central nervous system problems.

Other Nervous System Conditions

Fibromyalgia

Definition: What Is It?

Fibromyalgia syndrome (FMS) describes a multifactoral condition involving problems with neurotransmitter and hormone imbalances, sleep disorders, and ultimately chronic pain in muscles, tendons, ligaments, and other soft tissues. FMS is frequently seen with chronic fatigue syndrome, irritable bowel syndrome, migraine headaches, temporomandibular joint disorders, and several other chronic conditions.

Etiology: What Happens?

Fibromyalgia is a relatively common disorder, but it is not well understood. While the etiology of this condition is not clear, several issues are consistent among people who meet the diagnostic criteria for this disorder:

- *Neuroendocrine disruption.* The HPA axis is one line of connection between the autonomic nervous system and the endocrine system. Its dysregulation appears to be a factor for many fibromyalgia patients. This means they tend to secrete more stress-related hormones for longer periods of time than other people. HPA axis dysregulation is also a factor in several other disorders, including depression and

Fibromyalgia in Brief

Pronunciation: fy-bro-my-AL-je-ah

What is it?
Fibromyalgia syndrome (FMS) is a chronic pain syndrome involving neuroendocrine disruption, sleep disorders, and the development of a predictable pattern of tender points in muscles and other soft tissues.

How is it recognized?
FMS is diagnosed when other diseases have been ruled out, and when 11 active tender points are found distributed among all quadrants of the body, along with fatigue, morning stiffness, and poor quality sleep.

Massage risks and benefits
Risks: FMS patients tend to be hypersensitive and easy to overtreat. Care must be taken to stay within their tolerance for pain and adaptability.
Benefits: Fibromyalgia indicates massage, which can help reduce pain, improve sleep, and otherwise add to quality of life.

chronic fatigue syndrome—both of which are often seen in people with FMS.

- *Sleep disorder.* Most people with FMS seldom or never enter the deepest level of sleep, Stage IV. It is in this stage that adults secrete growth hormone, which stimulates the production of new cells and extracellular matrix for healing and recovery.
- *Central sensitization.* Fibromyalgia pain is perceived in muscles and soft tissues, but it is not generated there. The cerebrospinal fluid of many FMS patients has unusually high levels of two neurotransmitters: substance P and nerve growth factor. These substances are believed to stimulate nerve activity, cause vasodilation, and increase pain sensation. At the same time, FMS patients tend to have low levels of important inhibitory neurotransmitters, specifically norepinephrine and serotonin.
- *Tender points.* Fibromyalgia patients eventually develop tender points that are distributed all over the body, but they are most numerous around the neck, shoulders, and low back (Figure 4.21). Tender points themselves are not well understood. Histological studies of affected tissue have yielded no useful information about how these areas develop. Tender points are unique indicators of fibromyalgia, but not all patients experience them as a leading symptom.

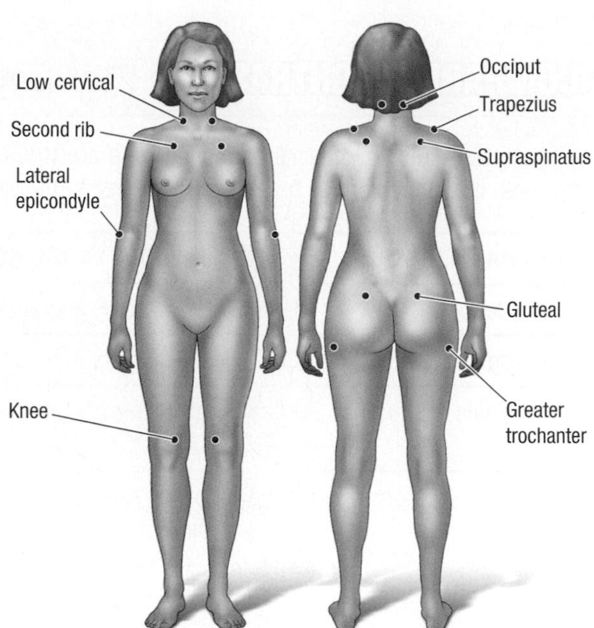

Figure 4.21. Fibromyalgia syndrome tender point map

While FMS is not a life-threatening disease, it certainly threatens quality of life. The pain it causes is "invisible": it doesn't show on imaging tests, in blood analysis, or by visible sign. A person with this syndrome may easily be discounted as a faker or malingerer by doctors, employers, even by friends and family. By the time a patient has reached a definitive diagnosis, the experience with the medical community has often been frustrating and overwhelmingly negative. It is not surprising, then, that anxiety and depression are common complications of FMS.

Signs and Symptoms

The signs and symptoms of FMS vary widely from one person to the next. Some of the most common indicators include the following:

- Stiffness after rest.
- Poor stamina.
- Fatigue.
- Memory problems and poor concentration; this is sometimes called "fibro fog."
- Widespread pain in shifting locations that is extremely difficult to pin down. The intensity

COMPARE & CONTRAST 4.1 Fibromyalgia vs. Myofascial Pain Syndrome

Fibromyalgia and myofascial pain syndrome are frequently confused. Because they call for quite different treatment options, it is important to be able to recognize both their similarities and their unique qualities.

CHARACTERISTICS	FIBROMYALGIA SYNDROME	MYOFASCIAL PAIN SYNDROME
Prevalence	Up to 3% of the US population	Unknown
Demographics	85%–90% of all diagnoses are in women	Women and men are equally affected
Prognosis	Lifelong problem; can be managed	Can be a short-term problem that is permanently solved
Primary symptoms	Tender points: predictable areas; light touch elicits intense, diffuse pain at the site	Trigger points: predictable areas in muscles; may be nodular or appear as a taut band that generates a twitch response with pressure. Manual pressure elicits pain locally and at distant areas
Implications for massage	Careful massage can help, but patients are often hypersensitive and easy to overtreat	Responds well to massage: rhythmic pressure and release can interrupt dysfunctional signals at trigger point sites

of the pain can be inconsistent, and it can range from a deep ache to burning and tingling.

- Tender points. Nine predictable pairs of these are distributed among all quadrants of the body. Tender points are painful, and that pain may appear to be diffused around the area, but they do not refer pain to distant sites.
- Sensitivity amplification and low pain tolerance. All kinds of sensation become more intense and likely to cause pain. This includes light, sound, and smells, but is true especially of cold, texture, and pressure.

Treatment

Treatment for FMS begins with a good diagnosis, which is a challenge (see Sidebar 4.15). This condition is typically diagnosed by ruling out other diseases with similar signs and symptoms, including Lyme disease, multiple sclerosis, rheumatoid arthritis, lupus, hypothyroidism, candidiasis, and several others. Several of these diagnostic differentials are also made by ruling out similar-looking conditions, and it is quite possible for a person to more than one of these conditions at a time. Further, a long history of confusion between FMS tender points and myofascial pain syndrome (MPS) trigger points continues to cloud the issue. A side-by-side comparison of FMS and MPS is provided in the table in Compare & Contrast 4.1.

For most people, FMS is a lifelong condition. Treatment focuses on finding ways to manage the disorder, so that the patient may lead as normal a life as possible. This includes patient education, careful exercise, and often cognitive-behavioral therapy.

Drug therapies for FMS include mild antidepressants to reduce levels of depression, manage pain, to improve the quality of sleep. Painkilling drugs are generally avoided, because they interfere with sleep and can be habit forming. An antiseizure drug has been successful with pain management without some of the side effects that this class of drugs often involve.

Medications

- Analgesics, including NSAIDs (have varying effectiveness)
- Antidepressants to aid with sleep, pain, and mood
- Antiseizure drugs to help with pain
- Anti-Parkinson drugs

Massage?

RISKS People with fibromyalgia live with chronic, invisible, widespread, and unpredictable pain. It is important that their pain not be exacerbated by massage that is insensitive or too aggressive.

BENEFITS Massage has much to offer fibromyalgia patients in terms of pain relief, sleep quality, improved mood, and reduced anxiety. Massage as part of an emphasis on good self-care is frequently part of a successful treatment strategy.

OPTIONS Research suggests that while many kinds of massage improve fibromyalgia symptoms, lighter and gentler work is more effective than deeper, more intrusive types of bodywork, especially for clients new to massage.

SIDEBAR 4.15 Diagnosing Fibromyalgia Syndrome

The history of fibromyalgia syndrome (FMS) identification and diagnosis is long and confusing. In its history, it has been called myositis, fibromyositis, myofibrositis, and several other names. It wasn't until the mid-1980s that tissue biopsies revealed that no inflammation was present in tender point tissue, so the suffix "-tis" was a misnomer. More recently, histological studies of fascial wrappings around painful tender points do show signs of inflammation, so this understanding continues to evolve.

In 1990, The American College of Rheumatology determined this set of diagnostic criteria:

- The patient reports chronic pain for a minimum of 3 months.
- The patient shows at least 11 of 18 mapped tender points to be active (i.e., they must elicit significant diffuse pain with digital pressure of about 4 kg).
- The active tender points are widely distributed, with some from each quadrant of the body.
- The patient reports persistent fatigue.
- The patient reports nonrefreshing sleep, and awakens with morning stiffness.

It is important to point out that these are guidelines only: they help with FMS research as a way to determine which subjects have FMS and which ones do not. A person who falls short of these criteria can still be diagnosed with this condition, and can still experience relief with appropriate treatment.

Headaches

Definition: What Are They?

Headaches are one of the most common physical problems in the range of human experience. Although they can indicate some serious underlying problems, most headaches are self-contained temporary problems.

Many experts discuss headaches as primary or secondary. Primary headaches are unrelated to serious underlying pathology, while secondary headaches are symptoms of other problems, some of which may be serious.

Tension-type headaches are the most common version of primary headaches. They are typically triggered by musculoskeletal issues: bony misalignment, eyestrain, myofascial trigger points, or temporomandibular joint disorders. Migraine headaches usually have different triggers than tension-type headaches, and they involve some unique symptoms, but they have some physiologic features in common. Cluster headaches have some issues in common with migraine, but they present very differently. Rebound

Headaches in Brief

What are they?
Headaches are pain caused by any number of factors. Muscular tension, nerve irritation, vascular spasm and dilation, and chemical imbalances can all contribute to headache. They can sometimes indicate a serious underlying disorder.

How are they recognized?
Headache pain can range from being mild to debilitating; it can involve the whole head or be isolated to a particular area; it can be described as dull, aching, or sharp, electrical and agonizing.

Massage risks and benefits
Risks: Headaches due to infection or central nervous system injury contraindicate massage. Many clients with migraine avoid massage and other stimulus during a headache, but might pursue it as a way to reduce frequency or intensity when the condition is not acute.
Benefits: Tension-type headaches, which are the most common variety of headaches, often respond beautifully to massage, which can address both stress and the mechanical imbalances in muscle tension that are so often involved.

headaches are specifically related to medicine use and disuse.

Secondary headaches are related to an underlying problem that requires attention: fever and general infection as seen with flu or cold can cause headaches, for example. Other secondary headaches are much more serious. They can be related to TBI, stroke, arteriovenous malformation, aneurysm, tumor, or some other threatening problem.

Etiology: What Happens?

Headaches have been organized into 150 subtypes of primary and secondary phenomena. Among primary headaches, some unifying features that are frequently observed include hypersensitivity among specific nerve pathways, irritability of the trigeminal nerve complex, and a tendency toward dilation of cranial blood vessels with subsequent edema. The most important differences between types of headaches, therefore, may simply be the triggers and the presence or absence of a throbbing sensation.

Types of Primary Headaches

- *Tension-type headaches*. The average head weighs about 18 to 20 lbs, and the area of bone-to-bone contact between the occipital condyles and the facets of C_1 is about the same as two pairs of fingertips touching. The whole mechanism is kept in balance by tension exerted by muscles and ligaments around the neck and head. The muscles primarily responsible for the stability of the cranium form two small inverted triangles just below the occiput (Figure 4.22). It is not surprising, then, that when this delicate balance is a little off, the resulting pain reverberates throughout the whole structure.

  Similarly, when postural or movement patterns elsewhere in the body exert force on the spine, the end result can be tension at the occipital connection. In this way, a foot that strikes the ground too hard on the lateral side may pull on the knee, which may then demand compensation in the hip. The sacrum moves to adjust to the tip in the os coxae. This creates a slight twist in the lumbar vertebrae, which reverberates all the way up the spine to the head. The result: headaches because the feet are not in alignment or shoes are worn down.

  Tension-type headache triggers can include soft tissue injury, muscle tightness and trigger points, subluxation or misalignment of cervical vertebrae, eyestrain, poor ergonomics, and ongoing mental or emotional stress that exacerbates inefficient postural and movement patterns.

  Tension-type headache can be episodic or chronic. It is often bilateral or nonfocused in area. Many patients describe a tight band

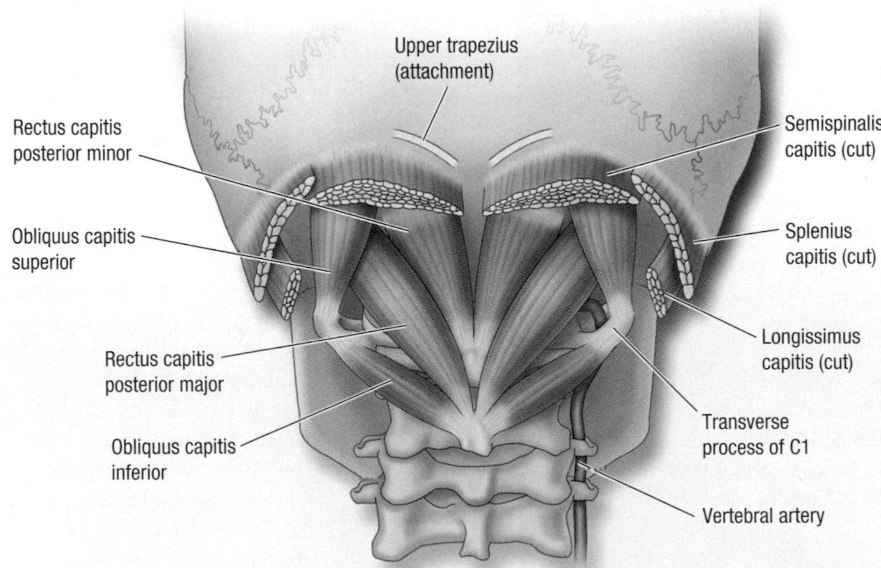

Figure 4.22. Muscular imbalance at the suboccipital triangle is a contributing factor in many headaches

around the head, or a deep, dull ache rather than a precise focal point for pain.

- *Migraine Headaches*. The word migraine originated from the Greek "hemikrania" to describe pain in one-half of the head. Migraine headaches, like tension-type headaches, involve hyper-excitability within pain-sensitive nerves of the cranium. When these nerves are irritated, a complex cascade of reactions occurs that lead to vasoconstriction followed by vasodilation. Common triggers include hormonal shifts with pregnancy or menstruation; food sensitivities, especially to red wine, aged cheese and chocolate; excessive exercise; too much or too little sleep; and stress.

  Many subtypes of migraine have been identified, but the two most common are called migraine with aura (which accounts for about 20% of all diagnoses) and migraines without aura (which is much more common). Migraine with aura may involve blurred vision, the perception of flashing and jagged lights or auras, and auditory hallucinations.

  All migraine patients experience throbbing pain on one side of the head, which may cause the ipsilateral eye and nostril to water. Hypersensitivity to light and noise, along with nausea, and vomiting are all possible. Some patients have tingling or other sensation changes in their extremities. Migraine pain can persist for several hours to several days.

- *Cluster Headaches*. These are a fairly rare, not well-understood variety of headache. Like migraines, they involve unilateral pain that can cause the eye and nostril of the affected side to water. They may also cause facial swelling and unilateral sweating. Each headache lasts a few moments to several hours, and in an episode a person may have one to four headaches every day for 4 to 8 weeks. They may occur seasonally, once or twice in a year, or just once in a lifetime. Cluster headaches affect men much more often than women. They usually occur at night, with pain severe enough to wake a person out of a sound sleep. Unlike migraines, which tend to make patients want to rest in a dark quiet room, cluster headaches tend to cause restlessness; stillness seems to exacerbate the pain.
- *Rebound Headaches*. These are caused by overuse of medication—often to relieve headaches. They are related to increasing tolerance for headache medication, which means more painkiller is needed to achieve the same level of relief. Rebound headaches can be present on waking in the morning, and they can include nausea, anxiety, restlessness, and irritability. The only way to eradicate them is to stop taking headache medication altogether, which can be a daunting prospect.

Signs and Symptoms

The signs and symptoms of headaches are self-evident, but they may have specific characteristics like location, triggers, duration, severity, and frequency, as discussed above. Symptoms indicate a serious underlying condition when headaches are severe, repeating, and have a sudden onset ("thunderclap headache"), when they appear in a new pattern after age 50, or when they have a gradual onset but no remission. This is true particularly if the headache is accompanied by slurred speech, numbness anywhere in the body, and difficulties with motor control. The first things to investigate in cases like these are encephalitis, meningitis, stroke, tumor, or aneurysm.

Treatment

Occasional headaches respond well to rest and NSAIDs, but if they are a recurring problem, then avoiding or managing headache triggers is the most proactive and least invasive solution. People who have recurrent headaches of any type are often encouraged to keep a headache journal to try to pin down specific triggers.

Medication for headaches falls into two categories: prophylactic treatment, which works to prevent the headache from beginning, and abortive treatment, which works to end the headache once it has begun.

Prophylactic Medications

- NSAIDs
- Beta blockers, calcium channel blockers
- Antidepressants, including tricyclics and SSRIs
- Serotonin (5 HT1) agonists (triptans)
- Antiseizure medications
- Injections of Botox

Abortive Medications

- Serotonin (5 HT1) agonists (triptans)
- Ergot alkaloids
- Analgesics
- NSAIDs
- Antiemetics to manage nausea

Massage?

RISKS Any headache that is accompanied by fever, confusion, numbness, or other CNS signs contraindicates massage, and may be a medical emergency. Many migraine or cluster headache patients don't seek massage until after the pain has subsided.

BENEFITS Tension-type headaches indicate massage, which can help to address the musculoskeletal and stress-related holding patterns that contribute to inefficient movement and pain.

OPTIONS It is important to be cognizant of all the factors that can contribute to headaches, including distortions that occur far away from the head. Massage therapists are in a better position than many care providers to untangle the clues that can lead to long-term improvement.

Ménière Disease

Definition: What Is It?

Ménière disease is a group of signs and symptoms that center on inner ear dysfunction, leading to vertigo, tinnitus, and hearing loss. It was first described and documented by French physician Prosper Ménière in 1861.

Etiology: What Happens?

The inner ear is composed of several structures that conduct sound and provide a sense of position in relation to gravity. The bony labyrinth forms the semicircular ducts leading to the ampulla, the vestibule, and the snail-shaped cochlea. The bony labyrinth is filled with a sodium-rich fluid called perilymph. Inside the bony labyrinth, the membranous labyrinth floats in the perilymph. The membranous labyrinth is filled with a potassium-rich fluid called endolymph (Figure 4.23). Together the endolymph and perilymph, separated by the membranous labyrinth, help to conduct sound vibrations.

Ménière Disease in Brief

What is it?
Ménière disease is an idiopathic condition that affects the inner ear, leading to problems with vertigo, tinnitus, and hearing loss.

How is it recognized?
Signs and symptoms of Ménière disease include episodes of extreme vertigo, tinnitus, a sensation of pressure in the middle ear, and hearing impairment. Episodes last anywhere from 20 minutes to 24 hours.

Massage risks and benefits
Risks: Ménière disease has no inherent contraindications for massage, as long as clients are comfortable lying down.
Benefits: If clients are comfortable on the table and techniques do not trigger symptoms, massage can be safe and supportive for a person with this condition.

Nerve endings from the vestibulocochlear nerve terminate in the ampulla, an enlarged space where the semicircular canals converge. These nerve projections are suspended in endolymph, and move like seaweed in water whenever the head changes position. Signals from the vestibulocochlear nerve coordinate with the eyes and proprioceptors throughout the body to help orient us in space.

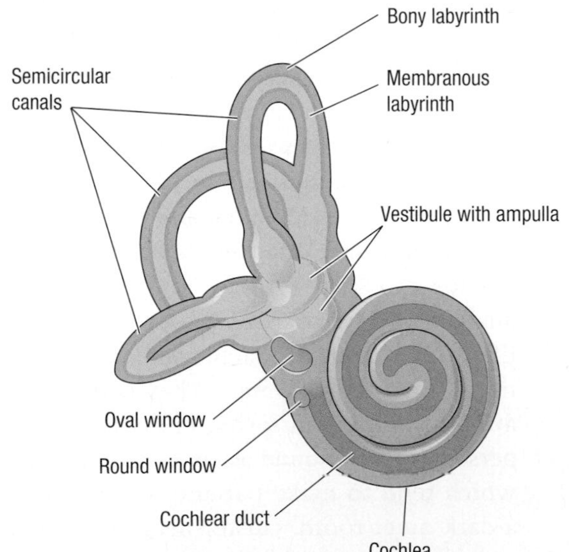

Figure 4.23. Semicircular canals. Perilymph fills the bony labyrinth, and endolymph fills the membranous labyrinth

The exact causes or sequence of events that lead to Ménière disease are not well understood. Most specialists agree that it has to do with the accumulation of excess fluid in the endolymph inside the membranous labyrinth. This is called **idiopathic endolymphatic hydrops**, a synonym for Ménière disease. Possible factors in the accumulation of excess endolymph include allergic reactions, head trauma, genetic predisposition, autoimmune activity, or viral infection.

Signs and Symptoms

Ménière disease has three classic symptoms, all of which appear intermittently and in any combination. It usually affects only one ear, but it can progress to affect the other ear as well. Onset of an episode is typically fast and unpredictable, and any given attack can last 20 minutes to 24 hours. Many patients find that their symptoms fluctuate in frequency, duration, and severity.

- *Hearing loss*. Hearing loss typically involves low-frequency sound. It is worst during flares, but eventually becomes permanent.
- *Tinnitus*. This is a collective term for any unexplained ringing, whistling, or pounding noise in the ear. Patients often describe noise like a million crickets or like the whine of a jet engine. It can feel loud enough to interfere with the ability to sleep or concentrate. It is often associated with a feeling of fullness in the inner ear.
- *Rotational vertigo*. This may be the most disabling symptom of Ménière disease: the person perceives that the world is spinning, or the floor is sloping. **Nystagmus** (an abnormal rhythmic oscillation of the eyes) is observed as well. Nausea and vomiting are common results. This can last for several minutes or hours, and is aggravated by any movement of the head.

Treatment

Because Ménière disease is an idiopathic condition, treatment options focus on symptomatic control. Some patients are able to identify triggers that increase their risk of having an episode. Many people are counseled to avoid foods and habits that raise blood pressure and increase fluid retention. A low-salt diet, avoiding monosodium glutamate, limiting caffeine and alcohol, and quitting smoking are usually recommended as early interventions. Medications to manage vertigo and nausea may be prescribed.

If diet and medications are unsuccessful, some patients explore more intrusive options to interfere with the sensation of vertigo. This can be accomplished by essentially disabling the vestibulocochlear nerve and relying on the unaffected side to compensate for the lost function. This is an option only when Ménière disease has not progressed to affect the contralateral side.

Medications

- Antiemetics for nausea control
- Steroidal anti-inflammatories
- Diuretics
- Antihistamines
- Anticholinergics to suppress nerve activity
- Benzodiazepines for vertigo and nausea

Massage?

RISKS Massage has no specific risks for clients with Ménière disease, as long as they are comfortable getting on and off a table, and lying down. Any bodywork that exacerbates symptoms must be avoided, of course.

BENEFITS While massage is unlikely to improve Ménière disease, it can certainly add to the quality of life of a person who lives with it.

Seizure Disorders

Definition: What Are They?

A seizure disorder is any kind of problem that causes seizures. Estimates suggest that up to 10% of the US population will have a seizure at some point, but seizure disorders are only diagnosed when they are a recurring problem. Epilepsy is a subtype of seizure disorders.

Etiology: What Happens?

When interconnecting neurons in the brain are stimulated in a certain way, a tremendous burst of excess electricity may stimulate the neighboring neurons. The reaction is repeated, and soon millions of neurons in the brain are giving off electrical discharge. This is

Seizure Disorders in Brief

Pronunciation: SE-zhur dis-OR-derz

What are they?
Seizure disorders are any condition that causes seizures. They may be related to neurological damage in the shape of tumors, head injuries, or infection, although it may be impossible to delineate exactly what that damage is. Epilepsy is a subtype of seizure disorder.

How are they recognized?
Seizures can range from barely noticeable "checking out" to life-threatening convulsions.

Massage risks and benefits
Risks: Massage is not appropriate for a person who is mid-seizure, and therapists should determine how best to minimize the risk of triggering an event during a session.
Benefits: While massage may not change the course of a client's seizure disorder, it can add to the quality of life for the person who has it.

the CNS "lightning storm" of a seizure, and it affects the rest of the body in a number of ways.

Seizure triggers vary from person to person. They can include sudden changes in light levels; flashing or strobe lights, or the effect created by a ceiling fan or the sun shining through moving leaves; watching television or playing video games; certain sounds, or even particular notes of music. Anxiety, sleep deprivation, hormonal changes, and fever can also lead to seizures.

NOTABLE CASES Russian novelist Fyodor Dostoyevsky had epilepsy and used his experience in the development of various characters. Actor Danny Glover, musician Neil Young, and track and field athlete Florence Griffith Joyner were all diagnosed with epilepsy. "Flo-Jo" died in 1998 when she asphyxiated during a tonic-clonic seizure in her sleep.

Whatever the trigger, the result is uncoordinated neuronal activity that allows electrical signals to become increasingly extreme, sometimes to the point of collapse and loss of consciousness. Some seizures are linked to underactive inhibitory neurotransmitters, overactive excitatory neurotransmitters, or both. The permeability of nerve cell membranes may also be a factor, as this has influence on the speed and strength of electrical signals.

In some cases, the cause of seizures can be definitively linked to a mechanical or chemical problem in the brain. Birth trauma, traumatic brain injury, stroke, brain tumors, and penetrating wounds can all cause seizures, as can some types of metabolic disturbances, infections, exposure to some toxins (lead, carbon monoxide, and others), and extreme hypotension or hemorrhage. Alcoholism and drug abuse are risk factors. Alzheimer disease is a leading cause of seizures among the elderly. Some seizures can be traced to a hereditary issue. Even with all these possible factors, about half of all seizures are idiopathic, untraceable to any identifiable problem.

Types of Seizure Disorders

- *Epilepsy*. This is identified as a specific disorder when a person has two or more seizures at least 24 hours apart. These seizures can be a complication of another disorder or injury. Epilepsy is one of the oldest conditions recorded in medical history. It was first described about 2,000 years BCE, but it was not studied as a specific problem other than "demonic possession" until the mid-19th century.

Signs and Symptoms

Seizures take very different forms in each person they affect. More than 30 classes of seizures have been identified, according to the parts of the brain they affect. Generalized seizures affect the whole brain, while partial seizures involve abnormal activity in isolated areas. Partial seizures can sometimes spread throughout the brain to become generalized. The most common types of seizures are described here.

- *Partial seizures*. These seizures involve abnormal activity only in isolated areas. The motor cortex and the temporal lobes are the sites most often affected. Partial seizures come in two subtypes:
  - *Simple partial seizures*. In this type of seizure, the patient doesn't lose consciousness. He or she may become weak or numb, may smell or taste things that aren't present, and may have some changes in vision or temporary vertigo along with some muscular tics or twitching.
  - *Complex partial seizures*. This type of seizure is specifically associated with temporal lobe dysfunction. The patient may exhibit

repetitive behaviors such as pacing in a circle, rocking, or smacking the lips. He or she may laugh uncontrollably or experience fear. Visual and olfactory hallucinations are other symptoms of complex partial seizures.

- *Generalized seizures*. These seizures involve electrical signals that occur all over the brain. They may be very subtle or dramatic. These are the major types:
  - *Absence seizures*. These involve very short episodes of loss of consciousness. The patient may simply "check out" for 5 to 10 seconds and have no memory of the lapse.
  - *Clonic seizures*. These consist of jerking movements with or without loss of consciousness in both upper and lower extremities.
  - *Tonic seizures*. These show a sudden onset of tight muscles leading to flexion of the head, trunk, and extremities for several seconds.
  - *Tonic-clonic seizures*. These are what have traditionally been called grand mal seizures. They involve uncontrolled movement of the face, arms, and legs followed by loss of consciousness, loss of bladder control, and loss of all muscle tone. Events may last for 5 to 20 minutes, and the patient is usually tired and disoriented after an episode.
  - *Myoclonic seizures*. These involve bilateral muscular jerking, which may be very pronounced or almost unnoticeable. They are usually seen among very young patients.
  - *Atonic seizures*. These involve a brief but complete loss in muscle tone, leading to falls and a risk of injury.
  - *Status epilepticus*. These are a life-threatening variation of tonic-clonic seizures; they last for a long period and can put such a strain on the body that they can cause brain damage or death. Status epilepticus, or static seizures, are a medical emergency.

Treatment

Seizures are treated with antiseizure medication, which acts to make neurons in the brain harder to stimulate. It can be difficult to find the right dosage of these powerful medications, and while most patients can find a strategy that works for them, some patients don't tolerate them well.

Some epilepsy patients find that their seizures are less frequent and less extreme when they follow a strict high-fat, low-fiber ketogenic diet.

Surgical intervention for seizure disorders is reserved for when an isolated and expendable mass (i.e., a tumor or clump of scar tissue) can be determined to be the cause of the seizures. Some patients with tonic-clonic seizures can control them when their corpus callosum is severed.

One device that is successful for some patients for whom medications don't work is a vagus nerve stimulator. This mechanism is implanted in the vagus nerves in the neck and sends pulses of electrical stimulation to the vagus nerve. It is believed that stimulating the vagus nerve in this way helps to activate some of the inhibitory neurotransmitters that seizure disorder patients lack.

Medications

- Antiseizure drugs
- Barbituates and tranquilizers

Massage?

RISKS It is inappropriate to try to massage someone who is in the midst of a seizure of any kind, and it is important to try to minimize the chances of triggering a seizure for clients who know they are vulnerable. This may mean adjusting lighting, turning off a ceiling fan, or being careful what kinds of scents or music are present in the treatment room. It is wise to discuss ahead of time how a client with seizure disorders would like an episode to be managed.

BENEFITS While massage is unlikely to change the course or prognosis for a client with a seizure disorder, bodywork can certainly add to his or her quality of life. Someone recovering from a tonic-clonic seizure is likely to be sore, and may have soft tissue injuries that massage can help to address.

OPTIONS Antiseizure medication may make a client feel fatigued or dizzy; massage must accommodate for that, with extra time to recover, or stimulating strokes to finish, or both.

Sleep Disorders

Definition: What Are They?

Sleep disorders are any disorders that interfere with the ability to fall asleep, to stay asleep, or to wake up

Sleep Disorders in Brief

What are they?
Sleep disorders are a collection of problems including insomnia, sleep apnea, restless leg syndrome, narcolepsy, circadian rhythm disruption, and others that make it difficult to get enough sleep or to wake up feeling rested and refreshed.

How are they recognized?
The primary symptom of sleep disorders is excessive daytime sleepiness. If this continues for a long period, a weakened immune system, memory and concentration loss, an increased risk of automotive or on-the-job accidents, and other complications may occur.

Massage risks and benefits
Risks: Massage has no particular risks for clients with sleep disorders.
Benefits: Sleep disorders indicate massage. Bodywork may not correct a mechanical or psychological dysfunction that leads to sleep deprivation, but it can improve the quality of sleep and can reduce the mental and physical stresses that may interfere with sleep.

feeling refreshed. More than 70 sleep disorders have been defined. This discussion covers the most common varieties: insomnia, sleep apnea, restless leg syndrome, narcolepsy, and circadian rhythm disruption.

Etiology: What Happens?

Most healthy adults sleep about 8 to 8.5 hours per night if not interrupted by an alarm clock or other disruption. The need for sleep is determined partly by the accumulation of metabolic byproducts in the blood and by the hormone **melatonin**, a secretion of the pineal gland, deep within the brain. Melatonin contributes to a feeling of drowsiness. A standard rotation of wakefulness and sleepiness usually runs on a 24- to 25-hour cycle called the **circadian rhythm**.

Chronic sleep deprivation can lead to a multitude of short-term and long-term problems, including higher pain sensitivity, slowed reflexes, lower cognitive skills, poor immune system efficiency, fibromyalgia syndrome, depression, hallucinations, and psychosis. Poor sleep is now linked to weight gain, high blood sugar, and an elevated risk of developing heart disease and type 2 diabetes. Sleep apnea is associated with an increased risk for stroke. Drowsy driving now rivals drunk driving for causes of motor vehicle accidents. In addition, fatigue and sleep deprivation contribute dangerously to on-the-job injuries that affect not only the sleep-deprived person but many others as well.

Stages of Sleep

Sleep occurs in five distinct phases or stages:

- *Stage I.* In this light sleep a person is easily wakened. Eye movement is slow. A phenomenon called **hypnic myoclonia**, the feeling that a person is suddenly starting to fall, occurs in this stage.
- *Stage II.* The eyes stop moving. Brain waves slow down but still show occasional bursts of activity called sleep spindles.
- *Stage III.* Brain waves are much slower. A deep-sleep pattern called delta waves are intermixed with slightly faster brain waves during this stage.
- *Stage IV.* Only delta waves are emitted from the brain. The body secretes growth hormone that enables new growth for children and adolescents and repair and regeneration for adults during this stage.
- *REM sleep.* In REM (rapid eye movement) sleep breathing is rapid, shallow, and irregular. Eyes move quickly, but muscular activity in the limbs is usually absent. Heart rate and blood pressure approach waking levels. REM sleep is the stage in which dreams occur.

During normal sleep, a person cycles through each of the five stages and then starts over again at stage I. It takes about 90 to 100 minutes to complete a sleep cycle, although the amount of time spent in each stage varies according to the time of night. Overall a healthy, organized sleep session allows an adult to spend 20% to 25% of his time in REM sleep, 50% of his time in stage II, and 30% of his time in the other stages.

Types of Sleep Disorders

Sleep disorders are loosely classified as **parasomnias** (disruptions of the sleep state) and **dyssomnias** (problems with initiating and maintaining sleep: the subject of this discussion). Parasomnias include conditions such as night terrors, sleep talking, sleepwalking, and REM sleep behaviors: the person essentially acts out dreams. The most common dyssomnias among adults are the following:

- *Insomnia*. Literally, this means lack of sleep. Insomnia can involve difficulty falling asleep, difficulty staying asleep, or difficulty sleeping long enough for the body to get the rest it needs. Insomnia can be transient, in which case it occurs for less than 4 weeks at a time, or chronic, in which a person can't sleep most nights for more than a month at a time.

  Transient insomnia is usually attributable to habits or environmental issues that are controllable. Caffeine taken too close to bedtime, alcohol, and some medications, including diet pills, antihistamines, and antidepressants, can interfere with sleep or reduce the time spent in REM stage. Cigarette smoking can cause a person to wake up too early from nicotine withdrawal.

  Unhelpful environmental conditions include having a room that is too cold, too hot, too loud, or too light; having a bed partner who snores or moves around a lot in the night; exercising too late in the day, or not exercising at all.

  Emotional stress is of course another major contributor to sleep loss. Ironically, the longer a person lies in bed feeling the need to sleep, the less likely he or she is to drop off: the stress of being impatient for sleep ensures that it doesn't come.

  Chronic insomnia is usually examined as a sign of a medical or psychological problem. Hyperthyroidism, fibromyalgia, depression, kidney failure, heart problems, and chronic fatigue syndrome are all possible factors when a person doesn't sleep well or long enough.

- *Obstructive sleep apnea*. Obstructive sleep apnea is a mechanical problem in which the air passage collapses when muscles relax, so that oxygen cannot enter during inhalation. When oxygen levels fall sufficiently, muscles tighten slightly, and air reenters the passageway with a loud snort or gasp. Repeated episodes may occur dozens or even hundreds of time each night. People with obstructive sleep apnea tend to have excessive daytime sleepiness and morning headache from oxygen deprivation.
- *Central sleep apnea*. Central sleep apnea is a neurologic problem involving decreased respiratory drive. A rise in carbon dioxide in the blood is the signal to waken and breathe again. In some extreme cases, central sleep apnea has caused brain damage or even death from respiratory arrest during sleep. This condition is often linked to heart disease.
- *Restless leg syndrome*. This disorder often runs in families, and it can also be associated with several other conditions, including pregnancy, diabetes, anemia, fibromyalgia, and ADHD. It involves a constant crawling, prickling, tingling sensation in the extremities, especially the legs, that is relieved only by rubbing and movement. It is closely related to another disorder called **periodic limb movement disorder**, in which a person experiences repeated involuntary jerking movements of the legs every 20 to 40 seconds.

  Although restless leg syndrome is present at all times, its symptoms are most pronounced when a person lies still in an effort to sleep. It is relieved by movement, massaging the affected areas, or warm baths. Symptoms tend to subside in the morning.

- *Narcolepsy*. This chronic neurological dysfunction gets its name from the Greek narco for stupor and lepsis for seizure. It involves unpredictable "sleep attacks" at inappropriate times, often in response to intense emotional reactions such as laughing or anger.

  Narcolepsy has three basic symptoms, which can appear in any combination for a positive diagnosis. **Cataplexy** refers to a sudden loss of muscle tone, even during waking hours. These events can last anywhere from several seconds to 30 minutes. Sleep paralysis is a phenomenon in which a person temporarily cannot speak or move while dozing. **Hypnagogic hallucinations** occur while drifting off to sleep. Narcolepsy patients often have poor nighttime sleep, which adds to a general problem with drowsiness during the day.

- *Circadian rhythm disruption*. The circadian rhythm is the normal cycle of drowsiness and wakefulness that all humans experience. Most people run through this cycle every 24 to 25 hours. They feel drowsy as the sun goes down, and wider awake as it rises. When people are forced to be physically or mentally active in a different cycle, their circadian rhythms are disrupted and the quality of their sleep, as well as the quality of their waking hours, is compromised.

Circadian rhythm disruption can occur in response to variable shift work, losing a night's sleep, or changing time zones through travel. Short-term difficulties associated with this problem are excessive sleepiness along with the degenerating reflexes and mental functioning that accompany exhaustion. Longer term problems can include depression and other physical and psychological disorders brought about by sleep deprivation.

Signs and Symptoms

The primary sign of a sleep disorder is excessive daytime sleepiness. Chronic sleep deprivation can also cause irritability, decreased ability to focus or concentrate, mood changes, and poor short-term memory. Other symptoms are associated with specific disorders, as described above.

Treatment

Cases of transient insomnia are treated with lifestyle changes that better support healthy sleep, including changes in diet and exercise habits, quitting smoking, adjusting temperature or sound levels in the bedroom, or other simple interventions.

The active ingredient in many over-the-counter sleep aids is usually an antihistamine, which has a diminishing effect over time. Prescription sleep aids can be helpful for short periods, but several of them are habit forming, so short-term use to reestablish a healthy sleep cycle is the preferred strategy.

Sleep apnea can be treated in a variety of ways. A mask to provide oxygen or continuous positive airway pressure may be used, or surgery to keep airways open may be conducted. Apnea patients should not sleep on their back, and if they are overweight, they should work to lose weight and reduce their risk of apnea complications. It is especially important that sleep apnea patients not drink alcohol or use sleep aids at night; these substances may interfere with their already challenged breathing mechanisms.

Restless leg syndrome is believed to be associated with dopamine deficiencies in certain brain areas. It is managed with dopamine agents, tranquilizers, and for very extreme cases, opioids and anticonvulsants. Less severe cases of restless leg syndrome can be managed with mild exercise, warm baths, and massage.

Narcolepsy is treatable with some medications and increasing exercise, which has been seen to reduce the number of sleep attacks.

Medications

- Over-the-counter sleep aids
- Benzodiazepines
- Nonbenzodiazepines
- Antianxiety medications
- Antidepressants
- Barbituates (rarely)
- Parkinson drugs for restless leg syndrome
- Stimulants and depressants for narcolepsy

Massage?

RISKS Massage has no particular risk for clients with sleep disorders.

BENEFITS Massage has been shown to assist people who are anxious or in pain to get to sleep, and to increase the amount of time spent in deep sleep. In addition, a massage therapist may be able to identify the risk of obstructive sleep apnea through the characteristic lack of breath followed by a gasping snore pattern in dozing clients.

Vestibular Balance Disorders

Definition: What Are They?

Vestibular balance disorders (VBD) are a group of conditions that can cause the vestibular branch of Cranial Nerve VIII to dysfunction, leading to debilitating vertigo that may last anywhere from a few seconds to many hours. They are most common in elders, for whom the risk of accidental death from balance-related falls is high.

Etiology: What Happens?

The vestibulocochlear nerve (CN VIII) terminates in the inner ear in two segments. The cochlear branch goes to the cochlea, where sound vibrations are transmitted to the brain for interpretation. The vestibular

Vestibular Balance Disorders in Brief

Pronunciation: ves-TIB-yu-lar BAL-ens dis-OR-derz

What are they?
Vestibular balance disorders (VBD) are problems with the vestibulocochlear nerve (CN VIII). They can be related to infection, inflammation, tiny calcium deposits, or other causes.

How are they recognized?
Vertigo, a sensation that the world is spinning, is the leading symptom of VBD. This may be accompanied by nausea, vomiting, and nystagmus.

Massage risks and benefits
Risks: The main risk for a client with any kind of VBD is that getting on, getting off, or rolling over on a table may exacerbate symptoms. Any bodywork session must be designed to minimize this possibility.
Benefits: As long as they are comfortable with positioning and any movements called for during a massage, bodywork is safe and appropriate for clients with VBD.

branch goes to the vestibule, an area of the inner ear where the semicircular canals converge. Vestibular nerve endings are suspended in fluid, and they sway like seaweed whenever the head moves or tilts in any direction. This information, when correlated with sensation from the eyes and general proprioceptors all over the body, provides our sense of position in relation to gravity and the horizon. Although CN VIII is encased within the cranium, technically it is part of the peripheral nervous system.

Changes in the vestibule or other problems with the vestibular branch of CN VIII can lead to vertigo: a sensation of uncontrollable spinning. These changes can be related to fluid pressure as seen with Ménière disease, which is discussed elsewhere, or to inflammation, injury, calcium deposits that fall out of place, or other factors.

Less common causes of VBD focus on the CNS. These include stroke, tumors, multiple sclerosis, aneurysm, or migraine headaches. Allergies that block the eustachian tubes can interfere with fluid in the inner ear. Drugs, including alcohol, barbiturates, antihypertensives, diuretics, and cocaine, can also cause vertigo.

Types of Vestibular Balance Disorders

- *Benign paroxysmal positional vertigo.* In this common condition, small grains of calcium called otoconia that are normally held within the vestibule are displaced into the semicircular canals. This causes a sudden onset of extreme vertigo that may last a few seconds to a few minutes. Special maneuvers of the head allow the otoconia to move back into the vestibule.
- *Labyrinthitis.* This is inflammation within the bony or membranous labyrinth. It is usually related to a self-limiting viral infection, sometimes with herpes zoster (the same virus seen with shingles and Ramsay-Hunt syndrome). This condition typically lasts a few days or weeks and then gradually subsides.
- *Acute vestibular neuronitis.* This is inflammation of the vestibular portion of CN VIII. If the cochlear branch is affected, hearing loss may develop along with vertigo. This can be a complication of a viral or bacterial infection, or of autoimmune activity.
- *Perilymph fistula.* Blows to the head, violent sneezing, or whiplash-type accidents can cause inner ear fluid to leak into the middle ear in a condition called perilymph fistula. This can also occur while scuba diving, when it is called barotrauma.

Signs and Symptoms

VBD cause vertigo (a sensation of spinning), dizziness (a sensation of disequilibrium), lightheadedness (a sensation of floating or faintness), blurred vision, and sometimes nausea and gastrointestinal upset. Nystagmus (abnormal rhythmic oscillations of the eyes) is predictable as well. Changes to blood pressure and heart rate sometimes occur.

Treatment

Treatment for VBD depends on what the contributing factors are determined to be. Benign paroxysmal positional vertigo is treated with appropriate head maneuvers; medication is usually not necessary. Labyrinthitis and acute vestibular neuronitis are treated with drugs to control nausea and vomiting and exercises to help the CNS adapt to changes in sensation. These exercises have been found to be extremely helpful in managing vertigo and have the added benefit of giving elders more confidence to avoid falls. Other forms of vertigo are treated according to underlying causes.

Medications

- Benzodiazepines to suppress vertigo symptoms
- Antiemetics to manage nausea
- Antivirals for viral infection
- Antibiotics for bacterial infection
- Steroidal anti-inflammatories for autoimmune dysfunction

Massage?

RISKS The biggest threat for a person with vestibular balance disorders who wants to get a massage is getting on and off the table, and rolling over. Any of these postural changes may trigger an attack, so the client and therapist must work together to strategize how to minimize this risk.

BENEFITS People who live in fear of "dizzy spells" may develop postural habits that are inefficient and that cause pain. Massage, as long as it doesn't threaten to cause an episode of vertigo, can help with some of these compensatory patterns.

OPTIONS Trigger points in neck muscles have been seen to create symptoms of vertigo; this is treatable with focused massage.

CHAPTER REVIEW QUESTIONS: NERVOUS SYSTEM CONDITIONS

1. What is the difference between spastic and flaccid paralysis? Where in the nervous system does each indicate damage?
2. Why is amyotrophic lateral sclerosis safe for some types of massage?
3. What are the key organs involved in the HPA axis? What conditions have a dysfunctional HPA axis as a feature?
4. Why is massage indicated for Bell palsy when it is contraindicated for most other types of paralysis?
5. Is postpolio syndrome contagious? Why or why not?
6. How can a person who has spinal cord damage at C6 still have control of his or her head and neck?
7. A client is recovering from a major stroke. What are some of the key criteria on which to base a judgment about the appropriateness of Swedish massage?
8. Can a person who has had chickenpox catch herpes zoster from another person? Why or why not?
9. A person with CRPS may have poor circulation and bluish skin in the affected area. Is it appropriate to massage him or her here? Why or why not?
10. What is the main risk for a client with a vestibular balance disorder who wants to receive massage?

References

1. Sapolsky RM. Why Zebras Don't Get Ulcers, 3rd ed. (c) 2004 by Robert M. Sapolsky. p 272.
2. CRPS RSD Overview. (c) 1997-2011 American RSDHope. URL: http://www.rsdhope.org

5

Circulatory System Conditions

Chapter Objectives

After reading this chapter, you should be able to . . .

- Name two deficiencies that may cause nutritional anemia.
- Name the most likely final destination for loose blood clots on the venous side of the systemic circuit.
- Name three possible destinations for loose blood clots or other debris on the arterial side of the systemic circuit.
- Identify the most likely consequence of untreated hemophilia.
- Name two signs or symptoms of deep vein thrombosis.
- Name the tissue that is damaged first in chronic hypertension.
- Name three controllable risk factors for the development of atherosclerosis.
- Name the difference between primary and secondary Raynaud syndrome.
- Name two factors that determine the severity of a heart attack.
- Describe how right-sided heart failure can develop as a result of left-sided heart failure.

Introduction

The body's cells are highly specialized and complex. Most of them are fixed: unable to move toward nutrition or away from wastes. They depend on the circulatory system for constant delivery of food and fuel, and the carrying away of garbage. Suppose a person needed hired help to get to the grocery store and to flush the toilets and take out the trash. What would happen if that service was interrupted? That is the scenario behind many circulatory system disorders. Massage may promote circulatory health, but under certain circumstances it can also interrupt or interfere with this service: it is the therapist's job to determine which modalities are likely to be a help or a hindrance for clients with circulatory dysfunctions.

General Function: The Circulatory System

Diffusion, the random distribution of particles throughout an environment, is the main mechanism for the exchange of nutrients and wastes at the cellular level. Diffusion requires that substances be able to move freely: blood and lymph comprise the perfect medium for this process. An average adult human body contains about 23 L of combined blood and lymph. In every milliliter of it particles flow, chemicals react, and life happens.

The circulatory system, through the medium of the blood, works to maintain **homeostasis**: the tendency to maintain a stable internal environment. It does this in a number of different ways:

- *Delivery of nutrients and oxygen.* The blood carries nutrients and oxygen to every cell in the body. If for some reason the blood can't reach a specific area, cells there starve and die. This is the situation with many disorders, including stroke, heart attack, pulmonary embolism (PE), renal infarction, and decubitus ulcers.
- *Removal of waste products.* While dropping off nutrients, the blood, along with lymph, picks up the waste products generated by metabolism. These include carbon dioxide and more noxious compounds that can cause problems if left in the tissues. Again, if blood and lymph supply to an area is limited, the affected cells can drown in their own waste products.
- *Temperature.* Superficial blood vessels dilate when it's hot, and they constrict when it's cold. Furthermore, blood prevents the hot places (the heart, the liver, working muscles) from getting too hot by distributing the heated blood throughout the body. In this way, the circulatory system helps to maintain a stable internal temperature.
- *Clotting.* Every time a rough place develops in the endothelium of a blood vessel, a complicated chain of chemical reactions results in the spinning of tiny fibers from plasma proteins. These nets catch cells to plug any possible gaps. Unfortunately, in certain circumstances, this reaction causes more problems than it solves.
- *Protection from pathogens.* Without white blood cells we would have no defense against the hordes of microorganisms that try to gain access to the body's precarious internal environment. This is discussed in more detail in the introduction to Chapter 6.
- *Chemical balance.* The body has a narrow margin of tolerance for variances in internal chemistry. Happily, blood components, including red blood cells (RBCs), are supplied with enzymes and other buffers specifically designed to keep pH balance within the safety zone.

Structure and Function: The Heart

The heart is divided by the **septum** into left and right halves. The right half pumps blood to the lungs (the pulmonary circuit), and the left half pumps to the rest of the body (the systemic circuit). Each half of the heart is further divided into top and bottom. The small top chambers, where blood returning from the lungs and body enters, are called the **atria** (the singular form is **atrium** from the Latin for entrance hall), and the larger bottom chambers are the **ventricles** (from the Latin for belly). The two-part "lub-dup" of the heartbeat is the closing of the valves that separate the chambers from each other and the ventricles from the arteries leaving the heart.

The cardiac muscle of the atria is much thinner and weaker than that of the ventricles. This is because the atrial contraction has to push blood only a few centimeters downhill into the ventricles. The cardiac muscle of the ventricles is thicker and stronger than that found in the atria because the ventricular contraction pushes blood into the circulatory system—through the pulmonary circuit to the lungs from the right ventricle, and through the systemic circuit to the rest of the body from the left ventricle. The differences in the workload of various parts of the heart have great implications for the seriousness of **myocardial infarctions** (heart attacks); the location of the damaged tissue determines how well the heart will function without it.

Structure and Function: Blood Vessels

The vessels leaving the heart are called arteries and arterioles; the vessels going toward the heart are called venules and veins; the vessels that connect them are called capillaries. Ideally this should be a closed system. That is, although white blood cells are free to come and go through capillary walls, the RBCs should never be able to leave the 60,000 miles of continuous tubing that constitutes the circulatory system. If they do leak out, it means that the system has an injury, and a blood clot should be forming.

Arteries and veins share the basic properties of most of the tubes in the body. They have an internal layer of epithelium (it's called endothelium here because it's on the inside); this layer is called the **tunica intima**, or inside coat. The middle layer (**tunica media**) is made of smooth muscle; and the external layer of tough, protective connective tissue is called the **tunica externa**, or the **adventitia**. This combination of tissues makes these tubes strong, pliable, and stretchy.

Capillaries are delicate variations of basic tube construction. As the arteries divide into smaller arterioles, their outer layers get thinner and thinner. Finally, all that is left is one layer of simple squamous epithelium wrapped with smooth muscle cells. This construction is ideal for the passage of substances back and forth, because most diffusion happens readily through single-cell layers. But because capillaries lack the tougher muscle and connective tissue layers of the larger tubes, they are much more vulnerable to injury.

Blood cells leave the heart through the thick-walled arteries, crowd into arterioles, and line up one by one to squeeze through the capillaries. Once they've dumped their cargo of oxygen and picked up some carbon dioxide, they have more room; now they're in the venules. Again the three-ply construction design is present, but with a difference. Much of the venous system operates against gravity. Blood flows upward in the legs, the arms, and the trunk, partly by indirect pressure exerted by the heart on the arterial system, but also with the help of hydrostatic pressure and muscular contraction. To help the blood move against gravity, small epithelial flaps called valves line the veins. The smooth muscle layer here is thinner and weaker than in the arteries, which have to cope with much higher pressure coming directly from the heart. Veins get wider, bigger, and stronger as they approach the heart, but they are never as strong as arteries.

When blood returns from the body to the heart (the systemic circuit), it goes to the lungs to be oxygenated (the pulmonary circuit) (Figure 5.1).

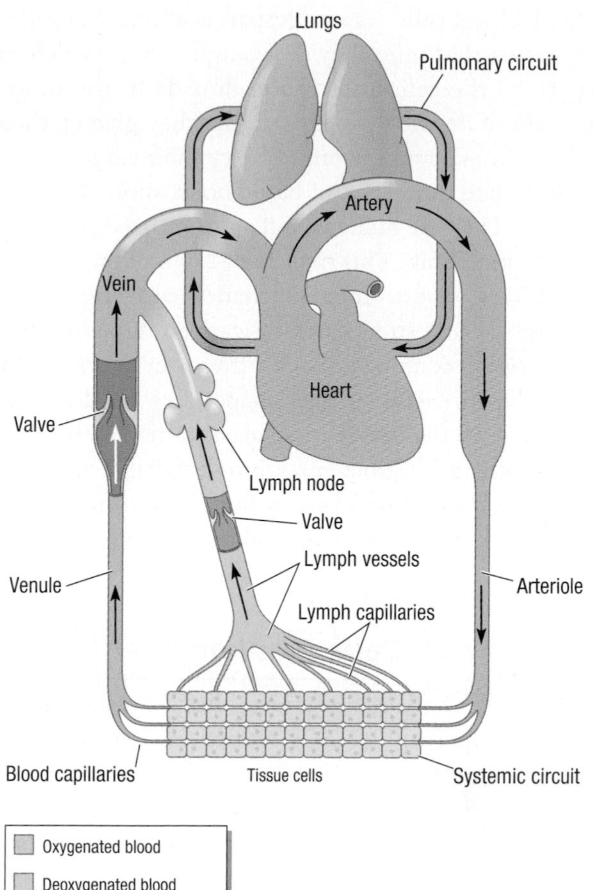

Figure 5.1. The circulatory and pulmonary circuits

Structure and Function: The Blood

Red Blood Cells (Erythrocytes)

Almost all blood cells, red and white alike, are made in the red bone marrow. RBCs are created at the command of a hormone secreted by the kidneys called **erythropoietin** (EPO). They are in constant turnover, some being released and others dying at a rate of about 2 million per second. They comprise

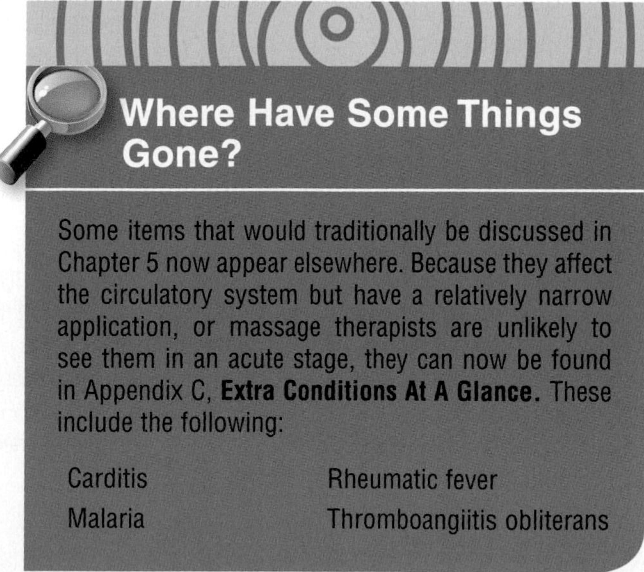

Where Have Some Things Gone?

Some items that would traditionally be discussed in Chapter 5 now appear elsewhere. Because they affect the circulatory system but have a relatively narrow application, or massage therapists are unlikely to see them in an acute stage, they can now be found in Appendix C, **Extra Conditions At A Glance.** These include the following:

Carditis	Rheumatic fever
Malaria	Thromboangiitis obliterans

98% of blood cells. Their lifespan is about 4 months, and during that time they do a single job: they deliver oxygen to the cells and carbon dioxide to the lungs. They are so devoted to this task that they give up their nuclei to make more room to carry their cargo.

RBCs are tiny; 1 mL of blood holds about 5 million of them. They are built around an iron-based molecule called hemoglobin. This molecule (250 million of them in each RBC) is extremely efficient at carrying oxygen and slightly less so at carrying carbon dioxide; most CO_2 is dissolved in plasma. Another characteristic feature of healthy RBCs is their shape: they are discs that are thinner in the middle than around the edges. They are smooth and flexible enough to bend and distort to get through the tiniest capillaries. If for some reason they are not round, smooth, and flexible, big problems ensue.

White Blood Cells (Leukocytes)

Leukocytes aren't really white; they're more or less transluscent. Unlike RBCs, which are all identical, different classes of white blood cells fight off different types of invaders in different stages of infection; this is discussed further in Chapter 6. White blood cells include neutrophils, basophils, eosinophils, monocytes, and lymphocytes (Figure 5.2).

Platelets (Thrombocytes)

Thrombocytes are not whole cells, but fragments of huge cells that are born in the red bone marrow. They are usually smooth, but when they are stimulated, they quickly become spiky and sticky. Thrombocytes travel the system looking for leaks or rough places in the blood vessels. If they find one, they secrete chemicals that trigger tiny threads of fibrin to be woven from plasma proteins in the injured area. These fibers act as a net to catch passing RBCs, forming a crust on the skin or a clot (thrombus) internally.

Blood Disorders

Anemia

Definition: What Is It?

While the term "an-emia" suggests lack of blood, it actually means shortage of red blood cells (RBCs), or

Circulatory System Conditions

Blood Disorders

- Anemia
  - Idiopathic anemia
  - Nutritional anemia
  - Hemorrhagic anemia
  - Hemolytic anemia
  - Aplastic anemia
  - Secondary anemia
- Embolism, thrombus
  - Pulmonary embolism
  - Arterial thrombus
  - Arterial embolism
- Hemophilia
  - Type A hemophilia
  - Type B hemophilia
  - Von Willebrand disease
- Leukemia
  - Acute myeloid leukemia
  - Chronic myeloid leukemia
  - Acute lymphoid leukemia
  - Chronic lymphoid leukemia
- Myeloma
  - Multiple myeloma
  - Solitary myeloma
  - Extramedullary plastocytoma
- Sickle cell disease
- Thrombophlebitis, deep vein thrombosis

Vascular Disorders

- Aneurysm
  - Saccular aneurysm
  - Fusiform aneurysm
  - Berry aneurysm
  - Dissecting aneurysm
- Atherosclerosis
  - Coronary artery disease
  - Carotid artery disease
  - Peripheral artery disease
- Hypertension
  - Essential hypertension
  - Secondary hypertension
  - Malignant hypertension
- Raynaud syndrome
  - Raynaud disease
  - Raynaud phenomenon
- Varicose veins
  - Esophageal varices
  - Hemorrhoids
  - Telangiectasias
  - Varicoceles

Heart Conditions

- Heart attack
- Heart failure
  - Left-sided heart failure
  - Right-sided heart failure
  - Biventricular heart failure

Anemia in Brief

Pronunciation: ah-NE-me-ah

What is it?
Anemia is a symptom rather than a disease in itself. It indicates a shortage of red blood cells (RBCs), hemoglobin, or both.

How is it recognized?
Symptoms of anemia include pallor, shortness of breath, fatigue, and poor resistance to cold. Other symptoms accompany specific types of anemia.

Massage risks and benefits

Risks: Anemia can sometimes cause neurological damage; this has implications for massage. Any anemia due to bone marrow suppression, inflammation, or premature destruction of RBCs requires that massage be adjusted to meet any limitations set by the underlying pathologies.

Benefits: Massage for idiopathic or nutritional anemia may be safe, but it is unlikely to change the course of this condition.

shortage of hemoglobin. Either way, oxygen-carrying capacity is limited. Anemia by itself is not a diagnosis; it is a description. The diagnosis is made when it is determined why a shortage of RBCs or hemoglobin has developed.

Etiology: What Happens?

RBCs are the most plentiful cells in the body, and healthy erythrocytes are packed full of a molecule called hemoglobin. Hemoglobin, built around iron, binds well with oxygen. This allows RBCs to pick up oxygen from the lungs, and deliver it to the tissues. When anemia develops, either a shortage of RBCs or a shortage or dysfunction of hemoglobin interrupts this important process.

Several kinds of anemia exist, depending on underlying conditions or other factors. Some of the most common varieties are discussed here.

Types of Anemia

- *Idiopathic anemia.* This condition, which has no well-understood cause, may be due to poor nutritional uptake due to stress, or other factors.
- *Nutritional anemias.* These occur because the body is missing something vital in its diet. Iron deficiency may be the most common version, affecting women much more often than men because women need about twice as much iron, but take in fewer calories (Figure 5.3). Folic acid is a nutrient found in green leafy vegetables that is critical for the formation of RBCs. Because it is water soluble, folic acid can't be stored; a steady supply is necessary.

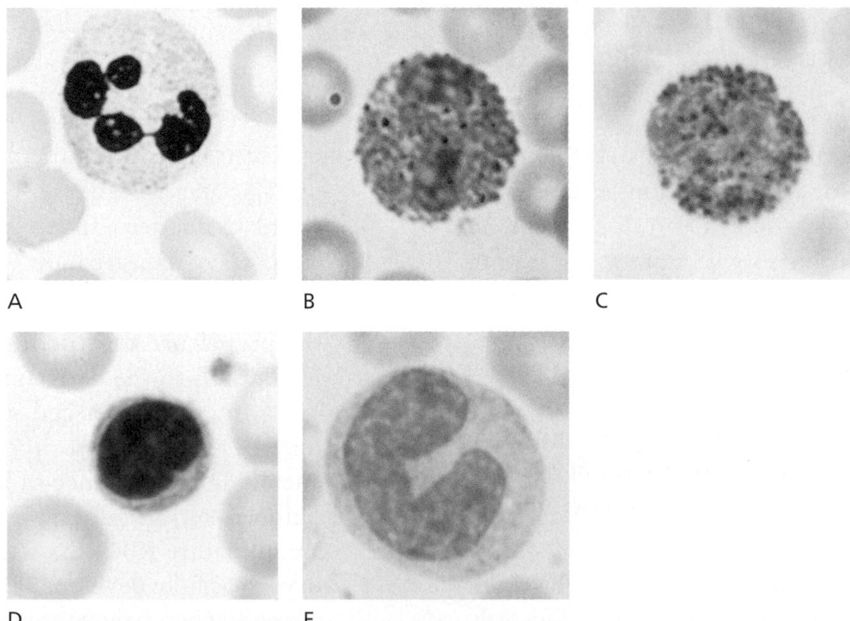

Figure 5.2. Different types of white blood cells

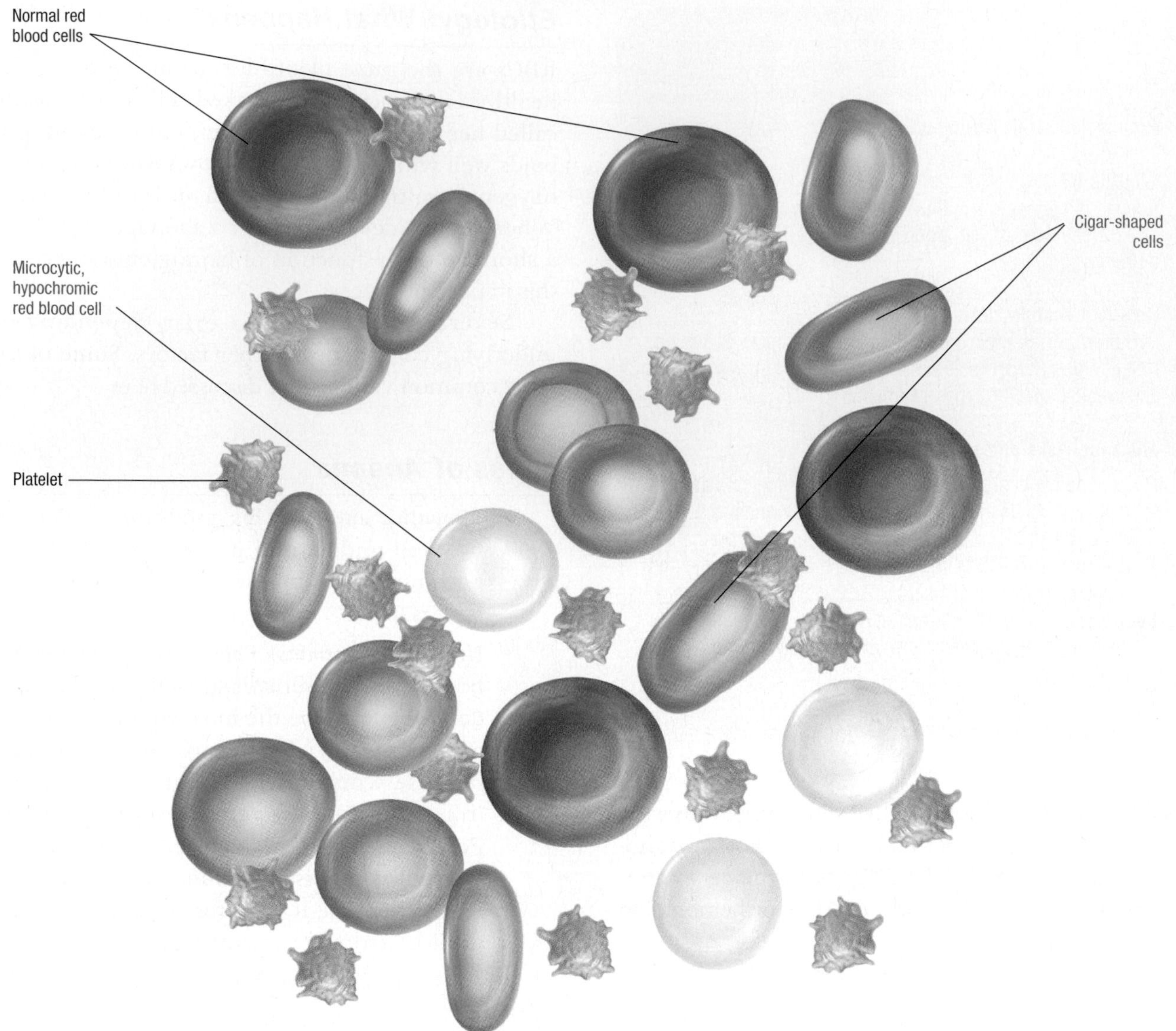

Figure 5.3. Iron deficiency anemia

Folic acid anemia is usually related to dietary insufficiency or malabsorption. Vitamin B_{12} is also necessary for RBC production. A B_{12} shortage or problems with uptake can lead to a serious complication called **pernicious anemia**. Because B_{12} is also critical to the maintenance of the central nervous system, a person with this deficiency experiences the slow onset of paralysis, loss of proprioception, and brain damage. Anemia can also be the result of shortages of several other substances, notably copper and protein.

- *Hemorrhagic anemias.* These are brought about by blood loss. Often the bleeding is a slow leak, but it can also be from trauma; this is acute hemorrhagic anemia. The most common causes are gastric or duodenal ulcers, chronic kidney problems, heavy menstruation, and large wounds.
- *Hemolytic anemias.* These are characterized by the premature destruction of healthy RBCs. In addition to the basic symptoms of anemia, **splenomegaly** (enlarged spleen) and jaundice may be present. Another sign of hemolytic anemia is the presence of higher than normal numbers of **reticulocytes** in the blood. These are immature RBCs that cannot carry as much oxygen as fully developed RBCs; their numbers increase when oxygen-carrying capacity is low.

- *Aplastic anemia*. In aplastic anemia, bone marrow activity is sluggish or nonexistent. The production of every kind of blood cell is slowed or suspended. Anemia develops with low RBC count, along with impaired immunity and bleeding problems that develop with insufficient thrombocytes. Aplastic anemia can be caused by autoimmune attack against bone marrow, renal failure, folate deficiency, certain viral infections, exposure to radiation, and exposure to some environmental toxins, including lead and benzene.

  Myelodysplastic anemia is closely related to aplastic anemia, but in this case, the bone marrow makes multitudes of abnormal cells rather than being suppressed altogether. This can be a precancerous condition that indicates a risk of leukemia or myeloma.
- *Secondary anemias*. Anemia is a frequent complication of other disorders. Sometimes a direct cause-and-effect relationship is obvious, and sometimes the association is a less clear. A partial list of the conditions that anemia frequently accompanies includes the following:
  - *Ulcers*. Gastric, duodenal, and colonic ulcers can all bleed internally. This may not be very obvious, but it results in a steady draining of RBCs, which can impair general oxygen uptake and energy levels. This is a type of hemorrhagic anemia, discussed earlier.
  - *Kidney disease*. When kidney capillaries are damaged, they can leak RBCs into the urine. The kidneys also secrete a hormone that stimulates bone marrow to produce RBCs (**erythropoietin**). When the kidneys are not functioning well, EPO levels drop and RBC production goes down.
  - *Hepatitis*. The liver contributes vital proteins to the blood, and it is responsible, with the spleen, for breaking down and recycling the iron from dead erythrocytes. If liver function is disrupted for any reason, the quality and amount of hemoglobin available to new RBCs may decline.
  - *Acute infection*. Anemia is sometimes an indicator that the body is under attack. It is a frequent follower of pneumonia, tuberculosis, or other infection. Anemia in these cases usually clears up spontaneously, once the primary condition has been resolved.
  - *Leukemia, myeloma, lymphoma*. In these conditions, masses of nonfunctional white blood cells are produced in bone marrow or in lymphatic tissues. These white blood cells essentially crowd out functional RBCs.

Signs and Symptoms

No matter what the cause of anemia is, some signs and symptoms are consistent. These include the following:

- *Fatigue*. Often this is the first noticeable symptom of anemia. Less oxygen is available, so muscles tire sooner and stamina is compromised.
- *Pallor*. Pallor is present because of a reduced number of RBCs, or a reduced amount of hemoglobin to carry the oxygen that gives the RBCs their color. Pallor is visible in the skin and in mucous membranes, gums, and nail beds. In dark-skinned people, pallor shows as an ashy-gray appearance on the skin.
- *Dyspnea, rapid breathing*. Dyspnea is a symptom of anemia because with less oxygen-carrying capacity, a person has to breathe more rapidly.
- *Rapid heartbeat*. Another term for this is tachycardia. This allows blood to travel faster through the body in an attempt to deliver adequate oxygen.
- *Intolerance to cold*. Without adequate oxygen for rapid or sustained muscle contractions (i.e., shivering), cold becomes overwhelming very quickly.
- *Heart problems*. Aplastic anemia can cause arrhythmia, cardiomegaly, and heart failure as the circulatory system tries to cope with fewer blood cells of all types.

Treatment

Anemia is treated according to its cause. Anemia triggered by exposure to a specific substance is treated by removing the offending agent. Other interventions range from nutritional supplements to medications, transfusions, stem cell transplants, or other strategies to correct the underlying conditions.

Medications

- Oral or injected nutritional supplements for nutritional anemias
- Steroidal anti-inflammatories for autoimmune hemolytic anemias
- Synthetic EPO to boost RBC production

Massage?

RISKS Anemia contraindicates massage when it accompanies other disorders that may be negatively affected. Specifically, if pernicious anemia has resulted in a decrease in sensation, or if anemia is due to acute infection, cancer, or other serious diseases, bodywork must be conducted with caution and as a part of an integrated healthcare strategy.

BENEFITS Massage may help with the fatigue that anemia brings about, but it makes no lasting changes in blood cell production or nutrition. A client who manages anemia successfully can enjoy the same benefits from massage as the rest of the population.

Embolism, Thrombus

Definition: What Are They?

An embolism is a traveling clot or collection of debris, and thrombus is a lodged clot (Figure 5.4). Thrombi and emboli that form on the arterial side of the systemic circuit are usually part of a wider cardiovascular disease picture that includes hypertension, atherosclerosis, and a risk of heart attack.

Thrombi that form on the venous side of the systemic circuit are discussed in detail in the *Thrombophlebitis, Deep Vein Thrombosis* section of this chapter.

Etiology: What Happens?

Blood leaves the left ventricle of the heart via the aorta and goes to its destination through smaller and smaller vessels: arteries, arterioles, and finally capillaries. Nutrient-waste exchange happens at the capillary level, and then the vessels get bigger and bigger as they lead back toward the heart: from venules to veins to the vena cava. The same telescoping action happens in the pulmonary circuit: de-oxygenated blood leaves the right ventricle through the huge pulmonary artery, and vessels going into the lungs get smaller and smaller. Oxygen and carbon dioxide are exchanged in capillaries in the lungs, and the freshly oxygenated blood goes back toward the heart through venules, veins, and finally the large pulmonary vein.

Platelets constantly flow through the whole system looking for rough spots, which indicate injury. If they find any disruption in the walls of the blood vessels, they quickly develop spikes and stick to that spot. Then they release the chemicals that cause blood proteins to weave fibers, making a net to catch other blood cells: a clot is formed. Clots can also form anywhere blood doesn't flow quickly; clotting factors thicken nonmoving blood, even without an injury to initiate the action. Tiny clots are constantly formed

Embolism, Thrombus in Brief

Pronunciation: EM-bo-lizm, THROM-bus

What are they?
Thrombi are stationary clots; emboli are clots that travel. Emboli are usually composed of blood, but may also be fragments of plaque, fat globules, air bubbles, tumors, or bone chips.

How are they recognized?
If venous thrombi embolize (break loose), they can only land in the lungs, causing pulmonary embolism (PE). Symptoms of venous thrombi may be subtle or nonexistent. Symptoms of PE include shortness of breath, chest pain, and coughing up blood-streaked sputum.

Arterial side clots can travel anywhere their artery carries them, until the vessel becomes too small to let them pass, leading to damage as cells waiting for oxygen and nutrition die. Some of the most common sites are the coronary arteries (heart attack), the brain (transient ischemic attack or stroke), kidneys (renal infarction), and the legs.

Massage risks and benefits
Risks: Any disorder associated with the potential for lodged or traveling clots contraindicates massage that intends to push fluid or significantly manipulate tissue. Medications used by these patients may also carry cautions for massage.
Benefits: Types of bodywork that invite rather than impose change are most appropriate for clients with the risk of emboli or thrombi. A client who has survived and successfully treated a blood clotting problem can enjoy the same benefits from massage as the rest of the population, as long as cautions for activity levels and medications are respected.

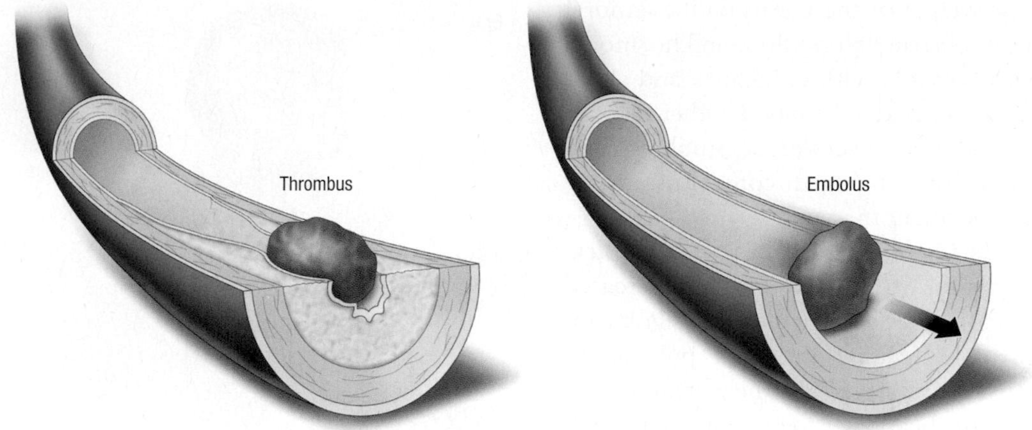

Figure 5.4. A thrombus is a lodged clot; an embolus is a moving piece of debris

and melted, especially on the venous side of the circuit, but sometimes clot-forming mechanisms outwork clot-melting mechanisms.

The construction of the circulatory system does not allow clots to pass through capillaries; clots form, they may break into fragments and travel, but they stay either on the arterial side of the systemic circuit or on the venous side. The damage that ensues depends on the origin of the clot, its size, and where it finally gets stuck.

Types of Thrombus and Embolism

- *Venous thrombosis.* This is discussed in detail in *Thrombophlebitis, Deep Vein Thrombosis.*
- *Pulmonary embolism.* Clots or debris anywhere on the venous side of the systemic circuit can only travel to the lungs (unless the heart has a structural defect called a patent foramen ovale, which allows communication between the left and right sides). When a clot forms and some event—a sudden movement after prolonged immobility, for instance—knocks any debris loose, it travels toward the heart in increasingly large tubes. It goes through the right atrium and ventricle, enters the pulmonary artery, and ends up in the lungs (Figure 5.5). Most pulmonary emboli are fragments that lodge in multiple places in both lungs simultaneously. The extent of damage can vary from a temporary loss of a tiny bit of lung function to total circulatory collapse.

  Risk factors for pulmonary embolism (PE) include other types of cardiovascular disease, recent trauma, extended bed rest, and any kind of surgery: PE is a leading cause of death in hospitals. Women who are pregnant or who have recently given birth are at high risk for

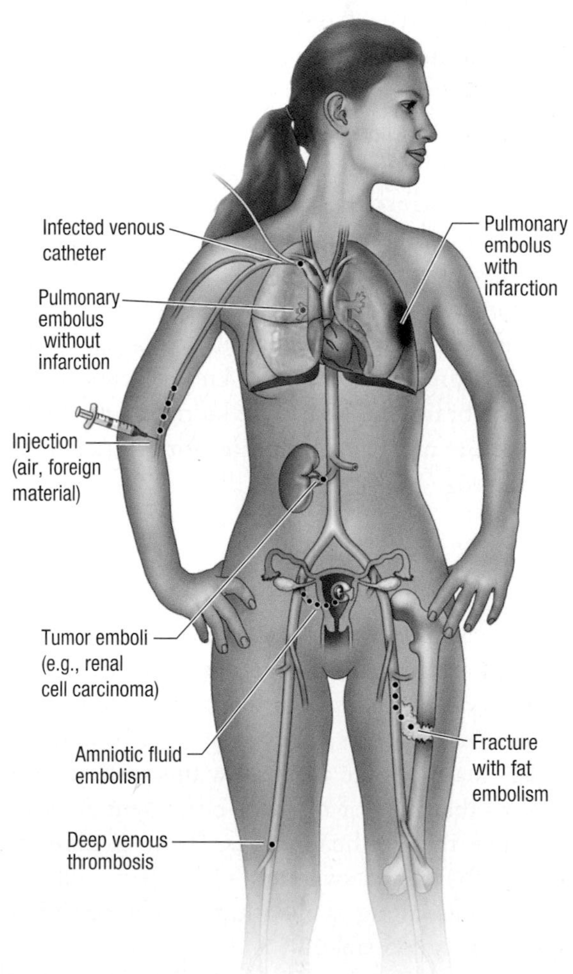

Figure 5.5. Sites of origin for pulmonary emboli

PE, as the weight of the uterus on the femoral vessels can obstruct blood flow, and hormonal changes associated with pregnancy and childbirth can also thicken the blood. Other risk factors include being overweight, smoking, and taking hormones for birth control or as hormone replacement therapy.

PE has some serious possible complications. A person with this history is at increased risk for another event. Further, if a significant amount of lung function is lost, pulmonary hypertension and right-sided heart failure may develop as the heart tries to push blood through the damaged, restricted pulmonary circuit.

- *Arterial Thrombus.* This is one of the many complications of atherosclerosis. Any roughness in the normally smooth artery or arteriole wall can trigger the production of a clot. Chronic inflammation, stress, and other factors can contribute to this as well. Clots can progressively grow to completely obstruct the lumen of the artery, or they can fragment to travel further along the system: this is an arterial embolism.
- *Arterial Embolism.* Arterial emboli can originate as clots or plaques that form with atherosclerosis, or they can be related to atrial **fibrillation** or rheumatic heart disease. Emboli are often composed of clotted blood, but they can be any foreign object in the bloodstream such as a bit of plaque, a bone chip, an air bubble, or a knot of cancer cells. The brain, the heart, the kidneys, and the legs are the most common sites for arterial emboli to lodge (Figure 5.6).

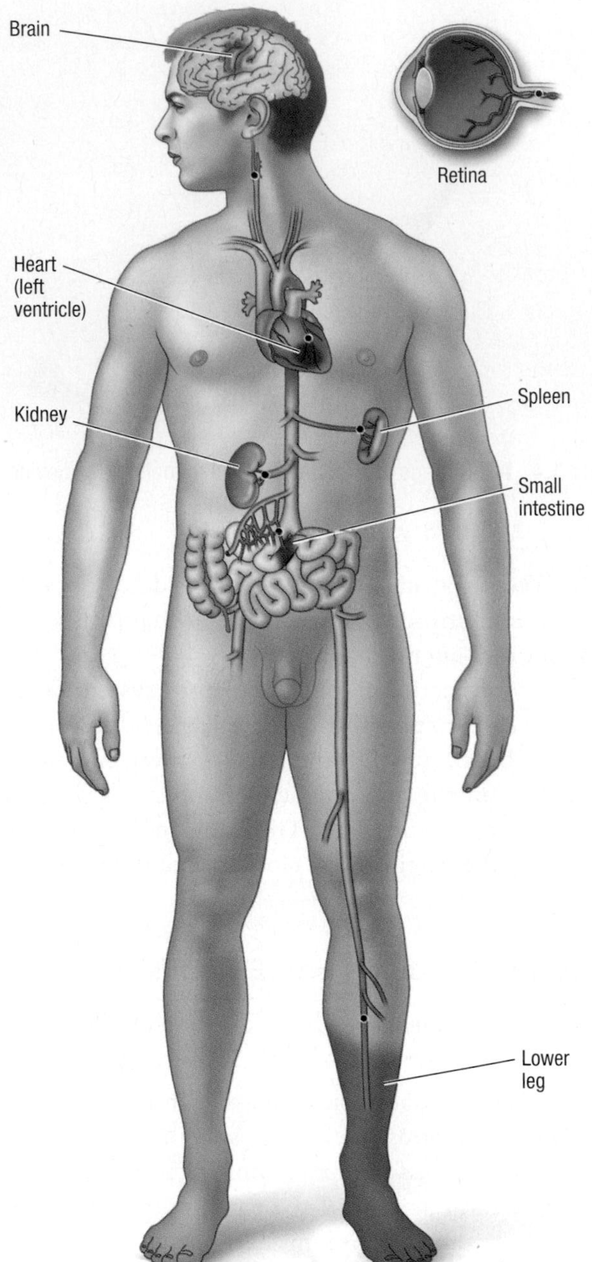

Figure 5.6. Arterial infarction sites

Signs and Symptoms

Many PE cases show no discernible signs or symptoms until after lung damage has occurred. Classic symptoms of PE include difficulty breathing, chest pain, and **hemoptysis** (coughing with bloody sputum), but many people don't show this pattern. Other symptoms that may or may not be present are shortness of breath, lightheadedness, fainting, dizziness, rapid heartbeat, and sweating. Chest pain and chest wall tenderness along with back, shoulder, or abdominal pain are also possible.

Symptoms of arterial emboli in organs may be nonexistent until the affected tissue has significant damage: this is called an **infarction**. This is particularly dangerous in the kidneys, where many tiny clots can come to rest somewhere in the renal arteries, leading to renal failure. If clots lodge in the legs, however, symptoms are sharp pain followed by numbness, weakness, coldness, and blueness. Left untreated, this tissue may become necrotic in a matter of hours; immediate medical attention is necessary.

If the embolus lodges in the brain and the symptoms are short lived, it is called a transient ischemic attack. A more serious brain embolism can cause an ischemic stroke. And finally, if debris lodges in a coronary artery, it's called a heart attack. Stroke and heart attack are discussed in detail elsewhere.

Treatment

The mainstay of treatment for thrombi or emboli is blood thinners, anticoagulants, and thrombolytics. A large clot lodged in the lung may be surgically extracted. When a thrombus in the lower extremity is threatening, a vena cava filter may be surgically implanted to prevent emboli from traveling to the lungs. Patients with damage from pulmonary emboli may supplement oxygen while their lungs heal. People at high risk for clots are counseled to stay well hydrated, and sometimes to use compression stockings that assist in blood flow from the legs back to the abdomen.

Medications

- Blood thinners to reduce the production of new clots
- Anticoagulants to reduce the production of new clots (use is suggested for up to 6 months following an event)
- Thrombolytics to help dissolve existing clots (these carry a high risk of bleeding and so are used sparingly)

Massage?

RISKS The tendency to form clots is a caution for mechanical types of bodywork, both because of the risk of life-threatening emboli and because the medications to treat these disorders have bruising as a possible side effect. Whether that caution is for the whole body or local regions depends on how carefully the condition is being watched and treated, and what kind of bodywork is being given.

BENEFITS Nonmechanical forms of bodywork may be soothing and supportive for clients at risk of thrombus or embolism. It is important that they be under treatment, however.
Clients who have a history of clotting issues but who have no lingering problems can enjoy the same benefits from massage as the rest of the population.

SIDEBAR 5.1 DVT + PE = VTE

The link between deep vein thrombosis (DVT) and pulmonary embolism (PE) is hard to overstate. When the two occur together (which probably happens more often than is officially recognized), the combined condition is called venous **thromboembolism** (VTE). The signs and symptoms for both DVT and PE can be subtle and easily missed: many people with DVT have a mild PE without realizing it, and for 25% of the people who die from PE, death is the first symptom ever recognized. VTE is considered a leading public health issue, killing about 200,000 to 300,000 people each year.

Hemophilia

Definition: What Is It?

Hemophilia is a collection of genetic disorders characterized by the absence of some plasma proteins that are crucial in the clot-forming process.

The mutations that cause most forms of hemophilia are carried on the X chromosome, so males with hemophilia pass the chromosome along to their

Hemophilia in Brief

Pronunciation: he-mo-FELE-e-ah

What is it?
Hemophilia is a genetic disorder in which certain clotting factors in the blood are either insufficient or missing altogether.

How is it recognized?
Hemophilia can cause superficial bleeding that persists for longer than normal, or internal bleeding into joint cavities or between muscle sheaths with little or no provocation.

Massage risks and benefits
Risks: Any bodywork that can accidently stretch or injure delicate tissues (including blood vessels) is risky for clients with severe hemophilia.
Benefits: Very gentle or energetic types of bodywork can help with pain and ease anxiety for clients with severe hemophilia. Clients with mild forms of the disorder who are otherwise healthy can enjoy any massage that fits within their typical daily challenges for physical activity.

daughters, who become carriers. These female carriers pass the mutation on to about half of their sons. It is possible for a girl to have a typically male form of hemophilia, but she would need positive X chromosomes from both her father and mother, and this is very rare.

Etiology: What Happens?

Thrombocytes constantly travel around the circulatory system looking for signs of damage. When they encounter any kind of rough spot inside a blood vessel, they stick to that spot and secrete a series of chemicals that cause plasma proteins to weave nets of fibers called fibrinogen. These nets catch passing platelets and RBCs, forming a plug to limit loss of blood through the damaged vessel. The plasma proteins that weave the fibrinogen have been identified as 12 distinct factors. Hemophilia occurs when a genetic mutation causes a deficiency in one or more of these clotting factors.

A person who is deficient in clotting factors has difficulty in forming a solid, long-lasting clot. Hemophiliacs don't bleed faster than average, but they do bleed longer. Hemophilia is rated as mild, moderate, or severe, depending on what percentage of normal levels of clotting factors the patient has. Severe hemophiliacs, who account for 60% of hemophilia patients, have lower than 1% of normal levels of clotting factors.

While hemophilia is a manageable disease, it has serious potential complications. The leading cause of death for children with this condition is intracranial bleeding: even minor head trauma can cause major bleeding episodes in and around the brain, and this risk continues into adulthood. Bleeding into joint cavities is also a significant problem: unless clotting factors are administered quickly, the blood inside the joint may lead to an inflammatory response that damages cartilage and articulating bones. This condition is called **hemophilic arthritis**, and it occurs most often at the ankles, knees, and elbows.

Bleeding into muscles can cause pain and numbness as nerve endings are compressed. If the pressure is not quickly resolved, the muscle may develop a compartment syndrome or contracture, with a permanent loss of range of motion. The muscles most at risk for **hematomas** are in the calf, thigh, upper arm, and forearm. The psoas is also at risk for deep bleeds and stiffness.

Infected blood products used to be another major worry for people with hemophilia. It is recommended that hemophiliacs and other people who regularly use blood products be vaccinated for hepatitis A and B.

Types of Hemophilia

- *Type A Hemophilia.* This is the most common form of hemophilia, accounting for about 80% of all cases. It is characterized by a deficiency in clotting factor VIII.
- *Type B Hemophilia.* Also called Christmas disease, this is characterized by insufficient levels of factor IX. Hemophilia B accounts for about 15% of hemophilia cases.
- *Von Willebrand disease.* Rather than a shortage of clotting factors from the liver, von Willebrand disease is a dysfunction of **von Willebrand factor**: a substance secreted by damaged endothelium. This substance normally helps platelets to clump together, and helps Factor VIII to do its work. Like Type A or B hemophilia, von Willebrand disease is the result of a genetic mutation. Patients have bleeding problems that range from mild to severe, although the vast majority of cases are very mild, and may go unrecognized. Unlike other forms of hemophilia, von Willebrand disease is not an X-linked disorder, so men and women are affected equally.

Signs and Symptoms

Hemophilia usually appears at birth, when the umbilical cord bleeds excessively, or in early childhood, as babies begin to engage in physical activities that involve minor bangs and bumps. These toddlers are subject to excessive bruising and bleeding with very mild irritation, and small scrapes and lesions tend to bleed for a long time.

As the person matures, he finds that he is prone to subcutaneous bleeding (bruising), intramuscular hemorrhaging (hematomas), nosebleeds (**epistaxis**), blood in the urine (**hematuria**), and severe joint pain brought about by bleeding in joint cavities. Bleeding episodes may follow minor trauma, or they may occur spontaneously.

Treatment

Progress in the production and packaging of clotting factors in a form that can be stored at home and self-administered has radically changed the quality of life for patients with severe hemophilia. Instead of being dependent on whole blood transfusions or the use of blood products, recombinant factors allow patients to be independent enough to be able to work and travel.

Clotting factors can be administered after an injury takes place to limit bleeding into a joint or between muscles. They can also be taken prophylactically on a regular basis or before a procedure like surgery or dental work to limit anticipated bleeding.

People with mild hemophilia A can also treat themselves with an injected or inhaled form of the hormone desmopressin, which stimulates production of extra clotting factor in response to an injury.

In addition to managing bleeding, people with hemophilia are counseled to exercise (although they must obviously avoid contact sports) and to keep their weight under control; both of these can limit the risk of arthritis and muscle contracture.

Medications

- Concentrated clotting factors from donated blood
- Recombinant clotting factors
- Desmopressin to promote clotting factor production
- Antifibrinolytics to slow clot breakdown

Massage?

RISKS Severe hemophilia contraindicates any rigorous bodywork or massage that might cause bruising or bleeding. If a client has this condition, it is wise to consult with his healthcare team to identify other risks.

BENEFITS Gentle or energetic massage is appropriate for clients with severe hemophilia, and this may be a potent way to help with the pain and stress of this complicated condition. For clients with milder forms of the disease, massage may be more rigorous, as long as it fits within their capacity for pressure without bruising.

Leukemia

Definition: What Is It?

Leukemia, or "white blood," is a cancer that affects bone marrow function. Some overlap has been established between types of leukemia that affect lymphoid cells and lymphoma: cancer associated with lymph nodes. Lymphoma is discussed in Chapter 6.

Dozens of types of leukemia have been identified, but this discussion focuses on the four most common classifications. These types of leukemia have much in common, but each has some unique features that are examined under individual headings.

Leukemia is diagnosed in about 38,000 Americans every year. Although this disease is the leading cause of death from cancer in children, it is much more common in adults. Over 200,000 leukemia patients and survivors are living in the United States today.

Leukemia in Brief

Pronunciation: lu-KE-me-ah

What is it?
Leukemia is a collection of blood disorders characterized by overproduction of nonfunctioning white blood cells in bone marrow.

How is it recognized?
Different types of leukemia have unique profiles, but all varieties include signs brought about by low production of normal blood cells: anemia, bruising, bleeding, and poor resistance to infection.

Massage risks and benefits
Risks: Leukemia and its treatments all take a toll on the immune system and blood clotting function. Clients with this disorder are extremely vulnerable to infection, bruising, and other complications.
Benefits: Gentle and noninvasive forms of bodywork can be extremely helpful for pain, anxiety, improved sleep, and other quality-of-life issues for leukemia patients.

Etiology: What Happens?

Two types of stem cells, **myeloid** cells and **lymphoid** cells, manufacture most of our white blood cells in bone marrow. Leukocytes are classified as myeloid or lymphocytic, depending on their origin. Leukemia occurs when a mutation in the DNA of one or more stem cells in the bone marrow causes the production of multitudes of nonfunctioning leukocytes. These cells crowd out the functioning cells in the bone marrow and in the blood. Leukemia can be aggressive and quickly progressive, releasing immature cells into the circulatory system (acute), or it can be slowly progressive, leading to the release of mature but nonfunctioning cells (chronic). In either case, the mutated cells do not function as part of the immune system, and they live far longer than normal cells, leading to dangerous accumulations of nonfunctioning cells.

Studies of cell lineage have revealed that the lymphocytic leukemias that affect T cells, B cells, and natural killer cells are essentially the same as associated forms of lymphoma; the only difference is in whether the targeted cells are stationary or circulating.

The genetic mutations seen with leukemia are usually acquired rather than inherited. Exposure to environmental toxins and radiation are cited most often as contributing factors. Electromagnetic fields are being studied as possible risk factors for leukemia, but results so far are inconclusive. Some forms of leukemia are linked to a congenital problem: Down syndrome and some other genetic anomalies can increase the risk for these diseases.

Untreated leukemia results in death from excessive bleeding or infection.

Types of Leukemia

- *Acute myelogenous leukemia* (AML). This is aggressive cancer of the myeloid cells that mainly affects people over 60 years old. The targeted immature cells are called blast cells, leading to the synonym acute myeloblastic leukemia. Other synonyms are acute myelocytic leukemia and acute granulocytic leukemia. The genetic damage that causes AML has been linked to certain environmental factors. High doses of radiation, chemotherapy for other types of cancer, and exposure to benzene all increase the risk of developing AML in later years. AML cells can congregate to form a tumor outside the bone marrow.
- *Chronic myelogenous leukemia* (CML). This is slowly progressive cancer of the myeloid cells. It is also called chronic granulocytic leukemia and chronic myeloid leukemia. Unlike other forms of leukemia, CML has been traced to a specific dysfunctional chromosome, called the Philadelphia chromosome. It involves the myeloid cells, which include neutrophils, eosinophils, basophils, and monocytes. These faulty cells can interfere with and slow down normal immune system activity, but they do not usually bring it to a halt.

  CML patients often have abdominal pain and an enlarged spleen, as the cancerous cells congregate in this organ. Night sweats, unexpected weight loss, and a decreasing tolerance for warm temperatures are other signs and symptoms common to CML patients. CML occasionally changes its pattern and becomes more aggressive, in which case it is approached as AML.
- *Acute lymphocytic leukemia* (ALL). This is aggressive cancer of the lymphocytes: B cells, T cells, and natural killer cells. ALL is the type of leukemia found most often among children. Synonyms for ALL include acute lymphoid leukemia and acute lymphoblastic leukemia. It usually involves B cell production, although T cells may also be affected.

  The proliferation of cells in a person with ALL is so overwhelming that all other bone marrow activity is suppressed, and immune system function is effectively crippled. Cancerous lymphocytes are released into the blood before they are fully mature. These lymphocytes may gather in lymph nodes, or they may cross into the central nervous system, where they can cause severe headaches, vomiting, and seizures.
- *Chronic lymphocytic leukemia* (CLL). This is slowly progressive cancer of the lymphocytes. Although it can involve T cells or natural killer cells, most cases involve B-cell malignancies. These mutated cells can accumulate in bone marrow and lymph nodes. CLL is especially common among veterans of the Vietnam War who were exposed to Agent Orange. In some cases, CML transforms into an aggressive form of lymphoma.

  Sometimes CLL is so stable and so nonthreatening that no treatment is recommended. If numbers of functioning blood cells drop to dangerous levels, chemotherapy may be recommended, along with radiation to shrink enlarged lymph nodes or other tissues.

Signs and Symptoms

Signs and symptoms of all types of leukemia point to bone marrow dysfunction. When the marrow is sabotaged by a genetic mutation that causes overproduction of nonfunctioning cells, functioning cells are then produced in smaller numbers. A leading sign of leukemia is fatigue and low stamina due to anemia: low numbers of RBCs are available to deliver oxygen to working tissues. A person with leukemia bruises easily, and small cuts and abrasions may bleed for long periods. Unusual bleeding or bruising comes about because platelet production is suppressed (**thrombocytopenia**) and the person has limited ability to make blood clots. Finally, a person with leukemia is susceptible to chronic infections because they are lacking in white blood cells, especially neutrophils: a condition called **neutropenia**. This can manifest as skin infections like hangnails or pimples, or respiratory infections like colds and flu, or chronic urinary tract infections. Whatever the infectious agent is, the person with leukemia has very limited resources to fight it off.

Other general symptoms include fever, headache, weight loss, abdominal pain, and enlarged lymph nodes.

Treatment

Leukemia treatment depends on what types of cells have been affected, how aggressive the disease is, and what kinds of treatments the patient has already had. Treatment usually begins with chemotherapy: administration of chemicals that are highly toxic to any cells that reproduce rapidly. Chemotherapy is usually administered in cycles of treatment followed by recovery. The goal is to suppress cancer cell growth, so that the patient enters remission. Exactly which chemotherapy drugs are used, and how they are administered, depends on the type of cancer that is present.

If a person doesn't respond well to chemotherapy, or if the cancer keeps recurring (**refractory** leukemia), it is necessary to explore other treatment options. This can include adding radiation therapy or surgery, especially if cancerous cells have aggressively invaded a particular organ or location.

Bone marrow transplants with preserved marrow of the patient (**autogenic** transplants) or closely matched donors (**allogenic** transplants) are useful for some leukemia cases, but the incidence of complications is high. It is also possible to harvest stem cells from the bloodstream, bone marrow, or umbilical cords of healthy people and to transplant these "cellular blanks" into leukemia patients, so that they can make healthy, functioning blood cells.

New treatments for leukemia also include the use of interferon or other biologic agents to slow the production of cancerous cells and the use of manufactured antibodies that are designed to identify and destroy cancer cells.

The treatment for leukemia, especially the acute varieties, can take as hard a toll on the body as the disease itself. Chemotherapy introduces substances whose function is to kill off any rapidly reproducing cell. Unfortunately, this doesn't just mean cancer cells; it also means epithelial cells in the skin and the digestive tract and, ironically, healthy blood cells. The side effects of chemotherapy on epithelial tissues include development of ulcers in the mouth, nausea, and diarrhea from gastrointestinal irritation, and hair loss as the epithelial cells in follicles are killed. One of the difficulties with digestive system disturbances is that if the patient can't eat well, the whole system becomes weaker and less able to cope with the stresses of both the disease and its treatment.

Medications

- Chemotherapeutic agents
- Biologic therapy agents, including interferon and monoclonal antibody therapy
- Drugs to mitigate side effects of cancer treatment, including blood cell growth factors to stimulate RBC production

Massage?

RISKS Leukemia and its treatments involve a high risk of bruising, bleeding, and infection. Any bodywork that increases these risks is of course not appropriate. A massage therapist should consult the client's healthcare team to assess the best timing for bodywork in the context of leukemia treatments.

BENEFITS The benefits that gentle bodywork can offer leukemia patients (reinforcing a parasympathetic state, improving sleep and appetite, reducing pain and anxiety) can be enjoyed with a minimum of risk if simple precautions are taken to allow for the client's fragility and medications. For more guidelines about massage in the context of cancer and cancer treatments, see Chapter 12.

Myeloma

Definition: What Is It?

Myeloma (literally, "marrow tumor") is a blood cancer involving maturing B cells that are found in bone

Myeloma in Brief

Pronunciation: my-eh-LOE-mah

What is it?
Myeloma is a type of blood cancer that targets certain B cells in bone marrow.

How is it recognized?
The earliest sign of myeloma is usually pain associated with damage from tumors invading bone tissue. Other signs can include low red blood cell count, low numbers of functioning white cells, kidney damage, and the presence of indicator proteins in the urine.

Massage risks and benefits
Risks: Myeloma patients require special care due to the fragility of affected bones. Other cautions are related to kidney damage, treatment options, and general adaptability.
Benefits: Gentle massage for pain, anxiety, sleep, and other issues related to cancer and cancer treatment can be wonderfully supportive for myeloma patients.

marrow. It is almost exclusive to people over 50 years old, and is twice as common among African Americans as it is among the general population.

Etiology: What Happens?

B cells are born and mature in bone marrow. During this phase, it is possible for some cells to undergo a mutation that causes them to do several things: they proliferate into tumors; they secrete cytokines that stimulate osteoclast activity; and they produce faulty antibodies. A relatively common condition among mature people is called **monoclonal gammopathy of undetermined significance**: this points to some dysfunctional B cells and the production of abnormal antibodies, but it does not always develop into myeloma.

Under normal circumstances, bone marrow holds only a few maturing B cells. When the healthy cells are ready, they migrate to lymph tissue, where they operate as **plasma cells**, producing antibodies. But when immature B cells become cancerous in the bone marrow, they rapidly proliferate into tumors. These usually grow in bone tissue (typically the spine, pelvis, ribs, or skull), but occasionally tumors form elsewhere: these are called **plastocytomas**. Tumors inside bone marrow can interfere with normal blood cell production, leading to the signs and symptoms of other blood cancers: anemia, poor clotting, and reduced resistance to infection. But myeloma cells also secrete cytokines that signal osteoclasts to dismantle bone tissue. This makes more room for the growing

COMPARE & CONTRAST 5.1 Blood Cancers

Blood cancers are a confusing collection of conditions because they seem to overlap each other. Indeed, it has been found that some forms of leukemia are essentially the same as some forms of lymphoma, because they affect the same cells. The only difference is that when the cells circulate, it is called leukemia, and when cells are fixed inside lymph nodes, the disease is called lymphoma.

FEATURES	LEUKEMIA	MYELOMA	LYMPHOMA
Cells affected	Any white blood cell: myeloid (monocytes, neutrophils, basophils, eosinophils) or lymphoid (T cells, B cells, natural killer cells)	Nearly mature B cells in bone marrow only	B cells, T cells natural killer cells, in lymph nodes or spleen
Earliest signs and symptoms	Anemia, thrombocytopenia, poor immune function	Bone pain from corroding tumors in marrow	Painless enlargement of lymph nodes, especially at jaw, axilla, and groin

tumor, and it leads to pathologic thinning or spontaneous fractures in bone tissue.

Healthy B cells produce many types of functioning antibodies (also called immunoglobulins) that work in different ways to neutralize pathogens. Myeloma cells, on the other hand, produce massive numbers of nonfunctioning antibodies, called **monoclonal immunoglobulins**: monoclonal because they are all alike, and immunoglobulins because they are technically antibodies, even though they don't offer any protective properties. Another name for monoclonal immunoglobulins is M-proteins.

Normal antibodies are Y-shaped proteins, and they are too big to pass through the kidneys into the urinary system. M-proteins have branches that sometimes break off during formation. These fragments, called **Bence Jones proteins**, are small enough to pass through the filters in the kidney to be excreted in the urine. The good news about this is that myeloma can be detected and to a certain extent tracked through urinalysis. The bad news is that if the disease is rapidly progressive, the kidneys can sustain extensive damage and even fail altogether.

Types of Myeloma

- *Multiple myeloma.* This form produces tumors at several sites simultaneously. It is the most common form, accounting for 90% of myeloma diagnoses.
- *Solitary myeloma.* This is the development of a single myeloma tumor in the bone marrow.
- *Extramedullary plastocytoma.* This is the growth of myeloma tumors outside of bone tissue. These growths can develop in the skin, muscle, lungs, or other areas.

Signs and Symptoms

Myeloma can be silent in early stages; it is sometimes found during a routine medical examination. The earliest symptom for most people is pain or even fractures that occur as tumors corrode bone tissue. Other signs include anemia, frequent and persistent infections, kidney problems related to the excretion of Bence Jones proteins, hypercalcemia as bone tissue is dismantled, and the risk of **amyloidosis**: the accumulation of inflammatory proteins in organs like the heart or lungs, where they can do significant damage.

Treatment

Myeloma is often not responsive to treatment. If it is slow growing and especially if the patient is elderly and in poor health, a period of watchful waiting is recommended to delay difficult procedures as long as possible. A combination of chemotherapy and bone marrow stem cell transplantation is usually suggested, but even with these intrusive interventions, the 5-year survival rate is relatively low.

Medications

- Chemotherapeutic agents
- Thalidomide and similar drugs to slow angiogenesis
- Corticosteroids, especially when amyloidosis occurs
- Bisphosphonates to promote healthy bone density
- Synthetic EPO to promote RBC production

Massage?

RISKS Myeloma patients are very much at risk for spontaneous fractures of the affected bones. It is imperative that any bodywork in this context respects that possibility with adjustments in pressure, positioning, and any other adaptive demands. Cancer treatments carry their own set of complications and cautions for massage. As always in this context, it is wise to work as part of a fully informed healthcare team.

BENEFITS Gentle, noninvasive massage can be a helpful adjunct to care for a myeloma patient, through pain relief, anxiety reduction, improved sleep, and other benefits. For more information on massage in the context of cancer, see Chapter 12.

Sickle Cell Disease

Definition: What Is It?

Sickle cell disease (SCD) is an autosomal recessive genetic condition that results in production of abnormal hemoglobin, the protein that carries oxygen in RBCs. Blacks, Hispanics, and people from Italy, Greece, Turkey, and the Middle East are most likely to be carriers of the gene. Roughly 2 million people in

Sickle Cell Disease in Brief

What is it?
Sickle cell disease (SCD) is a disorder in which the gene that controls hemoglobin production is faulty. The result is short-lived, misshapen red blood cells (RBCs) that cannot pass through tiny blood vessels.

How is it recognized?
The primary sign of SCD is the pain that occurs when abnormal erythrocytes block blood vessels. This can lead to organ damage, bone pain, kidney infarction, stroke, lung problems, and blindness. Other signs include a high risk of infection because the spleen is typically disabled, and anemia with jaundice because the abnormal RBCs die off faster than they can be replaced.

Massage risks and benefits
Risks: Because this condition drastically affects capillary circulation, it is important not to overchallenge the ability of clients with sickle cell anemia to adapt to the changes that massage brings about.
Benefits: Work that focuses on stress and pain relief without circulatory challenge can be well received and helpful for clients with SCD.

the United States have the sickle cell trait, and about 30,000 people have SCD.

Etiology: What Happens?

The gene for SCD is recessive; this means if a person has only one copy of the gene, he or she has the sickle cell trait but not SCD. If two people who have the sickle cell trait have children together, each child has a 25% chance of inheriting a copy of the gene from each parent. This is the only way SCD is spread.

Being positive for the sickle cell trait carries no health consequences for the carrier and in fact may be beneficial if that person lives in an area where malaria is endemic—interestingly, those areas also happen to be the places where sickle cell genes are most common (Sidebar 5.2). But having two copies of the sickle cell gene means that hemoglobin production is abnormal and many RBCs adopt a characteristic sickle shape (Figure 5.7). This prevents erythrocytes from squeezing through the smallest blood vessels and shortens their lifespan from about 4 months to about 10 days.

Some subtypes of SCD have been identified, depending on the exact nature of the genetic mutations, but their presentation and treatment options are all essentially the same.

SIDEBAR 5.2 Malaria and Sickle Cell Disease: A Close Connection

A person has sickle cell disease if he or she inherits a gene for it from both parents. If only one gene is present, a person has the sickle cell trait but not the disease. This is a crucial distinction, because the sickle cell trait usually doesn't create any symptoms, although some people have mild anemia. But the presence of this single gene does limit the rupturing of erythrocytes during an attack of malaria. Sickle cell genes are mostly found in populations (and descendants of populations) from the Mediterranean, subtropical Africa, and Asia, otherwise called the malarial belt. Isn't it an amazing world?

SCD can lead to many serious and potentially life-shortening complications:

- *Sickle cell crises*. A sickle cell crisis occurs when sickle cells block a capillary, causing an infarction (Figure 5.8). **Hand-foot syndrome** is an example. This is often the first indicator of SCD in a young child. The hands and feet are vulnerable to sickle cell crises, and they swell and become extremely painful.
- *Organ damage*. The spleen, as a collection site for dead and damaged RBCs, is often lost early in the disease process. Other organs that are frequently damaged include the liver, kidneys, and brain: even young children are vulnerable to ischemic strokes.

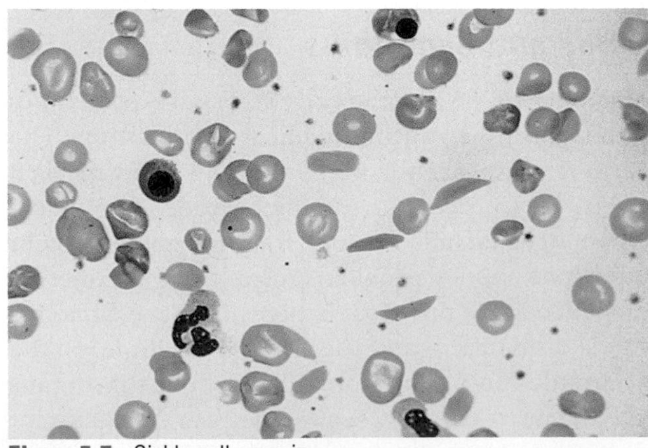

Figure 5.7. Sickle cell anemia

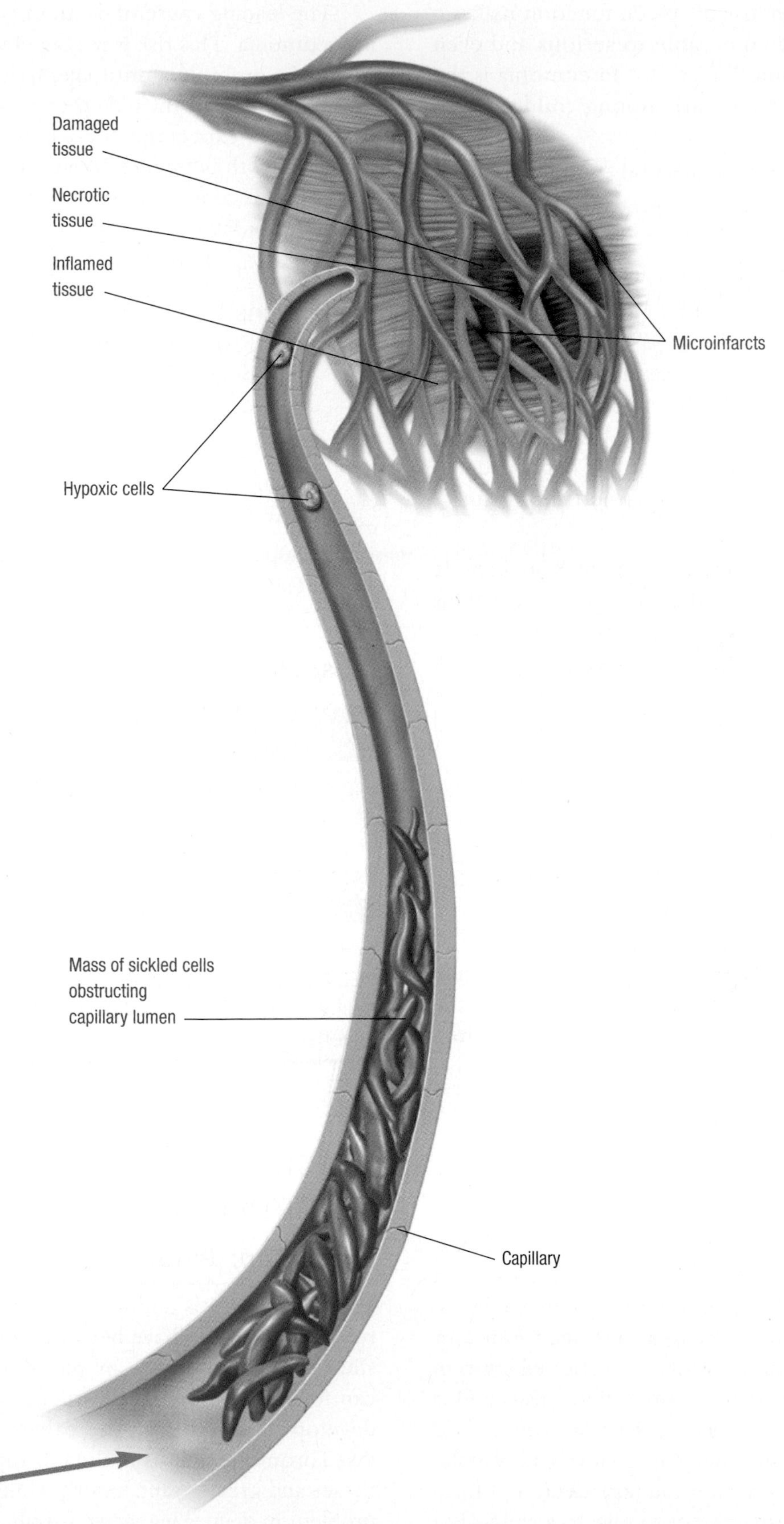

Figure 5.8. Sickle cell crisis

- *Infection*. The loss of spleen function makes a SCD patient vulnerable to serious and even life-threatening infections. Pneumonia is the leading cause of death among children with SCD.
- *Gallstones*. Accumulated bilirubin in the liver can concentrate into crystals that build up in the gallbladder.
- *Vision loss*. The accumulation of fragile RBCs in the arterioles that supply the retina can lead to blurred vision, hemorrhage, and blindness.
- *Acute chest syndrome*. Damaged cells accumulate in the lungs, leading to inflammation and pneumonia-like symptoms. This puts excessive strain on the right side of the heart and can lead to pulmonary hypertension and right-sided heart failure.
- *Others*. Other complications of SCD include delayed growth in children; chronic ulcerations of the skin, usually at the lower legs; and priapism, a painful and long-lasting erection of the penis that occurs because the vessels that would allow blood to flow out are blocked with damaged RBCs.

Signs and Symptoms

Having dysfunctional hemoglobin and brittle, fragile RBCs produces many consequences in the body. The symptoms of SCD include fatigue, shortness of breath, and pallor related to anemia. Jaundice may develop as RBCs die and bilirubin accumulates in the liver and backs up into the bloodstream. Other symptoms are also complications, as already described.

Treatment

SCD is treated by trying to limit the severity and frequency of sickle cell crises. Mild episodes can be treated at home with over-the-counter pain medications and hot packs, but more severe attacks are often treated in the hospital with intravenous opioid drugs. One cancer drug, hydroxyurea, has been found to limit the frequency and severity of sickle cell crises in adults, but it carries many serious side effects and is not approved for use in children. Families with a child who has SCD often use many alternative and complementary strategies for pain management, and massage—often taught to a parent to give to a child—is a popular choice.

The leading cause of death in children with SCD is pneumonia. This risk is managed with doses of prophylactic antibiotics until age 5, along with careful immunizations for flu and other possible infections.

The life expectancy of a person with SCD has increased with better treatment options; today a person with this condition can expect to live well into his or her 40s or later.

Medications

- Analgesics (nonprescription and prescription, including opioids) for pain management
- Prophylactic antibiotics in childhood for protection from infection
- Chemotherapeutic agent (hydroxyurea), which slows sickling
- Supplements of folate to support healthy new RBC production

Massage?

RISKS Clients with sickle cell disease (SCD) have severely compromised circulation, especially in the extremities. Any bodywork that demands circulatory adaptation may be simply too challenging for them to receive safely.

BENEFITS Massage for the purpose of pain relief and anxiety reduction but without the intent of mechanically pushing fluids may be welcomed by SCD patients as a noninvasive way to deal with pain and to have a safe and positive physical experience.

Thrombophlebitis, Deep Vein Thrombosis

Definition: What Is It?

Thrombophlebitis and deep vein thrombosis (DVT) refer to veins that have become obstructed and possibly inflamed because of blood clots. These clots can form anywhere in the venous system, but they develop most often in the calves, thighs, and pelvis. Thrombophlebitis is clots in superficial leg veins (lesser and greater saphenous), while DVT is a similar problem in deeper leg veins, specifically the popliteal, femoral, and iliac veins.

Thrombophlebitis, Deep Vein Thrombosis in Brief

Pronunciation: throm-bo-fleh-BI-tis

What is it?
Thrombophlebitis and deep vein thrombosis (DVT) describe veins obstructed by blood clots.

How is it recognized?
Signs and symptoms of thrombophlebitis may or may not include pain, heat, redness, swelling, local itchiness, and a hard cordlike feeling at the affected vein, and distal edema. Signs and symptoms of DVT may be nonexistent or more extreme: possibly pitting edema distal to the site with discoloration and intermittent or continuous pain that is exacerbated by activity or standing for a long time.

Massage risks and benefits

Risks: If a blood clot in a leg or pelvic vein fragments and travels, the ultimate destination is the lung, causing a potentially life-threatening pulmonary embolism. Any type of bodywork in the context of diagnosed clots in the legs must be done with the utmost caution for this risk.

Benefits: A client who has survived a venous clot with no long-lasting contraindications can enjoy the same benefits from massage as the rest of the population.

Etiology: What Happens?

Thrombophlebitis and DVT involve thrombi: stationary clots in the venous system, where, if they break loose, nothing stops them from traveling up the vena cava, through the right side of the heart, into the pulmonary artery, and finally to the lung, causing pulmonary embolism.

The clotting mechanism is an important function, but sometimes we form clots faster than we can melt them. In the mid-1800s, a pioneer in pathology, Rudolf Virchow, first outlined three key factors in clot formation. The Virchow triad—injury to endothelium, hypercoagulability, and venous stasis, or slowed blood flow—is used today to describe the risk factors leading to the formation of blood clots in veins.

Here are a few of the most common precipitators of thrombophlebitis or DVT:

- *Physical trauma*. Being kicked or hit in the leg can damage the delicate venous tissue, which is then prone to clot formation. Any fracture of bones in the leg can also increase risk (Case History 5.1).
- *Varicose veins*. These involve damaged tissue and the risk of clot formation. The clots that form in superficial veins tend to embolize much less frequently than those in deeper veins, but many people with varicose veins also have DVT.
- *Local infection*. This can cause an inflammatory reaction leading to clot formation. These infections are often related to surgical procedures involving catheters.
- *Physical restriction*. Too tight socks or leg braces can cause the clotting factors in the blood to accumulate, even without damage to a vessel wall.
- *Immobility*. Sitting for long periods can contribute to DVT. This phenomenon has given rise to the layman's term for this condition: "coach class syndrome."
- *Pregnancy and childbirth*. The weight of the fetus on femoral vessels slows blood return, and hormonal changes and stress can cause the blood to thicken and become more viscous.
- *Certain types of cancer*. Some cancers can lead to excessive clotting, either because of changes in the blood or because of irritation at the site of a catheter.
- *Surgery*. Thrombosis and subsequent PE are a leading cause of death following orthopedic surgery, especially for knee and hip replacements. Heart and any kind of pelvic surgery also hold high risks of thrombosis.
- *Hormone supplements*. High-estrogen birth control pills or hormone replacement therapy increase the risk of developing blood clots.
- *Other factors*. Cigarette smoking, hypertension and other cardiovascular diseases, paralysis, and some genetic conditions lead to excessive coagulation in the blood.

Most blood clots causing DVT or thrombophlebitis form in the lower legs, but they can develop elsewhere with surgery or other trauma. Sudden movement or change in position is often the factor that causes part of a clot to detach and travel to the lungs.

One further twist occurs when a person has a defect in the cardiac septum. Many people have a small hole in the wall between the left and right sides of the heart, usually at the atrium. This condition is called **patent foramen ovale**. If clots from damaged

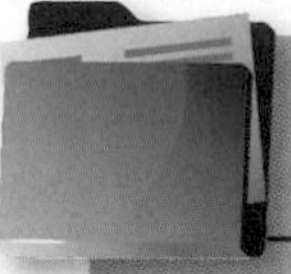

CASE HISTORY 5.1 Deep Vein Thrombosis

ANNE, AGED 67: "It was just a broken knee!"

Anne was a retired schoolteacher who spent her winters in Arizona and summers in the mountains of Colorado. In May, a week after she moved to her summer home, she took a bad fall over a curb and sustained a lateral plateau fracture to the tibia of her left leg, with which she had a history of varicose veins and phlebitis.

Because her health maintenance organization was out of state, it was reluctant to cover any treatment for conditions not considered life threatening. For that reason Anne, a mildly overweight moderate smoker, spent 3 days sitting in a chair all day at 10,000 ft of altitude (which thickens the blood, because less oxygen is in the air). She was unable to move except with the use of a walker. Her broken knee was never set or seen by an orthopedist.

By the third day, the swelling in the leg became so severely painful that she sought out a general practitioner in the Colorado town. He sent her to a local hospital for an ultrasound, which revealed a blood clot from her ankle to her groin. She immediately checked in, and began receiving anticoagulant medication.

Four days later, she was sent home. Still basically immobile but taking anticoagulants, she returned to sitting in her chair with her leg elevated for 12 to 14 hours a day. On her second night home she woke in the night with severe chest pains and shortness of breath. The emergency medical team took her back to the hospital, where it was revealed that she had thrown a large clot to the lung. At this point, her condition was too severe to be treated at a small rural hospital. After 2 days in the intensive care unit, she was transferred to a larger facility about 100 miles. away, where a filter was inserted into her vena cava to prevent any further clots from reaching her lungs.

When she checked out of the second hospital, she was prescribed supplemental oxygen to compensate for the loss of lung function and the high altitude. She used an oxygen tank for several weeks, but began smoking again after that time. Now many years later, Anne is still active, but her breathing and stamina have never recovered. ■

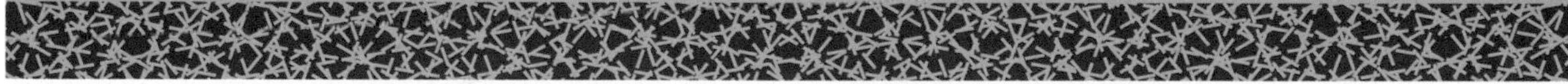

veins that travel to the right side of the heart cross into the left side, they can go on through arteries to the brain as a stroke, to the cardiac muscle as a heart attack, or anywhere else as an arterial embolism.

Thrombophlebitis and DVT may do permanent damage to leg veins, including destruction of valves that assist with blood return to the heart. These patients are at risk for chronic venous insufficiency, which can include permanent edema, skin discoloration or ulcers, and very slow healing in the affected area.

Signs and Symptoms

Thrombophlebitis can show the major signs of inflammation: pain, heat, redness, and swelling. Sometimes itchiness, a hard cord where the vein is affected, and edema with discoloration distal to the area are present (Figure 5.9). Thrombophlebitis that has become a chronic problem may result in poor blood flow to the skin, leading to flaking, discoloration, and skin ulcers. If it is caused by a local infection, fever and general illness may also be present.

DVT is considered the more dangerous of these two conditions because the clots in deeper veins can be big enough to do serious damage in the lungs. Unfortunately, fewer than one-half of all DVT patients experience significant symptoms. If DVT does show any signs, it may show more swelling and edema than thrombophlebitis, because the clot inhibits more blood flow back to the heart. The backup forces extra fluid out of the capillaries and into the interstitial spaces, thus adding general edema to any swelling of the vein. The capillary exchange may become so sluggish that the edema pits or leaves a dimple wherever it is touched.

Treatment

The goals for a patient with thrombophlebitis or DVT are to stop clots from growing, to prevent clots from fragmenting and embolizing, and to prevent future clots from forming. The most common strategy is to supplement anticoagulants: drugs that prevent new clots from forming. Thrombolytics ("clot busters") have much more serious risks and are only used in the most extreme cases.

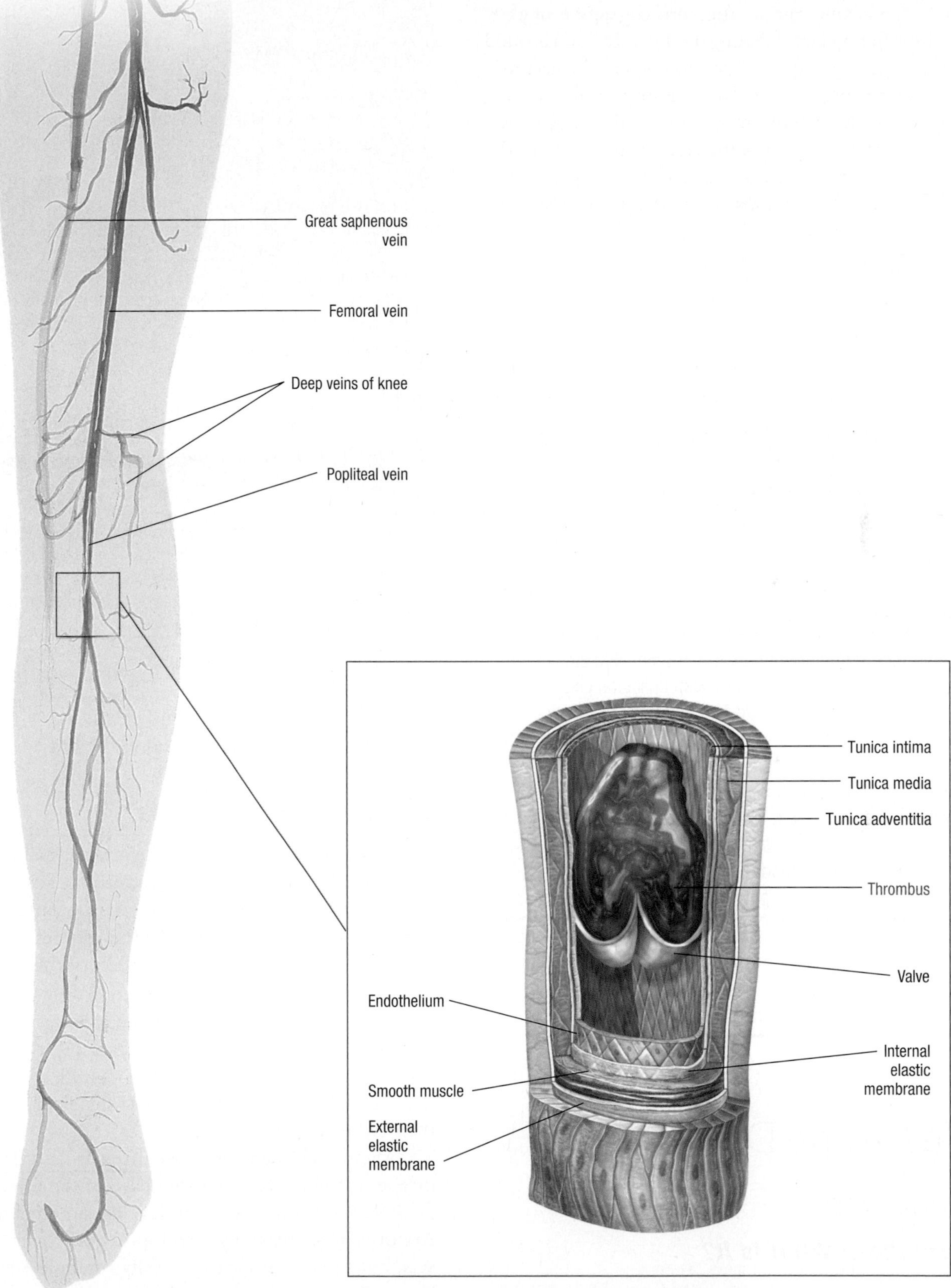

Figure 5.9. Deep vein thrombosis

A bedridden patient may be given pneumatic compression to reduce the risk of thrombophlebitis or DVT. A machine mimics the pumping action of exercise by inflating and deflating a tubular balloon around the affected leg. Support hose to prevent the accumulation of postoperative edema is also recommended.

High-risk patients may have a filter implanted in the vena cava to prevent clots from reaching the lungs. Surgery to remove a clot is sometimes performed, but other options are typically explored first.

Medications

- Aspirin (not well tolerated by some patients)
- Anticoagulants, including warfarin and heparin
  - Heparin is giving through injection or intravenously; it is fast acting.
  - Warfarin is taken orally for up to six months following an event.
- Thrombolytics in extreme cases

Massage?

RISKS A client with a diagnosed blood clot is not a candidate for any rigorous massage until that situation has completely stabilized. A client with signs of a blood clot (which can be simply deep unilateral calf pain) is likewise not a good candidate for circulatory massage until the source of the pain has been definitively determined not to be related to a blood clot. The risk, of course, is that a clot could fragment, embolize, and land in the lung.

Clients who are using anticoagulants are at significantly increased risk for bleeding and bruising. Any bodywork performed during this time must accommodate for those possibilities.

BENEFITS A client who has successfully treated and recovered from thrombophlebitis or deep vein thrombosis can enjoy all the benefits from bodywork as the rest of the population.

Vascular Disorders

Aneurysm

Definition: What Is It?

An aneurysm is a permanent bulge in the wall of a blood vessel or the heart. They happen most often at the aorta (aortic aneurysm) and in the brain (cerebral aneurysm).

Aneurysm in Brief

Pronunciation: AN-yur-izm

What is it?
An aneurysm is a bulge in a vein, an artery, or the heart. They usually occur in the thoracic or abdominal aorta or in the arteries at the base of the brain.

How is it recognized?
Symptoms of aneurysms are determined by their location. Thoracic aneurysms may cause chronic hoarseness; abdominal aneurysms may cause local discomfort, reduced urine output, or severe backache. Cerebral aneurysms may be silent or may cause extreme headache when they are at very high risk for rupture.

Massage risks and benefits
Risks: A person who has been diagnosed with an aneurysm typically has to take care not to challenge his or her circulatory system. Massage should also be gauged not to present excessive challenge.
Benefits: A person with a stable aneurysm that is under observation is a good candidate for calming, relaxing bodywork that stays within his or her capacity for adaptation. A person who has successfully treated an aneurysm can receive any massage that is appropriate to his or her activity levels.

Etiology: What Happens?

The three-ply construction of the arteries includes the endothelial inside layer, the smooth muscle middle layer, and the tough connective tissue outer layer. Blood pressure in the aorta and the arteries that supply the brain is very high. If the walls of these vessels lose their elasticity, they can bulge wide with blood. This bulge is an aneurysm. As the aneurysm grows, the walls stretch and weaken, increasing the risk of rupture and death. Aneurysms are identified when the diameter of the affected section of the artery is more than 150% of normal.

Aneurysms happen most often in the thoracic or abdominal aorta and at the base of the brain. It is possible for multiple sites to develop simultaneously. Aneurysms sometimes develop in more distal vessels, but those cases are generally much less serious because the blood pressure drops with distance from the heart.

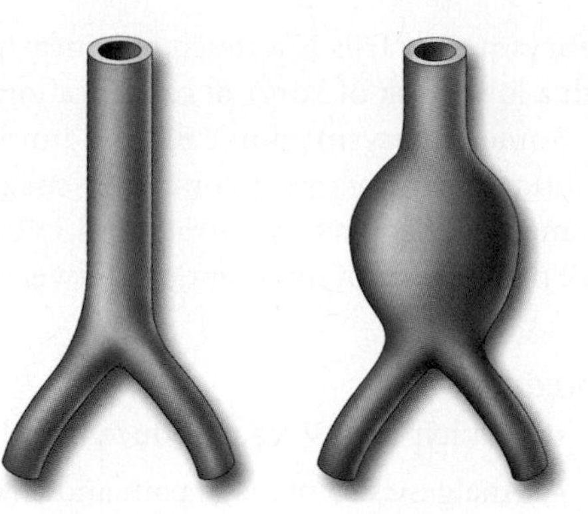

Common types of aneurysms

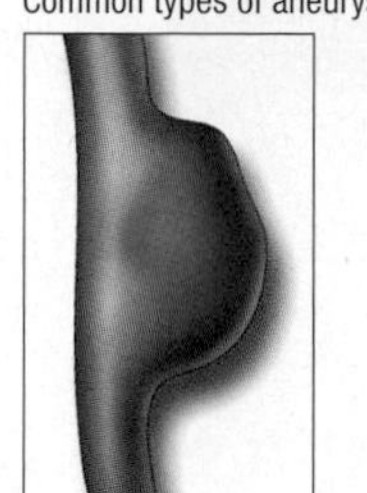

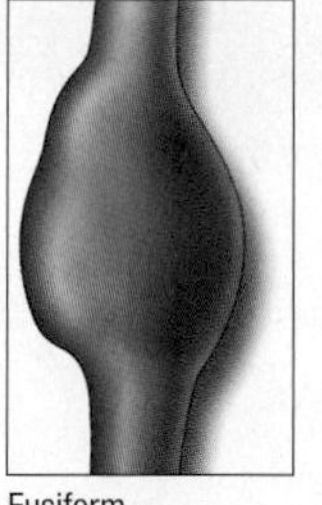

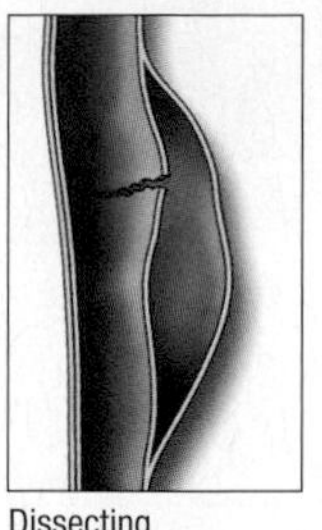

Figure 5.10. Types of aneurysm

An occasional complication of a major heart attack is an aneurysm in the left ventricle of the heart itself. The damage to myocardium reduces elasticity to the point that chronic pressure causes the whole wall of the ventricle to bulge. This is discussed further in the article on heart failure.

Several factors can contribute to the chances of developing an aneurysm:

- *Compromised smooth muscle.* Atherosclerotic plaques invade and weaken aortal muscle. Aortic aneurysms are a serious and common complication of atherosclerosis and high blood pressure.
- *Smoking.* The damage incurred to endothelium by carbon monoxide from cigarette smoke and a rise in blood pressure from nicotine makes smoking a leading risk factor for aortic aneurysm.
- *Congenitally weak arterial wall.* Sometimes the tissue simply isn't strong enough to manage normal blood pressure, and with no warning an aneurysm can rupture. Inherited connective tissue diseases such as Marfan syndrome and Ehlers-Danlos syndrome can contribute to this kind of event.
- *Inflammation.* A few diseases, such as polyarteritis nodosa and bacterial endocarditis, can cause inflammation and weakening of the arterial tissue.
- *Untreated syphilis.* This can lead to damage in the aorta, sometimes decades after the initial infection.
- *Trauma.* Mechanical trauma, such as a car accident in which a person is injured by a steering wheel, may sometimes damage the outer layers of the aorta while leaving the inner one intact. This results in the characteristic bulging and stretching of the most delicate arterial tissue.

For the rare aneurysms that are not in the aorta or the brain, no serious complications may develop unless the aneurysm gets large enough to impede blood flow, which can lead to gangrene. But more typically, aneurysms press against nearby structures, which can interfere with function. If blood pools inside an aneurysm for any length of time, clots may form and enter the bloodstream again. And of course, a rupture leads to hemorrhaging in the best case, and shock followed by circulatory collapse in the worst case. A ruptured cerebral aneurysm is fatal about 50% of the time; ruptured aortic aneurysms are fatal much more often than that: they lead to about 13,000 deaths each year.

Types of Aneurysm

- *Saccular aneurysm.* These usually occur with thoracic or abdominal aortic aneurysms. The aortal wall bulges like a rounded sack, which throbs and pushes against neighboring organs and other structures (Figure 5.10).
- *Fusiform aneurysm.* This is a common type of aortic aneurysm; in this case, the bulge is less round and more tubular, as if the aorta were widened like a sausage for a few inches.
- *Berry aneurysm.* These small aneurysms are usually in the brain (Figure 5.11).
- *Dissecting aneurysm.* Also called false aneurysm, this is the least common and most painful type of aortic damage. The blood pressure actually splits the layers of the aorta between the tunica intima (innermost layer) and the tunica media (muscular

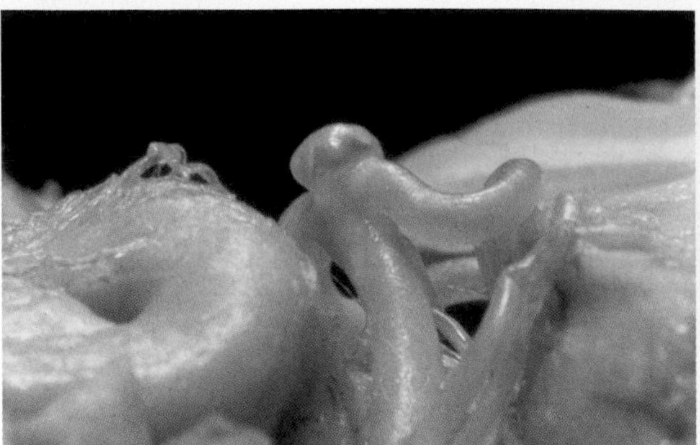
Figure 5.11. Cerebral aneurysm

layer). In some cases, this type of bulge can seal itself off when the blood trapped inside the split coagulates and solidifies. It is possible to have a dissecting aorta without an aneurysm.

Signs and Symptoms

Aneurysms can be difficult to identify early, because they often aren't painful until they become a medical emergency. With aortic aneurysms, the swelling might create some warning signals; this usually happens when the bulge is pressing on another organ. A pulsating mass may be palpable in the abdomen: this is pertinent for massage therapists doing abdominal work.

Thoracic aneurysms sometimes cause difficulty with swallowing (dysphagia), chest pain, hoarseness, and coughing that is not relieved with medication, because the protrusion presses on and irritates the larynx. Abdominal aneurysms sometimes show as a throbbing lump near the umbilicus, loss of appetite, weight loss, reduced urine output, and if it's pushing against the spine, severe backache. Aneurysms in the brain may have no signs, but if they suddenly change, they may cause headache, numbness, weakness, or other symptoms, depending on what they press on.

Treatment

Aneurysms don't spontaneously retreat, because the pressure that causes them is unrelenting. They must be repaired, either with open surgery or with endovascular surgery. Open surgery involves clamping off the artery above and below the lesion and attaching either a replacement graft or a Dacron substitute to the two ends. This is usually successful, but it has to be done before a rupture. Endovascular surgery involves inserting a catheter through the femoral artery and threading it up to the aorta to insert a patch or stent at the aneurysm site. This is a much less invasive procedure with a lower risk of surgical complications.

Some aneurysms don't require immediate intervention. Many doctors recommend checking the size of small aneurysms by ultrasound every 6 months until the benefits of intervention outweigh the risks.

Medications

- Antihypertensives to reduce blood pressure
- Analgesics to manage pain and anxiety

Massage?

RISKS Massage has been seen both to increase and decrease blood pressure. It causes superficial capillary dilation, which reroutes blood from elsewhere. It also appears to shift functions toward a parasympathetic state, which may be positive for a person with an aneurysm, but all of these internal changes must be within that client's ability to adapt.

BENEFITS A client with a stable aneurysm who is receiving medical care can receive any massage that is within his or her capacity for adaptation.

OPTIONS Any bodywork focused on dropping blood pressure without putting emphasis on fluid movement is probably appropriate for an aneurysm patient.

Atherosclerosis

Definition: What Is It?

Arteriosclerosis is hardening of the arteries from any cause. Atherosclerosis is a subtype of arteriosclerosis. It is a condition in which deposits of cholesterol, calcium, and other substances infiltrate and weaken layers of large and medium-sized blood vessels, particularly the aorta and coronary arteries. It is compounded by local spasm, and blood clots form at the site of these deposits. These features contribute to occlusion of the diameter, or lumen, of the arteries (Figure 5.12) and to the risk of forming and releasing blood clots on the arterial side of the systemic circuit.

Etiology: What Happens?

Development of atherosclerosis is a complex multifactorial process that varies according to gender, age,

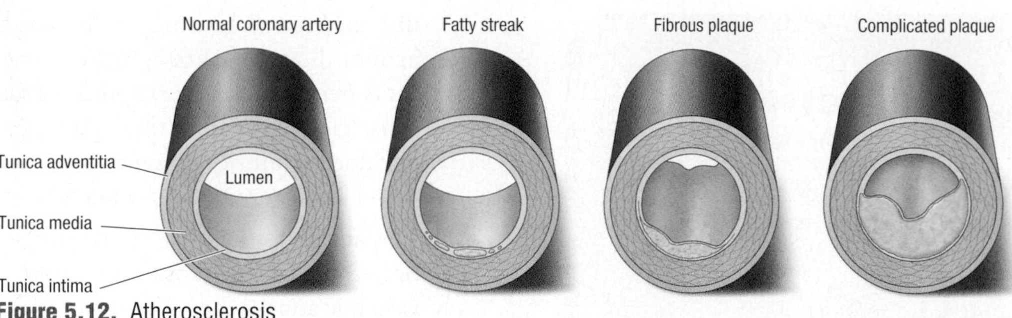

Figure 5.12. Atherosclerosis

race, diet, and other factors. At this point, the most widely accepted idea of how atherosclerosis develops includes the following steps:

1. *Endothelial damage*. The inside layer of arteries, also called the tunica intima, is made of delicate epithelial tissue and subject to a lot of abuse. A variety of things may hurl the first insult at the tunica intima: constant hypertension in the aorta and arteries surrounding the heart, carbon monoxide from cigarette smoke, high levels of oxidized low-density lipoproteins (LDL) and triglycerides, or high blood sugar can begin endothelial erosion. Damage occurs most readily at branches or sharp curves in the arteries, where turbulence in blood flow most severely affects endothelium.
2. *Monocytes arrive*. These small white blood cells are attracted to any site of damage in the body. The monocytes infiltrate the epithelial layer, and become fixed macrophages, or big eaters. See Animation at http://thePoint.lww.com/Werner5e.
3. *Macrophages take up LDL*. LDLs (low-density lipoproteins) are the "bad guys" of the cholesterol world. Their job is to escort usable cholesterol to the cells in the body. But when those cells don't need any more cholesterol, they stop accepting it. This leaves LDLs with nowhere to go. White blood cells in the tunica intima take them up, which is why they are sometimes called "foam cells" at this stage (see Sidebar 5.3).
4. *Foam cells infiltrate smooth muscle tissue*. Foam cells secrete growth factors; this causes the smooth muscle cells in the arterial wall to proliferate all around them. The grayish white lumps of plaque that are inside dissected arteries are made of these extra muscle cells and cholesterol-filled macrophages. Furthermore, these foam cells release enzymes that damage arterial walls and cause bleeding and clot formation.
5. *Platelets arrive*. Attracted by the changing texture of the arterial wall, platelets come and release their chemicals, which do three counterproductive things:
    a. Growth factors are secreted, and they reinforce the proliferation of new smooth muscle cells.
    b. Clots form, and they can further restrict the lumen of the artery.
    c. Vascular spasm occurs because the chemical that inhibits it can't get through all the plaque. This leads to a temporary lack of oxygen in the myocardium, and the gripping chest pain called **angina pectoris.**

Atherosclerosis in Brief

Pronunciation: ath-er-o-skler-O-sis

What is it?
Atherosclerosis is a condition in which arteries become inelastic and brittle as a result of the deposit of plaques.

How is it recognized?
Early atherosclerosis is silent. However, it is connected to several other types of circulatory problems, including hypertension, arrhythmia, aneurysm, coronary artery disease, cerebrovascular disease, and peripheral vascular disease.

Massage risks and benefits
Risks: Atherosclerosis is so common in this country that it is safe to assume that most adults have some plaque accumulation in major arteries. Massage for a client with diagnosed atherosclerosis must be gauged to stay within the physical challenges presented by that person's normal daily activities. Medications used to control the complications of atherosclerosis may also have implications for bodywork.
Benefits: Massage, as a form of self-care that is noninvasive and carries the reward of both feeling good and being good for health, can be a powerful aid for a person who lives with atherosclerosis, and who wants to adopt a lifestyle that is more conducive to overall good health..

SIDEBAR 5.3 A Brief Digression on Cholesterol

Cholesterol is a fatty substance produced in the liver and available in any animal product. Saturated fats are particularly rich in easily absorbable cholesterol.

Cholesterol by itself has no access to the body's cells. Just as glucose must be escorted into cells by insulin, cholesterol must be escorted by lipoproteins. When a cholesterol measurement is taken, it is actually the lipoproteins that are being counted.

Three varieties of lipoproteins are involved with the movement of cholesterol: **low-density lipoproteins** (LDL), **high-density lipoproteins** (HDL), and **triglycerides**. The LDLs ("bad cholesterol") deliver cholesterol to the body's cells. They are bad only when the body's cells have no more need for their cargo. At that point, the LDLs deposit the cholesterol in artery walls. The HDLs ("good cholesterol") are involved in reverse cholesterol transport. In this process, cholesterol is moved out of the arteries and back to the liver for metabolic processing. The third variety, triglycerides, are chemicals that help to convert fats and carbohydrates into energy for muscles. Studies have shown that elevated triglyceride levels contribute to plaque formation, so it is desirable to keep their numbers down.

When a person gets a cholesterol reading, it's useful to know not just what the overall levels are but in what ratios the fat types occur. An ideal reading would find total levels below 200 mg/dL, with a relatively high proportion of HDLs (over 35 mg/dL) and lower numbers of LDLs and triglycerides (less than 130 mg/dL combined).

6. *Plaques form.* These are made of cholesterol, calcium, and fibrin, with a fibrous cap. Inside the plaque, clots may form and tissue may die. Inflammation causes the fibrous cap to loosen, and the plaque ruptures. This releases the core of lipid and necrotic material into the blood.

The complications of atherosclerosis are sometimes the first symptoms of the disease. Several of them are also topics discussed elsewhere in this chapter. They include but are not limited to these issues:

- *High blood pressure.* Hypertension is both a cause and a result of this disease; it contributes to the original damage to the tunica intima, and it is made worse when the arterial walls are too brittle to adjust to the constant changes in blood volume flowing through them.
- *Aneurysm.* When the wall of an artery is rendered inelastic and defective, it can bulge and become thin, weak, and susceptible to rupture.
- *Arrhythmia.* Advanced atherosclerosis can contribute to the development of irregular or uncoordinated beating of the cardiac muscle as blood supply through the coronary arteries is periodically interrupted. Arrhythmia can cause clots to form in the atria when the chamber doesn't empty completely. These clots can travel anywhere the aorta takes them.
- *Thrombus or embolism.* Thrombi are the link between atherosclerosis and stroke or transient ischemic attack when they travel to the brain, and between atherosclerosis and heart attack when they develop or lodge in the coronary arteries.
- *Angina pectoris.* The process of developing atherosclerotic plaques also creates a higher risk of short-term vascular spasm, which leads to heart and chest pain.
  - Stable angina pectoris means that chest pain is predictable with exercise or exertion and subsides during rest.
  - Unstable angina pectoris means that chest pain varies in intensity, is not associated with exercise, and is unpredictable. Unstable angina is related to the rupture of a plaque: it is associated with a high risk of heart attack (see Compare & Contrast 5.2).
- *Heart attack.* When rough plaques form on smooth artery walls, they attract thrombocytes. If a clot or fragment of plaque breaks off in the coronary artery, or if a plaque and clot completely occlude a section of coronary artery, all of the myocardium that should have been supplied then dies. This is a myocardial infarction, or heart attack.

Risk Factors

Risk factors for atherosclerosis can be divided into modifiable and nonmodifiable types.

Nonmodifiable risk factors

- *Heredity, genetics.* Heart disease certainly runs in families, but genetics are only one among many risk factors for atherosclerosis.
- *Gender.* While both men and women are affected by atherosclerosis, the average onset for men is typically around age 45, and for women it is around age 55. This reflects the shift in hormones that occurs after menopause.
- *Age.* The incidence of heart disease rises with age, but it is not a disease exclusively of the elderly.

- *Kidney disorders*. Atherosclerosis can sometimes lead to kidney problems. But if the kidney problems predate the circulatory ones, high blood pressure brought about by kidney failure can be a precipitator for atherosclerosis.

Modifiable risk factors

- *Smoking*. Carbon monoxide from cigarette smoke is corrosive to endothelium. Furthermore, nicotine causes vasoconstriction and high blood pressure.
- *High cholesterol levels*. A predictable statistical link has been established between high cholesterol levels and the development of pathological atherosclerosis.
- *High blood pressure*. Chronic uncontrolled high blood pressure contributes to endothelial damage, which opens the door to the formation of plaques.
- *Sedentary lifestyle*. Regular moderate cardiovascular exercise, perhaps more than any other factor, can reduce the risk of atherosclerosis. It keeps arteries elastic and pliable, reduces weight, raises high-density lipoprotein (HDL) levels for the reduction of plaques, reduces the risk of diabetes, and lowers blood pressure.
- *Diabetes*. People with uncontrolled diabetes are especially susceptible to atherosclerosis because of the way their body metabolizes food. However, if the diabetes is controlled, the risk of atherosclerosis is much lower.

Other risk factors

Continued study into who develops atherosclerosis and what makes them different from the rest of the population has yielded some additional risk factors. It is unclear whether these are modifiable or not, and the exact relationship between these issues and heart disease is not thoroughly understood. However, identifying these issues early and controlling them may improve the outcome for many people.

- **C-reactive protein** is a liver enzyme secreted in the presence of a systemic inflammatory response. It is a dependable predictor for heart attack, stroke, and other conditions related to atherosclerosis, although the mechanism is not clearly understood.
- **Homocysteine** is an amino acid in the blood. A small part of the population tends to have very high levels of homocysteine, which can contribute to endothelial damage. People with high levels are usually counseled to try to control this imbalance with folic acid and vitamins B_6 and B_{12}.
- Other risk factors that continue to be studied include body mass index, levels of fibrinogen, and subtypes of lipoproteins, some of which may be more involved with plaque formation than others.

Types of Atherosclerosis

- *Carotid artery disease*. This is the formation of atherosclerotic plaque in the carotid artery where blood pressure is high, and where, if a fragment breaks off, the only direction it can travel is into the brain, where a transient ischemic attack or a stroke is the ultimate result (Figure 5.13).
- *Coronary artery disease*. This is atherosclerosis in the coronary arteries that supply the myocardium. Occlusion here—either from a clot that forms onsite or from a fragment that travels—can lead to the death of heart muscle (Figure 5.14, Animation 4 at http://thePoint.lww.com/Werner5e).
- *Peripheral artery disease*. This is the development of atherosclerosis away from the neck or heart. The abdomen or legs are the most frequent sites. If a clot builds or lodges in the renal artery, kidney damage occurs. In the legs, they can cause temporary pain and cramping (called **intermittent claudication**), erectile dysfunction, stasis dermatitis, gangrene, and skin ulcers (Figure 5.15).

Signs and Symptoms

Until the damage has progressed to dangerous levels, atherosclerosis is completely silent, partly because the body doesn't depend on any single artery to do a job. Most areas have two or three alternative vessels, or the body can generate new vessels that can be pressed into service if one of them gets clogged up.

Once signs of atherosclerosis begin to develop, they arise from poor delivery of oxygen to the tissues. If the starved cells are in the heart, low stamina and shortness of breath are the earliest signs.

Treatment

Treatment for atherosclerosis starts simply with adjustments in eating and exercise habits.

More advanced cases may require drugs and/or surgery. The drugs are generally designed to influence blood pressure, cholesterol levels, and platelet activity. Surgical intervention can include angioplasty, endarterectomy, or bypass surgery. Angioplasty is a procedure in which the artery may first be treated with a laser, which vaporizes plaques (laser angioplasty), and then a small balloon is inflated to widen the artery (balloon angioplasty). Unfortunately, the scarring that occurs when the balloon is removed (**restenosis**) can be a dangerous complication of this procedure; new cells rapidly proliferate where the endothelium was scraped. In an endarterectomy, a tiny rotating drill is inserted into clogged arteries to shave off plaque, and the shavings are trapped and removed. This is sometimes used for carotid arteries when the risk of stroke is high. In bypass surgery, surgeons remove the damaged piece of artery and replace it, often with a graft from the internal mammary artery or a piece of saphenous vein. A "single, double, triple, etc. bypass" refers to the number of sections of artery being replaced.

NOTABLE CASES Former President Bill Clinton underwent quadruple bypass surgery in 2004 to correct plaque accumulation associated with high cholesterol. While atherosclerosis is understood to be tied to a fatty diet, sedentary lifestyle, and smoking, evidence of it has been found in Egyptian mummies, who probably did not indulge in these modern temptations.

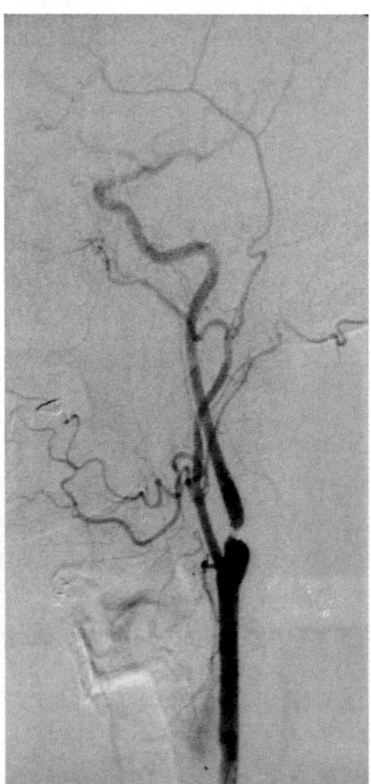

Figure 5.13. Carotid artery disease. Note the point of stenosis just past the bifurcation

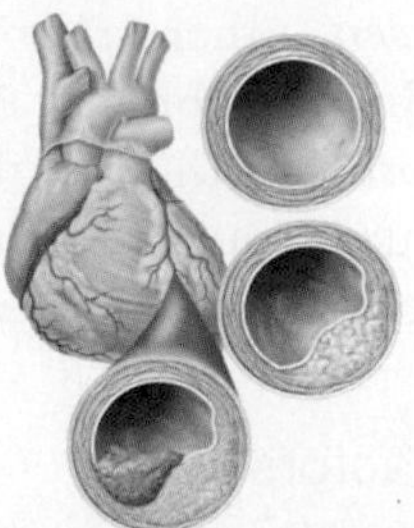

Figure 5.14. Coronary artery disease

Medications

- Cholesterol management drugs, including reductase inhibitors, fibric acid derivatives, and bile sequestering drugs
- Antihypertensive drugs, including beta blockers, calcium channel blockers, and ACE (angiotensin-converting enzyme) inhibitors
- Anticoagulants, including aspirin
- Antiangina drugs, including nitroglycerin

Massage?

RISKS Many people, perhaps the majority of adults in the united states, have a subclinical accumulation of plaque in major arteries. Those with atherosclerosis severe enough to threaten other complications of heart disease (heart attack, heart failure, aneurysm, etc.) may not have the adaptive capacity to keep up with the challenges of rigorous circulatory massage. Choices must be made based on the client's resilience, his or her normal levels of activity, and what kinds of medications are used to control this condition.

BENEFITS For a person with atherosclerosis who wants to support better health, careful massage along with dietary changes, exercise, and other self-care strategies can make a huge difference.

OPTIONS While a person with any kind of heart disease may not be a good candidate for most types of massage, it is a wonderful feature of human construction that no major blood vessels run close to the surface on the upper back or between the scapulae. This means it is possible to give a wonderful massage, without having a profound or direct impact on the circulatory system. The only caution here is to remember that the anterior aspect of the trapezius muscle runs dangerously close to the carotid artery, and this is an endangerment site for carotid artery disease.

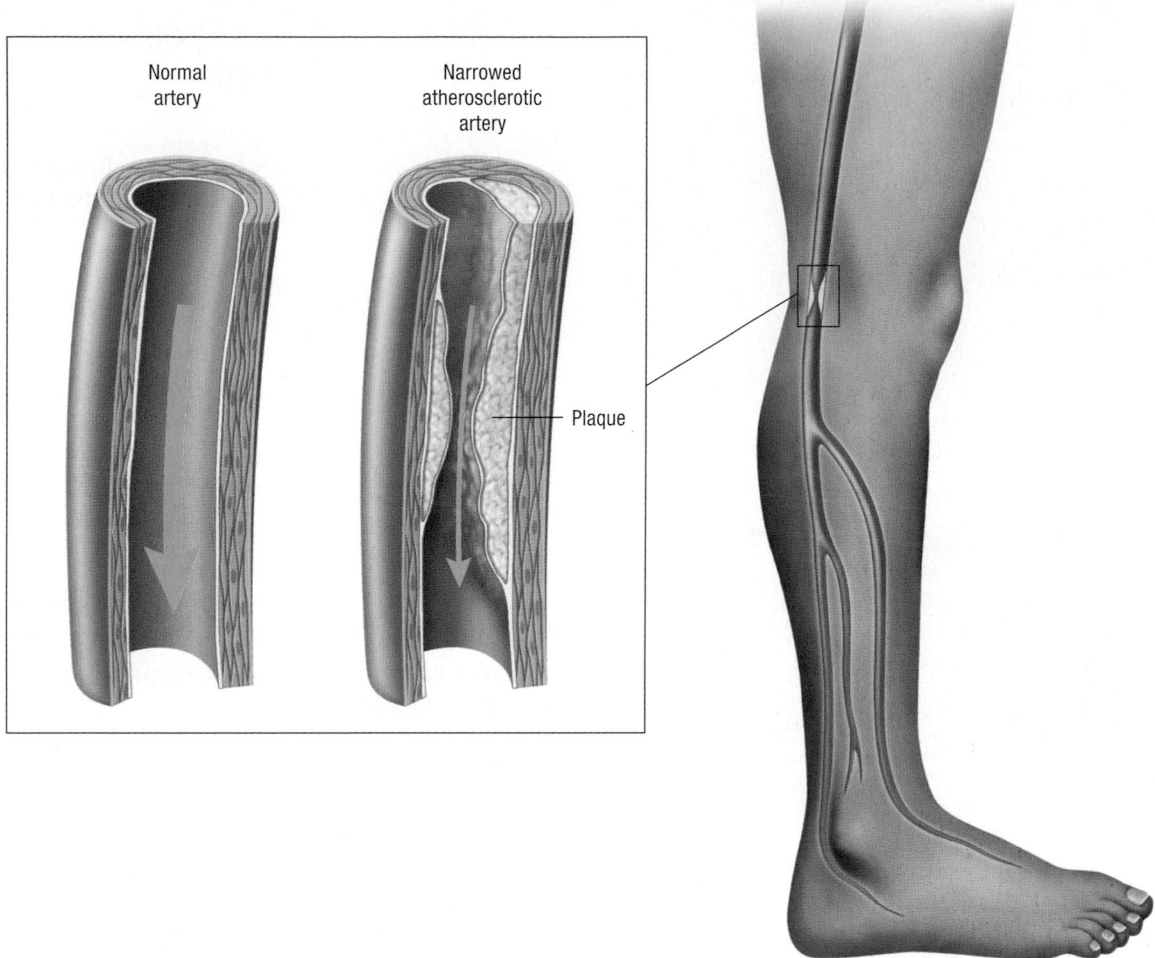

Figure 5.15. Peripheral artery disease

Hypertension

Definition: What Is It?

Hypertension is a technical term for high blood pressure. It is defined as blood pressure persistently elevated above 140 mm Hg systolic and/or 90 mm Hg diastolic. It is estimated that about one-third of all adults in the United States have high blood pressure. It is seen in men more often than women until women reach age 65; then it evens out and affects both genders equally. Age is a predisposing factor; about half of those over 60 years of age have high blood pressure. African Americans have higher hypertension rates than other races.

Etiology: What Happens?

In hypertension, internal and external forces put pressure on the arteries. To understand how these forces can cause damage, it is necessary to take a brief look at exactly what blood pressure is.

A sphygmomanometer is an instrument that measures the pressure blood exerts against arterial walls at two moments: contraction (**systole**) and relaxation (**diastole**). The blood pressure cuff converts the pressure in the arteries to millimeters of mercury see Animation at http://thePoint.lww.com/Werner5e.

The standard scale for hypertension in adults is based on how measurements correspond to the risk of developing cardiovascular disease, stroke, kidney disease, or heart failure. While a reading of 120/80 has traditionally been considered normal, the risk of secondary disease increases significantly when the systolic reading is over 115 or when the diastolic reading is over 75. A person's blood pressure is based on the averages of two or more readings taken at each of two or more doctor visits, because blood pressure

Hypertension in Brief

Pronunciation: hy-per-TEN-shun

What is it?
Hypertension is the technical name for high blood pressure.

How is it recognized?
High blood pressure is usually silent. The only way to identify it is by taking several blood pressure readings over time.

Massage risks and benefits
Risks: High blood pressure that accompanies other cardiovascular disease suggests that the client may have trouble adapting to changing environments, and bodywork must be adjusted accordingly. Medications that manage hypertension may also require some accommodation.
Benefits: For borderline or mild high blood pressure, massage may be a useful tool in healthcare management.

can change significantly from hour to hour. It's fairly common to see it shoot up from anxiety while a person is in a doctor's office; this is known as "white coat hypertension." Blood pressure ratings are shown in Table 5.1.

TABLE 5.1 Blood Pressure Ratings

Category	Systolic BP (mm Hg)	Diastolic BP (mm Hg)
Optimal	<120	<80
Pre-hypertension	122–139	80–89
Hypertension		
Stage 1 (mild)	140–159	90–99
Stage 2 (moderate)	160+	100+

High blood pressure quietly and progressively corrodes the major arteries, leading to a host of vicious circles that create threatening complications, including the following:

- *Edema.* High blood pressure forces fluid out of the capillaries at the nutrient-waste exchange sites. This adds to overall levels of interstitial fluid, causing edema. In a typically vicious circle, edema further raises blood pressure by putting external force on blood vessels.
- *Atherosclerosis.* Having blood pushing against arteries in an unceasing torrent simply wears

SIDEBAR 5.4 Heart Disease in the United States: Sobering Statistics[1]

The statistics for all varieties of cardiovascular disease are not generally separated from each other, since most of these conditions have a circular relationship. A person is unlikely to have atherosclerosis without high blood pressure, for instance, and a person is unlikely to have a heart attack without the predisposing factor of atherosclerosis, even if it never produces any symptoms.

Statistics for cardiovascular disease (this includes stroke, hypertension, heart failure, heart attack, angina, and congenital defects) in this country are sobering. These conditions collectively account for about 2,200 deaths every day, or a death every 39 seconds. About 33% of United States adults over 20 years of age have hypertension. Over 33 million adults over 20 years old have total serum cholesterol above 240 mg/dL, and more than 67% of US adults are overweight. The combined consequences of these facts lead to the finding that cardiovascular disease is the cause of death for about 2.4 million Americans each year; that is one in every three deaths.

Behaviors that limit the risk of heart disease have been identified to include not smoking, maintaining healthy weight, eating at least five servings of fruit and vegetables each day, and exercising for at least 30 minutes most days of the week. Other risk-lowering behaviors include having a diet that is low in trans fats, with a low glycemic load, high in fish oils, and high in folate. Studies consistently find that people for whom major risk factors are low in middle age, have a greatly increased possibility of living to age 85 years or older without severe illness.

[1] Heart disease and stroke statistics—2011 update. A report from the American Heart Association. © 2011 American Heart Association, Inc.URL: *http://circ.ahajournals.org/cgi/content/full/123/4/e18.* Accessed spring 2011.

out the walls, especially when the arteries have naturally lost some of their resiliency from age. As damage develops, the atherosclerotic process begins. This reinforces high blood pressure by narrowing arterial diameters.

- *Stroke*. Someone with hypertension is more likely to have a stroke than someone who does not have hypertension. The stroke may be from an embolism or it may be from ruptured arteries in the brain.
- *Enlarged heart, heart failure*. Pushing against narrowed arteries causes the left ventricle to grow considerably, but the coronary arteries do not grow with it to handle the extra load. The muscle fibers also lose elasticity. Therefore, the contractions are actually weaker, because the muscle is not well supplied with blood and it can't contract fully. This can also cause angina, or heart pain. When the ventricles of the heart are so overtaxed that they simply cannot keep up with the workload, the patient risks heart failure.
- *Aneurysm*. This is the result of high blood pressure causing a bulge in the arteries.
- *Kidney disease*. This complication of high blood pressure demonstrates the circular relationship between hypertension and kidney dysfunction. If problems start with the circulatory system, hypertension causes atherosclerotic plaques to form in the renal arteries, which are subject to huge blood pressure. This causes changes in blood flow to the kidney, which impairs kidney function, leading to kidney damage, systemic edema, and yet more pressure exerted against vessel walls from that edema. If the problem starts in the kidneys, decreased kidney function causes fluid retention. This is often accompanied by extra release of **renin**, the kidney-based hormone that regulates some electrolyte balance. Excess renin results in vasoconstriction, water and salt retention, increased edema, increased blood volume, and high blood pressure.
- *Retinopathy*. Chronic high blood pressure can damage the blood vessels that supply the eyes, causing them to thicken and lose elasticity. Reduction of blood flow to eyes results in permanent visual distortion.

High blood pressure is the most important modifiable risk factor in the development of coronary artery disease, stroke, congestive heart failure, end stage renal failure, and peripheral artery disease.

Types of Hypertension

- *Essential hypertension*. This is the focus of this discussion: it is not wholly dependent on some underlying factor. Essential hypertension accounts for about 95% of all diagnoses of high blood pressure.
- *Secondary hypertension*. This is a temporary complication of some other condition, such as pregnancy, kidney problems, adrenal tumor, or hormonal disorder.
- *Malignant hypertension*. This could be essential or secondary, but it involves diastolic pressure that rises very quickly, over a matter of weeks or months. It is extremely damaging to the circulatory system, a high risk for ischemic or hemorrhagic stroke. Left untreated, malignant hypertension is often fatal.

Signs and Symptoms

Hypertension, which is often called the silent killer, has few recognizable symptoms. When subtle signs are occasionally observed, they include shortness of breath after mild exercise; headaches or dizziness; swelling of the ankles, especially during the daytime; excessive sweating, anxiety, and occasional nosebleeds.

Treatment

Hypertension is a highly treatable disease, but because it has virtually no symptoms until it has progressed to very dangerous levels, it is frequently untreated or incompletely treated. Only about a third of the people who treat their hypertension at all are successful at getting their blood pressure below 140/90.

Exercise and diet are the first strategies to manage this condition. The National Heart Lung and Blood Institute (NHLBI) has created the DASH (Dietary Approaches to Stop Hypertension) diet: a combination of high-fiber, low-fat foods that provide higher than average levels of calcium, magnesium, and potassium while cutting sodium by about 20%. Following the

DASH diet (which is useful for anyone, not just hypertension patients) has been found to be as effective as treatment with any single type of blood pressure medication, without side effects or long-term health risks.

Exercise is also crucial for the development of healthy new blood vessels and for weight control. Losing even a small percentage of body weight for obese or overweight patients can have a profound effect on blood pressure and cardiovascular health.

Medication, if it's called for, includes diuretics, vasodilators, and beta blockers, which decrease the force of ventricular contraction. Medicating high blood pressure can be challenging. Because the disease itself has no strong symptoms, and because the medicines often have mild but unpleasant side effects (including dizziness, insomnia, impotence, and others), it can be difficult for hypertension patients to be consistent with their medications.

Medications

- Diuretics for fluid management and kidney support
- Vasodilators (calcium channel blockers, ACE inhibitors, angiotensin-receptor blockers) to reduce cardiac load
- Beta blockers, alpha blockers to decrease the force of ventricular contraction

Massage?

RISKS Clients with unmanaged or poorly managed hypertension may have complications that have cautions for massage, including kidney disease, atherosclerosis, and a risk of heart attack. All of these are concerns for massage therapists and bodywork practitioners. Further, clients who take medication for hypertension may feel dizzy or lethargic—this means they may need more time after a massage to make the transition back to full speed.

BENEFITS Any client with mild or borderline hypertension who is encouraged to exercise is a good candidate for most kinds of bodywork. Clients with more advanced cases but who manage their hypertension successfully require some caution, but if they can exercise safely, they can probably also receive massage safely: judgments about massage must be made by comparing the challenges of bodywork with activities of daily living. Bodywork has been seen to have at least a short-term effect on blood pressure, but the overall stress-reducing effects may be more useful in the long run.

Raynaud Syndrome

Definition: What Is It?

Raynaud syndrome is a condition involving the status of the arterioles in the hands and feet, although it can also affect the nose, ears, and lips. Primary Raynaud disease is a vasoconstriction disorder, while secondary Raynaud phenomenon is a complication of an underlying problem.

Etiology: What Happens?

Raynaud syndrome affects the arterioles in the extremities, so that they develop vasospasm, or contraction of smooth muscle tissue, followed by vasodilation. It occurs in temporary episodes at first, but especially if it is a secondary complication, the vasoconstriction can become long lasting. It can happen as a primary condition, or as a symptom of an underlying disease.

Types of Raynaud Syndrome

- *Raynaud disease.* This is primary Raynaud syndrome; it occurs without an identified underlying pathology. It may be due to emotional

Raynaud Syndrome in Brief

Pronunciation: ray-NO SIN drome

What is it?
Raynaud syndrome is a condition defined by episodes of vasospasm followed by dilation of the arterioles, usually in fingers and toes, and occasionally in the nose, ears, and lips.

How is it recognized?
Affected areas go through marked color changes of white, or ashy gray for dark-skinned people, to blue, to red. Attacks can last for less than a minute or several hours. Pain, numbness, and/or tingling may follow during recovery.

Massage risks and benefits
Risks: When Raynaud syndrome is attached to an underlying pathology, cautions must be followed for that condition.
Benefits: Raynaud syndrome that is not associated with underlying pathology indicates careful massage, even in the midst of an acute episode.

stress, cold, or a mechanical irritation, such as operating machinery that influences blood vessel dilation. Raynaud disease generally has a slow onset, and the attacks are less severe than when the symptoms occur as a secondary problem. If a person is prone to Raynaud disease, both the feet and hands tend to be affected.

- *Raynaud phenomenon.* This is a secondary reaction to an underlying condition. It generally has a much faster onset than Raynaud disease, the age at onset is typically older, and the risk of serious complications is much higher. Some conditions associated with Raynaud phenomenon include the following:
  - Arterial diseases that involve occlusions, such as diabetes, atherosclerosis, and Buerger disease (a rare disease marked by inflammation and blood clots in the arteries)
  - Autoimmune connective tissue diseases, such as scleroderma, lupus, and rheumatoid arthritis
  - Sensitivity to some drugs, including beta blockers and ergot compounds

Signs and Symptoms

Raynaud syndrome is usually bilateral. During an attack, patches of skin go through a characteristic cycle of colors: white as the blood is shunted away from the area (on dark-skinned people the skin looks ashy gray); blue as the cells are starved for oxygen; and red as the attack subsides, the arterioles reopen, and the blood returns to the affected area (Figure 5.16). Some people only shift between blue and red; others show only pallor or blueness (cyanosis) during an episode. It usually affects distal fingers and toes, not the thumb or the rest of the hand. Sometimes only one or two digits are affected, and these may change from one episode to another.

While Raynaud disease episodes are typically short, attacks of Raynaud phenomenon can last anywhere from less than a minute to several hours. These can be so extreme and long lasting that atrophy and ulcerations on the starved skin may develop. Arterioles in the nail beds can become thickened and distorted, the fingers may taper, and the skin can become thin, smooth, and shiny. Gangrene is a rare but possible complication for these extreme cases.

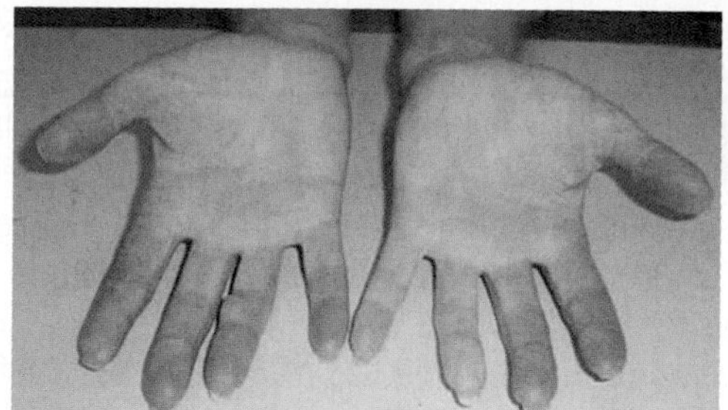

Figure 5.16. Raynaud syndrome

Treatment

Treatment depends on whether the patient has primary or secondary Raynaud syndrome. For primary Raynaud disease, a noninvasive approach is taken first. Quitting smoking, avoiding vasoconstrictors such as nicotine and caffeine, soaking in warm water, dressing appropriately for the weather, protecting the hands when working with cold or frozen foods, making sure that shoes aren't too tight, even moving to a warmer climate are all suggested before more intrusive intervention is suggested. In addition, because primary Raynaud disease can be exacerbated by emotional upset, patients are often encouraged to find productive ways to manage stress. This can range from learning biofeedback techniques, to exercising regularly, to receiving massage.

If results are unsatisfactory or if tissue damage from chronically impaired blood flow is a risk, the next step is medication to dilate the blood vessels.

Secondary Raynaud phenomenon often doesn't respond to medication. Surgery to interfere with sympathetic motor neuron stimulation of local capillaries may be conducted; this procedure, called a sympathectomy, is used only when no other options work, and it tends to be a temporary measure.

Medications

- Calcium channel blockers, ACE inhibitors for vasodilation
- Selective serotonin reuptake inhibitors for dilation of peripheral blood vessels

Massage?

RISKS Raynaud phenomenon can be a symptom of lupus, scleroderma, or other serious problems that compromise the blood vessels. In this situation, the underlying condition must dictate the choices for bodywork.

Clients with Raynaud disease may use vasodilating medications that have dizziness or lethargy as side effects. These clients may need adjustments in bodywork to deal with those changes.

BENEFITS Raynaud disease indicates massage as long as the skin is intact and healthy and the medications that the client uses are accommodated.

OPTIONS Many clients with Raynaud disease enjoy hydrotherapy applications, including warm baths or paraffin baths for the affected areas.

Varicose Veins

Definition: What Are They?

Varicose veins are permanently distended, often twisted or ropy superficial veins (**varix** means "twisted"). They occur when the veins of the legs are not strong enough to keep up with a person's needs. The valves that support blood flow against gravity are compromised. As blood collects, the affected vein is stretched, distorted, and further weakened. Women are more vulnerable to varicose veins than men for a variety of reasons, but anyone can develop them. About one-half of all people over 50 years old have varicose veins. Distended veins can develop in a few locations, but most often they are in the legs (Figure 5.17), which is the focus of most of this discussion.

Varicose Veins in Brief

Pronunciation: VARE-ih-kose vanez

What are they?
Varicose veins are distended veins, usually in the legs, caused by venous insufficiency and retrograde blood flow.

How are they recognized?
Varicose veins are ropy, bluish, elevated veins that twist and turn out of their usual course. They are most common in branches of the great saphenous veins on the medial side of the calf, although they are also found on the posterior aspects of the calf and thigh. Varicose veins can also develop at other locations, in which case they have other names.

Massage risks and benefits
Risks: Extreme varicose veins, especially with compromised skin, contraindicate any massage that might disrupt or irritate them. Milder varicose veins locally contraindicate deep specific work, but are safe for superficial massage as long as the skin is healthy. It is important to note that people with varicose veins are at increased risk for deep vein thrombosis, so massage therapists need to be knowledgeable about both conditions.
Benefits: Massage is unlikely to change or improve varicose veins. As long as they are accommodated, clients with varicose veins can enjoy the same benefits from bodywork as the rest of the population.

Etiology: What Happens?

The veins in the legs are constructed in a way that helps to move blood from the toes all the way back to the heart. Small veins pick up the blood from the internal muscle capillaries. These veins tend to run on the superficial aspect of muscles. They feed into larger veins that perforate the muscle bellies and then into the large deep veins that run under the muscles, close to the bones. When the leg muscles contract, the perforating veins are squeezed, sending their contents to the deep veins. When the leg muscles relax, the perforating veins draw in new blood from the smaller veins. The contraction and relaxation of the leg muscles (especially the soleus—"sump pump of the leg") is crucial to blood return. The valves inside the perforating veins and the deep veins ensure that blood does not collect in the smaller, weaker superficial veins.

When valves in the superficial veins become weak, problems ensue. Weakness can develop because of simple wear and tear: being on one's feet for many hours a day for instance, especially if the leg muscles are not allowed to fully contract and relax during that time. It could also be due to a mechanical obstruction to returning blood: knee socks that are too tight, a knee brace, or a fetus that presses on the femoral vein. Systemic problems from kidney or liver congestion have been seen to cause problems too. And finally, it could be simply congenitally weak veins or a structural anomaly at the junction between the great saphenous vein and the femoral vein.

Once a vein begins to widen, blood puts pressure on the inferior valves. Vascular incompetence ultimately causes the weakest superficial veins to become

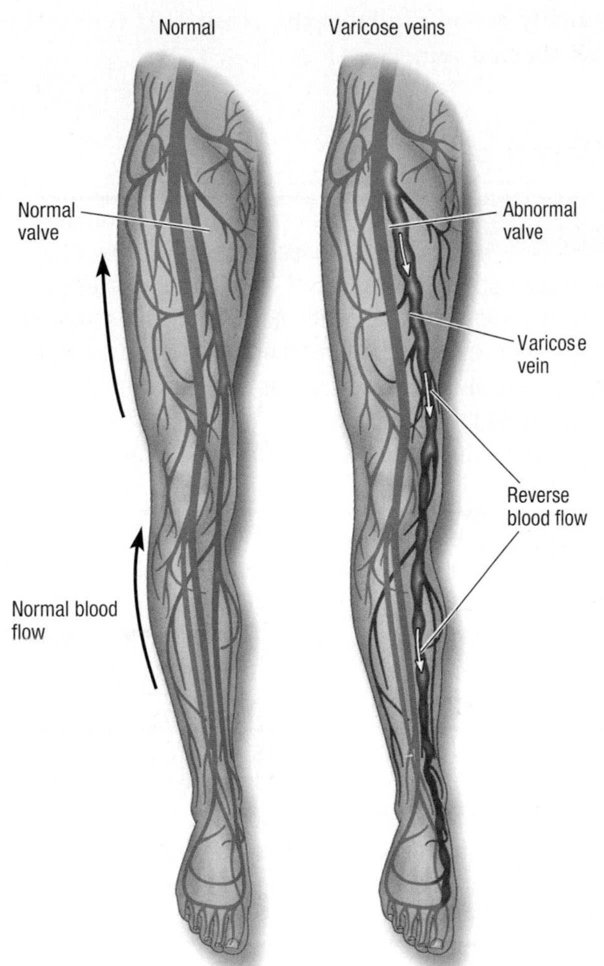

Figure 5.17. Varicose veins

distorted, dilated, and twisted off their regular pathway. Deeper veins are protected from this process because they have the external support of muscle tissue.

Although varicosities are seldom more than annoying, they can create some unpleasant or even dangerous complications. Chronic venous insufficiency may result in varicose ulcers, which don't heal until circulation is restored. Skin irritation from poor circulation occasionally leads to a type of dermatitis that isn't resolved until the varicosity is relieved. Interruptions in blood flow increase the likelihood of night cramps. And stagnant blood in a distended vein may coagulate, raising the possibility of clotting. However, most clots that form in varicose veins are superficial and melt easily, so they are usually a lesser threat than clots that form in deeper leg veins. Be aware, however, that the presence of grossly distended varicose veins may indicate an increased risk of DVT. This is true especially when the varicosities have a sudden onset or change in size and quality very rapidly.

Types of Varicose Veins

In addition to the varicose veins that frequently develop in the legs, veins in other structures are vulnerable to distension and structural dysfunction.

- *Esophageal varices.* These are large, distended veins at the distal part of the esophagus. Esophageal varices are most common in people who struggle with advanced liver disease or with bulimia. This situation carries a risk of dangerous internal bleeding. If it is determined that these varices are threatening, they may be surgically corrected.
- *Hemorrhoids.* Technically speaking, hemorrhoids are clusters of vascular tissue around the anus. They can contain veins, capillaries, and small arterioles. Distended vessels can develop inside the rectum, where they are typically silent, or externally, where they can cause pain, itching, and bleeding with bowel movements. Hemorrhoids are usually associated with constipation and straining during bowel movements. If they are severely swollen or prolapsed, they can be surgically removed. Otherwise, they are typically treated by including more fiber and water in the diet and using soothing ointment.
- *Telangiactasias.* These are the very small permanently dilated capillaries and venules sometimes called spider veins. They can appear around the ankles, on the legs, or on the face. A new pattern of **telangiectasias** can sometimes indicate a deeper circulatory problem, but these phenomena are usually harmless.
- *Varicoceles.* These are dilated venous structures that supply the spermatic cord. They are often painless, but they can interfere with fertility and testosterone production. Varicoceles are treated by surgery.

Signs and Symptoms

Varicose veins look like lumpy bluish wandering lines on the surface of the skin on the legs (Figure 5.18). They are often visible on the back of the calf, where they affect the lesser saphenous vein, but more often they affect the great saphenous vein, where they show up anywhere from the ankle to the groin on the medial side. They may itch, throb, or cause cramping, especially when the person is tired.

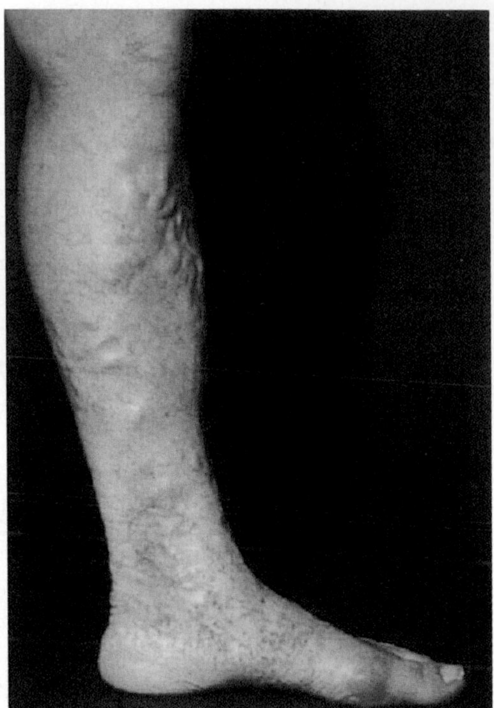

Figure 5.18. Varicose veins, photo

Treatment

Support hose or elastic bandages can give extra help to damaged veins, and avoiding long periods of standing up without full contraction and relaxation of the muscles is often recommended. Clothes that constrict at the leg, the groin, or the waist should be avoided. Reclining with the feet slightly elevated also reduces symptoms.

Surgery for mild varicose veins is not generally recommended as a purely cosmetic intervention. However, varicose veins are a progressive condition; they don't usually spontaneously reverse, and if they are left untreated, their complications can be serious. Therefore, a certain number of patients eventually seek treatment for health rather than cosmetic concerns.

Several strategies for reducing varicose veins have been developed. Vein stripping, ambulatory phlebectomy (ministripping), and sclerosing (injections of chemicals that cause the vein to close down completely) are all options, but using laser energy or radiofrequency through a catheter to large veins is usually successful with less risk of complications. In all of these treatments, the body's remarkable ability to generate new blood vessels quickly accommodates the closure or removal of the affected vein.

Massage?

RISKS If a client has very extreme distorted twisting varicose veins, and especially if their skin shows any signs of circulatory problems, this condition at least locally contraindicates massage. It is important to remember that people with varicose veins have an increased risk for deep vein thrombosis, some massage therapists must be aware of the subtle signs and symptoms that can accompany this condition.

BENEFITS While massage is unlikely to change the prognosis for varicose veins, if the skin is intact and healthy, then gentle gliding pressure is safe. Clients with varicose veins can enjoy the same benefits of bodywork as the rest of the population as long as locally affected areas are respected.

OPTIONS If varicose veins are very mild, they can sometimes respond well to hydrotherapy. Alternating hot and cold application can provide exercise for the smooth muscle inside the superficial vein. This can be done in a massage setting, but clients can also do this for themselves at home.

Heart Conditions

Heart Attack

Definition: What Is It?

A heart attack is a process that damages some portion of cardiac muscle tissue through ischemia, or lack of blood flow and oxygen supply (Figure 5.19). Atherosclerosis in the coronary arteries (coronary artery disease) is usually the cause, although extreme vasospasm without plaque can also damage the heart. The starved cells do not grow back; they are replaced by inelastic, noncontractile scar tissue. The damaged area is referred to as an **infarct**. Another term for heart attack is myocardial infarction.

About 1.5 million people have a heart attack in the United States each year. Heart attack is the leading cause of death for both men and women in this country, claiming over half a million lives every year.

Heart Attack in Brief

What is it?
A heart attack, also called myocardial infarction, is damage to the myocardium caused by an obstruction in blood flow through the coronary arteries, which results in permanent myocardial damage.

How is it recognized?
Symptoms of most heart attacks include a sensation of pressure on the chest, spreading pain, lightheadedness, dizziness, and nausea. Sometimes symptoms vary, and occasionally a heart attack may occur with no symptoms at all.

Massage risks and benefits
Risks: Recent heart attacks contraindicate rigorous massage until the patient has come back to normal levels of activity.
Benefits: Clients who have survived a heart attack but have no long-term impairments in function can enjoy any bodywork that stays within their limits for adaptation.

Etiology: What Happens?

A heart attack occurs when a portion of the cardiac muscle dies from lack of oxygen: an ischemic attack. It usually comes from a blockage in the coronary artery that grows until it completely obstructs blood flow. It could also be from a loosened blood clot or a broken or torn piece of atherosclerotic plaque that travels until it blocks the coronary artery. Rarely, a heart attack may occur when a coronary artery goes into prolonged spasm; this is seen most often in cocaine or other drug overdose.

Risk factors for heart attack are similar to those for other cardiovascular diseases. They include age, gender (men with heart disease outnumber women until menopause, and then both genders are affected equally), family history of cardiovascular disease, diabetes, hypertension, high cholesterol, obesity, lack of exercise, and stress.

Atherosclerotic plaques are important predisposing factors for heart attack risk. Older, harder plaques are relatively stable, but newer, softer plaques have a higher risk of rupturing to let go of clots or other debris that then block the coronary artery.

When a portion of the cardiac muscle is killed off by ischemic attack, the ability to contract with coordination and efficiency is badly damaged. If a heart attack is severe enough to trigger ventricular fibrillations, the risk of sudden death is very high.

The seriousness of a heart attack is determined by the size and location of the blockage, the length of time blood supply is deprived, and the metabolic needs of the cells that are affected. If it is relatively small and the affected area doesn't have to work especially hard, the heart attack is a mild one. But if the infarct is large enough to weaken the heart's ability to contract, or if the damaged tissue involves the electrical conduction system for the heart, major intervention is necessary to aid in recovery.

The chronology of heart problems is often circular rather than linear, which means that several heart attack complications are also heart attack contributors.

- *Atrial and ventricular fibrillations*. These are rapid, incomplete, weak attempts at contraction of the chambers. They occur most often if any part of the sinoatrial node, the heart's electrical pacemaker, has been damaged. These inefficient contractions allow blood to pool and thicken in the chambers of the heart and may contribute to the risk of embolism. Ventricular fibrillations, because they interfere with blood flow to the entire body, may result in death if they are not treated quickly.
- *Arrhythmia*. This is a potentially permanent consequence of losing some heart muscle function.
- *Embolism*. A heart attack can cause blood clots to form inside the chambers of the heart. Clots from the left side exit through the aorta, and travel to wherever the bloodstream takes them; they can land in the brain, causing a stroke, or the renal arteries, where they can contribute to renal failure. Clots on the right side or prolonged bed rest can also promote the risk of pulmonary embolism.
- *Aneurysm*. Weakened cardiac tissue can create a bulge in the heart muscle itself similar to aortic aneurysms.
- *Heart failure*. In heart failure, the muscle is no longer strong enough to do its work. A heart with patches of scar tissue is particularly

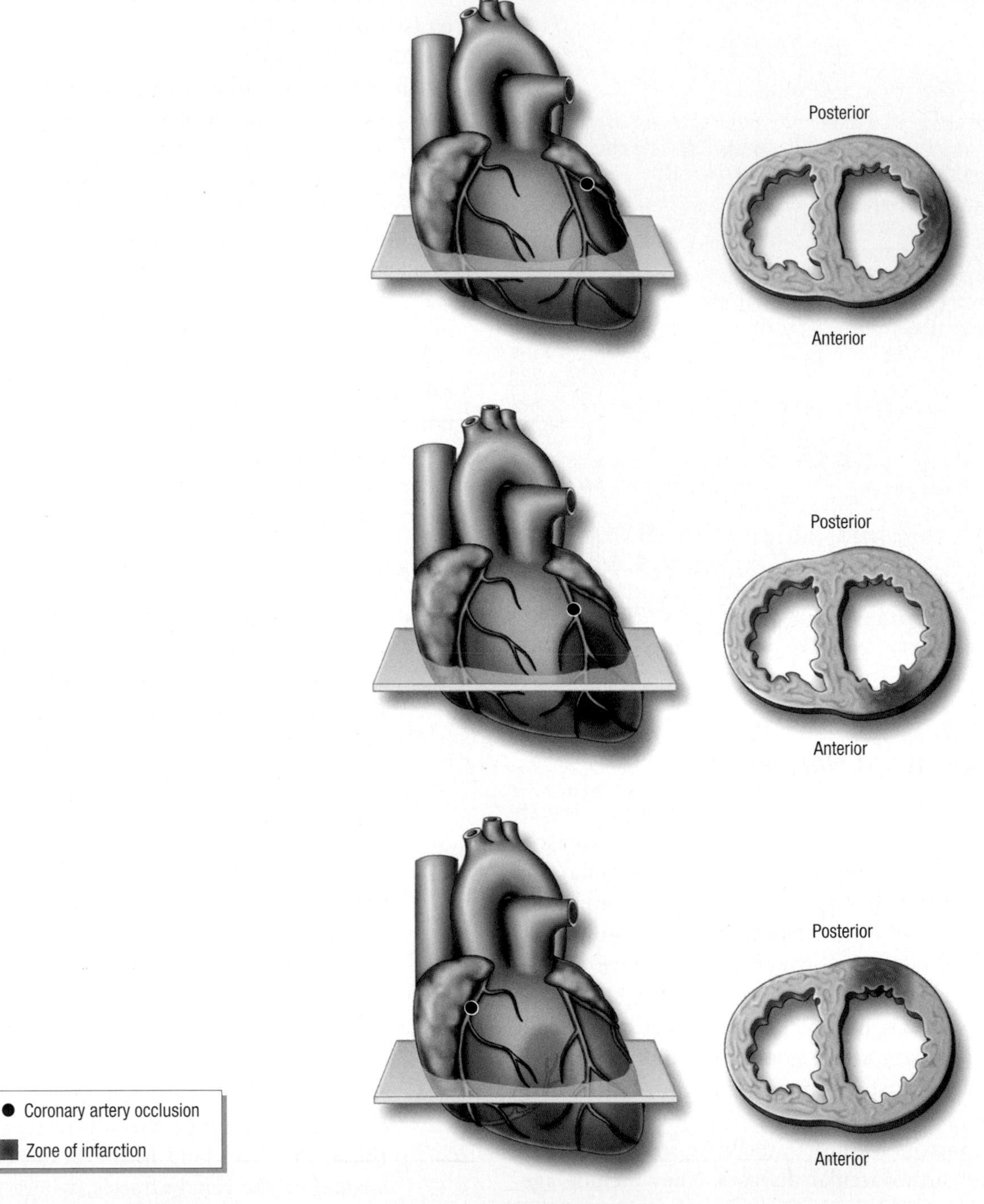

Figure 5.19. Myocardial infarctions

vulnerable. This condition is discussed further elsewhere in this chapter.

- *Shock.* In shock, the circulatory system swings reactively from a sympathetic to a parasympathetic state, opening the arteries to a maximum diameter in the process. The main danger with shock is loss of oxygen to the brain from radically decreased blood pressure.

Signs and Symptoms

Heart attacks have a variety of signs and symptoms, some of which are extremely subtle and some of which are very severe. Some of the most common and dependable signs are these:

- Angina pectoris (literally, "chest pain"). This is one of the few early warning signs for the risk of heart attack. Not all people have this symptom, but those who do should pay close attention. Pain may spread to the shoulder, arm, neck, and jaw of the left side of the body. This is the referred pain pattern for the dermatome shared by the heart. Angina can be stable or unstable.

- Stable angina is the simplest and most common form of angina. In this situation, the heart can get enough oxygen to perform regular tasks, but any extra effort, such as carrying something heavy or running up a flight of stairs, demands too much of the clogged coronary arteries. The result is moderate to severe chest pain that is relieved with rest and/or angina medication.
- Unstable angina can occur without unusual physical activity. It often appears in the night, with very extreme but short-lived chest pain. It is caused by vascular spasm at or near the site of atherosclerotic plaques, or by plaques rupturing.
- Spreading pain. Lightheadedness, nausea, sweating. These usually occur along with chest pain. When they occur without chest pain, they may still indicate a heart attack, but this is a less common presentation.
- Shortness of breath with or without chest pain; unexplained nausea, anxiety, or weakness; fainting; palpitations; and cold sweat.
- Stomach and abdominal pain.

A heart attack is a dynamic process. The critical blockage of the coronary artery may take place over several hours. This means that early intervention can preserve much of the myocardium: survival rates for heart attacks are better than ever because treatment is instituted quickly. But this is also bad news if people

COMPARE & CONTRAST 5.2 Chest Pain, Chest Pain, Chest Pain

Not all chest pain means heart attack, although in a culture in which almost 40% of deaths are related to cardiovascular disease, it seems logical to jump to that conclusion. What follows is a comparison of types of chest pain with some indications of what might be heart attack and what probably is not. However, heart attack symptoms are notoriously variable, and it is always a good idea to consult a healthcare professional when the source of chest pain is not clear.

FEATURES	ANGINA	HEART ATTACK	PULMONARY EMBOLISM	OTHER
Duration	Chest pain lasts several minutes, subsides.	Chest pain progressively worsens.	Chest pain progressively worsens.	Chest pain subsides in <1 min.
Trigger	Usually triggered by activity.	May or may not be immediately triggered by activity.	May or may not be immediately triggered by activity.	May or may not be immediately triggered by activity.
Activity	Stops when activity stops.	Doesn't stop when activity stops; continues to worsen.	Doesn't stop when activity stops; continues to worsen.	Stops when a person drinks water, changes position, or takes a deep breath.
Causes	Caused by transient ischemia; heart muscle temporarily doesn't get enough oxygen to function.	Caused by permanent ischemia; blockage deprives cells of oxygen, and heart is irrevocably damaged.	Caused by blood clot in lung. Small clot may have little impact. Large clot may lead to pulmonary and circulatory collapse.	Caused by any number of factors, e.g., musculoskeletal injury, gastroesophageal reflux.

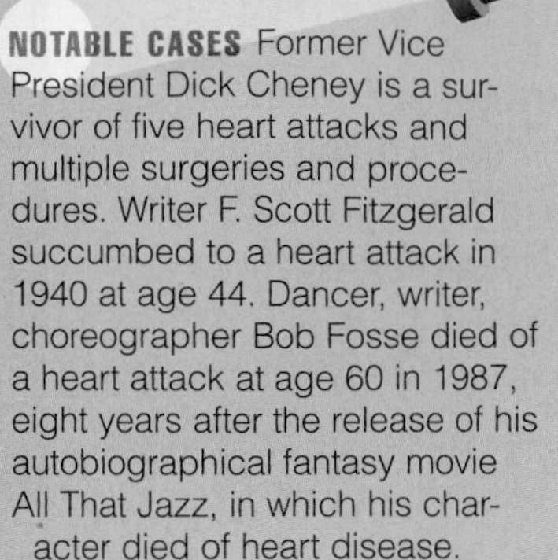

NOTABLE CASES Former Vice President Dick Cheney is a survivor of five heart attacks and multiple surgeries and procedures. Writer F. Scott Fitzgerald succumbed to a heart attack in 1940 at age 44. Dancer, writer, choreographer Bob Fosse died of a heart attack at age 60 in 1987, eight years after the release of his autobiographical fantasy movie All That Jazz, in which his character died of heart disease.

tend to ignore early warning signs and don't seek attention until symptoms have been present for many hours or even days.

It is important to point out that while heart attack symptoms can be severe, and heart attacks are part of a large and complex group of heart and circulatory problems, up to one-half of all the people who have a heart attack have no medical history of problems, and no memory of warning symptoms.

Treatment

The first priority with heart attack patients is to determine where the blockage is and to get rid of it as quickly as possible. This is done with clot-dissolving drugs, which can take effect in 90 minutes or less, and with immediate balloon angioplasty, which can open up most clogged arteries in about an hour. The technical term for this procedure is **percutaneous transluminal coronary angioplasty**. Other immediate-care options include the administration of oxygen and pain management with nitroglycerin and/or morphine.

Later care usually includes more clot dissolvers and nitroglycerin, which work to relax the smooth muscle tissue in the arteries. After the emergency has passed, a barrage of tests is conducted to determine the location and extent of damage to the cardiac muscle. These tests indicate one of three future courses of action: that the infarct was minor and requires no further medical intervention; that prescription anticoagulants are indicated; or that a serious and permanent narrowing of a coronary artery requires surgery to repair it. This surgery may be a more complete version of the angioplasty, or it may be coronary bypass surgery, in

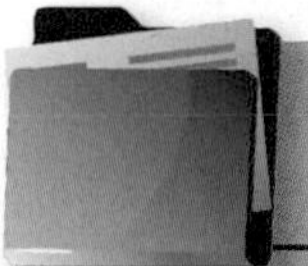

CASE HISTORY 5.2 Heart Attack

After watching my mother go through heart disease and stent surgery, I began to seriously think about my own health. I talked to my doctor, and he set me up with a low-cost, onsite stress test that just used an exercise bike. He said if I could pass that I'd be okay. I took it, and in the words of the technician, "My heart was not happy with what I was doing to it." So my doctor scheduled me with a cardiologist for a full treadmill test.

I didn't last long on the treadmill. When it was over, my blood pressure dropped and I had some really unpleasant symptoms, like dizziness, nausea, and a general feeling of crappiness. My doctor called my wife in from the waiting room, and with both of us together he said, "My recommendation is to put you in the hospital now. We'll do an angiogram along with anything else that needs to be done."

I checked right in.

The next day they found that the main section of the left coronary artery was 100% blocked. They had trouble pushing a wire through it, but when they got that done, they put in the balloon and then a titanium stent.

BOB, AGE 49
The wake-up call.

They also told me that they found evidence of a recent heart attack—one that was a fraction of an inch away from what they call a "widow maker." This was amazing to me, because I have no memory of any chest pains.

Three days after the angioplasty I went home. They started my cardiac rehab right away. I have to exercise under supervision, next door to an emergency room. My doctors tell me if I ever let my heart rate get over 120 beats per minute, I run the risk of forming clots around the stent.

This episode was a real wake-up call for me. I'm the youngest man at my job, and the last one they expected to have heart trouble. My identical twin went in for his own stress test and came back fine, but he was a couple of years later than me in developing his diabetes too, so he'll still have to keep an eye on it. I did some research about my situation, and I found that what I had—silent ischemia—is especially common in diabetic men over 40. I hope any man with type 2 diabetes over 40 or 45 will be sure to get his heart checked. You never know what you might find.■

which damaged sections of the coronary artery are replaced with grafts of healthy vessels from elsewhere in the body.

Treatment in heart attack and heart surgery recovery must also embrace the lifestyle changes that will support a healthier future: eating sensibly, exercising regularly, controlling high blood pressure, and quitting smoking are the most important factors.

Some studies have indicated that taking aspirin regularly can decrease the chance of a repeat heart attack for people with a history of heart disease. This intervention is not risk free, however, so it should be undertaken under a doctor's oversight.

Medications

- Emergency care:
  - Aspirin for antiplatelet activity to prevent blockage from getting bigger
  - Analgesics
  - Nitroglycerin for smooth muscle relaxation
  - Thrombolytics and anticoagulants to lower blood clot risk
- After-care
  - Nitroglycerin
  - Anticoagulants, antiplatelet drugs
  - Cholesterol management drugs
  - Hypertension management drugs

Massage?

RISKS The safety of massage for a heart attack survivor depends on how easily the client can withstand the changes in internal environment that this work will bring about. Anyone who is fragile or must exercise with great care may not be able to adapt to the changes that rigorous massage demands.

BENEFITS Gentle, supportive bodywork of most kinds is appropriate for heart attack patients; this is an option that is now used in some hospital settings to help mitigate the pain and anxiety that goes along with heart disease surgery. A client with a history of heart attack but who is physically active can probably adapt to any changes that massage may bring about.

Heart Failure

Definition: What Is It?

Heart failure is a term for the progressive loss of cardiac function that accompanies age and a history of cardiovascular disease. It does not mean that the heart has stopped working altogether (that would be cardiac arrest); it simply means that the heart cannot keep up with the needs of the body.

About 5 million people in the United States have heart failure, usually as a result of other cardiovascular diseases. This condition causes about 300,000 deaths each year. The prevalence of heart failure approximately doubles with each decade of life.

Etiology: What Happens?

A healthy heart pumps 2,000 gallons of blood each day. If resistance in the cardiovascular system

Heart Failure in Brief

What is it?
Heart failure is a condition in which the heart can no longer function well enough to keep up with the needs of the body. It is usually slowly progressive, developing over a number of years before any changes in function may be noticeable.

How is it recognized?
The symptoms of heart failure depend on which side of the heart is working inefficiently. Left-sided heart failure results in fluid congestion in the lungs with general weakness and shortness of breath. Right-sided heart failure results in fluid backups throughout the system, which shows as edema, especially in the ankles and legs. Both varieties of heart failure lead to chest pain; cold, sweaty skin; a fast, irregular pulse; coughing, especially when the person is lying down; and poor stamina.

Massage risks and benefits
Risks: Heart failure contraindicates any bodywork with the intention of mechanically pushing fluid through a system that is severely compromised.
Benefits: Massage or bodywork that does not demand an overwhelming adaptive response is appropriate for heart failure patients, as long as they are comfortable on a massage table.

increases (usually from atherosclerosis, hypertension, and other manifestations of cardiovascular disease), the heart compensates in various ways. Any of these mechanisms works for short-term challenges, but over the long term, they add to the problem rather than helping to solve it.

In one compensation strategy, the heart muscle cells respond to chronic stress by growing larger. The ventricles appear to become bigger and thicker, allowing the heart to push harder against resistance in the pulmonary or systemic circuits. Ultimately, however, this cardiac hypertrophy causes the ventricles to become stiff, so they don't fill or contract normally.

Some chemicals that influence heart function can also help to compensate for short-term problems but exacerbate long-term ones. Resistance in the system or injury to the heart causes the release of stress hormones, especially epinephrine and norepinephrine. These make the heart work harder. Shifts in hormones also cause the body to retain salt and water. Both these features compensate for weakness in the short run, but end up increasing blood pressure and adding to the workload of the overburdened heart.

Finally, the muscle simply wears out, and functions so inefficiently that blood flow to the rest of the body is insufficient for the most basic kinds of activities: climbing stairs, walking across a room, even getting out of bed. Left untreated, the failed heart muscle goes into fibrillations and the circulatory system collapses.

Most cases of heart failure are related to underlying cardiovascular disease. A history of atherosclerosis or heart attack with resulting scar tissue in the heart muscle increases the risk of developing heart failure. High blood pressure, untreated diabetes, smoking, and alcohol and drug abuse can all be contributing factors as well. An especially potent setup for heart failure is any combination of these risk factors: uncontrolled high blood pressure along with smoking, for instance.

A smaller number of heart failure patients do not have a history of cardiovascular disease but have sustained damage to the heart muscle for other reasons. **Cardiomyopathy**, valve diseases, infections of the valves or heart muscle, and congenital problems may all be factors in these cases.

Types of Heart Failure

- *Left-sided heart failure*. In this situation, the left ventricle is impaired, and blood backs up into the pulmonary circuit. This allows seepage of fluid back into the alveoli, causing pulmonary edema (Figure 5.20). Symptoms of left-sided heart failure include severe shortness of breath and stubborn coughing, perhaps with bloody sputum. Symptoms are worst when a person is active or lying down. One serious complication of this condition is the risk of pneumonia in the functionally impaired lungs.

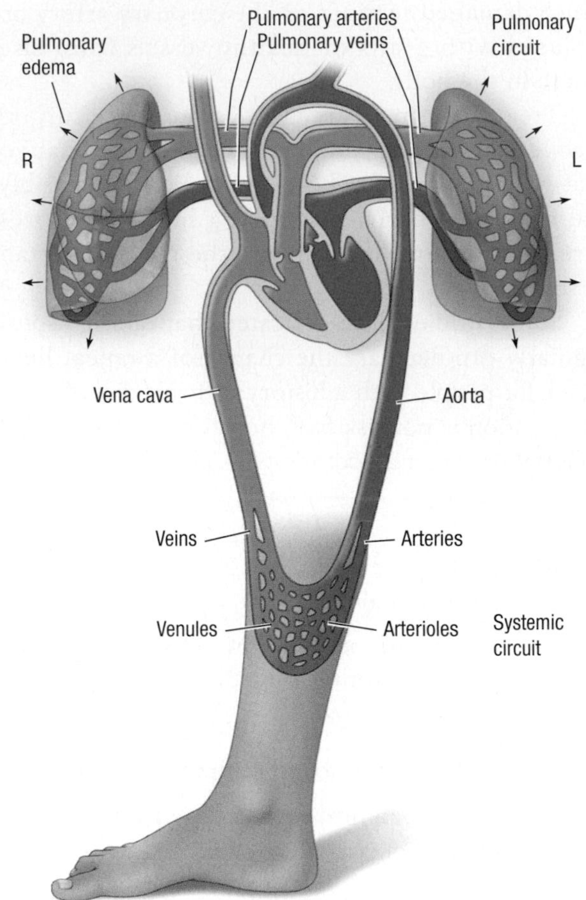

Figure 5.20. Left-sided heart failure

- *Right-sided heart failure*. Also called **cor pulmonale**; this commonly results from pulmonary disease and high vascular resistance in the lungs—often as a complication of the pulmonary edema that accumulates with left-sided heart failure. Consequently, it becomes difficult for the right ventricle to pump blood through the pulmonary circuit, and the backup is felt through the rest of the body. Symptoms include severe edema, especially in the legs (Figure 5.21). Someone with this

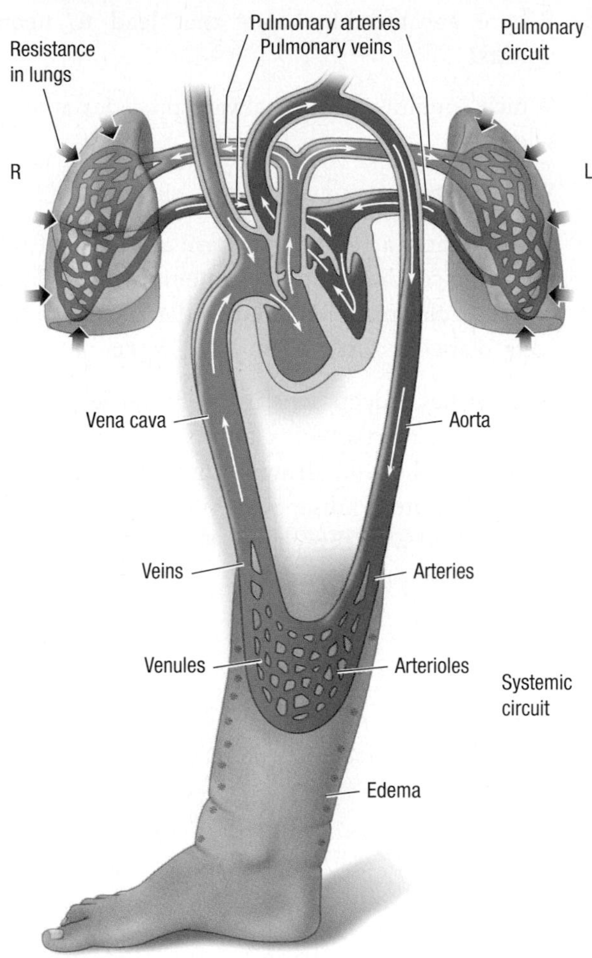

Figure 5.21. Right-sided heart failure

type of heart failure has ankles that look like they're spilling over the sides of the shoes. If the patient is bedridden, the edema may occur in the abdomen (**ascites**) or in the pelvis—wherever gravity is pulling most. Right-sided heart failure is also closely linked to enlarged liver (**hepatomegaly**) and renal failure. As blood flow to the kidneys is reduced, the kidneys begin to retain water, which systemically increases blood pressure and makes the heart work even harder to push blood through narrow tubes.

- *Biventricular heart failure.* This is left- and ride-sided failure simultaneously. It is the end stage of the disease, and if the patient doesn't respond to medications, he or she may be a candidate for a heart transplant or other surgery.

See Animation and video at http://thePoint.lww.com/Werner5e.

Signs and Symptoms

Signs of heart failure depend on which side of the heart is dysfunctional, as already described. Along with shortness of breath (often exacerbated by lying down), low stamina, and edema, heart failure patients may also have chronic chest pain, indigestion, arrhythmia, visibly distended veins in the neck, cold, sweaty skin, and restlessness.

Heart failure symptoms typically develop over a long period. If they have a sudden onset, they present a medical emergency.

Treatment

The treatment options for heart failure depend on how severe it is, and which side of the heart has been affected. Early interventions include rest, changes in diet (especially moving toward a low sodium diet), and modifications in physical activity so that the heart can be exercised without being overly stressed.

If a patient doesn't respond well to these noninvasive treatment options, surgery may be considered. Surgery can range anywhere from repair to damaged valves, to wrapping a strong mesh bag around the heart, to a complete heart or heart and lung transplant.

Medications

- Anticoagulants to prevent excessive blood clotting
- Beta blockers and ACE inhibitors to reduce the heart's workload
- Digitalis to slow and strengthen the heartbeat
- Diuretics to help shed excess fluid
- Statins to limit cholesterol levels

Massage?

RISKS Most heart failure patients have a history of cardiovascular problems that contribute to their problems. Any massage that requires them to adapt to changing environments may be too challenging to receive safely. Accommodations must also be made for heart failure medications, many of which have dizziness and lethargy as side effects.

BENEFITS Gentle or energetic bodywork that invites rather than imposes change may help to reduce blood pressure and perceived stress. This can be beneficial to heart failure patients in the short run, although it is unlikely to change their prognosis.

CHAPTER REVIEW QUESTIONS: CIRCULATORY SYSTEM CONDITIONS

1. Why are fatigue and low stamina symptoms of anemia?
2. What is the difference between an embolism and thrombus?
3. Name two types of blood cancer.
4. How does sickle cell disease lead to severely reduced immunity?
5. Which blood vessel outside the brain is most vulnerable to developing an aneurysm?
6. Where are the blockages that lead to heart attacks?
7. Which condition almost always precedes atherosclerosis?
8. Why is hypertension called the "silent killer"?
9. Describe how a person may have any three of the following conditions at the same time: high blood pressure, chronic renal failure, edema, atherosclerosis, diabetes, aortic aneurysm, stroke.
10. A client has a deep ache in the lower leg. Distal to the knee the tissue is clammy and edematous. Pressing at the ankle leaves a dimple, which takes several minutes to disappear. What cautions must be exercised with this client?

6

Lymph and Immune System Conditions

Chapter Objectives

After reading this chapter you should be able to…

- Describe the difference between an allergy and an autoimmune disease.
- Describe a circumstance in which an allergy can become life threatening.
- Identify one type of edema that indicates circulatory massage.
- Explain why lymphoma causes anemia.
- Describe one risk of working with clients who have mononucleosis.
- Describe two central nervous system components seen with many chronic fatigue syndrome patients.
- Explain three benefits of not interfering with fever.
- Describe the four phases of HIV infection.
- Identify four different autoimmune diseases.
- Describe why medications for autoimmune diseases may carry cautions for massage therapists.

Introduction

The lymphatic system is a bit peculiar among the other systems: its components are not even vaguely symmetrical, and it functions as a sort of subsystem to both the circulatory and immune systems. The conditions listed under this heading may be influenced by either of the other two systems. Here is a brief overview of how the lymphatic system works.

Lymph System Structure

As blood travels away from the heart, it goes through progressively smaller tubes—the aorta branches into the arteries, which branch into arterioles, which finally divide into the very tiny and delicate capillaries. The pressure and speed with which blood travels decrease as blood gets further away from the heart. Still, everything keeps moving at a good pace; a blood cell can complete its tour of the systemic circuit in about 60 seconds.

The walls of the capillaries are made of one-cell-thick squamous epithelium, designed to allow diffusion of substances through the walls. Capillaries are so tiny that the red blood cells must line up one by one to pass through. This is the moment for the transfer of nutrients and wastes in the tissue cells. This is also where, having dropped off oxygen and picked up carbon dioxide, the blood vessels turn from arterial capillaries into venous capillaries. And finally, this is the moment when plasma from the arterial blood is squeezed out of the capillaries. In other words, this is the origin of interstitial fluid (Figure 6.1).

Interstitial fluid is absolutely vital. It is the medium in which all of the body's nutrients and wastes travel. But it must keep moving; if it stagnates, waste products or pathogens can accumulate and cause problems. Interstitial fluid keeps moving through the system by flowing into a different type of capillary, a lymphatic capillary. Lymphatic capillaries are similar to circulatory capillaries in construction, with one major difference: they are part of an open system. That is, interstitial fluid and small particles can flow into lymphatic capillaries at almost any point along the length of that capillary. By contrast, circulatory capillaries are closed to the extent that red blood cells are not able to come and go unless the vessel has been damaged.

When interstitial fluid is drawn into a lymphatic capillary, it is called lymph. Lymph is composed mainly of plasma that has been pressed out of the bloodstream, loads of metabolic wastes that have been exuded by hardworking cells, and some chunks of particulate waste as well.

The new lymph is routed to a series of cleaning stations called nodes, where the wastes are neutralized and any small particles are filtered out. The nodes are also home to most of the body's specific immune-response cells, so if any pathogens have been picked up and marked by macrophages in the lymph, this is where the specific immune response gets started. The newly cleaned fluid reenters the circulatory system just above the right atrium of the heart, where the right and left thoracic ducts empty into the right and left subclavian veins, respectively.

Lymph System Function

Lymph flows through the lymphatic capillaries into bigger and bigger vessels, usually against the pull of gravity and without the aid of the heart's direct pumping action. Several processes help to move it along:

- Gravity helps to move lymph if the limb is elevated.

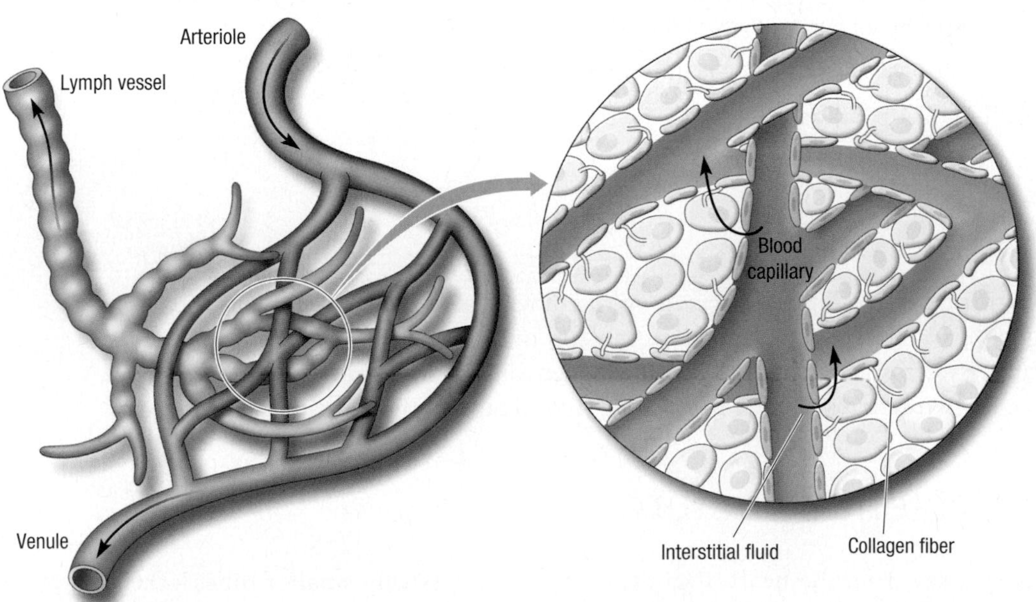

Figure 6.1. Lymphatic capillaries

- Muscle contractions push fluid through lymphatic vessels just as a hand squeezes around a tube of toothpaste. The larger lymphatic vessels also have smooth muscle tissue in their walls that contract rhythmically.
- Alternating hot and cold hydrotherapy applications can increase contractions in the smooth muscle tissue of lymphatic vessels to move fluid along.
- Deep breathing draws lymph up the thoracic duct like an expanding bellow during inhalation and squeezes it out during exhalation.
- Massage with big mechanical manipulative strokes such as petrissage and deep effleurage can increase lymph flow, but small, extremely superficial reflexive strokes can also cause fluid to be drawn into lymphatic capillaries. This is the mechanism employed with lymph drainage modalities.

If everything works well, fluid levels in the tissues are constant but not stagnant. The amount of fluid squeezed out of circulatory capillaries should be almost equal to the amount being drawn into lymphatic capillaries, with about 10% left over to become interstitial fluid; this is called the **Starling equilibrium**. But a backup anywhere in the system can result in major changes in fluid balance. If veins, lymph vessels, or nodes are blocked, fluid accumulates between tissue cells. The stagnant fluid quickly becomes a hindrance to diffusion and other chemical reactions rather than the transfer medium it is designed to be. This is the problem with many of the diseases of the lymph system, and it is a serious concern for massage practitioners, who generally should not be trying to push fluid through a system that is already overtaxed.

Immune System Function

The immune system is unique in that it is not composed of a collection of organs performing a task for a coordinated total effort, like other systems in the body. Instead, it is a nebulous, incredibly complex collection of cells and chemicals whose coordinated function is to keep the whole organism safe.

The primary function of the immune system is to distinguish what is self from what is non-self, and to eradicate anything that is non-self as quickly as possible. Immune system devices range from very general to highly specific in identifying exactly which antigens they attack (Sidebar 6.1). Some white cells attack anything; others simply ignore a pathogen if it's not their particular target. Most of the nonspecific immune devices, such as intact skin and the acidity of the gastric juices, are not discussed here. However, it is worthwhile to look at some of

SIDEBAR 6.1 Different White Blood Cells for Different Functions

White blood cells come in various sizes, classes, and strengths. Each type of leukocyte has a specific role in the immune system and inflammatory response. As researchers learn more about how these cells work and communicate with each other, we gain ability to influence their activities.

Neutrophils
Neutrophils are the smallest, fastest, and most common of the white blood cells. They are produced in bone marrow, and chemicals that leak from damaged cells stimulate their production in even greater numbers. Neutrophils typically have a short lifespan; they are the first to sacrifice themselves to disable potential invaders.

Monocytes
Monocytes begin as small white blood cells, but they have the power to change. When they are released into the bloodstream from the bone marrow, they circulate until they reach a target tissue. Then they leave the circulatory system to infiltrate that tissue and grow into macrophages, "big eaters" that can devour pathogens and display bits of cell membrane that begin the specific immune response.

Monocytes and macrophages move slowly; they are usually involved in the subacute or chronic phases of inflammatory response.

Eosinophils and Basophils
These inflammatory agents are observed most often in the context of allergic reactions and responses against invading parasites.

Lymphocytes
Lymphocytes include B cells, T cells, and natural killer cells. These are manufactured in both bone marrow and lymphoid tissue and are most often engaged in specific immune system responses to pathogens. These are the agents that allow us to develop immunity to infections.

the specific immune machinery, because when it's working well it's positively miraculous, and when it's not working well or when it makes mistakes, things can go terribly wrong.

T-cells and B-cells

The two interlocking branches of the specific immune responses are cellular immunity (T-cells) and humoral immunity (B-cells). Neither of these extremely complicated systems can work at all unless their target pathogen is displayed by a nonspecific white blood cell. So that is the first step in fighting off an infection: a white blood cell must find, destroy, and display a piece of the microorganism in question. Fortunately, white blood cells are distributed generously all through the blood and interstitial fluid, and they are concentrated in the superficial fascia, lymph nodes, lungs, and liver, where the chance of meeting pathogens is especially high.

Consider the sequence of events when someone touches a contaminated doorknob and then wipes his or her eye: rhinovirus 14 has just been introduced into the body. A passing monocyte eats the pathogen, and it is drawn through lymphatic capillaries into a nearby lymph node. A T-cell is waiting there. It just happens to be specially designed to recognize the flag of rhinovirus 14. The T-cell gets very busy, replicating itself into several forms that go out into the bloodstream in search of more viruses to attack. In the process, the original T-cell stimulates its B-cell partner. This B-cell clones, and the new cells start producing out rhinovirus 14–specific antibodies at a mind-boggling pace: 2,000 antibodies per second. Antibodies are not alive. They are Y-shaped chemicals forged especially to lock onto their target pathogen and retire it. This can happen in any of several ways, depending on the pathogen and the antibodies involved. See Animation at http://thePoint.lww.com/Werner5e.

Back when the T-cells and B-cells were first becoming active, they each made a few copies of themselves that would outlive the infection and circulate through the body on the lookout for future attempts by the same pathogen to invade. These are memory cells, and thanks to them, people very seldom get sick with the same pathogen twice. If rhinovirus 14 gains access to the body again, an immune attack can mobilize against it so quickly that a person might never know he was even exposed.

Immune System Mistakes

The immune system is miraculous. Most of the time, T- and B-cells can somehow recognize their own special pathogen and launch exactly the right attack against it. But the immune system occasionally makes mistakes. Sometimes it launches a full-scale attack, with an inflammatory response, antibody production, and collateral damage to nearby cells, against an antigen that's not dangerous: cat dander, oak pollen, or peanuts, for instance: this is called an allergic reaction. Allergies can range in severity from mildly annoying to life threatening.

The other slip the immune system can make is to mistake a part of the body for a dangerous pathogen. That is, it fails to distinguish self from non-self. Conditions involving this type of mistake are called autoimmune disorders. This group of diseases includes multiple sclerosis (MS), lupus, scleroderma, rheumatoid arthritis, myasthenia gravis, and several other chronic, incurable problems that are discussed in this chapter. Both allergies and autoimmune dysfunction are sometimes discussed as hypersensitivity reactions.

Four types of hypersensitivity reactions have been classified. Because two of them can involve the skin and the other two can involve systemic disorders, it's useful for massage therapists to be familiar with them.

- *Type I hypersensitivity reactions*. These are an immediate reaction to an antigen, or particle

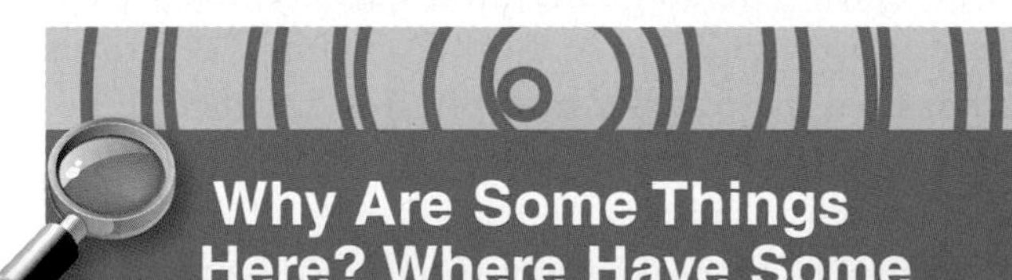

Why Are Some Things Here? Where Have Some Things Gone?

Autoimmune conditions that used to appear with the affected systems have been grouped here as part of the immune system disorder discussion. These include ankylosing spondylitis, Crohn disease, and several others. At the same time, some items that would traditionally appear in Chapter 6 now appear elsewhere. Because they have a relatively narrow application, or because massage therapists are unlikely to see them in an acute stage, they can now be found in Appendix C, **Extra Conditions At A Glance.** These include the following:

Polymyalgia rheumatica   Myasthenia gravis

Lymph and Immune System Conditions

Lymph System Conditions

- Edema
- Lymphangitis
- Lymphoma
  - Hodgkin lymphoma
  - Non-Hodgkin lymphoma
- Mononucleosis

Immune System Conditions

- Allergic reactions
  - Angioedema
  - Anaphylaxis
- Chronic fatigue syndrome
- Fever
- HIV/AIDS

Autoimmune Disorders

- Ankylosing spondylitis
- Crohn disease
- Lupus
  - Systemic lupus
  - Discoid lupus
  - Drug-induced lupus
- Multiple sclerosis (MS)
  - Benign MS
  - Relapse/remitting MS
  - Primary progressive MS
  - Secondary progressive MS
  - Progressive/relapsing MS
  - Malignant MS
- Psoriasis
  - Plaque psoriasis
  - Guttate psoriasis
  - Pustular psoriasis
  - Inverse psoriasis
  - Erythrodermic psoriasis
- Rheumatoid arthritis
  - Juvenile rheumatoid arthritis
- Scleroderma
  - Local scleroderma
    - Morphea s.
    - Linear s.
  - Systemic scleroderma
    - Limited
    - Diffuse
    - Sine
- Ulcerative colitis

of non-self. In this situation, immunoglobulin-E (IgE), a specific class of antibody, quickly sensitizes nearby mast cells to the presence of an "enemy," which may be a fragment of pollen, the proteins from peanuts or shellfish, or a droplet of bee venom. The alerted mast cells then release histamine and other chemicals that create dramatic changes in vascular permeability and that attract other white blood cells to the area. This inflammatory response produces the symptoms that are associated with typical allergic reactions: redness, swelling, itching, weepy eyes, and runny nose with hay fever; or nausea, vomiting, and diarrhea with certain food allergies. One version of a type I reaction occurs on the skin in response to certain massage oils; this is discussed in Sidebar 6.2.

- *Type II hypersensitivity reactions*. These are far less common than type I. They involve inflammatory cytotoxic (cell killing) reactions against a specific substance that may or may not belong to the body. Examples of type II reactions include hemolytic anemia, penicillin allergies, and reactions to the transfusion of mismatched blood.

SIDEBAR 6.2 Hypersensitivity Reactions and Massage Oil

Type I hypersensitivity reactions typically occur within severalseconds to a few minutes of exposure to an irritating substance. However, a late-phase type I reaction can sustain allergic symptoms long after the irritation has been removed. Arachidonic acid is a substance associated with late-phase type I reactions, especially in the form of bronchial asthma. The significance of this for massage therapists is that some types of massage oils can break down into arachidonic acid on the skin. A client who is sensitive to this type of reaction may have no immediate skin symptoms but may wonder several hours later why he is coughing, wheezing, and feeling short of breath.

Oils that are particularly prone to breaking down into arachidonic acid are composed mostly of omega-6 molecules. These include safflower, soy, almond, sunflower, and corn oils. Although they can be pleasant and convenient to use for massage, they are the most likely to cause skin irritation and allergic reactions. Therefore, when it is important to avoid potentially irritating oils for certain conditions, these are the ones to eliminate first.

- *Type III reactions*. These involve antibodies that bind with antigens, but the particles they form cannot be phagocytized. These conglomerates, called granulomas, are eventually caught in the body's most delicate fluid filters: in the kidneys, the eyes, the brain, and the serous membranes surrounding the heart, lungs, and abdominal cavity. There they stimulate an aggressive response, which results in inflammation and damage to these very delicate structures. Examples of type III reactions include systemic lupus erythematosus (SLE), a specific type of kidney damage called glomerulonephritis, and possibly rheumatoid arthritis.
- *Type IV reactions*: These delayed reactions are cell mediated; they rely on T cells to stimulate an immune response to an irritant. Contact dermatitis is an example of a type IV hypersensitivity reaction. In this case, an inflammatory reaction appears on the skin after exposure to an irritating substance such as plant toxins, certain dyes, soaps, metals, or latex. This usually delayed reaction may occur 24 to 48 hours after an initial exposure.

By contrast, several conditions that use to appear in other chapters are now discussed here, because they are autoimmune diseases that indicate dysfunction in the body's ability to distinguish "self" from "non-self."

To hear the author discuss autoimmune diseases and massage, go to http://thePoint.lww.com/Werner5e.

Edema in Brief

Pronunciation: eh-DEE-mah

What is it?
Edema is retention of interstitial fluid due to electrolyte or protein imbalances, or because of mechanical obstruction in the circulatory or lymphatic systems.

How is it recognized?
Edematous tissue is puffy or boggy in early stages. It may become hard (indurated) if it is not resolved quickly. The area may be hot if associated with local infection, or quite cool if local circulation is impaired.

Massage risks and benefits
Risks: Most forms of edema contraindicate massage, especially when the tissue is indurated or nonresilient. In these situations, a chemical imbalance or physical obstruction must be resolved before most types of bodywork are safe.
Benefits: Acute edema that is not related to infection may be appropriate for lymphatic types of massage. Subacute or postacute musculoskeletal injuries may be edematous and respond well to various bodywork approaches.

Lymph System Conditions

Edema

Definition: What Is It?

Edema is accumulation of excessive fluid between cells. It may be a local or systemic problem, and it is usually associated with chemical imbalance, inflammation, or poor circulation.

Etiology: What Happens?

The Starling equilibrium states that the forces that cause fluid to leave blood capillaries should almost equal the forces that cause fluid to be reabsorbed by blood capillaries, and that anything left over (which should be about 10%) should be processed by the lymph system. Lymph capillaries are perfectly designed to pick up excess interstitial fluid: each squamous cell is anchored to surrounding tissue by a collagen filament. When excess fluid accumulates in any area, these anchoring filaments pull back on the squamous cells, increasing the lymph capillary's ability to take in fluid. Sometimes, however, more fluid builds up in the tissues than the circulatory and lymph systems combined can take in, and this is called edema. Edema isn't generally noticeable until interstitial fluid volume is about 30% above normal.

Edema can have any of several causes; most of them are a combination of chemical and mechanical factors. Mechanical factors may involve a weakened heart, a dysfunctional liver, serious kidney problems, or an obstruction to venous or lymphatic return in the form of a blood clot, or removed nodes. Even socks or knee braces that are too tight can cause distal edema. Chemical causes of edema usually have to do with accumulation of salts or proteins in the interstitial fluid, which causes the area to retain water. Other chemical factors include inflammatory responses to infection or allergens. Many cases of edema have both chemical and mechanical factors.

Lymphedema is different from simple edema; this is the result of damage to lymphatic structures and accumulation of proteins in the interstitial fluid. It is discussed in Chapter 12.

Signs and Symptoms

Edema varies in presentation according to the source, the duration, and the area that is affected. Tissue is often soft, puffy, or boggy. The area may be hot if the edema is related to a recent injury or infection, or cool if the edema is long standing and related to poor circulation.

When blood or lymphatic movement is chronically impaired, pitting edema may develop: a pit or dimple remains in the tissue for several minutes after it is gently compressed (Figure 6.2). Tissue that is edematous because of chronic problems such as heart failure or lymph node loss may become indurated or hardened.

Treatment

Edema is treated by addressing the underlying cause. This may mean treatment for something as complex as liver failure, or as simple as a sprained ankle. Medications are likewise gauged to treat the contributing factors.

A person who experiences chronic or repeating edema may be counseled to follow a low-salt diet and to sit or recline with legs elevated whenever possible.

Medications

- Antihistamines for allergic reactions
- NSAIDs
- Steroidal anti-inflammatories
- Diuretics for heart, liver, or kidney dysfunction

Massage?

RISKS Most types of edema contraindicate all but the lightest forms of bodywork, because the delicate lymphatic capillaries are already working past capacity.

BENEFITS Subacute or postacute musculoskeletal injuries may have long-term edema that hydrotherapy and massage can help to resolve safely.

OPTIONS Lymphatic work from a highly trained practitioner is appropriate for edema in any stage that is not connected to an infection or other contraindicating condition.

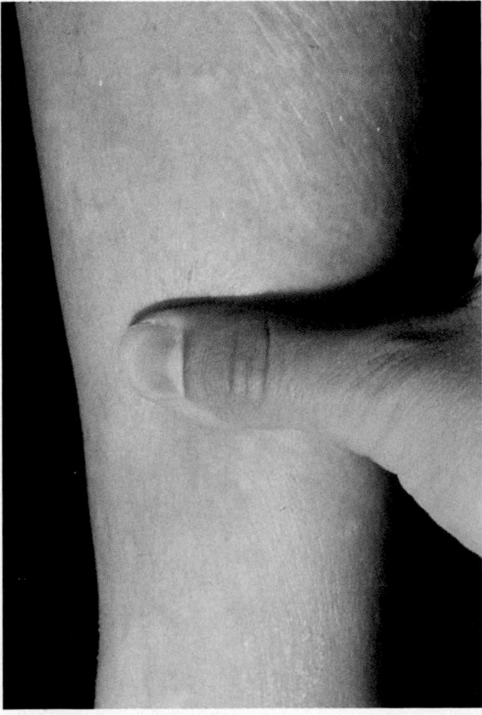
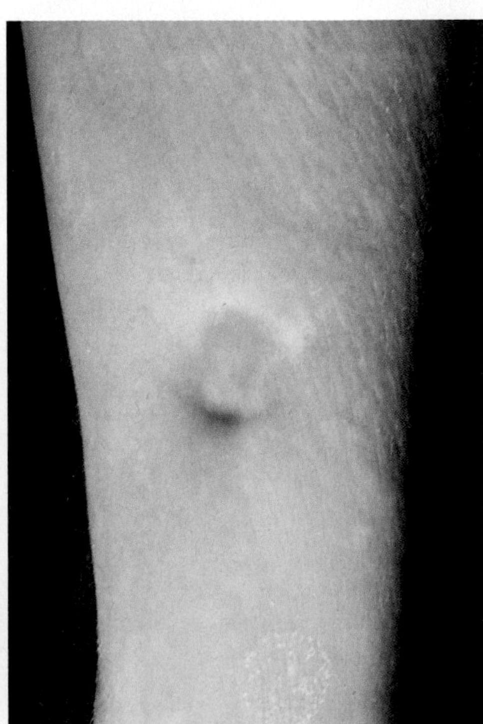
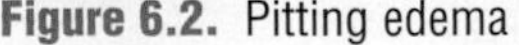

Figure 6.2. Pitting edema

Lymphangitis

Definition: What Is It?

Lymphangitis is an infection with inflammation in the **lymphangions**, or lymphatic capillaries. It is a particular risk for people with depressed immunity or poor circulation, because their white blood cell activity is sluggish. This allows any available bacteria the opportunity to establish a stronghold in the lymphatic system. Massage therapists are also at risk, because tiny lesions may be present on their hands. These are vulnerable to invasion by the bacteria that reside on the skin of even the healthiest clients.

Etiology: What Happens?

In lymphangitis, the lymph capillaries become infected, usually with *Streptococcus pyogenes*, although other pathogens, including Staphylococcus, can also be the cause. This condition usually arises from a small injury on the skin. It can be a complication of cellulitis or of a viral or fungal infection such as herpes simplex or athlete's foot.

When the pathogens gain entry, they set up an aggressive infection in the lymph vessel before macrophages or other white blood cells can stop them. Infections that invade the lymph nodes are called **lymphadenitis**. If even a few bacteria get past the filtering action of the lymph nodes, the infection can enter the bloodstream at the right or left subclavian vein. Then the situation is much more serious: the person has **septicemia**, or blood poisoning, which is potentially life threatening. This is why, if lymphangitis is a possibility, medical intervention is advisable at the earliest possible opportunity.

Lymphangitis in Brief

Pronunciation: lim-fan-JY-tis

What is it?
Lymphangitis is an infection of lymph capillaries. If the infection invades the nodes, it is called lymphadenitis. If it gets past the lymphatic system and enters the bloodstream, it is called blood poisoning (septicemia), and it can be life threatening.

How is it recognized?
Lymphangitis has all of the signs of local infection: pain, heat, redness, and swelling. It may also show red streaks from the site of infection running toward the nearest lymph nodes. Fever and malaise are often present as well.

Massage risks and benefits
Risks: Lymphangitis contraindicates any bodywork with the intention of impacting fluid movement until the infection has been eradicated.
Benefits: Clients who have fully recovered from lymphangitis can enjoy the same benefits from bodywork as the rest of the population.

Signs and Symptoms

Lymphangitis starts with signs of local infection: pain, heat, redness, and swelling, all focused around the initial site of infection. The infected lymph vessel often shows a visible scarlet track running proximally from the portal of entry, which is usually some lesion in the skin such as a hangnail, a knife cut, or an insect bite (Figure 6.3).

If the infection is unchecked by white blood cells, it quickly moves deeper into the lymph system, leading to swollen nodes, fever, and a general feeling of misery. Blisters may develop along the line of infection. Depending on the virulence of the bacteria, extensive tissue damage may also occur. This can happen surprisingly quickly; lymphangitis can become a systemic infection in a matter of hours.

Treatment

Lymphangitis is usually treated successfully with antibiotic therapy. Treatment must begin as soon as possible after the infection has been identified to avoid the risk of blood poisoning. Any abscesses may need to be drained.

Medications

- Antibiotics for bacterial infection
- Analgesics for pain
- Anti-inflammatories for inflammation

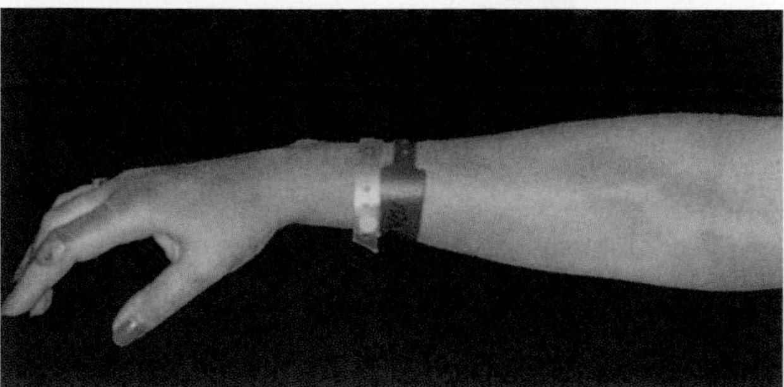

Figure 6.3. Lymphangitis

Massage?

RISKS A client with acute lymphangitis is unlikely to want to keep a massage appointment because he or she probably has a fever and general malaise along with throbbing pain and edema at the site of infection. This condition contraindicates massage locally because of the threat of communicable pathogens, and systemically because of the threat of complication to septicemia.

BENEFITS A client who has fully recovered from lymphangitis can enjoy the same benefits from massage as the rest of the population.

OPTIONS This condition can be an occupational hazard for massage therapists and bodywork practitioners whose hands may have open hangnails or other wounds that serve as a portal of entry. For this reason, it is important to cover any compromised skin with a liquid bandage, a finger cot, or another device that will prevent this risk.

Lymphoma

Definition: What Is It?

Lymphoma is a collective name for cancer that starts in the lymph nodes. Like leukemia and myeloma, lymphoma involves a mutation of the DNA in specific white blood cells. Some types of lymphoma affect the same cells as some types of lymphocytic leukemia, so the delineations between these cancer labels are no longer clear-cut.

Etiology: What Happens?

Lymphoma is cancer that originates in lymph tissues. It begins with a mutation of the DNA of the affected cells, usually some type of B cell (these account for about 80% of cases) or of T cells or natural killer cells. The mutated cell begins to replicate, producing massive numbers of nonfunctioning lymphocytes. This causes the lymph tissues to enlarge, and it initiates the other symptoms associated with lymphoma, namely, anemia, night sweats, itchy skin, and fatigue, among others.

Mutated cells may travel through the lymphatic system to begin tumors elsewhere: this can occur in other lymph node regions, or in organs like bones, the spleen, or the liver. In some cases, cells can gain access to the central nervous system and begin growing tumors there.

Lymphoma in Brief

Pronunciation: lim-FOE-mah

What is it?
Lymphoma is any variety of cancer that grows in lymph tissues. Many types have been identified, some of which are aggressive and very threatening, others that may progress more slowly.

How is it recognized?
The cardinal sign of lymphoma is painless swelling of lymph nodes, along with anemia, fatigue, low-grade fever, night sweats, itchiness, rashes, abdominal pain, and loss of appetite.

Massage risks and benefits
Risks: Rigorous massage that challenges adaptation is inappropriate for lymphoma patients who are currently dealing with their disease.
Benefits: Any bodywork strategy works best as part of an integrated healthcare plan for lymphoma and other cancer patients. The benefits of anxiety reduction, sleep improvement, pain relief, and others can be useful tools during a very demanding process.
Clients who have recovered from lymphoma and who have no long-term complications that contraindicate massage can enjoy the same benefits from bodywork as the rest of the population.

The increasing incidence of lymphoma in the last 30 years has raised the possibility that this cancer can be linked to environmental exposure. A statistical relationship exists between lymphoma and exposure to insecticides, herbicides, fertilizers, and black hair dye, but the direct cause-and-effect sequences have not been established. Lymphoma risk is increased with some infections, including HIV, hepatitis B and C, Epstein-Barr virus, human T-cell lymphotropic virus, and *Helicobactor pylori*. Other risk factors for lymphoma include the presence of autoimmune disease, using immunosuppressant drugs, and genetic predisposition.

The seriousness of lymphoma depends on what type of cell has mutated, and how quickly it replicates. This disease is sometimes described by the behavior of its cells:

- Low-grade or indolent lymphoma grows slowly. It is often nonresponsive to treatment and may change to a more aggressive form later.

- Intermediate grade lymphoma is aggressive, but responsive to treatment.
- High-grade lymphoma is aggressive and grows rapidly, but it may be resistant to treatment.

Types of Lymphoma

- *Hodgkin lymphoma (HL).* This involves the mutation of B cells into large, malignant, multinucleate cells called Reed Sternberg cells. It is seen most often in the submandibular nodes, but can also occur at the axillary and inguinal nodes. Eventually the growths metastasize to organ tissues, particularly the liver or bone marrow. Several subtypes of HL have been identified, but their patterns of progression are similar. The process of metastasis tends to be predictable and organized, which distinguishes HL from non-Hodgkin lymphoma (NHL), and which makes HL a very treatable form of cancer.
- *Non-Hodgkin lymphoma (NHL).* This group comprises many subtypes of lymphoma that affect B cells, T cells, and natural killer cells. NHL is much more common than HL. It tends to be less predictable than HL, and it can be harder to treat successfully.

NOTABLE CASES In 2009, cofounder of Microsoft Paul Allen was diagnosed with non-Hodgkin lymphoma (NHL) approximately 25 years after successful treatment for Hodgkin lymphoma. Jacqueline Kennedy Onassis was diagnosed with NHL in 1993, and died in 1994 at age 64. "Lucky Lindy" Charles Lindbergh, who first flew across the Atlantic in 1927, died of lymphoma at age 72 in 1974.

Signs and Symptoms

The primary symptom of any kind of lymphoma is painless, nontender swelling of lymph nodes, especially in the neck, axilla, and inguinal area (Figure 6.4). Other symptoms include anemia, fatigue, weight loss, night sweats, itchy skin, and loss of appetite. These symptoms typically have a relatively fast onset, and persist for two weeks or more. Indolent varieties of lymphoma may have symptoms that come and go; this is problematic, because it may cause a person to delay in getting an important diagnosis.

In later stages, lymphoma may show easy bruising and skin discoloration as platelet numbers drop, along with decreased resistance to cold, flu, or other infections.

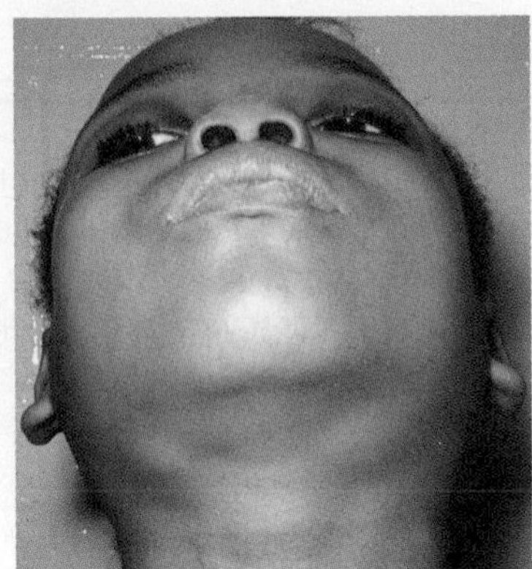

Figure 6.4. Hodgkin lymphoma

Treatment

Treatment choices for lymphoma depend on several factors, including exactly which type of cells are affected, the stage of the disease, and whether the stage is qualified by an A, B, E, or S finding (see Sidebar 6.3).

SIDEBAR 6.3 Staging Lymphoma

Lymphoma is staged by its degree of progression, and by the microscopic appearance of the affected cells.

Stage I. The cancer is found in only one nodal region, or it has invaded only one nearby organ.

Stage II. Two or more nodal regions are affected, and they are on the same side of the diaphragm; or multiple nodal regions along with one organ all on the same side of the diaphragm are affected.

Stage III. Nodes on both sides of the diaphragm are invaded, along with organ involvement; the spleen may or may not be affected.

Stage IV. The cancer is disseminated throughout the body, affecting nodes, organs, bone marrow, and/or in the central nervous system.

Recurrent. Recurrent lymphoma is cancer that reappears after a full course of treatment.

In addition to a numerical stage, lymphoma is also described by letters A, B, E, and S:

A. No symptoms other than painless enlarged lymph nodes.

B. Fever, weight loss, and night sweats accompany enlarged lymph nodes.

E. Extranodal tumors are found.

S. Tumors are found in the spleen.

Chemotherapy and radiation are the usual choices, but some other options are finding success in dealing with lymphoma, including allogenic and autologous bone marrow transplants, stem cell transplants, and various types of biologic therapy involving radioactive antibodies, cancer vaccinations, and other strategies.

Medications

- Chemotherapeutic agents
- Medication to mitigate chemotherapy symptoms
- Biologic therapy agents

Massage?

RISKS Lymphoma involves lymph nodes and possibly the spleen, so any bodywork that focuses on lymphatic or other fluid movement may be too demanding for patients to comfortably and safely receive.

BENEFITS Massage can be a useful strategy to deal with the physical and emotional demands of dealing with both cancer and cancer treatments, as long as work is within a client's capacity to adapt, and when bodywork is integrated into the rest of the treatment plan.

Clients who have fully recovered from lymphoma and who have no long-term complications can enjoy the same benefits from bodywork as the rest of the population.

Mononucleosis

Definition: What Is It?

Mononucleosis is a viral infection of the salivary glands and throat that then moves into the lymphatic system. The causative agent in about 90% of all cases is the Epstein-Barr virus, a member of the herpes family. Other pathogens that can cause mononucleosis include other members of Herpesviridae, specifically cytomegalovirus, herpes zoster, human herpes virus 6 and 7, and others.

Epstein-Barr virus is extremely common in the United States, but not everyone who is exposed develops mononucleosis. The people most often diagnosed are young adults between 15 and 25 years old.

Mononucleosis in Brief

Pronunciation: mon-o-nu-kle-O-sis

What is it?
Mononucleosis is an infection, usually with the Epstein-Barr virus but occasionally with cytomegalovirus or other agents. The virus first attacks the epithelial tissue in the salivary glands and throat, and then invades B-cells in lymph nodes, the spleen, and elsewhere.

How is it recognized?
The three leading signs and symptoms of mononucleosis are fever, swollen lymph nodes, and sore throat. Others may include profound fatigue, low stamina, enlarged spleen, and enlarged liver.

Massage risks and benefits
Risks: Mononucleosis contraindicates rigorous massage while it is acute and the client is working hard to conquer this stubborn infection. Any kind of bodywork must accommodate the risk of lymphatic congestion.
Benefits: If circulation is healthy and the spleen and liver are not compromised, circulatory massage may improve recovery time. Clients who have fully recovered from mononucleosis can enjoy the same benefits from bodywork as the rest of the population.

Etiology: What Happens?

Epstein-Barr virus, the pathogen most often associated with mononucleosis, is fragile outside of a human host. While it may remain viable for a short time on a dish or suspended in a droplet of mucus in the air, the most dependable way to catch it is through direct saliva-to-saliva contact; this is why it is often called the "kissing disease."

Mononucleosis moves through the body in two stages. In the first stage, the virus invades cells in the epithelial tissue of the throat and salivary glands. It takes an unusually long time for the infection to get established; incubation can take up four to six weeks, during which time the patient is infectious but not strongly symptomatic. Once well established in the epithelial tissue of the throat, the virus moves on to infect B-lymphocytes, which carry it to the lymph nodes, liver, and spleen.

As infected B-cells proliferate, the body responds by producing high numbers of cytotoxic (killer)

T cells. These T cells eventually establish control over the rogue B-cells, and ultimately the virus becomes dormant in epithelial cells of the throat.

Once a person is infected with Epstein-Barr virus, the virus is present forever, although usually dormant. It may intermittently reactivate, however. During these episodes, it is likely to be contagious but asymptomatic. This makes the spread of mononucleosis virtually impossible to control.

For most people, mononucleosis is an unpleasant but basically benign, self-limiting infection. It can significantly disrupt a person's life because it has such a powerful effect on stamina, resiliency, and general strength, but it is seldom life threatening. A very small number of patients, however, do develop serious complications. These include infection of the central nervous system leading to Bell palsy, seizures, or meningitis; enlargement of the heart; temporary anemia and thrombocytopenia; and breathing problems when lymph nodes and tonsils get so inflamed that they block air passageways.

One fairly common complication of mononucleosis is a streptococcal infection of the throat ("strep throat"). It is important to be clear about what infection is causing which symptoms in this case, since while strep throat is easily treatable with antibiotics, mononucleosis is not. Further, the antibiotics used for strep throat can sometimes cause a rash in patients who also have mononucleosis.

Perhaps the greatest danger for most mononucleosis patients is the potential for damage to the spleen. This gland can become dangerously enlarged with lymphocytic activity. Since the spleen also breaks down and recycles dead red blood cells, it has a generous blood supply. If the enlarged organ should be injured by a fall or other trauma, it could rupture, which could lead to internal hemorrhage and rapid circulatory collapse. Persons recovering from mononucleosis are counseled to avoid contact sports for several weeks to reduce their risk of this kind of injury.

Signs and Symptoms

Mononucleosis is notorious for presenting different symptoms in different patients. The younger a person is at exposure to Epstein-Barr virus, the subtler the symptoms tend to be. Young children often go through exposure, infection, and recovery with no discernible symptoms at all.

In older patients, particularly adolescents and young adults, the signs and symptoms are more dependable. The prodromic stage, as the infection is becoming established but creates no strong symptoms, may be marked by general fatigue and malaise; the patient often does not feel well but may not feel sick, either. This may last anywhere from a few days to several weeks. Then as the infection becomes more aggressive, the leading triad of symptoms appears: fever of 102°F to 104°F (38.9°C to 40°C), an extremely sore throat, and lymph nodes that are swollen from the production of massive numbers of B-cells and T cells. The cervical lymph nodes are usually affected most, but submandibular, axillary, and inguinal lymph nodes may also be palpably swollen and tender. Swelling around the throat can be severe enough to affect breathing.

Puffy, swollen eyelids are a common complaint among mononucleosis patients. **Splenomegaly** (enlargement of the spleen) occurs in about half of patients. Many also have inflammation of the liver and jaundice. Some mononucleosis patients develop a splotchy, measly rash, especially if they are taking amoxicillin or ampicillin, two penicillin-family antibiotics that are prescribed for strep throat.

Signs and symptoms of acute mononucleosis tend to last approximately 2 weeks before subsiding, but the whole infection is so wearing on the body that it can take several weeks or even months before a patient feels fully functional again.

Treatment

Although it is a viral infection, mononucleosis does not respond to antiviral medications. The typical approach is to treat the symptoms (acetaminophen to reduce fever and pain, rest, good nutrition, and generous hydration) and wait for it to be over. Patients may need to curtail activities to avoid exhaustion, and avoid situations like contact sports that could put them at risk for damaging the spleen.

Medications

- Acetaminophen or ibuprofen for fever, muscle aches
- Steroidal anti-inflammatories for inflammation of the throat and tonsils

Massage?

RISKS A client with fever, inflamed lymph nodes, and general malaise is not a good candidate for rigorous Swedish or circulatory types of bodywork. Lymphatic congestion and fatigue may linger for weeks or even months after the acute phase, and these also require adaptation in bodywork choices.

BENEFITS Energetic work that supports healing properties without taxing the lymph or immune systems may be a valuable addition to the lengthy healing process for mononucleosis. A client with a history of this infection and no lingering weakness or illness can enjoy all the benefits from massage as the rest of the population.

Immune System Conditions

Allergic Reactions

Definition: What Are They?

Allergies are immune system reactions against stimuli that are not inherently hazardous. The immune system behaves as though an allergen, which could be oak pollen, cat dander, peanuts, or another essentially benign substance, were a potentially dangerous threat.

Allergic Reactions in Brief

What are they?
Allergic reactions are immune system mistakes in which an inflammatory response becomes irritating or dangerous as it reacts inappropriately to a variety of triggers.

How are they recognized?
The most dangerous acute sign of an allergic reaction is swelling around the face and throat that may obstruct airflow. This may be accompanied by decreased blood pressure and bronchospasm. Other signs include hives and other rashes, gastrointestinal discomfort with food allergies, and in the case of multiple chemical sensitivity, headache, disorientation, cognitive difficulties, joint pain, and other symptoms.

Massage risks and benefits
Risks: Most hypersensitivity reactions contraindicate massage in the acute stage, since increasing blood flow to areas that are already congested is counterproductive. Between episodes, persons with allergies who want to receive massage need to be careful about massage lubricants, essential oils, perfumes, candles, and other equipment that therapists often use that may trigger a reaction.
Benefits: A client with a tendency toward allergies can enjoy all the benefits of massage as the rest of the population, as long as the practitioner can provide an environment that is free from allergic triggers.

Etiology: What Happens?

Antibodies are the Y-shaped proteins manufactured by activated B cells against specific pathogens. Some classes of antibodies and some types of T cells are particularly reactive to noninfectious antigens, causing acute or chronic allergic symptoms. These hypersensitivity reactions have been classified as having four distinct types. For details on types of hypersensitivity, see the introduction to this chapter.

Different types of allergies affect different parts of the population, depending on what substances people are exposed to and how often. The "hygiene hypothesis" suggests that rates of allergic rhinitis ("hay fever"), asthma, eczema, and some other allergies are on the rise in the United States because children are overprotected from exposure to allergens in early childhood, and this interferes with proper immune system development.

Alternatively, repeated exposure to some substances, especially latex, can lead to dangerous allergic reactions later in life. This is a particular problem for people with spina bifida or other medical problems that require frequent surgeries, and for healthcare professionals who use latex gloves or latex-based equipment (e.g., catheters, syringes) on a regular basis. Allergies to latex are triggered by natural latex made from derivatives of rubber trees; synthetic latex does not appear to be a potent allergen.

Multiple chemical sensitivity syndrome (MCS) develops most often in people who undergo exposure to toxic substances and who consequently develop progressively more extreme reactions to other substances as well. MCS is discussed in Sidebar 6.4.

Several conditions involving allergic reactions are discussed elsewhere in this book, in the chapter dedicated to the system that is most significantly affected. Eczema and dermatitis affect the skin, asthma and

SIDEBAR 6.4 Multiple Chemical Sensitivity Syndrome

Multiple chemical sensitivity syndrome (MCS) is also called idiopathic environmental intolerance. It is a condition in which a history of exposure to a trigger (usually an environmental toxin) results in a variety of possible reactions that become increasingly severe with repeated exposures. It is seen most often in people who have been exposed to chemical spills or other toxic exposures, who work in poorly ventilated buildings, or who have had other long-term toxic exposures. Military personnel have MCS more commonly than the rest of the population and people who served in the first Gulf War have a higher incidence still.

The accepted description of MCS is as follows:

- A set of objectively observable signs and symptoms is acquired after documentable exposure to a triggering substance.
- Multiple body systems are affected.
- Severity of symptoms is in relation to measurable (but not usually toxic) levels of chemical triggers.
- Chemically unrelated substances can trigger a reaction.
- Episodes leave no objective evidence of permanent organ damage.

A few of the most common triggers of MCS include cigar and cigarette smoke; colognes, perfumes, and deodorants; diesel and gasoline exhaust; household and laundry detergents and cleaners; varnish, shellac, and lacquer; and tar fumes from roof or roadwork.

MCS symptoms vary widely, including chronic headaches, joint pain, cognitive difficulties, weakness, dizziness, and heat intolerance. Exposure to one trigger may permanently exacerbate responses to future exposures, even to different chemical triggers.

A massage therapist whose client has MCS must ensure that the work space is a safe and comfortable place. Detergents or bleach used to launder massage linens may be a trigger, as may be any candles, scents, incense, or the perfume worn by the client who just left. Any lubricant must be evaluated carefully not only for allergenic ingredients but for the risk of contamination from pesticides or the plastic bottle in which it is stored. If these hurdles can be overcome, or if the client with MCS can tolerate whatever levels are present in a massage room, bodywork willbe a supportive, strengthening, and preciously rare time for a person to feel that his or her body is a good place in which to live.

allergic sinusitis affect the respiratory system, and allergic gastroenteritis affects the digestive system. The rest of this article addresses two more general examples of hypersensitivity reactions: anaphylaxis and angioedema.

Types of Allergic Reactions

- *Anaphylaxis*. This is an acute, severe systemic allergic reaction leading to the release of massive amounts of histamine from previously sensitized mast cells. The result is a sudden drop in blood pressure (hypotension) and accumulation of fluid in the tissues (edema). If the reaction centers in the respiratory tract, it can interfere dangerously with breathing. Some of the most common triggers include antibiotics; blood products; the contrast medium used in diagnostic imaging; latex; stings of wasps, ants, and honeybees; and some foods, including peanuts and other nuts, soybeans, cow's milk, eggs, fish, and shellfish. The first exposure to a trigger may not cause a significant allergic reaction, but repeated exposures lead to increased antibody activity, complement activation, and mast cell activity, which causes and reinforces inflammation. Anaphylaxis is distinguished from angioedema because it occurs both at the site of exposure and systemically through the body.
- *Angioedema*. This is the rapid onset of localized swelling. The swelling can occur in the skin, genitals, extremities, or gastrointestinal tract. If it occurs in the tongue, larynx, or pharynx, angioedema can interrupt airflow, which is life threatening. Allergens commonly associated with angioedema include peanuts or tree nuts, chocolate, fish, tomatoes, eggs, fresh berries, milk, and food preservatives. Medicines associated with this condition include aspirin, angiotensin-converting enzyme (ACE) inhibitors, and some other hypertension medications. Exposure to poison ivy, poison oak, or poison sumac can also create this kind of reaction (Sidebar 6.5).

Signs and Symptoms

Typical respiratory allergies cause itchy eyes, nose, and throat. This is covered in more detail in Chapter 7 under the sinusitis article.

Anaphylaxis in the skin creates hives, itchiness, and flushing. Excessive edema can cause respiratory symptoms, including shortness of breath, coughing, and wheezing. A person may have so much swelling around the throat that swallowing becomes difficult; this is **dysphagia**. Gastrointestinal symptoms include nausea, vomiting, cramps, bloating, and diarrhea. In extreme

SIDEBAR 6.5 Poison Ivy, Poison Oak, Poison Sumac

Poison ivy, poison oak, and poison sumac all have a chemical in their sap called **urushiol**. Urushiol is a highly allergenic substance in leaves, stems, and roots that causes a type IV delayed reaction on the skin involving inflammation, itchiness, and blisters. Up to 85% of the population has an allergic reaction to urushiol.

Poison ivy, poison oak, and poison sumac reactions occur in three ways: through direct contact with the sap, indirect contact with equipment or a pet that has been running through the woods, or through the air when plants are burned.

Many people are familiar with the signs of poison ivy: the rash is red, hot, and very itchy. It can appear to spread after the initial exposure, but this is often due to the fact that some areas of skin tend to react more quickly than others. Blisters may form and crust over. The rash can take up to 10 days to heal fully. Poison sumac and poison oak produce the same symptoms because the allergen is the same chemical. Occasionally, a rash leads to a very extreme allergic reaction in the shape of angioedema or anaphylaxis; this is a risk especially when swelling takes place around the face or neck, where it can obstruct the airway.

Poison ivy and its relatives are of particular interest to massage therapists because they usually cause a delayed reaction: an exposed person may have no symptoms for 24 hours or more after contacting the plants, although the toxin is present on the skin. This means a massage therapist working with a client who had a pleasant walk in the woods that morning may spread the urushiol further or even pick up some of the toxin.

circumstances, a person may have a slowed heart rate, hypotension, fainting, and shock. Anaphylaxis may take several hours to develop, and symptoms can appear to subside before returning in a more extreme form.

Signs of angioedema depend on where the inflammation takes place. The skin may be puffy and hot, although if it appears without hives, it may not be itchy. It is often asymmetrical, affecting only one part of the lip, for instance, or one side of the face. It has a rapid onset but usually resolves within 72 hours (Figure 6.5).

Treatment

Antihistamines are usually recommended to treat mild allergies. These block the release of histamine that triggers many allergy signs: itchy skin, runny nose, and irritated eyes.

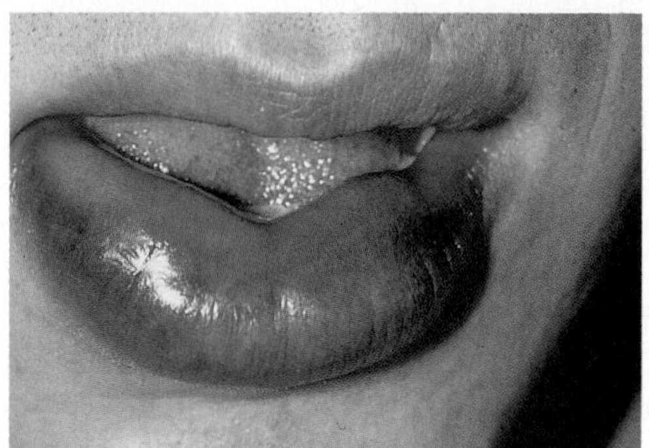

Figure 6.5. Angioedema

Angioedema and anaphylaxis are more serious, and they are typically treated in the short term with epinephrine and oxygen if breathing is impaired and steroidal anti-inflammatories after the crisis has passed. People at risk for anaphylactic reactions are taught how to avoid triggers and trained to keep medication, usually injectable epinephrine (an EpiPen), close at hand in case of emergency.

When a person has dangerous allergic reactions to insect stings, a long-term course of desensitization may be recommended; this process can reduce the risk of dangerous anaphylactic reactions.

Medications

- Antihistamines to block histamine activation sites
- Epinephrine for severe angioedema or anaphylaxis
- Steroidal anti-inflammatories

Massage?

RISKS A person with acute swelling, especially in a location that inhibits breathing, needs medical intervention more than massage. Practitioners must have hypoallergenic lubricants and be able to create a session room that is free from allergens like perfume and other heavy scents for clients who live with the possibility of severe allergic reactions.

BENEFITS Chronic allergies can leave a person feeling exhausted. Massage that does not exacerbate symptoms can be a helpful restorative, as long as positioning and other environmental factors can be controlled for maximum comfort.

OPTIONS Any massage that works to reduce inflammation in the sinuses and throat may provide symptomatic relief from respiratory allergies.

Chronic Fatigue Syndrome

Definition: What Is It?

Chronic fatigue syndrome (CFS) is a collection of signs and symptoms that affect multiple systems in the body. It varies in severity from mildly limiting to completely debilitating.

CFS was named in 1988 by scientists at the Centers for Disease Control, and its definition continues to evolve. The name is vague on purpose because this disease affects different people in very different ways. Nonetheless, some people feel this title trivializes their condition, and CFS is therefore also called chronic fatigue immune dysfunction syndrome. In Europe and Canada, a condition called **myalgic encephalomyelitis** is sometimes referred to as a synonym for CFS.

NOTABLE CASES It is thought that Florence Nightingale, who pioneered modern nursing practices during the Crimean War, had chronic fatigue syndrome. Author Laura Hillenbrand (Seabiscuit: An American Legend) is an active spokesperson for patients with this condition.

Etiology: What Happens?

The etiology of CFS is not well understood. It seems clear that it arises from a combination of factors that may or may not involve infectious agents, mentally or emotionally stressful events, neuroendocrine dysfunction, and other factors.

For many years, the leading theory was that a person was infected with a common virus (probably Epstein-Barr, the herpesvirus that causes most cases of mononucleosis) and then the body simply continued to behave as though the infection were acute long after the danger had passed. Although blood studies of patients with CFS often show some immune system abnormalities (levels of the inflammatory cytokine interleukin-1 are very high, while natural killer cell levels tend to be unusually low), it now seems clear that not all CFS cases begin with mononucleosis.

Other pathogenic exposures have been implicated in CFS, specifically candida, mycoplasma (a bacteria-like pathogen), some enteroviruses and retroviruses, *Chlamydia pneumoniae*, and other infectious agents. No single pathogen has been found to be present in most CFS patients, however, and most people who have been exposed to these agents do not develop CFS symptoms.

Two central nervous system components seem to be consistent problems for many CFS patients:

- *Hypothalamus-pituitary-adrenal (HPA) axis dysfunction*. This can lead to a sluggish but tenacious stress response and eventually to adrenal dysfunction. Interestingly, the HPA axis appears to be a factor in both fibromyalgia and depression, and both of these conditions commonly appear with CFS. The differences lie in cortisol secretion. A problem with the HPA axis typically leads to excessive cortisol secretion, but people with CFS usually have lower-than-normal levels of circulating cortisol. Whether this is because of adrenal depletion or simply poor adrenal regulation is still an unanswered question. Low cortisol levels mean that many CFS patients experience very extreme allergies.
- *Neurally mediated hypotension*. In this situation, impulses from the brain to the circulatory system do not keep the blood vessels contracted enough to maintain a normal blood pressure. Unlike the more common **orthostatic hypotension**, episodes of **neutrally mediated hypotension** are not always triggered by a sudden change in position. This condition is connected to an inappropriate response to adrenaline.

Chronic Fatigue Syndrome in Brief

What is it?
Chronic fatigue syndrome (CFS) is a collection of signs and symptoms that affect many systems in the body and result in potentially debilitating fatigue.

How is it recognized?
The central symptom to CFS is fatigue that is not restored by rest. It may be accompanied by cognitive problems, swollen nodes, fever, muscular and joint aches, headaches, and excessive pain after mild exercise.

Massage risks and benefits
Risks: Bodywork has few risks for CFS patients, other than the possibility of overtreatment for a person who is already fatigued.
Benefits: CFS indicates massage, which can help with sleep quality, stress perception, mood, and pain.

TABLE 6.1 Chronic Fatigue Symptoms

Poor short-term memory, concentration: mental fog	Changes in sleep quantity and quality	Muscle and joint pain without inflammation	Headache
Tender lymph nodes	Low-grade fever	Sore throat	Postexertional pain out of proportion to the amount of exercise

Signs and Symptoms

Fatigue is the central symptom of CFS. The fatigue is unending and not restored by sleep or rest. The basic diagnostic criterion for CFS includes unrelenting fatigue that persists for a minimum of 6 months, along with at least four of the symptoms listed in Table 6.1.

Of these, poor memory and concentration, along with significant postexertional pain, are the most consistent CFS symptoms. Patients may also report extreme allergies, abdominal bloating, nausea, diarrhea, cramping, chest pain, irregular heartbeat, coughing, dizziness, fainting, dry eyes and mouth, weight loss, jaw pain, morning stiffness, night sweats, and psychological problems related to living with chronic illness, especially depression and/or anxiety.

This list of symptoms points to an important feature of CFS: it closely resembles two other chronic stress-related conditions: fibromyalgia syndrome and irritable bowel syndrome, and it frequently occurs along with them. In fact, so much overlap exists between these conditions that many people with aspects of all three disorders are simply diagnosed with whatever syndrome's primary features appear first: irritable bowel syndrome for gastrointestinal discomfort, fibromyalgia syndrome for predominant muscle and joint pain, or CFS if the leading symptom is unrelenting fatigue.

One of the most difficult issues for CFS patients is that symptoms are variable and unpredictable. They may come and go with no connection to activity or other triggers. When a person enters a period of remission, the tendency to over-exert can then put them back into an exhausted state.

Treatment

The primary treatment for CFS is making lifestyle choices that support the body as fully as possible. This means managing stress (any stimulus, emotional or physical, that requires the body to adapt to a change) as well as possible. It also means avoiding stimulants (caffeine, sugar) and depressants (alcohol) as much as possible, and exercising consistently and gently, so as not to exacerbate symptoms.

An important part of treatment for CFS patients is education; the more they learn about their condition, the better equipped they are to handle its challenges. Some evidence indicates that cognitive behavioral therapy can be effective as CFS patients seek coping skills to live with this condition.

Medical intervention may include low-dose antidepressants, but many experts suggest that these drugs are not particularly effective for CFS patients. Other medications are geared toward symptomatic treatment.

Medications

- NSAIDs for muscle and joint pain
- Anxiolytics
- Antiallergy medication to control allergic symptoms

Massage?

RISKS Chronic fatigue syndrome (CFS) patients tend to have low stamina, and may not welcome a rigorous, long, full body demanding massage that could leave them more fatigued after their treatment than before.

BENEFITS Evidence shows that massage can help with pain, sleep, and perceived anxiety: all issues for CFS patients. Gentle massage is a safe and appropriate choice for clients with this condition.

Fever

Definition: What Is It?

Fever, also called pyrexia, is an abnormally high body temperature, usually brought about by bacterial or viral infection, but sometimes stimulated by other types of tissue damage. Exactly when fever is identified is a bit of a moving target: most people vary in internal temperature by a degree Fahrenheit or more throughout the day. Generally, fever is identified when an undertongue thermometer registers 101°F (38.3°C) or more. Fever is a controlled change in temperature, which distinguishes it from other types of hyperthermia (Sidebar 6.6).

Etiology: What Happens?

Several steps are involved in the development of an infection-based fever:

1. A person is infected with some microorganism, such as bacteria, viruses, or fungi.
2. White blood cells find and eat those invaders.
3. Some pieces of the pathogens cell membranes are displayed by the macrophages. They stimulate other white blood cells to secrete interleukin-1 and other pro-inflammatory cytokines.

Fever in Brief

What is it?
Fever is a controlled increase in core temperature, usually brought about by immune system reactions, often in response to pathogenic invasion.

How is it recognized?
Fever is identifiable by readings on a thermometer, but other symptoms can include shivering, flushing, and sweating.

Massage risks and benefits
Risks: Fever contraindicates any massage that requires an adaptive response that may challenge a body while it is fighting a pathogenic invasion. Further, the practitioner must take pains not to pick up a new infection.
Benefits: Gentle reflexive or very light massage may help a person with a fever sleep better. A person who has fully recovered from a fever with no lingering complications can enjoy the same benefits from massage as the rest of the population.

SIDEBAR 6.6 Types of Hyperthermia

Fever is a systemic rise in body temperature that is carefully controlled by the hypothalamus. It has the advantages of speeding up immune system activity while slowing and starving infectious agents. Fever is an extraordinarily efficient mechanism to fight infection.

Sometimes, however, a person's core temperature rises without hypothalamic control. This generally occurs when a person generates more heat than he or she can release. In this case, the body temperature continues to rise until external factors work to cool off the person. If environmental factors don't allow this to happen, the person is at risk for brain damage or death.

The three levels of hyperthermia are heat cramps, heat exhaustion, and heat stroke. They are most commonly seen in people who are physically very active in warm, humid environments. Massage therapists who work at summertime sporting events can expect to see any of these manifestations of hyperthermia. A fourth condition, malignant hyperthermia, is a genetic condition that may be triggered by exposure to anesthesia.

- *Heat Cramps.* Muscle cramping is a frequent result of the dehydration that accompanies excessive heat production. The body sweats in an attempt to lower its temperature, and the result is a deficit in interstitial fluid. This makes it more difficult for the calcium ions that stimulate muscle contractions to be reabsorbed into their storage containers. Consequently, muscle contractions are sustained and uncontrolled. Fortunately, massage along with rehydration is an excellent way to move fluid back into the muscle bellies and stimulate the chemical and neurological reactions that reduce the spasm.
- *Heat Exhaustion.* Heat exhaustion occurs when muscular activity generates more heat than a person can release. It is marked by excessive sweating, headache, vasodilation, and dehydration. Excessive sweating may lead to low blood pressure, lightheadedness, and fainting. Fast hydration is the best recourse for this situation.
- *Heat Stroke.* Heat stroke is the final stage of hyperthermia. In this condition, body temperature rises to dangerous levels (~104°F, or 40°C, for adults). Prolonged dehydration may lead to lack of sweating and circulatory shock from loss of water and electrolytes. The person may become confused or delirious. Heat stroke can be fatal if the core temperature is not quickly but carefully reduced to safe levels.
- *Malignant Hyperthermia.* This is not a sports-related problem but rather a genetic anomaly that allows the body temperature to rise to dangerous, even fatal, levels with a minimum of muscular work. It is sometimes seen as part of an allergic reaction to anesthesia. Many people don't know they are at risk for this disorder until they have a dangerous episode.

4. Interleukin-1 circulates through the system, including the brain. It causes a series of chemical reactions involving prostaglandins that tell the hypothalamus to reset the body's thermostat to a higher level. In this situation, interleukin-1 is acting as a **pyrogen**, a fever starter.
5. Orders from the hypothalamus ripple through the body, setting up the muscular and glandular reflexes that raise the core temperature. These reflexes include shivering, constriction of superficial capillaries, and increased metabolism.

The characteristic shivering and chills that go along with a rising fever are part of the mechanism to increase the core temperature: this is called the chill phase. Once that goal has been met, the shivering stops, but processes keep working to maintain the increased temperature until the stimulating chemicals have been removed. This peak is called the crisis of the fever. When the crisis has passed, the body's cooling mechanisms, sweating and capillary dilation, take over: the flush phase. At this point, the worst is over, and the fever is broken.

Pathogenic invasion is the causative factor of most but not all fevers. Severe injury can upset the hypothalamic thermostat, as can poison, certain cancers, and some autoimmune diseases.

This culture has a strange and troubling discomfort with discomfort. Often people would rather hide a symptom than feel it and figure out what it's trying to tell them. This is true particularly with fever, which can be disagreeable and inconvenient. In rare cases, it can get high enough to do some serious damage, but most of the time fever is a sign that the body is working in the most efficient possible way to get rid of invading pathogens. Some of those mechanisms include the following:

- Interleukin-1 and other **cytokines** not only help to reset the body's thermostat, but also stimulate T-cell production. Increased T-cell production stimulates B cells and the production of antibodies.
- Interferon, a powerful antiviral agent, becomes much more active in the presence of fever.
- Increased temperature limits iron secretion from the liver and spleen, slowing bacterial and viral activity.
- Increased temperature raises the heart rate (10 beats per minute per degree), which in turn increases the distribution of white blood cells throughout the body.
- Increased temperature increases cell wall permeability and speeds chemical reactions. This promotes faster recovery for damaged tissues.

Fever occasionally presents a danger, particularly when the temperature rises over 104°F (40°C) for adults; this is called **hyperpyrexia**. The most common complications are dehydration (from prolonged sweating), **acidosis**, and brain damage. Death from fever occurs somewhere around 112°F to 114°F (44.4°C to 44.5°C) for adults. If a fever comes down too fast, it can quickly dilate blood vessels. This can lead to shock, which can be dangerous, especially to older patients.

Signs and Symptoms

The primary sign of fever is self-evident: it is a body temperature that is higher than normal. It is important to remember that many individuals have a "normal" temperature that is not exactly 98.6°, and also our temperature varies throughout the day, so small fluctuations without other symptoms like headache or malaise may not be significant. Other symptoms include the chills and shivering that go with raising internal temperature, and the flushing and sweating that go along with lowering it.

Treatment

Experts don't agree about the best time to treat simple fevers in adults. Suppressing symptoms may prolong an infection, and allowing a person to go back to work or school puts them in contact with other people who may subsequently become infected. On the other hand, fevers are uncomfortable and inconvenient, and it is natural to try to interrupt their course.

Medications

- Aspirin, ibuprofen, or acetaminophen to interrupt hypothalamic control of internal temperature
- Note: aspirin is not appropriate for use with children

Massage?

RISKS Fever systemically contraindicates most types of bodywork for the dual reason that the client is already challenged, and the practitioner shouldn't run the risk of exposure to a contagious condition.

BENEFITS Gentle or reflexive bodywork may help a client with a fever feel better, although it may have no impact on the fever itself. Any client who has fully recovered from a condition involving fever can enjoy the same benefits from bodywork as the rest of the population.

HIV/AIDS

Definition: What Is It?

AIDS (acquired immune deficiency syndrome) was first recognized as a specific disease in the United States in 1983. The causative virus, HIV (human immunodeficiency virus), attacks various agents of the immune system with disastrous results.

Etiology: What Happens?

HIV enters the body by way of body fluids: blood (including contaminated transfusions and shared needles), semen, vaginal secretions, and breast milk are the most efficient carriers of the virus.

HIV can attach to cells in mucosal epithelium to gain entry to the body. Any other sexually transmitted infection, such as syphilis, genital herpes, chlamydia, or gonorrhea, can significantly increase the risk of transmitting the virus. Once in the tissue, the virus invades a target cell through a molecular portal of entry on the membrane called CD4, along with coreceptor sites, which vary. Monocytes, macrophages, T cells, stem cells for blood, fibroblasts, and several cells found in the central nervous system all have this molecular doorway, and so are called CD4+ cells. HIV often invades circulating monocytes and macrophages, and uses these hosts as transport to concentrations of CD4+ cells in the bone marrow, lymph nodes, spleen, tonsils, adenoids, and central nervous system.

These targets are significant for a couple of reasons. First, when the virus pools in macrophages before moving up in the immune system hierarchy, its presence does not immediately trigger the production of antibodies, which makes it difficult to identify in a blood test (Sidebar 6.7). Second, consider the consequences of a virus that targets immune system cells: the entire immune system collapses and leaves the body vulnerable to a wide array of opportunistic diseases.

Blood-borne HIV can move from one CD4+ cell to another, and it can pool in the core of lymph nodes, where it eventually causes the cells to break down and the lymph node to lose all function. HIV has also been found in astrocytes and microglial cells in the central nervous system. This breaks down the **blood-brain barrier**, so toxic accumulations in the brain can lead to neurological symptoms.

HIV is composed of RNA rather than DNA, which holds the blueprints for our own cells (see Sidebar 6.8). Once inside a CD4+ cell, this retrovirus uses the enzyme **transcriptase** to convert its RNA to DNA in order to replicate. In the process, the virus is often minutely altered—just enough to make it resistant to identification or treatment. Ultimately, CD4+ cells die through membrane rupture or **apoptosis**, where the cell essentially self-destructs (Figure 6.6).

HIV/AIDS in Brief

What is it?
Acquired immune deficiency syndrome (AIDS) is a disease caused by human immunodeficiency virus (HIV), which attacks and disables the immune system. This leaves a person vulnerable to a host of diseases that are usually not a threat to people without HIV.

How is it recognized?
Most people with HIV have several days of flu-like symptoms within a few weeks of being infected, followed by an interval with no symptoms. When the virus has successfully inactivated the immune system, infection by opportunistic infections or characteristic types of cancer appear.

Massage risks and benefits
Risks: It is possible, although not typical, that a person with HIV can carry an infection that is communicable through casual contact, and this is something massage therapists need to know about. But in most cases, the main risk when working with the client is HIV positive or has AIDS is that the client may be vulnerable to whatever pathogens the therapist carries into the session.
Benefits: All stages of HIV infection indicate massage as long as the practitioner is healthy and doesn't pose any risk to the client, and the practitioner can adjust modalities to meet the client's needs.

SIDEBAR 6.7 Diagnosing HIV

Infection with HIV is determined by the presence of antibodies in the blood. This is a bit problematic, since the peculiar nature of this pathogen prevents the body from tagging it and initiating antibody production until the virus is widespread. To get a truly dependable diagnosis, HIV tests must be conducted up to 6 months after the last incidence of high-risk behavior: sharing intravenous drug needles, unprotected sex with a possibly infected partner, or the use of blood or blood products.

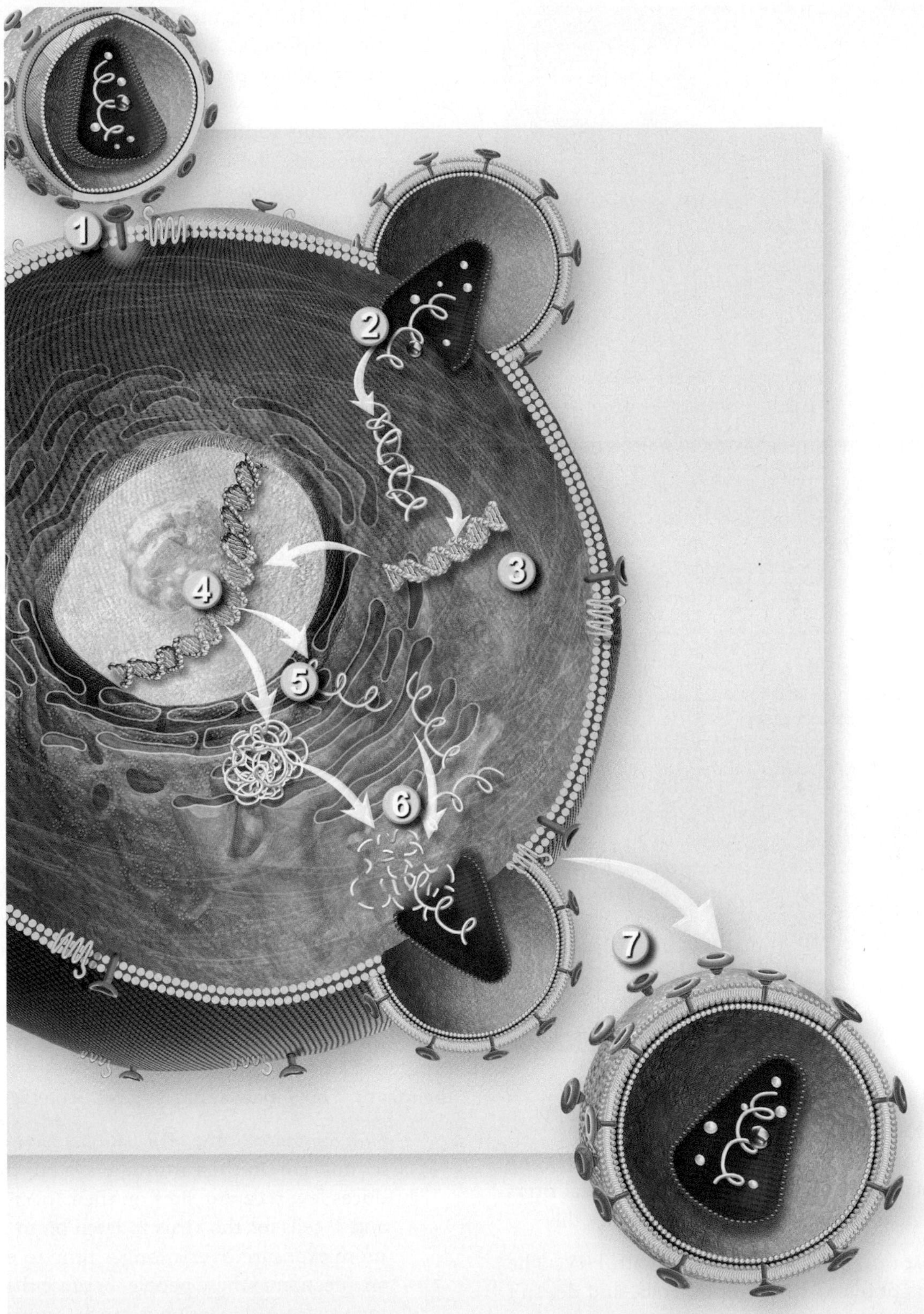

Figure 6.6. HIV/AIDS. 1. The virus attaches to a CD4 site on a target cell.2. RNA enters the cytoplasm. 3. RNA uses transcriptase to become DNA. 4. The virus reprograms the cell's function. 5. The cell now manufactures many copies of HIV. 6. Viruses are manufactured in the cell and leave to find new targets.

SIDEBAR 6.8 A Virus Primer

Viruses consist of a protein coat of variable complexity wrapped around a core of DNA or RNA. Outside a host cell, viruses have no metabolic functions and cannot replicate. Inside a host cell, the virus reprograms the functions of that cell to replicate more viruses. In other words, the host cell becomes a virus factory. When the factory is full of inventory, it either seeps virions (viral particles) from its membrane or ruptures, releasing hordes of new viruses in search of other hosts. Enormous amount of damage occurs with any viral infection, not just to the cells attacked by the virus but also to the cells the body sacrifices to fight back.

Most viruses cause short-term acute infections that spread easily. The coughing and sneezing seen with respiratory tract infections such as cold and flu are remarkably efficient distributors of virus. Likewise, the diarrhea that occurs with intestinal infections is an effective way to spread virus through fecal contamination. The immune system response to these viruses is severe and usually successful; most infections are curtailed, and the viruses are expelled in short order.

A few viruses, however, cause long-term chronic infections instead of short-term acute illness. Hepatitis B and C, herpes viruses, and HIV are notorious among these. For a virus to live in a body for a long time, it must be able to hide from immune system cells to escape attack and destruction. It is precisely the ability of HIV to hide from typical immune system activity that makes it so difficult to fight. In addition to being good hiders, chronic infectious viruses have been seen to produce decoy particles that draw antibody attack away from themselves and to secrete fake cytokines, chemical messengers that confuse and slow down immune system response.

As we learn more about how chronic infectious viruses pool in hidden reservoirs in the body, our ability to fight back will improve. We may someday be able to eradicate these hidden invaders permanently.

Progression

Each stage of HIV/AIDS is associated with decreasing numbers of active CD4+ cells and increased viral **titers** (counts of virus). The typical pattern looks like this:

- *Phase 1.* A person is infected with HIV. The virus pools in white blood cells, and doesn't elicit an immune response. Consequently, tests are negative, and no symptoms are present, but the person can transmit the disease because the viral load is high. This incubation phase can last a year or more, although the average is 3 weeks to 6 months in sexually transmitted cases.
- *Phase 2.* In the acute primary phase, HIV infection antibodies become detectable in blood tests. Many people have fatigue, swollen glands, fever, weight loss, headaches, drowsiness, and confusion within several weeks of exposure. These signs and symptoms usually last about 2 weeks and are often mistaken for flu or mononucleosis.
- *Phase 3.* No signs, symptoms, or opportunistic diseases are obvious. Although immune system cells are being destroyed in lymphatic tissue, the body is able to produce some antibodies against the virus. It is during this phase that medical intervention inhibits viral replication and prolongs life expectancy. The length of the asymptomatic phase varies widely, lasting anywhere from 1 to 20 years or more, with a median of 10 years.
- *Phase 4.* Signs and symptoms of opportunistic diseases or AIDS-related cancers become apparent and eventually debilitating. A normal T-cell count is 800 to 1,000 cells per milliliter of blood. AIDS is diagnosed when these levels drop to 200 cells per milliliter or below, and **indicator diseases** begin to develop.

HIV Resistance

Some HIV-AIDS research has focused on the variables that determine how long an infected person can stay healthy. Some people who are infected with HIV never develop symptoms, or develop them much more slowly than most people. These "long-term nonprogressors" can provide important clues to ways the virus may be fought once infection has been established. It seems clear that most long-term nonprogressors or very slow progressors have a combination of factors working in their favor. Three main variables have been identified:

- *Host resistance.* Some HIV patients have a genetic mutation in their immune system that produces few receptor sites on their macrophages and T cells for the virus to latch on to. It takes more exposure over a longer time to establish an infection in these people, because the chance for a successful invasion is much lower.
- *Immune system response.* When most cells are invaded by a virus, they display a fragment of that virus on their membrane. This serves as a signal to immune system agents that the cell is compromised and should be destroyed. HIV is

capable of slowing down this display reaction or of hiding from it altogether by mimicking normal cell membranes. If the efficiency of the display mechanism is improved, immune system response is more aggressive.

- *Virulence of the virus.* Sometimes HIV is partially weakened by medication or an immune system response but remains transmittable to another person. Infection with a weakened virus generally means the new host is better able to control it. Relative virulence of individual viruses is difficult to measure, however.

Communicability

HIV is spread from one person to another through the exchange of intimate fluids. These include blood (as from contaminated blood products, shared needles, or maternal-fetal circulation), semen, vaginal secretions, and breast milk. HIV does not accumulate in concentrations high enough to cause infection in other body fluids, such as sweat, saliva, or tears. The virus is unstable outside a human host, so it is not considered to be transmissible through contaminated surfaces or insect vectors such as mosquitoes, ticks, or bedbugs.

Complications

When HIV has virtually disabled normal immune function, the body is incapable of fending off attacks from pathogens that are not threatening to healthy people. A group of formerly obscure diseases that are now so closely associated with AIDS are called **indicator diseases**. Here are some of the most common and serious ones:

- *Pneumocystis carinii pneumonia.* This is a fungal infection of the lungs. It is now also called *Pneumocystis jiroveci.*

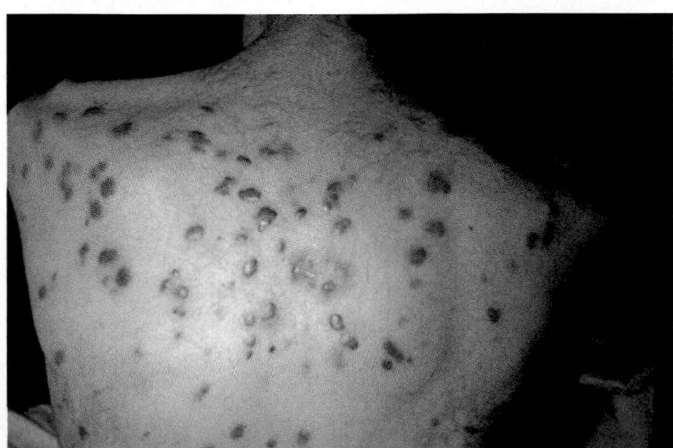

Figure 6.7. Kaposi sarcoma

- *Cytomegalovirus.* This member of the herpes family can cause retinitis and blindness, colitis, pneumonia, and infection of the adrenal glands.
- *Kaposi sarcoma.* This is a type of skin cancer (Figure 6.7) related to infection with human herpesvirus 8. Kaposi sarcoma is much more common in men with AIDS than in women.
- *Non-Hodgkin lymphomas.* HIV has been found to specifically initiate cancer cell replication with a variety of lymphomas. They tend to be aggressive, frequently metastasize to the central nervous system, and are highly resistant to treatment.

Other opportunistic indicator diseases include toxoplasmosis, a protozoan that can cause encephalitis or pneumonia; candidiasis, a yeast infection that can cause thrush or esophagitis; and *Cryptococcus neoformans*, a fungal infection that can cause meningitis and pneumonia.

In addition to these indicator diseases, people with AIDS are highly susceptible to gastrointestinal disturbances, herpes simplex, meningitis, shingles, cervical cancer, hepatitis C, and many other conditions. When tuberculosis occurs simultaneously with HIV, the risk of having tuberculosis become an active, contagious condition rises with each year of coinfection.

It is important to point out that while it is difficult to catch HIV from an infected person without some kind of intimate contact, it is not difficult to catch some of the contagious complications of AIDS. Tuberculosis, herpes, and other infections don't discriminate between HIV positive and other persons.

Signs and Symptoms

Signs and symptoms of HIV depend on the stage of infection; these are described earlier in this section.

Treatment

One of the things that makes finding a cure for AIDS so difficult is that when it reproduces, the virus can minutely change—just enough to make it resistant to drugs as well as to immune system activation. The solution to that problem has been to combine various drugs to anticipate the mutations of the virus. This has been highly successful in laboratory settings, but these drug combinations are often prohibitively toxic to the actual patients. The other challenge is that once the virus is hiding inside the genetic material of a target cell, it cannot be extracted without killing that cell.

The most successful AIDS treatments so far have involved using multiple strategies to interrupt viral replication. The use of highly active antiretroviral therapy (**HAART**) has been seen to slow progression in many patients, but it can't eradicate the virus. Although the goal of eliminating the virus from an infected person is still a long way off, studies of patients who manage to control their infection efficiently continue to point the way to better treatment options, and the life expectancy for a person with HIV today (who can afford to treat it) is better than it has ever been.

NOTABLE CASES The list of important and influential people lost to AIDS is too long to attempt. Perhaps the first "big name" to go public with this disease was actor Rock Hudson, but he was only one of thousands, including actor Tony Perkins ("Psycho") and tennis grand slam winner Arthur Ashe. Basketball legend Magic Johnson may be the public figure with the longest history of being both healthy and HIV positive; he was diagnosed in 1991 and continues to be an activist for AIDS prevention and accessibility of treatment.

The biggest controversy in HIV treatment currently is deciding when it is best to initiate antiviral therapy. It is clear that drugs prolong the lives of AIDS patients, but they are also highly toxic and have many serious side effects, including low blood cell count, peripheral neuropathy, pancreatitis, insulin resistance, chronic diarrhea, liver inflammation, kidney stones, and many others. One of the most visible side effects of HIV medication is **lipodystrophy**: fat in the cheeks and the buttocks degenerates, but fat in the upper back, breasts, and around the belly accumulates. Furthermore, many AIDS patients live in isolation, and they are more likely than most to be depressed and/or substance abusers, which increases the risk of their not taking their medication according to prescription: this gives rise to ever more resistant strains of the virus.

Treatment recommendations vary. If HIV is identified during the primary phase of flu-like symptoms, some research suggests the best prognosis if therapy is started right away. Healthcare workers who get needle sticks with a risk of contamination are treated immediately to reduce the risk that the virus can take hold. But if the virus isn't identified until the person is asymptomatic, many experts recommend holding off on aggressive treatment until CD4+ levels drop to below a specific threshold.

SIDEBAR 6.9 HIV-AIDS Statistics

Recent advances in reporting practices and statistical analysis suggest that the incidence of HIV/AIDS in the United States is significantly higher than previously thought, at about 56,000 new cases each year. About 53% of those new infections occur as a result of homosexual activity between men; 31% occur as a result of heterosexual intercourse; and 12% are among injected drug users. (The remainders are among people who do multiple high-risk behaviors.)

The good news is that this doesn't actually reflect an increase in new cases; it is simply a more accurate snapshot. Furthermore, the new infection rate has remained essentially stable since the late 1990s. Obviously, far too many people are being infected with HIV, but those numbers are at least not rising. Earlier detection and better treatment access can help to reduce both death rate and the rate of transmission, because a person whose infection is treated is less likely to spread it to others. For this reason, the Centers for Disease Control now recommends testing for all sexually active adults, regardless of their self-perceived risk of infection.

Medications

- Anti-retroviral drugs

Massage?

RISKS It is possible (although not typical) for a person who is HIV positive to have an opportunistic disease that is potentially contagious through casual contact. This is obviously a caution for massage therapists working with HIV-positive clients, but in most cases, the person most at risk for getting sick when an AIDS patient receives massage is not the therapist; it's the client. Therefore, care must be taken that the practitioner does not carry active pathogens that may put a client with AIDS at risk.

BENEFITS Asymptomatic HIV indicates massage. Some studies indicate that massage boosts immune system activity and efficiency for clients who are HIV positive. Clients with advanced AIDS can also benefit from massage that is specifically adjusted to meet their special needs. Bodywork can be a wonderful treatment option and an important source of support and comfort for people who are often rejected, ignored, or actively persecuted by society.

Autoimmune Disorders

Ankylosing Spondylitis

Definition: What Is It?

Ankylosing spondylitis (AS) is spinal inflammation (spondylitis) leading to stiff joints (ankylosis). In this condition, the joints between and around vertebrae can become permanently fused. AS is a progressive inflammatory arthritis of the spine. It is sometimes called rheumatoid spondylitis.

A specific gene (HLA-B27) has been identified with an increased risk for AS, but it is not a definitive marker. Unlike most autoimmune diseases, AS affects males more often than females; the ratio is about 3:1.

Etiology: What Happens?

AS is generally recognized as an autoimmune disease, but the blood of people with AS shows no sign of the **antinuclear antibodies** (ANA) that are typical of other autoimmune diseases. For this reason, it is classified as a **seronegative spondyloarthropathy**. Other seronegative autoimmune diseases include inflammatory bowel disease (IBD) (Crohn disease and ulcerative colitis), psoriasis, and psoriatic arthritis. Interestingly, these conditions are frequently seen in people with AS or in the family members of AS patients.

AS typically begins with chronic inflammation at the sacroiliac joint on one or both sides. Inflammation affects points of connection between bone and ligament or tendon, in a condition called **enthesitis**. Cartilaginous discs ossify, and bony deformation leads to the squaring of vertebral bodies. These fusions are called **syndesmophytes**. Although it is usually limited to intervertebral and costal joints, the heels, hips, shoulders, toes, and sternoclavicular joints may be affected too.

The pattern of inflammation and damage proceeds up the spine, leaving in its wake a trail of injured vertebrae that may eventually fuse sometimes with a flattened lumbar curve and an exaggerated thoracic curve (Figures 6.8 and 6.9). If the progression reaches all the way up to the neck, the cervical vertebrae may fuse with the head in a permanently flexed position as well. Fusions may also occur at the vertebrocostal joints, resulting in a locked rib cage and difficulty breathing.

AS carries a high risk of osteoporosis and vertebral fracture. Poor support from damaged ligaments means a greater chance of peripheral nerve pressure or **cauda equina syndrome** (loss of bowel and bladder control due to pressure on the cauda equina).

Ankylosing Spondylitis in Brief

Pronunciation: ang-kih-LO-sing spon-dih-LY-tis

What is it?
Ankylosing spondylitis (AS) is a progressive inflammatory arthritis of the spine.

How is it recognized?
AS usually begins as stiffness and pain around the sacrum, with occasional referred pain down the back of the buttocks and into the legs. It runs in cycles of flare and remission. In advanced AS, the vertebrae fuse in flexion or lateral flexion. Signs and symptoms may also include inflammation of the iris, inflammatory bowel disease, and other issues.

Massage risks and benefits
Risks: When AS is in flare, inflammation in the spine and other tissues is acute. This contraindicates any bodywork that might exacerbate inflammation.
Benefits: Between flares massage that promotes range of motion and pain-free movement can be helpful along with exercise and physical therapy to maintain flexibility.

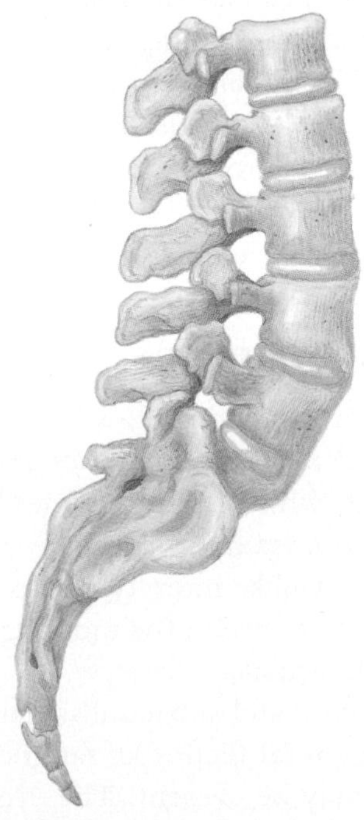

Figure 6.8. AS: vertebral fusions

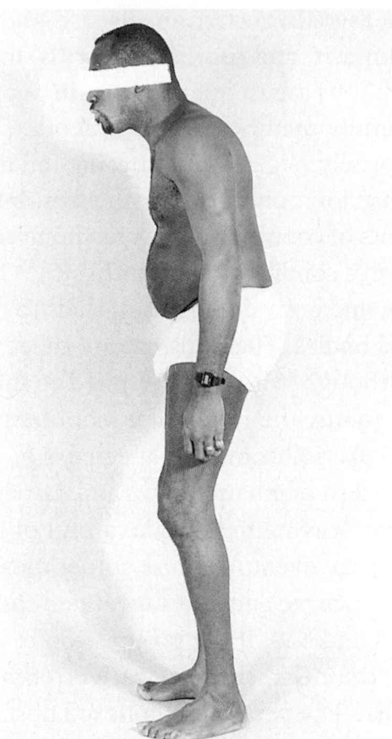

Figure 6.9. AS: postural distortion

Loss of lung capacity is an important complication of AS. Fusions at the costovertebral joints interfere with lung capacity, which results in constant shortness of breath, low stamina, and reduced resistance to chest infections such as pneumonia. Further, rib rigidity and limited lung capacity may contribute to right-sided heart failure.

Inflammation outside of joints may affect the eyes, heart, aorta, prostate, and kidneys. inflammatory bowel disease, (ulcerative colitis and Crohn disease) is often seen in AS patients.

Signs and Symptoms

AS usually starts as chronic low back pain. Often pain is felt in the buttocks, sometimes all the way down into the heels, which can sometimes lead to a misdiagnosis of herniated disc. The spine and hips feel stiff and immobile. Unlike more typical low back pain, AS is usually much worse in the morning or after rest; it improves with activity.

AS has acute and subacute stages. During acute episodes, a general feeling of fatigue, illness, and a slight fever may be present. The eyes may become dry, red, and uncomfortable; this is called **iritis**. Pain and stiffness gradually spread up the spine. When the inflammation subsides, the fever and acute pain are resolved, but stiffness and pain may continue to be present. Usually, the disease is limited to the low back, but it can progress to the neck or other joints in the body: hips and shoulders are most often affected.

Treatment

The first option for dealing with AS (which has no known cause and therefore no cure) is exercise. Physical therapy is recommended to preserve the suppleness of the spine and the strength of the paraspinals without aggravating the condition. Maintaining correct posture is the primary goal, since the vertebrae tend to fuse in a flexed position.

If exercise alone doesn't help, painkillers and anti-inflammatories are usually prescribed. Drugs that suppress immune system activity (DMARDs, or disease-modifying antirheumatic drugs) might be recommended. In very extreme cases, surgery may be suggested: an osteotomy is a procedure that fuses joints in a straightened position. If the knees, shoulders, or hips have been impaired, joint replacement surgery may also be suggested.

Medications

- Analgesics
- NSAIDs
- Oral and injected steroidal anti-inflammatories
- DMARDs to alter immune system activity
- Biologic agents to alter immune system activity

Massage?

RISKS Ankylosing spondylitis is a progressive, inflammatory condition that spreads up the spine and may affect other tissues as well. For these reasons, massage or bodywork during periods of flare must be gauged not to promote inflammation of any kind.

BENEFITS Between flares, massage for pain and relaxation can be helpful not only to preserve function but also to deal with the stress that inevitable accompanies a chronic, painful, progressive disease.

OPTIONS Careful range of motion, proprioceptive work, and massage that focus on deep breathing may be especially helpful for AS patients who place a high priority on preserving freedom of movement for as long as possible.

Crohn Disease

Definition: What Is It?

Crohn disease is a progressive inflammatory disorder that can affect any part of the GI tract, from the mouth to the anus. Advanced cases may also involve tissues outside the digestive system.

Crohn disease and ulcerative colitis are often described together under the umbrella term **inflammatory bowel disease**, but they have some important differences. Although Crohn disease can and often does affect the large intestine, it also affects the upper GI tract; this is not seen with ulcerative colitis. For more information on how these two conditions are alike and different, see Compare & Contrast 6.1.

Etiology: What Happens?

Crohn disease involves the development of inflamed areas in the large and small intestine. Many cases begin in the distal portion of the small intestine, the ileum, but this progressive disease can

Crohn Disease in Brief

Pronunciation: krone dih-ZEZE

What is it?
Crohn disease is a progressive inflammatory condition that may affect any part of the gastrointestinal tract. It is characterized by deep ulcers, scarring, and the formation of fistulas around the small and large intestines.

How is it recognized?
The primary symptom of Crohn disease is abdominal pain, especially in the lower right quadrant at the distal end of the ileum. Cramping, diarrhea, and pain with fissures or abscesses at the anus may also accompany active flares of this disease.

Massage risks and benefits
Risks: A client in a Crohn disease flare is likely to find a typical rigorous circulatory massage too challenging for comfort.
Benefits: Light, reflexive work that helps the body to organize its responses to stimuli may be welcomed during a Crohn disease flare. Any massage that is well tolerated is appropriate for a patient in remission.

COMPARE & CONTRAST 6.1 Crohn Disease and Ulcerative Colitis

Crohn disease and ulcerative colitis are two conditions linked under the description inflammatory bowel disease, or IBD. This may create the impression that these two disorders are slightly different manifestations of the same problem, but they are significantly different in etiology, progression, and long-term prognosis. Although differentiating between these conditions has little impact on a massage therapist's decision, it may have big impact on the life of the client.

CHARACTERISTICS	CROHN DISEASE	ULCERATIVE COLITIS
Area affected	Often begins in ileum but can spread to colon or to rest of small intestine.	Almost always begins in rectum. May spread up colon but never to small intestine.
Pattern of progression	Unpredictable, disconnected patches may appear anywhere along GI tract.	Contiguous connected series of lesions.
Depth of lesions	Ulcers may burrow through mucosa, into muscular or serous wall of GI tract. Perforation fairly common.	Ulcers penetrate only mucosa or submucosa of colon; seldom perforate.
Complications	Can lead to liver problems, skin and mouth ulcers, eye inflammation, peritonitis, bladder infections, colorectal cancer.	Significantly raises risk of colon cancer; other complications: liver inflammation, arthritis, skin rash, anemia.
Surgery	Surgery can remove affected areas, but disease often continues to attack healthy tissue; surgery often must be repeated.	Surgery to remove affected area is curative.

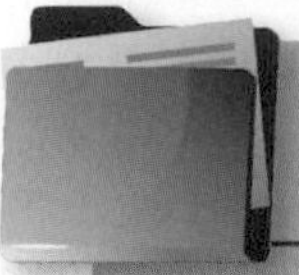

CASE HISTORY 6.1 Crohn Disease

Karen was diagnosed with Crohn disease when she was a young adult, but she has had stomach pain as long as she can remember. "When I was a kid, my mother literally had to hold my head and put food in my mouth. She wasn't being mean, it's just what the doctors told her to do because I wouldn't eat. All I knew was, food hurt."

Karen's doctor was convinced that there was nothing wrong with her. "It's all in your head," he told her. The Thanksgiving she was 22, she collapsed on a trip to California. She had a fever of 105°F. She had formed an abscess on her intestine, and the infection had invaded her bloodstream: she had sepsis and was hospitalized in Los Angeles for a week. After the attack subsided, she had her first colonoscopy, and the evidence of Crohn disease was clear.

After her diagnosis, Karen tried two medications to control the disease, but one gave her severe headaches and another, a sulfa drug, caused some breathing problems. Fortunately, she went into remission and had no problems for several years. Then in 1995, she developed severe stomach pain with diarrhea. Unable to absorb adequate nutrition from food, she developed bone pain, and her hair began to fall out. At this time, she began treating her disease with stronger medication.

KAREN, AGED 41
"ALL I KNEW WAS, FOOD HURT."

Karen's first surgery was conducted in 1997. Her small intestine was resected where a stricture had obstructed it; a fistula was repaired, adhesions between abdominal organs were released, and her appendix was taken out. She had remarkable relief after this, but it was short lived. "Most Crohn disease patients go about 4 years between surgeries; I go more like 2 years."

Karen's Crohn disease involves a tendency to build up scar tissue in the small intestine, leading to strictures, fistulas, and obstruction. She took infliximab (Remicade) to control symptoms, but several months ago it seemed to stop working. She finds that prednisone controls most of her symptoms, but she can use it only for about 6 weeks before developing serious side effects.

One of Karen's challenges is monitoring the progress of her disease. A colonoscopy goes only to the ileocecal valve, and a barium swallow shows problems only in the esophagus and stomach; Karen's problems are between the two points. She tried to use a new technology, a tiny camera in a pill-sized capsule, called a capsule endoscopy, that takes hundreds of pictures as it travels through the GI tract, but the camera got caught at an intestinal stricture, and she needed surgery to have it removed.

When she is in remission, Karen finds she doesn't have to be especially careful about her diet, but she doesn't tolerate caffeine well. When her disease is active, she has to avoid any roughage; she needs a low-fiber diet. She takes vitamins to make up for some lost absorption in her small intestine.

Karen works out 4 days a week in a gym, which she says is very helpful for managing her stress. A massage therapist visits her office once a month. She enjoys this, but she reports that when her disease is active, she has a hard time receiving massage: "Obstructive pain is intense! The intestines are twisting and turning, trying to shove the stuff through. I get terrible spasms in my back, and the therapist says the muscles in my back are stiff as a board."

Karen had five surgeries between 1997 and 2006, and she says she now recognizes the symptoms of another stricture forming, just 6 months since her last surgery. She gets along well with her doctor, who she calls GI Joe, and she enjoys interaction with other Crohn disease patients. She is happy to "share my agonies" with anyone who asks, and she does so with laughter and good will. "You have to laugh," she says. "What else are you gonna do?"

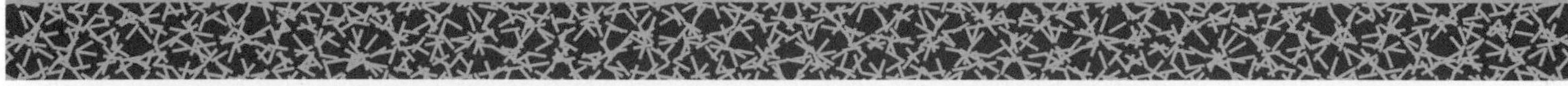

affect upper regions of the GI tract as well as the colon and the anus.

Crohn disease is an idiopathic disease. It is considered to be a multifactorial problem, with aspects of pathologic invasion, genetic predisposition, immune system dysfunction, environmental influences, and dietary triggers. An inappropriate inflammatory response against bacteria in the gut is part of the picture, but it is unclear whether that response is the cause or the result of the disease.

One of the distinguishing features of Crohn disease is that the areas it affects are not contiguous; the inflamed regions appear in an unpredictable patchwork anywhere in the GI tract. Eventually, these ulcers can cause accumulations of scar tissue that partially block the intestine (**stenosis**), or they can stimulate the development of abnormal connecting tubes from the colon to other organs, for instance the bladder or to the surface of the skin. These tubes are called **fistulas**, and they allow intestinal contents to exit the GI tract (Figure 6.10).

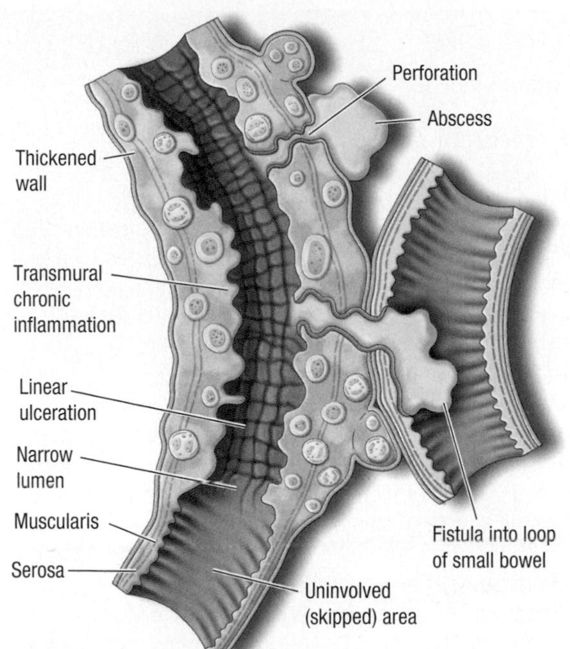

Figure 6.10. Crohn disease

Crohn disease disrupts normal digestion in several ways. Inflammation in the intestines interferes with absorption; this means a patient is at risk for serious malnutrition, gallstones, and a specific type of kidney stone. When Crohn disease occurs in young children, it can lead to stunted growth and delayed development. This disease can also cause bowel obstruction, at first by swelling and spasm, and eventually by scar tissue strictures. Deep ulcers may bleed into the GI tract, or perforate, leading to peritonitis. Adhesions can form between layers of the peritoneum. Abscesses can form in the GI tract or around the anus. If fistulas into the bladder form, leaking fecal material can cause serious bladder infections. Chronic irritation to epithelial cells in the GI tract also increases the risk of colon cancer.

Crohn disease is linked to problems outside the GI tract as well. It can cause inflammation at the bile duct, leading to cirrhosis, jaundice, and gallstones. It can lead to acute inflammation affecting the liver, eyes, and joints. It can cause ulcers called **aphthae** in the mouth and lesions on the skin as well; these open sores most often appear around the ankles and lower legs.

Signs and Symptoms

Crohn disease occurs in periods of flare and remission. During periods of remission, a patient may have no symptoms at all, but during a flare, the most common symptoms include abdominal pain, especially at the distal end of the ileum in the lower right quadrant, along with cramping, diarrhea (often with blood), and bloating. Weight loss, fever, joint pain, small ulcers in the mouth and throat, and lesions on the skin may also accompany acute flares. Many Crohn disease patients also have severe pain around the anus, along with anal fissures and abscesses.

NOTABLE CASES In 1956, just 9 months after a major heart attack, President Dwight D. Eisenhower had an emergency ileotransverse colostomy. The 30 cm of removed tissue showed signs of Crohn disease. He was back at his desk 5 days after his surgery.

Treatment

The damage to the whole length of the digestive system that Crohn disease can cause is serious, so it is usually treated aggressively. Treatment during flares usually begins with a class of drugs called aminosalicylates: these quell inflammation and immune system activity in the GI tract. Antibiotics may be necessary for abscesses or infections. Steroidal anti-inflammatories and other immune modifiers are used if other drugs are unsuccessful. Most Crohn disease patients eventually have surgery to remove affected sections of intestine or open blockages, but this is not curative; new patches of inflamed tissue may arise in other places, requiring further surgery.

Crohn disease patients have to be extraordinarily careful about their diet, especially during flares. High-fiber, bulky foods can exacerbate symptoms and create obstructions if scar tissue has narrowed the passageway. Sometimes, a high-calorie liquid diet is recommended during these episodes. In extreme cases, the patient may take in all nutrients intravenously to give the whole system a break from the stress of digesting food.

Medications

- Aminosalicylates by mouth, enema or suppository to suppress inflammation in the GI tract
- Antibiotics as needed
- Oral, injected, or topical steroidal anti-inflammatories to limit inflammation and scarring
- Immune-modifying drugs to interfere with immune system response

Massage?

RISKS During a Crohn disease flare, a person may not be at ease with some positions on the table, and rigorous bodywork may be too challenging to be comfortable. Further, the medications that Crohn disease clients take may carry some cautions for massage therapists.

BENEFITS When Crohn disease is in remission, massage can be supportive and safe choice. Deep abdominal work should probably be avoided, but any strategy that can establish a parasympathetic state can support efficient digestion.

OPTIONS Extremely gentle work or simply holding on the abdomen can help the body to "organize" its responses to stimuli. This can be especially important to help incorporate this problematic area for a client who struggles with digestive discomfort.

Lupus

Definition: What Is It?

Lupus is an autoimmune disease in which various types of tissues are attacked by the immune system. Lupus can be mild, but has the potential to be life threatening. In extreme cases, this disorder can attack the heart, the lungs, the kidneys, and the brain, with devastating results.

Like many autoimmune disorders, many more women are affected by lupus than men; in this case, the ratio is about 9:1.

Lupus in Brief

Pronunciation: LU-pus

What is it?
Lupus is an autoimmune disease in which antibodies attack various types of tissue throughout the body. Several distinct types of lupus exist, but systemic lupus erythematosus is both the most common and the most serious.

How is it recognized?
A group of 11 specific signs and symptoms have been determined for a diagnosis of lupus; a patient must have at least four of them. They include, among other things, arthritis in two or more joints, pleurisy, pericarditis, kidney disease, and nervous system dysfunction.

Massage risks and benefits
Risks: Lupus during a flare is an inflammatory disease that can affect the skin, heart, lungs, joints, and kidneys. Challenges to these systems present special cautions for massage therapy.
Benefits: During flare, clients with lupus may appreciate gentle or reflexive work that focuses on pain and anxiety relief without the risk of exacerbating inflammation or promoting fluid flow through challenged systems. During remission, clients with lupus can enjoy any kind of bodywork that is within their capacity for adaptation.

Etiology: What Happens?

Lupus is a condition with a wide range of presentations, but the common factor is immune system attacks against a variety of tissue types throughout the body. These attacks often begin in small blood vessels, which can cause inflammation, clotting, and nutrition supply problems to all the affected tissues.

The precise cause or causes of lupus are unknown; it seems to be a combination of racial predilection, genetic predisposition, hormones, and environmental exposures. A genetic link is clearly a factor, but a child of a parent with lupus has only a small risk of developing the disease. Further, when one identical twin develops lupus, the other twin may not. This indicates that although a genetic susceptibility may be inherited, other factors must also contribute to the development of the disease. Another indicator that genetics is not the primary issue is that while lupus in the United States and the United Kingdom has the highest incidence among Black women, lupus is practically unheard of among women in Western or Central Africa.

Environmental contributors may include exposure to certain viruses, ultraviolet light, certain medications, and high levels of estrogen. Women with lupus often report a change in symptoms with their menstrual cycle, and estrogen replacement therapy that is employed to reduce the risk of osteoporosis can increase the risk of lupus for some women.

Types of Lupus

- *Drug-induced lupus.* This is brought on by some prescribed medications for high blood pressure, heart arrhythmia, psychosis, and epilepsy. These symptoms resolve when the medications are discontinued.

- *Neonatal lupus.* This occurs when a mother with lupus or another autoimmune disease transfers antibodies to a newborn baby. The baby sustains a skin rash, liver problems, or a low blood count for a few weeks or months until the antibodies are no longer active. At that time, the symptoms disappear, usually with no long-term consequences.
- *Discoid lupus erythematosus (DLE).* This is a chronic skin disease. It can involve small scaly red patches with sharp margins that don't itch, or the characteristic butterfly or **malar** rash of redness over the nose and cheeks (Figures 6.11 and 6.12). The skin can become very thin and delicate, or lesions may become permanently discolored and thickened. DLE is sometimes described as a subset of skin disorders called **subacute cutaneous lupus**. A small number of people with DLE go on to develop SLE.
- *Systemic lupus erythematosus (SLE).* This is caused by antibody attacks against a variety of tissues throughout the body. This can result in arthritis, renal failure, thrombosis, psychosis, seizures, coronary artery disease, inflammation of the heart, and pleurisy. SLE can be very serious. It can usually be controlled, but at this time, it cannot be cured. SLE sometimes begins as DLE, but not always.

Signs and Symptoms

Lupus can look like a lot of different diseases. While it does have some markers in the blood that can help to identify it, those markers are sometimes present in people without lupus, so they can't be used as a definitive diagnosis. Along with blood markers, lupus usually involves four or more of the following, not necessarily simultaneously:

- Debilitating fatigue
- Mental confusion, cognitive dysfunction, short-term memory loss
- **Alopecia** (unexplained hair loss)
- Malar rash
- Discoid skin rash that can cause permanent scarring
- Photosensitivity
- Mucous membrane ulcers, particularly in the mouth, nose, or throat
- Arthritis in more than two joints, specifically in the hands or feet (not in the spine)
- Pleurisy and/or pericarditis
- Kidney problems: blood or protein in the urine
- Brain irritation: headaches, seizures, or psychosis
- Blood count abnormalities: low red blood cell count, white blood cell count, or platelet count
- Immunologic disorders: special antibodies and/or lupus anticoagulants are present in the blood
- Antinuclear antibodies in the blood

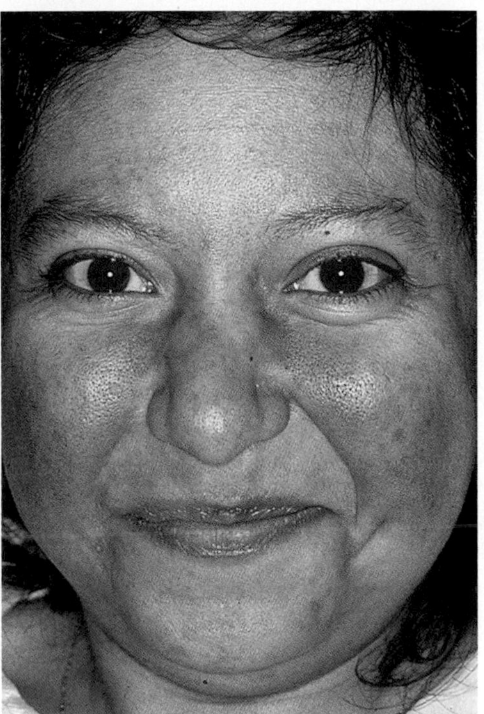

Figure 6.12. Lupus: malar rash

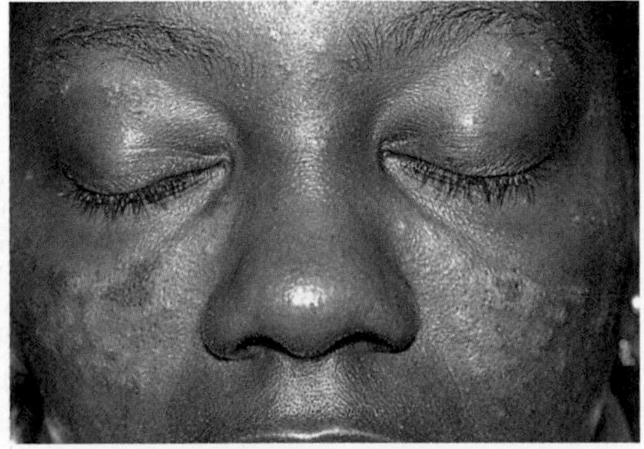

Figure 6.11. Lupus

Lupus flares are exacerbated by certain kinds of stimuli. Excessive exposure to ultraviolet light, emotional stress, injury, infection, or trauma can be triggers. Pregnancy is a trigger for some women, while for others it may suppress flares. Someone who has lupus must identify the stimuli that are particularly potent for her and avoid them carefully.

One of the challenges in identifying lupus is that symptoms fluctuate and may change entirely over time. In addition, other connective tissue diseases may occur simultaneously with lupus to further cloud the issue (Sidebar 6.10).

Lupus can affect virtually every system in the body (Figure 6.13). Because some of the features of this disease make profound changes in health, it is worth looking at how SLE affects several systems.

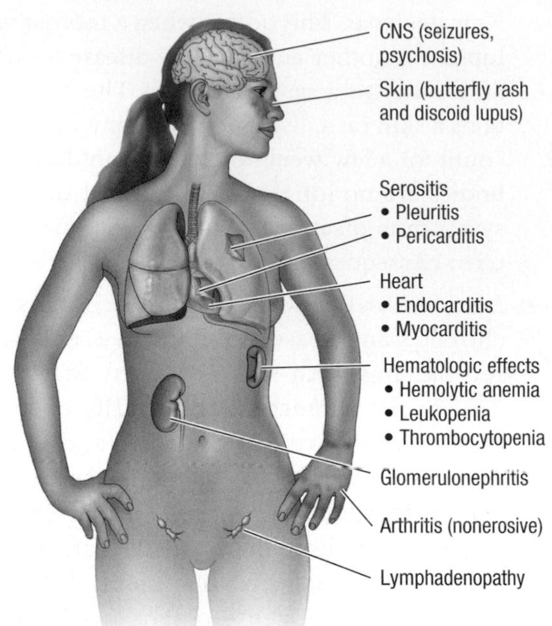

Figure 6.13. Lupus: systemic effects

- *Integumentary system.* The characteristic rashes seen with lupus have already been described. These rashes may be exacerbated by sunlight in a condition called **photosensitivity**. Lupus can also cause ulcers in the mucous membranes, particularly in the nose, throat, and mouth. When SLE causes superficial blood vessels to become inflamed, symptoms may appear on the skin in the shape of telangiectasias ("spider veins"), welts, red lines, and painful bumps.
- *Musculoskeletal system.* Most people with lupus eventually develop painful, swollen, but nonerosive arthritis. Joint pain usually occurs asymmetrically at the hands or knees, but seldom in the spine. Nonspecific muscle pain is another common symptom, and many lupus patients also meet the diagnostic criteria for fibromyalgia.
- *Nervous system.* Nervous system complications can range from extreme headaches to psychosis (including paranoia and hallucinations), to fever or seizures, depending on which part of the brain is adversely affected by blood vessel inflammation. When the clotting disorders that may accompany this disorder occur in the brain, the result is a transient ischemic attack or stroke.
- *Cardiovascular system.* Lupus can lead to inflammation of major blood vessels, opening the door to rapidly progressive atherosclerosis and the risk of heart attack, even in young people.

SIDEBAR 6.10 Mixed Connective Tissue Disease: The Combination Platter

About 10% of people diagnosed with lupus have it simultaneously with other autoimmune diseases. This combination of conditions is sometimes called mixed connective tissue disease.

The autoimmune diseases that are most often a part of mixed connective tissue disease include scleroderma, rheumatoid arthritis, lupus, polymyositis, and dermatomyositis. Rheumatoid arthritis and lupus occur together so often that a new name has been coined for this condition: **rhupus**.

In many cases, a person presents over a long period with a range of fluctuating symptoms that are not specific to any particular autoimmune disease. These usually include fatigue, muscle weakness, joint pain and swelling, swollen fingers, mild fever, and bouts with Raynaud phenomenon. Much later, the symptoms often narrow down to point to just one condition, which is usually scleroderma.

The role of massage for a client with mixed connective tissue disease is to work conservatively, being supportive but not challenging during flares, and working to improve function during remission. Communication with a client's healthcare team is important to maximize benefits (e.g., reducing stress, improving attitude, easing pain) while minimizing risks (exacerbating inflammation, irritating damaged tissues).

Lupus is also associated with slow clot formation and slow clot dissolving. This problem can lead to thrombophlebitis or pulmonary embolism. In addition to blood vessel damage, lupus inflames the serous membranes of the heart, leading to arrhythmia and severe chest pain. Anemia is a frequent complication of long-term inflammation and bone marrow suppression. Thrombocytopenia, or a shortage of platelets, may occur when lupus antibodies have attacked thrombocytes. Finally, Raynaud phenomenon is a sign of **vasculitis**.

- *Respiratory system.* A common complication of lupus is **pleurisy** or inflammation and fluid accumulation in the serous membranes that line the lungs. This causes pain on inhalation and restricted movement of the lungs. If enough resistance in the lungs develops, a lupus patient may be at risk for pulmonary hypertension and right-sided heart failure.
- *Urinary system.* Tissue damage in the kidneys leads to a specific type of **glomerulonephritis**. Kidney damage can accumulate without symptoms until the kidneys are on the brink of renal failure.
- *Reproductive system.* The clotting disorder associated with lupus can make it difficult to carry a child to term. Repeated spontaneous miscarriages are sometimes the first sign of the disease that will lead to a diagnosis. Pregnant women with lupus face special challenges, as some of the medications that control symptoms are not safe for the baby.

Treatment

The treatment strategy for lupus is to minimize the negative impact of inflammation during flares. If the case is not very severe, it may be managed with nonsteroidal anti-inflammatories. These drugs are inexpensive and easily accessible, and they are often effective against inflammation. Unfortunately, they are also associated with chronic stomach irritation, and long-term use can irritate and damage the kidneys—a special point of concern for lupus patients.

Steroidal anti-inflammatories (especially prednisone) are sometimes prescribed for short-term use, especially during flares. These are very powerful anti-inflammatories, but they are also associated with many dangerous side effects, including mood changes, weight gain, liver damage, bone thinning, and osteonecrosis, or death of bone and joint tissue, especially in the hips and shoulders.

Antimalarial drugs have found success in treating some of the symptoms of lupus, especially skin rashes and ulcers of mucous membranes, and reducing the needed dose of corticosteroids. Some antimalarial drugs cause changes in eye function, so an ophthalmologist must closely monitor their use.

NOTABLE CASES Singer Michael Jackson was diagnosed with lupus shortly after his signature album, *Thriller*, was released. Singer Seal carries the facial scars from the malar rash associated with discoid lupus.

In very severe cases, immune-suppressant drugs may be recommended. This of course leaves the patient vulnerable to secondary infections.

Other treatment options for lupus depend on the presenting symptoms. Acute rashes may be treated with topical steroid creams or ointments. If a patient has blood clotting problems, anticoagulants may be administered. It is a high priority to treat lupus symptoms quickly as they arise; early intervention can reduce the amount of damage that accrues during flares and keep the body functioning at normal levels during periods of remission.

Medications

- NSAIDs for low-grade pain and inflammation
- Steroidal anti-inflammatory during flare
- Antimalarial drugs for skin rashes
- Immune-suppressant drugs
- Drugs for symptomatic and side effect treatment: steroid cream, anticoagulants, bisphosphonates for osteoporosis, etc.

Massage?

RISKS Active flares of lupus mark periods of inflammation that can damage the skin, heart, lungs, and kidneys, and cause painful swelling at joints. Rigorous massage during these acute episodes may exacerbate symptoms and put undue stress on an inflamed cardiovascular system.

BENEFITS Gentle and reflexive massage may be soothing during flares, and more rigorous massage during remission (within tolerance of course) may help to deal with pain and stiffness, allowing the client with lupus to be more active when it is possible.

Multiple Sclerosis

Definition: What Is It?

MS is a condition characterized by inflammation and degeneration of myelin sheaths in the spinal cord and brain. It is thought to be an autoimmune disease, but the triggering pathogens or other stimuli appear to vary.

Etiology: What Happens?

The word sclerosis means hardened scar or plaque. In MS, T cells, B-cells, antibodies, and destructive cytokines attack and destroy myelin in patchy areas of the CNS. **Oligodendrocytes**, the myelin-producing cells in the CNS, multiply and attempt to repair the damage, but eventually they fail.

As attacks progress, normal myelin is replaced with scar tissue. Electrical impulses are either slowed or completely obstructed. If flares are persistent and repetitive, the damage may affect the neuron itself. In this case, lost function is more likely to be permanent. The result is loss of motor control, cognitive changes, or motor and sensory paralysis.

MS, like many autoimmune diseases, often works in cycles of inflammatory flares followed by periods of remission. During flares, the myelin is under attack and is replaced by scar tissue. During remission, inflammation subsides and some myelin regenerates. In this way, MS patients may lose some neurological function during flares but regain some or all of it during remission.

At present, the leading theories behind MS point to immune system attacks against some component of myelin sheaths in the CNS. This leads to an inflammatory response that destroys the protective myelin sheath and may eventually attack the nerve tissue itself (Figure 6.14).

It also seems clear that a genetic predisposition raises the risk of developing MS, but this seems to be a relatively small factor. The population-wide risk of developing MS is less than 1%. People with a first-degree relative who have the disease carry a risk of only 1% to 3%. If one identical twin has the disease, the other twin has only a 30% chance of developing MS.

Further, epidemiologists have examined why the incidence of MS appears to increase with distance from the equator. The key factor here appears to be the availability of vitamin D: this nutrient, which is manufactured with the stimulus of exposure to sunlight, decreases proinflammatory cytokines. People with high vitamin D levels appear to have a lower-than-average risk of developing MS. The issue appears to be where a person spends the majority of their adult life; if she is born in the tropics, but moved to the extreme northern or southern hemisphere by age 15, the risk of her developing MS is the same as for the rest of the population for that area.

This collection of information indicates that MS is probably an autoimmune disease to which some people are genetically predisposed, but that requires some combination of environmental triggers to initiate the disease process.

Types of Multiple Sclerosis

- *Benign MS.* This version of MS shows virtually no progression after a single episode.

Multiple Sclerosis in Brief

Pronunciation: MUL-tih-pul skler-O-sis

What is it?
Multiple sclerosis (MS) is an idiopathic disease that involves the destruction of myelin sheaths around both the motor and sensory neurons in the CNS.

How is it recognized?
MS has many symptoms, depending on the nature of the damage. These can include fatigue, eye pain, spasticity, tremors, and a progressive loss of vision, sensation, and motor control.

Massage risks and benefits
Risks: When MS is in flare, it can involve numbness, tingling, weakness, and extreme pain. Rigorous bodywork may be overwhelming for a client in this condition to receive, but very gentle work that focuses on symptomatic relief may be safe.
Benefits: When a client with MS is in an acute stage, he or she may benefit from extremely gentle, reflexive work that focuses on relieving pain and anxiety, without trying to create specific change. A client with MS who is in remission can receive any bodywork that is within his or her capacity for adaptation. Depending on the severity of disease, clients with full or close to full function may choose massage as part of a coping strategy.

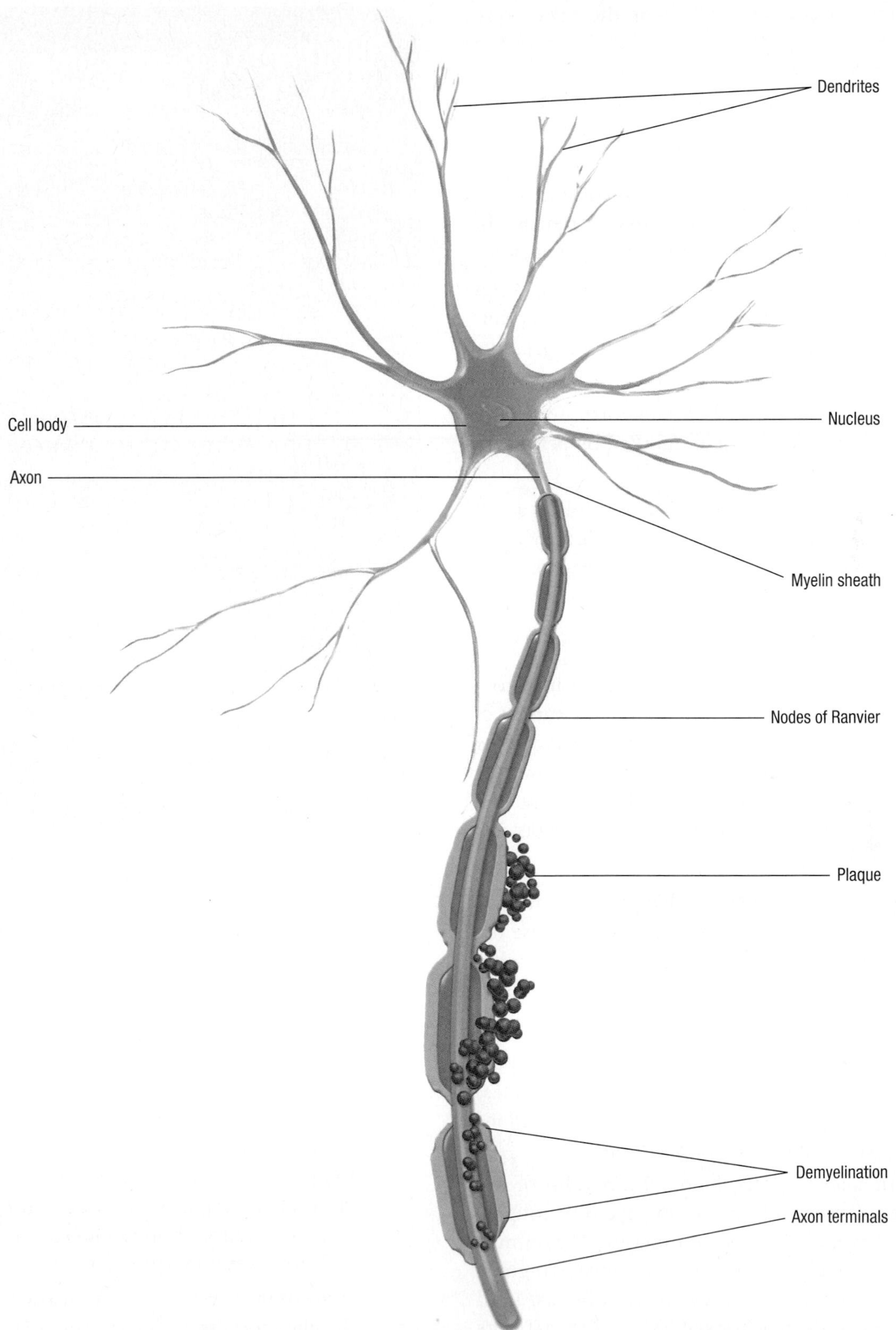

Figure 6.14. Myelin destruction with MS

- *Relapse/remitting MS.* This is the most common form of MS, involving cycles between flare and remission. While some recovery of the myelin sheath can occur during remission, ultimately some level of damage is usually permanent.
- *Primary progressive MS.* This version involves a chronic, low-grade progression that is not marked by periods of acute flare or remission.
- *Secondary progressive MS.* In this version, cycles of flare and remission occur, but recovery during remission is only partial. A progressive decline in function is observed.
- *Progressive/relapsing MS.* This form involves a slow but steady decline, marked by periods of extreme flare.
- *Malignant MS.* This rare form involves a fast and relentless decline, leading to disability and death within weeks or months of diagnosis.

SIDEBAR 6.11 Diagnosing Multiple Sclerosis

Multiple sclerosis (MS) is notoriously difficult to diagnose, because the signs that appear on tests (including various types of MRIs and a spinal tap to look for fragments of damaged myelin) often don't correspond to the severity of symptoms.

The medical convention is to describe a person's disease as possible, probable, or definite MS. To achieve a conclusive diagnosis, a patient must have these findings:

- Objective evidence of at least two episodes. (This can be determined through MRI, examination of cerebrospinal fluid, or evoked potential tests that show the speed of nerve transmission in the brain.)
- Episodes of flare that are separated by at least a month and by location of affected function.
- No other explanation for symptoms that can be found.

Several conditions can produce MS-like symptoms. Part of a thorough diagnosis is ruling out the following:

Lyme disease	HIV/AIDS	Scleroderma
Vascular problems in the brain	Disc disease	Lupus
CNS tumors	Fibromyalgia	Encephalitis
B_{12} or folic acid deficiency		

Signs and Symptoms

This disease is sometimes called "the great imitator" because its initial symptoms can look like a variety of other diseases, depending on what area of nerve tissue has been affected (Sidebar 6.11). The order with which symptoms appear also varies greatly from one person to the next. Some of the most dependable signs and symptoms include these:

- *Weakness.* The onset of this problem may be gradual or sudden. It comes about because the loss of myelin makes nerve transmission slow.
- *Spasm.* This can take the form of chronic muscle stiffness or active acute cramping.
- *Changes in sensation.* MS patients often report numbness or **paresthesia** (pins and needles) in various parts of the body. These sensations may last for hours or days at a time.
- *Optic neuritis.* Attacks on the myelin of the optic nerve result in extreme eye pain coupled with progressive loss of function. Vision may be minimally impaired (for instance, red-green color distortions) or it may be fully lost until the episode has passed. Most MS patients recover full or close to full vision when they go into remission.
- *Urologic dysfunction.* MS patients may find it difficult to urinate, or they may be incontinent.
- *Sexual dysfunction.* Difficulty maintaining an erection for men or having an orgasm in women are sometimes early signs of this disease.
- *Difficulty walking.* This problem can be a product of several factors, including muscle stiffness, numbness, dizziness, balance problems, and loss of coordination.
- *Loss of cognitive function.* A frequently overlooked issue for many MS patients is a change in mental ability. Short-term memory and the ability to learn and perform complex tasks are often challenged. A small percentage of MS patients undergo severe changes in cognitive skills that result in dementia.
- *Depression.* This is a complication of many chronic progressive diseases, especially in situations as unpredictable as those of MS.
- *Digestive disturbances.* Many MS patients have severe digestive disturbances (nausea, diarrhea, constipation) that vary greatly from day to day.

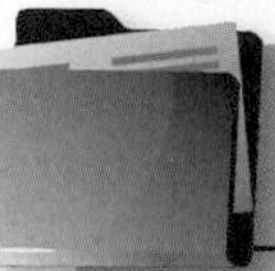

CASE HISTORY 6.2 Multiple Sclerosis

About a year and a half ago, we had just moved into a new house and my youngest child had just started school. For the first time in 15 years, I was looking forward to having some time, to getting on with my life. Then there was a pain in my left heel that felt like a stone bruise. We were just back from a long vacation, so I thought it was from too much walking. Two weeks later my foot went numb, and it traveled up my leg to my knee. It began affecting my right leg too. Then there was numbness and tingling in my left hand. It felt like I had just had a shot of Novocain, it was that kind of tingling.

My doctor sent me to a neurologist who checked me out and watched me walk. Then while I was sitting there, he went out into the hall with another doctor and they started speaking in medical jargon that I couldn't understand; it made me really nervous. When he came back he asked me, "Will you come in for a spinal tap?"

TRICIA, AGE 36
"IT TAKES ALL THE COURAGE I CAN MUSTER JUST TO STAND UP IN THE MORNING."

"Why?"

"There are some things we want to check out."

"What do you think I have?"

"I think you have MS."

"Excuse me?"

I never dreamed it would be something like this.

They started me on intravenous steroids. The next morning I got up after a bad night, and for the first time in 2 months I could walk normally. I was so excited, I woke my family and called my mom on the phone. But by the end of that morning I was already beginning to feel tired.

The head of the department was prepared to tell my family I had progressive MS, and I could be dead in a matter of weeks. I finally decided that I needed to be home, I needed to be with my family, so I checked out even though they didn't want me to.

I continued physical therapy at a local clinic. At first, they would have me sit in a warm pool with jets of water after I exercised, and I would go home feeling so drained and worn out, it was awful. Finally, they adjusted that part of it and I did better.

Today I still don't have much sensation below my knees. It takes all the courage I can muster just to stand up in the morning. I never know what kind of day I'll have, whether I'll be able to walk without a cane, whether I'll be tied to the house because my digestive system is unpredictable. I have terrible headaches that begin on the lower half of one side of my face and go up into my ear. I have days when I can't eat at all. I've had episodes of dizziness and double vision. I'm not on steroids now, but I take an antidepressant for the headaches. We're still struggling to find the right dose. My greatest fear, even more than being in a wheelchair, is that I will lose bladder or bowel control or go blind.

But my doctor says my scenario is good. It's been a year and a half without any exacerbations and he says I'm in remission. The only thing that's worse is my headaches, which are more painful and happen more often.

I think everything depends on your attitude. A major thing for me is to feel needed. If I have a purpose, I feel better. I have five wonderful children and a husband who loves me. My doctor thought I was going to die, and here I am in remission. I just feel so lucky to be here.

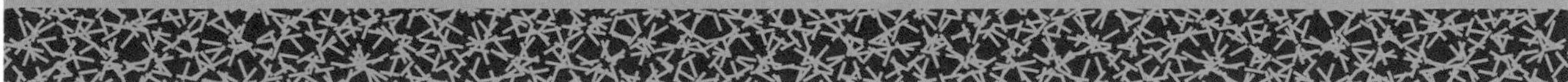

- *Sensitivity to heat.* Many MS patients find that warm temperatures, especially rapid changes from cool to warm, trigger painful spasms.
- *Fatigue.* Perhaps the most common symptom for MS patients is debilitating fatigue, which is particularly exacerbated by heat. The fatigue may be a result of slower or impaired nerve transmission (requiring fewer muscle fibers to work harder), muscle spasm, and other factors.

Treatment

The mainstay of current MS treatment is a class of drugs called **DMAMS**: disease-modifying agents for MS. These include several types of interferons, which can shorten the periods of flare and prolong periods between episodes; and methotrexate and similar drugs, which slow cell growth and quell immune system activity. Steroidal anti-inflammatories are also used, but it is important to point out that all these medications carry strong side effects, some of which can be life threatening.

Other medications are used to control symptoms like fatigue, constipation, bladder control, cognitive difficulties, and other problems.

Nonpharmacological options for people living with MS include careful exercise and physical or occupational therapy designed to maintain strength and function as long as possible. Eating well and getting adequate amounts of high-quality sleep are important for maintaining health and prolonging remissions. Stress management techniques, including massage, are often recommended for the same reasons.

NOTABLE CASES Actress Teri Garr, comedian Richard Pryor, talk show host Montel Williams, and Mouseketeer Annette Funicello comprise a short list of notable celebrities diagnosed with multiple sclerosis.

Medications

- DMAMS, including interferons, methotrexate, and others
- Steroidal anti-inflammatories
- Medication for symptomatic control:
  - Anticholinergics for bladder control
  - Laxatives for constipation
  - Amantadine for fatigue
  - Analgesics for pain
  - Antidepressants as necessary

Massage?

RISKS Massage that is too deep or two fast can sometimes stimulate painful and uncontrolled muscle spasms, even for clients with MS who are in remission. Sudden changes in environment, including pressure, temperature (especially heat) and other variables, appear to be difficult for many MS patients to process.

BENEFITS Massage may help MS patients to sleep better, to manage stress and depression, and thereby to reduce the frequency of flares.

OPTIONS Some MS patients experience weakness or spasm in the extremities. Massage can be used to slow or minimize this, as long as sensation is present.

Psoriasis

Definition: What Is It?

Psoriasis is a chronic skin disease in which cells, which normally replicate every 28 to 32 days, are replaced every 3 to 4 days. Instead of sloughing off, they accumulate into itchy, scaly plaques on the skin, usually on the trunk, elbows, and knees. It could be classified as an autoimmune disease, and in that pattern, it runs in cycles of flare and remission, and it is treated with immune-suppressant drugs.

Etiology: What Happens?

Normal skin cells are produced at the stratum basale, and then move toward the surface as new ranks are formed underneath. The process from birth to exfoliation typically takes 28 to 30 days. (It is interesting that this pattern is found in other cyclical processes in the body!) When a person has psoriasis, however, changes in function cause skin cells to replicate faster and they don't slough off as readily.

Recent research on psoriasis and other inflammatory skin diseases has yielded a lot of fascinating new

Psoriasis in Brief

Pronunciation: so-RY-uh-sis

What is it?
Psoriasis is a noncontagious chronic skin condition involving the excessive production of skin cells that pile up into lesions.

How is it recognized?
Plaque psoriasis (the most common variety) looks like red circular lesions, often with a silvery scale on top. Other forms look like shiny patches in skin folds or noninfectious pustules.

Massage risks and benefits
Risks: Psoriasis can be itchy, and massage may exacerbate that symptom.
Benefits: As long as skin is intact so the risk of secondary infection is low, clients with psoriasis can receive any kind of bodywork that doesn't make itching worse, and the dry skin and flaking that accompanies this condition may improve. Using a hypoallergenic lubricant may be important for this population.

information. It is now clear that this is a multifactorial condition that involves a genetic anomaly with immune system dysfunction and susceptibility to certain triggers.

The immune system dysfunction seen with psoriasis focuses on the presence of certain types of T cells that can stimulate inflammation and new capillary growth in the epidermis. This revelation has opened the door to new treatment options that interfere with these T-cell activities.

The genetic patterns seen with this condition have to do with a tendency to produce abnormally high levels of certain proinflammatory chemicals. Interestingly, this anomaly is also associated with insulin resistance, and the overlap between psoriasis and metabolic syndrome (a collection of issues that increases the risk for heart disease and diabetes) is high enough that people diagnosed with psoriasis are often counseled to test for heart disease and diabetes as well.

Triggers for psoriasis flares are fairly predictable. Emotional stress ranks high on this list, and because the disease and its treatment are both extremely challenging, this can become a self-fulfilling prophecy. Other triggers include viral and bacterial infections, reactions to medications, weather (especially dry cold winter air), and skin injuries. A psoriasis flare that develops 10 to 14 days after a minor skin wound is so predictable that this has a name: **Koebner phenomenon**. Smoking and hormonal fluctuations are also risk factors for psoriasis flares.

Signs and Symptoms

Signs and symptoms of psoriasis vary with the type. They often run in cycles of flare and remission. The lesions tend to have well-defined edges, and if they have been present for a prolonged time, they may be covered with a silvery flaky scale. Small lesions close together may converge into larger ones.

Most psoriasis lesions develop on the trunk, scalp, elbows, or knees, but they can be found on the palms, soles, and under nails, where lesions can destroy the whole nail: this is called onycholysis. More rarely, it can develop in skin folds, inside the mouth, or on the genitals.

Types of Psoriasis

- *Plaque psoriasis.* This is by far the most common presentation, affecting about 80% of all psoriasis patients. It involves small to large lesions (Figures 6.15 and 6.16) in a symmetrical distribution that itch and flake. Plaque psoriasis sometimes progresses to a more severe form.
- *Guttate psoriasis.* This is often triggered by a viral or bacterial infection. It involves multiple round shallow lesions that are small and regular ("guttate" comes from the Latin for "drop," as in raindrop) (Figure 6.17).
- *Pustular psoriasis.* This involves small pus-filled noninfectious blisters. These can appear anywhere, but palms and soles are especially vulnerable. It can be quite serious because the risk of secondary infection is high.

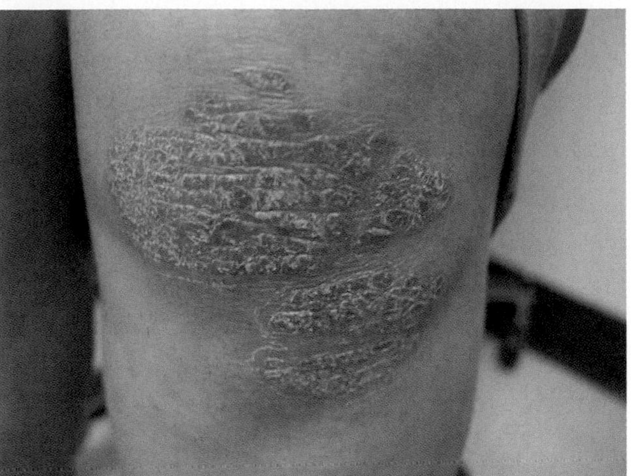

Figure 6.15. Plaque psoriasis, mild

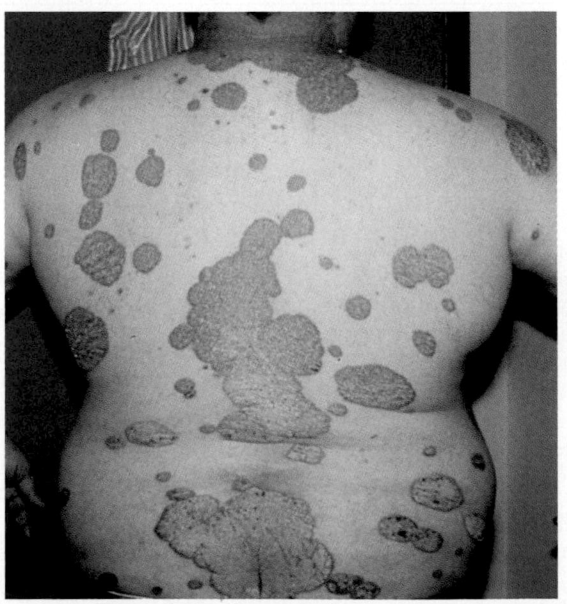

Figure 6.16. Plaque psoriasis, severe

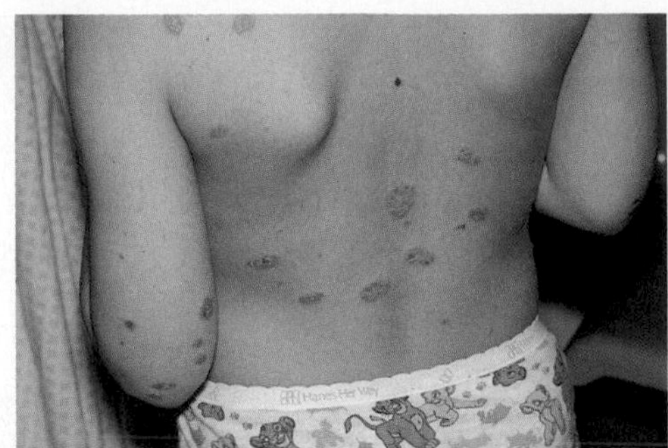
Figure 6.17. Guttate psoriasis

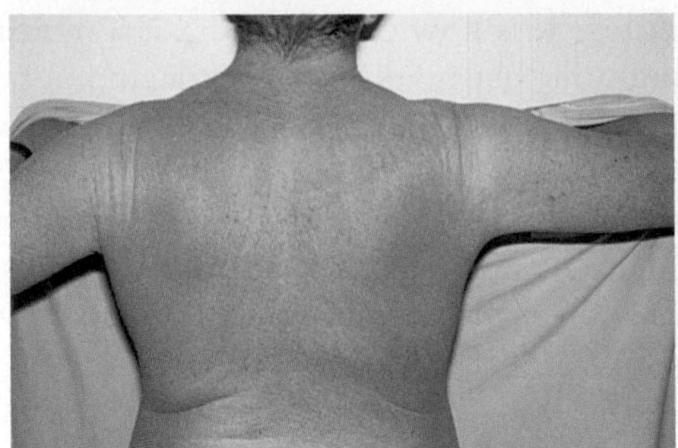
Figure 6.18. Erythrodermic psoriasis

- *Inverse psoriasis.* This condition appears at skin folds. The skin is red and shiny, and vulnerable to secondary yeast or fungal infection.
- *Erythrodermic psoriasis.* This serious condition is often triggered by sun exposure or topical steroidal anti-inflammatory use or cessation. It can involve extensive damage, infection, and fluid loss, and may become a medical emergency (Figure 6.18).

Psoriasis is rarely life threatening, but because it can be at least temporarily uncomfortable and disfiguring, it can certainly interfere with quality of life. Additionally, 10% to 30% of patients develop joint pain in an associated condition called psoriatic arthritis. This situation is complex and has several subtypes, but in many ways it resembles rheumatoid arthritis, and can be addressed by bodywork practitioners in the same way.

Treatment

Psoriasis has no permanent cure, and treatment options tend to be only temporarily successful or carry potentially dangerous side effects. Consequently, a person with a moderate to severe case may need to alternate his or her treatments on a regular cycle. To complicate things further, some treatment options react negatively with others, so this is a situation that requires careful oversight.

NOTABLE CASES Five-time pro-bowl football player Mark Gastineau, musicians Art Garfunkel and Tom Waits, and "the Beaver" Jerry Mathers are all psoriasis patients.

Psoriasis treatment typically begins with topical applications, then careful doses of UV radiation. If these are unsuccessful, then biologic therapies that impact immune system function might be applied. A limited amount of research into psoriasis and herbal remedies has been conducted. Topical applications of capsaicin and aloe vera have tested well. Oral doses of Dong Quay and milk thistle also showed some good responses, but these carry a risk of negative interactions with other medications.

Medications

- Topical applications of soothing lotion or medicated creams, including steroidal anti-inflammatories, retinoins, or coal tar extract
- Vitamin D analog cream (calcipotriene): note, this is not Vitamin D, and rubbing Vitamin D on lesions is ineffective
- Injections of steroidal anti-inflammatories directly into plaques to help dissolve them
- PUVA: psoralen (a systemic drug that heightens photosensitivity) along with UV radiation.
- Biologics to alter immune system activity

Massage?

RISKS Massage may make itchy lesions itchier. Of course any open lesion is a possible portal of entry for infectious agents. Otherwise, psoriasis carries no specific contraindications for massage.

BENEFITS Massage can be a welcome experience for someone who has trouble with their skin. Stress is seen to be a significant trigger, and massage may help to modulate that. Because this condition isn't contagious and doesn't spread through touching, massage anywhere the skin is intact and not irritated is safe and appropriate.

OPTIONS Choose a hypoallergenic lubricant for clients with psoriasis.

Rheumatoid Arthritis

Definition: What Is It?

Rheumatoid arthritis is an autoimmune condition in which the synovial membranes of various joints are

Rheumatoid Arthritis in Brief

Pronunciation: RUE-mah-toyd arth-RY-tis

What is it?
Rheumatoid arthritis is an autoimmune disease in which immune system agents attack synovial membranes, particularly of the joints in the hands and feet. Other structures, such as muscles, tendons, skin, blood vessels, and serous membranes may also be affected.

How is it recognized?
In the acute phase, affected joints are stiff, swollen, hot, and painful. They often become gnarled and distorted. RA tends to affect the body symmetrically, and it is not age related.

Massage risks and benefits
Risks: If a client with RA is in the midst of flare, not only will his or her joints be inflamed and painful but inflammation may be system wide. This is a situation that indicates only the gentlest and least intrusive types of bodywork, although many people report a decrease in pain with gentle heat and manipulation during this phase. RA medications may increase the risk of infection or other problems that can inform decisions about bodywork.
Benefits: Clients with RA who are in remission can receive more rigorous massage, of course always within tolerance. Passive range of motion at the affected joints may be useful to help maintain freedom of movement. Some clients may use massage to help manage stress, and thereby reduce the frequency or severity of their flares.

attacked by immune system cells. Unlike other forms of arthritis, rheumatoid arthritis can also involve inflammation of tissues outside the musculoskeletal system.

This disease affects about 3.1 million people, or about 1% of all Americans. Like many autoimmune diseases, women are affected more often than men; in this situation, the ratio is about 3:1.

Etiology: What Happens?

Rheumatoid arthritis is an autoimmune disease in which the immune system attacks the synovial membranes of certain joints, but other areas (blood vessels, serous membranes, the skin, eyes, lungs, liver, and heart) may also be affected.

When a synovial membrane is under attack, all the signs of inflammation develop: heat, pain, redness, swelling, and loss of function. Studies of joint tissues show that B cells, T cells, antibodies, and many proinflammatory chemicals are present during a flare. In response, the synovial membrane thickens and swells. Fluid accumulates inside the joint capsule, which causes pressure and pain. The inflamed tissues release enzymes that erode cartilage and bone; tendons and ligaments may also be affected. This causes the telltale deformation of the joint capsules and gnarled appearance of rheumatoid arthritis (Figure 6.19).

Synovial membranes are just one of the types of tissue that may be attacked. Other possibilities include:

- Rheumatic nodules on the sclera (whites) of the eyes
- Sjögren syndrome (pathologically dry eyes and mouth)
- Pleuritis, which makes breathing painful and increases vulnerability to lung infection
- Carditis or pericarditis, that is, inflammation of the heart or pericardial sac
- Hepatitis or inflammation of the liver
- Vasculitis or inflammation of blood vessels. This complication carries another set of risks: Raynaud syndrome, skin ulcers, bleeding intestinal ulcers, and internal hemorrhaging.
- Bursitis and anemia, especially when onset of the disease occurs in childhood

Advanced structural damage brings a different set of complications. Deformed and bone-damaged joints

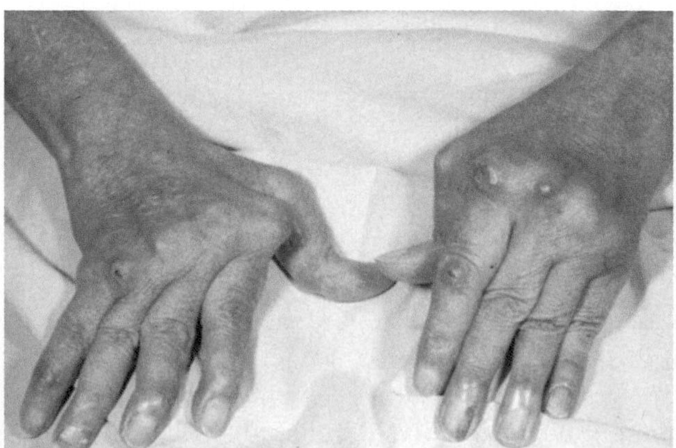

Figure 6.19. Rheumatoid arthritis

may dislocate or collapse, rendering them useless. The tendons that cross over distorted joints sometimes become so stretched that they snap. If the disease is at the C1-C2 joint and the joint collapses, the resultant injury to the spinal column may result in problems with sphincter control or paralysis.

Types of Rheumatoid Arthritis

- *Juvenile Rheumatoid Arthritis (JRA)*. JRA is a group of chronic arthritic conditions that affect children. Three main subtypes have been identified: pauciarticular JRA affects fewer than five joints; polyarticular JRA affects five or more joints; and systemic JRA sometimes called "Still's disease" can affect the whole body with arthritis, fevers, rashes, and secondary organ involvement. The treatment goals for JRA are to help the patient live as normal a life as possible using diet, exercise, and pain management strategies along with drugs.

Signs and Symptoms

Symptoms of rheumatoid arthritis vary considerably at the onset of the disease. Most patients have a period of weeks or months with a general feeling of illness: lack of energy, lack of appetite, low-grade fever, and vague muscle pain, which gradually becomes sharp, specific joint pain. A few patients have a sudden onset with joint pain alone. **Rheumatic nodules**, small, painless bumps that appear around fingers, elbows, and other pressure-bearing areas, are also common indicators of the disease.

In the acute stage, the affected joints are red, hot, painful, and stiff, although they improve considerably with heat and moderate amounts of movement and stretching. The joints rheumatoid arthritis most often attacks are the knuckles in hands and toes. It frequently develops in ankles and wrists; knees are less common. One of the most serious places to get it is in the neck, where it can lead to dangerous instability. It generally affects the body bilaterally, although it is sometimes worse on one side than the other.

NOTABLE CASES French impressionist painter Renoir struggled with rheumatoid arthritis, and used to paint from a wheelchair with a brush jammed into his twisted fingers. Actress Kathleen Turner is an outspoken advocate for rheumatoid arthritis research and treatment.

Like many autoimmune diseases, rheumatoid arthritis appears in cycles of flare followed by periods of remission. Some patients have only a few flares in their life and are never affected again. Moderate cases involve cycles of flare and remission up to several times a year. Severe rheumatoid arthritis involves chronic inflammation that never fully subsides.

Treatment

It is a high priority to correctly diagnose RA as quickly as possible, because it has been found that delaying treatment, even for just a few months, radically increases the risk of permanent joint damage. The goals of treatment are to reduce pain, to limit inflammation, to halt joint damage, and to improve function. Medications that help to achieve these goals include DMARDs (disease-modifying antirheumatic drugs), biologic agents, steroids, NSAIDs, and analgesics. Most of these have serious potential side effects and some are extremely expensive, so working out a drug strategy is an important part of RA treatment.

Nonmedical intervention for rheumatoid arthritis can include adjustments to diet, exercise, and stress reduction techniques, including massage. Splints, orthotics, canes, or other devices that make it easier to get through the day may become necessary.

Surgery can be a successful option for rheumatoid arthritis patients, if the disease has affected joints that can be easily treated. Joint fusion or replacement is sometimes an option, along with surgery to rebuild damaged or ruptured tendons and to remove portions of affected synovial membranes.

Medications

- NSAIDs, including Cox-2 inhibitors
- Analgesics
- Steroidal anti-inflammatories
- DMARDs, including gold salts, antimalarial medications, methotrexate, and others
- Biologic agents, including Tumor Necrosis Factor-alpha inhibitors, IL-1 inhibitors, and others

Massage?

RISKS In its acute (flare) phase, rheumatoid arthritis is an inflammatory condition that affects not just joints but possibly the entire body. Rigorous circulatory massage during this phase is not appropriate, but gentle, soothing, reflexive work may help ease this experience. Many patients appreciate heat and gentle manipulation of painful joints. Be aware that the medications a client with RA takes may also have an impact on decisions about bodywork.

BENEFITS Massage can be effective for pain, stress, and muscle tension. All these benefits can be specifically applied for RA patients, especially between episodes of flare.

OPTIONS Painless passive range of motion exercises can be helpful for RA patients who are trying to maintain flexibility at their affected joints. Special attention to the muscles and tendons that cross the painful joints may also be extremely effective.

Scleroderma in Brief

What is it?
Scleroderma is an autoimmune disorder involving damage to small blood vessels. It leads to abnormal accumulations of collagen in the skin, blood vessels, and other tissues.

How is it recognized?
Scleroderma has varied symptoms, depending on which tissues are involved. The most common outward signs are edema followed by hardening and thickening of the skin, usually of the hands and face. Lesions may be oval or linear. Other symptoms are determined by what other organs are affected.

Massage risks and benefits
Risks: Scleroderma can involve damage to the skin, kidneys, and other tissues. Any bodywork must be gauged to stay within whatever limitations these complications create.
Benefits: Massage as a strategy to manage stress and painful symptoms may be useful, as long as client's limitations are respected.

Scleroderma

Definition: What Is It?

Scleroderma is an autoimmune disease in which inflammation stimulates fibroblasts in small blood vessels to produce abnormal amounts of collagen. This frequently occurs in the skin, hence the name: sclero (Greek for hard)–derma (Greek for skin), but other tissues and organs may also be affected.

Scleroderma is relatively rare, affecting about 300,000 people in the United States. As with other autoimmune diseases, women are affected more often than men, at a ratio of about 3 or 4 to 1.

Etiology: What Happens?

Scleroderma is the result of an immune system attack against the lining of small blood vessels: the arterioles, capillaries, and venules. Damage to these tiny vessels causes local edema and stimulates nearby fibroblasts to spin out huge amounts of type I and III collagen, the basis for scar tissue. Eventually the edema subsides, but the scar tissue deposits remain hard and unyielding for years at a time.

The cause of scleroderma is unknown, but several contributing factors have been identified. Abnormal immune responses and chronic inflammation stimulate the fibroblasts to produce excessive collagen. Some patients have accumulated chimeric cells that contain genes not only of the affected person but of someone else as well; probably they are leftover fetal material from pregnancies that may date from many years previously. These cells, which are "non-self" may stimulate an immune system response.

Other factors associated with scleroderma include exposure to chemicals, including silica, vinyl chloride, epoxy resins, uranium, and aromatic hydrocarbons. Organic solvents and viral infections (especially with cytomegalovirus or human herpesvirus 5) may also be environmental triggers.

Complications of the most serious forms of scleroderma are serious and potentially life threatening. Blood clots, pulmonary fibrosis, renal failure, and heart failure are all possible for people with systemic diffuse scleroderma.

Types of Scleroderma

- *Local scleroderma.* In this form of scleroderma, the areas of damage are limited to the skin. The initial edema may last for several weeks or months, the thickening of the skin may accumulate over a course of about 3 years, and then the symptoms gradually stabilize or even reverse. Local scleroderma is often discussed in two forms:

- *Morphea scleroderma*. **Morphea** scleroderma takes the shape of discrete oval patches that develop on the trunk, face, or extremities. The lesions first appear as areas where the skin seems dry and thick. Eventually they become pale in the center and purplish around the edges.
- *Linear scleroderma*. This appears as a discolored line or band on a leg or arm or over the fore head. In this location, it may be called "coup de sabre," because it resembles a sword-fight scar (Figure 6.20).

- *Systemic scleroderma*. This has a slow onset that begins as CREST syndrome (described below), but may eventually infiltrate internal organs. Tissues most at risk are in the digestive tract, the heart and circulatory system, the kidneys, lungs, and various parts of the musculoskeletal system, especially synovial membranes in joints and around tendons. This disease may stabilize and even reverse itself, but it can also be fatal. Systemic scleroderma is also called "systemic sclerosis." It occurs in three major subtypes.
  - *Limited systemic scleroderma*. This version begins with CREST syndrome, and it is only slowly progressive.
  - *Diffuse scleroderma*. This has a more sudden onset and earlier involvement of internal organs.
  - *Sine scleroderma*. This doesn't involve the skin at all; it only involves internal organs. (**Sine** means without.)

Signs and Symptoms

Scleroderma can produce a huge variety of symptoms, depending on which blood vessels are under attack. The term **CREST** syndrome has been coined as a mnemonic for the most common scleroderma symptoms:

- C. **Calcinosis** refers to accumulation of calcium deposits in the skin, especially in the fingers.
- R. Raynaud phenomenon is a result of impaired circulation and vascular spasm in the hands.
- E. Esophageal dysmotility refers to sluggishness of the digestive tract and chronic gastric reflux.
- S. **Sclerodactyly** is hardening of the fingers, a result of the accumulation of scar tissue in the hands (Figure 6.21).
- T. Telangiectasia is a discoloration of the skin caused by permanently stretched and damaged capillaries. It is also known as "spider veins."

Other symptoms of scleroderma include tight, hardened skin, usually on the hands or face; skin ulcers in which circulation prevents normal nutrition for healthy cells; changes in pigmentation; and hair loss in the affected patches. Muscles may become weak, while tendons and tendinous sheaths become painful and swollen. Trigeminal neuralgia and carpal tunnel syndrome may develop as a result of nerve entrapment. **Sjögren syndrome** (pathologically dry mucous

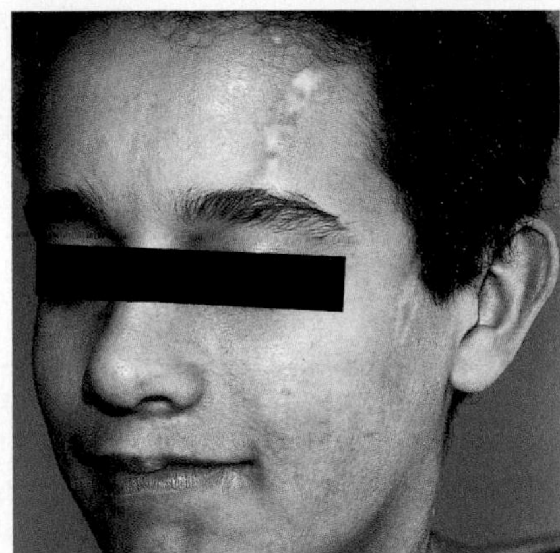

Figure 6.20. Scleroderma: coup de sabre lesion

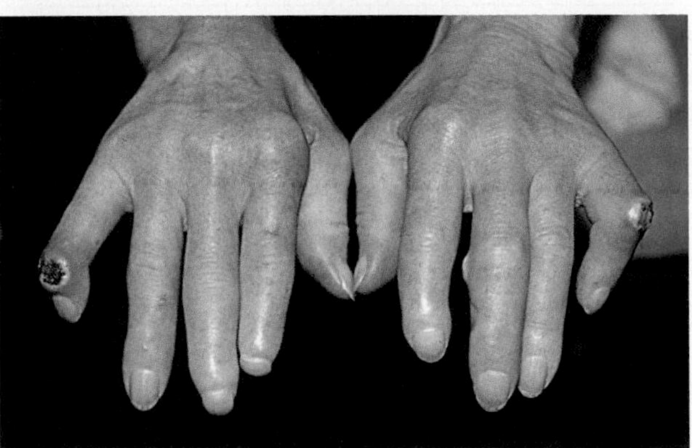

Figure 6.21. Scleroderma: hard, tight skin with ulcerations

membranes) may also be a part of the picture. Lungs may accumulate edema or fibrosis where blood vessels are under attack, opening the door to pneumonia. Heart pain, arrhythmia, and heart failure may develop as the heart tries to push blood through a system that cannot accommodate it. And kidneys, working under high blood pressure and with damaged arterioles, may fail.

Treatment

Treatment for scleroderma is directed at managing the symptoms and complications of the disease. In addition, immune system modifiers are finding increasing use to help control this autoimmune condition. Physical or occupational therapies are employed to maintain flexibility in the hands. Patients are usually advised to avoid smoking, cold conditions, and spicy foods to minimize symptoms.

Medications

- Immune system modifiers to suppress immune system overactivity
- Steroidal anti-inflammatories (with the caution that these may stress the kidneys)
- Calcium channel blockers for Raynaud phenomenon
- ACE inhibitors for kidney function
- Diuretics for kidney function
- Antacids and proton pump inhibitors for gastric reflux
- NSAIDs for muscle and joint pain

Massage?

RISKS Because scleroderma can involve permanent damage to blood vessels as well as skin lesions, lung, and kidney problems, any kind of massage must be done with extreme caution. Decisions must be based on the resilience of the client; this can be a moving target that changes from one day to the next. Be aware that some medications used to control scleroderma may have side effects that impact decisions about bodywork.

BENEFITS Any bodywork that can be done to restore parasympathetic balance without overchallenging a damaged circulatory system could prove beneficial for scleroderma patients.

Ulcerative Colitis

Definition: What Is It?

Ulcerative colitis is a disease involving inflammation and shallow ulcers in the colon (Figure 6.22). Ulcerative colitis and Crohn disease are sometimes referred to collectively as inflammatory bowel disease. The inflammation with ulcerative colitis is limited to the large intestine, however, which distinguishes it from Crohn disease. For more information on the connections between Crohn disease and ulcerative colitis, see Compare & Contrast 6.1.

Etiology: What Happens?

The initial cause of ulcerative colitis is a subject of some debate, although most specialists agree that it is an autoimmune disease, possibly triggered by an abnormal response to colon-dwelling bacteria. It almost always begins in the rectum when immune system cells attack the most superficial layer of the

Ulcerative Colitis in Brief

Pronunciation: UL-ser-ah-tiv ko-LI-tis

What is it?
Ulcerative colitis is a condition in which the mucosal layer of the colon becomes inflamed and develops shallow, contiguous ulcers.

How is it recognized?
Symptoms of acute ulcerative colitis include abdominal cramping pain, chronic diarrhea, blood and pus in stools, weight loss, and mild fever.

Massage risks and benefits
Risks: Acute ulcerative colitis contraindicates any massage that might exacerbate symptoms. A client in the flare stage of this disease is already under great challenge, so any bodywork must be adjusted to accommodate for the client's discomfort or other limitations. During remission, abdominal work may be safe, but only done with the most extreme care.
Benefits: During remission, a client with ulcerative colitis can receive any massage that is comfortable. Clients who have had surgery for ulcerative colitis and fully recovered can enjoy the same benefits from bodywork as the rest of the population, with respect for whatever adjustments are required by their colostomy bag.

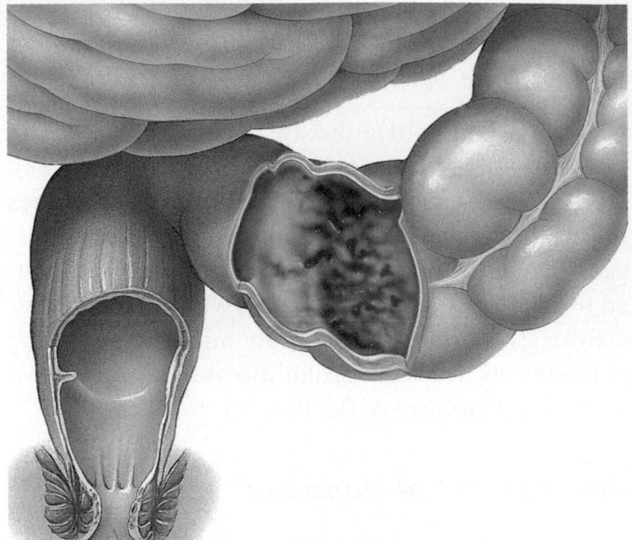

Figure 6.22. Ulcerative colitis

colon. The resulting inflammation kills tissue and results in the formation of shallow ulcers: open sores that may never fully heal. Colon function is extremely limited, and the patient has chronic bloody diarrhea. The sores may become infected, leading to the release of blood and pus in the stools.

Ulcerative colitis is classified by what part or parts of the colon are affected. Disease that is limited to the rectum is called ulcerative **proctitis**, left-sided colitis involves the descending colon, and **pancolitis** describes inflammation of the entire colon. The most extreme and dangerous form of ulcerative colitis is **fulminant** colitis. In this condition, the whole colon is acutely inflamed and ulcerated, and the risk of life-threatening complications from a condition called **toxic megacolon** is high.

About half of all ulcerative colitis patients have it in a mild form that doesn't become threatening. Patients with ulcerative colitis that involves the whole colon are at significantly more risk for developing colorectal cancer than the general population. This risk goes up significantly 8 to 10 years after diagnosis of ulcerative colitis.

Signs and Symptoms

Symptoms of ulcerative colitis depend largely on how much of the bowel is affected: the greater the extent of inflammation, the worse the symptoms tend to be. Symptoms run in cycles of flare and remission. During flares, the primary symptom is painful chronic diarrhea with blood and pus in the stools. Abdominal cramping, loss of appetite, and mild fever may also occur during acute episodes.

The inflammatory nature of this disease often affects other systems in the body. A person with ulcerative colitis may also have inflammation of the liver or gallbladder ducts, arthritis, osteoporosis, anemia from blood loss, and kidney stones from the disruption in electrolyte balance and chronic dehydration that accompanies long-term diarrhea. **Uveitis**, or inflammation of structures in the eye, may result in permanent vision loss if it is not treated. Some skin disruptions are also associated with ulcerative colitis; these may occur in connection with flares or may outlive a flare to be a chronic infection.

Between acute episodes, the ulcerative colitis patient may have only minimal abdominal pain but must be careful to avoid any triggers of abdominal cramping or discomfort.

Treatment

Treatment options for ulcerative colitis begin with aminosalicylates: a class of medications that lessen the severity of flare-ups and prolong periods of remission. If these don't control the inflammation satisfactorily, corticosteroids may be prescribed for short periods. Immunosuppressive drugs and, surprisingly, nicotine patches have also been found to improve symptoms.

If these options are not satisfactory, or if inflammation of the colon has progressed to a dangerous degree, surgery is the only permanent solution. Several surgical options have been developed, but all of them involve the removal of the bowel. External **colostomy** bags, internal colostomy bags, and the joining of the small intestine to the muscles of the rectum are options for replacing the main functions of the colon.

Medications

- Oral, suppository, or by enema application of aminosalicylates to control inflammation and immune system response
- Oral or injected corticosteroids to suppress inflammation
- Immune-modifying drugs to alter immune system response

Massage?

RISKS Ulcerative colitis in a flared stage contraindicates local intrusive massage. Even during remission, it's important to remember that the colon sustains permanent damage; consequently, deep abdominal work must be done with extreme caution. Clients who use colostomy bags may require some special positioning adjustments in order to receive massage comfortably.

BENEFITS When a client with ulcerative colitis that is in remission can receive any massage that is well tolerated, although of course abdominal work must be done with care. A client who has fully recovered from ulcerative colitis surgery can enjoy all the benefits from massage as the rest of the population, with adjustments for a colostomy bag.

OPTIONS Clients with ulcerative colitis or other conditions that cause digestive discomfort can especially benefit from reflexive work or gentle holding that focuses on the abdomen in order to help incorporate this problematic part of the body into the whole.

CHAPTER REVIEW QUESTIONS: LYMPH AND IMMUNE SYSTEM CONDITIONS

1. Briefly describe where interstitial fluid comes from.
2. Identify an important feature that distinguishes lymphatic capillaries from circulatory capillaries.
3. What is pitting edema?
4. Why are massage therapists particularly at risk for lymphangitis?
5. What is the causative agent for most cases of mononucleosis?
6. Name four fluids that carry HIV in high enough concentrations to be communicable.
7. What is the difference between anaphylaxis and angioedema?
8. Your client has been diagnosed with systemic lupus. Her symptoms are acute, and she's using steroidal anti-inflammatories to help control her disease. She would like to receive massage for pain and anxiety. What are some cautions were concerns about bodywork in this situation?
9. What do MS, scleroderma, and myasthenia gravis all have in common?
10. Your 62-year-old client has extreme low back pain due to his advanced ankylosing spondylitis. Is it appropriate to plan a session with deep massage and extensive stretching in flexion, extension, and side flexion? Why or why not?

7

Respiratory System Conditions

Chapter Objectives

After reading this chapter, you should be able to . . .

- Name what percentage of calories a healthy person invests in the act of respiration while at rest.
- Identify the oxygen saturation of an average inhaled breath compared with the oxygen saturation of an exhaled breath.
- Identify triggers of acute bronchitis.
- Explain why no single vaccine can currently protect against colds or flu.
- Identify a synonym for the common cold.
- Name three causative agents for pneumonia.
- Identify which form of sinusitis is most appropriate for massage.
- Describe the difference between tuberculosis exposure and active disease.
- Name the group of conditions to which chronic bronchitis and emphysema belong.
- Explain why persons with asthma, chronic bronchitis, or emphysema are often encouraged to be vaccinated against flu.
- Name what kinds of glands are affected by cystic fibrosis.

Introduction

Respiratory System Structure

The easiest way to discuss the structure of the respiratory system is to follow a particle of air through it (Figure 7.1). Take a deep breath. Air drawn in through the nose encounters mucous membranes. Various types of mucous membranevs line any cavity in the body that communicates with the outside world, specifically the respiratory, digestive, reproductive, and urinary systems. In the respiratory system, the mucous membranes start inside the nose and mouth, and they line the sinuses and throat all the way down into the small tubes in the lungs. The wet, sticky mucous membranes in the respiratory system are responsible for warming, moistening, and filtering the air that passes by.

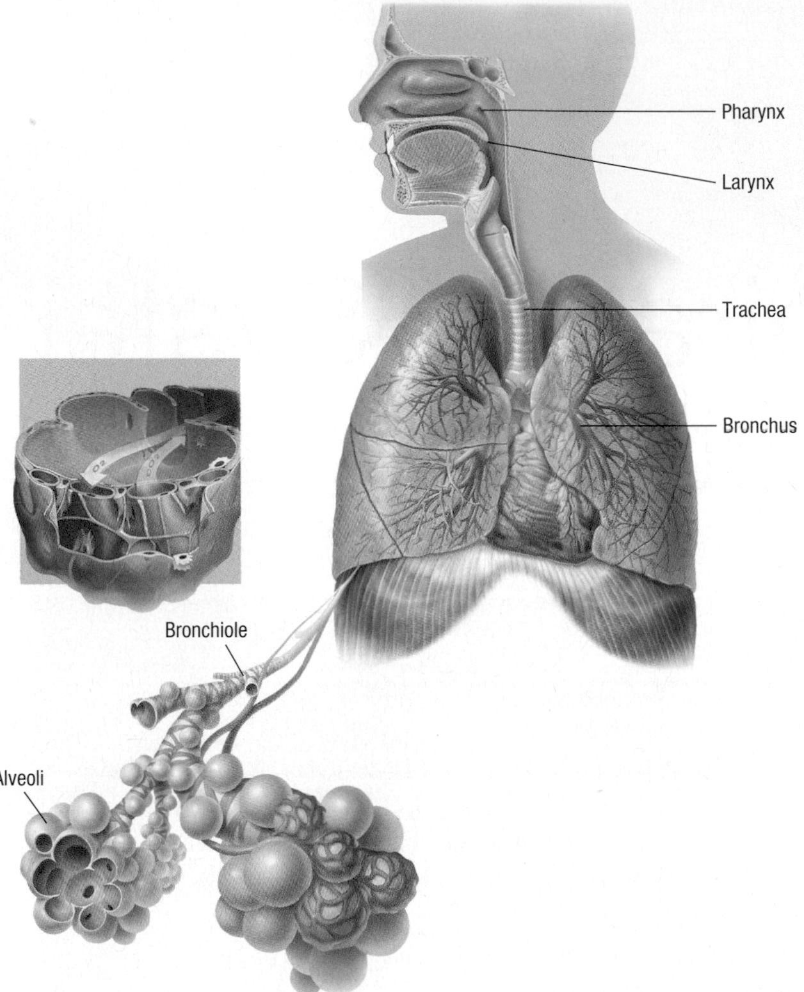

Figure 7.1. Respiratory system

Once past the nose and mouth, air enters first the pharynx, then the larynx, the trachea, and the bronchi. The bronchi are asymmetrical. The right bronchus is bigger, wider, and straighter, leading into the three lobes of the right lung. The left bronchus is smaller in diameter, and it curves off to the side to reach the two lobes of the left lung. This is significant if a foreign object is inhaled into the lungs; it almost always follows the path of least resistance to the right side.

The bronchi divide into the bronchioles, which then separate out 23 times until they terminate in microscopic alveoli. These grape-shaped clusters of epithelial bubbles are like tiny balloons surrounded by blood capillaries. Gaseous exchange occurs through the permeable surfaces between the alveoli and the capillaries. If the alveoli are impaired or not functioning correctly, the body cannot make an efficient trade of carbon dioxide for oxygen.

The structure of the lungs themselves is well suited for fighting off infection. Each lung has two or three separate lobes (two on the left and three on the right), and each of these lobes has smaller separate

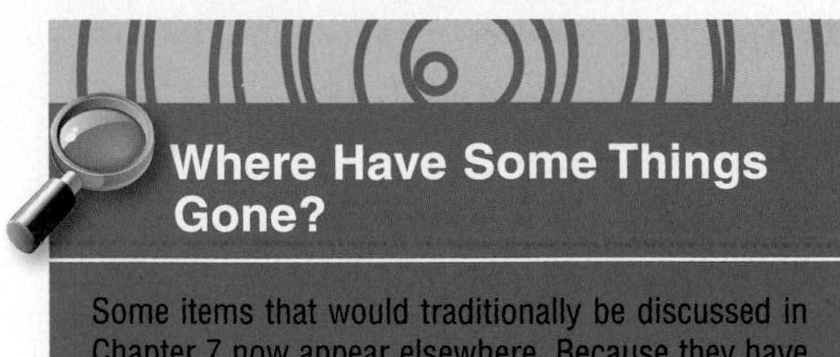

Where Have Some Things Gone?

Some items that would traditionally be discussed in Chapter 7 now appear elsewhere. Because they have a relatively narrow application, or massage therapists are unlikely to see them in an acute stage, they can now be found in Appendix C, **Extra Conditions at a Glance**. These include the following:

- Bronchiectasis
- Pleurisy

Respiratory System Conditions

Infectious Respiratory Disorders

- Acute bronchitis
- Common cold
- Influenza
  - Seasonal flu
  - H5N1 Avian flu
  - H1N1 Swine flu
- Pneumonia
  - Bronchopneumonia
  - Lobar pneumonia
  - Community-acquired pneumonia
  - Nosocomial (hospital-acquired) pneumonia
  - Aspiration pneumonia
- Sinusitis
  - Noninfectious sinusitis (Hayfever)
  - Infectious sinusitis
- Tuberculosis
  - Drug-susceptible TB
  - Multi-drug resistant TB
  - Extensively drug resistant TB

Chronic Obstructive Pulmonary Diseases

- Chronic bronchitis
- Emphysema

Other Respiratory Disorders

- Asthma
  - Bronchial asthma
  - Exercise-induced asthma
  - Silent asthma
  - Cough variant asthma
- Cystic fibrosis
- Laryngeal cancer
- Lung cancer
  - Small cell lung cancer
  - Non-small cell lung cancer
  - Other types of lung cancer

segments called lobules. This isolation of areas makes it difficult for pathogens to infect the whole structure. All of the tubes are lined with mucous membrane, which traps pathogens and other particles. Then the cilia in the tract help move the **mucus blanket** toward the mouth and nose for expulsion. Smooth muscle tissue lines all of the tubes down to the smallest bronchi; when an irritant is trapped in these tubes, a healthy cough reflex quickly moves it out of the body.

Respiratory System Function

Air cycles through the lungs 12 to 20 times per minute. The lungs themselves do not have any muscle tissue to make them fill up or empty; they are simply limp-walled sacs that inflate or deflate according to the air pressure inside and outside of them. A change in air pressure is brought about by a change in the shape of the thoracic cavity. If the cavity is made larger, the air pressure inside the lungs is low until air rushes in to equalize it. In other words, the act of inhaling is simply filling a vacuum. When the pressure inside and outside the lungs has been equalized, air eases out again: exhalation. Exhalation is mostly a passive process; elastic connective tissue fibers in the lungs pull them back to their original size, so relaxed exhalation doesn't involve muscular activity unless a person specifically tries to remove air from the lungs.

The efficiency of this mechanism is astonishing. Even though oxygen-carbon dioxide exchange is only partial with each breath (a typical inhalation contains roughly 21% oxygen, while a typical exhalation still contains about 16% oxygen), the respiratory system supplies the entire body with enough oxygen to function with minimal effort. In fact, a healthy person invests only 5% of resting calories in the act of breathing.

The conditions examined in this chapter mostly have to do with the vulnerability of the respiratory system to infection. Fortunately, thanks to the sticky mucous membranes and lungs with isolated segments; those infections seldom get a strong enough grip to do lasting damage.

Infectious Respiratory Disorders

Acute Bronchitis

Definition: What Is It?

Acute bronchitis is a self-limiting inflammation of the respiratory tract, specifically of the bronchial tree. It

Acute Bronchitis in Brief

Pronunciation: ah-KYUTE brong-KY-tis

What is it?
Acute bronchitis is inflammation of the bronchial tree anywhere between the trachea and the bronchioles. If inflammation extends into the bronchioles and alveoli, it is called bronchopneumonia.

How is it recognized?
The hallmark of acute bronchitis is a persistent, productive cough along with sore throat, nasal congestion, fatigue, and fever. Although other symptoms generally subside within 10 days, the cough may last for several weeks while the bronchi heal.

Massage risks and benefits

Risks: When a bronchial infection is acute, rigorous massage is not the best choice: not only because of the risk of communicability from the client to the practitioner but also because the person with an infection is metabolically dedicated to solving this problem—the extra challenge of a massage that demands an adaptive response is an unnecessary addition. Even when a person is in recovery, being flat on a table may be irritating, so accommodations may need to be made in positioning.

Benefits: During acute bronchitis, gentle, supportive bodywork may be helpful for improving sleep. When a person is in recovery, massage may be useful in dealing with tension in the breathing muscles and improving general energy levels.

is usually a complication of the common cold or flu. Acute bronchitis typically resolves within 10 days to several weeks of onset. This helps to distinguish it from chronic bronchitis, which is an irreversible condition with a very different etiology.

Etiology: What Happens?

When the bronchi are irritated or infected by any kind of pathogen, an inflammatory response ensues. The tubes swell, the cilia are damaged, excessive mucus is produced, and the result is coughing and wheezing as air moves through passageways that are obstructed with swelling and excessive mucus. Most cases of acute bronchitis are complications of a cold or flu in which the viruses simply move from the upper respiratory system to the bronchial tubes. Other causative agents include a variety of bacteria, fungi, and noninfectious irritants, such as fumes, air pollutants, and other contaminants. Chronic reflux from the esophagus can also irritate the bronchi.

An important feature of acute bronchitis is that it is self-limiting and results in no permanent changes to the bronchi, cilia, or mucous membranes. This distinguishes acute bronchitis from chronic bronchitis (Compare & Contrast 7.1).

Signs and Symptoms

The primary sign of acute bronchitis is a persistent cough. It often starts dry, but within a few days becomes productive. Sputum may be clear or opaque. Wheezing, nasal congestion, headache, low fever, muscle aches, chest pain, and fatigue may also be present. Most of the symptoms of acute bronchitis subside within about 10 days of onset, but the cough may persist for several weeks while the delicate lining of the bronchial tubes heals.

If fever persists or exceeds 101°F (38.3°C), or if the sputum becomes greenish, yellow, or blood streaked, the possibility of pneumonia must be considered. This is a more serious condition that usually needs medical intervention.

Treatment

The best treatment options for most cases of acute bronchitis include rest, fluids, and warm, humid air to liquefy mucus and aid in its expulsion. Antibiotics are not effective in most cases of acute bronchitis, but they are appropriate when the causative agent has been identified as bacterial.

Bronchodilators and cough suppressants can help to ameliorate some of the symptoms of acute bronchitis, but they do not eradicate the infection or speed recovery.

Medications

- NSAIDs for general discomfort and fever reduction
- Cough suppressants (for dry cough—productive cough is often left untreated to help the body shed contaminated mucus)
- Bronchodilators
- Antibiotics if necessary

COMPARE & CONTRAST 7.1 Acute Bronchitis, Chronic Bronchitis, or Bronchiectasis: Which Is Which?

The lungs are particularly vulnerable to infection, stationed as they are at the receiving end of everything that enters the body through the nose. They have some structural features that make it easy to isolate sites of infection, and they are well stocked with immune system cells to fight off incoming invaders, but they are susceptible to a variety of disorders that can cause both short-term and long-term damage. Three lung problems have similarities and differences that make it useful to examine them side by side:

- *Acute bronchitis* often accompanies upper respiratory infections or flu. This is a viral attack directly on the bronchi, although it can also complicate into a bacterial infection.
- *Chronic bronchitis* involves long-term irritation to the bronchial lining, all the way down to the terminal bronchioles. This irritation can cause the lining to become permanently thick with excessive mucus production that can make it difficult to breathe. Chronic bronchitis raises the risk for lung infections, but it doesn't start with a pathogenic invasion.
- *Bronchiectasis* is a disorder brought about by repeated lung infections that cause structural changes to the bronchial tubes: they become permanently widened. When the bronchi become unable to move mucus out of the body, it pools in the lungs, creating a risk of further infection and more structural damage. Bronchiectasis is discussed further in Appendix C, Extra Conditions at a Glance.

If a lung disorder is present, it is useful for the massage therapist to have a clear idea of the situation so that the client may be made as comfortable as possible on the table and that the risk of spreading infection is minimized.

CHARACTERISTICS	ACUTE BRONCHITIS	CHRONIC BRONCHITIS	BRONCHIECTASIS
Cause	Viral attack on lungs; often accompanies cold or flu.	Long-term lung irritation, e.g., cigarette smoke, pollution, particles in air.	History of multiple lung infections, including acute bronchitis, pneumonia.
Symptoms	Productive cough with clear sputum (colored sputum: suspect secondary bacterial infection); fever, aches, pains.	Productive cough with clear sputum (colored sputum: suspect secondary bacterial infection). Excessive mucus production, frequent throat clearing. Susceptibility to lung infections. Wheezing, shortness of breath, cyanosis.	Frequent cough with green or yellow sputum, especially when lying down.
Prognosis	If basically healthy, full recovery with no long-term problems.	If irritation to lungs halts, may not progress but is not reversible. If it progresses, may develop into right-sided heart failure, respiratory failure, and emphysema.	Patient must avoid lung irritants and possibility of further lung infections, which may further damage bronchi.
Implications for massage	Should not receive rigorous massage until infection resolves.	May receive massage if positioned on table so as not to exacerbate symptoms. Essential to rule out possibility of circulatory weakness.	May receive massage if positioned on table so as not to exacerbate symptoms.

Massage?

RISKS Any massage that demands a significant adaptive response should be delayed until the acute phase of a bronchial infection has passed. At any point during acute bronchitis, accommodations may have to be made for a client who is uncomfortable lying supine on a table.

BENEFITS Gentle reflexive or energetic bodywork may be appropriate for someone with acute bronchitis, as long as precautions are taken to protect the therapist from infection. When the client is in recovery, massage may be helpful for improving energy levels.

OPTIONS Within client tolerance, focus on the breathing muscles may improve efficiency of breathing function.

Common Cold

Definition: What Is It?

The common cold is an infection of the respiratory tract brought about by any of hundreds of viruses.

Common Cold in Brief

What is it?
The common cold is a viral infection from any of hundreds of types of viruses.

How is it recognized?
The symptoms of colds are nasal discharge, sore throat, mild fever, dry coughing, and headache. Symptoms last anywhere from 2 days to 2 weeks.

Massage risks and benefits
Risks: Common cold is easily contagious, so a therapist working with a client who has a cold needs to take precautions against transmission. Someone who is recovering from a cold may benefit from massage with the caveat that anecdotal evidence suggests that massage may temporarily exacerbate symptoms.
Benefits: Gentle reflexive or energetic work could be helpful if a person is having trouble moving past the peak of a cold. Massage in the subacute stage may help speed recovery (although symptoms may be temporarily exacerbated). Any person who has fully recovered from a cold can enjoy the same benefits from massage as the rest of the population.

Over the course of a lifetime, people are exposed to multitudes of cold viruses. They get sick, establish immunity to that particular pathogen, and move on to the next infection. Much of this happens in childhood; by adulthood, people have encountered most of what they are likely to see, and the frequency of infections generally subsides. But no single infectious agent causes the so-called common cold. Consequently, no effective single vaccine against common cold may ever be developed.

Etiology: What Happens?

The common cold, also known as an upper respiratory tract infection (URTI), **coryza**, or viral rhinitis, is caused by any of hundreds of viruses. Rhinoviruses cause approximately half of colds; this group has about 110 subtypes and is most active in autumn and spring. Other pathogens include coronaviruses (these are the group that also cause severe acute respiratory syndrome, or SARS), adenoviruses, and respiratory syncytial virus. Most of these viral infections are low grade and not dangerous, but some can cause very severe infections, especially in infants and young children.

The viruses that cause the common cold enter the nose, where the temperature is about 91°F (32.8°C), a perfect growth environment. The cilia in the mucous membrane carry the viruses to the back of the throat, where they have access to their target cells in the lymphoid tissue of the adenoids. When a virus gains access to its target, it infiltrates that cell and takes over its processes until the cell literally bursts with new viruses. Cold viruses act fast: the incubation period between being exposed and developing symptoms can be as short as 12 hours.

While the damage that cold viruses cause is substantial, it pales in comparison with the damage caused by the immune system when it is fighting off a cold virus. Signals released by infected cells trigger an aggressive response, which causes the area to be flooded with inflammatory chemicals and aggressive immune system cells. It is the immune system response to a viral threat that causes most of the discomfort associated with common cold symptoms.

Cold viruses can stay viable for up to 3 hours outside the body. The viruses are airborne after an infected person coughs or sneezes, but they are even more readily spread when someone gets a virus on the hand, and it finds access to the body through a portal of entry: the mouth, the eyes, or the nose. Picking up a virus from a light switch, a doorknob, a keyboard, or a piece of money and then rubbing the nose is a very efficient way to spread the disease.

The best way to prevent the spread of colds and other infectious diseases is by frequently washing the hands, focusing on the cuticles and nails, using soap or detergent and scrubbing for 30 seconds or more before rinsing. Using paper tissues and disposing of them carefully, avoiding contact with people who are sick, and employing good judgment about sleep, diet, and exercise can also help to prevent the spread of colds.

Colds are seldom dangerous, except when they complicate into a secondary infection. The compromised integrity of the membranes and the accumulations of mucus, a perfect growth medium, leave the body vulnerable to secondary infections that can include ear infection, laryngitis, acute bronchitis, sinusitis, and pneumonia. People with asthma also frequently find that colds exacerbate their respiratory symptoms.

Signs and Symptoms

The symptoms of a cold are probably familiar to everyone: runny nose, sneezing, sore throat, dry coughing, headache, and perhaps a mild fever. Symptoms generally last less than 2 weeks, although the cough may linger for 3 weeks or more.

Treatment

Because they are viral infections, antibiotics are useless for treating colds. Getting extra rest, drinking lots of fluids, and isolating oneself from family, classmates, and coworkers who could get infected are all high priorities. Using a humidifier may relieve some of the irritation to mucous membranes, although some types of humidifiers can be breeding grounds for fungi or bacteria, so it's important to keep them scrupulously clean.

Over-the-counter drugs can relieve the symptoms of a cold, but they do not reduce recovery time. In fact, by inhibiting the ways a body fights off infection (reducing fever, drying up the sinuses), over-the-counter drugs may actually increase the amount of time the infection is present in the body.

Medications

- NSAIDs for fever and pain
- Cough suppressants
- Decongestants
- Zinc lozenges (note: zinc nasal sprays have been associated with a risk of permanent anosmia—loss of the sense of smell)

Massage?

RISKS Anecdotal reports suggest that clients who receive a rigorous circulatory massage while a cold or flu infection is taking hold may get sicker than if they had delayed. By contrast, clients who receive massage while in recovery from a respiratory tract infection often find that their symptoms are temporarily exacerbated, and then their recovery is shortened. No rigorous research has been published on this issue, however.

Rigorous massage that demands an adaptive response is best delayed until the acute phase of a cold has passed. Cold viruses are contagious through casual contact, so therapists must take precautions on behalf of their own health.

BENEFITS Gentle reflexive work may be soothing and effective to promote good sleep at any stage of a cold. A client who has fully recovered from a cold can enjoy the same benefits from bodywork as the rest of the population.

Influenza

Definition: What Is It?

Influenza, or flu, is a viral infection of the respiratory tract. Seasonal flu is usually a relatively benign, self-limiting infection, but it can become life threatening if an aggressive virus invades a vulnerable patient. A flu infection with a particularly virulent virus, or in a person with limited immune resources, can be a deadly situation. Flu and its complications hospitalize 200,000 people and kill an average of 23,000 to 36,000 Americans each year.

A synonym for flu is grippe, from the French *gripper*, to seize.

Etiology: What Happens?

Flu viruses work in the usual way of infectious agents: they gain access to the body, usually by inhalation or touch from a contaminated surface that carries the virus to a portal of entry: the nose, mouth, or eye. Then the viruses invade their target cells: mucus-producing cells that line the respiratory tract.

Once the infection is established, the immune system response causes most of the extreme symptoms.

Influenza in Brief

Pronunciation: in-flu-EN-zah

What is it?
Influenza (flu) is a viral infection of the respiratory tract.

How is it recognized?
The symptoms of flu include high fever and muscle and joint achiness that may last for up to a week, followed by a runny nose, coughing, sneezing, and general malaise.

Massage risks and benefits
Risks: Influenza is highly contagious through airborne droplets as well as via hands touching contaminated surfaces. For this reason, it is generally preferable to delay a bodywork session until the acute phase has passed.
Benefits: Gentle, reflexive or energetic bodywork may be appropriate to support a person who is fighting a flu infection, with respect for the fact that this condition is highly contagious and contact may put the therapist at risk. After the acute phase has passed, massage may help to restore energy and vitality.

White blood cells attack infected mucous cells, causing sore throat and coughing. They also release the chemicals that stimulate fever. It can take 2 or 3 days for symptoms to appear, but the person is shedding virus in oral and mucous secretions during that time. The peak of communicability is usually around day 4 of the infection. The person continues to shed virus throughout the acute and subacute stages.

Three classes of flu virus have been identified. The type A viruses are the most virulent, responsible for major epidemics that can claim millions of lives (Sidebar 7.1). Type A viruses mutate quickly and so can cause repeated infections in the same person. Type B flu viruses can also spread, but they are not as aggressive or widely spread as type A viruses. Type C flu viruses are not associated with epidemics, and they are relatively stable. They create much less severe symptoms than the other types.

Type A flu viruses are remarkably adaptable. They can infect several species besides humans, including birds, pigs, ferrets, seals, whales, and horses. It appears that when flu passes from one species to another, it undergoes some minor changes to its enzymes that allow it to invade its new host. In some cases, it may move directly from animals to humans without mutation. Type A flu viruses also have the ability to mutate as they develop resistance to attack. This makes it impossible for the body to establish permanent immunity, because each time it is exposed, the pathogen is different.

SIDEBAR 7.1 We Are All under the Influence: The History of Flu

Symptoms of the infectious disease now called flu have been documented since the fifth century BCE. It was observed in those early days of medicine that this disorder could spread throughout a population, but symptoms sometimes wouldn't appear for a few days after exposure, and it continued to spread for several days after all symptoms were gone among the original patients. Because its course seemed so mysterious, it was assumed to be controlled by the influence of the planets and stars. In the early 1500s, the Italian term for influence (influenza) became the common name for this disorder.

The first recorded pandemic of flu virus is known from records from Europe from 1580. The 20th century saw three pandemics of flu infections and a strong threat of a fourth. So far the 21st century has seen one pandemic.

- 1918 to 1921. The "Spanish Lady" was a flu virus that in the course of 3 years killed half a million people in the United States and more than 20 million people worldwide. It is credited with helping to end WWI because so many soldiers were lost to this pandemic.
- 1957. Asian flu.
- 1968. Hong Kong Flu.
- 1977. Russian flu. These flu viruses killed a total of 1.5 million people worldwide.
- 1997. In Hong Kong, a new flu virus was identified that was directly communicable from birds to people. It infected 18 people and killed 6, but if it had escaped Hong Kong, it could have killed millions more. It was controlled by an aggressive public health effort that ended in the slaughter of all of Hong Kong's domestic poultry to limit the spread of the virus. The flu that appeared in 1997 is the same virus (H5N1) that now called "bird flu"; it is closely related to the virus that caused the "Spanish Lady" pandemic of 1918.
- 2009. H1N1. An alarming outbreak of "swine flu" began in April, and by June it was labeled a pandemic. It was especially virulent among adults under 65—a population that is not usually threatened by flu infections. It killed 12,000 Americans in 2009, but coverage for H1N1 in subsequent flu vaccines has made it a much less threatening infection.

Type A viruses are labeled according to the presence of certain proteins, called **hemagglutinin** and **neuraminidase**, on their outer coat. Researchers have identified 15 subtypes of hemagglutinin and 9 subtypes of neuraminidase, and individual strains of virus are named for the subtypes they carry. For instance, the most common forms of human flu are H2N2 and H3N1.

Flu can become life threatening because it can allow the possibility of an opportunistic secondary infection in the shape of pneumonia or acute bronchitis. This is a particular danger for high-risk populations: those under 2 to 5 years old; those over 65 years old; smokers; diabetics; and people who are immunosuppressed, living in long-term care facilities, or affected by chronic lung or heart problems. One alarming feature of the H1N1 version of flu is that it appears to be especially virulent among people under 65 who are normally not endangered by flu.

Types of Influenza

- *Seasonal flu*: This is the most common form of flu, and it can involve several different subtypes of type A viruses. It is most active from fall through early spring.
- *H5N1* (Avian flu): Also called "bird flu"; this is a variety that passes from wild water birds (swans, geese, ducks) to domestic poultry with devastating results. In rare cases, it has passed from birds to humans (typically when people are working or living with infected poultry), and very rarely from person to person. Since 2003 only about 500 people have been diagnosed with bird flu worldwide. This strain is extremely virulent, with a mortality rate of close to 30% among humans, so it is being watched closely. If it mutates with a more communicable form of seasonal flu, the results could be very dangerous (see Sidebar 7.1).
- *H1N1* (Swine flu): This variety was recognized in a fast-moving international outbreak in 2009. H1N1 is unique among flu viruses in that it appears to target people under 65 years old with very extreme and sometimes fatal consequences.

Signs and Symptoms

Flu symptoms can range from subtle to fatal within hours or days. For most common infections, the symptoms look like a bad cold: respiratory irritation with runny nose and dry cough, sore throat, headache, chills, and a long-lasting high fever. While not all flu patients develop a fever, it is not unusual for flu-related fever to go over 102°F (38.9°C) in adults, and it may last for 3 days or more. Most flu infections cause symptoms that affect more than the upper respiratory tract, however. Many patients have aching muscles and joints and debilitating fatigue. For more information on how flu differs from the common cold, see Compare & Contrast 7.2.

COMPARE & CONTRAST 7.2 Is it a Cold? Is it the Flu? Does It Matter?

Colds and flu are both caused by viral attacks on cells in the respiratory tract. They have similar symptoms, and they carry similar cautions about working with clients who have these infections. Still, flu can be much worse than a cold. Flu is more contagious, and it can linger in the body much longer, and it can occasionally be lifethreatening. Therefore, it's useful to have a clear idea of which pathogen a client is battling.

PRESENTATION	COMMON COLD	INFLUENZA
Duration	Usually less than a week.	Could be 10 days or more.
Fever	Usually low (under 102°F, 38.9°C) and short term (resolves within 48 hours).	Usually high (over 102°F, 38.9°C) and long term (may persist for 3 days or more).
Location	Symptoms strictly in upper respiratory tract.	Possible systemic muscle and joint pain, inflamed lymph nodes, debilitating fatigue.
Complications	Complications usually involve sinus or ear infection.	Complications affect the lower respiratory tract as bronchitis or pneumonia.
Communicability	Usually spread by hands touching contaminated surfaces. Contagious, but not usually epidemic.	Usually spread by inhalation of airborne virus. Often highly virulent; may infect high proportion of population.
Resolution	Quickly eliminated; when symptoms are over, no longer contagious.	May linger several days after symptoms abate, still communicable.

One area that flu viruses generally don't attack is the gastrointestinal tract. What is commonly referred to as "stomach flu" is far more likely to be infection with Norovirus or a case of food poisoning. Flu infections can involve vomiting and diarrhea, but this is related to systemic stress and inflammation rather than a specific attack in the GI tract.

Flu symptoms usually appear about 3 days after exposure to the virus, and they may persist for up to 2 weeks. If they persist longer than that, or if the coughing begins to produce a lot of streaked or opaque phlegm, it may be that the original viral infection has complicated to a secondary infection of the lungs: pneumonia.

Treatment

As a viral infection, flu is unaffected by antibiotics. Good-sense measures include rest and liquids. Over-the-counter drugs may abate the symptoms but do not speed healing. They can be useful, however, if the symptoms are preventing a person from getting the sleep necessary to heal.

Some antiviral medications are finding use among flu patients. **Amantadine** can reduce the duration of symptoms of flu caused by a type A virus, but it is associated with central nervous system side effects, including sleeplessness, restlessness, and confusion, especially among elderly patients. A closely related medication, **rimantadine**, usually has fewer side effects. Neither amantadine nor rimantadine is effective against type B or C virus, and both medications have been seen to allow the mutation of flu virus into more dangerous drug-resistant strains. Further, they must be administered within 2 days of exposure to have any efficacy.

Another class of drugs, called **neuraminidase inhibitors**, includes the name brands Tamiflu and Relenza. These drugs have some advantages in that they tend to cause fewer side effects than amantadine and rimantadine. However, they are expensive and not suitable for use in children.

Every year the Food and Drug Administration distributes a vaccine to fight a combination of type A and type B viruses. These vaccines are formulated about 9 months ahead of flu season. Because viruses mutate quickly, flu vaccines must be updated every year. Flu vaccines are recommended for high-risk populations, including those who are immune suppressed and who have chronic respiratory illnesses.

Medications

- NSAIDs for general malaise and fever
- Antivirals
- Neuraminidase inhibitors

Massage?

RISKS A lot of anecdotal evidence (backed by experience but not formal research) has been gathered about massage for clients with cold and flu. Experience suggests that if a person receives a massage while these infections are still becoming established, then he or she may be more extremely ill than otherwise. By contrast, many people have experienced that getting a massage after a cold or flu has peaked makes them feel sick again for a day or so, and then the rest of their recovery appears to be very much shortened: they come back to full energy and vitality quickly. For this reason, it is important to inform clients that massage may temporarily exacerbate symptoms so that they can make an informed choice about whether it is a good time for them to receive bodywork.

BENEFITS Influenza viruses are highly communicable through airborne droplets as well as by way of contaminated surfaces. Practitioners must be aware that working with clients who have flu puts them at risk for contracting this infection. Clients in an acute stage of flu are engaged in fighting off an aggressive infection. While gentle bodywork that doesn't demand an extensive adaptive response may be soothing and promote good sleep, any more intrusive bodywork may be unnecessarily challenging.

OPTIONS Gentle, nondemanding bodywork during an acute phase of flu may be highly relaxing, as long as the practitioner takes appropriate precautions. After the acute phase has passed, massage to promote good sleep and rebounded energy may be useful.

Pneumonia

Definition: What Is It?

Pneumonia is a general term for inflammation of the lungs, usually due to an infectious agent. Because it is an opportunistic infection that takes advantage of weak immune systems, it is the leading cause of death by infectious disease in the United States. The

Pneumonia in Brief

Pronunciation: nu-MO-ne-ah

What is it?
Pneumonia is an infection in the lungs brought about by bacteria, viruses, or fungi.

How is it recognized?
The symptoms of pneumonia include coughing that may be dry or productive, high fever, pain on breathing, and shortness of breath. Extreme cases may show cyanosis, or a bluish cast to the skin and nails.

Massage risks and benefits
Risks: Pneumonia can be a life-threatening event, so a person with an acute infection is not a good candidate for any kind of rigorous massage that demands an adaptive response. Further, pneumonia can be contagious, so a therapist working with a client who is ill must take appropriate precautions.
Benefits: A client who is in recovery from pneumonia may benefit from percussive massage that aids the expulsion of mucus from the lungs. Gentle massage that promotes relaxation and sleep is also useful during this time. A client who has fully recovered from pneumonia can enjoy the same benefits from bodywork as the rest of the population.

severity of pneumonia ranges from being not much worse than a bad cold to being a cause of death within 24 hours.

Etiology: What Happens?

The alveoli are the tiny hollow balloons with walls made of squamous epithelium found at the very end of the bronchioles in the lungs. Each alveolus is surrounded by a net of capillaries of the pulmonary circuit so that oxygen and carbon dioxide can be exchanged. When an infectious agent enters the lungs, the alveoli fill with dead white blood cells, mucus, and fluid seeping back from the capillaries (Figure 7.2). Eventually diffusion of gases is impossible. Abscesses may form, and capillary damage may occur, allowing bleeding into the alveoli and eventually into the sputum.

In extreme infections, the pleurae may be affected as well. Scar tissue can develop between layers, leading to pain and limited movement with each breath; this is called pleurisy. Alternatively, the pleural fluid itself can host infection in a condition called empyema.

Several infectious agents can cause pneumonia, and more than one type of pathogen may be present at a time: a fact that sometimes makes diagnosis and treatment of this condition a challenge.

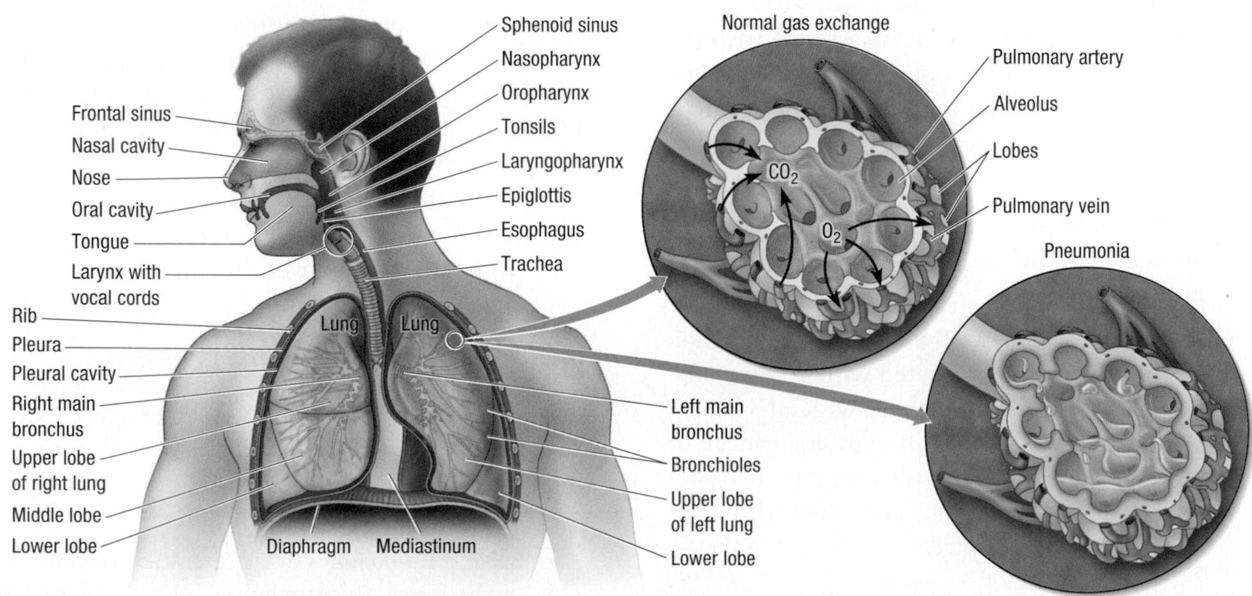

Figure 7.2. Pneumonia: alveoli fill and gaseous exchange cannot take place

- *Viruses*. Viral infections account for about half of pneumonia cases. Influenza and syncytial virus are the most common culprits. Other viruses include cytomegalovirus, herpes simplex, and adenovirus. The incubation period of viral pneumonia is 1 to 3 days. Viral pneumonia tends to be short lived and not serious. It appears most frequently in children.
- *Bacteria*. Varieties of staphylococci and streptococci often live harmlessly in the nose and throat, but when resistance is low, they may invade the lower respiratory tract to set up an infection in the lungs. The toxins released by the bacteria initiate an inflammatory response, leading to edema in the alveoli and a reduced ability to draw oxygen into the system. This kind of infection usually responds well to antibiotics. *Streptococcus pneumoniae*, also called **pneumococcus**, is the most common form of bacterial pneumonia. Another infection is caused by *Legionella pneumoniae*, named for the Legionnaires' convention where it was first identified in 1977. Chlamydia (a different pathogen from the chlamydia that causes sexually transmitted infections) and tuberculosis (TB) bacilli can also cause bacterial pneumonia.
- *Mycoplasma*. Often described as tiny bacteria, **mycoplasma** are the smallest free-living infectious agents ever found. The incubation period for mycoplasma pneumonia is 1 to 4 weeks, and because it tends not to be as severe as bacterial or viral types of infection, it is sometimes called "walking pneumonia" or "atypical pneumonia." Fortunately, like bacterial pneumonia, mycoplasma pneumonia responds well to antibiotics.
- *Fungi*. Some fungi that are endemic to certain areas of the United States are associated with pneumonia.
- *Pneumocystis jiroveci*. *P. jiroveci* is an infection almost exclusively associated with immunosuppressed patients, such as those with HIV/AIDS; people receiving chemotherapy for cancer or immunosuppressive drugs to prevent the rejection of organ transplants; and those who don't have a functioning spleen.

Considering the delicacy of the epithelium in the lungs, it is amazing that if a pneumonia infection is short lived, it is completely reversible. The body can liquefy and absorb the consolidated matter in affected alveoli, and it can reabsorb the fluid from any inflamed part of the lung. A basically healthy patient who gets appropriate treatment can expect to recover fully within 2 weeks. Untreated pneumonia, however, has a high mortality rate. It can also complicate into meningitis, respiratory failure, and bacteremia (the presence of bacteria in the blood, a type of blood poisoning); these situations are nearly always fatal.

In long-standing cases with accumulation of fibrosis and scar tissue, permanent damage to the elasticity of the epithelial tissue may occur, or the freedom with which the lungs move in the pleural cavity may be compromised. This can raise the risk of future infections.

When people develop pneumonia as a complication of a more serious underlying disorder, this infection can be life threatening. Secondary pneumonia is an opportunistic disease. It is often the final complication of other serious conditions, even noninfectious ones. People who have had a stroke, heart failure, alcoholism, or cancer die of pneumonia more often than any other disease. People who are bedridden or paralyzed are susceptible too, because their cough reflex is often impaired; they cannot expel mucus easily. Having a preexisting respiratory problem such as flu, bronchitis, emphysema, or asthma is an open invitation. And finally, being immunosuppressed because of tissue transplant, AIDS, sickle cell disease, steroid use, leukemia, or cytotoxic drug use makes a person particularly vulnerable to pneumonia.

Many cases of pneumonia could be prevented through appropriate vaccine use. The annual flu vaccine, if it is effective against the circulating viruses, prevents flu infections from complicating into viral or bacterial pneumonia. Pneumovax, a vaccine against pneumococcus, is also available. This vaccine is recommended for high-risk patients and for people who live or work in long-term care facilities or hospitals.

Types of Pneumonia by Location

- *Bronchopneumonia*: This starts as a bronchial inflammation and spreads into the lungs. It appears in a patchy pattern all over the lungs, not segregated to a specific area.
- *Lobar pneumonia*: This is restricted to one lobe of the lungs. Eventually the whole lobe may be affected.
- *Double pneumonia*: This affects both lungs. It can be bacterial or viral (Figure 7.3).

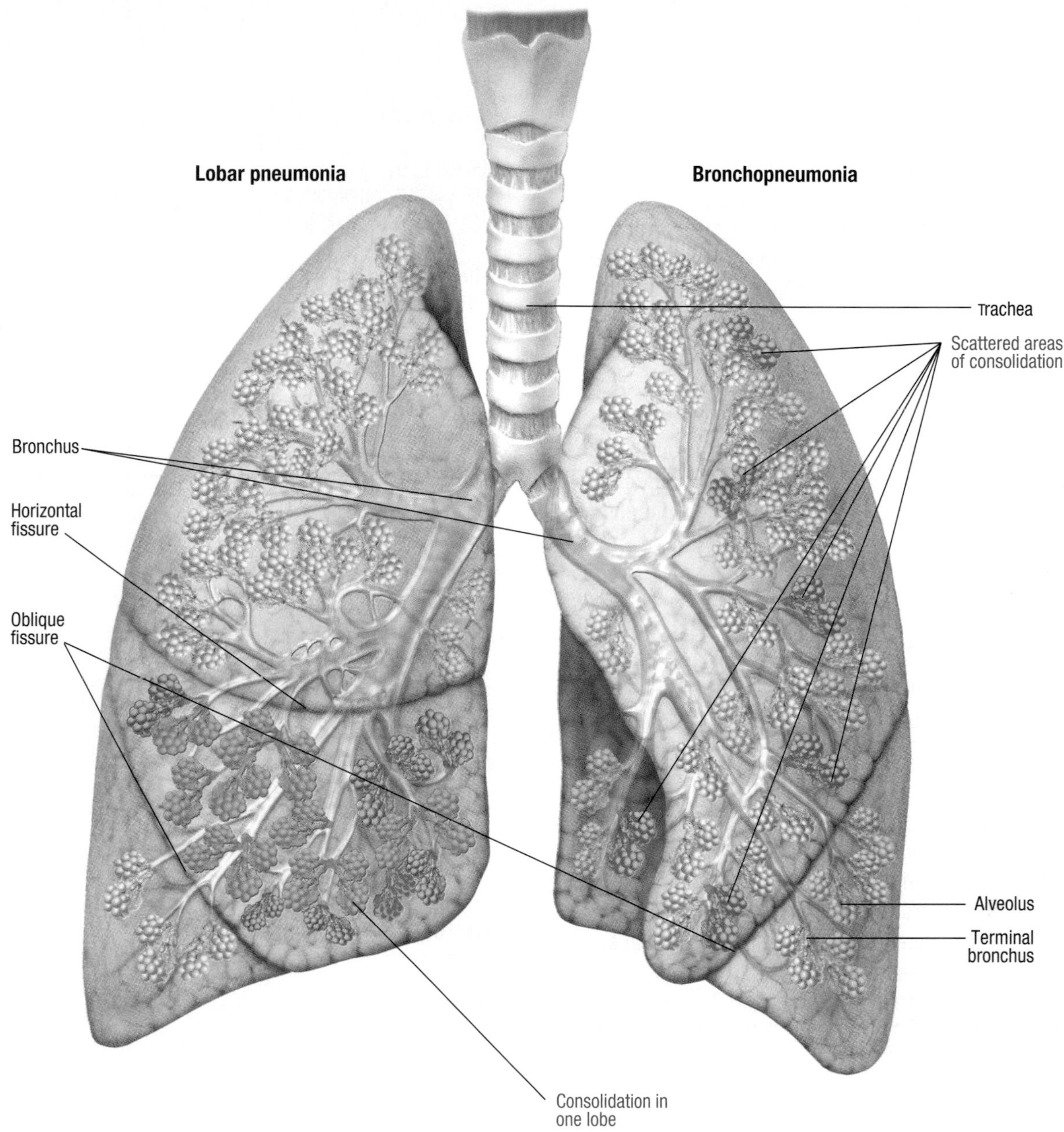

Figure 7.3. Types of pneumonia

Types of Pneumonia by Source of Infection

- *Community-acquired pneumonia*: This is the most common form. It is usually a bacterial infection or a complication of flu.
- *Nosocomial, or hospital-acquired pneumonia*: This is an infection in that develops within 48 hours of being in a hospital or other health care setting.
- *Aspiration pneumonia*: This is an infection brought about when a person accidentally inhales food, liquid, or other substances into the lungs. It is a particular risk for anyone with swallowing difficulties or with a weakened cough reflex.

Signs and Symptoms

Signs and symptoms of pneumonia vary widely, depending on the causative factor and how much of the lung is affected. They include coughing, very high fever, chills, sweating, delirium, chest pains, cyanosis, thick and colored sputum, shortness of breath, muscle aches and pains, and pleurisy.

Pneumonia can have a sudden or gradual onset. Very often it follows the same course as flu, but instead of getting better, the respiratory symptoms get rapidly worse and are accompanied by fever up to 104°F (40°C).

Treatment

Treatment depends entirely on what type of pneumonia is present. Bacterial and mycoplasma pneumonias generally respond well to antibiotics, but these do not apply for viral infections. Cough suppressants are generally discouraged because they interfere with the ability to move contaminated mucus.

Symptomatic relief and supportive therapy include breathing humidified air, drinking ample fluids, and supplementing oxygen if necessary. If damage to the pleurae is extensive, surgery to drain the pleural space may be conducted.

Medications

- Antibiotics if necessary
- Antiviral medication if necessary
- NSAIDs for fever reduction and general malaise

Massage?

RISKS Pneumonia is a serious and complicated condition that frequently accompanies other serious disorders. A client with this condition should not be challenged by rigorous massage. Gentle, reflexive work may be supportive, as long as the therapist is safe from the risk of infection.

BENEFITS When the acute phase of pneumonia has passed, massage can be helpful for a person undergoing a long and slow recovery. A person who has fully recovered from pneumonia can enjoy all the benefits from bodywork as the rest of the population.

OPTIONS Although today this is typically done by machine, manual percussion on the chest to loosen mucus can be helpful for a person recovering from pneumonia.

Sinusitis

Definition: What Is It?

Sinusitis, as the name implies, is a condition in which the mucous membranes that line the sinuses become inflamed and swollen. It can be due to infectious or noninfectious causes.

Sinusitis in Brief

Pronunciation: sy-nus-I-tis

What is it?
Sinusitis is inflammation of the paranasal sinuses from infection, allergies, or physical obstruction.

How is it recognized?
Signs and symptoms include headaches; tenderness over the affected area; runny or congested nose; facial or tooth pain; headache; fatigue; and, if it's related to an infection, thick, opaque mucus, fever, and chills.

Massage risks and benefits

Risks: Acute sinus infections contraindicate any bodywork that could exacerbate symptoms. If the client has fever, chills, and other signs of systemic infection, it is best to delay any rigorous massage until this has passed. A client with a tendency toward inflamed sinuses may have problems lying flat on a table, especially, face down. It is important to be able to make accommodations for this problem.

Benefits: Very gentle massage around the face, as long as no infection is present, may help the sinuses to drain, and for sinus pain to diminish. A client with inflamed sinuses who does not have an infection can benefit from bodywork as long as he or she is comfortable on the table.

Etiology: What Happens?

Sinuses are hollow areas lateral to, above, and behind the nose (Figure 7.4). They provide resonance for the voice, and they lighten the weight of the head. The mucous membranes lining sinuses are provided with cilia, tiny hairs that move the mucus along, so that trapped pathogens and particulate matter can be expelled or swallowed and destroyed instead of reaching the lower respiratory system.

When the cilia break down or are paralyzed, often as a result of viral infection or environmental irritants, pathogen-laden mucus lingers over delicate epithelial cells, stimulating an inflammatory response. Soon the hollow areas fill with sticky, pus-filled mucus that cannot drain. This forms an ideal growth medium for bacteria that normally live in small numbers in the sinuses.

Alternatively, the cilia remain intact and highly functional, but the mucous membranes are stimulated to respond to oak pollen or other allergens as if they were life-threatening organisms. Inflammation ensues, with the production of huge amounts of thin, runny

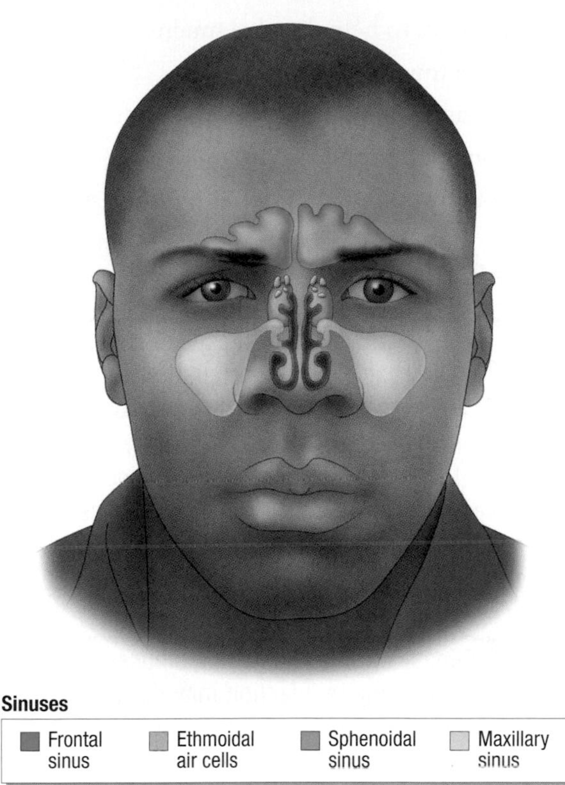

Figure 7.4. Sinusitis

mucus; puffy, itchy eyes; and all of the symptoms associated with allergic rhinitis, or hay fever. This can also provide a hospitable environment for local bacteria, so a person with hay fever has a significantly higher than normal risk of intermittent sinus infections.

Many different factors can cause inflamed sinuses, including the following:

- *Viruses and bacteria.* The most common types of infectious sinusitis begin as viral infections such as cold or flu. When defense mechanisms are low, the bacteria that normally colonize the skin and mucous membranes take and begin to multiply. The bacteria most commonly associated with these infections are *S. pneumonia*, *Haemophilus influenza*, or *Moraxella catarrhalis*.
- *Fungi and bacteria.* Some people with chronic sinusitis have significant amounts of fungal growth in their sinuses. One theory is that sensitivity to fungi stimulates an inflammatory response that allows naturally occurring bacteria to grow and cause a chronic infection. This is a problem particularly for persons with diabetes, HIV/AIDS, or other immunosuppressive disorders.
- *Structural problems.* A deviated septum or the growth of nasal polyps can obstruct the flow of mucus out of the sinuses. Structural anomalies in the shape of the facial bones can also block drainage. This is not an infection to begin with, but mucus held back from normal flow is an inviting growth medium for bacteria, so what begins as a simple structural anomaly can become a true infection.
- *Environmental irritants.* Exposure to cigarette smoke (first- or second-hand), indoor and outdoor pollutants, cocaine, or other irritants can destroy cilia and increase the risk of infection.
- *Other conditions.* Acute or chronic sinusitis is frequently seen with other conditions. Severe dental caries (cavities) raise the risk of sinusitis, probably from the availability of local bacteria. Asthma is closely associated with sinusitis, as both conditions have to do with excessive mucus production and a hyperreactive inflammatory response.

Types of Sinusitis

- *Noninfectious sinusitis*: Also called allergic rhinitis or hay fever, this causes inflammation of the sinus membranes without underlying infection. Hay fever is often distinguished from infectious sinusitis by the lack of congestion and the quality of the nasal discharge. It tends to be thin and runny rather than thick and sticky. People with hay fever do have inflamed sinuses, however, which put them at risk for secondary infections.
- *Infectious sinusitis*: This is a pathogenic invasion followed by an inflammatory response that creates a vicious circle: the body creates excessive mucus to help remove infectious agents, but the inflamed tissues make drainage of that mucus (which can harbor bacteria and other pathogens) difficult or impossible. Sinus infections are often complications of upper respiratory tract infections like colds or flu.

Signs and Symptoms

Signs and symptoms of sinusitis vary according to the cause of the inflammation and which sinuses are involved. Severe headache is a key feature, especially upon waking. Bending over makes it much worse, because that position increases pressure on already stressed membranes. The affected area may be extremely painful to the touch, and swelling or puffiness around the eyes or cheeks may be visible. Fever and chills may accompany an acute bacterial infection. Sore throat, coughing (caused by postnasal drip), and congestion or runny nose may appear with any type of sinus irritation, and regardless of whether it's infectious or allergic, people with sinusitis are likely to experience fatigue and general malaise because the body is fighting hard to cast off an invader.

The mucus expressed with a sinus infection is likely to be streaked or opaque, in shades that range from pale green to yellow to brown. It tends to be thick and sticky. The mucus expressed with hay fever, on the other hand, tends to be thin, runny, and clear.

Treatment

Treatment for sinusitis begins with self-help measures: staying in humid air or breathing steam to help moisturize and liquefy clogged mucus is an important step. Increasing daily water intake and reducing the use of alcohol, caffeine, and other diuretics may also help to soften and loosen thick, sticky mucus. Many experts recommend using a saline wash to rinse the sinuses regularly. Using air filters to remove irritating particles from the air can also help.

Drugs prescribed for this disorder begin with antibiotics if the infection is bacterial. Sinuses are difficult to access, and the bacteria associated with most cases of sinusitis tend to be drug resistant, so this condition often requires a long-term course of specialized antibiotics.

Decongestants are sometimes recommended to shrink the mucous membranes, but these are only appropriate for short-term use because they can create a significant rebound effect when usage is stopped. Corticosteroids in nasal spray form can reduce swelling, but they can take several weeks to become effective.

In very extreme cases, surgery is recommended. This involves inserting a tube through the nose and enlarging sinus passages, removing polyps, repairing a deviated septum, and doing anything else that may assist the mucus to drain freely. Using tiny balloons on catheters (balloon **sinusotomy**) tends to have fewer risks than traditional endoscopy, and it can also be used with children.

Medications

- Antibiotics, if necessary, along with acidophilus to reduce the risk of yeast infections
- Mucolytics to help dissolve mucus
- Antihistamines
- Antifungal medication if necessary
- Decongestants and antihistamines
- Steroidal anti-inflammatories by nasal spray

Massage?

RISKS Acute sinus infections, especially with fever, headache, and general malaise, contraindicate any bodywork that might exacerbate symptoms. While gentle or reflexive work away from the face is unlikely to make this problem worse, a person running a fever is better off delaying rigorous massage until this crisis has been resolved. Clients with an acute infection are also likely to be uncomfortable lying flat on the table.

BENEFITS Clients who have inflamed sinuses that are not due to infection may derive benefits from bodywork, as long as they are comfortable on the table. Gentle work on and around the face may help the sinuses to drain, which can help to relieve symptoms.

OPTIONS Therapists trained in lymphatic work find that this approach is often particularly successful for allergic sinusitis.

Tuberculosis

Definition: What Is It?

"Tubercle" means bump, as in the greater tubercle of the humerus. Tuberculosis (TB) is a disease involving pus- and bacteria-filled bumps, usually in the lungs but sometimes in other locations as well.

The World Health Organization reports that TB affects about one-third of the world's population, and it causes about two million deaths each year.

TB used to be considered virtually conquered in the United States, because in the 1940s effective antibiotics were developed. Its incidence steadily declined until the early 1980s, when suddenly it began to rise again. When public health efforts became more focused, rates of new TB infection began to decline again. It is still declining, but at a much slower rate.

The distribution of TB in the United States is not demographically even. It occurs in highest numbers among the poor, people of color, people with limited

Tuberculosis in Brief

Pronunciation: tu-ber-kyu-LO-sis

What is it?
Tuberculosis (TB) is a bacterial infection that usually begins in the lungs but may spread to bones, kidneys, lymph nodes, central nervous system, or elsewhere in the body. It is a contagious airborne disease.

How is it recognized?
Exposure to the TB bacterium may produce no initial symptoms. If the infection turns into the active disease, symptoms may include coughing, bloody sputum, fatigue, fever, weight loss, and night sweats.

Massage risks and benefits
Risks: Active TB disease contraindicates massage unless the client has been on appropriate antibiotics for at least 2 weeks and has medical clearance. This disease is spread through airborne contaminants, so it presents a risk for massage therapists.
Benefits: A client who is under treatment for active TB disease, or who has been exposed to TB but does not have active disease, can enjoy the same benefits from bodywork as the rest of the population.

access to health care, people in prisons or homeless shelters, and recent immigrants.

Etiology: What Happens?

TB is an airborne disease caused by *Mycobacterium tuberculosis*. This is a bacterium with a waxy coat that allows it to survive outside of a host. When a person with an active infection coughs or sneezes, thousands of infective droplets are released into the air. The tiny bacteria, protected from drying out by their waxy covering, drift in the air until another host comes along and takes a deep breath.

TB moves in the body in two phases:

- *Primary phase.* A person inhales some bacteria that travel all the way to the alveoli, where they are engulfed by macrophages. Their waxy coating makes them resistant to the macrophages' digestive enzymes. Instead, the bacteria slowly build up whole colonies inside the alveoli. Unable to expel these invaders, the body builds a protective fibrous wall around the site of infection: a tubercle. Tubercles are usually found in the lungs, but if some of the bacteria seep out into the bloodstream or lymph, the same process happens elsewhere. Kidneys, the spine, and the central nervous system are the most common other locations.

A single, tiny, undetectable cyst in the lung is where TB stops for most people. This is TB exposure, but not the active disease; it is also called a latent infection. Within 10 to 12 weeks, T-cells are activated, and a specific immune response ensues. The body is prepared to react to another contact with the bacillus, which is the mechanism behind the skin test that looks for past exposure. The inhaled bacteria remain contained inside their tidy fibrous package. They may stay there forever unless something happens to set them free: this is usually a depression in immune system function.

- *Secondary phase.* About 10% of the people exposed to TB eventually develop the active disease. This usually happens within the first year after exposure, but it can be decades later. The bacteria escape and spread into other areas in the lungs or wherever else in the body they may be stationed. The body attempts to surround the new sites with bigger and bigger fibrous capsules, which can cause permanent scarring. Pleurisy, the scarring and sticking of the pleurae, is a frequent complication of active TB. Inside the capsules, the bacteria destroy cells, and the tissue is necrotic, or dead (Figure 7.5).

New tubercles eventually erode enough lung tissue to impede function. A cough begins, and gradually produces bloody sputum; this phlegm actually contains detached pieces of the bacteria-infested tubercles, which

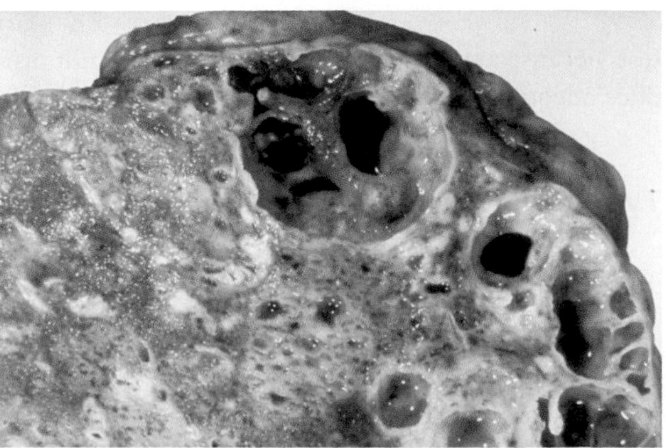
Figure 7.5. Tuberculosis

is why active TB is so very contagious. If several of the tubercles join together, their necrotic centers can cause a large cavity in the lung. Surrounding blood vessels may hemorrhage into the cavity, leading to coughing up blood, or **hemoptysis**. Similar cavities can develop in the kidneys if the tubercles form there. Infections in the bones tend to destroy articular cartilage.

The major risk factor for TB infection is exposure to someone with active disease. Travelers to parts of the world where TB is most common are at risk, as are people who spend time with immigrants from those areas, hospital workers, or residents of close living quarters where the disease may be rampant, such as prisons, nursing homes, and homeless shelters.

Once a person has been exposed to TB, the question is whether he or she will develop an active infection. Several risk factors for this process have been identified, including HIV status, socioeconomic standing, the use of injected illegal drugs, alcoholism, the presence of other immunosuppressive diseases or medications, age, and a history of not completing TB medication.

Coinfection with HIV is a major risk factor for TB making the transition from latent to active disease. The risk that latent TB will become active increases each year that a person carries both infections. It is estimated that about 10% of all people who are HIV positive are also at risk for TB disease; that is about 400% higher than for the general population. Furthermore, having HIV and TB simultaneously can interfere with an accurate TB skin test, because a damaged immune system may not produce adequate antibodies to create a normal reaction.

NOTABLE CASES The list of historical and current public figures who have had tuberculosis is impressive indeed. It includes King Tutankhamen; writers John Keats, Emily Bronte, Fyodor Dostoevsky, and Robert Louis Stevenson; artist Paul Gaugin; First Lady Eleanor Roosevelt, and former President of South Africa and Nobel Peace Prize winner Nelson Mandela.

Types of Tuberculosis

- *Drug-susceptible tuberculosis*: This is the regular type of TB that is the main focus for this discussion. It is sensitive to first-line antibiotics, and the prognosis for a fully treated patient is excellent.
- *Multidrug resistant tuberculosis (MDR-TB)*: This is a mutation that occurs when a patient does not fully treat drug-susceptible TB. The bacteria are resistant to all first-line antibiotics, so it requires much more expensive, aggressive treatment with potentially dangerous side effects. A person with active MDR-TB in an active form spreads this mutation of the bacteria to others.
- *Extensively drug-resistant tuberculosis (XDR-TB)*: This relatively rare strain of TB is resistant to most antibiotics, so its treatment is limited to less effective drugs. Since 1993, 83 cases of XDR-TB have been identified in the United States. It is most common in the former Soviet Union, parts of Asia, and among HIV-positive populations in South Africa.

Signs and Symptoms

The primary phase of TB is so benign a person may never know about the exposure; the symptoms, if any develop at all, are the same as for a mild flu. But the active disease shows much more severe symptoms. They include fever, sweating, weight loss, and exhaustion. Chest pain and shortness of breath are common. A stubborn cough that starts dry and becomes productive of bloody or pus-filled phlegm is a cardinal sign. Other symptoms arise if other organs have been infected as well: bone pain, blood in the urine, or central nervous system symptoms, for instance.

Treatment

In the old days, wealthy TB patients were sent to sanitaria, where it was hoped that sunlight, rest, and good food would enable them to outlive their infection. Many of those facilities are now modern-day spas. Fresh air, rest, and good nutrition are still good ideas, but they work even better when they are combined with the right antibiotics.

Anyone who has drug-susceptible TB, whether the infection is latent or active, can successfully treat it, including people who are HIV positive. People identified with latent TB are recommended to treat it with a single medication called isoniazid (INH) alone. People with active TB need INH along with several other medications for 6 to 9 months in order to prevent mutation to a drug-resistant form. Common side effects include sensitivity to sunlight and yellow or orange tears, sweat, and saliva. More serious side effects include liver damage, neuropathy, joint pain, dizziness, tinnitus, and other problems. These are most likely to develop if a person takes TB medication while consuming alcohol.

SIDEBAR 7.2 A Tuberculosis (TB) Vaccine?

A vaccine against TB has been developed and is in use in some countries, but because of some inherit difficulties, it is not used in the United States. It is called the BCG, or bacille Calmette-Guérin, vaccine.

BCG vaccine can reduce the risk of contracting TB, but it comes with some problems. It is most effective for infants and young children; it is only sporadically effective for adults. And because it initiates an immune response to TB, a person vaccinated with BCG shows positive on all TB tests. This means that if the vaccine fails and a person is truly infected, the infection is impossible to identify while it is still latent.

Work on a more effective TB vaccine is under way. This, along with better means of delivering drugs, working with governments to educate patients and doctors, and many public outreach programs to limit the spread of TB around the globe, may eventually mean that this disease will be a thing of the past.

Medications

- Antibiotics: one for latent TB or up to four for active TB

Massage?

RISKS Tuberculosis (TB) is contagious through indirect casual contact. For this reason, active untreated disease contraindicates massage. Clients treating TB may have side effects that impact massage choices.

BENEFITS A client who is treating TB and who has received clearance risk of communicability can receive massage safely. A client who tests positive for TB exposure, but who has no active disease can also enjoy all the benefits from bodywork as the rest of the population, as long as drug side effects don't interfere with nerve, liver, or kidney function.

Chronic Obstructive Pulmonary Disorders

Chronic Bronchitis

Definition: What Is It?

Chronic bronchitis is part of a group of the closely connected lung problems called chronic obstructive pulmonary disease (COPD). Chronic bronchitis, as its name implies, is a long-term irritation of the bronchi and bronchioles, which may occur with or without infection. It is a progressive disorder that may be halted or slowed but not reversed. It often occurs simultaneously or as a predecessor to emphysema.

Chronic Bronchitis in Brief

Pronunciation: KRAWN-ik brong-KY-tis

What is it?
Chronic bronchitis is one of the lung disorders classified as chronic obstructive pulmonary disease. It involves long-term inflammation of the bronchi with or without infection, leading to permanent changes in the bronchial lining. Chronic bronchitis frequently occurs before or simultaneously with emphysema.

How is it recognized?
Chronic bronchitis is diagnosed when a person has a productive cough that occurs most days for 3 months or more for at least 2 consecutive years. Other common signs are susceptibility to respiratory tract infections, cyanosis, and edema.

Massage risks and benefits

Risks: people with chronic bronchitis are at very much increased risk respiratory infections. If this is the case, any intrusive bodywork that demands an adaptive response must be delayed until the infection has resolved. Chronic bronchitis can lead to heart failure, so this complication, plus the drugs that it may involve, must be considered in making decisions about massage.

Benefits: Massage can be appropriate for chronic bronchitis patients, as long as their heart is healthy, they are not fighting an acute infection, and they can be made comfortable on a massage table or chair. Focused work on and breathing muscles may reduce resistance, improve efficiency, and reduce fatigue.

Etiology: What Happens?

The act of breathing is a deceptively simple process. The muscles of inhalation lift and separate the ribs, which creates a vacuum in the thoracic cavity. Air rushes in to fill the empty space. When tissues are stretched the impulse to inhale stops, and elastin fibers embedded in the lungs and all the membranes of the thorax essentially snap the rib cage back to its original shape. The lungs themselves do not dilate or contract; they are passively filled by muscles contracting to expand the rib cage, or emptied by the action of elastin fibers.

Chronic bronchitis is the result of long-term irritation to bronchial tubes. When the delicate lining of the respiratory tract is chronically insulted with cigarettes (first-hand, second-hand, or sidestream smoke), air pollutants, industrial chemicals, or other contaminants, an inflammatory response follows. Attacks against the bronchial lining destroy elastin fibers and cause overgrowth of mucus-producing cells, excessive production of mucus, and increased resistance to the movement of air in and out of the (Figure 7.6). Eventually, the damage to the bronchioles is permanent; chronic bronchitis is an irreversible progressive disorder.

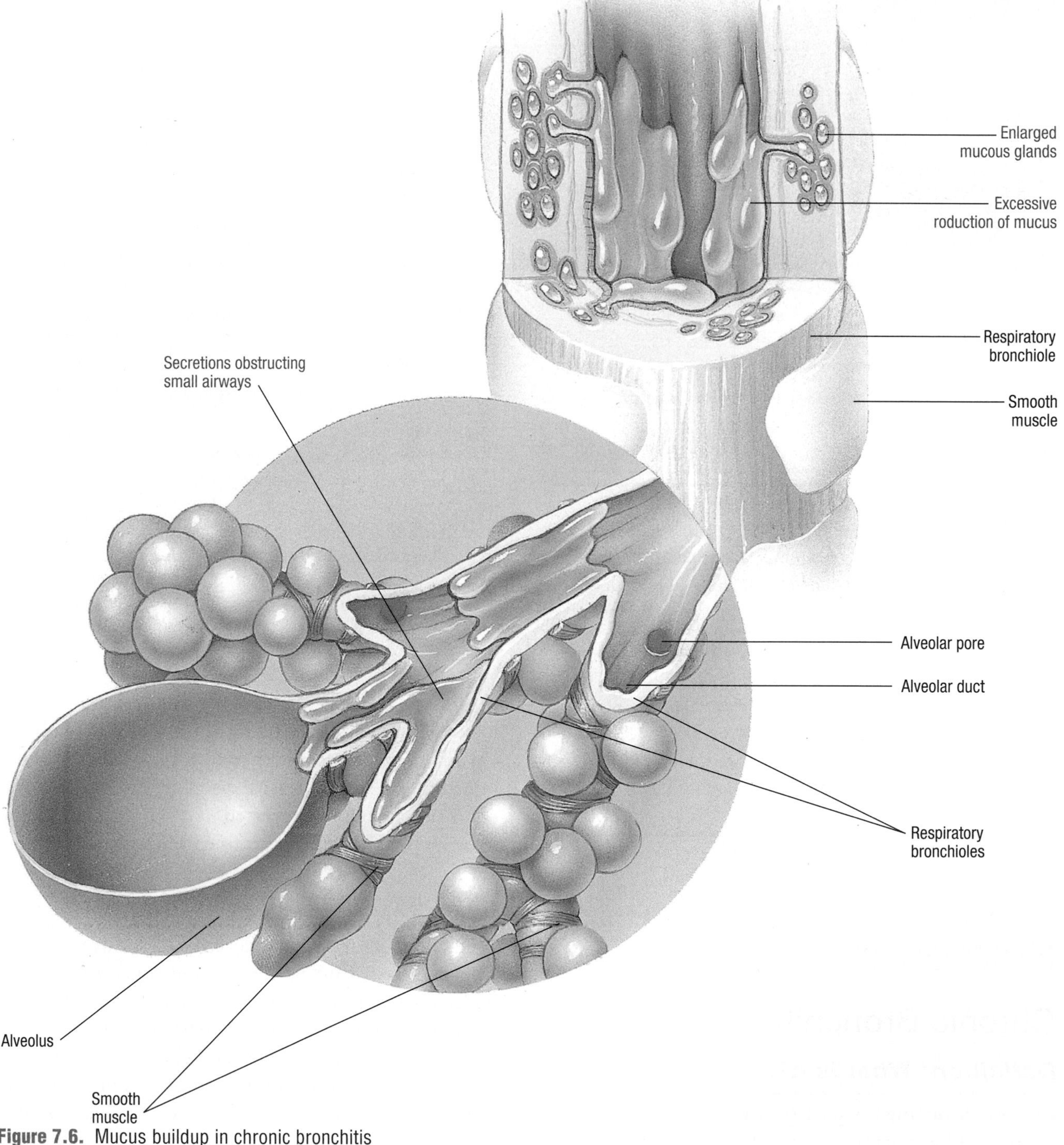

Figure 7.6. Mucus buildup in chronic bronchitis

As elastin breaks down, it requires more muscular work to exhale. At the same time, resistance in the airways means that less oxygen enters the body with each breath. The heart has to work harder to push enough blood into the lungs to supply the body with fuel. At the same time, red blood cell production may increase in an effort to provide more access to any oxygen that can seep into the capillaries. The blood may become thicker with excess erythrocytes (polycythemia), so the heart has to work even harder to push it through the pulmonary circuit. As oxygen levels in the blood drop, acidosis develops; this contributes to vasoconstriction in the pulmonary arteries and worsens pulmonary hypertension. Eventually right-sided heart failure may develop and lead to edema, especially in the legs and ankles.

Complications of chronic bronchitis are serious. Bronchi that are chronically inflamed and producing a lot of mucus are highly vulnerable to viral or bacterial infection. A person with chronic bronchitis can develop life-threatening pneumonia from cold or flu viruses much more easily than the general population. In addition, the risk of right sided heart failure is significant. This serious prognosis is the reason it is important to stop the progression of chronic bronchitis as soon as it can be recognized.

Signs and Symptoms

Signs and symptoms of chronic bronchitis develop slowly, often taking months or years before they are severe enough to attract attention. The process usually begins with a mild cough, perhaps following a typical flu or cold infection. But the cough lingers long after the infection has cleared. It is present most days for 3 months or more, producing thick, clear sputum. This pattern occurs for at least 2 years in a row.

Patients may have to clear their throat very often, especially in the morning; this reflects the excessive production of mucus in the lungs. Shortness of breath progresses, and people become highly vulnerable to respiratory infections.

Later in the process, chronic bronchitis patients may develop signs of oxygen deprivation, including cyanosis and eventually edema related to right-sided heart failure.

Treatment

People with chronic bronchitis are especially susceptible to viral and bacterial infections of the respiratory tract. If a bacterial infection arises, aggressive treatment with antibiotics may be recommended to prevent life-threatening pneumonia. Chronic bronchitis patients are encouraged to be vaccinated against pneumococcus pneumonia and to get yearly flu shots for the same reason.

Other than preventing secondary infections, treatment for chronic bronchitis focuses on halting the progression of the damage and keeping the patient as comfortable as possible. Quitting smoking, if that is an issue, is the single most important step a chronic bronchitis patient can take. Patients should avoid polluted air and known triggers of bronchial spasm. Oxygen may be provided in a medical emergency, but most chronic bronchitis patients don't need to supplement oxygen on a regular basis.

Balancing short-acting bronchodilators with longer acting anti-inflammatories is often a successful strategy; manage this irreversible condition. Ultimately, a combination of medication, education, and careful exercise to rehabilitate underused tissues may slow or even stop the progression of chronic bronchitis.

Medications

- Bronchodilators to clear the airways
- Inhaled and oral corticosteroids to control inflammation
- Expectorants to assist in the clearing of mucus
- Antibiotics as necessary to fight bacterial infection

Massage?

RISKS Chronic bronchitis patients may be dealing with heart problems and discomfort lying flat on a table. These require adjustments for bodywork to take place. Further, clients with chronic bronchitis are especially prone to respiratory infections that can rapidly become life threatening. Any client in this situation should delay bodywork until the infection has resolved.

BENEFITS Gentle, reflexive massage can be supportive for clients who are quite frail with chronic bronchitis, but any work that requires an adaptive response should be reserved for people who are more resilient.

OPTIONS Bodywork that addresses the intercostal muscles, the scalenes, the serratus posterior, and the diaphragm—all within tolerance, of course—can improve the efficiency in the way these muscles work, which has profound impact on fatigue and energy levels for the client.

Emphysema

Definition: What Is It?

The name emphysema means "blown up" (as in inflated, not exploded); this describes what happens to the alveoli as part of this disease process. Emphysema, along with chronic bronchitis, involves irreversible destruction of the respiratory system. The collective name for chronic bronchitis and emphysema is COPD: chronic obstructive pulmonary disease. Because chronic bronchitis and emphysema or so often seen together, some specialists do not delineate between these two diseases. COPD is the third leading cause of death in the United States, and it is involved in about 125,000 deaths a year. For more on COPD statistics, see Sidebar 7.3.

Etiology: What Happens?

During a normal breathing cycle, muscles contract to increase the size of the thoracic cavity, and air rushes in to fill the vacuum, stretching the lungs. When those muscles relax, elastin in the epithelium of the lungs pulls them back to their original size. In this way, exhalation is mainly a passive process that doesn't require muscular contraction. To expel extra air from the lungs (this is called expiratory reserve volume), the internal intercostals and transversus abdominus contract to compress the thoracic cavity.

Normal, healthy lungs can be compared to a new balloon: filled with air it is stretched tight, and when it is released, the elastic walls force air out. If we want that to happen faster or more completely, we can squeeze the balloon from the outside. But when the balloon gets old and stretched out, it doesn't snap back to its original size. Its elastic walls don't compress well, and air can linger inside and become stale. This is essentially what happens to the alveoli in emphysema.

The lungs have 300 million alveoli that provide sites for oxygen-carbon dioxide exchange. Each one forms a tiny cup with its own circulatory capillary to allow the exchange of oxygen and carbon dioxide. All healthy alveoli are coated with alpha 1-antitrypsin, a protein that protects elastin from breaking down. Long-term exposure to cigarette smoke or other

SIDEBAR 7.3 Statistics on Chronic Obstructive Pulmonary Disease (COPD)[1]

It can be difficult to separate statistics for emphysema and chronic bronchitis, the two main conditions that make up the group called COPD, because many people have both conditions and many more have them in silent stages that aren't identified until their lungs have accrued extensive damage. Over 13 million people in the United States have been diagnosed with COPD, but about 24 million adults have signs of impaired lung function, so COPD may be underdiagnosed. This disease spectrum costs the United States about $50 billion a year in direct health care expenses and indirect morbidity and mortality expenses.

The single greatest contributing factor to COPD is cigarette smoking; smoking causes 85% to 90% of COPD deaths. Men with COPD outnumbered women for many years; but for the last several years, mortality rate has been higher for women than men.

COPD kills (usually with overwhelming infection and respiratory failure) about 125,000 people every year, making it the third leading cause of death in the United States.

[1] Chronic Obstructive Pulmonary Disease (COPD) Fact Sheet. American Lung Association ©2011. URL: http://www.lungusa.org/lung-disease/copd/resources/in-depth-resources.html. Accessed summer, 2011.

Emphysema in Brief

Pronunciation: em-fih-ZEE-mah

What is it?
Emphysema is a condition in which the alveoli of the lungs become stretched out and inelastic. They merge with each other, decreasing surface area, destroying surrounding capillaries, and limiting oxygen-carbon dioxide exchange.

How is it recognized?
Symptoms of emphysema include shortness of breath with mild or no exertion, a chronic dry cough, rales, cyanosis, and susceptibility to secondary respiratory infection.

Massage risks and benefits

Risks: Emphysema patients may have serious circulatory complications, difficulty lying flat, and a high risk of respiratory infection. All of these require adjustments in bodywork choices.

Benefits: If an emphysema patient is resilient enough to receive massage, attention to the breathing muscles can help with anxiety, fatigue, and efficiency of function. Gentle, reflexive work is always appropriate, as long as the client is comfortable and no-one is at risk for picking up a communicable infection.

pollutants overcomes the protective abilities of alpha 1-antitrypsin, resulting in destruction of the alveolar elastin fibers. The alveoli lose their recoil ability, and they fill up with mucus, which interferes with their ability to exchange oxygen and carbon dioxide. Instead of emptying and filling with every breath, they only partially empty or stay altogether full. This usually begins in a small area, but if the irritation continues, proinflammatory chemicals excreted by damaged cells can cause structural damage throughout the lung. The alveolar walls eventually break down and merge with each other, forming larger sacs, called **bullae** (Figure 7.7). These sacs have less volume and less surface area for gaseous exchange than the uninjured alveoli did.

As the alveoli fuse and surface area for gaseous exchange is lost, the emphysema patient has to work much harder to move air in and out of the lungs. A person with healthy lungs expends about 5% of resting energy in the effort of breathing. A person with advanced emphysema puts closer to 50% of resting energy into this job and must do this every minute, 24 hours a day. For this reason, both eating and sleeping become extremely challenging for emphysema patients.

When alveoli lose function, gaseous exchange is impaired, leading to reduced oxygen levels in the blood, or **hypoxia**. This is not only toxic to brain cells, but it triggers several vicious circles that affect respiration and cardiovascular function. Hypoxia causes the epithelial walls of the alveoli to thicken into tough fibrous connective tissue, which allows even less diffusion than before. As breathing becomes more difficult, respiration rate slows. This leads to even higher concentrations of carbon dioxide in the blood: hypoxia is exacerbated. The blood vessels supplying the damaged alveoli also sustain damage, and hypoxia can cause vascular spasm, so it becomes harder to pump blood through the pulmonary artery.

In addition to cardiovascular challenges, emphysema patients lose much of their ability to resist secondary infection, so they are extremely vulnerable

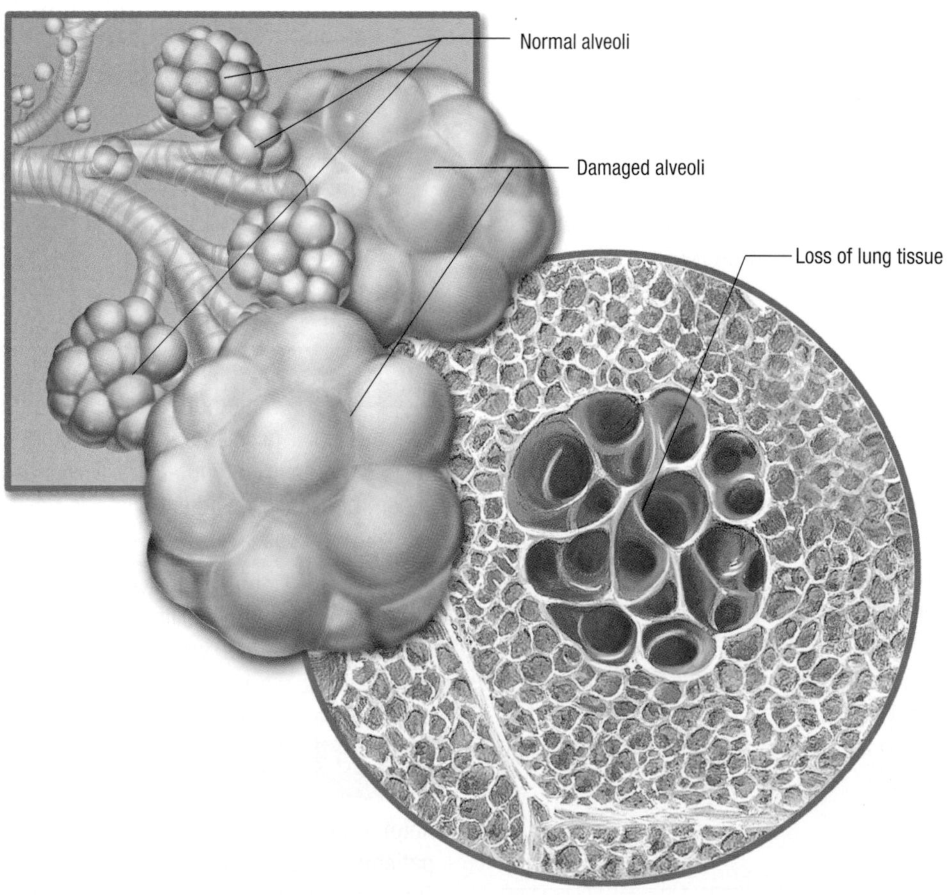

Figure 7.7. Emphysema

to influenza and pneumonia. Another complication occurs if the bullae rupture: this allows air into the pleural space (which is supposed to be completely closed) and ends in total lung collapse, or **pneumothorax**. And finally, the stress to the circulatory system is very great. The right ventricle, trying to pump blood through the partially collapsed pulmonary circuit, enlarges and eventually develops right-sided heart failure, or **cor pulmonale**. The risk of blood clots forming in the circuit is also high, which results in pulmonary embolism. Eventually an untreated emphysema patient undergoes respiratory and circulatory collapse.

The leading cause of the damage seen with both chronic bronchitis and emphysema is exposure to cigarette smoke, although genetic predisposition also clearly plays a role. A small percentage of emphysema patients have an inherited condition in which they are deficient in alpha-1 antitrypsin, so the elastin in their lungs tends to break down early, regardless of whether they smoke.

Signs and Symptoms

It can take many years for emphysema to advance to a stage where symptoms demand that a person seeks medical help. Because it usually affects people over 65 years old, early symptoms are often assumed to be normal signs of aging. These include pain with breathing, shortness of breath, a dry cough, and wheezing. Weight loss often occurs, as a person who must exert so much energy in breathing has little interest in eating. **Rales**, a characteristic bubbling, rasping sound of air moving through a narrowed passage, may occur. Exhalation is labored, and the patient may develop a habit of pushing air out through pursed lips. This is an attempt to push against increasing back pressure in the lungs. Because the lungs no longer deflate normally with each breath, the diaphragm becomes permanently flattened. The emphysema patient often develops "barrel chest"; that is, the intercostals lock into a position that holds the rib cage out as wide as possible.

NOTABLE CASES A short list of influential people whose lives were shortened by chronic obstructive pulmonary disease includes poet T.S. Eliot, talk show host Johnny Carson, the original "Frankenstein" Boris Karloff, founder of Alcoholics Anonymous Bill Wilson, and iconic American painter Norman Rockwell.

Treatment

Emphysema is irreversible. If it is found and treated early, further progression can be slowed or stopped. But once the alveoli have begun to break down, they don't recover. The first course of action is to remove any irritating stimulus; usually this is cigarette smoke.

Medication for emphysema can dilate the bronchi and take pressure off the alveoli, remove mucus and edema from the lungs, and ward off potential lung infections. Emphysema and other COPD patients are often strongly urged to be vaccinated against pneumococcus pneumonia and to get a yearly flu shot, because they are at higher risk for serious lung infections than the general population.

Oxygen supplementation may be recommended during sleep or following exercise.

Lung volume reduction surgery removes only damaged portions of the lung. This increases thoracic capacity for the diaphragm to work and improves circulation. Lung transplants are a last-ditch option that has been successful for some patients: emphysema is the leading reason for lung transplants.

Medications

- Nicotine patches or gum to aid in quitting smoking
- Short-acting and long-acting bronchodilators to reduce airway resistance
- Inhaled and oral corticosteroids, to manage inflammation
- Mucolytics and expectorants to help clear the lungs of mucus
- Antibiotics as necessary

Massage?

RISKS The major risks for working with a client with emphysema include the possibility of cardiovascular problems, difficulty lying flat, and secondary respiratory infection. These can be accommodated with adjustments to positioning and modality choices.

BENEFITS Gentle, reflexive massage (with respect for the possibility of infection) is appropriate for emphysema patients, who often feel debilitating fatigue. More specific work on muscles of the chest, shoulders, and neck can be beneficial if the client can tolerate it.

OPTIONS Massage that focuses on the muscles of inspiration and expiration can be especially helpful for chronic obstructive pulmonary disease patients and anyone who has breathing difficulties. Reducing the effort that it takes to breathe can allow patients to feel energized and less fatigued.

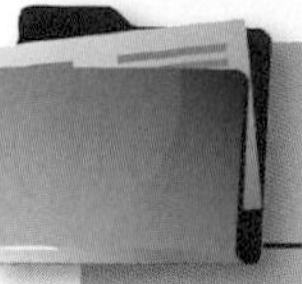

CASE HISTORY 7.1 Emphysema

Roberta started smoking in 1947 and quit in 1984. In the mid 1980s, she noticed that she was frequently short of breath, had low energy, and had consistent headaches on rising each morning. She was unable to walk far or fast. In an effort to catch her breath, she hyperventilated easily, which only made matters worse. She had a lot of stress and frustration because breathing was so difficult and she could no longer accomplish the things she wanted to do.

Roberta's primary care physician diagnosed chronic obstructive pulmonary disease and chronic bronchitis. She also saw a pulmonary specialist who diagnosed emphysema. This finding was based on a number of tests, including chest radiography, spirometry, an analysis of arterial blood gases, and measurement of the air volume she was able to expel.

Emphysema makes it hard for Roberta to do anything. The activities of daily living are difficult, and every daily routine has to be altered to accommodate the disease. Stairs and hills are especially challenging. Emphysema dulls the thinking by depriving the brain of oxygen. It reduces appetite, and the lack of oxygen reduces the benefit from what food is eaten. It also strains the heart, because the heart has to work harder to push more blood, which contains less oxygen, through the body.

ROBERTA F., AGE 68: "Emphysema makes it hard for Roberta to do anything... every daily routine has to be altered."

Roberta also has osteoporosis. This condition, in combination with her breathing difficulties, has significantly altered her posture. Her shoulders rise to her ears as she attempts to get more air, and her chest is compressed because of her spine.

Another aspect of Roberta's experience with emphysema is how it has seriously affected her resistance to disease.

In June 1997, she had a bad cold, which put her in the hospital for 4 days.

In January 1998, Roberta contracted pneumonia, which was confirmed by chest radiography. She was in the hospital for 5 days. The pneumonia cleared up with antibiotics, and she returned home.

Roberta is now feeling improved. She still supplements oxygen, and her daily activities have become a little easier. She tries to keep up with her exercises, eat properly, and reduce stress. She also attends Better Breathing Club meetings sponsored by the American Lung Association to keep up with new information about techniques to deal with her disease, and she sees her pulmonary specialist regularly.

Author's note: Roberta passed away from pneumonia in 2002. Many thanks to her and her family for generously sharing her story.■

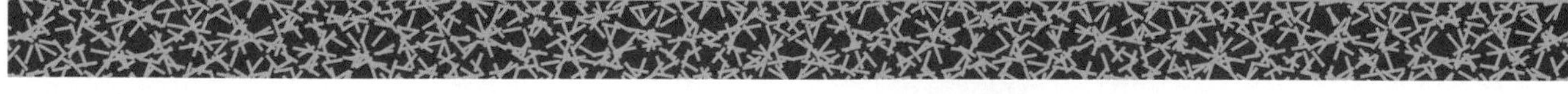

Other Respiratory Disorders

Asthma

Definition: What Is It?

Asthma is a chronic disorder of the airways that interferes with breathing. It may be triggered by external factors such as allergens or pollutants, but it is also linked to internal factors such as emotional stress.

Etiology: What Happens?

All bronchioles are sensitive to foreign debris, but asthmatics' bronchioles are extremely irritable and hyperreactive. Furthermore, the bronchial tubes of a person with asthma appear to be in a state of ongoing inflammation, always poised to begin an attack. When they encounter a trigger, the irritated membranes lining these tubes swell and secrete extra mucus (Figure 7.8). Some small passageways may become completely obstructed by mucous plugs during an attack. People with asthma find it very difficult to breathe, especially to exhale, during an episode; this is called respiratory distress.

Pet-related allergens, cockroach wastes, cigarette smoke, and dust mites have been found to be especially potent asthma triggers. The high rate of asthma among young children supports the "hygiene hypothesis": infants and toddlers, especially in industrialized countries, are generally more protected from immune system challenges than those of previous generations. This appears to set up the immune system to be more

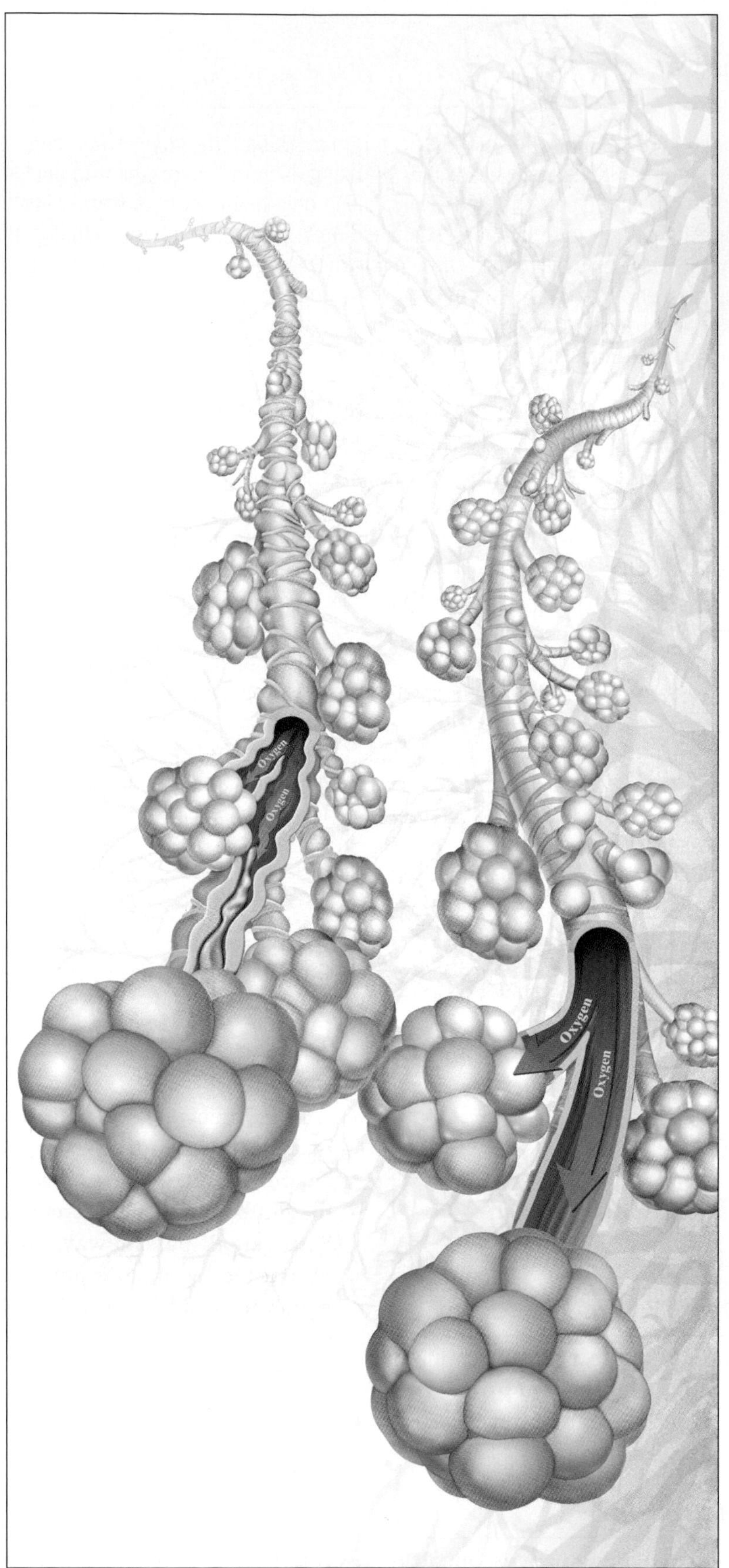

Figure 7.8. Asthma. *To see a video of the author discussing asthma and the massage room environment, go to http://thePoint.lww.com/Werner5e.*

Asthma in Brief

Pronunciation: AZ-muh

What is it?
Asthma is the result of airway inflammation, intermittent airflow obstruction, and bronchial hyper-responsiveness.

How is it recognized?
Asthma attacks are sporadic episodes involving coughing, wheezing, and difficulty with breathing, especially exhaling.

Massage risks and benefits
Risks: A client in the midst of an acute asthma attack is not a good candidate for massage. It is important to prepare the session room for clients with a tendency toward asthma by avoiding scents, candles, and essential oils that might exacerbate symptoms, and by using a hypoallergenic lubricant.
Benefits: Clients with asthma or other breathing problems, who are not in the midst of an acute episode, typically have extremely tight breathing muscles: the diaphragm, intercostals, and scalenes can benefit run any work that improves their efficiency.

reactive to potential allergens. Among adults, gastroesophageal reflux disorder (GERD), sensitivity to aspirin, and some occupational exposures have been seen to exacerbate asthma.

Asthma is typically rated by severity and pattern. These labels help to determine the best balance of treatment options to control symptoms.

- Mild, intermittent asthma means that episodes occur less than twice a week, and between episodes breathing is normal. This variety may have little impact on activity.
- Mild, persistent asthma means that episodes occur more often than twice a week, up to once a day. Nighttime episodes might happen once a month. Frequency and severity may affect activities.
- Moderate, persistent asthma is characterized by episodes every day and nighttime attacks at least once a week.
- Severe, persistent asthma means that attacks occur most days and nights, and activity is severely limited.

Types of Asthma

- *Bronchial asthma.* This is a typical form with tight bronchioles and excessive mucus production and wheezing during episodes.
- *Exercise-induced asthma.* This version occurs with physical exertion, although symptoms are sometimes delayed for several hours. It is probably a multifactoral problem, but hard-working athletes may not be able to adequately condition the air that is taken into their lungs, leading to a higher risk of irritation.
- *Silent asthma.* In this situation, no symptoms warn of an impending episode, but then the patient suddenly is dangerously short of breath.
- *Cough variant asthma.* This form shows coughing alone as its primary symptom. It is frequently worst in the middle of the night.

Signs and Symptoms

Symptoms of asthma include **dyspnea** (shortness of breath), wheezing (the sound of air moving through tightened and clogged bronchioles), and coughing that may or may not be productive. While inhaling is not difficult, exhaling is extremely li mited: the bronchioles are constricted, so the alveoli don't empty easily. Even with deep inhalation, oxygen levels drop because the stale air in the lungs cannot be replaced; hyperinflation of the lungs is the result.

If the symptoms are extreme and prolonged, the asthmatic person may start to feel panicky. This may add sweating, increased heart rate, and anxiety to the list of symptoms. In emergencies, the lips and face may take on a bluish cast (**cyanosis**) when access to oxygen is severely restricted.

NOTABLE CASES Many elite athletes report that they live with asthma. Among them are the following Olympic medalists: Greg Lougainis (diving), Tom Dolan (swimming), Bill Koch (crosscountry skiing), and Jackie Joyner-Kersee (track and field).

Asthma attacks are sporadic, lasting anywhere from a few minutes to a few days, but between attacks the lungs are normal. Eventually, however, some airway remodeling may become evident. Hypertrophy of smooth muscle cells and fibrosis of the epithelial membranes can leave a permanent mark of asthma affects.

Treatment

Treatment for asthma begins with limiting exposure to the stimuli that are known to trigger attacks. Drugs are typically prescribed to manage this chronic disorder, in order to reduce the risk of acute attacks. Patients are also taught to recognize the warning signs of an attack, so it can be treated as quickly as possible.

Medical intervention is available in several forms with two basic goals: immediate relief and long-term control. Short-term intervention is administration of beta agonist inhalers that act as bronchodilators. Inhaled or orally taken steroids can be used for long-term control.

When asthma attacks are directly related to a respiratory allergy, patients are often advised to take allergy medication and to consider immunotherapy: allergy shots to help desensitize the system to a particular allergen.

Medications

- Bronchodilators to reduce airway resistance
- Inhaled or oral corticosteroids as long-term anti-inflammatories
- Antihistamines for allergy control

Massage?

RISKS For clients who have asthma and other hypersensitivity situations, it is important to create an environment that is as free from allergens as possible. This means avoiding any heavy scents, essential oils that are irritating, and lubricants that are not hypoallergenic. Clients with asthma may use medication that demands adaptation for massage.

BENEFITS Massage can be soothing for a person who lives in anxiety about being able to draw a deep breath, and it can help make profound changes in the ease with which breathing happens.

OPTIONS Specific attention to the muscles of inhalation and exhalation (intercostals, scalenes, serratus posterior, and diaphragm) can make a dramatic difference in the resting tension and overall efficiency of these muscles.

Cystic Fibrosis

Definition: What Is It?

Cystic fibrosis (CF) is an autosomal recessive genetic disorder. This means that a person must inherit

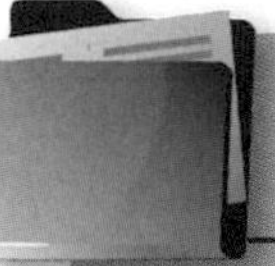

CASE HISTORY 7.2 Asthma

RICHARD L., AGED 52: "Do you have any pets?"

I didn't contract asthma until I was 22, after I got back from Vietnam. I was living in Los Angeles, and I got real bad bronchitis. I was diagnosed then with just a common smog problem.

Then I moved to Corvallis, Oregon, and ran into the Willamette Valley crud: they have pollination 10 months of the year there. I saw an allergist who gave me skin tests, and I came up positive to 95% of the things he tested me for. I realized it wasn't just the smog; I had a lung problem.

When I moved to Seattle, I wound up with an asthma specialist who's been really good for me. I've had a few bouts here; one time a cold put me in the hospital for about a week.

I've been doing massage since the 1960s but just recently went to school and got licensed. I'm really sensitive to perfumes, and massage school students are 90% female, so I'd always choose where to sit away from anyone wearing perfume. But I never thought about massage oils until we got into it. I knew to stay away from oils and lotions that are scented at all. When I got a massage with almond oil, I noticed my skin would turn really red, but it wasn't until someone worked on my chest and back that I noticed about an hour later my breathing was affected.

Asthma affects my life in all kinds of ways. My lung capacity is only about 65% of normal. I like to go listen to music, but the venues where the good bands play are always too smoky. I have to stay away from flower shops. It was almost impossible to go into a mall because you have to walk past the perfume counter to get through the big department stores. Asthma really limits my social life too. When someone asks us over to dinner, our first question has to be, "Do you have any pets?"■

Cystic Fibrosis in Brief

Pronunciation: SIS-tik fy-BRO-sis

What is it?
Cystic fibrosis (CF) is a congenital disease of exocrine glands that causes their secretions (mainly mucus, digestive enzymes, bile, and sweat) to become abnormally thick and viscous.

How is it recognized?
CF is a multisystem disease, but its effects on the respiratory system are typically the most common and most serious. Signs and symptoms include chronic lung infections, shortness of breath, productive cough, digestive difficulties, and failure to thrive in very young children.

Massage risks and benefits
Risks: People with CF are extremely vulnerable to respiratory infections. This obviously presents a caution for most kinds of bodywork.
Benefits: CF patients receive therapy to help dislodge mucus from the lungs; massage can be used in this context as well. As long as clients are not dealing with respiratory infection, any bodywork that fits within their capacity for adaptation can improve their quality of life.

one faulty gene from each parent. It affects exocrine glands, causing production of thick, viscous secretions. The digestive, integumentary, and reproductive system glands are all involved with this disease, but the greatest impact is on the respiratory system.

It is estimated that about 12 million people in the United States carry the CF gene, although many don't know. About 30,000 people in the United States have CF at any given time. Before the 1950s, the life expectancy for a person with CF was under 10 years. Today, about 45% of CF patients today are over 18 years old, and the median life expectancy is about 35 and getting higher with the development of new treatment options.

Etiology: What Happens?

Several hundred slightly different mutations can lead to CF, but the net result is that the transmembrane conductance regulator gene is altered so that cell membranes in secreting tissues can't conduct chloride. This changes how these cells use water and leads to abnormally thick, sticky secretions in many exocrine glands but most particularly in the respiratory tract, digestive tract, skin, and reproductive tract (Figure 7.9).

- *Respiratory system.* CF usually has its most profound effects on the respiratory system. The changes in mucous membrane function cause

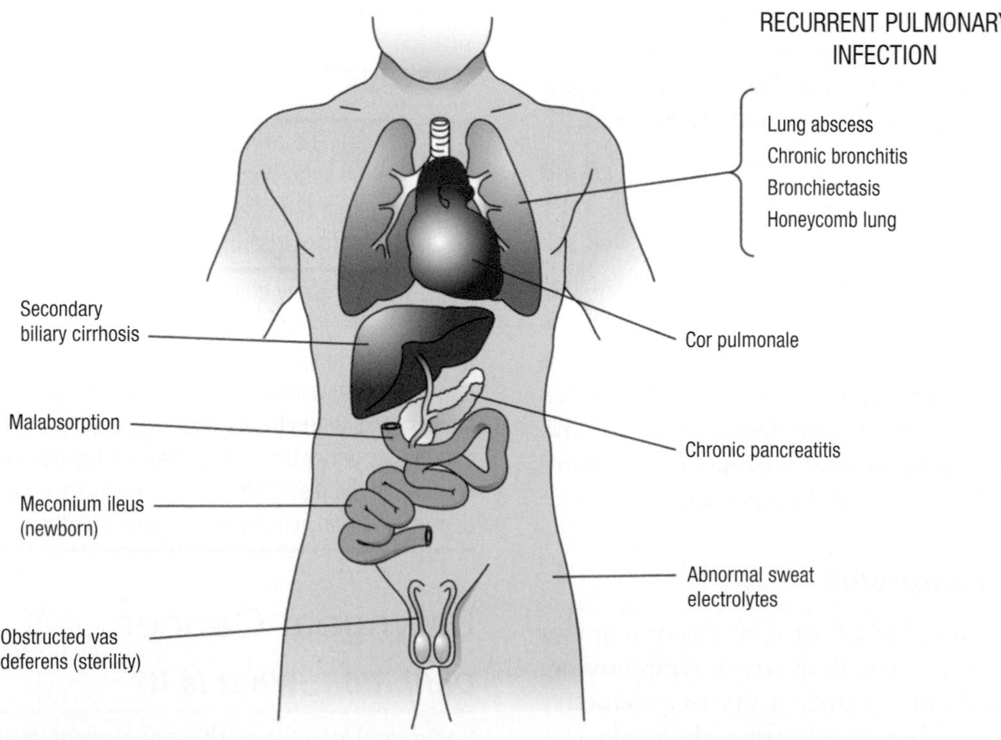

Figure 7.9. Cystic fibrosis

mucus in the respiratory tract to become thick, gluey, and difficult to dislodge. This provides a rich growth medium for bacterial infection. Because of the genetic dysfunction, immune system action against pathogens reinforces the inflammatory response, which causes more damage and supports rather than suppresses infection. A variety of bacterial agents may create chronic infection, but the one that is the most difficult to eradicate is *Pseudomonas aeruginosa*. Other respiratory system changes include the growth of nasal polyps and the development of chronic rhinitis. Ultimately, congestion in the lungs can alter the pulmonary circulation and lead to the possibility of right-sided heart failure.

- *Digestive system*. Digestive system dysfunction can affect both the gastrointestinal tract and the accessory organs. A warning sign for CF is a baby born with an intestinal obstruction; this happens because the mucus in the small and large intestines doesn't move well. Poor absorption in the small intestine also leads to greasy, bulky stools and failure to thrive. Limited access to vitamins and minerals can cause important deficiencies. Adults with CF are vulnerable to osteoporosis. CF can interfere with the normal production of bile and drainage of bile into the small intestine, leading to an enlarged spleen, gallstones, portal hypertension, liver congestion, or cirrhosis. Poor secretion of bicarbonate and digestive enzymes from the pancreas can lead to diabetes and peptic ulcers in the duodenum and pancreatitis.
- *Integumentary system*. CF affects sweat glands in the skin, leading to abnormally thick, salty perspiration and the risk of heat stroke and salt depletion, especially in infants.
- *Reproductive system*. Almost all men with CF are sterile. This occurs because the epididymis cannot secrete normally or because the vas deferens doesn't form completely. Women with CF often have normal reproductive systems and can have successful pregnancies.

Signs and Symptoms

Signs and symptoms of CF vary by the system that is affected most severely. Respiratory symptoms are most common. They include a dry or productive cough, shortness of breath, wheezing, chest pain, cyanosis, hemoptysis (coughing up blood), and clubbing of fingers, which occurs with oxygen deprivation in the extremities.

Signs and symptoms of other affected systems are discussed in the etiology section.

Treatment

CF is not curable; treatment options focus on symptoms and complications. Devices to help break up congestion in the lungs, along with breathing exercises to maintain and improve function, are often suggested. Taking food in easily digestible forms, supplementing vitamins and enzymes, and exercising to increase or maintain lung function are recommended for people who are not fighting acute infection or intestinal blockages.

Bronchodilators, mucolytics, antibiotics to fight infection, and anti-inflammatories are typical medical interventions for CF patients. Patients with advanced cases may be candidates for lung transplants, although this procedure has a high rejection rate.

Medications

- Inhaled bronchodilators to reduce resistance in airways
- Inhaled mucolytics and saline to help dissolve mucus
- Inhaled and oral antibiotics as needed for bacterial respiratory infection
- Anti-inflammatories

Massage?

RISKS The primary risk for working with a client who has cystic fibrosis (CF) is respiratory infection: either the client may be ill, or the therapist may be inadvertently carrying pathogens that put a client at risk.

BENEFITS Many children and adults with CF undergo intense physiotherapy to dislodge deposits of mucus in the lungs, and when no acute infection is present, they are recommended to exercise within tolerance to build stamina and strength. Massage is probably safe and appropriate under these circumstances as long as the therapist works with the rest of the health care team, is healthy, and doesn't share any virulent pathogens with the client.

Laryngeal Cancer

Definition: What Is It?

Laryngeal cancer is the development of malignant growths on and around the larynx. It is a relatively

Laryngeal Cancer in Brief

What is it?
Laryngeal cancer is the development of malignant cells somewhere in the larynx. These cells may metastasize to other locations in the head or neck, or may migrate to the lungs.

How is it recognized?
Hoarseness, a feeling that something is constantly stuck in the throat, and a persistent cough are some of the signs of laryngeal cancer.

Massage risks and benefits

Risks: The side effects of laryngeal cancer treatment can be severe. In addition, many laryngeal cancer patients may have a temporary or permanent stoma: an opening into the trachea that bypasses the soft tissues of the throat. This device is vulnerable to being disturbed or contaminated. Any bodywork must accommodate for these challenges.

Benefits: As with other types of cancer, massage can be a useful strategy to help improve sleep and appetite, reduce anxiety and depression, minimize postsurgical pain, and generally add to the quality of life.

common disease, diagnosed about 12,000 times a year in the United States, and leading to about 4,000 deaths.

Etiology: What Happens?

The larynx is the portion of the throat where the division of the digestive and respiratory tracts occurs. This 2-in long, 2-in wide structure is often discussed as three subparts: the supraglottis, which connects to the pharynx; the glottis, which holds the vocal cords; and the subglottis, which connects the larynx to the trachea. A small flap called the epiglottis forms a protective shield over the respiratory tract to prevent the aspiration of liquids or solids into the lungs.

A healthy larynx is vital for speech, swallowing, protection of the respiratory tract, and breath control. When the larynx is compromised, any of these functions may be impaired, and the risk for a life-threatening lung infection from aspirated material is very high.

The larynx is vulnerable to several types of growths, including polyps, nodules, and tumors (Figure 7.10). When tumors are cancerous, they almost always begin in the squamous cell lining of the glottis and may spread from there through the throat to the tongue and into other structures of the neck,

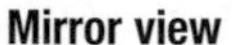

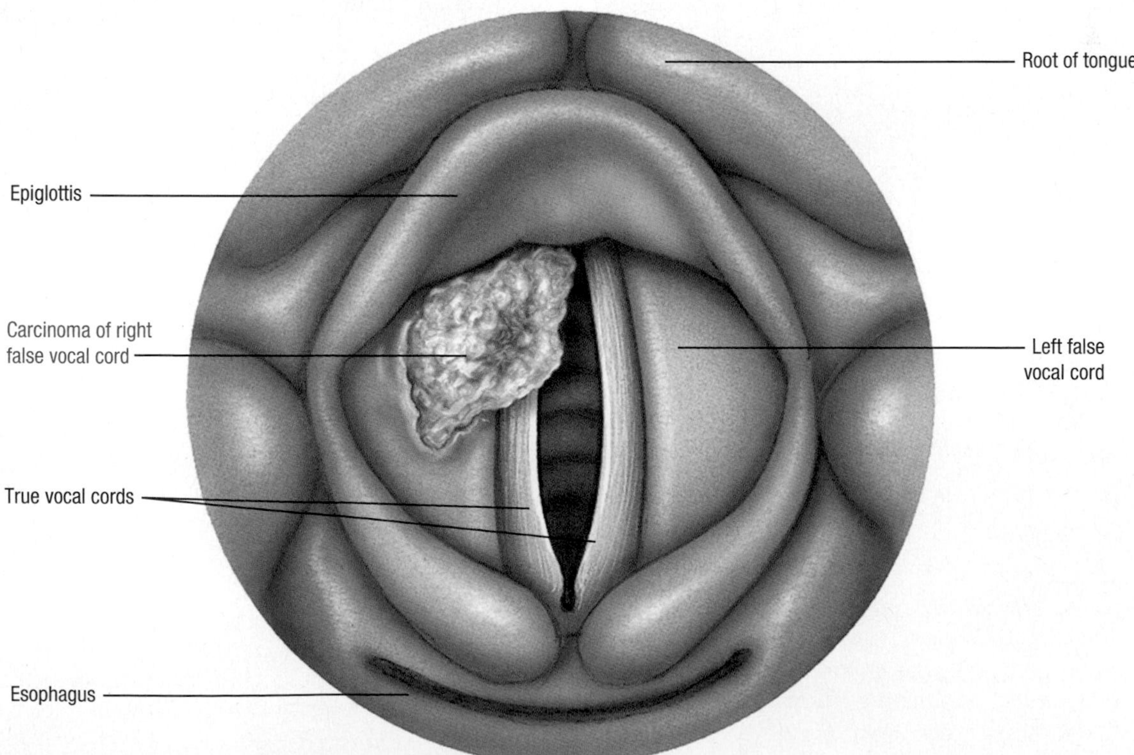

Figure 7.10. Laryngeal cancer affecting the vocal cords

including the cervical lymph nodes. Metastasis to the lungs is common for this form of cancer.

A specific cause for laryngeal cancer has not been identified. Rather, as with many types of cancer, risk factors appear to accumulate to increase the possibility that a person will develop this disease. The main risk factors for laryngeal cancer include using tobacco of any kind, and drinking excessive alcohol, and these two habits tend to potentiate each other. That is, the risk associated with drinking *and* smoking is greater than for the risks of each behavior accrued separately. Other risk factors include age (laryngeal cancer is seldom identified in people under 55), gender (it is four times more common in men than in women), exposure to human papilloma virus, poor dental hygiene, a diet poor in Vitamin A and beta-carotene, having a history of GERD, a history of radiation to the neck for other reasons, and a history of exposure to nickel, sulfuric acid, or asbestos.

Signs and Symptoms

Early signs and symptoms of laryngeal cancer may be subtle. They typically include a chronic cough, hoarseness, sore throat, and a feeling of something being "stuck" in the back of the throat. Bad breath, problems breathing, and ear ache are also frequently reported. Later in the process, a person with laryngeal cancer may have blood in their sputum and unintentional weight loss.

Treatment

Laryngeal cancer is treated aggressively, but the larynx performs such vital functions that oncologists

SIDEBAR 7.4 Staging Laryngeal Cancer

Laryngeal cancer staging identifies three major factors to predict the prognosis and to determine the best treatment options: the number of subsites on the larynx where the cancer is found, the mobility or fixedness of the vocal cords, and the presence of metastases to the cervical lymph nodes and beyond. Laryngeal subsites are identified as the supraglottis, the glottis, and the subglottis.

Here is a simplified version of the laryngeal cancer staging protocol, first in the TNM format, and then translated into the Stage 0 to IV format:

(T) Tumor assessment

Tx	Tumor cannot be assessed
T0	No evidence of primary tumor in situ
T1	One subsite affected; vocal cords are mobile
T2	Invasion into nearby tissues; vocal cord mobility is mildly impaired
T3	Invasion into nearby tissues, vocal cords are fixed
T4	Invasion throughout larynx, local cartilage, and soft tissues of the anterior neck

(N) Node assessment

Nx	Node involvement cannot be assessed
N0	No node involvement
N1	1 node is invaded with a growth <3 cm
N2	1 node is invaded with a growth 3 to 6 cm, or multiple nodes on the same side with growths <6 cm, or multiple nodes on both sides with growths <6 cm
N3	Any growths in nodes >6 cm

(M) Metastasis

Mx	Metastasis cannot be assessed
M0	No distant metastasis is found
M1	Distant metastasis is found

Stage 0 to IV

Stage 0	Tis, N0, M0
Stage I	T1, N0, M0
Stage II	T2, N0, M0
Stage III	T3, N0, M0 or T-1-3, N1, M0
Stage IV-a	T4, N0, M0 or T4, N1, M0 or T-any, N2, M0
Stage IV-b	T4, N-any, M0 or T-any, N3, M0
Stage IV-c	T-any, N-any, M1

consider preserving the best function possible as a high priority. Consequently, radiation and chemotherapy, which spare the larynx, are often pursued before surgery to remove cancerous tissue. Surgical procedures also emphasize preserving the best possible function, so that the risk of future problems with speech or accidental aspiration of solids or liquids into the trachea can be minimized.

Medications

- Chemotherapeutic drugs
- Analgesics following surgery

Massage?

RISKS As with other cancers, risks for working with laryngeal cancer patients center more on the treatments than on the cancer itself. Radiation, chemotherapy, and surgery must all be accommodated with modality choices.

BENEFITS Massage can reduce anxiety and depression, improve appetite and sleep, and generally add to the quality of life for a person with laryngeal or other types of cancer.

OPTIONS Laryngeal cancer patients may have a temporary stoma placed in their neck: this is vulnerable to disruption and contamination. More information about massage in the context of cancer patients is found in Chapter 12.

Lung Cancer

Definition: What Is It?

Lung cancer is the growth of malignant cells in the lungs. These cells eventually form tumors, but because they have extremely easy access to both the circulatory and lymph systems, they are capable of spreading to other tissues (metastasizing) before tumors are detectable.

Lung cancer is an example of epithelial cancer that tends to grow where tissue is vulnerable to repeated irritation and damage.

It is estimated that about 203,000 people are diagnosed and 157,000 people die of this disease each year. About 370,000 lung cancer patients are alive in the United States today. The average lung cancer patient is a person in the sixth to seventh decade of life who has smoked for 20 years or more.

Lung Cancer in Brief

What is it?
Lung cancer is development of malignant cells in the lungs. These cells have easy access to blood and lymph vessels, and can quickly spread to other organs in the body.

How is it recognized?
The early symptoms of lung cancer are difficult to distinguish from irritation related to tobacco use: a chronic cough, bloodstained sputum, shortness of breath, chest pain, and recurrent bronchitis or pneumonia.

Massage risks and benefits
Risks: Lung cancer patients are likely either to be undergoing very aggressive treatment, which carries several cautions for bodywork, or looking for palliative care for symptomatic relief at the end of life. In this situation, bodywork practitioners must be mindful of positioning, pressure, and medical equipment that may be disrupted. Any work that puts a client at risk for exacerbating pain or other complications must be avoided.
Benefits: Massage has been seen to offer several benefits for cancer patients, including reducing pain, anxiety, fatigue and depression, and improving sleep and appetite.

Cancer is the second leading cause of death in the United States, and lung cancer accounts for 28% of cancer deaths. It causes more deaths than breast, colon, and prostate cancers (the next three runners up) combined.

Etiology: What Happens?

Lung cancer occurs in epithelial cells that are chronically irritated by environmental contaminants. Although cigarette, pipe, and cigar smoke are responsible for 85% to 90% of cases of lung cancer, other causes have also been identified, including exposure to **radon**, asbestos, uranium, arsenic, and air pollution. These are all much more potent carcinogens when they are paired with smoking.

When the epithelial cells that line the respiratory tract have a long history of exposure to highly toxic substances, their orderly pattern of replication and repair is eventually disrupted. Abnormal cells accumulate in uncontrolled and disorganized patches (Figure 7.11). A rich supply of blood and lymph vessels allows mutated cells to travel out of their immediate area before a detectable tumor appears; this is why lung cancer is seldom found before metastasis.

The lymph nodes around the lungs and in the mediastinum are often the first site of metastasis for lung cancer. From there the cells have access to distant places in the body. The liver, bone tissue, adrenal glands, and brain are frequently invaded.

The most obvious risk factor for lung cancer is smoking. Cigarette smoke contains multiple known carcinogens, and the tar in cigarettes holds the damaging chemicals close to the delicate linings of the lungs. In addition to airborne toxins, lung cancer is a risk for people who have had radiation to the chest for breast cancer or other treatments or a history of tuberculosis, chronic obstructive pulmonary disease, or severe lung infections.

Every year thousands of people who were never smokers die of lung cancer. These cases are often linked to second-hand or sidestream smoke or other risk factors, but the potential for inherited predisposition is now being actively pursued through genetic research. This may eventually yield ways to identify people at particularly high risk for lung cancer, along with ways to identify it early and treat it more successfully.

SIDEBAR 7.5 Staging Lung Cancer

The staging protocol for lung cancer depends on whether the diagnosis is for small cell or non–small cell lung cancer. It is important to stage any kind of cancer accurately to choose the best possible treatment options. Patients may also choose to volunteer for clinical trials to add to the body of knowledge about best options according to stage.

Small cell lung cancer, because it is so aggressive and is usually inoperable, is described as being either limited or extensive. Limited small cell lung cancer means that it is found in only one lung and local lymph nodes; extensive small cell lung cancer means that it is found in both lungs, multiple nodes, and in distant areas as well.

Non–small cell lung cancer comes in several forms; but they are similar in presentation and treatment protocols, so they are all staged together using a combination of the TNM and stage 0 to IV classifications. These staging protocols are described in detail in Chapter 12. Here is a simplified version of non–small cell lung cancer staging:

These delineations are then translated into stages 0 to IV in this way:

Tumor (T)	Node (N)	Metastasis (M)
T X: positive findings on tests; no lesion found	N 0: no nodes involved	M 0: no metastasis found
T IS: cancer in situ, limited to endothelial cells	N 1: some nodes involved near affected lung	M 1: distant metastasis found
T 1: tumor <3 cm in diameter	N 2: nodes in mediastinum on side of affected lung	
T 2: tumor is 3–7 cm in diameter; may involve pleura or bronchi	N 3: Nodes on opposite side of involved lung	
T 3: tumor >7 cm, extensions into nearby structures		
T 4: tumor invasion of mediastinal structures		

Stage	Tumor	Node	Metastasis
I A	T 1	N 0	M 0
I B	T 2	N 0	M 0
II A	T 1–2	N 1	M 0
III A	T 1–3	N 1–2	M 0
III B	T 1–4	N 1–3	M 0
IV	T any	N any	M 1

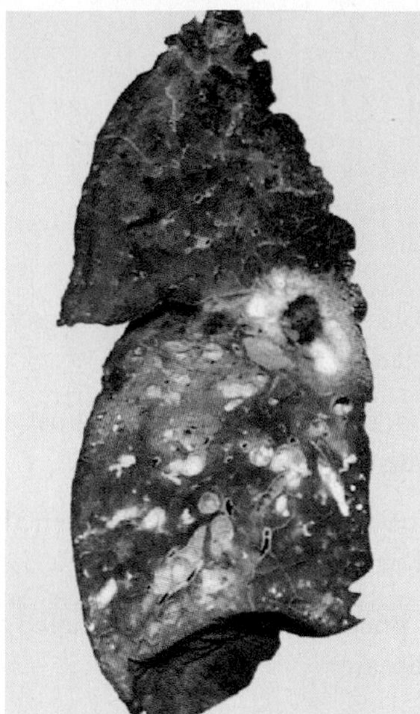

Figure 7.11. Lung cancer

Types of Lung Cancer

- *Small cell lung cancer.* This is also called "oat cell" carcinoma. It accounts for 20% of lung cancers. Small cell lung cancer grows fast, spreads quickly, and is rarely operable.
- *Non–small cell lung cancer.* This includes several types of cancers, depending on which cells they affect first. Non–small cell carcinomas account for about 85% of lung cancers. They include squamous cell carcinoma, adenocarcinoma, large cell carcinoma, and several others. Most of these grow more slowly than small cell carcinoma, but the symptoms they produce are so subtle that diagnosis doesn't usually happen until long after the cancer has spread beyond its original area.
- *Other types of lung malignancies.* Small cell and non–small cell lung cancers account for most types of cancer, but a few cases of other types are identified as well. These include carcinoid tumors, adenoid cystic carcinoma, sarcomas, and others. **Mesothelioma** is a type of cancer that arises in the pleural sac that surrounds the lung; this is closely associated with asbestos exposure.

Signs and Symptoms

One of the most challenging problems with lung cancer is that it is extremely difficult to identify early. The growth of abnormal cells in alveoli, bronchial linings, or mucous membranes stimulates virtually no changes in function or sensation. A persistent smoker's cough is one early sign, along with bloodstained phlegm, chronic chest pain, wheezing, and possibly shortness of breath. None of these symptoms seems cause for alarm, since a smoker or someone who works with irritating chemicals often has them regardless of the health of their respiratory tract cells.

NOTABLE CASES The list of influential lives that have been cut short by lung cancer is too long to contemplate. Among them are musician George Harrison; water lilies painter Claude Monet, singer Rosemary Clooney, animator and innovator Walt Disney, actor and director Paul Newman, and Dana Reeve ("Superman" Christopher Reeve's wife), who never smoked.

Later signs of lung cancer may be more revealing. If a tumor grows near the apex of the lung, it may put mechanical pressure on the brachial plexus, leading to symptoms that mimic thoracic outlet syndrome. A tumor that presses on the superior vena cava may cause facial swelling and dilated blood vessels in the neck and face; this is called **superior vena cava syndrome**. If a tumor protrudes on the esophagus or larynx, a person may have chronic hoarseness. Tumors that press on the phrenic nerve can paralyze the diaphragm.

Treatment

Treatment for lung cancer depends on what kind of cancer is growing and how far it has progressed. For the lucky few who find non–small cell lung cancer while it is still local, surgery followed by radiation may be adequate. The surgery could involve the removal of a small section of lung tissue (a wedge resection), the removal of an entire lobe (a **lobectomy**), or even the removal of an entire lung (a **pneumonectomy**).

Small cell carcinoma grows so fast and spreads so quickly that it is generally treated with radiation and chemotherapy alone; surgery usually has no chance of containing the growth. While this can be successful in the short run, most small cell lung cancer patients have a recurrence within 2 years, and the cancer tends to become unresponsive to treatment.

Targeted therapies for lung cancer include the use of biologically engineered antibodies that deliver drugs or radiation to cancer cells; drugs that interfere with angiogenesis; drugs that inhibit cancer cell growth factors; drugs that make cancer cells sensitive to light; and a cancer "vaccine" that essentially introduces a substance that makes immune system cells more sensitive to cancer cells. All of these are still in experimental use, and they all carry serious potential side effects, but they may eventually be both more effective and less risky than traditional cancer treatments.

Medications

- Chemotherapeutic agents to kill fast-growing cells
- Targeted therapies to
  - Deliver treatment to cancer cells
  - Interfere with angiogenesis
  - Suppress local growth factors
  - Use light to kill cancer cells
  - Stimulate immune system responses against cancer cells
- Medication to ameliorate the side effects of chemotherapy

Massage?

RISKS A person with lung cancer may be undergoing extremely aggressive treatment to manage this disease; chemotherapy, radiation, and surgery all have specific cautions for massage. Alternatively, he or she may be at the end of life and seeking strictly palliative care, in which case bodywork must be adjusted for frailty, the risk of problems with bones or major organs, and any medical equipment that can be disrupted.

BENEFITS Massage can be a supportive strategy for a person going through a challenging time. It can help with insomnia, pain, fatigue, anxiety, and depression—all of which can make both the cancer and the side effects of medication seem worse.

OPTIONS Details about massage in the context of cancer are covered in Chapter 12.

CHAPTER REVIEW QUESTIONS: RESPIRATORY SYSTEM CONDITIONS

1. How does the structure of the lungs work to limit the spread of infection?
2. What is the best strategy against catching or spreading a cold virus?
3. Are antibiotics effective to shorten the duration of cold or flu? Why?
4. Why is pneumonia sometimes called an opportunistic disease?
5. What is MDR-TB? What is XDR-TB? How did these types of infection arise?
6. Why is cystic fibrosis associated with a high risk of lung infection?
7. What is the relationship between chronic bronchitis and acute bronchitis?
8. How does emphysema lead to right-sided heart failure?
9. A client has sinusitis. Her mucus is thick, opaque, and sticky. She has had a headache and a mild fever for several days. Is she a good candidate for massage? Why or why not?
10. Your client, a smoker, reports a mild cough and shortness of breath. She gets colds easily, and they often disable her for several days or even weeks. You notice that she clears her throat very frequently. What condition is probably present? What strategies might serve her best in a bodywork session?
11. Your client has asthma. Name three ways to minimize the risk of his having an attack as a result of visiting your session room.
12. Why is it difficult to find lung cancer in early stages?

8

Digestive System Conditions

Chapter Objectives

After reading this chapter, you should be able to . . .

- Name what structures are damaged with celiac disease.
- Name the most dangerous complication of gastroesophageal reflux disorder.
- Identify the aggressive and defensive factors that contribute to peptic ulcers.
- Identify the precancerous condition associated with colorectal cancer.
- Explain why irritable bowel syndrome can also be called functional bowel syndrome.
- Name three possible complications of ulcerative colitis.
- List symptoms or complications of cirrhosis.
- Name the primary modes of communicability for hepatitis A, hepatitis B, and hepatitis C.
- Name three risk factors for liver cancer.
- Identify two types of pancreatitis and the behavior that is common to both.

The Digestive Tract: Structure and Function

The best way to discuss how the digestive tract works is to follow a piece of food through the system (Figure 8.1).

When the teeth grind a morsel of food, it is broken into small pieces so that the digestive enzymes in saliva and the rest of the gastrointestinal (GI) tract have access to the nutrients. The food moves from the mouth down the esophagus, through the lower esophageal sphincter, and into a wide place in the tube: the stomach. Here it is further pulverized by powerful muscular contractions and exposed to more corrosive chemicals. When the former food, now referred to as **chyme**, moves through the pyloric valve into the small intestine, the gallbladder and pancreas add their secretions. By now the barrage of digestive enzymes has reduced the meal into its most primitive building blocks: sugars, fats, and proteins.

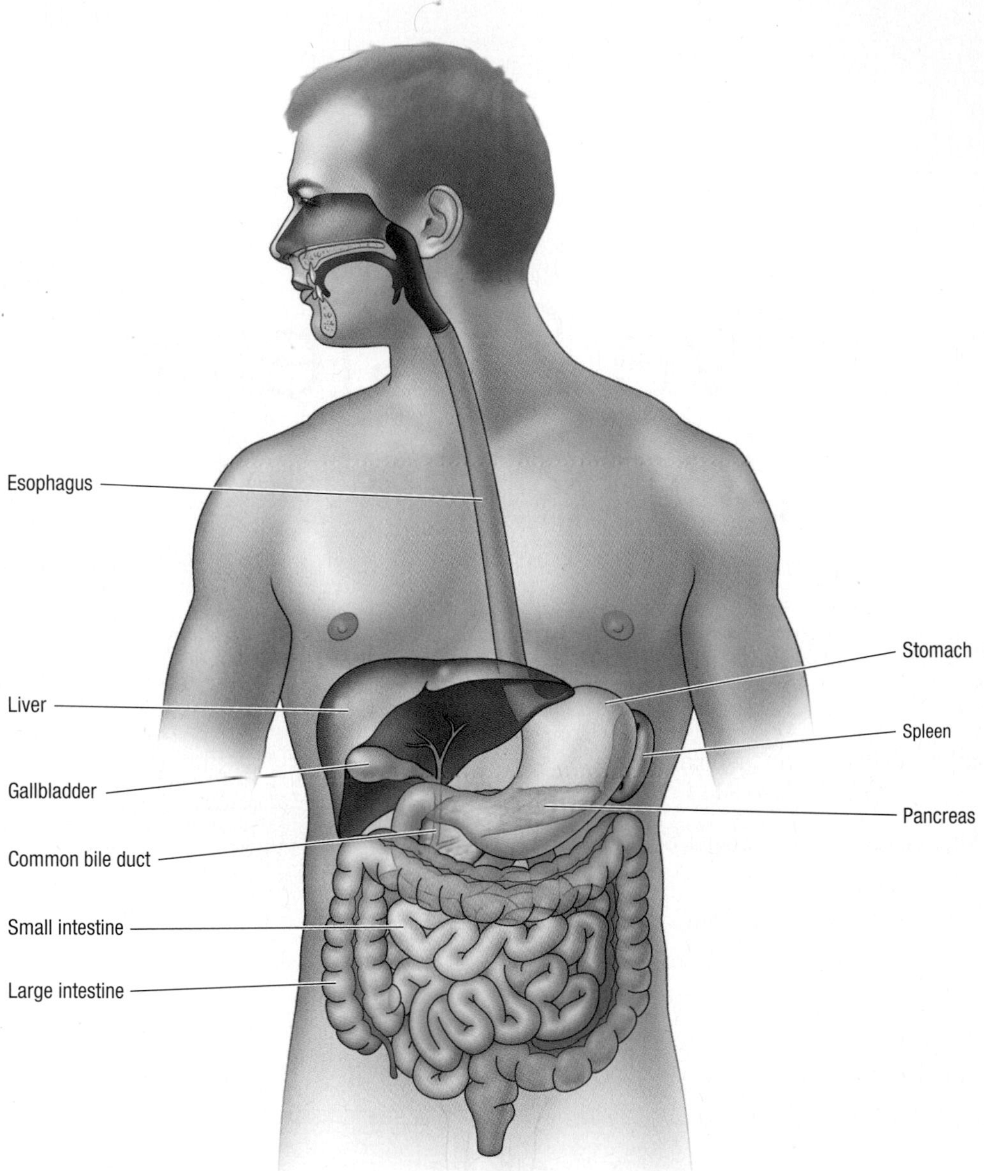

Figure 8.1. Digestive system overview

The secretion of digestive enzymes anywhere in the upper GI tract is largely a function of the vagus nerve, the biggest contributor to the parasympathetic nervous system. In this way, the efficiency of digestion depends on whether a person is in a sympathetic or parasympathetic state.

The small intestine loops and twirls around the abdomen, secured by sheets of connective tissue membrane called the **mesentery**, a part of the peritoneum. It is lubricated on the outside by other layers of the peritoneum, which allow it to move freely as a person twists, squirms, and changes positions. The inside of a healthy small intestine looks like velvet or velour, with millions of tiny **villi**, each one supplied with blood and lymph capillaries for the absorption of nutrients and fats. This is where amino acids and glucose enter the bloodstream, and fats are drawn into the lymph system. Rhythmic waves of smooth muscle contraction gently ease the chyme along the tube until at the distal end of the small intestine the leftovers pass through the ileocecal valve, the entryway to the colon.

The colon is a much shorter and wider section of tubing than the small intestine, and it differs also in the absence of villi and the presence of anchoring pieces of connective tissue that bind the colon down at the four flexures, or corners, of the abdomen. A healthy colon has segments called **haustra**. In this part of the tube, water is squeezed out of the fecal matter and reabsorbed back into the body. This is also the site of vitamin K synthesis. The colon functions like a trash compactor; everything left of a meal that makes it this far is condensed and excreted.

The Accessory Organs: Structure and Function

The continuous tube that winds from mouth to anus is only one part of the digestive system; the accessory organs contribute to the process of turning food into energy or building blocks as well. These organs include the liver, gallbladder, and pancreas, each of which produces or releases chemicals into the digestive tract. Here is a brief review of each of these organs.

The Liver

The liver is an organ of immense complexity, with literally hundreds of functions. One of the things that makes the liver unique is its power of regeneration; hepatocytes are remarkably adaptable. Livers that have been partially removed can recover full functional size soon after surgery, and small pieces of liver that have been transplanted into other hosts can grow to full function within a similar short period. The liver also has twice the blood supply of most other organs: between the hepatic artery delivering oxygen-rich blood and the portal vein delivering blood with the products of digestion from the small intestine, it's no wonder that this organ is hot and dark red.

The liver is the largest organ in the body. It is the destination of the portal system detour, receiving all of the vitamins, amino acids, and glucose that are extracted from the small intestine and not immediately needed in the body. By storing glucose as glycogen until it is called for, the liver also acts as a sugar buffer, preventing the radical swings in blood glucose levels that would happen without an intermediate stop for sugar. The liver is also the site for much protein synthesis. Many of the enzymes that support cellular activity are made here, as are the blood proteins that regulate intracellular fluid and blood clotting.

Detoxification functions of the liver are well known. The liver alters many drugs into forms that are less toxic than the original, or that can be excreted. A functioning liver prevents many substances, including alcohol, from reaching toxic levels in the bloodstream. It also processes the poisonous wastes generated by protein digestion, changing them to uric acid to be excreted by the kidneys.

In addition to these functions, the specialized leukocytes in the liver called Kupffer cells are constantly watching for any pathogens that they can eradicate. Finally, the liver helps to recycle the **heme** from dead red blood cells into **bilirubin**, a major component of bile, which is vital for the digestion of fats. The liver produces up to three cups of bile each day. Bile leaves the liver via the cystic duct and enters the gallbladder.

The Gallbladder

The gallbladder is a small green sac that hangs off the liver about halfway along the right costal angle. Its function is fairly simple: it receives bile from the liver, stores it, and concentrates it. The gallbladder can hold up to one cup of bile at a time. On hormonal command, it releases the bile into the duodenum via the common bile duct. There the bile helps to emulsify fats, that is, separate them into tiny separated globules to make them easier to digest. The gallbladder and its ducts are susceptible to dysfunction, which can have serious repercussions.

The Pancreas

The pancreas is a fascinating gland that holds the distinction of being both an exocrine gland, releasing digestive juices into the intestine via the pancreatic duct, and an endocrine gland, releasing hormones directly into the bloodstream. Its exocrine secretions are potentially corrosive. Any blockage in the pancreatic duct can lead to very serious tissue damage, as the pancreas is quite capable of digesting itself.

Digestive System Problems and Massage

Most of the digestive system problems that respond well to massage are related to autonomic imbalance; when a person is under stress, digestion is a low priority. If this state of affairs goes on for a long time, problems inevitably develop. The most common disorders of this type are spastic or flaccid constipation, indigestion, and gas.

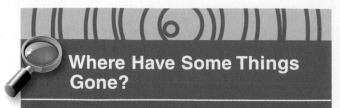

Where Have Some Things Gone?

Some items that would traditionally be discussed in Chapter 8 now appear elsewhere. Crohn disease and ulcerative colitis have been moved to Chapter 6 because they are autoimmune diseases, and peritonitis and jaundice now appear in Appendix C, Extra Conditions at a Glance.

The first concern, however, is to eliminate the possibility of more serious conditions that contraindicate circulatory massage. Red flags include severe local pain, bloody stools, anemia, bloating, and fever; any of these along with digestive pain constitute a good reason to visit the doctor. In addition, any new pattern of milder digestive pain persisting for 2 weeks or more should be investigated.

Problems in the digestive system are impossible to pin down without diagnostic tests, which are outside the scope of practice of massage therapy. Massage should not be performed when the client has any unexplained or undiagnosed pain. Any temporary relief that a massage provides may delay the client getting medical assistance for a serious and acute illness. Although spastic constipation is not inherently dangerous, colon cancer is— and massage therapists are not equipped to tell the difference.

Disorders of the Upper Gastrointestinal Tract

Celiac Disease

Definition: What Is It?

Celiac disease is a condition in which the intestinal villi are flattened or destroyed altogether as part of a reaction in the presence of gluten, a group of proteins present in many types of grains. It is also known as **celiac sprue**, nontropical sprue, or **gluten-sensitive enteropathy**.

Celiac disease occurs in about 1% of the United States population, although the majority of people with this condition are undiagnosed. Comparisons to tissue samples from previous decades suggest that the

Digestive System Conditions

Disorders of the Upper Gastrointestinal Tract

- Celiac disease
- Esophageal cancer
- Gastroenteritis
- Gastroesophageal reflux disorder
- Peptic ulcers
- Stomach cancer

Disorders of the Large Intestine

- Colorectal cancer
- Diverticular disease
- Irritable bowel syndrome
  - IBS-D
  - IBS-C
  - IBS-M
  - IBS-A

Disorders of the Accessory Organs

- Cirrhosis
- Gallstones
- Hepatitis
  - Hepatitis A
  - Hepatitis B
  - Hepatitis C
  - Other forms of hepatitis
- Liver cancer
- Pancreatic cancer
  - Adenocarcinoma of the pancreas
  - Neuroendocrine tumors of the pancreas
- Pancreatitis
  - Acute pancreatitis
  - Chronic pancreatitis

Other Digestive System Conditions

- Candidiasis
  - Mucocutaneous candidiasis
  - Vulvovaginitis
  - Internal candidiasis

Celiac Disease in Brief

Pronunciation: SEE-le-ak dih-ZEZE

What is it?
Celiac disease is a condition in which an inflammatory response follows the consumption of any food with gluten. This leads to the destruction of intestinal villi and poor access to any ingested nutrients.

How is it recognized?
Celiac disease can develop in childhood or adulthood, and its symptoms can range from mild to severe. Most symptoms are related to malabsorption (many nutrients are not absorbed and so pass through to the stools) or malnutrition (complications related to vitamin and nutrient deficiencies develop).

Massage risks and benefits
Risks: Massage has no particular risks for a person with celiac disease, except for offering temporary relief from digestive pain that may contribute to a delay in getting an important diagnosis.
Benefits: Massage may offer some temporary relief for people with celiac disease, but it has no direct effect on the condition itself. Clients who successfully manage this condition can enjoy the same benefits from bodywork as the rest of the population.

rate of celiac disease has increased dramatically from fifty years ago.

Etiology: What Happens?

Gluten is a name for a group of proteins found in many grains, including wheat, rye, barley, spelt, and others. When gluten is consumed by a person without celiac disease, digestive enzymes break it down into small chains of amino acids that are absorbed into the intestinal villi. When celiac disease is present, gluten is broken into its component pieces, including a long chain of amino acids called **gliadin**, but this substance resists enzyme action to break it up any further. For reasons that are not completely clear, gliadin is absorbed into the villi of people with celiac disease, where it triggers a mild or severe inflammatory response.

Eventually, repeated inflammatory attacks on intestinal villi cause them to degenerate, lie flat, or disappear altogether. The person then loses access to absorbable nutrition not only from sources of gluten but from other sources as well. Glucose from dairy products is often particularly difficult to digest, which leads to symptoms of lactose intolerance, although the problem isn't with the lactose itself but with the villi that are meant to absorb it. Fats become similarly unavailable, and they pass through the digestive system to be expelled in the stools. Poor uptake leads to signs of malabsorption and malnutrition, although the diet of a person with celiac disease may be identical to that of an unaffected person.

Celiac disease is at least partly related to immune system hyperactivity, and it frequently occurs concurrently with autoimmune disorders, including type 1 diabetes, hypothyroidism, hyperthyroidism, lupus, rheumatoid arthritis, and Sjogren syndrome. A genetic link in celiac disease is easy to trace, since the incidence within families is significantly higher than that in the general population. Age at onset varies significantly, however. Some people develop symptoms in early childhood, and others develop symptoms after a significant stressful trigger in adulthood, such as surgery, childbirth, or trauma. Still others may go throughout life with symptoms so mild that they are ignored or misdiagnosed as other GI disorders.

Some people with celiac disease don't have significant GI symptoms, but they develop a painful, itchy rash called **dermatitis herpetiformis**. It usually clears when gluten is eliminated from the diet.

Complications of celiac disease have to do with malabsorption and malnutrition. Young children with celiac disease have delayed growth and development, and many never reach their projected height. Poor uptake of iron and vitamins leads to anemia, folic acid deficiency, and a high risk of miscarriage or neural tube defects in a growing fetus. Poor uptake of calcium leads to osteomalacia (weak bones) in children or osteoporosis in adults. Muscle weakness, chronic spasm, and joint pain may develop. Behavioral changes, irritability, peripheral neuropathy, and a risk of seizures can be linked to a vitamin B12 deficiency.

Constant irritation and inflammation of the GI tract also raises the risk of adenocarcinoma or lymphoma in the small intestine. Non-Hodgkin lymphoma is a significant cause of death for persons whose celiac disease is never identified.

Signs and Symptoms

Signs and symptoms of celiac disease typically center on malabsorption of nutrients and malnutrition. While some patients have pain or discomfort in the GI tract, many others have only the results of poor vitamin and nutrient uptake. Symptoms may be determined by the section of the small intestine that is affected. Damage to the duodenum, for instance, results in different nutritional deficiencies from those of damage to the jejunum.

GI symptoms include gas, bloating, and diarrhea. Stools are often high volume, pale, and foul smelling, as they contain much of the fat and other material that would normally have been absorbed in the small intestines. It can be difficult to differentiate between symptoms of celiac disease and those of irritable bowel syndrome. Furthermore, these conditions can occur simultaneously. It is useful to have a full clinical picture, however, because each of them responds to a different treatment strategy.

Other symptoms include weight loss (or failure to gain weight in children), anemia, irritability, depression, behavior changes, muscle cramps and weakness, poor stamina, tooth discoloration, and dermatitis.

Treatment

No reliable treatment exists for celiac disease, except to avoid gluten in any form. Gluten is present in many grains, including wheat, rye, barley, spelt, triticale, and kamut. Many (but not all) people with celiac disease are also sensitive to oats, although whether this grain actually contains gluten or is frequently contaminated with it is somewhat questionable. Gluten is also used in many other products, including vitamins and other pills, cosmetics (especially lipstick), and as a thickener in many processed foods.

Gluten is not present in corn, quinoa, potatoes, beans, nuts, rice, or soy; flour made from these foods can frequently be substituted to help comprise a gluten-free diet. Other gluten-free foods include fruits, vegetables, and meats. It is possible to have a varied and well-balanced gluten-free diet, but eating processed foods or at restaurants may be problematic.

The majority of celiac disease patients who avoid all sources of gluten for months or years can heal completely, and achieve the complete rebuilding of their intestinal villi. However, this reconstruction can easily be undone if gluten-rich foods are consumed; a person with celiac disease must commit to a lifelong dietary adjustment.

Medications

- Short-term steroidal anti-inflammatories if restricting gluten does not improve symptoms quickly enough
- Vitamin and mineral supplements as necessary
- Topical medication for dermatitis herpetiformis

Massage?

RISKS Any relief that follows massage may cause a client to delay getting an important diagnosis, so therapists need to support clients in pursuing nagging digestive symptoms. Abdominal work for a client with diagnosed celiac disease must be conducted conservatively and with ample client feedback for comfort. The characteristic skin rash that many celiac disease patients have locally contraindicates massage.

BENEFITS A client who has been diagnosed with celiac disease and manages it successfully can enjoy all the benefits of bodywork as the rest of the population.

OPTIONS Many celiac disease patients find that lotions or shampoos with wheat germ oil or other gluten-containing ingredients exacerbate their symptoms. Whether this is from a skin reaction to a topical application or the substance ends up inadvertently gaining access to the bloodstream through mucous membranes is moot: it is important to have nongluten topical oil or lotion to work with clients who have celiac disease.

SIDEBAR 8.1 Where is Crohn Disease?

Crohn disease, an autoimmune disorder of the whole digestive tract, used to be discussed in this section. It now appears in Chapter 6.

Esophageal Cancer

Definition: What Is It?

Esophageal cancer is the development of malignant cells in the esophagus. It typically appears in either of two forms: cancer that grows in the thoracic area of the esophagus (squamous cell carcinoma) or cancer that grows at the distal end (adenocarcinoma).

Worldwide, squamous cell esophageal cancer is quite common. In the United States, adenocarcinoma is the most common form of esophageal cancer, and it is one of the few types of cancer with an increasing rather than decreasing incidence.

Etiology: What Happens?

The esophagus is a tube about 10 inches long running from the throat to the lower esophageal valve, which opens into the stomach. It is composed of four layers of tissue: the mucous membrane, which lines the tube; the submucosa, which provides blood and lymph support for the active mucus-producing cells; the muscularis, which provides strong wavelike contractions to move a food bolus from the throat into the stomach; and the adventitia, a connective tissue outer layer. The esophagus does not have a serous membrane covering.

When malignant cells grow in the upper or middle parts of the esophagus, they tend to appear in squamous epithelial cells; this is called squamous cell carcinoma of the esophagus. This condition is closely related to smoking or alcohol use; smoking in combination with alcohol use increases the risk of malignancies by a large margin.

When malignant cells grow in glandular tissue, the growth is called adenocarcinoma. This is the case when esophageal cancer originates at the distal end of the tube, close to the lower esophageal valve. A condition called **Barrett esophagus** is a complication of gastroesophageal reflux disease (GERD), and it is considered a precancerous state for adenocarcinoma. Barrett esophagus is the result of exposure to a chronic, repeated barrage of gastric juices from reflux that causes cells of the esophageal mucosa to mutate. This raises the risk of malignancy so significantly that many physicians recommend surgery or other interventions before cancer is confirmed.

Malignant cells from esophageal cancer can invade other tissues in several ways. Because the esophagus has no serous membrane cover, any tumor that penetrates through all four layers of the esophagus can spread easily to nearby structures. The trachea, diaphragm, aorta, vena cava, and laryngeal nerve are most susceptible. Because the esophageal submucosa has a generous supply of lymphatic capillaries, lymphatic spread of the disease is also a risk. The lymph system can carry malignant cells to nearby nodes and other tissues, including the lungs, liver, and bones. Esophageal cancer can also spread through the bloodstream, although this appears to happen more rarely than other routes for metastasis.

Smoking and alcohol use increase the chance of developing upper esophageal cancer, and GERD increases the risk of lower esophageal cancer. Other risk factors include obesity (this may contribute to GERD), a history of any other head or neck cancer, exposure to toxic substances (i.e., ingesting lye or other poisons), exposure to human papillomavirus in the throat, and a lifetime habit of drinking extremely hot beverages. Worldwide studies also reveal that a shortage of vitamins A, B, and C, beta carotene, and selenium are common among esophageal cancer patients.

Esophageal Cancer in Brief

Pronunciation: e-sof-uh-JE-ul KAN-sur

What is it?
Esophageal cancer is the growth of malignant cells in the esophagus. It is classified as either squamous cell carcinoma, which usually occurs in the thoracic portion of the esophagus, or adenocarcinoma, which occurs at the distal end, near the lower esophageal valve.

How is it recognized?
Esophageal cancer is rarely recognized in early stages. In later stages, a growth may obstruct the esophagus, leading to a feeling of food or liquid "getting stuck" on the way to the stomach. Pain and difficulty swallowing, along with unintended weight loss, are the symptoms that usually prompt people to seek a diagnosis.

Massage risks and benefits
Risks: Esophageal cancer patients may undergo chemotherapy, radiation, and surgery; all of these require adjustments in massage therapy or bodywork.
Benefits: Massage has many benefits to offer esophageal cancer patients, as long as accommodations are made for the challenges of the disease and its treatments.

Signs and Symptoms

Early signs and symptoms of esophageal cancer are practically nonexistent, which is why this disease has such a high mortality rate; it is often undetected until a tumor is large enough to create a mechanical obstruction, and metastasis to other nearby organs and/or lymph nodes has already occurred.

The symptoms that most often cause people to go to the doctor include **dysphagia**, a feeling of food or liquid "getting stuck" on its way to the stomach, pain with swallowing, and unplanned weight loss. A chronic cough, with or without blood, may also occur. Hoarseness may be related to mechanical irritation of the trachea or to damage at the laryngeal nerve. Hiccups may indicate damage to the phrenic nerve.

Other signs suggest that the cancer has spread or that complications have developed. Deep pain indicates possible metastasis to bones. Fever and lung infection may be connected to a tracheo-esophageal fistula, which allows materials into the respiratory tract that shouldn't be there.

Treatment

Treatment for esophageal cancer could include surgery, chemotherapy, radiation therapy, or photodynamic therapy, in which specially designed drugs are absorbed into cancerous cells, and exposure to a laser destroys them. Surgery may be conducted to remove the affected section of the esophagus, or simply to create a more function passageway. Radiation may be externally or internally applied. Chemotherapy is not generally successful by itself, but may be used as part of a larger treatment strategy.

Treatment options are determined by the stage of cancer at diagnosis. Staging protocols are provided in Sidebar 8.2.

Recovery from treatment for esophageal cancer is often problematic, since good nutrition is essential to heal from such invasive procedures, and eating is often very difficult.

Medications

- Chemotherapeutic agents
- Photodynamic therapy

Massage?

RISKS As with other cancers, massage for esophageal cancer patients must be adjusted according to the client's general resilience and the treatment options (along with commensurate side effects) that are in use. This client may have a reduced ability to adapt to changing environments, so bodywork must be carefully accommodated.

BENEFITS Massage for cancer patients has been seen to improve sleep and appetite, reduce depression and anxiety, and help with pain. All of these can benefit esophageal cancer patients, with appropriate accommodations. More information on massage in the context of cancer appears in Chapter 12.

Gastroenteritis

Definition: What Is It?

Gastroenteritis is inflammation of the GI tract, specifically the stomach or small intestine. By convention, gastroenteritis is usually discussed as a result

SIDEBAR 8.2 Staging Esophageal Cancer

The staging of esophageal cancer is determined by how deeply the esophagus has been penetrated and whether lymph nodes have been affected or metastasis has developed. Esophageal cancer is staged using both the TNM (tumor, node, metastasis) technique and numerical staging from 0 to IV. Here is a simplified version of esophageal cancer staging.

Tumor (T)	Node (N)	Metastasis (M)
T IS: cancer in situ, limited to superficial mucosa	N 0: no nodes involved	M 0: no metastasis found
T 1: mucosa and/or submucosa invaded	N 1 a–c: some nearby nodes involved	M 1a: distant lymph nodes involved
T 2: muscularis invaded		M 1b: distant organs involved
T 3: adventitia invaded		
T 4: nearby structures invaded		

These delineations are then translated into stages 0 to IV in this way:

Stage	Tumor	Node	Metastasis
0	T IS	N 0	M 0
I	T 1	N 0	M 0
II A, B	T 2–3	N 0–1	M 0
III	T 3–4	N any	M 0
IV A, B	T any	N any	M 1a, b

Gastroenteritis in Brief

Pronunciation: GAS-tro-en-ter-I-tis

What is it?
Gastroenteritis is any form of GI inflammation.

How is it recognized?
The symptoms of gastroenteritis are nausea, vomiting, and diarrhea. Fever, blood in the stools, and other signs may be present, depending on the cause.

Massage risks and benefits
Risks: Acute gastroenteritis, especially when related to an infectious agent, contraindicates most massage because the client is unlikely to be comfortable receiving bodywork.
Benefits: If gastroenteritis is fully diagnosed and under control, and the client is comfortable on a massage table or chair, then massage may be helpful to improve symptoms and general quality of life. Clients who have fully recovered from gastroenteritis can enjoy the same benefits from massage as the rest of the population.

of an infection with bacteria, viruses, or parasites. Noninfectious problems can also cause inflammation of the GI tract, however, and it can sometimes be difficult to identify the cause of a person's symptoms.

Etiology: What Happens?

Damage to the intestines can occur in a variety of ways. Some pathogens produce toxins that damage the intestinal mucosa. Others directly invade mucosal cells to destroy them. When peristalsis is slowed or delayed, which can occur with diabetes and some other diseases, pathogens that would normally be expelled can linger and overpower protective mechanisms.

When the GI tract is damaged or inflamed, absorption of nutrients and water is severely limited. Both water and valuable electrolytes are lost through diarrhea and vomiting. Gastroenteritis can have several causes:

- *Viruses*. The most common cause of GI inflammation among adults in the United States is with Norwalk virus (one of a group called noroviruses). Any of the hepatitis viruses can cause GI inflammation, as can any member of the enterovirus family. Viral gastroenteritis is highly communicable and can reach epidemic levels.
- *Bacteria*. Common bacterial pathogens include *Salmonella*, *Shigella*, *Campylobacter*, and several varieties of *E. coli*. Bacterial gastroenteritis is usually spread through improperly stored or prepared food or contaminated water or ice. "Traveler's diarrhea" is almost always from *E. coli* or *C. jejuni*. *H. pylori*, the pathogen associated with gastric ulcers is a common source of gastroenteritis. One increasingly common bacterial infection of the GI tract is caused by *C. difficile* (C-diff). It is particularly dangerous, because C-diff produces toxins that can seriously damage the wall of the colon. It is sometimes called necrotizing colitis or pseudomembranous colitis. It is resistant to most antibiotics, and is seen frequently in hospital patients.
- *Parasites*. Microscopic animal parasites can invade the GI tract, causing typical symptoms of gastroenteritis. Among the most common are Giardia, cryptosporidium, and *E. histolytica*.
- *Others*. Other causes of inflammation in the GI tract include fungal infections, (i.e., candidiasis), toxins (i.e., poisonous mushrooms or shellfish, or seafood from red tide areas), dietary problems (i.e., food allergies), medications (i.e., antibiotics or magnesium-containing laxatives or antacids), and other conditions that interfere with absorption. These include celiac disease, appendicitis, Crohn disease, ulcerative colitis, IBS, and diverticulitis. Weakness at the pyloric valve may allow contents of the duodenum to back up into the stomach, causing local irritation. This is called bile reflux.

Pathogenic forms of gastroenteritis are highly communicable. They can spread through an environment via oral-fecal contamination or via contaminated water or ice. Food prepared on contaminated surfaces can carry viruses or bacteria. For these reasons, travelers to places where gastroenteritis is common are advised to use only bottled water for drinking and brushing teeth and to avoid raw fruits and vegetables that may have been rinsed in contaminated water.

The most serious complication of gastroenteritis is dehydration from the massive fluid and mineral loss that goes along with diarrhea and vomiting. The loss of critical fluid and electrolytes can be fatal; gastroenteritis is a leading cause of death in many developing nations. In the United States, the people most at risk for this extreme reaction are infants, immunocompromised persons, and elders, whose systems are not capable of coping with this extreme change in internal environment. Signs of dangerously progressed dehydration include sunken eyes, lack of urination, and skin tenting: when the skin is pinched it does not immediately go back to its original position.

Some gastroenteritis factors can cause other problems as well. *Campylobacter* has been linked with Guillain-Barré syndrome, and *Salmonella* can complicate into meningitis or blood poisoning. Some forms of *E. coli* are highly toxic and can lead to renal failure.

Most cases of gastroenteritis resolve within 2 or 3 days without medical intervention. If symptoms persist longer than 2 to 3 weeks, it is no longer considered an acute infection, but a chronic condition. This leads medical professionals to look for an underlying condition such as food allergy, IBS, diverticulitis, Crohn disease, ulcerative colitis, hepatitis, or HIV/AIDS.

Signs and Symptoms

Different causative factors of gastroenteritis can lead to varying signs and symptoms, but the basic trio of intestinal inflammation includes nausea, vomiting, and diarrhea. These are appropriate responses to infection, as they are efficient methods of clearing out the GI tract, but several of these diseases are spread through oral-fecal contamination, so hygiene is critical when dealing with these symptoms.

Other signs that may develop with gastroenteritis include bloating, cramps, gas, and mucus or blood in the stools.

Treatment

Gastroenteritis is much easier to prevent than to treat. When it occurs in large outbreaks, it is often due to a specific source of contamination: a shipment of infected vegetables, a contaminated well, or shellfish harvested from contaminated water. Since foodstuffs are now shipped quickly all over large areas, it is a constant public health challenge to track down the source of infection and to limit its spread among the rest of the population.

Gastroenteritis is usually an acute, self-limiting condition and is generally treated with rest, fluid and electrolyte replacement. Viruses do not respond to antibiotics, and antibiotics for bacterial infections are problematic because they may make intestinal inflammation worse. The use of antidiarrhea medications is often discouraged because they interfere with the process of shedding pathogens, and so may prolong the infection.

Treatment focuses on preventing dehydration. If taking fluids by mouth aggravates vomiting, it may be necessary to use intravenous fluid replacement in a hospital setting.

Medications

- An oral vaccine for Norovirus is available
- Antibiotics, if tolerated
- Antiemetics to control vomiting

Massage?

RISKS Acute gastroenteritis contraindicates massage mainly because the client is unlikely to be comfortable. Pathogenic infections may also be communicable if surfaces are contaminated.

BENEFITS If a client has a digestive system irritation that is unrelated to infection, cancer, or other dangerous causes, bodywork could be helpful in promoting a parasympathetic state that can improve function and comfort.

Gastroesophageal Reflux Disease

Definition: What Is It?

GERD is a condition involving damage to the epithelial lining of the esophagus when it is chronically exposed to digestive juices released from the stomach. It is usually associated with a weakness at the lower esophageal sphincter, but several other factors may contribute as well.

Etiology: What Happens?

Most cases of GERD are connected to some combination of four problems: the lower esophageal sphincter is too relaxed; the lower esophageal sphincter doesn't allow appropriate clearing of acids in the esophagus; the diaphragmatic hiatus has trapped a portion of the stomach; or the stomach is slow to empty, adding to back pressure at the lower esophageal sphincter.

Any one of these problems allows stomach contents, including highly corrosive hydrochloric acid (and occasionally bile and pancreatic enzymes that have backed up from a weak pyloric valve), to enter the esophagus, which lacks the thick layer of mucus that protects the stomach from acid exposure (Figure 8.2).

Gastroesophageal Reflux Disease in Brief

Pronunciation: gas-tro-e-sof-a-JE-ul RE-flux dih-ZEZE

What is it?
Gastroesophageal reflux disease (GERD) describes chronic splashing of acidic stomach secretions into the unprotected esophagus.

How is it recognized?
Most people occasionally have heartburn, the sensation of corrosive gastric juices entering the esophagus. GERD is diagnosed when backsplash of gastric juices causes structural changes to the esophageal lining, which can lead to serious complications.

Massage risks and benefits
Risks: Because lying flat may promote GERD, and because massage may stimulate a parasympathetic response that triggers digestive activity, clients with this condition may be more comfortable scheduling their massage appointment for several hours after the last time they ate.
Benefits: Massage has no specific benefits for GERD, but if the condition is well controlled, a client can enjoy all the benefits from bodywork as the rest of the population.

Risk factors for GERD include pregnancy, obesity, smoking, a diet high in fatty or spicy foods, caffeine and alcohol use, and connective tissue disease like lupus or scleroderma. A hiatal hernia, which is an enlargement of the opening in the diaphragm where the esophagus passes through the stomach, may catch and irritate the superior part of the stomach. Most people with hiatal hernias have GERD, although not all GERD patients have hiatal hernias. Some diseases, including diabetes, ulcers, and spinal cord injuries, cause reduced peristalsis and sluggish movement of substances through the GI tract. When stomach contents linger too long, the accumulation of pressure and gastric juices can cause them to put back pressure on the esophagus.

Chronic irritation of the esophageal lining can cause several reactions:

- *Respiratory injury*. This may occur if gastric secretions reach up to the larynx where these substances can be aspirated into the lungs. GERD is now being investigated as a risk factor for laryngeal cancer.
- *Decay of tooth enamel*. This may develop as acidic juices are increasingly present in the mouth.
- *Esophageal ulcers*. These lesions may become infected, or they may bleed into the GI tract.
- *Stricture*. This is a thickening of the esophageal wall with scar tissue in response to irritation. Strictures may make it difficult to swallow normally.
- *Barrett esophagus*. This is a pathological change in the normal esophageal cells; they mutate into cells that resemble the stomach lining. **Barrett esophagus** has been identified as a precancerous condition, opening the door to adenocarcinoma, an increasingly common and dangerous type of esophageal cancer.

Signs and Symptoms

Signs and symptoms of GERD are largely produced by the action of gastric juice on the delicate esophageal lining. A bitter taste, a feeling like some food has been regurgitated, gas, indigestion, bloating, and pain in the chest behind the sternum are common symptoms. The pain of GERD can be mistaken for heart attack or angina. Symptoms are reliably aggravated by bending over or lying down.

Other GERD symptoms that occur less frequently include trouble swallowing, along with coughing, wheezing, and coughing up blood if ulcers in the esophagus have eroded into a blood vessel.

Treatment

Treatment for GERD falls into two categories: management and repair. Managing GERD so that it doesn't progress includes strategies like losing weight; eating smaller portions; not lying down within 2 hours after a meal; avoiding caffeine, alcohol, and nicotine; raising the bed about 6 in at the head; loosening clothing that puts pressure around the waist; and putting a heating pad on the stomach when it is painful.

Medications for GERD can work in a variety of ways. Antacids neutralize stomach acid, but over-the-counter brands may also cause the stomach to expand with gas, putting more pressure on the esophageal valve. Other medications can block receptors in the stomach that stimulate acid production, increase stomach motility to assist in sluggish movement, and block the release of hydrogen ions that contribute to the stomach's acidic environment.

Surgery usually focuses on strengthening the esophageal sphincter and taking pressure off the stomach. If the esophagus is limited by the development of a

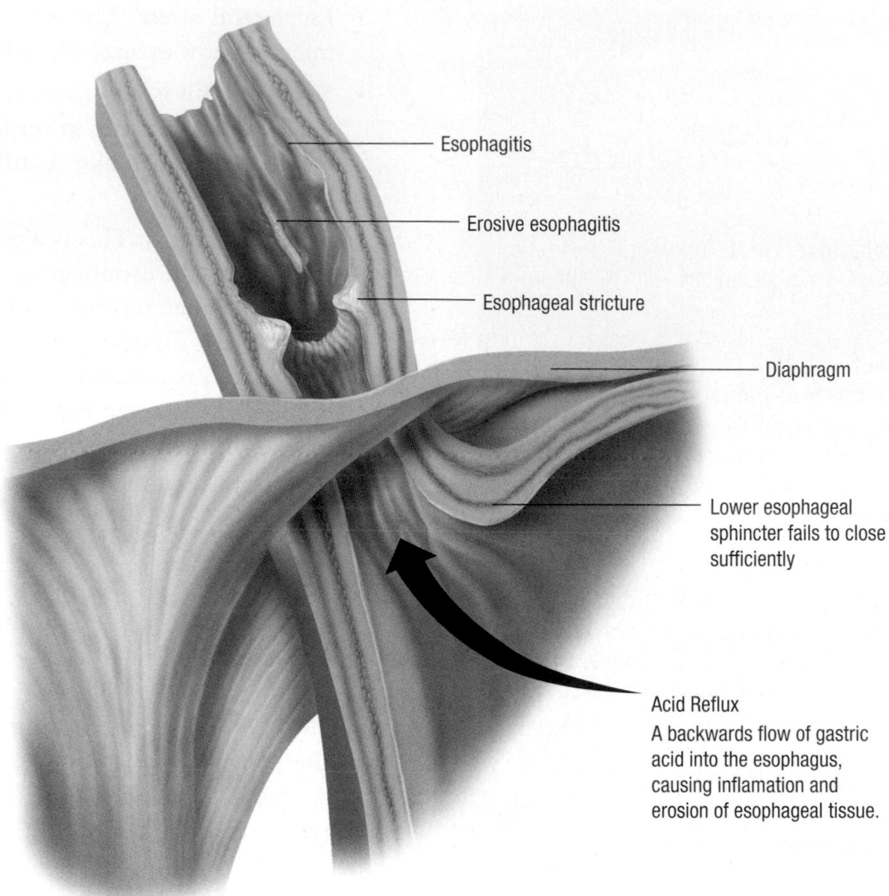

Figure 8.2. Gastroesophageal reflux disorder: backsplash from the stomach enters the esophagus

scar tissue stricture, this may be dilated. A portion of the stomach may be wrapped around the sphincter to give it external support in a procedure called a fundoplication. And of course, if a hiatal hernia puts pressure on the stomach, surgery may be performed to correct it.

Medications

- Antacids to reduce the acidic environment in the stomach
- H2 blockers to reduce histamine activity and acid production
- Proton pump inhibitors to reduce acid production
- Coating agents to protect tissues from acid
- Promotility agents to promote peristalsis and tighten the lower esophageal valve

Massage?

RISKS It is important to work with GERD patients in a way that does not exacerbate their symptoms. This may mean not working with them lying flat on a table, or delaying a massage appointment until several hours after the last time they ate.

BENEFITS Clients who successfully treat this condition can enjoy the same benefits of massage as the rest of the population, although work around the superior aspect of the abdomen should probably be conservative.

OPTIONS Clients with GERD may accept massage most comfortably if they can sit in a recliner or a massage chair.

Peptic Ulcers

Definition: What Are They?

An ulcer is the result of progressive tissue damage due to constant irritation or some impediment to the healing process. Cells in the lesion die, and a crater erodes into deep layers of tissue. An ulcer is a perpetually open sore, and an invitation to infection. This section focuses on peptic ulcers of the inner surfaces of the esophagus, stomach, and duodenum, but an ulcer has the same properties, whether it's in the GI tract or on the skin.

Etiology: What Happens?

Ulcers in the esophagus, stomach, or small intestine are called peptic ulcers, named for pepsin, the protein-digesting enzyme that contributes to their development (Figure 8.3).

Until fairly recently, ulcers have been assumed to be connected to too much stress and/or spicy or acidic food. Ulcer patients have historically been counseled to eat bland food, to drink lots of milk, and to avoid getting upset or overly excited. Many found that their ulcers eventually subsided, but would recur later; they were essentially a lifelong condition. A more current understanding of these lesions shows that they are multifactoral condition involving fluctuations in stress, bacterial infection, and some medications.

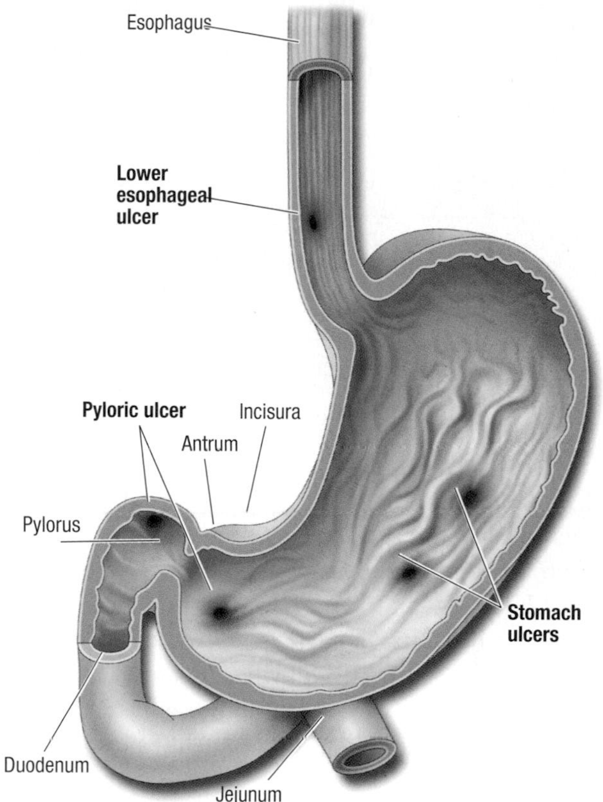

Figure 8.3. Sites of peptic ulcers

> **Peptic Ulcers in Brief**
>
> Pronunciation: PEP-tik UL-surz
>
> **What are they?**
> Ulcers are sores that for various reasons don't heal normally; they remain open and vulnerable to infection. Peptic ulcers occur on the inner surfaces of the esophagus, stomach, or duodenum.
>
> **How are they recognized?**
> The symptoms of peptic ulcers include general burning or gnawing abdominal pain between meals that is relieved by taking antacids or eating. Other symptoms include bloating, burping, gas, and vomiting after meals.
>
> **Massage risks and benefits**
> ***Risks:*** Specific or intrusive work on the abdomen may exacerbate symptoms of peptic ulcers. Also, because massage tends to stimulate digestive activity, clients may want to time their massage sessions around their eating schedule.
> ***Benefits:*** Massage has no direct impact on peptic ulcers, but the overall parasympathetic effect that usually accompanies bodywork may be a positive experience for a person who struggles with this condition.

Stress and Ulcers

The link between stress and ulcers is a significant factor, but the incidence of ulcers across the population doesn't follow demographics that are associated with high-stress situations, so some variables in stress-coping mechanisms have evidently never been identified.

The normal environment inside a stomach has some features that can be classified as aggressive and others that are defensive. Aggressive features include the production of hydrochloric acid and pepsin, which help to digest proteins. Defensive features include a generous blood supply to the stomach wall, which serves to help damaged cells regenerate quickly, and stimulates mucus production. Mucus protects the stomach wall from acid and pepsin. The acid is then neutralized in the first section of the small intestine by bicarbonate from the pancreas. These aggressive and defensive mechanisms work best when they keep each other in balance.

NOTABLE CASES Iconic Irish writer James Joyce (*Ulysses, The Dubliners*) died of complications related to a perforated ulcer at age 59. English writer Rudyard Kipling (*The Jungle Book, Gunga Din*) lost his life at age 70 to a perforated duodenal ulcer. And "Bird" jazz saxophone pioneer Charlie Parker was officially said to have died of a bleeding ulcer at age 34, but the recent heart attack, cirrhosis, and pneumonia that were all present at the same time might also have contributed.

Recall that when a person is in a sympathetic state, blood supply to the whole digestive tract is suppressed, and stomach activity is suspended. Lack of blood flow means that mucus production is slowed, but so is acid and pepsin production: the two mechanisms stay in balance. But when stress is lifted and a person shifts back into a relaxed, parasympathetic state, stomach secretions are stimulated again. The problem is that the stomach produces acid and pepsin much faster than it rebuilds a delicate mucus lining. This imbalance between aggressive and defensive features leaves the stomach wall vulnerable to damage. In other words, ulcers seem to be more related to the fluctuations in stress than to the perception of stress alone.

Helicobacter pylori and Ulcers

In 1984, a remarkable discovery revealed an unexpected phenomenon: a bacterium that can survive and thrive in the highly acidic environment of the stomach. This bacterium, *H. pylori*, is found in many biopsies of ulcers, especially those in the duodenum. It is an unusual bacterium, shaped like a bacillus (it can be rod shaped), but it also has spiral flagella (Figure 8.4). Identification of *H. pylori* led to the conclusion that imbalances in GI tract chemistry can initiate tissue damage to the mucosa, but bacterial infection makes the ulcer a long-term chronic problem. (For more information on *H. pylori*, see Sidebar 8.3.)

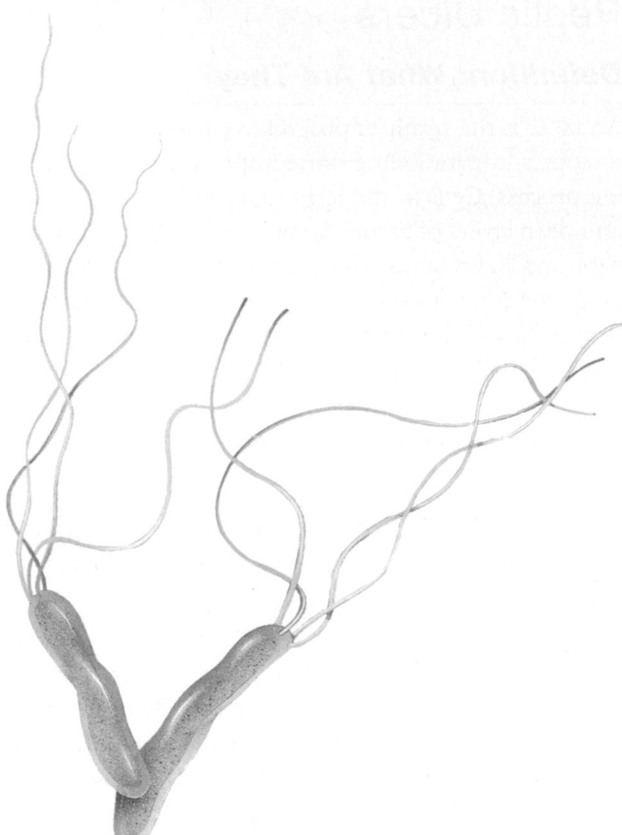

Figure 8.4. *Helicobacter pylori*

Anti-inflammatories and Ulcers

The use of nonsteroidal anti-inflammatory drugs (NSAIDs) for everything from headaches to back pain to heart disease and stroke prevention has led to significant disruption of stomach function for many patients. Aspirin, ibuprofen, and naproxen sodium all inhibit the cyclooxygenase-1 pathway, so they impede the production of prostaglandins that would otherwise support blood flow and healthy mucus production. Interestingly, these medications also inhibit the production of bicarbonate in the pancreas, which means the duodenum is especially vulnerable to corrosion.

Complications of ulcers can be serious. When they erode into capillaries, cumulative slow bleeding can lead to anemia. If the corroded blood vessel is a larger arteriole or artery, untreated hemorrhaging can lead quickly to shock and death. Ulcers can also perforate, or eat all the way through the organ wall, releasing bacteria and partially digested food into the peritoneal space, leading to peritonitis. Perforation happens more often with duodenal than stomach ulcers. Ulcers can create a combination of scar tissue and inflammation that causes the pyloric valve to spasm. If this is not quickly resolved, surgery can be required to reopen the digestive tract. Finally, having a peptic ulcer significantly raises the risk of developing stomach cancer. Although stomach cancer is on the decline in the United States, it is still the second leading type of cancer worldwide. Another type of cancer, mucosal-associated lymphoid-type lymphoma, is also associated with *H. pylori* and a history of peptic ulcers.

Signs and Symptoms

The primary symptom of peptic ulcers is a gnawing, burning pain in the chest or abdomen that can last anywhere from 30 minutes to 3 hours. When the pain occurs in relation to eating varies greatly from one

SIDEBAR 8.3 What is *Helicobacter pylori*?

H. pylori is a bacterium that is admirably designed to withstand and even thrive in the corrosively acidic environment of the stomach. The bacterium has several anatomical features that allow it to infect the mucous membranes of the stomach and duodenal wall.

Until 1984, it was never even considered that a bacterium could survive in the digestive tract. When pioneer researchers Barry Marshall and Robin Warren proposed the possibility and a scientific meeting, they were all but laughed offstage. But biopsies of lesions consistently revealed the presence of *H. pylori*. And when ulcer patients found that combining appropriate antibiotics with other acid-limiting medications led to a permanent cure for their ulcers—something that was unheard of at the time—the approach to treating this common condition completely changed. In 1994, the National Institutes of Health issued a statement that it was clear that *H. pylori* does indeed cause most peptic ulcers and is also a contributing factor to stomach cancer and lymphoma.

What is *H. pylori*, and where does it come from? Little is well understood about this pathogen. It is a short, microaerophilic gram-negative bacillus with spiraling flagella. Its presence can be easily determined by a blood test for antibodies, although this test does not indicate whether the infection is acute or longstanding. It is sensitive to common antibiotics such as tetracycline and amoxicillin.

The discovery of *H. pylori* and its role in peptic ulcers has raised as many questions as it has answered:

- How is the bacterium communicated? No one knows, but it could be through oral-fecal contamination or through salivary contact.
- How can it be prevented? It is impossible to prevent the spread of *H. pylori* without knowing how it gets from one person to another.
- If it is sensitive to common antibiotics, why isn't it eradicated when a person takes amoxicillin or tetracycline for something else? Antibiotics for *H. pylori* seem to work only when an ulcer has formed or when the infected person has acute gastritis from bacterial irritation.
- Does the presence of *H. pylori* contribute to general indigestion? It is unclear, but taking antibiotics for indigestion definitely doesn't clear up an *H. pylori* infection or relieve symptoms of dyspepsia.
- What diseases are associated with *H. pylori*? This bacterium has been definitively associated with an assortment of serious conditions, including chronic active gastritis, stomach cancer, peptic ulcers, and lymphoma that begins in the stomach.

person to the next (it can depend on the location of the ulcer), but it is generally relieved by antacids or eating more food.

Other signs of ulcers can include nausea, vomiting, loss of appetite, and bleeding into the GI tract.

Treatment

Treatment for most ulcers includes antibiotics for the *H. pylori*; bismuth, which protects the delicate stomach lining; and several medications that limit histamine release (H2 blockers) or acid production (proton pump inhibitors). When the treatment regimen is carefully followed, ulcers may be permanently healed.

Ulcers caused by the use of NSAIDs do not respond to antibiotic therapy. The only way to limit them is to suspend the use of the medications that damage the stomach lining.

Ulcers that don't heal satisfactorily or that continue to bleed, perforate, or cause strictures may be surgically corrected, either by removing damaged sections of the stomach or by severing the appropriate branch of the vagus nerve to limit acid secretion.

Medications

- Antibiotics for *H. pylori*
- Bismuth to protect the stomach lining
- H2 blockers to limit histamine release in the stomach
- Proton pump inhibitors to limit acidity in the stomach

Massage?

RISKS Because massage stimulates a parasympathetic press response, which can boost digestive activity, a person with ulcers may be most comfortable timing his or her massage appointments around his or her eating schedule for the least discomfort. If lying flat on a table exacerbates symptoms, massage may be better offered in a reclining chair or on a massage chair.

BENEFITS While massage has no direct impact on peptic ulcers, the general parasympathetic response that it brings about can be helpful for a person with this condition.

Stomach Cancer

Definition: What Is It?

Stomach cancer is the development of malignant tumors in the stomach that can block the passage of food through the digestive system, and can spread to other organs either through direct contact or through blood and lymph flow. It is relatively rare in the United States, but worldwide it is the second leading cause of death by cancer.

Etiology: What Happens?

Although several types of cancer have been observed to grow from stomach cells, most stomach cancers are adenocarcinomas, involving mutations of glandular cells (Figure 8.5). It is not always clear what triggers these mutations, but a comparison of eating habits and the history of both refrigeration and antibiotic use yields some clues.

NOTABLE CASES Actor John Wayne survived lung cancer in 1964 but succumbed to stomach cancer in 1979. Everybody's favorite neighbor Fred Rogers died of stomach cancer at age 74. At the opposite end of the personality spectrum, Napoleon Bonaparte's death may have been due to stomach cancer, although some speculate that he may have been the victim of arsenic poisoning.

Stomach Cancer in Brief

What is it?
Stomach cancer is the growth of malignant tumors in the stomach that may metastasize directly to other abdominal organs, or through lymph or blood flow to distant places in the body.

How is it recognized?
Symptoms of stomach cancer include a feeling of fullness after a small meal, unintentional weight loss, heartburn, abdominal pain above the navel, and occasionally vomiting, constipation, or diarrhea. Ascites may develop in advanced cases.

Massage risks and benefits

Risks: Stomach cancer patients are dealing with not only an aggressive form of cancer but also an aggressive strategy in cancer treatments. Any bodywork must accommodate these challenges.

Benefits: Massage has many benefits to offer stomach cancer patients, including improving sleep, and reducing anxiety, pain, depression, and other side effects of cancer treatment.

Stomach cancer rates in the United States began to decline in the 1930s, about the time that refrigeration became accessible for most Americans. The average diet shifted away from smoked, pickled, and salted foods and toward more fresh meats and fresh, canned, or frozen vegetables. In countries where stomach cancer is very prominent, the consumption of salted, smoked, or pickled foods is significantly higher than it is in the United States.

Most stomach cancer patients test positive for *H. pylori*. This bacterium, which is associated with peptic ulcers, converts the nitrates and nitrites in high-risk foods (mainly cured meats) into carcinogens. Infection rates of this not-well-understood bacterium are relatively low in the United States.

Any situation that impedes the production of gastric digestive secretions increases the risk of stomach cancer. This can include a history of *H. pylori* infection, atrophic gastritis (long-term inflammation that destroys acid-producing cells), stomach surgery, pernicious anemia, and other factors. When the environment in the stomach is insufficiently acidic, ingested materials don't break down properly and many become carcinogenic.

At its most complex, the stomach wall has five distinct layers: the mucosa, the submucosa, the muscularis, the visceral layer of the peritoneum, and the parietal layer of the peritoneum. In some areas, however, the serous membranes don't separate the stomach from adjacent organs.

As the mucosal layer of the stomach wall is assaulted with chronic exposure to carcinogens, tiny changes in the glandular cells may develop. These precancerous changes are virtually silent and are almost never detected. Malignant cells eventually grow into tumors large enough to obstruct the passage of food through the digestive tract, or they can invade and perforate the muscular layer and the serous membranes, allowing them to spread to nearby abdominal organs. By the time stomach cancer is detected, it has usually spread through the portal vein to the liver or into the lymph system.

Adenocarcinomas account for 90% to 95% of stomach cancer diagnoses. Other types of cancers in the stomach include a type of non-Hodgkin lymphoma, carcinoid tumors that arise from hormone-producing cells, and stromal tumors, which can occur anywhere in the GI tract.

The major risk factors for developing stomach cancer include *H. pylori* infection; a diet that is high

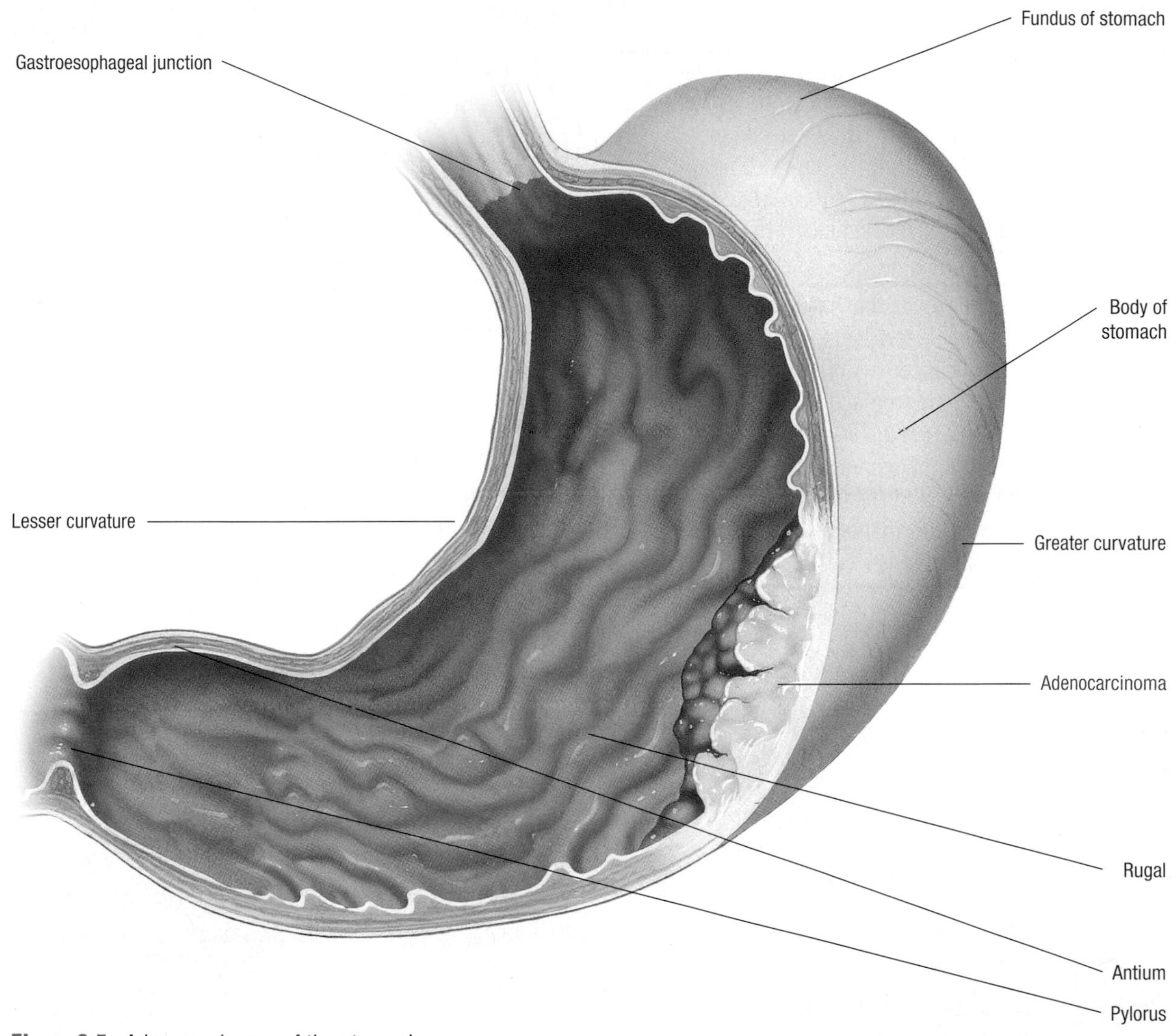

Figure 8.5. Adenocarcinoma of the stomach

in smoked, salted, or pickled foods; tobacco and alcohol use; having had previous stomach surgery; having type A blood; being male (men outnumber women with this disease by about 2 to 1); being between 60 and 80 years old; and having genes that are associated with breast or colorectal cancer.

Signs and Symptoms

Signs and symptoms of stomach cancer are mostly related to the sensation of having an obstruction in the digestive tract. They include a feeling of fullness after only a little food, vague abdominal pain above the navel, unintentional weight loss, heartburn and other ulcer symptoms, nausea and vomiting, and the development of ascites: the accumulation of excessive fluid in the peritoneal space. Tumors may bleed slightly, leading to small amounts of blood in the stool and possible anemia.

Treatment

Staging protocols for stomach cancer are discussed in Sidebar 8.4. This condition is treated with a combination of chemotherapy, externally applied radiation therapy, and surgery. Many patients undergo a course of chemotherapy both before and after surgery to improve the odds of success.

Medications

- Chemotherapeutic agents to limit neoplastic cell growth
- Biologic therapies, including monoclonal antibodies to target cancer cells

Massage?

RISKS Stomach cancer is usually treated very aggressively, which means clients with this condition will be dealing not only with cancer but with the challenges of surgeries, chemotherapy, and radiation as well. All of these require adjustments in bodywork, but with care, massage can be appropriate.

BENEFITS Because massage has been seen to ease pain, anxiety, depression, sleeplessness, and other side effects of cancer treatment, it has some well-defined benefits to offer stomach cancer patients any treatment must be gauged according to the resilience of the client and the cautions connected to the advancement of the cancer and treatment strategies that are being used. For more information on massage in the context of cancer, see Chapter 12.

Disorders of the Large Intestine

Colorectal Cancer

Definition: What Is It?

Colorectal cancer is the development of tumors anywhere in the large intestine from the ascending right side to the rectum. Although the two conditions are linked, malignant colon or rectal cancer is not the same thing as the presence of adenomas, or colon polyps.

Colorectal cancer is a relatively common form of cancer in this country, diagnosed about 101,000 times per year, and leading to about 49,000 deaths. It is the third leading cause of death by cancer in the United

SIDEBAR 8.4 Staging Stomach Cancer

Stomach cancer is usually staged using a combination of the TNM (tumor, node, metastasis) and numerical (0 to IV) protocols.

Tumor ratings

T x: tumor can't be assessed.

T 0: no evidence of primary tumor.

T IS: in situ cancer, affecting mucosa only.

T 1: affects submucosal layer.

T 2: affects muscularis.

T 3: affects subserosa.

T 4: whole serosa affected; adjacent organs may be involved.

Node ratings

N x: nodal involvement can't be assessed.

N 0: no nodal involvement.

N 1: 1–2 nearby nodes invaded.

N 2: 3–6 nearby nodes invaded.

N 3a: 7–15 nearby nodes invaded.

N 3b: >16 nearby nodes invaded.

Metastasis ratings

M x: metastasis can't be assessed.

M 0: no metastasis.

M 1: distant metastasis.

Stage	Tumor	Node	Metastasis
0	T IS	N 0	M 0
I A	T 1	N 0	M 0
I B	T 1–2	N 0–1	M 0
II A	T 1–3	N 0–2	M 0
II B	T 1–4	N 0–3	M 0
III A	T 2–4	N 1–3	M 0
III B	T 3–4 a or b	N 0–3	M 0
III C	T 4 a or b	N 2–3	M 0
IV	T any	N any	M 1

Colorectal Cancer in Brief

Pronunciation: ko-lo-REK-tal KAN-sur

What is it?
Colorectal cancer is development of malignant tumors in the colon or rectum. Growths can block the bowel and/or metastasize to other organs.

How is it recognized?
Signs and symptoms of colorectal cancer depend on what part of the bowel is affected. The most obvious symptoms are changes in bowel habits, including diarrhea or constipation lasting more than 10 days. Other symptoms include blood in the stool, iron deficiency anemia, and unintentional weight loss.

Massage risks and benefits
Risks: Risks for working with a client with colorectal cancer are the same as those for every other kind of cancer: the challenges presented by the cancer itself, cancer treatments, and any temporary or permanent medical devices that a person uses must all be accommodated for with any kind of bodywork.
Benefits: Massage has many benefits to offer cancer patients, as long as basic precautions are observed. A person who has successfully treated colorectal cancer can enjoy the same benefits from massage as the rest of the population, although the presence of a colostomy bag may require some adaptation in bodywork.

States. Colorectal cancer deaths have been declining because of better screening and earlier treatment.

Etiology: What Happens?

The colon, or large bowel, is the last and widest section of the digestive tract. In this 6-foot long tube the remnants of food are compacted, water is reabsorbed, and feces are stored in the rectum until they are expelled. The inner lining of the colon is composed of epithelium, which, as has been seen in other discussions of cancer, is particularly susceptible to uncontrolled cell growth.

Most colon cancers begin with the development of adenomas, small polyps in the bowel. Minor chromosome damage is believed to cause the formation of these polyps. The cells in the mucosa of the colon simply multiply without any reason and produce small pile-ups of excess tissue (Figures 8.6 and 8.7). But if the polyps are present for a long period, two things happen: **oncogenes** are activated and **tumor suppressor genes** are suppressed. The net result is that cells on the surface of the colon mucosa continue to replicate, and don't die off. They can invade the deeper layers of the bowel and even erode all the way through it to reach out to other pelvic organs. They can obstruct the movement of fecal matter through the GI tract. And they can metastasize through the lymph system to other places in the body, notably, the brain, liver, and lungs.

It is not clear why common colon polyps, which occur in up to 50% of older Americans, become malignant. One theory is that high-fat foods linger in the colon longer than other types of food, and some of their byproducts are carcinogenic. This theory also suggests that diets that are high in fiber help material to move through the colon faster and more completely, "scrubbing" the bowel walls of damaging or irritating materials.

NOTABLE CASES The list of notable personalities with colon or rectal cancer is extremely varied, ranging from French composer Claude Debussy to the original Cat Woman Eartha Kitt, to U.S. President Ronald Reagan, and "Peanuts" creator Charles Schulz. Football coach Vince Lombardi and early science fiction writer H.P. Lovecraft were also colon cancer patients.

Research into the influence of diet and colon cancer is sometimes contradictory. General associations can be made between a high-fat, low-fiber diet and an increased risk of colorectal cancer, but when it comes to individual cases, other variables appear to influence the development of polyps and cancer, so diet is just one factor among many.

As with many diseases, the risk factors for developing colorectal cancer include some that can be controlled and others that can't. Risk factors for colorectal cancer include the following:

- *Obesity, sedentary lifestyle*. People who are obese have a relatively high chance of developing colon cancer. People who get little exercise are also prone to this disease; regular exercise has been shown to be protective against colorectal cancer.
- *Genetics*. **Familial adenomatous polyposis** and **hereditary nonpolyposis** colorectal cancer syndrome are genetic conditions that predispose some people to the development of colorectal cancer. Although people with these genetic profiles have a 90% to 100% chance

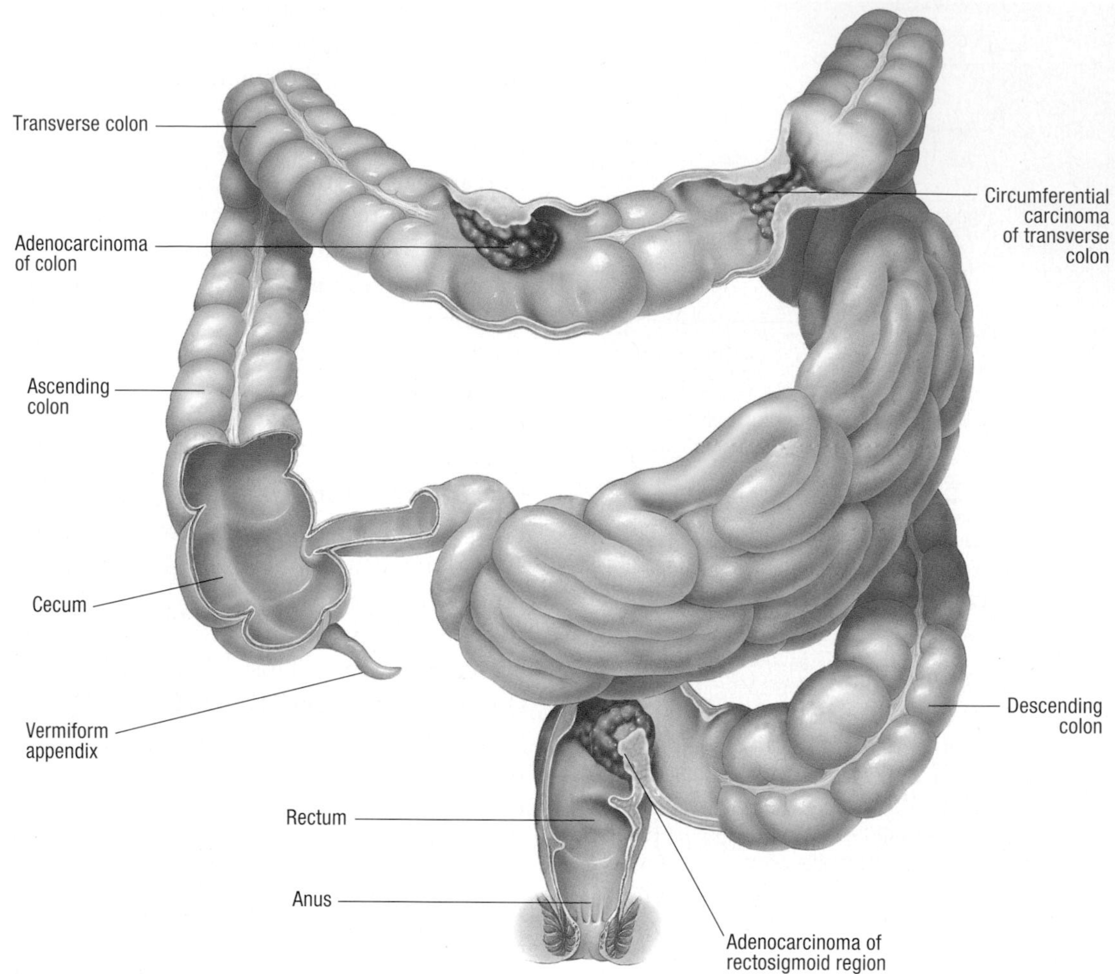

Figure 8.6. Colorectal cancer

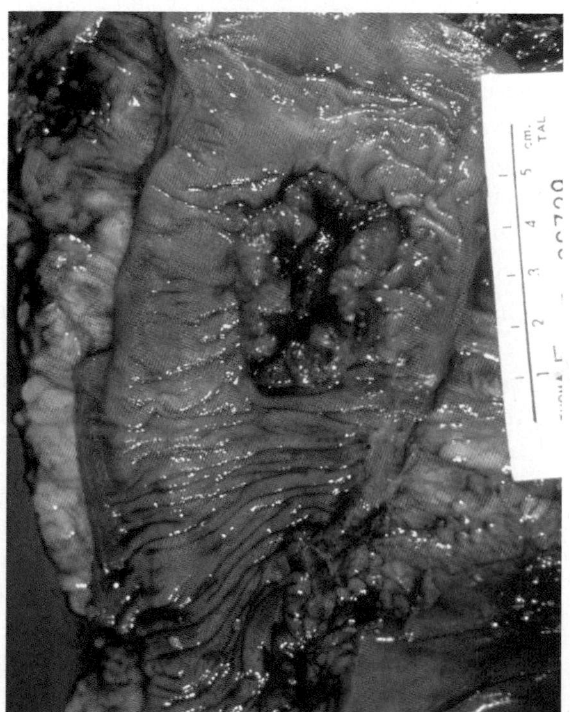

Figure 8.7. Colorectal cancer tumor

of developing the disease, they constitute only a small percentage of colorectal cancer patients.

- *Inflammatory bowel disease*. Ulcerative colitis and Crohn disease are very closely connected with colon cancer. The younger a person is when diagnosed with either of these problems, the greater the chances of eventually developing colon cancer. The risk is so high that for some people preventive surgery to remove the whole colon is suggested before the cancer has a chance to develop.
- *Age*. The chances of having colon cancer rise with age; 90% of colon cancer patients are over 50 years of age.

Signs and Symptoms

Like many other types of cancer, colon cancer often doesn't show distinctive symptoms until it has progressed to a dangerous stage. Symptoms vary according to where tumors grow. Cancer in the spacious ascending colon is often first manifested as unexplained anemia: tumors can bleed slowly but continuously into the colon, making less iron, and therefore less oxygen, available to body cells. Iron deficiency anemia, especially among men and postmenopausal women, is a warning sign for colon cancer.

Growths in the more constricted descending colon are experienced as constipation or narrowed stools. Other signs of colon cancer that a person may or may not be aware of include blood in the stools (sometimes it is obvious and bright red, sometimes it occurs in invisible, microscopic amounts), lower abdominal pain, a feeling that bowel movements are incomplete, and unintentional weight loss.

Treatment

Treatment for colon cancer depends on the stage at which it is identified. (Staging protocols for colorectal cancer are discussed in Sidebar 8.5.) Treatment typically involves a combination of surgery, internally or externally applied radiation, chemotherapy, and using monoclonal antibodies to attack cancer cells. For information about colorectal cancer prevention, see Sidebar 8.6.

Medications

- Chemotherapeutic agents to slow the growth of cancer cells
- Biologic therapies, specifically monoclonal antibodies that target cancer cells

SIDEBAR 8.5 Staging Colorectal Cancer

The TNM classification system identifies the progress of tumors, lymph node involvement, and the extent of metastasis. Here is a simplified version of the TNM system for colorectal cancer:

Tumor	Node	Metastasis
T x: can't be assessed	N x: can't be assessed	M x: can't be assessed
T 0: no evidence of tumor	N 0: no nodal involvement	M 0: no distant metastasis
T-IS: in situ tumor(affects mucosa only)	N 1: 1–3 nodes involved	M 1a: distant metastasis to one organ or site
T 1: submucosa invaded	N 2: ≥4 nearby nodes involved	M 1b: metastases to more than one site
T 2: muscularis invaded		
T 3: subserosa invaded		
T 4a: tumor penetrates through visceral serosa		
T 4: tumor invades or adheres to other organs and structures		

The TNM classifications are then applied to a numerical staging system as follows:

Stage	Tumor	Node	Metastasis
0	T-IS	N 0	M 0
I	T 1—2	N 0	M 0
II A	T 3	N 0	M 0
II B	T 4	N 0	M 0
III A	T 1–2	N 1–2	M 0
III B	T 3–4	N 1–2	M 0
III C	T any	N 2	M 0
IV A	Any	Any	M 1a
IV B	Any	Any	M 1b

SIDEBAR 8.6 Colorectal Cancer Prevention

While it has been difficult to prove specific diet and lifestyle causes of colorectal cancer, protective mechanisms have been somewhat easier to identify. The following habits are associated with a lower-than-average risk of developing this disease:

- Eat at least five servings of fruits and vegetables every day; choose whole-grain foods.
- Reduce fats in the diet, especially saturated fats.
- Get recommended vitamins and minerals, particularly calcium, magnesium, vitamin B_6, and folate.
- Limit alcohol consumption to two drinks a day for men and one per day for women.
- Don't smoke.
- Be physically active and maintain a healthy weight.

Massage?

RISKS Colorectal cancer patients may undergo any combination of surgery, radiation, chemotherapy, and other treatment strategies, all of which require some adaptation on the part of a massage therapist or bodywork practitioner.

BENEFITS Massage can be an important and useful addition to colorectal cancer treatment, as long as the challenges of treatment are respected. For more information about massage in the context of cancer, see Chapter 12.

OPTIONS Some massage therapists may be nervous about working with a client who uses a colostomy bag. Because these devices take many forms, it is best simply to consult with the client about how to make him or her most comfortable.

Diverticular Disease in Brief

Pronunciation: dy-ver-TICK-yu-lar dih-ZEZE

What is it?
Diverticulosis is the development of small pouches that protrude from the colon or small intestine. Diverticulitis is the inflammation that develops when these pouches become infected. Collectively, these disorders are known as diverticular disease.

How is it recognized?
Diverticulosis is often silent. When inflammation (diverticulitis) is present, lower left side abdominal pain, cramping, bloating, constipation, or diarrhea may occur.

Massage risks and benefits
Risks: If the client knows that he or she has diverticulosis, abdominal massage must be done with care because the colon is structurally compromised. During a flare of diverticulitis, it is safest to delay massage until the infection has passed.
Benefits: Massage has no specific benefits for diverticular disease, but if the condition is well controlled and care is taken not to exacerbate symptoms, a client with this condition can enjoy the same benefits from massage as the rest of the population.

Diverticular Disease

Definition: What Is It?

Diverticular disease is a condition of the small intestine or colon in which the mucosal and submucosal layers of the GI tract bulge through the outer muscular layer to form a sac, or **diverticulum**. It happens most often in the descending section or sigmoid bend of the colon. The presence of these bulges is called diverticulosis. If they become infected, this is called diverticulitis.

Diverticular disease is most common in countries where diets are based on animal fats and processed grains. Interestingly, it was first documented in the early 1900s, just when new technology had been developed to remove the bran from wheat and the American diet shifted to rely heavily on low-fiber white flour. It affects up to half of the U.S. population aged 60 to 80, and two-thirds or more of people over 85 years.

Etiology: What Happens?

Diverticular disease is a multifactoral condition involving a combination of inefficient colon motility, changes in the strength of the colon wall, and the lack of sufficient dietary fiber.

Contractions of the large intestine are very strong, but without adequate bulk supplied by soluble and insoluble fiber, internal pressure between areas of contraction causes colon walls to bulge. This is especially problematic if the collagen matrix of the muscularis is impaired (as with Marfan syndrome or Ehlers-Danlos syndrome) or weakened by age. In this situation, the mucosa and submucosa of the colon can herniate through the outer muscular layer to form small sacs, or **diverticula**. These sacs may fill with fecal matter and bacteria, and the potential for infection, called diverticulitis, is high (Figure 8.8).

Most diverticula form in the sigmoid flexure or descending colon, but they have been seen throughout the GI tract, all the way up to the esophagus.

Complications of diverticulitis are rare, but they can be serious enough to become life threatening very quickly. They can include the following:

- *Bleeding*. Sometimes capillaries get stretched over the dome of the protrusion, and they may tear open and bleed into the colon.
- *Abscess*. Infected diverticula may have tiny tears that allow contents to leak out. If this is small, an abscess develops. If an abscess ruptures, its contents may be released into the peritoneum, causing peritonitis.
- *Perforation and rupture*. Diverticula may tear open and release their contents into the peritoneum.
- *Blockage*. The accumulation of scar tissue where diverticula have formed and become infected may block the colon.
- *Fistula*. In the areas that have been damaged by long-term inflammation and scarring, small passageways or **fistulas** may develop between hollow organs, allowing the passage of fecal

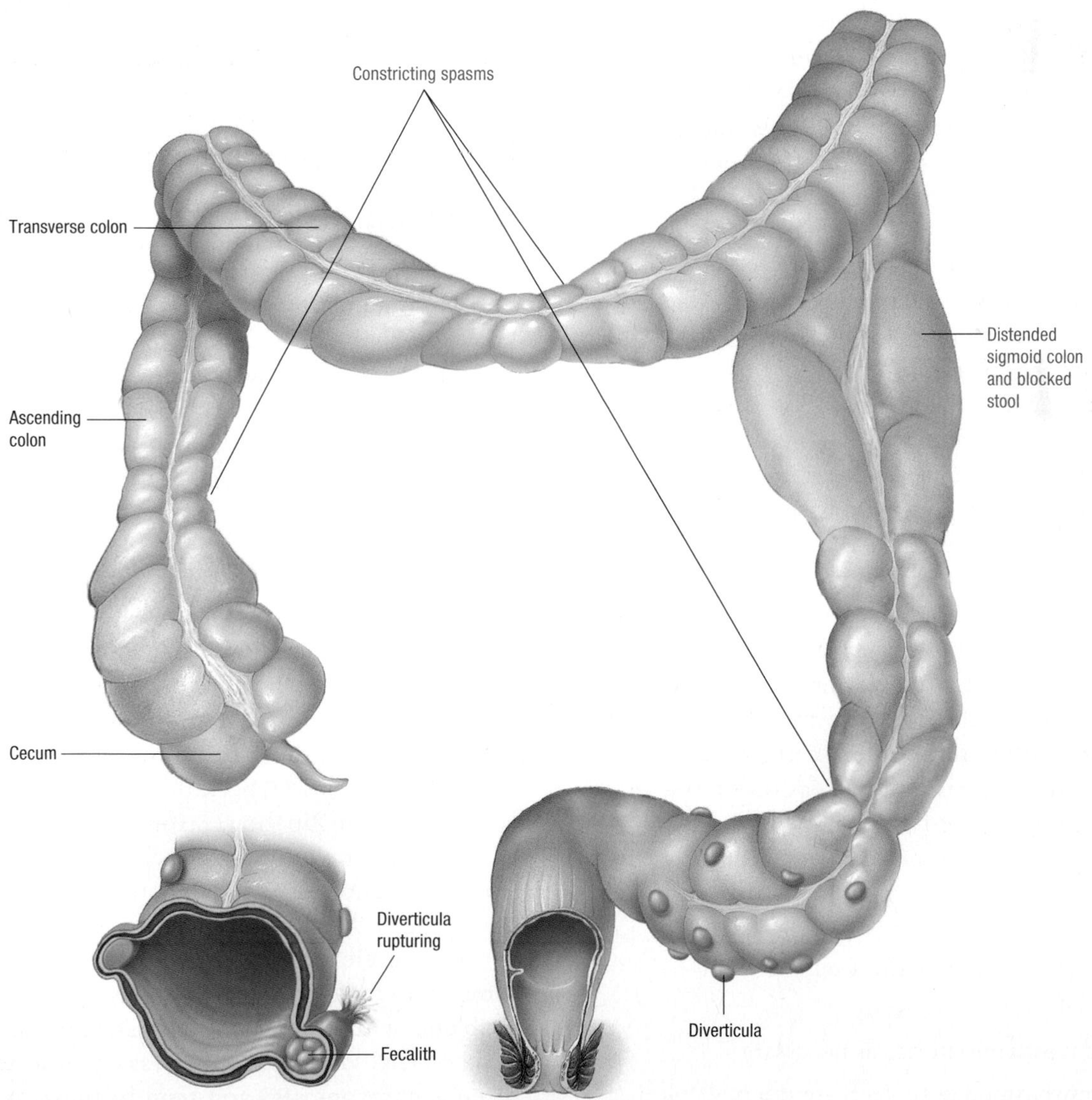

Figure 8.8. Diverticular disease

matter into spaces where it doesn't belong. In this situation, the colon may connect with the urinary bladder, small intestine, or uterus.

Signs and Symptoms

Symptoms of diverticulosis may be nonexistent. When infection is present however, symptoms include bloating, nausea, fever, cramping, and severe pain, usually on the lower left side of the abdomen. Diarrhea and/or constipation may also occur. Symptoms of diverticulitis often have a sudden onset and become rapidly worse, but some people have several days of mild discomfort before severe infection sets in.

Treatment

Diverticular disease is more easily prevented than corrected. Daily fiber intake is recommended to be 25 to 30 grams per day, along with 64 ounces of fluid. Without healthy amounts of soluble and insoluble fiber to create bulk in the colon, the smooth muscle has to work hard to compact fecal material and even harder to expel it from the body. The fact that vegetarians and people whose diets are built on whole grains, fruits, and vegetables seldom develop diverticular disease is an indication that healthy levels of dietary fiber can prevent this problem.

Treatment for diverticulosis isn't usually necessary because the symptoms are so mild or don't exist at all. Although the diverticula are not reversible, further growths can be prevented with changes toward a higher fiber diet and exercise.

Treatment for diverticulitis starts with antibiotics and a clear liquid diet for several days. If substantial tissue damage has occurred, including a bowel obstruction, uncontrolled bleeding, perforation, large abscesses, or fistulas, surgery may be performed. Depending on the seriousness of the condition, surgery may involve a simple resection of the colon, removing the infected or damaged area, or it may require a temporary or permanent colostomy.

Medications

- Antibiotics when infection is present
- Analgesics as necessary
- Anti-inflammatories as necessary
- Antispasmodics to decrease internal colon pressure

Massage?

RISKS It is important to realize that the signs and symptoms of diverticular disease can be similar to those of simple digestive upset. If massage temporarily eases these symptoms, it may delay the client in getting a very important diagnosis. Consequently, if symptoms persist for more than 2 weeks, it is important to advise clients to pursue a formal diagnosis.

When a client has been diagnosed with diverticular disease, care must be taken with abdominal work, because the colon is structurally compromised. During flares of acute inflammation (diverticulitis), it is best to delay any intrusive bodywork until the infection has passed.

BENEFITS Massage or bodywork is unlikely to improve the prognosis for a person with diverticular disease, but as long as care is taken not to exacerbate symptoms, bodywork may be a helpful strategy to deal with anxiety and abdominal pain.

Irritable Bowel Syndrome

Definition: What Is It?

IBS is a condition involving digestive system dysfunction without major structural changes. It has also been known as spastic colon, irritable colon, mucus colitis, and functional bowel syndrome.

It is considered a biopsychosocial disorder, involving aspects of basic health processes as they relate to mood and stress management.

Etiology: What Happens?

In a normal colon, fecal matter is squeezed and compacted, while water and salts are reabsorbed into the bloodstream. The shorter the transit time, the less water is reabsorbed; this leads to watery stools or diarrhea. The longer the transit time, the more water is absorbed, and stools become extremely dense and compacted: constipation. Strong contractions move the formed stools into the rectum, where they are stored until another wave of contractions moves them out of the body altogether.

The development of IBS symptoms is related to three main factors: hypersensitivity in the intestines, problems with **motility** or organized peristalsis, and psychosocial factors like depression or anxiety that often accompany IBS and tend to make symptoms worse (Figure 8.9).

Irritable Bowel Syndrome in Brief

What is it?
Irritable bowel syndrome (IBS) is a collection of signs and symptoms that indicate a problem with colon function. Symptoms are aggravated by stress and diet.

How is it recognized?
The symptoms of IBS include abdominal pain along with constipation or diarrhea (or alternating between the two); bloating or abdominal distension; and a sensation of incomplete emptying with defecation.

Massage risks and benefits
Risks: Massage poses no specific risks for clients with IBS as long as they are comfortable receiving bodywork.
Benefits: If the experience of touch feels safe to a client with IBS, massage can be a powerful aid to someone whose digestive comfort is related to stress.

While this syndrome is usually discussed as a digestive system disorder, it is also connected to a dysfunction of the brain-gut axis, that is, the link of continuous feedback between GI tract sensation and motor response from the central nervous system. Many people with IBS also have other smooth muscle tissue dysfunction. IBS frequently appears simultaneously with chronic fatigue syndrome and fibromyalgia: two chronic conditions that both have important central nervous system components.

One subset of IBS patients develops long-term symptoms after having an acute infection of the gut. Tissue studies of these patients reveal the possibility of low-grade inflammation, which may indicate the presence of infection. This is significant finding, as it suggests treatment options that are not successful with other IBS patients.

SIDEBAR 8.7 Where is Ulcerative Colitis?

Ulcerative colitis has been discussed as a disorder of the lower digestive tract, but because it is an autoimmune disease, it now appears in Chapter 6.

IBS is a common disorder, and responsible for significant lost quality of life. As specialists learn more about it, overlap with some food sensitivities have emerged as common phenomena. Sensitivity to gluten (i.e., low-grade or latent celiac disease) or mild lactose and fructose intolerance are seen more often in people who meet the diagnostic criteria for IBS than in the general population.

Types of Irritable Bowel Syndrome

- *IBS—D*: This describes irritable bowel syndrome, in which the primary symptom is a chronic diarrhea.
- *IBS—C*: This describes irritable bowel syndrome in which the primary symptom is chronic constipation.
- *IBS—M*: In this version, a person can experience both diarrhea and constipation within a short time span.
- *IBS—A*: This describes alternating irritable bowel syndrome, in which symptoms fluctuate between diarrhea and constipation.

Signs and Symptoms

Symptoms of IBS can range from occasionally inconvenient to severely debilitating, but it is not a life-threatening disease. It can mimic several serious digestive system conditions, however. In particular, diverticulitis, colon cancer, ulcerative colitis, and Crohn disease must be eliminated as possibilities.

An internationally recognized symptomatic profile for IBS identifies leading symptoms as recurrent abdominal pain at least 3 days every month, pain with defecation, changes in stool frequency, and changes in stool appearance. Other symptoms can include gas, bloating, headaches, and general malaise.

The changes brought about by IBS are purely functional; no structural anomalies like scar tissue, ulcers, polyps, or tumors develop because of this disorder. For this reason, if a person with IBS develops a fever or has blood in the stool, IBS is not the cause, and these new symptoms should be reported to a physician.

Treatment

Treatment for IBS depends on the individual. The first recourse is to consider dietary and stress

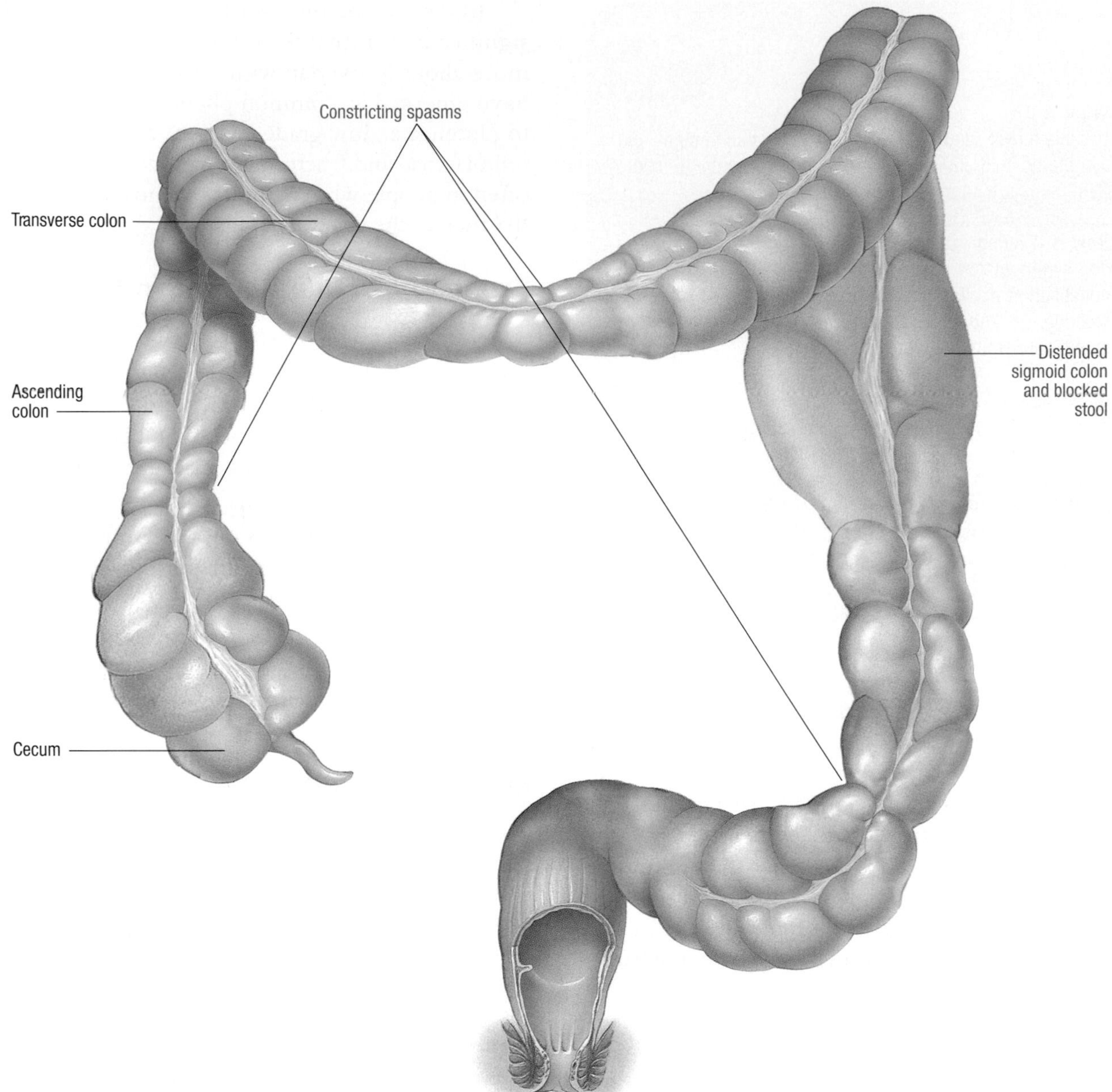

Figure 8.9. Irritable bowel syndrome

factors. Nicotine, caffeine, alcohol, the artificial sweetener sorbitol, and dairy products have been found to be particularly irritating, but no particular food or drink is a definitive trigger for IBS attacks for all patients. Somc doctors rccommend fiber supplementation; the addition of bulk to the diet can fill the colon more completely and help to limit spasm.

Complementary treatments for IBS have found some success. Acupuncture, peppermint, and the use of probiotics to restore normal intestinal bacteria have shown success with some patients.

Medications

- Antispasmodics to limit colon hyperreactivity
- Fecal binders for diarrhea
- Bulking agents
- Laxatives for constipation
- Antidiarrheals as necessary
- Antacids to limit digestive discomfort
- Antidepressants/antianxiety medications for stress management
- Antibiotics if low-grade bacterial infection is confirmed

Massage?

RISKS Some clients with Irritable bowel syndrome (IBS) are extremely self-conscious about passing gas during a massage appointment. This, or nervousness about touch in general, may make it difficult for a person to enjoy the experience of massage. If these challenges can be addressed, massage has no particular risks for a client who has IBS.

BENEFITS Because massage is an effective way to address anxiety and stress, clients with IBS welcome touch may find this a powerful tool to help manage their condition.

OPTIONS The key factor for someone who has IBS to derive benefit from massage is for them be able to relax and not worry about passing gas. To address this issue for all her nervous clients, I know one massage therapist who has a plaque up on her wall that states "It's not a good massage until somebody farts."

Disorders of the Accessory Organs

Cirrhosis

Definition: What Is It?

The word cirrhosis, from the Greek "kirrhos," means "yellow condition," referring to the jaundice that can develop as a complication of this condition. Cirrhosis is a result of long-term liver damage. It describes the crowding out and replacement of healthy liver cells with nonfunctioning scar tissue. This interferes with virtually every function of the liver, with potentially fatal repercussions.

Etiology: What Happens?

The liver is composed of highly organized layers of epithelial hepatocytes: cells that produce a myriad of vital chemicals for metabolism and survival. The liver produces bile, which helps to metabolize fats, and other enzymes that metabolize proteins and carbohydrates. Clotting factors, proteins that maintain the proper balance of tissue fluid, and cells that help filter and neutralize toxins and hormones are all produced in the liver.

Under normal circumstances, the liver has great powers of regeneration. But chronic long-term irritation or infection may suppress the growth of healthy, organized cells. Instead, collagen and other extracellular matrix components proliferate. Healthy cells are crowded into abnormal nodules (leading to a knobby, "hobnailed liver" appearance, Figure 8.10), and the tiny channels that are meant to direct fluid flow to the appropriate vessels become blocked.

Traditionally, alcoholism has been the leading cause of cirrhosis in the United States. Now hepatitis

Cirrhosis in Brief

Pronunciation: sir-OH-sis

What is it?
Cirrhosis is a condition in which normal liver cells become disorganized and dysfunctional; many of them are replaced or crowded out by scar tissue. Cirrhosis is often the final stage of chronic or acute liver disease.

How is it recognized?
Symptoms of cirrhosis are linked to progressive loss of liver function. Early symptoms include loss of appetite, nausea, vomiting, and weight loss. Later complications may include muscle wasting, jaundice, ascites, internal bleeding, vomiting blood, and mental and personality changes.

Massage risks and benefits
Risks: Advanced cirrhosis involves a fundamental problem with managing fluid flow. Rigorous massage that challenges this process is not appropriate in these circumstances.
Benefits: Bodywork that does not excessively challenge homeostasis or adaptive responses can be helpful for a person with this complex condition. Further, cirrhosis patients with muscle wasting as a complication of liver damage may be advised to exercise and pursue physical therapy. Massage in this context may support this effort.

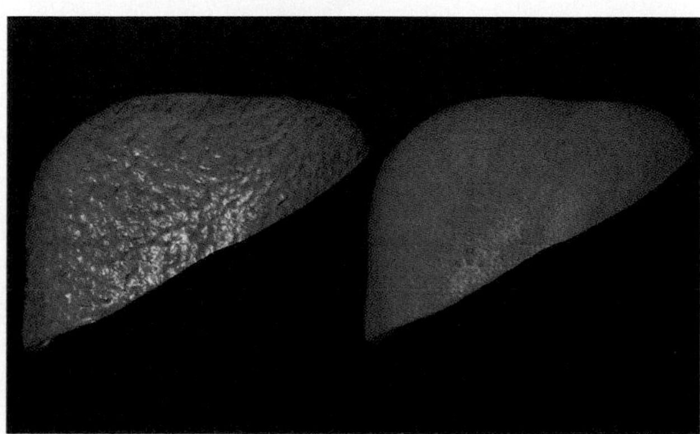

Figure 8.10. Cirrhotic liver compared to normal liver

C probably causes cirrhosis at least as often as long-term alcohol abuse. Cirrhosis can also arise from types B, D, drug-related, and autoimmune hepatitis. Nonalcoholic fatty liver disease (NAFLD) is also a significant contributor to cirrhosis: this is a complication of obesity, type 2 diabetes, and high triglycerides. NAFLD progresses to another condition, nonalcoholic steatohepatitis in some adults. Steatohepatitis is inflammation of fatty tissue in the liver. Chronic inflammation is linked to the formation of excessive connective tissue, the hallmark of cirrhosis.

Other causes for cirrhosis include any factor that can obstruct the complicated bile duct system (Figure 8.11), including gallstones, pancreatic tumors, and congenital malformation of the bile duct system. Long-term exposure to environmental toxins can contribute to cirrhosis, as can congestive heart failure and some congenital diseases. It is important to bear in mind that most people with cirrhosis have multiple factors that may contribute to this disease: hepatitis B along with obesity, for instance.

As the liver progressively loses function, many complications arise. At the center of several complications is portal hypertension. In this situation, the liver becomes so congested that it cannot freely accept blood delivered from the digestive and accessory organs, and pressure accumulates in the portal system veins. Other complications arise as the liver simply no longer produces enough vital blood components or inadequately filters and neutralizes hormones and toxic materials. Complications of cirrhosis include the following:

- *Splenomegaly* (enlarged spleen). The spleen enlarges because it can't drain through the portal vein. The danger with splenomegaly is that when fluid backs up in this organ, the risk of rupture and internal hemorrhage is high.
- *Ascites*. When pressure in the portal system increases, plasma seeps out of the veins and lymphatic vessels into the peritoneal space, causing the abdominal distension known as ascites (Figure 8.12). The bacteria that normally inhabit the GI tract may seep out to set up an infection in this fluid, causing spontaneous bacterial peritonitis, a potentially life-threatening infection.

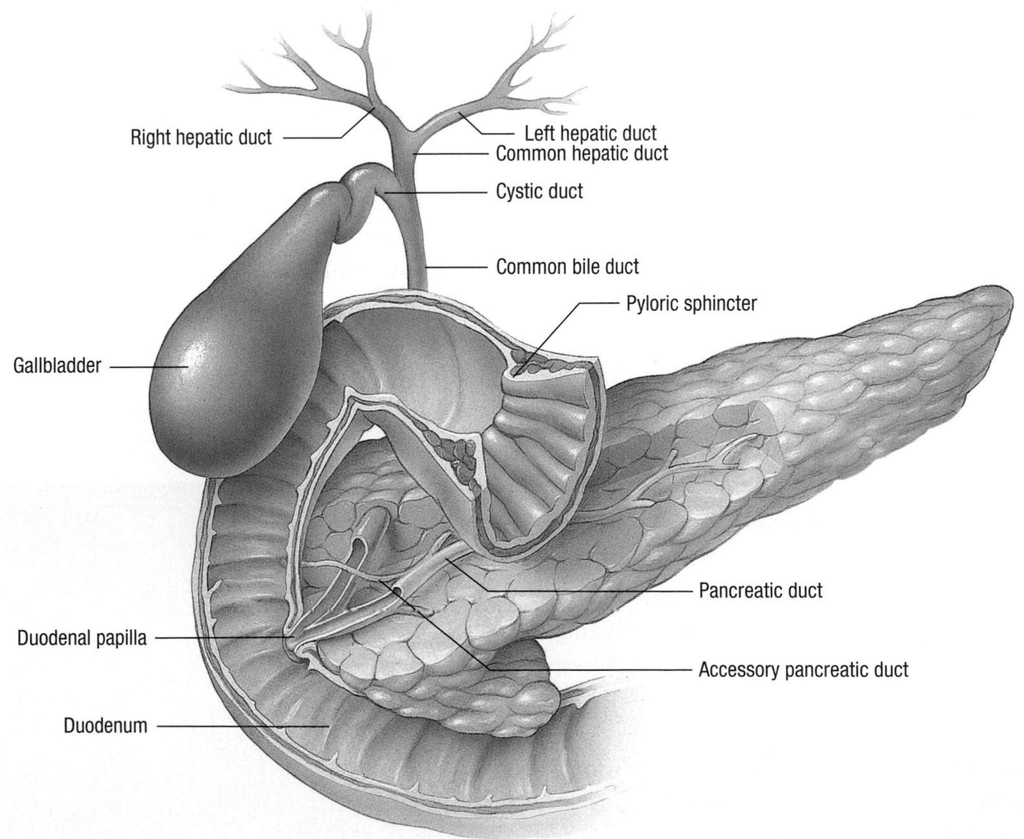

Figure 8.11. Cirrhosis: gallbladder and duct system

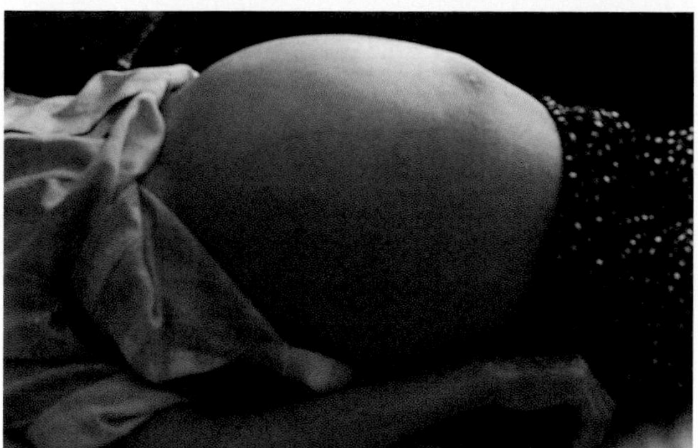

Figure 8.12. Cirrhosis: ascites

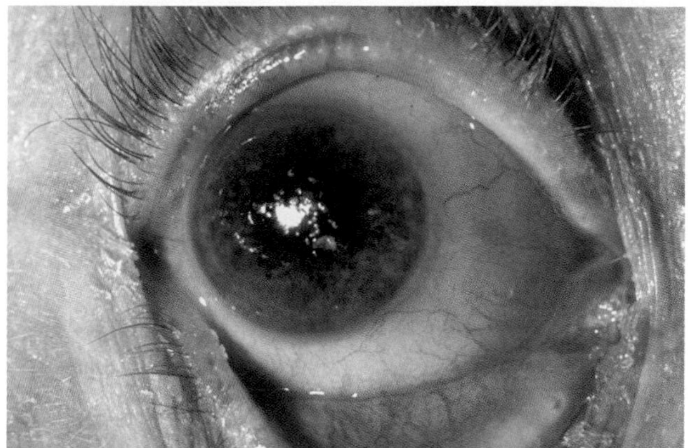

Figure 8.13. Cirrhosis: jaundice

Ascites in the peritoneum can also seep across the diaphragm to cause pleural effusion.

- *Internal varices.* Pressure in abdominal veins grows as fluid backs up through the system. This can lead to internal venous distensions and varicosities, especially in the esophagus and stomach. Varicose veins can hemorrhage during vomiting, leading to bloody vomit, internal bleeding, shock, or death.
- *Bleeding, bruising.* When the liver no longer produces adequate clotting factors, the ability to heal from minor injury is severely impaired. Cirrhosis patients may bruise extensively and bleed for abnormally long periods.
- *Osteoporosis.* The liver helps to process vitamin D. Without this function, it is impossible to absorb adequate calcium from the diet, so osteoporosis is likely to develop.
- *Muscle wasting.* When the enzymes that aid in protein metabolism are in short supply, a cirrhosis patient may undergo progressive atrophy of the skeletal muscles.
- *Jaundice.* **Bilirubin** (a byproduct of dead red blood cells) is produced in the spleen, and it is meant to be recycled in the liver to be a component of bile. When cirrhosis interferes with this process, water-soluble components of bilirubin accumulate in the bloodstream. Bilirubin is strongly pigmented, and it can turn the sclera of the eyes and skin a yellowish color. It can also cause rashes and itching, as some people have an extreme reaction to this unfamiliar chemical in their skin (Figure 8.13). Jaundice is discussed further in Extra Conditions at a Glance, Appendix C.
- *Systemic edema.* One of the critical proteins for maintaining fluid balance in the body, albumin, is significantly lowered in advanced cirrhosis. Without albumin, the body cannot maintain proper fluid levels, and edema accumulates systemically in all interstitial spaces.
- *Hormone disruption.* The liver of men with cirrhosis no longer inactivates their normal low levels of estrogen; feminizing characteristics such as breast development, loss of chest hair, impotence, and atrophy of the testicles soon follow. For women, hormonal changes include the cessation of periods, infertility, and the growth of body hair. Both men and women with cirrhosis can expect a decreased sex drive.
- *Encephalopathy.* When cirrhosis is very advanced, the detoxifying agents in the liver are out of commission. Protection from toxic metabolites is no longer provided. Furthermore, the blood-brain barrier, which usually keeps the central nervous system safe, becomes much less effective with cirrhosis. Toxic wastes accumulate in the blood and eventually cause brain damage. Symptoms include somnolence, confusion, tremors, hallucinations, and even coma and death.
- *Kidney failure.* Advanced cirrhosis can impair blood flow to the kidneys, resulting in kidney failure. **Hepatorenal syndrome** is an emergency that requires a liver transplant for survival.
- *Liver failure.* The progressive loss of liver function can lead to a failure of the liver to keep up with daily needs. A person with end-stage liver failure is a candidate for a liver transplant.

- *Liver cancer*. Chronic inflammation in the liver increases the risk of cellular mutation and liver cancer.

Signs and Symptoms

The liver readily compensates for slowly progressive losses in function. Consequently, by the time symptoms are observable without blood tests, cirrhosis is likely to be advanced. Early symptoms are vague and can be attributed to any number of other common disorders. They include nausea, vomiting, weight loss, and the development of red or itchy patches on the skin. Later symptoms are usually identified by the complications discussed above.

Treatment

The prognosis for someone in the early stages of cirrhosis caused by alcoholism or drug abuse is excellent, if the damage can be stopped. Medication is sometimes administered to counteract the complications of this disease: diuretics for edema, antacids for intestinal discomfort, levulose, an undigestible sugar, to bind with ammonia so that it can be excreted. Vitamins and minerals are recommended to guard against malnutrition. Cirrhosis due to hepatitis is treated with interferon as an antiviral measure. Steroids for inflammation due to autoimmune hepatitis are occasionally prescribed. Surgical repair of internal varicosities may be necessary, and if the kidneys are impaired hemodialysis can assist in their function until the crisis has passed.

When these interventions are inadequate, a liver transplant is considered. In this country, about 15,000 liver transplants are conducted each year. The liver regenerates so readily that a person can give about 60% of a healthy organ, and both the donor and recipient will have healthy functioning livers within a few months.

Medications

- Diuretics for water retention
- Beta blockers for portal hypertension
- Antacids for digestive discomfort
- Levulose to help eradicate ammonia
- Steroidal anti-inflammatories for autoimmune problems
- Interferon for chronic viral hepatitis

Massage?

RISKS Complications of cirrhosis can damage the skin, interfere with blood clotting, promote blood toxicity, and generally impair function of several systems. Clients with advanced cirrhosis do not have the adaptive capacity to manage rigorous massage or bodywork.

BENEFITS Gentle or reflexive work that invites calm and reduces anxiety can be helpful for any person with a complicated disease. If a client is encouraged to exercise to promote recovery of muscles, massage may fit into this context as well.

Gallstones

Definition: What Are They?

Gallstones are concentrated deposits of bile salts or pigments in the gallbladder. The technical term for gallbladder is **cholecyst**, because it is a cyst (holding tank) that collects, among other things, cholesterol. The formation of tiny crystals or stones

Gallstones in Brief

Pronunciation:

What are they?
Gallstones are crystallized formations of cholesterol or bile pigments in the gallbladder. They can be as small as a grain of sand, or as large as a golf ball.

How are they recognized?
Most gallstones do not cause symptoms. When they do, pain that may last several hours develops in the upper right side of the abdomen. Pain may refer to the back between the scapula and the right shoulder. Gallstones stuck in the ducts of the biliary system may cause jaundice or pancreatitis.

Massage risks and benefits
Risks: An acute gallbladder attack requires medical intervention, not massage. If a gallstone is causing problems, massage in the vicinity of the right costal angle may be painful. Gallstone pain can also refer to the back and shoulder, where clients may mistake it for muscle pain.
Benefits: Massage has no particular benefits for gallstone patients, but as long as no danger to the biliary system exists, a person with a history of gallstones can enjoy the same benefits from massage as the rest of the population.

in the gallbladder is called **cholelithiasis** ("lith" means stone). Inflammation of the gallbladder from a stuck stone or other cause is called **cholecystitis**. When stones become lodged in the common bile duct, the condition is called **choledocholithiasis**. Inflammation of any of the ducts in the biliary system (the exocrine ducts of the liver, gallbladder, and pancreas) is called **cholangitis**.

Gallstones are fairly common, leading to about 800,000 hospitalizations and 500,000 surgeries each year. Women are far more prone to developing gallstones than men are; depending on age, they outnumber men by about 2 to 1.

Etiology: What Happens?

Bile is produced in the liver and delivered to the gallbladder through the hepatic duct and the cystic duct (Figure 8.14). When a person eats a high-fat meal, hormonal commands cause the gallbladder to release its contents into the cystic duct. The bile flows into the common bile duct, and then into the small intestine. Pancreatic secretions also use the common bile duct for access to the small intestine.

The purpose of bile is to hold particles of fat in tiny, discrete pieces, so that they can be absorbed into the lacteals, that is, lymphatic projections in the intestinal villi. Without bile, fat particles tend to stick together in indigestible clumps. This reduces access to important fat-soluble vitamins and nutrients.

Bile is primarily made up of water, bile salts (which help in fat digestion), bilirubin from recycled red blood cells, and cholesterol, which is filtered out of the bloodstream by the liver. When either cholesterol or bilirubin occurs in higher-than-normal concentrations in bile, they can precipitate out of the liquid to become tiny granules called "bile sludge," or larger stones (Figure 8.15).

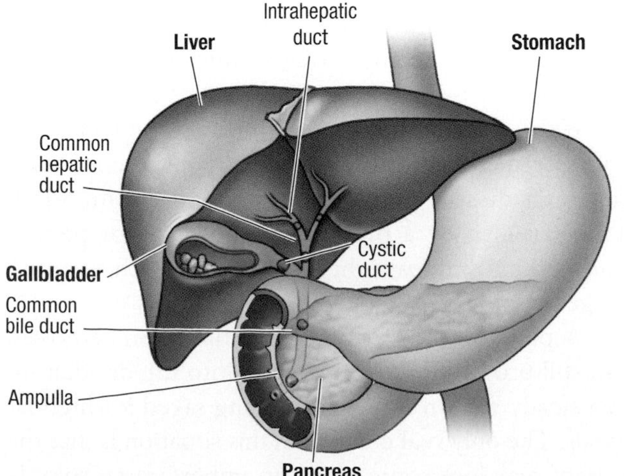

Figure 8.14. Gallstones in ducts

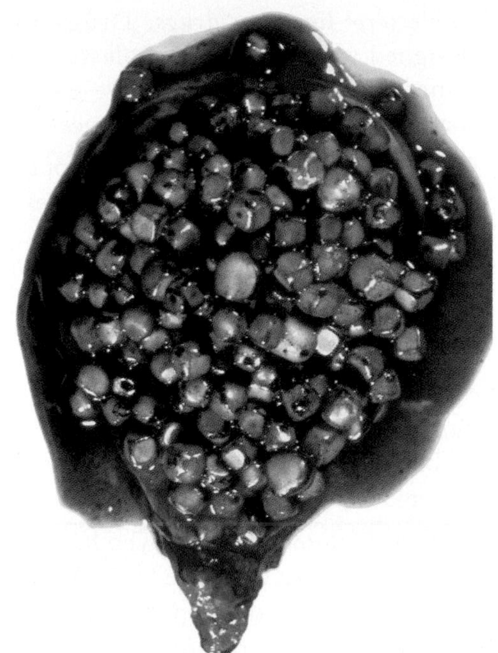

Figure 8.15. Gallstones

A relatively small percentage of gallstones (10% to 20%) are made of bilirubin, the coloring agent for feces. Bilirubin stones are also called "pigment stones." They are usually a sign of some type of blood dysfunction that causes premature destruction of red blood cells, resulting in abnormally high levels of bilirubin in the blood and in the liver. Most gallstones (80% to 90%) are composed of cholesterol. Several factors can increase the risk of developing cholesterol stones, including the following:

- *Obesity*. Obesity increases the amount of cholesterol manufactured by the liver and stored in the gallbladder.
- *Estrogen*. Estrogen tends to increase the amount of cholesterol in bile while decreasing gallbladder activity, which allows the cholesterol to crystallize. Estrogen levels may be related to pregnancy, birth control pills, or hormone replacement therapy.
- *Race*. Native Americans and Mexican Americans have the highest incidence of gallstones of any specific racial groups.
- *Gender*. Women aged 16 to 60 with gallstones outnumber men by about 2 to 1.

- *Cholesterol-lowering drugs.* Drugs that are designed to lower blood cholesterol help to concentrate cholesterol in the gallbladder, increasing the risk of forming stones.
- *Diabetes.* Diabetics have high levels of triglycerides, which raises the risk for gallstones.
- *Rapid weight loss.* Rapid weight loss causes the liver to metabolize fat for fuel, resulting in higher levels of cholesterol in the bile. Gallstones are a common complication of bariatric surgery.
- *Fasting.* Fasting reduces gallbladder emptying, so bile becomes concentrated and cholesterol precipitates out into stones.
- *History of gallstones.* People who have had gallstones in the past are more likely than the general population to develop them again.
- *Other diseases.* People with Crohn disease, cirrhosis, and diabetes have a higher incidence of gallstones, although the mechanisms for this are not clear.

Gallstones in themselves are not usually a serious threat, but they can create unpleasant or even life-threatening complications. The most obvious is an obstruction of the cystic or hepatic duct, which can lead to jaundice or acute pancreatitis. The pooling of stagnant bile can also lead to infection of the gallbladder, or cholecystitis. It is possible for an infected gallbladder to rupture, releasing its contents and causing abscesses or peritonitis. And a person with chronic gallbladder irritation has an increased risk of developing fibrosis and gallbladder cancer.

Signs and Symptoms

Most people who have gallstones never know, because symptoms are typically generated only when a stone becomes lodged in the hepatic duct, the cystic duct, in the common bile duct. This causes extreme local pain called biliary colic, which often lasts for hours, builds to a peak, and then gradually subsides when the stone moves back into the gallbladder or on to the duodenum. The pain may be intense enough to induce nausea and vomiting. If the stone is immovably stuck, the patient may require hospitalization to have it surgically removed.

The gallbladder refers pain between the scapulae and over the right shoulder. Although most patients have pain in the upper right quadrant of the abdomen, some feel it primarily in the back (where even the most gifted massage won't relieve it).

SIDEBAR 8.8 Lose the Gallbladder, Keep the Fat

Bile, manufactured in the liver and stored in the gallbladder, suspends consumed fats in tiny pieces, so the body can absorb and digest them in the small intestine. A person who loses her gallbladder has less access to incoming fat and so absorbs less fat from the diet.

Why, then, do gallbladder surgery patients not lose a lot of weight after surgery? It seems like gallbladder removal would be a popular form of elective surgery!

It turns out that to burn fat that is stored in the body's lipid cells, we must consume certain kinds of fats that will help to soften those lipid cells' membranes. When a person loses her gallbladder, hence access to incoming nutrition in the form of fats, it actually becomes harder to lose weight, because the body much more tenaciously retains whatever fat is in the lipid cells. Since obesity is a leading contributor to the formation of gallstones, losing one's gallbladder makes it doubly hard to resolve problems with being overweight.

Treatment

Laparoscopic surgery is the most common intervention to deal with gallstones. The whole gallbladder is removed in this procedure.

Another surgical option is **endoscopic retrograde cholangiopancreatography**. This is a scope on a thin tube that is inserted through the mouth, down the esophagus, through the stomach, and into the small intestine and biliary duct system. It may be used as a diagnostic tool, but in some cases, a device can be attached to the scope to remove or dislodge gallstones.

If the gallstones are determined to be small and cholesterol based, a long-term dosage of chemicals that can dissolve stones may be recommended. This can also be a preventive measure for people undergoing rapid weight loss, as seen with bariatric surgery.

A person whose gallbladder has been removed can still produce bile, but it drips into the duodenum in a steady stream rather than being saved for high-fat meals. The only real concern in this situation is that the patient may lose some access to important fat-soluble vitamins. Fortunately, digestive supplements can aid in the digestion of fats (Sidebar 8.8).

Medications

- Analgesics for acute gallbladder attacks
- Ursodeoxycholic acid or chenodeoxycholic acid for 6 to 18 months to dissolve small cholesterol-based gallstones

Massage?

RISKS Acute biliary colic (a gallbladder attack) contraindicates massage until the problem has been addressed. When gallstones have been identified but no symptoms are present, the right costal angle is a local caution.

BENEFITS A client with a history of gallstones but no current symptoms, or someone who has had uncomplicated gallbladder surgery, can enjoy the same benefits of massage as the rest of the population.

Hepatitis

Definition: What Is It?

Hepatitis means inflamed liver. It can be caused by drug reactions, autoimmune disease, or exposure to certain toxins, but it is most often one of a variety of viral infections that can mildly or severely impair liver function. Seven types of viral hepatitis have been identified to date: hepatitis A through G. Hepatitis A, B, and C cause about 90% of cases in the United States; they are the primary focus of this discussion.

To hear the author discuss the different types of hepatitis and implications for massage, go to http://thePoint.lww.com/Werner5e.

Hepatitis in Brief

Pronunciation: hep-ah-TY-tis

What is it?
Hepatitis is inflammation of the liver, usually but not always due to viral infection.

How is it recognized?
All types of hepatitis produce the same symptoms, with variable severity. Symptoms are often subtle, and include fatigue, abdominal pain, nausea, diarrhea, and jaundice.

Massage risks and benefits
Risks: Acute hepatitis of any kind contraindicates any bodywork that demands an extensive adaptive response. Hepatitis B can be communicable through indirect contact, which is why it is important to follow standard precautions for hygiene.
Benefits: Gentle massage that invites rather than imposes change can be appropriate for a person in recovery from hepatitis. A person with a history of hepatitis but no current symptoms or complications can enjoy the same benefits from bodywork as the rest of the population.

Etiology: What Happens?

Hepatitis A, B, and C all are viral attacks against liver cells. Each type of virus is unique, however. Exposure to one type of hepatitis does not impart immunity to any other type of hepatitis.

Once a hepatitis virus gains access to the body, it attacks liver cells and stimulates an immune system response. Hepatitis can be identified and diagnosed by the presence of antibodies in the blood, and also by the presence of enzymes that indicate liver damage.

Viral hepatitis of any kind may be described in four basic phases:

- Phase 1. New infection and viral replication. During this phase, the virus attacks cells in the liver, but the liver compensates for the damage, so no symptoms develop. Blood tests for indicator enzymes or antibodies are positive.
- Phase 2. Prodromal stage. Symptoms develop in this stage. Food aversion, nausea, vomiting, and malaise are the most common complaints.
- Phase 3. Icteric stage. At this point, the signs of jaundice develop, including yellowing skin (**icterus**), pale stools, dark urine, and hepatomegaly. For more information on jaundice, see Appendix C, Extra Conditions at a Glance.
- Phase 4. Convalescence. During this time, the liver heals, jaundice resolves, enzymes return to normal levels, and health is restored.

NOTABLE CASES Hepatitis C has affected a number of notable personalities, including Jim "Gomer Pyle" Nabors, and musicians Greg Allman, Natalie Cole, and David Crosby.

For information about communicability, prognosis, and prevention for various types of hepatitis, see Compare & Contrast 8.1.

Types of Hepatitis

- *Hepatitis A*: This used to be called infectious hepatitis. It is a short, acute infection (relative

COMPARE & CONTRAST 8.1 The ABCs of Hepatitis

The three most common types of hepatitis seen in developed countries are caused by viruses that, while they are unrelated to each other, share a common target: hepatocytes. Consequently, they tend to create a similar symptomatic picture with varying severity. This chart compares other important features of these viruses, namely communicability, prognosis, and the availability of a preventive vaccine.

	COMMUNICABILITY	PROGRESSION	VACCINE AVAILABLE?
Hepatitis A	Hepatitis A virus concentrates in the feces of an infected person; therefore, it is most easily transmitted through oral-fecal contact, often by way of contaminated food or water. Hepatitis A is the reason for "employees must wash hands before returning to work" signs in restaurant bathrooms. Raw or undercooked shellfish grown in contaminated water can spread the disease to humans. Hepatitis A can also be shared through sexual activity, but this does not appear to an efficient method of communication.	Hepatitis A usually develops over several weeks, spontaneously resolves, and does not cause long-term complications.	Yes; one vaccine is sufficient.
Hepatitis B	Hepatitis B virus occurs in high concentration in the blood, and is viable outside a host for many hours or days. It is communicable through exposure to intimate fluids, but doesn't necessarily require direct contact. Sharing a tattoo needle, body piercing equipment, an intravenous needle, or even a razor or a toothbrush with a person who has hepatitis B is a potent mechanism for communicating the virus from host to another. Infants born to mothers with hepatitis B are at very high risk for chronic liver disease unless they are treated immediately.	Hepatitis B infections can be long-lasting and silent, requiring treatment for many months before the virus is eradicated. About 5% of hepatitis B patients are long-term carriers, and resistant to treatment. Untreated hepatitis B patients and long-term carriers experience chronic liver inflammation. This can lead to the development of varicose veins on the stomach and esophagus, which may rupture and bleed. Liver failure, cirrhosis, and liver cancer are other possible complications.	Yes; a series of three vaccines over a period of 6 months needs to be repeated about every 20 years.
Hepatitis C	Hepatitis C is most communicable through blood-to-blood contact (i.e., accidental needle sticks in health care settings, transfusions, shared needles, tattoo or piercing equipment, or sexual activity with damage to mucous membranes). It does not appear to be easily communicable without direct contact, but many cases develop from unknown sources of exposure.	Only about 25% of hepatitis C patients recover spontaneously. Of those with chronic hepatitis C, many are at risk for chronic liver disease, including cirrhosis, liver failure, and liver cancer. The presence of other illnesses, specifically HIV, hepatitis B, or alcoholism, raises the risk of complications from long-term hepatitis C infections.	No vaccine is available for hepatitis C.

to other types of hepatitis), that usually causes no long-lasting damage. One exposure creates lifelong immunity. Hepatitis A virus (HAV) incubates for 2 to 6 weeks after exposure before symptoms appear, but it is contagious during this period. Once symptoms develop, the virus is present for another 2 to 3 weeks, although a person may not feel fully restored to health for up to 6 months.

Up to 30% of all adults in the United States test positive for exposure to hepatitis A, even if they have never had symptoms.

- *Hepatitis B*: Hepatitis B virus (HBV) is spread through exposure to intimate fluids: blood, semen, breast milk, or vaginal secretions. It causes long-term infections with subtle symptoms. In this case, the virus itself is not responsible for most liver injury; chronic inflammation is the cause of most of the damage. HVB incubates for 2 to 6 months before symptoms develop, but it is communicable during this time. Most adults who are exposed to hepatitis B recover fully within 15 months. However, infants who contract the disease from their mothers, and about 5% of exposed adults develop chronic infections. These individuals are long-term carriers of the virus, and their risk of developing other liver diseases is higher than that of the general population.

  Unlike many pathogens, HVB is sturdy outside of a host, and is communicable through indirect blood-to-blood contact with a contaminated surface. Furthermore, it occurs in high concentrations, so limited exposure can cause an infection. For this reason, it is especially important to sterilize any instruments that come in contact with human blood: tattoo needles, body piercing equipment, acupuncture needles, and professional medical and dental tools all fall into this category. Further, sharing household items that might contact blood, such as razors or toothbrushes, must be avoided.

- *Hepatitis C*: Before the viruses D, E, F, and G were discovered, hepatitis virus C (HCV) was called "hepatitis non-A, non-B."

  Hepatitis C has been called a "silent epidemic": although many people have never heard of it, it is carried by more than 3 million Americans, and of those, about three-quarters have it as a chronic infection, and those individuals are consequently at high risk for cirrhosis, liver failure, or liver cancer. HCV is unique in that it damages the liver so slowly that symptoms may not develop until decades after exposure. The individual is contagious all that time, however.

- *Other forms of hepatitis*: Liver inflammation may be caused by other viruses. Hepatitis D is a form that can only exist alongside hepatitis B. Types E, F, and G are rare pathogens that are uncommon in the United States. Two members of the herpes family, Epstein-Barr virus and cytomegalovirus, have also been seen to cause liver inflammation.

  Nonviral hepatitis is an occasional reaction to certain medications or an autoimmune attack launched against hepatocytes. Autoimmune hepatitis frequently accompanies other autoimmune diseases, including type 1 diabetes, Graves disease, and ulcerative colitis.

Signs and Symptoms

The severity of hepatitis symptoms varies widely from one person to another, depending on the phase of the infection, the general health of the patient, and the type of virus involved. The basic picture of hepatitis symptoms includes general malaise, weakness, fever, nausea, food aversion, and sometimes jaundice. Hepatitis A typically presents the most extreme symptoms for the shortest time; hepatitis B and C tend to be much subtler, developing symptoms only when so much liver function has been lost that it can no longer compensate for the damage. Blood tests for antibodies or liver enzymes can indicate infection long before symptoms suggest an illness. A person infected with any type of hepatitis who has any other form of liver disease is at risk for a much more serious case than someone who begins with a healthy liver.

Treatment

Hepatitis A is typically treated with a shot of immunoglobulin (usually equine antibodies) to begin fighting the virus while the patient establishes an immune response. Hepatitis B and C are treated with antiviral agents, rest, good nutrition, and patience during a long recovery period.

If significant liver function is lost due to hepatitis C, a liver transplant may be recommended; this is the leading reason for liver transplants in the United States.

Medications

- For hepatitis A: Immunoglobulin injection to boost active antibodies while the patient establishes an immune response
- For hepatitis B and C: Any combination of lamivudine, ribavirin, interferon, or other antiviral agents

Massage?

RISKS Acute hepatitis carries a risk of several serious complications, including jaundice, cirrhosis, and liver failure. Any bodywork that puts an extra adaptive stress on the body may be overwhelming rather than supportive during this time. Further, some types of hepatitis are communicable without direct contact with body fluids; this presents a risk to the therapists as well as the client.

BENEFITS Massage that is within the capacity of a client to adapt can be appropriate for client with hepatitis that is not acute. While it probably won't have a profound impact on the progress of the disease, it can improve the quality of life for a person dealing with a very challenging situation. Clients who have fully recovered from any type of hepatitis can enjoy the same benefits from bodywork as the rest of the population.

Liver Cancer

Definition: What Is It?

Primary liver cancer, also called hepatocellular carcinoma, is cancer that originates in the liver. This is distinguished from secondary liver cancer, or metastatic liver disease, which is a result of cancer that originates elsewhere and leads to tumors in the liver.

Liver cancer is relatively rare in the United States, affecting about 18,000 people each year. Rates have more than doubled in the past 20 years, however, probably because of links between cirrhosis and nonalcoholic fatty liver disease, and hepatitis B and C.

Etiology: What Happens?

Liver cancer develops when hepatocytes replicate out of control. A history of slow-acting viral infection, alcoholism, and cirrhosis are all contributing factors to uncontrolled cellular activity. This is true especially when any combination of these factors affects a single person.

Liver cancer tumors may develop singly, or they may occur in several disconnected areas throughout the left and right lobes. They tend to be highly invested with blood vessels, which raises the risk for distant metastasis (usually to the lungs) before signs and symptoms lead to a diagnosis. Interestingly, the tumors are supplied mostly by the hepatic artery, while the rest of the liver's tissues are supplied mostly by the portal vein. This means medication can be administered via the portal artery with minimal damage to nontumor cells.

Several risk factors for liver cancer have been identified. They are especially potent when they appear in combination.

- *Hepatitis B infection*. This virus has specifically been seen to cause, not just appear frequently with, a specific type of liver cancer. Genetic material from HBV can be found in the malignant cells of liver cancer. Hepatitis B is an especially high risk for liver cancer when the infection was contracted in infancy or childhood.
- *Hepatitis C infection*. The relationship between hepatitis C virus and liver cancer is not

Liver Cancer in Brief

What is it?
Primary liver cancer is the growth of malignant cells that begins with mutations in hepatocytes. Liver cancer is aggressive and usually silent in early stages, leading to late diagnoses and a generally poor prognosis.

How is it recognized?
Liver cancer is silent when it begins, but as tumors grow and interfere with function, signs and symptoms may include vague to intense abdominal pain, ascites, itchy rashes on the skin, psychological changes, muscle wasting, fever, unintended weight loss, and jaundice.

Massage risks and benefits
Risks: A person with liver cancer may undergo extensive and intrusive treatment options; any bodywork must be adjusted to respect the challenges of these treatments.
Benefits: Liver cancer is often terminal, and massage as a way to manage pain, anxiety, depression, and other consequences may be an important and welcome comfort measure in this situation.

completely understood; some research indicates that the virus may actually cause the cancer, while other studies suggest that liver cancer develops indirectly through the chronic inflammation associated with hepatitis C. Regardless, about 5% to 10% of people diagnosed with hepatitis C eventually develop liver cancer. Because Hepatitis C virus infects over 3 million people in the United States, liver cancer rates are expected to keep rising for the next several years.

- *Alcoholism*. Alcohol abuse, especially in combination with hepatitis B or C, greatly raises the risk of liver cancer. Ironically, it appears that it is the cessation of alcohol use that triggers the cellular mutation: when a person stops drinking and the liver begins to regenerate, cells are more likely to become malignant.
- *Hemochromatosis*. This is a genetic blood disorder, involving the production of too many red blood cells. Persons with untreated hemochromatosis are at high risk for cirrhosis, which may then progress to liver cancer.
- *Nonalcoholic fatty liver disease (NFALD)*. NFALD can lead to cirrhosis. This is a relatively new risk factor for liver cancer, but it is a potent one in a country where two-thirds of the adult population is overweight.
- *Cirrhosis*. This condition, the result of long-term liver damage, develops in the presence of chronic viral infection, alcoholism, toxic exposure, or other circumstances. It is possible, but unusual, for liver cancer to develop without cirrhosis.
- *Aflatoxin B1*. This is a chemical from a mold called *Aspergillus flavus* that grows on peanuts and grains stored in hot, humid conditions. Aflatoxin B1 is an extremely potent carcinogen, responsible for many liver cancer cases in Asia and sub-Saharan Africa.

Signs and Symptoms

Tumors in the liver can interfere with normal function, but because hepatitis and/or cirrhosis are probably also present, these signs are easily missed or ignored. The most commonly reported signs and symptoms of liver cancer include vague abdominal pain that becomes increasingly intense, unintended weight loss and food aversion, muscle wasting, ascites (which may obscure signs of weight loss), fever, an abdominal mass, and if the bile duct is blocked, jaundice. Blood tests may reveal signs of liver dysfunction. One specific substance, alpha fetoprotein, is present in the blood about 60% of the time when liver cancer is present. Other blood tests may show unusual hormonal activity, as cancerous cells secrete chemicals usually restricted to other cells.

Treatment

Even when liver cancer is caught in its earliest recognizable stages, survival for more than 5 years is rare. Staging protocols for liver cancer are discussed in Sidebar 8.9. Most survivors of liver cancer surgery have a recurrence within several months, unless they are lucky enough to receive a new liver in a transplant surgery before metastasis occurs. This cancer is aggressive and difficult to control, and most patients have serious underlying liver disease that makes them poor candidates for many types of surgery. Furthermore, liver cancer tends not to respond well to chemotherapy or radiation. Consequently, a number of treatment options have been developed that try to control the growth of the cancer without invasive surgery. These include techniques to burn or freeze tumors through laparoscopic or percutaneous instruments; injections of ethanol to destroy tumor cells; and the use of drugs or implements to block the blood vessels that supply tumors. No single treatment option shows outstanding promise for a long-term cure, however.

NOTABLE CASES Liver cancer was the cause of death for composer Johannes Brahms, musicians Ray Charles and John Coltrane, baseball great Mickey Mantle, and dancer/actor/director Gregory Hines.

Surgery typically entails a resection of the liver (removing the portion or portions in which tumors are present) or liver transplant. The fact that many liver cancer patients have a long history of cirrhosis and/or hepatitis makes both resections and transplant surgeries difficult.

Medications

- Chemotherapy administered by catheter to sections of the liver to kill off targeted cells
- Oral antiangiogenic agents to inhibit the growth of blood vessels supplying tumors
- Injections of ethanol to destroy tumor cells
- Medication to manage liver cancer complications, including pain, encephalopathy, and ascites

SIDEBAR 8.9 Staging Liver Cancer

Staging protocols for liver cancer have several variations. The typical TNM classification with numerical groupings follows this pattern:

Tumor (T)	Node (N)	Metastasis (M)
T 1: One tumor, no vascularization	N 0: no nodes involved	M 0: no metastasis found
T 2: One tumor with vascularization or multiple tumors < 5 cm	N 1: regional nodes involved	M 1: tumors found outside the liver
T 3: Multiple tumors >5 cm or one tumor involving portal vein or hepatic artery		
T 4: Multiple tumors with direct invasion of adjacent organs and/or perforation of visceral peritoneum		

These delineations are then translated into stages I to IV in this way:

Stage	Tumor	Node	Metastasis
I	T 1	N 0	M 0
II	T 2	N 0	M 0
III A	T 3	N 0	M 0
III B	T 4	N 0	M 0
III C	Any	N 1	M 0
IV	T any	N any	M 1

Liver cancer staging may be discussed in stages 0 through IV, as other cancers are, but it is also discussed in terms of best treatment options.

- *Localized resectable cancer.* This indicates that a single tumor smaller than 2 cm without signs of spreading to blood or lymph vessels has been found. The tumor can be fully removed surgically.
- *Localized unresectable cancer.* This means that although metastasis is not obvious, the liver is too damaged by cirrhosis or other factors to make surgery safe.
- *Advanced cancer.* This indicates that distant metastasis has occurred, and while chemotherapy and radiation may slow the progress, the cancer is probably not curable.
- *Recurrent cancer.* This is cancer that returns after previous treatments.

Massage?

RISKS Liver cancer often involves aggressive therapies including various types of surgery and surgical devices, which require adaptation in bodywork choices. For more information about massage in the context of cancer, see Chapter 12.

BENEFITS Because liver cancer is often terminal, massage may be welcomed as a way to provide comfort, pain relief, and other benefits at the end of life.

Pancreatic Cancer

Definition: What Is It?

Pancreatic cancer begins as mutation of certain genes that sponsor uncontrolled growth of cells in the pancreas. It usually grows in the exocrine ducts of this gland, but occasionally grows in the endocrine-producing cells. Pancreatic cancer is aggressive, metastasizes easily, and is difficult to detect in early stages; consequently it is the fourth leading cause of death from cancer in this country. About 43,000 people are diagnosed annually, leading to about 37,000 deaths.

Pancreatic Cancer in Brief

Pronunciation: pan-kre-AT-ik KAN-sur

What is it?
Pancreatic cancer is the growth of malignant cells in the pancreas. It is usually a cancer of the exocrine cells that produce digestive enzymes, but it occasionally grows in the islet cells, where hormones are produced.

How is it recognized?
Early signs of pancreatic cancer are subtle: abdominal discomfort, unintended weight loss, and loss of appetite are frequently reported. Later signs may include jaundice, hepatomegaly or splenomegaly, ascites, and signs of distant metastasis, which vary according to location.

Massage risks and benefits
Risks: Pancreatic cancer tends to be aggressive, painful, and terminal. Patients with this disease are likely to be facing end-of-life issues and treatments that require special sensitivity from massage therapists. For more information on massage and cancer, see Chapter 12.
Benefits: Massage as an end-of-life comfort measure for pancreatic cancer patients can be a wonderful tool to manage pain, anxiety, and other consequences of this disease.

Etiology: What Happens?

The pancreas is a small, spongy gland behind the stomach. It produces digestive enzymes that collect in an extensive duct system and eventually enter the duodenum. It also manufactures hormones for maintenance of blood sugar levels.

Pancreatic cancer comes about when mutations of cells lead to the growth of invasive, aggressive, life-threatening tumors. When these tumors arise in the exocrine ducts, they are adenocarcinomas. When they grow in the islet cells, they are neuroendocrine tumors. In either case, the tumors tend to grow quickly and easily invade nearby tissues simply by spreading out. The duodenum, stomach, and peritoneal wall are often affected by these local extensions. When cells invade the abdominal lymph system or large blood vessels, the liver is often the first site of metastasis.

Exact causes or triggers of pancreatic cancer have not been identified, but a number of risk factors have been seen to increase the chance that pancreatic cells may mutate. The primary risk factors for pancreatic cancer include the following:

- Age (most diagnoses are among people 60 to 80 years old)
- Race (it occurs slightly more frequently among African Americans)
- A history of smoking (this may be responsible for up to 30% of genetic mutations)
- A history of type 2 diabetes
- Chronic pancreatitis, especially when due to alcohol abuse
- Obesity and diet (high in animal fats, red meat and processed meat; low in fresh fruits and vegetables)
- Inherited characteristics, including a family history of pancreatitis, or a genetic predisposition to colorectal cancer, breast cancer, or melanoma

Types of Pancreatic Cancer

- *Adenocarcinoma of the pancreas.* This is cancer of the exocrine ducts. It affects the secretion of digestive enzymes, sometimes by blocking the pancreatic duct. Pancreatic adenocarcinoma is the most common form of pancreatic cancer.
- *Neuroendocrine tumors of the pancreas.* This is cancer of the endocrine cells of the pancreas, specifically the islet cells that produce insulin and other hormones. A problem with these cells leads to difficulties with regulating blood glucose.

Signs and Symptoms

Early pancreatic cancer creates such subtle symptoms that people rarely consult their doctor about them: abdominal discomfort, mid-back pain, loss of appetite, and unintended weight loss typically occur for 2 months or more before most people seek a diagnosis.

If a tumor obstructs the common bile duct, jaundice may develop, sometime with pruritis. Other late-stage signs of include difficulty with digestion, ascites, and enlargement of the liver and spleen. If the cancer affects the endocrine cells, difficulty with the regulation of blood glucose may arise.

Treatment

Because pancreatic cancer is so difficult to identify in early stages, the majority of patients have local or distant metastasis when they are diagnosed. Staging protocols for pancreatic cancer are discussed in Sidebar 8.10. A small percentage of patients are good candidates for resection, and those who are have a better prognosis than others. Nonetheless, surgery for this condition is invasive and often requires removing not only parts of the pancreas but also the gallbladder, part of the stomach, and some of the small intestine. The chance of recurrence after surgery is very high.

NOTABLE CASES This disease has shortened the lives of many notable personalities, including Apple Computer co-founder Steve Jobs, Dizzy Gillespie opera singer Luciano Pavarotti, and actor Patrick Swayze. As of this writing, Supreme Court Justice Ruth Bader Ginsburg is a pancreatic cancer survivor.

If it is determined that a person has inoperable cancer, various combinations of chemotherapy, targeted therapy, and radiation therapy may be used to slow the tumors' growth and prolong life. In some cases, the combination of chemotherapy and radiation can reduce a growth to the point that it can be surgically excised.

Surgery may be performed to relieve some of the symptoms of pancreatic cancer. This may include bypassing the exocrine ducts, inserting a stent to keep ducts open, or damaging the local nerves to reduce pain.

Ultimately the treatment options for pancreatic cancer probably include hospice care for a dying person. At this point, any comfort measures are appropriate and welcome.

SIDEBAR 8.10 Staging Pancreatic Cancer

Staging for pancreatic cancer follows the pattern for TNM classification and numerical assignments, but it can be difficult to evaluate the extent of lymph node involvement without surgery. Consequently, the true extent of the cancer progression may not be known before treatment options are chosen. Staging is as follows:

Tumor (T)	Node (N)	Metastasis (M)
T 1: Only pancreas involved; tumor <2 cm	N 0: no nodes involved	M 0: no metastasis found
T 2: Only pancreas involved; tumor >2 cm	N 1: regional nodes involved	M 1: tumors outside pancreas
T 3: Cancer has spread but not invaded large blood vessels		
T 4: Cancer has spread and invaded large blood vessels		

These delineations are then translated into Stages I to IV in this way:

Stage	Tumor	Node	Metastasis
I A	T 1	N 0	M 0
I B	T 2	N 0	M 0
II A	T 3	N 0	M 0
II B	T 1–3	N any	M 0
III	T 4	N any	M 0
IV	T any	N any	M 1

Because it can be difficult to assess pancreatic cancer without surgery, many experts simply discuss it in terms of possible treatment options:

- *Potentially resectable* means a growth is isolated to a particular area that is accessible through surgery for removal. Life expectancy is much better if it is caught while operable.
- *Locally advanced* means tumors reach out and invade local tissues such as the stomach, liver, and peritoneum. This often happens before distant metastasis.
- *Metastatic cancer* means that tumors have invaded the lymph system and may be growing far from their site of origin.

Medications

- Chemotherapy to kill fast-growing cells
- Biologic or targeted therapy to kill cancer cells
- Narcotic analgesics, sometimes with antidepressants and antiemetics to address pain and side effects of treatment

Massage?

RISKS Pancreatic cancer patients are likely to be fragile, in pain, and facing the end of life. Any bodywork offered in this context must be given with the utmost sensitivity and care. For more on massage and cancer, see Chapter 12.

BENEFITS Appropriate massage can help with pain, anxiety, depression, and general quality of life for a person who dealing with this often-terminal disease.

Pancreatitis

Definition: What Is It?

Pancreatitis is inflammation of the pancreas. Acute pancreatitis can be triggered by alcohol binging, gallstones, toxic exposures, blunt trauma, or other factors; chronic pancreatitis is usually related to long-term abuse of alcohol.

Etiology: What Happens?

The pancreas manufactures both endocrine and exocrine secretions. Its exocrine products are produced in **acinar** cells. They include bicarbonate to neutralize material exiting the highly acidic stomach, and digestive enzymes that break down carbohydrates, proteins, and fats into absorbable particles. If the ducts in the pancreas are blocked or if the gland develops cysts or abscesses, these functions are lost, and the secretions may even destroy the pancreas tissue itself; this is called **autodigestion**.

The main complications of chronic pancreatitis include pain, malabsorption of nutrients (which can lead to **steatorrhea**, or oily, foul-smelling stools), bleeding into the peritoneum, infection of cysts, and secondary diabetes mellitus. The pain associated with chronic pancreatitis can be so persistent and extreme that addiction to opioid painkillers is a significant risk for these patients.

Pancreatitis in Brief

Pronunciation: pan-kre-uh-TY-tis

What is it?
Pancreatitis is inflammation of the pancreas. It has an acute and a chronic form.

How is it recognized?
Constant or episodic pain high in the abdomen is the leading sign of pancreatitis. This pain often refers to the back. Other signs have to do with pancreatic dysfunction: poor absorption of food leading to weight loss, secondary diabetes mellitus, and jaundice are all possible signs of pancreatitis.

Massage risks and benefits
Risks: Pancreatitis is a potentially dangerous disease, and a client who has upper abdominal pain in a new pattern that persists for more than a few days is well advised to consult a doctor. If massage brings about temporary relief, that could delay an important diagnosis.
Benefits: A client who is actively managing pancreatitis can receive massage that does not exacerbate symptoms. A client who has fully recovered from pancreatitis can enjoy the same benefits of bodywork as the rest of the population.

Types of Pancreatitis

- *Acute pancreatitis*. This is a sudden onset of symptoms related to a blockage of the pancreatic ducts, so that corrosive secretions are trapped within the gland (Figure 8.16). This can be brought about by alcohol use, blunt trauma, a congenital malformation of the pancreas, gallstones lodged in the common bile duct, exposure to ethanol or other toxins, or cystic fibrosis. Acute pancreatitis is usually short lived with an uneventful recovery. But when it is severe, cysts, abscesses, necrosis, and the release of dangerous toxins into the bloodstream that can lead to circulatory shock, renal failure, or adult respiratory distress syndrome can occur.
- *Chronic pancreatitis*. In this situation, long-term wear and tear leads to permanent, irreversible damage to the delicate epithelial tissue of the gland. Chronic pancreatitis is almost always related to alcohol abuse. Ethanol can cause

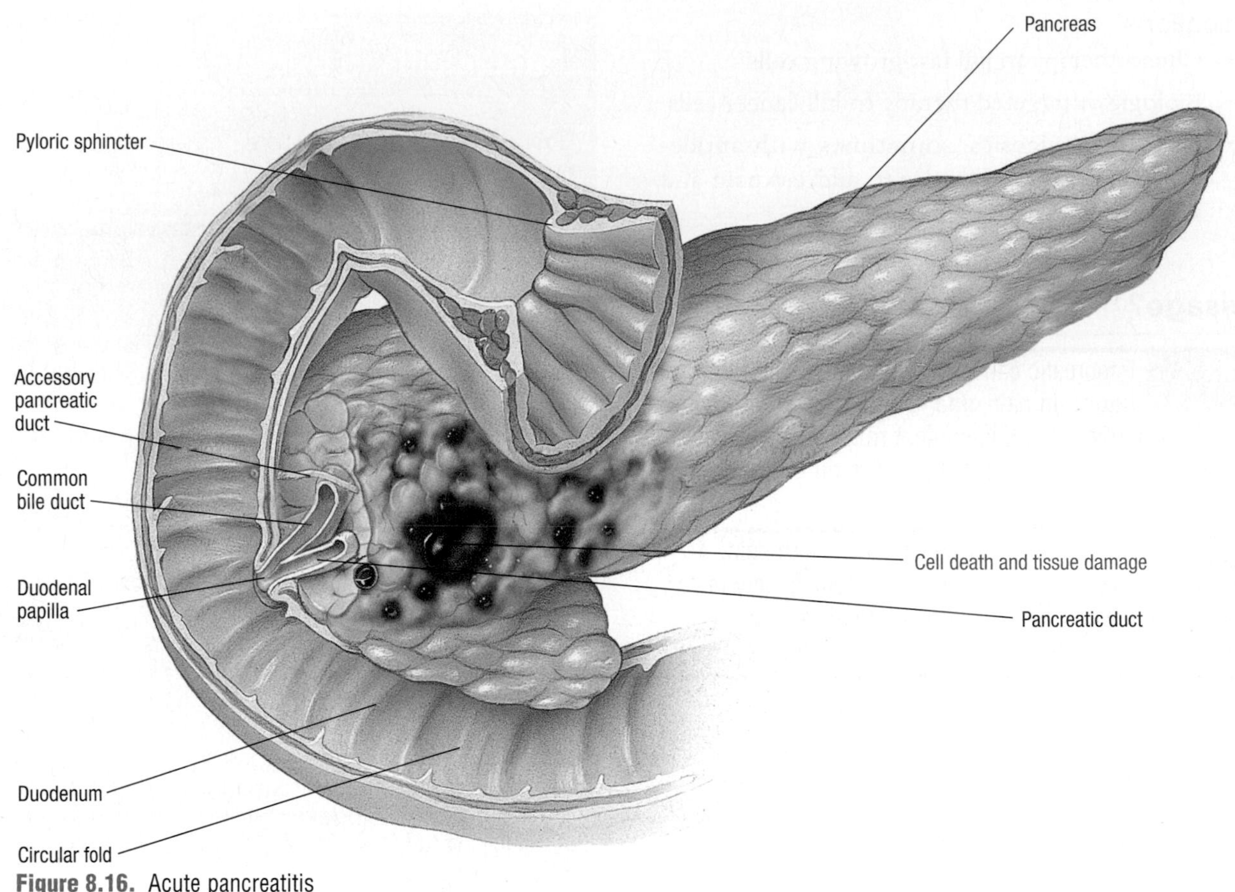

Figure 8.16. Acute pancreatitis

enzymes to be released prematurely, damaging the gland, promoting fibrosis, and forming protein plugs that may calcify to become pancreatic stones. Other causes of chronic pancreatitis include heredity, autoimmune dysfunction, and gallstones.

Signs and Symptoms

Dull upper abdominal pain is the leading symptom of acute and chronic pancreatitis. With acute pancreatitis, the pain has a sudden onset. It may appear with nausea, vomiting, fever, and rapid pulse.

In chronic pancreatitis, the pain may be episodic, lasting for many hours and then subsiding until the next attack. Episodes get closer together until the pain is unremitting. Pancreatic pain often refers into the back, which is an issue of concern for massage therapists, of course.

Other symptoms suggest the loss of pancreatic enzymes and hormones: unintended weight loss, difficulties with the regulation of blood glucose, and the possibility of jaundice if the obstruction of the pancreatic duct also affects the common bile duct.

Treatment

Pancreatitis is treated according to the cause. Most patients undergo a few days of taking no food by mouth to allow the organ to heal. If it is related to gallstones, these are removed, so the ducts can flow freely. If abscesses form, these are drained or removed. If tissue has died because of autodigestion, that is also removed. The pancreatic duct may be surgically reopened, or a stent may be inserted. Digestive enzymes may be taken orally to relieve the pancreas of the work of producing them. Finally, if the pain from chronic pancreatitis is unresponsive to any other interventions, surgery may be performed to sever the sensory nerves from the gland.

Medications

- Analgesics for pain management
- Supplementary digestive enzymes if necessary

Massage?

RISKS Pancreatitis, which is rare but potentially dangerous, can refer pain to the midback, which may push clients toward seeking massage rather than medical care: this is a situation where undiagnosed abdominal pain is a good reason to visit a doctor as soon as possible.

BENEFITS Clients who are appropriately treating pancreatitis can receive any massage that fits within their capacity for adaptation, and those who have fully recovered can enjoy all the benefits that bodywork offers the general population.

Other Digestive System Conditions

Candidiasis

Definition: What Is It?

C. albicans is one type of about 20 yeastlike fungi that inhabit the digestive tract, often from the mouth to the anus (Figure 8.17). They usually live in balance with other flora and fauna of the GI tract. Under certain circumstances, that balance is upset and candida replicates too easily, leading to a variety of problems. This condition of having normal levels of candida grow out of control is called candidiasis.

Etiology: What Happens?

Under normal circumstances, a balanced environment of flora (plantlike organisms) and fauna (animal-like organisms) peacefully coexist in the GI tract. The flora

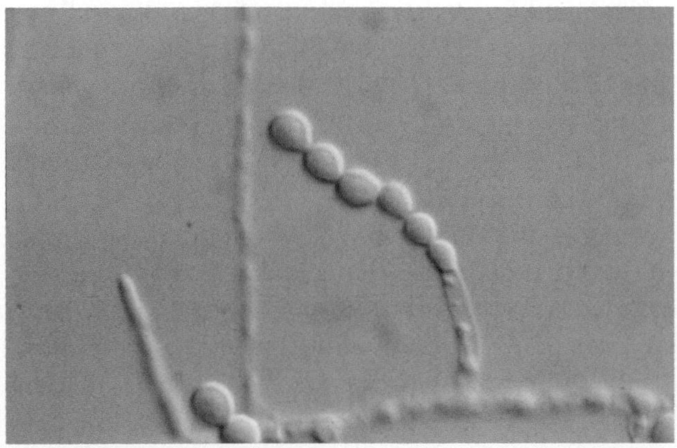

Figure 8.17. *Candida albicans*

Candidiasis in Brief

Pronunciation: kan-dih-DY-ah-sis

What is it?
Candidiasis is a condition in which *Candida albicans* or related fungi that colonize the GI tract become invasive and disrupt normal function of the digestive system and other systems in the body.

How is it recognized?
Signs and symptoms of candidiasis can be severe and acute, involving mouth and skin lesions as well as systemic blood and organ infections; or subtle and chronic, involving fatigue, impaired mental ability, food and chemical sensitivities, and several other symptoms in varying degrees of severity.

Massage risks and benefits
Risks: Candida is not contagious through skin-to-skin contact, but if a person has it severely enough to cause skin symptoms, he or she is also likely to have a systemic illness that impairs the immune system, and this is a caution for rigorous massage.
Benefits: Massage probably has little impact on mild or subtle candida overgrowth; clients with this condition may enjoy the temporarily improved digestion, alertness, and relief of fatigue that bodywork can provide.

keep the fauna from replicating too much, and the fauna do likewise for the flora. These organisms live in symbiosis: a mutually beneficial relationship with their human hosts.

When a disruption in the balance of the GI tract occurs, either plants or animals can dominate. When bacteria are suppressed, candida in the GI tract convert from benign, helpful yeastlike organisms to more aggressive fungi. In the absence of balancing bacteria, the fungi have more opportunity to reproduce and spread. Because candida are already present, the exact delineation between colonization and infestation is not always clear. Opinions vary about how extensive a candida colonization has to be before it causes symptoms (Sidebar 8.11).

Often the trigger for intestinal imbalance is use of antibiotics. These medications, designed to kill harmful bacteria, may also kill beneficial bacteria. This is why many health care providers recommend supplementing lactobacilli along with antibiotic prescriptions. Other well-accepted causes of candidiasis

SIDEBAR 8.11 Is it Candidiasis?

Two schools of thought dominate the discussion of candidiasis. The more conservative allopathic approach generally assumes that the overgrowth of candida isn't a problem until very severe symptoms occur, which may involve the skin, mucous membranes, or invasive candidiasis, a systemic infection of the blood.

Many naturopathic and holistic practitioners propose that milder overgrowths of candida can also cause many chronic, low-grade symptoms. The fungi may grow and spread throughout the intestines, sinking rootlike structures into the walls. They produce waste products that can be irritating to the host. Invasion of the intestinal wall may also allow other substances to enter the bloodstream, where immune system responses launched against incompletely digested material may be extreme. Between losing access to nutrition because the fungi get it first, dealing with their metabolic wastes, and immune system responses against digestive contents, a person with chronic, low-grade candidiasis may develop a number of subtle or severe symptoms.

Practitioners who deal with candidiasis as a contributor to many other chronic disorders often report success when helping their patients change their diet and lifestyle in ways that restore balance to intestinal flora and fauna. This clinical evidence has yet to be reproduced in a formal research setting, however, which leads to resistance to the acceptance of candidiasis as a common, chronic disorder responsible for symptoms that range from fatigue to menstrual pain to food allergies.

include immune suppression as seen with HIV/AIDS patients and people undergoing treatment for cancer, genetic immune system dysfunctions, thymus tumors, and hormonal imbalances.

Candidiasis is an emerging problem in hospital settings where patients undergo increasingly complex and prolonged treatments that leave them vulnerable to colonization. Pathogens that enter the body by way of a catheter, port, or open wound can invade the bloodstream and colonize organs, bones, and joints.

Types of Candidiasis

- *Mucocutaneous candidiasis*. This is yeast infections that appear in the mouth or on the skin. **Thrush** is an outbreak of whitish, usually painless lesions in the mouth, is one form that is commonly seen in infants and immunosuppressed people. This type of infestation can cause painful fissures to develop around the mouth (**angular cheilitis**), and ulcers to erupt in the digestive tract. Candida yeasts can also colonize fingernails and toenails. Other skin signs include **intertrigo** (yeast colonies in skin folds around the groin, axillae, and breasts) and the diaper rash and jock itch that appear when yeasts from the GI tract colonize the external skin around the anus.
- *Vulvovaginitis*. This is the development of candidiasis in and around the vagina. It is a common infection for women. It can cause itching and burning at the vagina, painful intercourse, and characteristic cottage cheese-like, yeasty-smelling vaginal discharge.
- *Internal candidiasis*. This is candida that has invaded the GI tract and possibly other organs as well (although this is rare in people whose immune systems are essentially healthy). It ranges from subtle to severe and potentially life threatening.

Signs and Symptoms

Candidiasis can show a variety of signs and symptoms depending on the severity of the condition, its location, and the underlying health of the affected person. Symptoms range from patchy, painless white lesions in the mouth (thrush) to yeasty vaginal discharge (vulvovaginitis), and can include variations like skin lesions, chemical sensitivities, and headaches on the mild end, to drug-resistant fever, chills, and organ failure on the severe end of the spectrum.

Treatment

Various topical antifungal medications may be recommended for severe versions of candidiasis. Some drug-resistant strains of fungi have emerged, but they appear to be sensitive to boric acid and some essential oils.

Oral antifungals can be effective for some versions of candidiasis.

For subtler versions of this condition, reestablishing internal flora to balance out the fungi is a high priority. This requires dietary changes that essentially rule out simple carbohydrates, sweet things, fermented foods, and many processed foods. Some clinicians suggest that most people would feel more energetic and less sluggish with a dietary change of this sort, so whether an overabundance of yeasts has been addressed or not may be moot.

Medications

- Topical antifungal medication for cutaneous or vaginal candidiasis
- Oral antifungal medications:
  - The "-azole" group to block essential materials in the yeast cell wall
  - The polyene group including nystatin or amphotericin B for more resistant infestations

Massage?

RISKS Extreme cutaneous candidiasis is usually seen in the context of significant immune system impairment, which carries its own cautions for massage therapy.

BENEFITS Mild candidiasis has no risks for massage, and clients with this condition can enjoy the same benefits from bodywork as the rest of the population.

CHAPTER REVIEW QUESTIONS: DIGESTIVE SYSTEM CONDITIONS

1. Your client has persistent low-grade abdominal pain in a new pattern. Massage relieves symptoms for a day or two, but then they return. What is the most appropriate course of action?
2. What are two main locations for esophageal cancer? Which one is becoming more common, and why?
3. What is the most serious complication of gastroenteritis?
4. What are the two leading risk factors for developing stomach cancer?
5. How can having gallstones cause pancreatitis?
6. Your client informs you that during her colonoscopy, her surgeon found pouches that protrude from the colon and contain hardened bits of fecal matter. What condition is she describing?
7. Name two conditions that are frequently comorbid with irritable bowel syndrome.
8. Why do most people who have gallstones never find out?
9. Your very large client informs you that he is not really overweight: he has been diagnosed with ascites. What organ dysfunction is most likely to be present?
10. Your client is recovering from hepatitis A. His skin and sclera are yellowish. What condition is present?

9

Endocrine System Conditions

Chapter Objectives

After reading this chapter, you should be able to . . .

- Describe why the pituitary gland is called the master gland.
- Identify the functions of the hormones calcitonin, parathyroid hormone, thyroxine, epinephrine, and cortisol.
- Identify the two most common types of diabetes.
- List two emergencies associated with extremes in blood glucose levels.
- Describe three possible complications of type 2 diabetes that affect organs outside the endocrine system.
- Explain why people who are treated for hyperthyroidism often develop hypothyroidism.
- Name three signs of hypothyroidism.
- Name five factors that contribute to metabolic syndrome.
- Identify two conditions for which metabolic syndrome is a predictor.
- Name three types of thyroid cancer.

Introduction

The endocrine system is a collection of glands that secrete hormones: chemical messages that instruct or stimulate other glands and tissues in the body to function in a variety of ways. Where the autonomic nervous system exerts electrical control over homeostatic body functions, the endocrine system exerts chemical control. Interestingly, the control center for both systems is the same structure, the hypothalamus.

The hypothalamus is a nondescript mass of tissue deep in the brain. It has a generous blood supply, which allows it to monitor functions of the body. The hypothalamus is primarily responsible for maintaining homeostasis, or a stable internal environment. It does so through electrical transmission to the brainstem to manage heart rate, blood pressure, temperature, and other functions, and also through electrical and chemical transmission to the pituitary gland, which then sends out signals to the targeted tissues. This is why the pituitary is sometimes called the "master gland" of the endocrine system. The hypothalamus is directly above and behind the pituitary, and it tells the pituitary what to secrete and when to secrete it. Sometimes the hypothalamus, via a stalk called the **infundibulum**, sends out its own hormones to be released into the blood by the pituitary gland.

Chemicals released by the hypothalamus and pituitary travel to their target glands through the circulatory system. They stimulate those glands to release their hormones. When those secretions reach appropriate levels in the blood, the hypothalamus and pituitary stop sending out signals; most endocrine regulation is operated via this **negative feedback loop**.

The cycle of hormone stimulation and suppression usually works best when it occurs in gentle, rhythmic fluctuation. For example, when a person's blood sugar gets low, two things happen: he perceives that he is hungry and his pancreas secretes glucagon, a hormone that stimulates the liver to release stored glucose. He eats, his digestive tract absorbs sugar from his meal, and his blood sugar rises. This stimulates the pancreas to release insulin to carry the sugar out of the blood and into cells, lowering blood sugar. When levels are low enough, the person gets hungry, beginning the cycle again. The blood sugar-insulin cycle takes place several times a day; it takes only a few hours to move from one state to another. Another endocrine cycle, the circadian rhythm, moves on a roughly 24-hour rotation. The menstrual cycle also depends on regular fluctuations, but this one lasts about 4 weeks. Other cycles, specifically those related to stress and perceived threat, depend on external circumstances to determine their frequency and duration.

Endocrine system glands secrete dozens of chemicals, each of which has specific target tissues and functions. Endocrine effects may also be determined by the frequency with which they are released into the bloodstream and the balance between each hormone and its antagonists.

Hormones fall into three chemical classes:

- Peptides are the most common type of hormones. They are made of chains of amino acids and are stored in various cellular holding tanks. Growth hormone, erythropoietin, and parathyroid hormone are peptide hormones.
- Amines are derived from a specific amino acid, tyrosine. They are also stored in cellular deposits. Adrenaline and thyroxine are examples of amine hormones.
- Steroids are lipids. They are not stored; steroid levels are maintained through constant production. Cortisol and testosterone are steroid hormones.

Major Hormones

It is useful for massage therapists to be able to recognize the names of most hormones and their actions, since this is a key feature of physiology. But a few hormones are so strongly implicated in basic health issues that massage therapists may benefit from more than just passing familiarity:

- Growth hormone is released from the pituitary gland and stimulates conversion of fuel into new cells. Infants, children, and teenagers secrete massive amounts of growth hormone; adults secrete less. When a person has finished growing, the primary purpose of growth hormone is to stimulate regeneration and repair of damaged tissue, in other words, healing. Growth hormone is secreted primarily in stage IV sleep. Sleep disorders can lead to a shortage of this important chemical.
- Epinephrine, also called adrenaline, is a steroid hormone. It comes from the adrenal gland medulla, along with a very similar hormone, noradrenaline. It is associated with short-term, high-grade stress and acts to reinforce the reactions initiated by the sympathetic nervous system. An inefficient connection between the pituitary gland and the adrenal glands can cause a sluggish stress response system; this is discussed in the article on depression in Chapter 4.
- Cortisol, another steroid hormone, is one of a group of glucocorticoids secreted by the adrenal cortex. It is the hormone secreted under long-term, low-grade stress. Cortisol is important for several reasons: it is a very powerful anti-inflammatory and is sometimes used systemically or locally for that purpose. It can damage

connective tissues, so people with systemically high levels of cortisol are prone to musculoskeletal injury and osteoporosis. It also suppresses immune system response to disease and infection. Chronically high levels of cortisol are a factor in many chronic stress-related disorders.

- Mineralocorticoids are adrenal cortex secretions that help to regulate electrolyte balance and control fluid retention. Aldosterone is a major mineralocorticoid.
- Insulin and glucagon work together to regulate blood glucose. Insulin decreases it, and glucagon increases it. Both are manufactured and released by the pancreas.
- Thyroid hormones are secreted by the thyroid gland in two molecular forms: triiodothyronine (T3) and thyroxine (T4). These hormones stimulate the metabolism of fuel into energy. Thyroid pathologies have to do with overproduction or underproduction of metabolic hormones.
- Calcitonin, another thyroid secretion, stimulates osteoblasts to extract calcium from the blood and add to bone density. In other words, it decreases blood calcium.
- Parathyroid hormone comes from the tiny parathyroid glands located deep to the thyroid gland. It is the antagonist of calcitonin, stimulating osteoclast activity and pulling calcium off the bones to raise blood calcium.
- Testosterone, estrogens, and progesterone are steroid hormones released mainly by the gonads (testicles for men and ovaries for women). They have to do with secondary sexual characteristics, menstrual cycle, maintaining pregnancy, and a host of other issues. Anabolic steroid supplements increase muscle mass; this is why they are sometimes employed by athletes, often with dangerous results. The negative feedback loops in these hormone relationships seem to be especially precarious, possibly because environmental exposures to various types of hormones (in medications, dairy products, meat, plastics, pesticides, and other environmental toxins) overbalance the scales.
- Other hormones have less implication for massage but a big impact on how well the body works. One is erythropoietin, secreted by the kidneys. Erythropoietin stimulates the production of red blood cells. It can be artificially supplemented to increase oxygen-carrying capacity of the blood, but this may also increase the risk of blood clots. Thymosin is a hormone from the thymus; it is involved with the maturation of T-cells. Melatonin comes from the pineal gland and helps to regulate wake-sleep cycles. Prostaglandins are hormones produced by almost any kind of cell for local action. Prostaglandins produce a myriad of effects in the body, including smooth muscle contraction and increased pain sensitivity.

Where Have Some Things Gone?

Some conditions that would have appeared in this chapter have been moved, either because they are relatively rare or because they are situations that massage therapists are unlikely to see in an acute or extreme form. Endocrine system conditions that can now be found in Appendix C, Extra Conditions at a Glance include

Acromegaly	Addison disease
Cushing syndrome	Diabetes insipidus
Hyperparathyroidism	Hypoparathyroidism

By contrast, both hyperthyroidism and hypothyroidism have stayed in this chapter. Although these conditions are often brought about by autoimmune activity, this is not always the case. This is why they are here and not with other autoimmune disease discussions in Chapter 6.

Endocrine glands release their secretions (often under direction of the pituitary-hypothalamus unit) directly into the blood. This distinguishes them from exocrine glands, which send their secretions into ducts for release into specific local areas. The hormones circulate systemically through the body but attach to specific receptor sites on their target tissues. Then they stimulate the target tissue to perform some function, such as making red blood cells (erythropoietin from the kidneys acting on bone marrow) or pulling calcium off the bones (parathyroid hormone acting on osteoclasts).

Most endocrine system disorders have to do with imbalances in the hormones being produced. Autoimmune attacks or tumors may stimulate or suppress certain glands, leading to problems with the negative feedback loop. When too much or too little of any hormone is present in the blood, symptoms can be felt throughout the body. Other endocrine disruptions occur when circulating hormone levels are normal but target tissues have developed resistance to their action.

To hear the author discuss the HPA axis, visit http://thePoint.lww.com.

Endocrine System Conditions

Diabetes Mellitus

Definition: What Is It?

The word "diabetes" comes from the Greek for "siphon" or to "pass through," referring to the tendency for diabetics to urinate very frequently. Mellitus is from Latin for "sweetened with honey." Diabetes mellitus essentially means sweet pee.

Diabetes is not a single disease, but rather a group of related disorders that all result in hyperglycemia, or elevated levels of sugar in the bloodstream. Two main varieties, type 1 and type 2 diabetes, are examined in this article. These account for about 98% of diabetes diagnoses.

Diabetes is the seventh leading cause of death in the United States, although this is probably underreported. Estimates vary, but most resources suggest that about 26 million Americans have diabetes, although about 7 million people don't know it yet. About 1.6 million people are diagnosed with diabetes each year. Researchers credit an aging population along with higher numbers of obese young people and sedentary lifestyles for these alarming figures.

Diabetes Mellitus in Brief

Pronunciation: di-ah-BE-tez meh-LY-tus

What is it?
Diabetes is a group of metabolic disorders characterized by problems with glucose metabolism.

How is it recognized?
Early symptoms of diabetes include frequent urination, thirst, and increased appetite along with weight loss, nausea, and vomiting. These symptoms can be subtle enough that the first indicators of disease are the complications it can cause: neuropathy, impaired vision, kidney dysfunction, or other problems.

Massage risks and benefits

Risks: If the circulatory and urinary systems are impaired, a client with diabetes may have limited capacity to adapt to the changes that rigorous massage demands. Advanced disease can result in skin damage and ulcers, especially to the legs and feet; these are cautions for bodywork as well. Numbness associated with diabetic neuropathy can interfere with a client's ability to give accurate feedback about pain and pressure. And massage has been seen to drop blood sugar; clients may experience hypoglycemia if they have a massage and supplement insulin without adequate food.

Benefits: A client with well-managed diabetes and no contraindicating complications can enjoy the same benefits from massage as the rest of the population, with the caveat that massage may temporarily cause a drop in blood sugar, so the client and therapist should anticipate that possibility.

Endocrine System Conditions

- Diabetes mellitus
  - Type 1 Diabetes Mellitus
  - Type 2 Diabetes Mellitus
- Hyperthyroidism
  - Graves disease
  - Toxic adenoma
  - Multinodular goiter
  - Thyroiditis
- Hypothyroidism
  - Hashimoto thyroiditis
  - Secondary hypothyroidism
  - Iodine deficiency hypothyroidism
  - Idiopathic hypothyroidism
  - Other types of hypothyroidism
- Metabolic syndrome
- Thyroid cancer
  - Papillary thyroid cancer
  - Follicular thyroid cancer
  - Medullary thyroid cancer
  - Anaplastic thyroid cancer
  - Thyroid lymphoma

Etiology: What Happens?

Many cells, especially those in muscles, do best when they can use glucose for fuel. Glucose is an efficient energy source, and the leftovers of this "burn" are easy to process; they are carbon dioxide and water. But glucose has no easy access to the cells that need it: insulin, a hormone produced by beta cells in the pancreas, is required to escort glucose across cell membranes. Insulin also aids in the removal of fat from the blood into storage lipid cells. Diabetes develops when insulin is in short supply, or because insulin receptor sites have developed resistance, or both. Consequently, glucose and fats accumulate in the blood, and cells must resort first to stored fat reserves and then to proteins for fuel sources. (See Sidebar 9.1 for more information on insulin resistance.)

Risk factors for type 1 diabetes are essentially noncontrollable: they include genetic background and childhood exposure to agents that might stimulate an immune system mistake. Risk factors for type 2 diabetes include being over 45 years old (although it is often diagnosed among young people); being 20% or more over desired weight; having a family history of diabetes; having a racial predisposition for diabetes (being Native American, Hispanic, a Pacific Islander, Asian American, or African American); having problems with glucose tolerance, hypertension, gestational diabetes, or polycystic ovarian syndrome.

Complications of diabetes are potentially serious, and they are often the first signs of the disease that cause a person to seek medical intervention.

- *Cardiovascular disease*. Diabetics are especially prone to these problems because high blood glucose and insulin resistance lead to chemical changes that damage endothelium, leading to atherosclerosis throughout much of the circulatory system. Diabetes more than doubles the risk of stroke, hypertension, and aneurysm, and cardiovascular disease is the leading cause of death for people with diabetes.
- *Edema*. Fluid retention develops in the extremities because of sluggish blood return. It can also give rise to stasis dermatitis.
- *Ulcers, gangrene, and amputations*. When the body's blood vessels are caked with plaque, even minor skin lesions don't heal well. Ingrown toenails, blisters, or pressure spots on the feet can become life threatening for diabetics: the tissue either dies of starvation or is infected with pathogens that are impossible to fight off, forming characteristic diabetic ulcers, usually on the feet (Figure 9.1). Diabetes is the leading cause of nontraumatic foot and leg amputations in this country.
- *Kidney disease*. Renal vessels are especially vulnerable to atherosclerosis, because they are one of the first diversions from the descending aorta. Excessive blood glucose, which acts as a powerful diuretic, is also hard on the kidneys, causing reduced formation of glomerular

SIDEBAR 9.1 Insulin Resistance: Silent and Dangerous

Insulin resistance is a condition in which a given concentration of insulin does not have the expected effect on cellular uptake of blood glucose. It is typically related to decreased numbers of insulin receptors on cell membranes, often in conjunction with postreceptor problems inside the cell. Blood sugar levels climb, stimulating the production of more insulin. In this way, hyperglycemia and hyperinsulinemia (the presence of excessive insulin in the blood) occur simultaneously. This situation, along with excessive release of glucose from the liver, opens the door to type 2 diabetes mellitus.

Insulin resistance is also considered a causative factor for another disorder, metabolic syndrome, which is associated with a dangerously increased risk of many forms of heart disease.

Insulin resistance is directly connected to overloaded abdominal fat cells. These fat cells are metabolically different from subcutaneous fat cells; they produce many chemicals that have adverse affects on body functions. Losing 5% or more of overall fat storage can reduce the risk of insulin resistance and its associated diseases.

Insulin resistance itself is often a silent disorder. Some patients develop a skin discoloration called **acanthosis nigricans**: velvety brown patches appear around skin folds, especially at the axilla. It is thought that excessive insulin interacts with skin cells to produce this sign. Episodes of hypoglycemia occasionally affect people with insulin resistance; this indicates that antibodies have destroyed damaged insulin receptor sites, temporarily causing a sudden uptake of blood glucose.

Insulin resistance may be identified by testing blood glucose and/or insulin after fasting, when levels should be low. Other experts suggest that a glucose tolerance test, which measures glucose in the blood 2 hours after a patient ingests 75 mg of sugar, is more indicative of the early stages of this disorder.

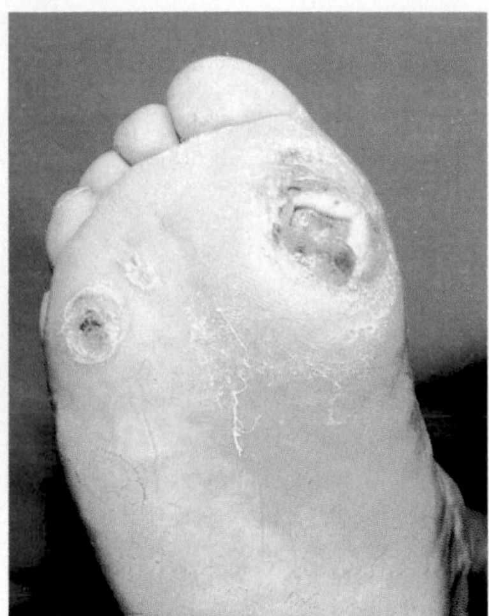

Figure 9.1. Diabetic ulcers

filtrate and a thickening of the basement membrane in the Bowman capsule. Consequently, diabetes is the leading cause of end-stage renal failure and of the need for kidney transplants.

- *Impaired vision*. The capillaries of the eyes of diabetes patients can become abnormally thickened, depriving eye cells of nutrition. Diseased capillaries leak blood and proteins into the retina. Microaneurysms can form that also cut off circulation. All of these contribute to diabetic retinopathy. Excessive glucose also binds with proteins in the lens, causing first cataracts, then blindness. This disease is the leading cause of new blindness among people 20 to 70 years old in the United States.
- *Neuropathy*. Lack of capillary circulation and excessive sugar in the blood both contribute to nerve damage. Symptoms of peripheral neuropathy include tingling or pain and eventual numbness. Neuropathy of the autonomic motor system (mainly the vagus nerve) can lead to an inability to maintain postural blood pressure, delayed or inefficient emptying of the stomach, diarrhea, constipation, and sexual impotency for both genders. One especially dangerous consequence of neuropathy is hypoglycemia insensitivity: a loss in the ability to sense when blood sugar is too low.
- *Others*. Diabetes affects every body system in some way. It is linked to urinary tract infections, candidiasis, birth defects, a mold infection of the nose and sinuses called mucormycosis, aggressive ear infections that can invade the cranial bones (malignant otitis externa), and higher-than-normal rates of gingivitis and tooth loss.

Types of Diabetes Mellitus

- *Type 1 diabetes mellitus*. Type 1 diabetes, formerly known as insulin-dependent diabetes mellitus (IDDM), is an autoimmune disorder. It can be brought about by a number of factors, including exposure to certain drugs and chemicals, or as a complication of some kinds of infections. Immune system cells of people with type 1 diabetes attack the beta cells in the pancreas where insulin is produced. The destruction of these cells leads to a lifelong deficiency in insulin.

  Type 1 diabetes usually shows symptoms before age 30, but one variety, called latent autoimmune diabetes in adults may not be identified until later. Type 1 diabetes is the rarer and more serious of the two basic types of diabetes. It accounts for 5% to 10% of diabetes in this country.
- *Type 2 diabetes mellitus*. This variety used to be called non–insulin-dependent diabetes mellitus, but since many patients do end up supplementing insulin, that name is no longer accurate. The exact cause of type 2 diabetes is probably a combination of prodiabetes behaviors along with genetic predisposition.

  Type 2 diabetes can be controllable with diet, exercise, and possibly some antidiabetes drugs, depending on how far advanced it is when treatment begins, but many patients eventually benefit from supplementing insulin.
- *Other types of diabetes*. Other types of diabetes include gestational diabetes and secondary diabetes. Gestational diabetes occurs when a woman develops a transient case during pregnancy. This condition can cause birth defects in the child, as well as changing fetal metabolism, which results in very high birth weights and a high incidence of cesarean sections. Women who have gestational diabetes and their babies also have an increased risk of developing type 2 diabetes later in life.

  Secondary diabetes may develop with damage or trauma to the pancreas or as a symptom of some other endocrine disorder, such as acromegaly or Cushing syndrome. And diabetes insipidus is a dysfunction of the pituitary gland and insufficient production of antidiuretic hormone. These conditions are discussed in Appendix C, Extra Conditions at a Glance.

Signs and Symptoms

Three defining "polys" are common to all types of diabetes. Polyuria, or frequent urination, results from elevated blood sugar, which acts as a diuretic; it pulls water from the cells in the body, and excess water is expelled in the urine. Polydipsia means excessive thirst, which accompanies the loss of water with polyuria. Polyphagia refers to increased appetite, since diabetics must get most of their energy from fats and proteins instead of carbohydrates, which are the most efficient kind of fuel. Other symptoms of diabetes include fatigue, weight loss, nausea, and vomiting.

Very often, signs of diabetes are missed until the disease has damaged other organs. It is estimated that an average adult diagnosed with diabetes has probably had the disease for 4 to 7 years by the time it is identified.

Diabetic Emergencies

People with diabetes are vulnerable to two classes of medical emergencies, both of which can be fatal if not treated promptly.

Ketoacidosis. This is a critical shortage of insulin and lack of glucose in the cells in type 1 diabetics; people with type 2 diabetes don't have this problem. The body partially metabolizes fats for fuel, and the acidic byproduct of that metabolism (ketones) dangerously changes the pH balance of the blood. Ketoacidosis is identifiable by a characteristic sweet or fruity odor to the breath. Diabetics can test themselves for ketoacidosis with test strips that look for signs of ketones in the urine. Ketoacidosis can be brought on by stress, infection, or trauma, and can lead to shock, coma, and death. An analogous condition in type 2 diabetics is hyperosmolality. This causes a change in the pH of the blood, which can lead to shock, coma, and death.

Insulin shock. This is an emergency at the other end of the scale. In this case, too much insulin is circulating, either because too much has been administered or because a skipped meal, sudden exertion, stress, infection, or trauma has resulted in the consumption of all available blood sugar. The consequence of having too much available insulin is

NOTABLE CASES The list of influential people with diabetes is long and varied. It includes Rania Al-Abdullah (Queen of Jordan), Anwar Sadat (President of Egypt), and Mike Huckabee (American politician). Johnny Cash had it, and as of this writing B.B. King is still going strong with his diabetes. MacDonald's founder Ray Kroc had diabetes, along with actors Halle Berry, James Cagney, and Mary Tyler Moore. Writers Ernest Hemingway and H.G. Wells had this disease, and so did inventor and innovator Thomas Edison.

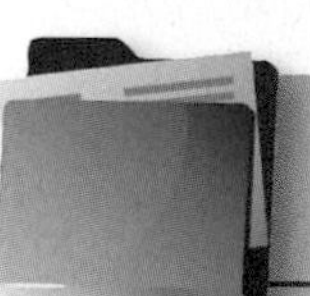

CASE HISTORY 9.1 Type 2 Diabetes

MAUREEN, AGE 43
"A do-it-yourself project."

Maureen had gestational diabetes while pregnant with two of her three children. At age 42, she began having chronic yeast infections, unintentional weight loss, blurred vision, and unusual thirst. When she went for her annual checkup, she was not happy but also not surprised to be diagnosed with type 2 diabetes.

At first Maureen was intimidated by the glucose testing equipment she had to use, and she was terrified by the long-term complications that often develop with diabetes. But as she did more research, she came to the conclusion that diabetes is very much a do-it-yourself project. She found that proper control can be achieved through education, hard work, and stress reduction.

She tests her blood frequently and sees immediate relationships between her glucose levels and how much stress she's going through and how much exercise she gets. Since her diagnosis, Maureen's diabetes medication has been cut in half, and she is able to maintain reasonable glucose levels by being proactive about her health. Although she is still upset about her disease, she is thankful that she was diagnosed early enough to take control of her situation and change it for the better.

a dangerously low blood sugar level, or hypoglycemia. Symptoms of insulin shock include dizziness, confusion, weakness, and tremors. It too can lead to coma and death if not treated (with sugar tablets, juice, milk, candy, or nondiet soda to replace blood sugar) quickly.

Treatment

Before the development of insulin in 1921, the diagnosis of diabetes was a death knell. Most people lived only a few years after the disease was identified. Now diabetes is a highly treatable disease, although not all diagnosed people treat it aggressively enough to prevent complications.

The goals for diabetes treatment are to improve insulin production in the pancreas when possible, to inhibit the release of glucose from the liver, to increase the sensitivity of target cells to insulin, and to decrease the absorption of carbohydrates in the small intestines. In addition to these measures, special care of eyes and feet can reduce the risk of blindness and amputations associated with the disease.

Type 1 diabetes is treated primarily with various forms of insulin. This can be delivered by injection; with an insulin pen, which delivers a measured dose under the skin without a hypodermic needle; or with insulin pumps, which feed a steady drip into the body through a plastic tube.

Type 2 diabetes is first addressed with changes in diet and exercise, but many patients are eventually treated with drugs that manipulate how insulin is used, and insulin supplementation. (See Sidebar 9.2 for more managing blood glucose.)

Many diabetes patients eventually develop renal insufficiency; their kidneys simply cannot keep up with their needs. **Hemodialysis** is a treatment in which the blood is routed through a filtering machine that removes excess water and waste products before returning the blood to the body. Dialysis of any kind is usually a stopgap measure while a person waits for a kidney to become available for transplant.

Medications

- Fast-acting and slow-acting insulin by injection, pen or pump (insulin cannot be administered orally) to reduce blood sugar for type 1 and some type 2 diabetes
- Medications including metformin to stimulate insulin release and insulin uptake
- Medications to address hyperlipidemia
- Antihypertensives, especially angiotensin converting enzyme inhibitors and angiotensin II receptor blockers
- Medications to address other complications of diabetes

SIDEBAR 9.2 Managing Diabetes: Blood Glucose

Keeping blood glucose within a limited range of variation can be a complicated undertaking. Normal fasting blood sugar (a measurement that is taken before eating in the morning) is 110 mg/dL of blood or less. Diabetes is diagnosed when fasting levels rise over 125 mg/dL for 2 or more consecutive days.

Another test, called the hemoglobin A1c test, measures how much sugar sticks to the hemoglobin in circulating erythrocytes. This is often considered a better long-term test, since it reflects general blood sugar levels for 3 months or more instead of in increments of several hours. A normal reading is 4% to 5.9%; diabetes is diagnosed when A1c tests show 8% or more glucose.

Massage?

RISKS The risks of massage for a person with advanced or poorly managed diabetes are complex. Cardiovascular disease, kidney disease, skin ulcerations, and neuropathy comprise a short list of common complications that alter bodywork choices. Injection sites or insulin pump attachment sites are local contraindications. In addition, timing bodywork choices around insulin doses is preferable, to avoid causing a hypoglycemic episode.

BENEFITS A client who has healthy, responsive tissue and well-controlled diabetes can enjoy the same benefits from bodywork as the rest of the population.

OPTIONS Because massage has been seen to drop blood sugar, it is a good idea to try to schedule massage or bodywork sessions when insulin is at its most stable: in the middle of a cycle, rather than just after or just before administering this treatment. It is also wise to ask a diabetic client ahead of time how he or she would want to handle a hypoglycemic episode. Some people keep sugar tablets with them; others prefer milk, juice, or other options.

Hyperthyroidism

Definition: What Is It?

Hyperthyroidism is a condition in which the thyroid gland produces excessive amounts of hormones that stimulate metabolism of fuel into energy. It falls under a larger heading of **thyrotoxicosis**, which describes any situation in which too much thyroid hormone is present in the blood (see Sidebar 9.3).

Hyperthyroidism is a common disorder, affecting between 1% and 2% of people in the United States at some time in their lives.

Etiology: What Happens?

Hyperthyroidism is usually caused by one of three things: an autoimmune attack against the thyroid gland that causes it to secrete excessive amounts of metabolic hormones, a nodule or group of nodules that become hyperactive for unknown reasons, or inflammation of the thyroid.

Hyperthyroidism in Brief

Pronunciation: hy-per-THY-roid-izm

What is it?
Hyperthyroidism is a condition in which the thyroid gland produces excessive levels of the hormones that stimulate the conversion of fuel into energy. It is often related to an autoimmune attack against the whole thyroid gland, but it can also be caused by small hyperactive nodules or local inflammation.

How is it recognized?
Signs and symptoms of hyperthyroidism are related to having too much energy. They include restlessness, sleeplessness, irritability, dry skin and hair, rapid heartbeat, tremor, unintended weight loss, and for women, irregularity of menstrual periods. Some hyperthyroid patients have eye problems or skin rashes. A severe and acute episode of hyperthyroidism can be life threatening; this is called a thyroid storm.

Massage risks and benefits
Risks: Massage has no direct affect on thyroid gland function or dysfunction, and it offers no specific risks for hyperthyroidism patients.
Benefits: If a client is comfortable on a table, massage may offer a welcome change from a hyperthyroidism patient's usual restlessness.

SIDEBAR 9.3 Hyperthyroidism Semantics

Hyperthyroidism is a condition in which the thyroid gland is overactive, and produces too much hormone, but it is not the only situation in which T3 and T4 can flood the system. **Thyrotoxicosis** describes any situation in which too much thyroid hormone is present. This includes hyperthyroidism, but also includes some forms of thyroiditis (which leads to stored hormones being released), oversupplementation of replacement hormones, active thyroid cells elsewhere in the body (with metastatic thyroid cancer or dermoid cysts, for instance), and the consumption of too much iodine, which can happen with some kinds of medications, cough syrups, or seaweed.

Under normal circumstances, secretions of thyroid-stimulating hormone (TSH) from the pituitary control thyroid activity. When hyperthyroidism is well established, circulating levels of TSH drop significantly, but the thyroid produces much more hormone than normal. The result is that the conversion of fuel into energy increases by 60% to 100%, and many body systems are affected (see Figure 9.2).

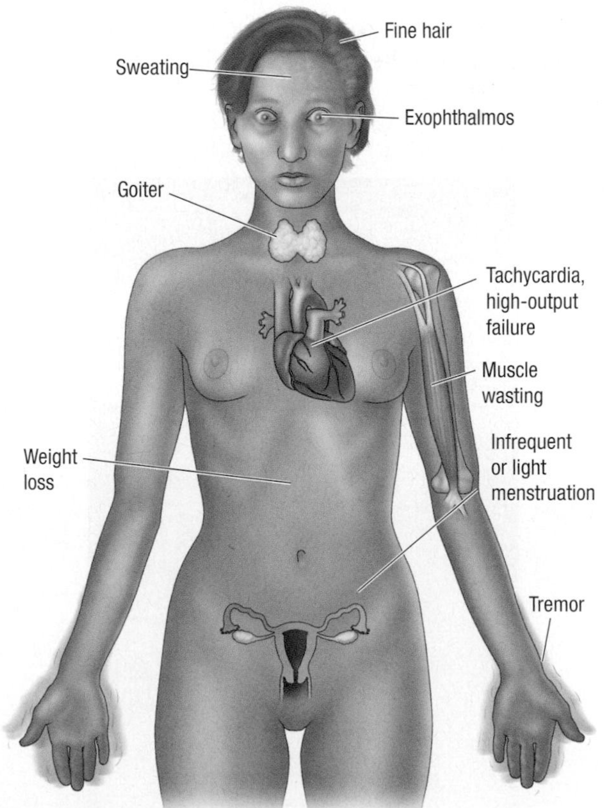

Figure 9.2. Hyperthyroidism

In addition to affecting the thyroid and associated hormones, hyperthyroid can cause problems in several other tissues. Hyperthyroidism is most common among mature adults, and osteoporosis is a risk for both genders, because the thyroid and parathyroids together normally secrete hormones that influence bone density. Eyes are affected in a couple of ways. One fairly common condition is elevation of eyelids in a way that makes the eyes seem to bulge. Protrusion of the eyes is known as **exophthalmos** or **proptosis** (Figure 9.3). Another eye problem is a rare disorder called **Graves ophthalmopathy**. This causes the eyeball to protrude beyond its protective orbit because tissues behind it swell. The front surface of the eye can dry out, causing light sensitivity, double vision, decreased freedom of movement within the orbit, pain, and excessive tearing.

NOTABLE CASES Marty Feldman (Igor in *Young Frankenstein*) built a comic career out of the exophthalmus that was a complication of his hyperthyroidism. Former President and First Lady George and Barbara Bush both have hyperthyroidism (as did their dog). Sprinter Gail Devers did not let hyperthyroidism interfere with her athletic goals: after treatment for her condition, she won multiple track and field Olympic and World Champion medals.

Some hyperthyroidism disease patients develop raised red patches of skin on their shins, feet, or elsewhere. These rashes, called **pretibial myxedema**, are caused by deposition of mucopolysaccharides in the dermis. They are generally not painful or dangerous. Another fairly rare complication is thyroid **acropachy**: the skin around the fingernails becomes swollen but is not typically painful.

In addition to eye and skin problems, some hyperthyroidism patients have occasional episodes of dangerously high metabolism called thyroid storms. In these episodes, symptoms suddenly become acute and may include rapid heartbeat, fever without infection, intolerance to heat, nausea, confusion, agitation, and finally shock. Thyroid storms are medical emergencies and require immediate intervention to slow the heart and bring down the fever.

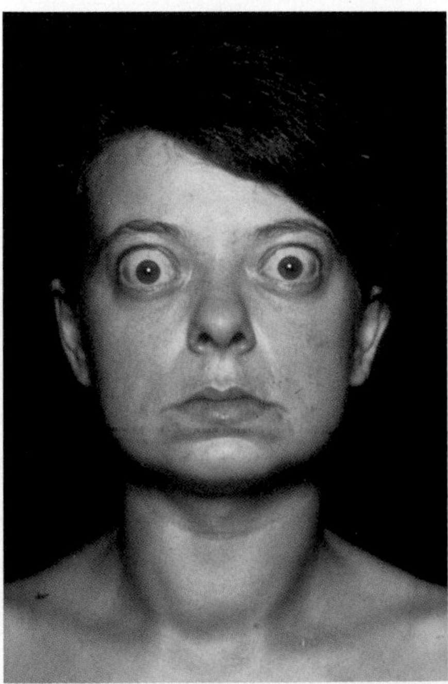

Figure 9.3. Hyperthyroidism: exophthalmus

Types of Hyperthyroidism

- *Graves disease.* This is autoimmune hyperthyroidism, the most common form of this condition. In this situation, antibodies called thyroid-stimulating immunoglobins attack the thyroid gland, causing it to grow to huge dimensions and to secrete excessive levels of thyroid hormones, especially thyroxine. While genetics clearly plays a major part in development of Graves disease, its onset often seems to be connected to a stressful trigger. Other risk factors for developing this disorder include exposure to x-rays and having taken antiviral medications such as interferon or interleukin.

SIDEBAR 9.4 Graves Disease and Autoimmune Polyglandular Syndrome: Why Have Just One?

A strong genetic link has been established in Graves disease; if one person has this disorder, it is likely that some kind of thyroid dysfunction will be present in some other first- or second-degree relative. In some families, Graves disease shows as one of several problems that are known collectively as **autoimmune polyglandular syndrome**. Related conditions in this syndrome include type 1 diabetes, systemic lupus erythematosus, pernicious anemia, and others.

- *Toxic adenoma*. This is the development of benign tumors, and it is related to chronic iodine deficiency.
- *Multinodular goiter*. The accumulation of small, nonfunctioning thyroid nodules is not unusual, but they sometimes become active, leading to excessive hormone production or mechanical impingement on the trachea or esophagus.
- *Thyroiditis*. This is inflammation of the thyroid leading to temporary hyperactivity. It is sometimes due to a viral infection but may also be a complication of childbirth.

Signs and Symptoms

Signs and symptoms of hyperthyroidism are mostly related to the excessive secretion of thyroid hormones. They include anxiety, irritability, insomnia, rapid heartbeat, tremor, increased perspiration, sensitivity to heat, frequent bowel movements, and unintentional weight loss. Skeletal muscles, especially in the upper arms and thighs, often become weak in a condition sometimes called **thyrotoxic myopathy**. Other symptoms may include light flow during menstrual periods, dry skin and brittle nails, and problems specifically with the skin and eyes. Many hyperthyroidism patients develop a **goiter**: the thyroid becomes enlarged enough to create a visible painless swelling in the neck.

Long-term hyperthyroidism can lead to dangerous changes in arterial and cardiac tissues. The ventricles become thickened, raising the risk for pulmonary edema and heart failure, and the heartbeat may be vulnerable to atrial fibrillations.

Treatment

Hyperthyroidism can be treated in a number of ways, depending on the underlying causes and the severity of the symptoms. Most treatment options eventually lead to hypothyroidism, which is treatable and much less threatening than hyperthyroidism.

Radioactive iodine can be used as a diagnostic tool to track iodine uptake, but it can also be used to kill off hyperactive thyroid cells. Some medications prevent the thyroid from producing too much T4, or they reduce its effect. These medications may be used to prepare a patient for surgery or radioactive iodine treatment, but they are occasionally successful by themselves. Beta-blockers may be recommended to reduce heart rate and the sense of palpitations. Patients who can't take antithyroid drugs or radioactive iodine may consider a thyroidectomy, a surgery in which most of the thyroid is removed. This is a risky procedure, however, because the parathyroids, which control calcium metabolism, are often damaged in the process, along with the vocal cords and laryngeal nerves.

Medications

- Radioactive iodine to identify and kill off overactive thyroid tissue
- Antithyroid medications to interfere with thyroid hormone production
- Beta-blockers for symptomatic relief

Massage?

RISKS If a client has skin damage as part of his or her hyperthyroidism, massage may be a local caution. Otherwise, it has no risks for this condition.

BENEFITS If a client's skin is healthy and intact, massage may be able to offer temporary relief from the frenetic pace of life that many people with hyperthyroidism experience, even though long-lasting changes to thyroid function are not a realistic expectation.

Hypothyroidism

Definition: What Is It?

Hypothyroidism is a condition in which circulating levels of thyroid hormones are abnormally low. This interferes with the body's ability to generate energy from fuel.

Etiology: What Happens?

The thyroid gland produces thyroid hormone in two forms, T3 (triiodothyronine) in small amounts, and T4 (thyroxine) in larger amounts. It does this under the direction of the pituitary gland, which releases thyroid-stimulating hormone (TSH). The liver and other tissues convert T4 to T3, which is more usable by the body. When adequate amounts of T3 and T4 are circulating in the blood, secretion of TSH is suppressed. This is the negative feedback loop that keeps thyroid and pituitary secretions in balance.

The purpose of thyroid hormones is to stimulate the conversion of fuel (oxygen and calories)

Hypothyroidism in Brief

Pronunciation: hy-po-THY-roid-izm

What is it?
Hypothyroidism is a condition in which the thyroid gland produces an inadequate supply of the hormones that regulate metabolism of fuel into energy. Some cases of hypothyroidism are the result of an autoimmune attack on the thyroid gland, but others are related to the long-term complications of treatment for hyperthyroidism or other factors.

How Is It recognized?
Symptoms of hypothyroidism are subtle and often missed. They include fatigue, weight gain, depression, intolerance of cold, an increased risk for cardiovascular disease, and, for women, heavy menstrual periods.

Massage risks and benefits
Risks: The risk of cardiovascular disease must be recognized in hypothyroidism patients, especially elders.
Benefits: While massage won't change the course of hypothyroidism, as long as the risk of cardiovascular disease is controlled, it can add to the quality of life of a client with this condition.

into energy or work. In hypothyroidism, inadequate amounts of T3 and T4 are produced, so incoming fuel is simply stored and not used. In a typical early case of hypothyroidism, the pituitary gland releases lots of TSH, and circulating levels of T4 are converted to T3 very quickly. Consequently, TSH levels are high, T4 levels are significantly low, but T3 levels are close to normal. In later stages, TSH remains high, but both T3 and T4 levels drop.

NOTABLE CASES Singer Linda Ronstadt and talk show icon Oprah Winfrey both struggle with hypothyroidism.

Whatever the cause of hypothyroidism, the net result is that a person has difficulty turning fuel into energy. Changes in thyroxine-sensitive cells lead to decreased contractility of the heart muscle, heart enlargement, low cardiac output, and high levels of low-density lipoproteins (the atherosclerosis-promoting form of cholesterol). Other consequences include slow gastrointestinal activity (gastric stasis), delayed puberty, menstrual changes, and infertility.

Types of Hypothyroidism

- *Hashimoto thyroiditis*. This is an autoimmune attack against the thyroid gland that results in suppression of thyroid secretions.
- *Secondary hypothyroidism*. Most hyperthyroidism patients who use radioactive iodine or surgery to suppress thyroid activity eventually develop hypothyroidism.
- *Iodine deficiency hypothyroidism*. Worldwide, this is the most common cause of hypothyroidism. In the United States it is rare, largely because of the use of iodized salt.
- *Idiopathic hypothyroidism*. Some cases of hypothyroidism don't seem to be related to any specific underlying disorder but simply arise without known cause. Because many patients exhibit the signs and symptoms of hypothyroidism without strongly indicative blood test confirmation, the identification and treatment of hypothyroidism for these patients is controversial.
- *Other types of hypothyroidism*. Thyroid suppression can be a side effect of some medications (especially the lithium-based drugs used for bipolar disease), a tumor or brain injury that interferes with the pituitary-thyroid axis, a birth defect, exposure to radiation, or a transient complication of childbirth.

Signs and Symptoms

Signs and symptoms of hypothyroidism are often subtle but steadily progressive (Figure 9.4). A person who cannot convert fuel into energy is likely to gain weight, feel fatigued and depressed, and have a sluggish digestive system with chronic constipation. Heart rate and basal temperature drops, and reflexes may become slow. A patient may have poor tolerance of cold, and her skin may be puffy but dry. Fluid retention in the extremities raises the risk of carpal tunnel syndrome and other nerve entrapment syndromes. Her hair becomes brittle and may even break off or fall out. For some reason, this is especially common at the lateral aspect of the eyebrows. Menstrual periods tend to be heavy and long lasting. Some hypothyroidism patients develop goiter, a painless enlargement of the thyroid.

Very severe or untreated cases may cause a person to become so cold and drowsy that she becomes

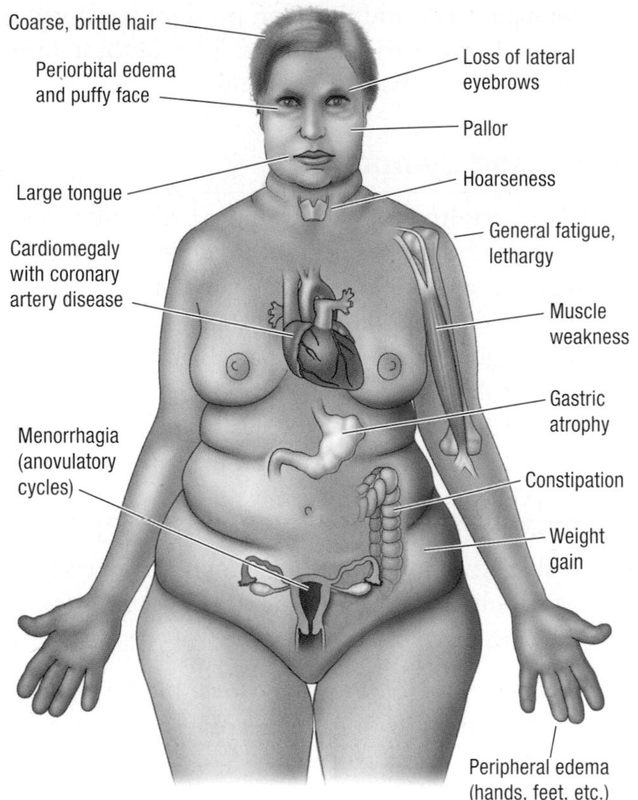

Figure 9.4. Hypothyroidism

unconscious. This is called myxedema coma, and it is a rare but dangerous complication of hypothyroidism, especially among elderly patients.

Treatment

Identifying the need to treat hypothyroidism can sometimes be a challenge. The symptoms of this condition are often vague; it can resemble depression, fibromyalgia, chronic fatigue syndrome, and several other chronic conditions. Also, whether standard scales of "normal" blood tests are accurate for all patients is controversial; subclinical hypothyroidism doesn't fit the typical tests, but can respond well to treatment. For these reasons, the identification and treatment of mild cases of hypothyroidism may vary from one professional to another.

It is especially important for pregnant women to be tested for thyroid function. Pregnancy can hide some symptoms of hypothyroidism, which can create serious repercussions for the unborn child. Most newborns are tested for thyroid function as a matter of course; early intervention in the rare cases when thyroid function is subnormal can prevent stunted growth and mental disability.

The usual treatment for hypothyroidism is to supplement thyroid hormones, usually in the form of synthetic T4, which most people can metabolize into adequate amounts of T3. While many people find relief with this treatment, others must explore other options to find the right supplement for both T3 and T4. This can be in the form of synthetic versions of these hormones or as desiccated porcine or bovine glands. Using animal products for hormone replacement is challenging, though, because the potency from one batch to another can vary greatly.

It is important to remember that hypothyroidism can be a progressive disease, and the appropriate dosage may change over time. Treatment is important not only to manage symptoms of fatigue and low energy but also to regulate cardiovascular function and decrease the risk of heart or artery disease complications.

Medications

- Synthetic T4 (levothyroxine)
- Synthetic T3
- Desiccated animal gland (Armor)

Massage?

RISKS Persons with hypothyroidism are at increased risk for cardiovascular disease, and that informs some choices about massage. However, this situation is so prevalent in the American population, it is safe to assume that most mature clients live with it.

BENEFITS Massage won't necessarily improve thyroid activity, but it may help to ameliorate some of the fatigue and depression that often accompanies this condition.

Metabolic Syndrome

Definition: What Is It?

Metabolic syndrome is not a freestanding disease. Instead, it is a group of problems that, when seen in combinations, have been identified as indicators for a high risk of developing type 2 diabetes and cardiovascular disease.

Estimates of the incidence of metabolic syndrome vary widely, but most agree that about 30% of adult

Metabolic Syndrome in Brief

Pronunciation: met-uh-BOL-ik SIN-drome

What is it?
Metabolic syndrome is a collection of signs that together indicate a high risk of several serious diseases, including diabetes, heart attack, atherosclerosis, and stroke.

How is it recognized?
Metabolic syndrome is recognized by its combined associated conditions, including hypertension, disruptions in cholesterol, central obesity, and others.

Massage risks and benefits
Risks: A person with metabolic syndrome may have compromised cardiovascular health; this obviously has implications for rigorous massage.
Benefits: If it is safe for a person with metabolic syndrome to exercise in order to lose weight and improve insulin function, massage is probably also safe and may be a helpful adjunct other health promoting activities.

Americans would fit the diagnostic criteria for this condition, although many do not know it.

Etiology: What Happens?

Metabolic syndrome is identified as a cluster of five main features, including high triglycerides, low high-density lipoproteins (the "good" cholesterol), hypertension, central obesity (fat retention in the omentum more than in superficial fascia), and high fasting blood glucose levels. Other possible features in metabolic syndrome include a high risk of blood clotting, high levels of C-reactive protein (an indicator of inflammation), and polycystic ovary disease in women.

These factors are not particularly alarming when they appear individually, but in combination, they set the stage for a high risk of type 2 diabetes, atherosclerosis, heart attack, heart failure, and stroke. Nonalcoholic fatty liver disease, early cognitive decline, and an increased risk for some kinds of cancers are also associated with metabolic syndrome.

The primary risk factors for metabolic syndrome are obesity and insulin resistance. Further, obesity tends to cause insulin resistance, and insulin resistance can cause obesity, forming a vicious circle. This is complicated by the fact that fat cells in the omentum are metabolically more active than those in subcutaneous fat, and they can produce proclotting and proinflammatory secretions. Both of these raise the risk for cardiovascular problems.

Signs and Symptoms

Metabolic syndrome typically appears as central obesity (much of the body weight is carried around the abdomen in an "apple" rather than a "pear" shape), along with disruptions in cholesterol, hypertension, and blood glucose. The point at which this is associated with risk varies by racial profile; Asian Americans are at risk for the consequences of metabolic syndrome with a smaller abdominal measurement than other races. Outside of excessive body weight, however, metabolic syndrome does not typically cause noticeable symptoms; its other components are silent.

Metabolic syndrome is identified when three of these five risk factors are simultaneously present:

- High fasting blood glucose (over 100 mg/dL after 9 hours of fasting) or needing medication to manage blood glucose
- Abdominal obesity: a waist measurement of over 88 cm (35 in) for women or over 102 cm (40 in) for men; for Asian Americans, the risk begins at 80 cm (32 in) for women and 90 cm (35 in) for men
- Elevated triglyceride levels (>140 mg/dL for men and >150 mg/dL for women)
- Low levels of high-density lipoproteins (<40 mg/dL for men and <50 mg/dL for women)
- Hypertension (systolic blood pressure >130 mm Hg; diastolic > 85 mm Hg)

Treatment

Treatment for metabolic syndrome is often divided into short-term and long-term goals. Short-term goals include lowering blood glucose and correcting cholesterol levels with diet, exercise, and medical intervention.

Long-term goals include increasing physical activity and losing weight. Reducing body weight by 5% to 7% (this is only 10 to 14 lb for a 200-lb person) reduces the risk of complications by about 60%, and exercise improves insulin action and decreases blood glucose. Limiting alcohol use and quitting smoking are other important steps.

Some of the remedies used in Traditional Chinese Medicine have shown promising results to manage aspects of metabolic syndrome, as has meditation as a relaxation technique.

Medications

- Metformin or other insulin-regulating medication
- Cholesterol-lowering drugs to manage hyperlipidemia
- Low-dose aspirin as needed for antiplatelet activity

Massage?

RISKS The safety of massage for clients with metabolic syndrome depends on their resilience and ability to adapt to homeostatic challenge. A person at high risk for cardiovascular disease or diabetes may have more trouble with rigorous massage than someone with a milder version of this condition.

BENEFITS While massage alone is unlikely to have a profound impact on metabolic syndrome, along with diet and exercise, it can be a part of a supportive change in lifestyle practices that can reduce the risk of this condition becoming a more serious problem.

Thyroid Cancer in Brief

Pronunciation: THY-royd KAN-ser

What is it?
Thyroid cancer is any type of cancer that arises from cells in the thyroid. It is derived from follicular cells that produce T3 and T4, from C cells that produce calcitonin, or from lymphocytes in the thyroid gland.

How is it recognized?
Most types of thyroid cancer cause enlargement of the gland, which may press on the trachea or esophagus, leading to hoarseness and difficulty with swallowing or breathing.

Massage risks and benefits
Risks: The risks of massage for clients with thyroid cancer and any cancer depend mainly on what kinds of treatments they are using and how bodywork might provide excessive challenge during this stressful time. Because a common treatment for thyroid cancer is radioactive iodine, close contact with the patient must be avoided until this protocol is concluded.
Benefits: Massage has many benefits to offer thyroid cancer patients, as long as care is taken to respect the challenges of both this disease and its treatments.

Thyroid Cancer

Definition: What Is It?

Thyroid cancer is any type of cancer that originates in the thyroid gland. Three types of thyroid cells can become cancerous: follicular cells, C cells, and lymphocytes. Most varieties of thyroid cancer are slow growing and easily treatable, but some forms are more aggressive.

Etiology: What Happens?

The thyroid gland is composed of two main types of epithelial cells: follicular cells, which normally produce T3 and T4, and parafollicular cells, also called C cells, which produce calcitonin, a hormone that pulls calcium out of the blood to increase bone density.

Cancer develops when DNA in thyroid cells is damaged and cell growth becomes uncontrolled and disorganized. Thyroid cancer is often related to a history of radiation exposure. People who were treated with radiation for acne, tonsillitis, or an enlarged thymus are at increased risk for this disease. Similarly, people exposed to radioactive fallout from nuclear testing or nuclear reactor accidents have a higher-than-normal risk for thyroid cancer; this is one of the long-term repercussions of the Chernobyl nuclear accident in 1986. Radiation from standard neck or dental radiography is not associated with an increased risk of thyroid cancer.

Other forms of thyroid cancer are related to inherited genetic characteristics. Children of people with the genetic mutation for thyroid cancer have a 50% chance of developing the disease themselves. Inherited forms of thyroid cancer tend to be more aggressive and harder to treat than other forms, so when this condition is discovered, all family members, especially children, are recommended for genetic testing.

Types of Thyroid Cancer

- *Papillary thyroid cancer.* This is the most common type of thyroid cancer, accounting for 70% to 80% of diagnoses. Papillary cells look like fern leaves, with many tiny extensions; they arise from follicular cells. This type of cancer usually stays local, and while it may intrude on local lymph nodes, it is usually extremely stable and doesn't tend to grow or invade other tissues. In rare cases, it does metastasize through the lymph system to the bones or the lungs.

- *Follicular thyroid cancer*. This form of thyroid cancer also arises from follicular cells. It is less common than papillary thyroid cancer, accounting for about 10% of thyroid cancer diagnoses. Follicular thyroid cancer is more likely to metastasize than papillary thyroid cancer, particularly if it is diagnosed in someone over 50 years old. **Hürthle cell carcinoma** is a subtype of follicular thyroid cancer. It tends to have a poor prognosis because it is harder to find early and less responsive to treatment than other forms of thyroid cancer.

NOTABLE CASES Film critic Roger Ebert had radiation treatment for an ear infection when he was young. He is now a survivor of papillary thyroid cancer. His multiple surgeries have led to the loss of his voice, but this does not keep him from being actively involved in his profession. Other thyroid cancer patients have included Supreme Court Chief Justice William Rehnquist and prolific science fiction author Isaac Asimov.

- *Medullary thyroid cancer*. This form of cancer arises from C cells that normally produce calcitonin. It is rare but it can be aggressive. It is often related to a group of identified genetic mutations.
- *Anaplastic thyroid cancer*. Also called undifferentiated thyroid cancer, anaplastic thyroid cancer is highly aggressive, metastasizing easily to the mediastinal lymph nodes, trachea, lungs, and bones. It originates from benign or low-grade thyroid tumors and usually affects people over 60 years old.
- *Thyroid lymphoma*. Lymphocytes in the thyroid gland are also vulnerable to DNA mutation. This is most likely to happen along with hypothyroidism in the form of Hashimoto thyroiditis.

Signs and Symptoms

Nonaggressive forms of thyroid cancer may be silent, especially in early stages. Later symptoms include painless enlargement in the throat. This may press on the esophagus or trachea, leading to problems with breathing, coughing, hoarseness, and difficulty with swallowing.

Later stages of aggressive thyroid cancers may include tumors in the lungs or on bones; symptoms may be related to these complications.

Treatment

Most cases of thyroid cancer are successfully treated with surgery to remove part or all of the thyroid gland. Thyroid hormones must be supplemented after this procedure. Lymph nodes in the neck are often dissected to look for signs of metastasis.

Surgery may be followed with doses of radioactive iodine or external beams of radiation at tumor sites. This regimen is successful for most cases of thyroid cancer, even if it recurs after surgery.

Aggressive forms of thyroid cancer are typically treated with radioactive iodine and other forms of chemotherapy, but not surgery, since the chance of getting all of the cancer cells is negligible.

Staging protocols for thyroid cancer are discussed in sidebar 9.5.

Medications

- Chemotherapeutic agents
- Radioactive iodine
- Thyroid hormones to stabilize blood levels and to inhibit the secretion of TSH

Massage?

RISKS As with other types of cancer, massage for thyroid cancer is based on the treatment options and the general resilience of the patient. One special caution for this population is that someone undergoing treatment with radioactive iodine must be kept in isolation until the treatment is complete. This means massage must be delayed as well. For more information about massage in the context of cancer, see Chapter 12

BENEFITS Because massage can offer relief of pain, anxiety, depression, and other problems that accompany cancer treatment, it can be helpful for someone living with this disease, as long as the challenges presented by the cancer and its treatments are respected.

SIDEBAR 9.5 Staging Thyroid Cancer

Staging protocols for thyroid cancer are tied to the type of cancer, the age of the patient, and the best treatment options in the circumstances. As new ways to identify thyroid cancer early are developed, these staging protocols may continue to evolve.

As with other types of cancer, thyroid cancer is staged using the TNM system, which is then translated into stages I to IV, as follows:

Tumor (T)	Node (N)	Metastasis (M)
T X: tumor cannot be assessed	N X: nodes cannot be assessed	M X: metastasis cannot be assessed
T 0: no evidence of primary tumor	N 0: no nodes involved	M 0: no metastasis found
T 1: tumor <2 cm, within the boundaries of the thyroid	N 1a: some nodes in neck involved	M 1: distant metastasis to lymph nodes, organs, or bones
T 2: tumor 2–4 cm, limited to thyroid	N 1b: some nodes in neck and mediastinum involved	
T 3: the tumor is >4 cm; or the tumor has invaded nearby tissue		
T 4a: tumor any size; has invaded anterior neck tissues		
T 4b: tumor any size; has invaded posterior neck, spine, or large blood vessels		

These delineations are translated into stages I to IV in this way:

For papillary or follicular thyroid cancer in patients under 45 years old

Stage I	any T, any N, M0
Stage II	any T, any N, M1

For anaplastic thyroid cancer

Stage IVa	T4a, any N, M0
Stage IVb	T4b, any N, M0
Stage IVc	any T, any N, M1

For papillary or follicular thyroid cancer in patients over 45 years old

Stage I	T1, N0, M0
Stage II	T2, N0, M0
Stage III	T1–3, N0–N1a, M0
Stage IVa	T1–4a, N0–1b, M0
Stage IVb	T4b, any N, M0
Stage IVc	any T, any N, M1

CHAPTER REVIEW QUESTIONS: ENDOCRINE SYSTEM CONDITIONS

1. What structure controls both the autonomic nervous system and the endocrine system?
2. How can diabetes contribute to heart disease? Kidney disease? Blindness?
3. Your client controls her diabetes with insulin injections. She wants to schedule her massage right after her injections, in the hope that this will enable her to use less insulin. Is this a good idea? Why or why not?
4. Why does a person with diabetes often feel thirsty?
5. What are three symptoms of abnormally high levels of T4?
6. What is the eventual prognosis for a person who treats hyperthyroidism by using radioactive iodine?

7. Your 43-year-old client is overweight, chronically cold, with poor stamina. She is puffy, and her hair is thin and dry. She says she is too tired to exercise, but she eats very little, and can't lose weight. What condition is probably present? Is massage likely to change the prognosis?

8. What are two leading risk factors for thyroid cancer?

9. Describe how successfully treating metabolic syndrome can prevent other serious health problems.

10. A 26-year-old client reports that she had papillary thyroid cancer 3 years ago. She had surgery to treat it and has had no further problems. What cautions might a massage therapist want to observe in this situation?

10

Urinary System Conditions

Chapter Objectives

After reading this chapter, you should be able to . . .

- Name the basic functional unit of the kidneys.
- Name a hormone secreted by the kidneys.
- List four types of kidney stones and identify the most common type.
- Identify what part of the kidney is affected with polycystic kidney disease.
- Explain the difference between uncomplicated and complicated pyelonephritis.
- List the stages of chronic renal failure.
- Define glomerular filtration rate.
- Identify the most common early symptom of bladder cancer.
- Explain why women are more prone to urinary tract infections than men.
- Name the causative agent of most urinary tract infections and uncomplicated pyelonephritis.

Urinary System Introduction

The urinary system is a relatively small system composed of the kidneys, ureters, bladder, and urethra (Figure 10.1).

The huge renal artery comes directly off the aorta and enters the kidneys. It rapidly decreases in diameter and splits up to form thousands of capillaries, terminating in tiny knots called **glomeruli**. Each of these is surrounded by a **Bowman capsule**, the entry point to the **nephron**. Blood pressure forces fluid from the glomeruli into the Bowman capsule. Nephrons and circulatory capillaries exchange water and waste products as they intertwine along the loop of Henle (Figure 10.2). By the time fluid enters the collecting tubules, any water, electrolytes, or other material the body needs has been reabsorbed, so that only waste products are left. This fluid is urine. The collecting tubules pour their contents into the renal pelvis, the renal pelvis empties into the ureters, they lead to the

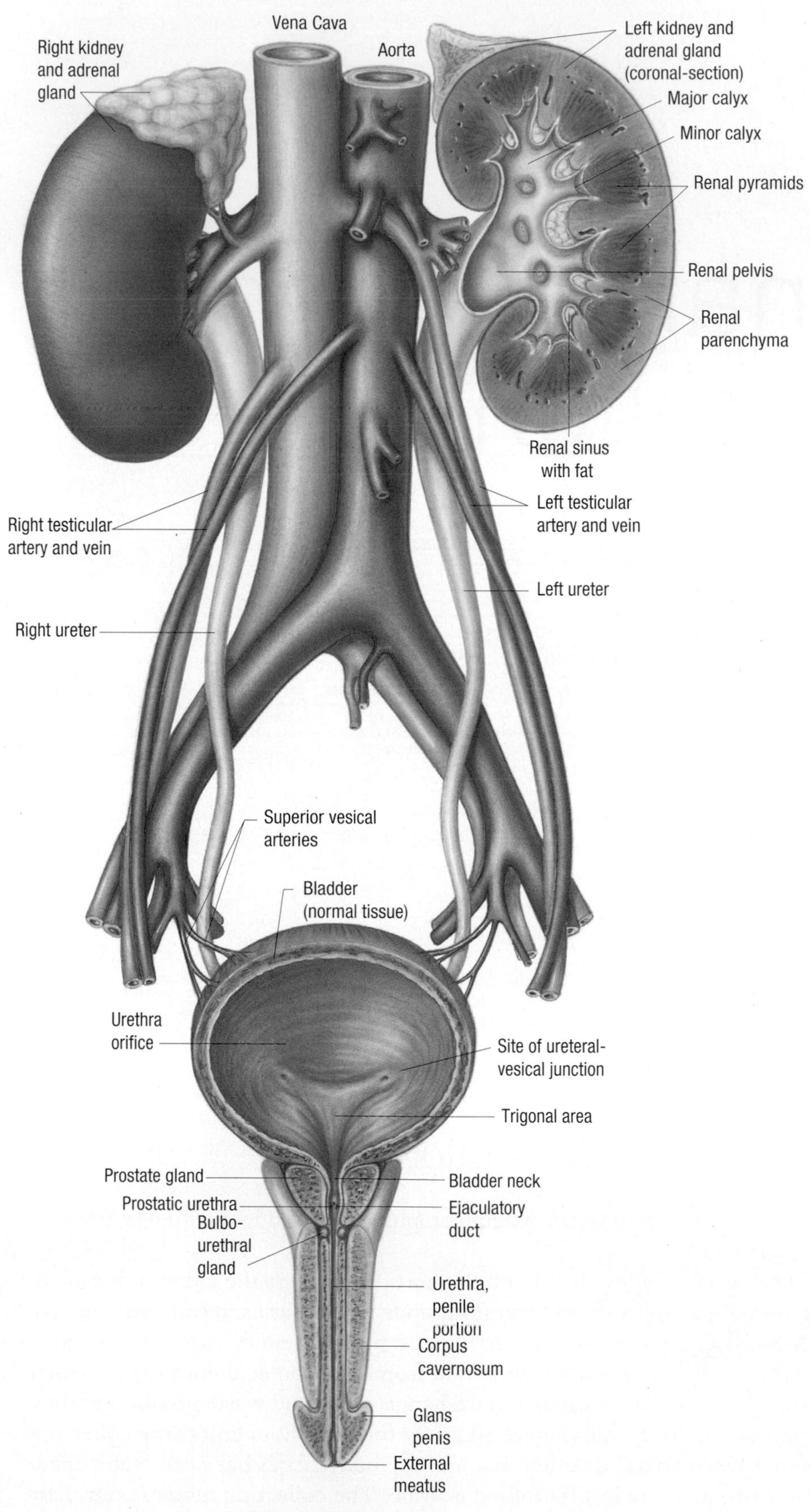

Figure 10.1. Urinary system overview

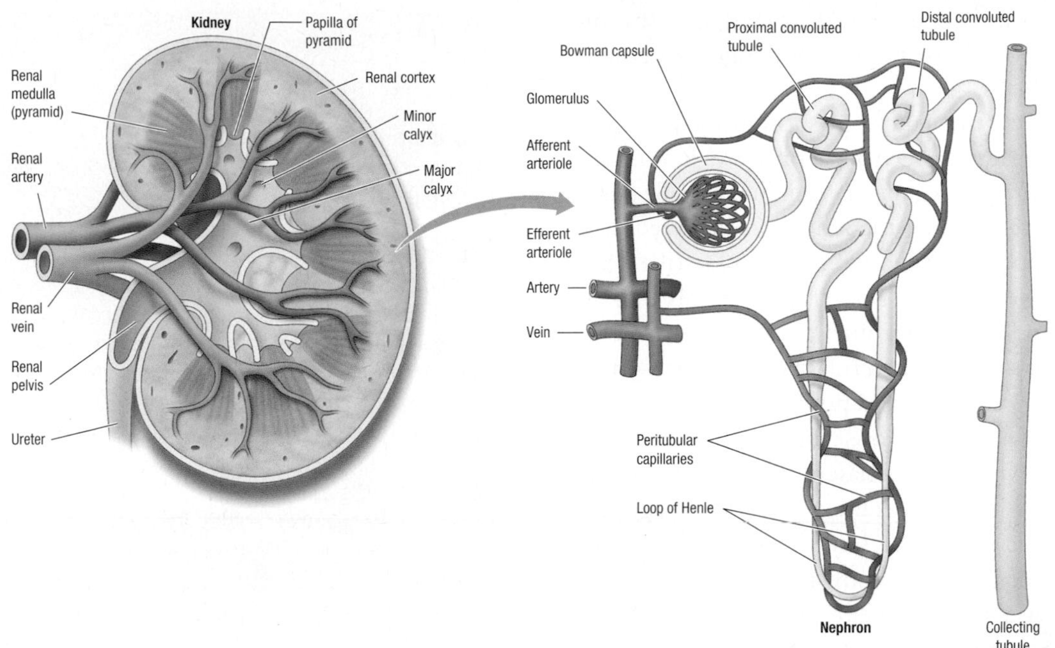

Figure 10.2. Kidney function

urinary bladder, and urine is excreted from the bladder through the urethra.

The kidneys have another function that is not directly involved in the removal of waste products from the blood. Erythropoietin (EPO), a hormone that stimulates red blood cell production, is produced in the kidneys. Damage to these delicate organs can therefore sometimes be identified by changes in red blood cell production.

Kidneys are constructed primarily of epithelial tissue, which makes them vulnerable to injury. When the kidneys have been damaged, red blood cells leak from capillaries into the nephrons. This shows as

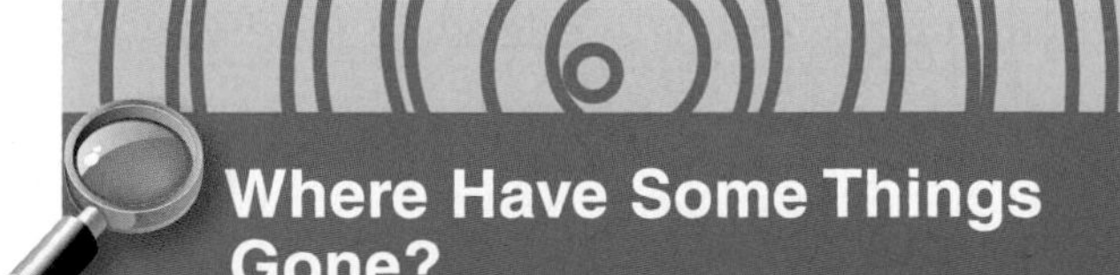

Where Have Some Things Gone?

Glomerulonephritis is the only urinary system condition that has been moved from this chapter. It is an inflammatory condition of the kidneys that can be freestanding or a symptom of a serious underlying problem. It can now be found in Appendix C, Extra Conditions at a Glance.

Urinary System Conditions

Kidney Disorders

- Kidney stones
  - Calcium stones
  - Struvite stones
  - Uric acid stones
  - Cystine stones
  - Other stones
- Polycystic kidney disease
- Pyelonephritis
  - Acute pyelonephritis
  - Chronic pyelonephritis
- Renal cancer
  - Renal cell carcinoma
  - Transitional cell carcinoma
  - Wilms tumor
- Renal failure
  - Acute renal failure
  - Chronic renal failure

Bladder and Urinary Tract Disorders

- Bladder cancer
  - Transitional cell carcinoma
  - Squamous cell carcinoma
  - Other types of bladder cancer
- Interstitial cystitis
- Urinary tract infection

blood in the urine (hematuria). It is evidence of trauma, infection, or another possibly dangerous condition in the kidneys.

Filtration, the movement of substances through a membrane by external mechanical pressure (in this case the blood pressure), is the mechanism that initially pushes waste-filled plasma into the kidneys. The speed with which this happens is called the **glomerular filtration rate**, or GFR. Normal GFR is 120 mL/min: this adds up to 180 L of fluid moving through the kidneys each day! (Of course, most of the glomerular filtrate is reabsorbed into circulatory capillaries and put back into the bloodstream.) It is clear then, how closely blood pressure and kidney health are interrelated. If blood pressure is consistently too high, the kidneys sustain damage and become less efficient. Conversely, if the kidneys are not functioning adequately, the body accumulates excessive fluid, which raises blood pressure. This vicious circle is a recurring theme in kidney dysfunction.

Kidney Stones in Brief

What are they?
Kidney stones are solid deposits of crystalline substances inside the kidney.

How are they recognized?
Small stones may cause no symptoms at all, but when larger stones enter the ureters, they can cause blood in the urine and extreme pain called renal colic. Renal colic may be accompanied by nausea and vomiting. Fever and chills indicate that infection is part of the problem. Pain may refer from the back into the groin.

Massage risks and benefits
Risks: Massage won't alter the progression of kidney stones, and if a client complains of extreme, severe back and flank pain with nausea and other symptoms, he or she is better off in the hospital than in a massage session.
Benefits: Clients who have fully recovered from kidney stones can enjoy the same benefits from massage as the rest of the population.

Kidney Disorders

Kidney Stones

Definition: What Is It?

Also called renal calculi or **nephrolithiases**, kidney stones are crystals that sometimes develop in the renal pelvis. The size of kidney stones varies widely, depending on how long they have been developing and what they are made of. Most stones range between the size of grains of sand to about 1 in in diameter. Some stones are much larger, growing into the cortex of the kidney, forming what is called a staghorn calculus (Figure 10.3).

Small stones may pass through the urinary tract with no symptoms, but larger ones may get stuck in the ureters. The technical name for them in this location is **ureterolithiases**.

Kidney stones usually form in the absence of adequate fluids. Thus, they are most common in hot environments, where people tend to lose more liquid through sweat than they replace. Peak months for the diagnosis of kidney stones in the United States are June through August, for the same reason.

Etiology: What Happens?

Several genetic anomalies raise the risk of kidney stones, along with the use of certain medications, a history of surgery or inflammation in the gastrointestinal tract, and urinary tract infections (UTIs) or blockages. Kidney stones can be composed of any of several substances, each one indicative of a different type of metabolic problem.

When a stone forms in the kidney, it may cause no symptoms or problems. But when it moves into the urethra, pressure builds up behind it, and the kidney can swell; this causes the characteristic grabbing pain associated with kidney stones.

Most kidney stones that are big enough to cause problems are excruciatingly painful but eventually pass into the bladder and out in the urine without causing long-lasting damage to the urinary system. Occasionally, however, a stone grows large enough to seriously disrupt kidney function. This may lead to chronic or acute renal failure.

Kidney stones are rarely once-in-a-lifetime event. Most people who pass one stone pass at least one more, possibly many years later.

Types of Kidney Stones

- *Calcium stones*: These account for most kidney stones. They are composed of calcium

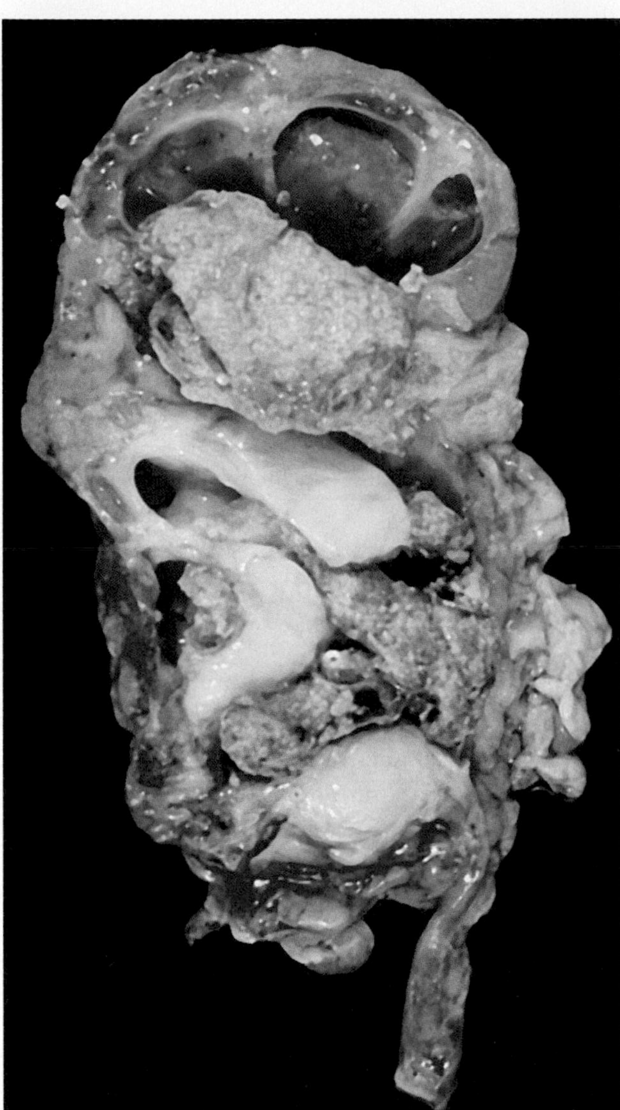

Figure 10.3. Staghorn calculus

oxalate or calcium phosphate, and associated with problems with calcium metabolism or too much incoming calcium, usually in the form of calcium supplements or calcium-based antacids.

- *Struvite stones*: These are composed of magnesium and ammonia and are associated with chronic UTIs.
- *Uric acid stones*: These form in the kidneys of people whose blood is abnormally acidic. They are associated with a diet high in meat and purines. People who have uric acid kidney stones are also at high risk for gout.
- *Cystine stones*: These are relatively rare. They are directly related to a genetic dysfunction with the metabolism of cystine, an amino acid.
- *Other stones*: These account for a tiny percentage of kidney stones. Genetic problems with metabolism and the use of protease inhibitors to treat HIV/AIDS are the primary causes of these stones.

Signs and Symptoms

Most kidney stones are completely silent, and they pass through the ureters without pain. If they get stuck or if they are large enough to scrape the delicate lining of the urinary tract however, they cause hematuria. In addition, the kidney may swell as it continues to produce urine that can no longer drain; this is extremely painful. The ureters contract in irritation, causing renal colic. The pain has a sudden onset, comes and goes in waves, and can be so severe that it causes nausea and vomiting as a sympathetic reaction. The pain often refers to the groin. Occasionally the stone may be caused by or may lead to an infection in the kidneys; in these instances, fever and chills accompany the severe pain.

Treatment

The pain of kidney stones is so intense that long ago people operated on them without anesthesia: "cutting for stone" was considered worth the pain just to get rid of them. Nowadays several other options are available, and only a small percentage of kidney stone patients have to go through major surgery. If a person is unable to pass a stone without help, three main interventions are available.

- **Percutaneous nephrolithotomy** is a surgery conducted through a tiny tunnel in the back leading to the stone, which is either extracted or subjected to sonic waves that break it up.
- Ureteroscopic stone removal uses a flexible tube that is inserted into the urethra and snakes up to where the stone is lodged to remove it from the ureters.
- **Extracorporeal shockwave lithotripsy** is the use of sound waves to break up stones into a size that can be passed through the ureters with minimal risk of getting stuck. This procedure can leave the patient feeling bruised and

battered from the extremity of the shock waves that are required to break up stones, but it can treat larger deposits than either of the other two options.

People who have passed a stone before will recognize the signs of another attack. They may be counseled to pass the stone at home, using over the counter painkillers, and urinating into a strainer, so the stone can be captured and analyzed later.

Prevention for persons susceptible to kidney stones depends on what the stones are made of. Possible interventions include removal of the parathyroid glands; medication to regulate metabolism, dietary adjustments; and most important: adequate hydration. Kidney stone patients need to drink up to one gallon of water every day to keep stones moving through the system before they become big enough to cause problems. Patients are also frequently advised to limit caffeine, alcohol, and oxalate-rich foods (dark leafy vegetables, nuts, and chocolate) to reduce the risk of future stones.

Medications

- For calcium or uric acid stones, alkalinizing agents, including allopurinol, to change the pH of fluid in the kidneys
- For struvite stones, possibly long-term low-dose prophylactic antibiotics
- For cystine stones, medication to bind cystine
- Analgesics, including ibuprofen or narcotics as necessary

Massage?

RISKS A person in the throes of a kidney stone attack is not a good candidate for massage; this is a medical emergency that needs appropriate attention.

BENEFITS A client who has fully recovered from kidney stones can enjoy the same benefits from massage as the rest of the population.

Polycystic Kidney Disease

Definition: What Is It?

Polycystic kidney disease (PKD) is a common inherited disorder that involves a genetic mutation in the cells that form tubules or collecting ducts in the kidneys, along with some other tissues. PKD affects about 600,000 people in the United States.

Etiology: What Happens?

PKD can be autosomal recessive (a person must inherit the gene from both parents for the disease to

CASE HISTORY 10.1 Kidney Stones

WALTER B. AGED 77
"Once you've had a kidney stone, you never forget it."

I've had kidney stone attacks all my life. In 1944, I had an attack at night in bed. Once you've had a kidney stone attack, you never forget what it feels like. I knew immediately what was happening, and they rushed me via command car to a military hospital, 20 miles away from the Battle of the Bulge. The renal surgeon authorized an attempt to remove the stone with a uretoscopic tube. Back in those days, the tube was metal, not flexible—hence the discomfort, which I've never forgotten. The procedure was unsuccessful because somehow I had already passed the stone.

Then, in the blizzard of '78, I had my last attack. Boston was digging out from a huge snowstorm. No one was allowed to drive; the streets had to be clear for ambulances and fire trucks. The pain was God-awful, just unbearable. They always say it's like having a baby—you just wouldn't believe it. I couldn't get to the hospital right away, so the doctor told me to drink some whiskey to dull the pain. Finally, I was given special dispensation to take a taxicab to the hospital.

When the stone was basketed at the hospital, it was sent to the kidney stone lab, where it was identified as a calcium stone. The medication consisted of allopurinol tablets and hydrochlorothiazide pills taken daily. There's been no sign of an attack since then.■

Polycystic Kidney Disease in Brief

What is it?
Polycystic kidney disease (PKD) is a genetic disorder leading to the formation of multiple cysts in the kidney and other organs. The cysts interfere with normal organ function, often leading to end-stage renal failure and the need for a kidney transplant.

How is it recognized?
Depending on the type of mutation, symptoms may appear in infancy or adulthood. Problems with urine production, enlarged liver, dangerously high hypertension, back pain, and headaches are among the signs and symptoms.

Massage risks and benefits
Risks: PKD involves problems with internal fluid management and a significant risk of other tissue anomalies that include liver cysts, diverticular disease, and cerebral aneurysms. Massage for a person with this condition must be gauged to fit within the challenges of their normal activities of daily living, which may be restricted.
Benefits: Massage may help to temporarily drop blood pressure, ease pain and anxiety, and add to general quality of life, as long as it doesn't overchallenge an impaired fluid management system.

manifest) or autosomal dominant (a person develops the disease if they inherit the gene from only one parent).

Autosomal recessive PKD is present at birth. It is often seen with extensive liver damage called **congenital hepatic fibrosis**. It is usually more severe than autosomal dominant PKD (ADPKD), and it is associated with a high risk of infant mortality.

ADPKD is the most common version of the disease. It usually doesn't cause problems until adulthood. Unusually high blood pressure is often the first indicator, followed by other symptoms that typically develop in a person's 30s or 40s.

In either form of PKD, a genetic anomaly causes certain cells in the kidneys to proliferate. They form hollow pockets that then fill with fluid (Figures 10.4 and 10.5). The cysts can be tiny or large, and both kidneys are affected. As the cysts increase in size and number, the rest of kidney function is seriously impaired. The unaffected tubules or collecting ducts can be physically obstructed or heavily invested with scar tissue. Ultimately, a person with PKD will probably develop renal failure, and about half of all PKD patients eventually become candidates for a kidney transplant.

PKD opens the door to several serious complications. The genetic anomaly that causes cysts to develop in the kidneys can also affect the liver, leading to hepatomegaly and loss of liver function. The constant high blood pressure seen with PKD contributes to atherosclerosis and other cardiovascular complications. In addition, blood vessels may be unusually weak; thoracic and cerebral aneurysms and hemorrhagic strokes are more common for PKD patients than for the general population. Heart valves are often abnormal, which raises the risk for arterial and pulmonary emboli. Even the colon appears to be affected by this disease: diverticular disease is common among PKD patients.

The progressive kidney damage seen with this disease also has direct impact on the health of the whole urinary system. Kidney stones, and infections in the cysts themselves, and in the rest of the urinary tract are all frequent complications.

The progressive loss of function with PKD means that many patients eventually develop end-stage renal failure. At this point, dialysis becomes necessary, and a kidney transplant may be a life-saving intervention. About one-half of all PKD patients will eventually seek a donor kidney. Fortunately, transplanted tissues do not develop cysts.

Signs and Symptoms

Hypertension that is unusually high for young adults is often the first indicator for ADPKD; this may develop even while kidney function is normal. A reduction in urine concentration is predictable, along with pain that is related to delicate kidney tissue that is stretched, compressed, and irritated. Headaches are a frequent complaint for PKD patients, along with extreme back and flank pain from kidney stones, urinary tract infections, and infected cysts.

Treatment

As a genetic disorder, PKD has no treatment to correct the core problem. Treatment focuses instead on controlling complications and symptoms to preserve function for as long as possible. Managing pain and

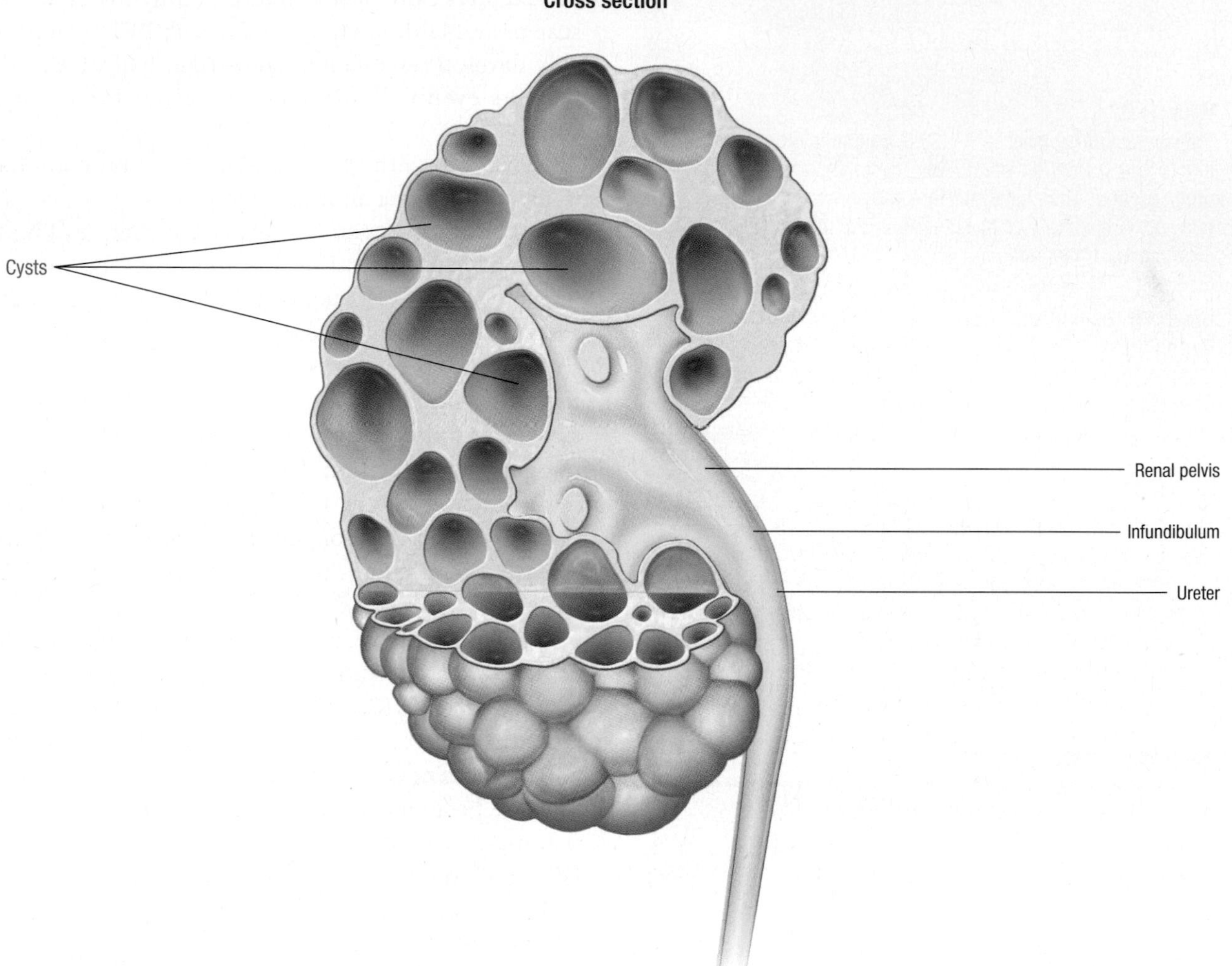

Figure 10.4. Polycystic kidney disease

high blood pressure are high priorities, of course. Needle aspiration of large cysts using ultrasound imaging as a guide can relieve symptoms for months at a time, but cysts do inevitably recur. Surgery may be considered for liver cysts.

Tracking the progress of PKD is important so that dialysis and kidney transplantation can be considered at the appropriate time.

Medications

- Antihypertensives, especially angiotensin-converting enzyme (ACE) inhibitors, but not calcium channel blockers
- Analgesics to manage headache and kidney-related pain; Nonsteroidal anti-inflammatory drugs must be avoided
- Antibiotics for infection

Massage?

RISKS A person with polycystic kidney disease (PKD) may have impaired ability to manage fluid, dangerously high blood pressure, and an increased risk for both liver damage and cerebral aneurysm, among other problems. All these factors may make rigorous circulatory massage a stimulus that is too challenging for their ability to adapt. Further, PKD patients may use particularly strong painkillers; this influences massage choices too, because pain sensation may be impaired.

BENEFITS Massage may help to drop blood pressure at least temporarily, and reduce some of the anxiety and fear that may accompany a serious chronic and progressive condition like PKD. As long as a bodywork session is designed not to overly challenge a client's homeostatic capacity, massage can be a safe and helpful choice for a person with PKD.

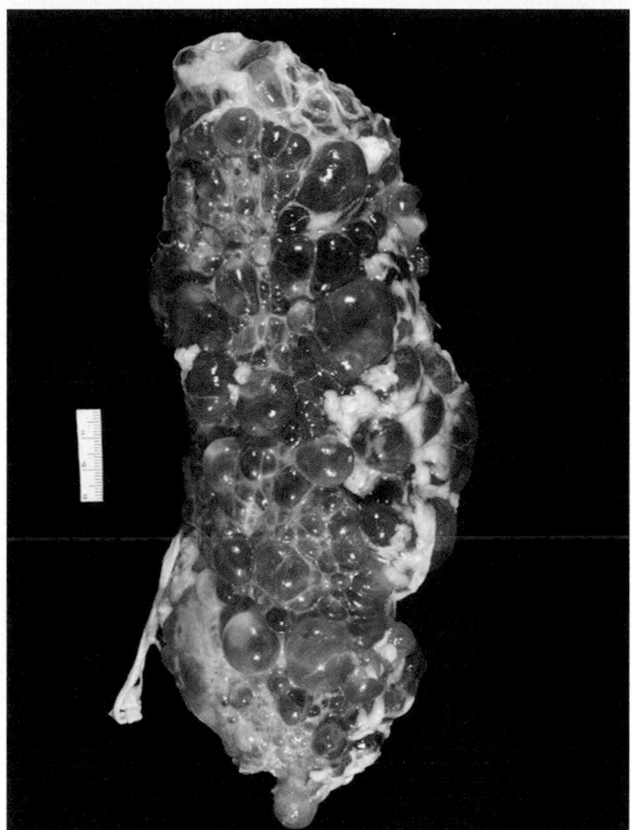

Figure 10.5. Polycystic kidney disease

Pyelonephritis in Brief

Pronunciation: py-el-o-neh-FRY-tis

What is it?
Pyelonephritis is an infection of the kidney and/or renal pelvis.

How is it recognized?
Symptoms of acute pyelonephritis include burning pain with urination, back pain, fever, chills, nausea, and vomiting. Chronic infections may show no or only very subtle symptoms.

Massage risks and benefits
Risks: Acute kidney infections contraindicate rigorous massage not only because the body is undergoing a major challenge but also because the patient is likely to be in pain and uncomfortable on a table.
Benefits: In the midst of an infection, gentle energetic or noncirculatory bodywork may be soothing. A person who has fully recovered from pyelonephritis can enjoy the same benefits from bodywork as the rest of the population.

Pyelonephritis

Definition: What Is It?

As the name implies, pyelonephritis is an infection of the nephrons in the kidney, although the renal pelvis may also be involved. They are usually a complication of a urinary tract infection, but can be related to other problems. Women hospitalized with pyelonephritis outnumber men by about 5:1.

Etiology: What Happens?

The most simple form of kidney infection is one in which bacteria have moved from the lower urinary tract into the upper urinary tract. In this situation, the pathogen is nearly always *Escherichia coli*. More complex infections involve structural anomalies, urethral blockage, pregnancy, diabetes, or a neurogenic bladder (a bladder that has no motor control and so empties passively into a bag). Contaminated surgical or medical instruments such as cystoscopes and catheters can also introduce pathogens into the urinary tract. The causative agent for these complicated situations may be *Pseudomonas*, *Klebsiella*, or many other pathogens.

Types of Pyelonephritis

- *Acute pyelonephritis:* This involves severe symptoms as the kidney is actively and aggressively attacked by bacteria. In some cases, bacteria can invade the capillaries of the kidney to lead to potentially life-threatening sepsis.
- *Chronic pyelonephritis:* This is usually the result of an incompletely treated infection. The bacteria continue to grow and destroy kidney tissue, but they do it slowly and painlessly. The net result is a risk of permanent damage and lost function.

Signs and Symptoms

Acute pyelonephritis usually involves the rapid onset of symptoms that begin with a UTI and ascend the urinary tract. They include fever, burning and frequent urination, cloudy and blood-tinged urine, extreme back pain, fatigue, nausea, and vomiting. In elderly patients, cognitive decline and disorientation are sometimes the leading signs of an infection. Symptoms typically develop over a day or two.

Chronic pyelonephritis symptoms in adults are often subtle. Therefore, many chronic kidney infections cause no symptoms, but damage in the kidney accumulates. When chronic pyelonephritis occurs in children, it is typically related to a structural anomaly at the vesicouretral valve. This condition, called vesicouretral reflux, allows urine to back up into the kidney, which creates a high risk of long-term, silent, cumulative damage.

Treatment

It is important to treat UTIs to prevent them from complicating to a kidney infection, which can result in permanent scarring, hypertension, and an increased risk for renal failure.

Most kidney infections clear up with antibiotic therapy, but it is important to ensure that the infection has been fully eradicated before ending treatment. If the infection is extreme, the patient may need to be hospitalized. People with pyelonephritis along with diabetes, spinal cord injury survivors, and kidney transplant recipients need to be monitored especially closely.

Medications

- Antibiotics for bacterial infection

Massage?

RISKS Acute kidney infections contraindicate most types of bodywork, largely because they are so painful that adding another adaptive challenge could be unpleasant. Chronic renal infections carry less risk, but still require that massage therapists be sensitive to the fact that this client has a compromised ability to process fluid.

BENEFITS Soothing, gently massage during an infection may be supportive but won't have much impact on the infection itself. Clients who have fully recovered from acute or chronic kidney infections can enjoy the same benefits from bodywork as the rest of the population.

Renal Cancer

Definition: What Is It?

Renal cancer is an umbrella term for any type of cancer that begins in kidney tissues. The vast majority of renal cancer cases are renal cell carcinoma (RCC). Synonyms for RCC include renal adenocarcinoma and hypernephroma.

Renal cancer is diagnosed about 32,000 times a year in this country; men outnumber women with this disease by a little less than two to one. The average age at diagnosis is about 64 years, but it can certainly appear at a younger age, especially if it is related to an inherited genetic predisposition.

Renal Cancer in Brief

What is it?
Renal cancer is any cancer that arises in the kidney. The most common type is renal cell carcinoma.

How is it recognized?
Signs and symptoms of renal cancer include blood in the urine, flank pain, unintended weight loss, and general malaise.

Massage risks and benefits

Risks: As with other cancers, renal cancer is treated aggressively with interventions that present specific cautions for massage therapists, including some skin problems.

Benefits: As with other cancers, massage has many benefits to offer as long as a session is designed to maximize the relaxing, anti-pain, anti-anxiety aspects of massage while minimizing any techniques that may overwhelm a client's ability to adapt to the changes that massage brings about.

Etiology: What Happens?

The kidneys are made primarily of epithelial cells, which grow fast, but are also more vulnerable to the genetic mutations that lead to cancer than other types of cells in the body. The kidneys are shielded by a layer of protective fat. They and the adrenal glands are all wrapped together by a dense layer of connective tissue called Gerota fascia.

In RCC, cellular mutations in the renal tubules lead to the formation of highly vascularized aggressive tumors (Figure 10.6). They begin in the renal cortex, but may extend into the renal fat, adrenal glands, the renal vein, and sometimes even the wall of the inferior vena cava.

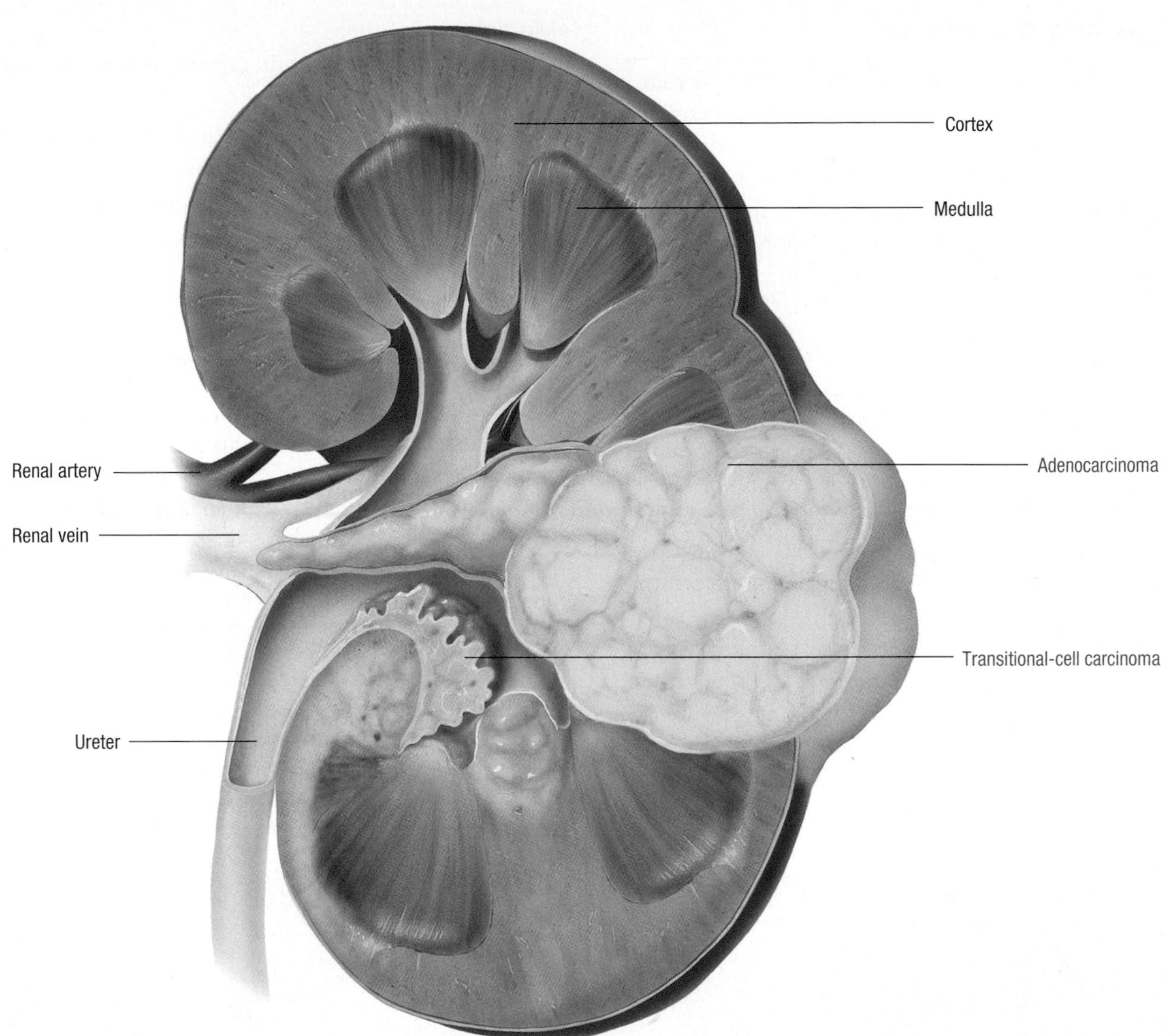

Figure 10.6. Renal cell carcinoma

Specific causes for RCC have not been identified, but a genetic condition called **von Hippel-Lindau syndrome** is associated with a high risk for the disease. Other risk factors include cigarette smoking (which essentially doubles the chances of developing this disease), obesity, chronic hypertension, long-term dialysis, and excessive exposure to cadmium, coke ovens, and asbestos.

Whether a person inherits this condition or experiences a spontaneous genetic mutation, the net result is that their kidneys are prone to excessive cell growth, angiogenesis to support that growth, excellent tumor cell survival, and the tendency for those cells to proliferate and then travel to other parts of the body. RCC metastasizes readily to the lungs, bones, and liver.

Types of Renal Cancer

- *Renal cell carcinoma*: This is the main focus of this discussion. It is the most common form of renal cancer, and can be due to genetic or environmental influences.
- *Transitional cell carcinoma*: This is cancer that arises in the renal pelvis. It is essentially identical to bladder cancer, with the same histology, risk factors, and treatment challenges.
- *Wilms tumor*: This is a rare subtype of renal cancer that affects young children, mostly between 2 and 6 years old. It is also called **nephroblastoma**. It is usually found before it metastasizes, and responds well to treatment, so the prognosis for this condition is usually very positive.

Signs and Symptoms

One of the distinguishing features of RCC is that it tends not to create any significant symptoms until it is advanced. Symptoms include blood in the urine, flank pain, a palpable mass in the abdomen, unintended weight loss, fever, fatigue, and malaise. In short, most of the signs of RCC mimic those of polycystic kidney disease or upper urinary tract infection.

Treatment

RCC is treated aggressively to achieve the best results. Surgery is often performed to remove the affected part of a kidney, the whole kidney, or the kidney plus adrenal gland and nearby lymph nodes. Arterial embolization (using a catheter to insert an instrument that shuts down feeder arteries) may be used to shrink tumors before surgery.

Unfortunately RCC is resistant to most types of chemotherapy and biologic therapy, so these are not first-line interventions. Instead, drugs called **multikinase inhibitors** are used: these interfere with angiogenesis at the tumor site, but they are also associated with a number of side effects that impact the health of the skin.

Medications

- Traditional chemotherapy (many cases of renal cancer are resistant)
- Biologic therapies to alter immune system activity (has low success rate)
- Multikinase inhibitors to interrupt angiogenesis that feeds tumor growth

Massage?

RISKS Renal cancer is treated aggressively with drugs and surgery that can be extremely challenging to receive. Some drugs are associated with skin problems, including dry skin, hair loss, discoloration, and problems with finger and toenails. Hand-foot reactions involving redness and peeling on the palms and soles may also happen. Any massage or bodywork choices must respect these challenges.

BENEFITS Massage has many benefits to offer cancer patients, including reductions in anxiety and pain, better sleep and appetite, improved immune system function, and general improvement in quality of life. For more information on massage in the context of cancer, see Chapter 12.

SIDEBAR 10.1 Staging Renal Cancer

The seriousness of renal cancer is identified by whether growths have penetrated outside the tough Gerota fascia that encloses the kidneys, renal fat, and adrenal glands. As with many cancers, renal cancer is staged using the TNM classifications, and then translating those into Stages 0 to IV. These stages are used to identify the best treatment options for patients.

Tumor (T)	Node (N)	Metastasis (M)
Tx: Tumor cannot be assessed	Nx: Node involvement cannot be assessed	Mx: Metastasis cannot be assessed
T0: No evidence of primary tumor in situ	N0: No node involvement	M0: No distant metastasis is found
T1: Tumor is <7 cm, within the kidney	N1: 1 regional node is involved	M1: Distant metastasis is found
T2: Tumor is >7 cm, within the kidney	N2: More than one regional node is involved	
T3: Tumor invades the renal vein, kidney fat, and/or adrenal glands		

The TNM classifications are translated into stages 0 to IV in this way:

Stage 0	**T0, N0, M0**
Stage I	T1, N0, M0
Stage II	T2, N0, M0
Stage III	T1–2, N1, M0 *or* T3, N0–1, M0
Stage IV	T any, N2, M0 *or* T any, N any, M1

Renal Failure

Definition: What Is It?

Renal failure means that for various reasons, the kidneys are not functioning adequately. If the kidneys slow down suddenly (e.g., in response to shock or systemic infection), it is acute renal failure. If they sustain cumulative damage over the course of many months or years, it is chronic renal failure. In either case, although the name implies that they have ceased functioning altogether, the truth is that the kidneys are still working, but they are unable to keep up with the body's demands.

Some researchers suggest that as many as eight million Americans are in early stages of kidney disease, although at this stage it is silent, so it usually goes undiagnosed. Statistics for end-stage renal disease are also alarming. This serious condition is diagnosed about 102,000 times each year, and about 453,000 people in the United States live with it. About 324,000 kidney failure patients are in dialysis, and 84,000 are on the waiting list for a new kidney.

Etiology: What Happens?

Although the kidneys are able to heal from most short-term abuse, any chronic or severe recurrent problems may eventually cause permanent damage to the delicate tissues, thereby interfering with kidney function. The two most common contributors to renal failure are long-term high blood pressure and untreated or undertreated diabetes. Both of these conditions damage the kidneys by exerting excessive mechanical pressure through the renal arteries, which is then focus that pressure into the delicate Bowman capsule. Fortunately, the human body is equipped with two million nephrons, about twice as many as it absolutely needs, so people can tolerate a lot of damage before problems develop.

Kidneys have several important functions: they produce EPO, the hormone that stimulates blood cell production; they manage electrolyte levels in the blood; they concentrate urine; and they manage overall fluid levels. Any of these functions may be lost during renal failure. This can lead to anemia; peripheral and pulmonary edema; pericarditis with fluid in the pericardial sac (**cardiac tamponade**); and dangerous changes in circulating levels of calcium, phosphorus, and potassium. This has important effects on bone density, digestive capabilities, the inflammatory process, and heart rhythms.

To hear the author discuss the connection between renal failure and hypertension, visit http://thePoint.lwww.com/Werner5e.

Renal Failure in Brief

What is it?
Renal failure involves the inability of the kidneys to function at normal levels. It may be an acute or a chronic problem, and it can be life threatening.

How is it recognized?
Symptoms of acute and chronic renal failure differ in severity and type of onset, but some things they have in common are reduced urine output, systemic edema, and changes in mental state brought about by the accumulation of toxins in the blood.

Massage risks and benefits
Risks: Massage that has the intention to mechanically influence fluid flow may be overwhelming for a person with chronic or acute renal failure.
Benefits: Gentler forms of bodywork that are gauged to fit within a limited capacity for adaptation may be helpful for the stress of dealing with a very challenging disorder.

Types of Renal Failure

- *Acute renal failure.* Acute renal failure is also called acute kidney injury. It is identified when kidney function suddenly drops to 50% or less of normal levels; this may take place over several hours or days. It is often a short-term problem that can be corrected, but it can be life threatening. Causes of acute renal failure usually fall into one of three categories:
  - Prerenal problems. In this situation, blood flow into the kidneys drops and the nephrons essentially collapse from lack of fluid volume. Causative factors include a blockage in the renal artery, low blood volume (i.e., bleeding out), and blood poisoning followed by shock.
  - Intrinsic problems. These are problems that arise within the kidneys. They include a local infection with *E. coli* (also called **hemolytic uremic syndrome**), drug allergies, an embolism inside the kidney, or others.
  - Postrenal problems. When fluid is prevented from leaving the kidneys, damage to the nephrons can accumulate to dangerous levels. Kidney stones, an enlarged prostate, or tumors can create this kind of problem.

- *Chronic renal failure.* Chronic renal failure is also called chronic kidney disease. This describes impairment in kidney function that may persist for months or years before it causes any symptoms. Kidney function is measured in terms of glomerular filtration rate (GFR), that is, how efficiently fluid moves from the glomeruli into the nephrons. Normal GFR is 120 mL/min. Renal failure is a progression along a continuum of lost function, and is discussed in these stages:
  - Stage I: Kidney damage is minor and GFR is above 90 mL/min.
  - Stage II: Mild reduction in function; GFR is 60 to 89 mL/min.
  - Stage III: Moderate reduction in function; GFR is 30 to 59 mL/min; chronic kidney disease is recognized at this stage.
  - Stage IV: Severe reduction; GFR is 15 to 29 mL/min; dialysis may be recommended at this stage.
  - Stage V: End-stage renal failure; GFR is less than 15 mL/min.

Signs and Symptoms

Because the kidneys have so many functions, symptoms of renal failure affect virtually every major organ system of the body. Symptoms include decreased urine output, systemic and pulmonary edema from salt and water retention, arrhythmia from potassium retention, anemia from the lack of EPO, and osteomalacia (bone thinning) from the lack of vitamin D, which is necessary for calcium metabolism. Rashes and skin discoloration arise from retention of toxic pigments in the blood. Other symptoms include lethargy, fatigue, headaches, loss of sensation in the hands and feet, tremors, seizures, easy bruising and bleeding, muscle cramps, and changes in mental and emotional states as the accumulation of wastes in the blood affects the brain.

Treatment

The treatment goal for acute renal failure is to restore renal blood flow as quickly as possible, so that a minimum of permanent damage accrues. Treatment goals for chronic renal failure are to control the symptoms, prevent further complications, and slow the progress of the disease. This often means aggressively controlling blood pressure and blood sugar levels (if diabetes is part of the picture). Medication to control potassium and phosphorus levels is important to avoid heart problems. Fluid, protein, and salt intake may be restricted until kidney function can keep up with the body's demands. Diuretics are sometimes prescribed to help the kidneys process fluids.

If a patient's kidneys are simply incompetent regardless of these interventions, dialysis may become necessary. This routes the blood through a machine or through the peritoneum to extract wastes. Dialysis can be a long-term intervention, but for many people it is a stop-gap measure to buy time while hoping for a suitable kidney to become available. For more information on kidney transplants, see Sidebar 10.2.

Medications

- Antihypertensive medication
- Antidiabetes medication, including glucose-lowering drugs and injected insulin
- Diuretics to shed excess fluid if necessary
- Phosphate and potassium lowering agents to manage arrhythmia
- EPO-stimulating drugs or analogues for anemia
- Iron salts for anemia

Massage?

RISKS Circulatory massage is not a good choice for clients with significant renal function loss. Clients undergoing dialysis are at increased risk for infection, especially where the equipment enters the body, so a massage therapist must accommodate this special situation.

Clients who have treated renal failure with a kidney transplant also take immune-suppressant drugs, so they are vulnerable to any pathogens carried by a massage therapist.

BENEFITS Gentle types of massage or bodywork that do not demand a great adaptive change may be helpful and supportive for a person who is going through a very difficult process. Clients who have successfully undergone a transplant may receive any bodywork that is within their capacity for adaptation, and that respects the fact that they are committed to a lifetime of immune-suppressant drugs.

SIDEBAR 10.2 Kidney Transplants: Many are on the Waiting List; Few are Chosen

The urinary system has about twice the capacity for urine production that any person actually needs. This is good news indeed, because it means that if it is necessary, we can get along with just one healthy kidney.

Kidney transplants replace a damaged organ with a healthy kidney from an appropriate donor. The new kidney is surgically implanted low in the abdomen, and the nonworking kidneys are usually left in place. Most kidney transplants use organs donated from people who have died, but if a good match is found, a kidney can be donated by a close relative or loved one.

Unfortunately, the shortage of suitable donated organs means that among the 84,000 people waiting for kidney transplants this year, only about 18,000 operations will be performed.

Bladder Cancer in Brief

What is it?
Bladder cancer is the growth of malignant cells in the urinary bladder. Most bladder cancer starts in the superficial layer of transitional epithelium.

How is it recognized?
The earliest sign of bladder cancer is painless blood in the urine, which may be red or rust colored. In later stages, the bladder may become irritable: painful urination, reduced urination, or increased urinary frequency may all occur.

Massage risks and benefits
Risks: As with most other types of cancer, the primary risk for bladder cancer patients receiving massage is that the challenges of both the disease and the treatment may reduce their capacity for adaptation. Most bladder cancer patients undergo surgery at some point, and this comes with risks as well.
Benefits: The soothing, anxiety-relieving effects of massage for bladder cancer patients can be enjoyed as long as the fragility of the client is respected.

Bladder and Urinary Tract Disorders

Bladder Cancer

Definition: What Is It?

Bladder cancer is the growth of malignant cells in the urinary bladder. Transitional cells are most often affected. For this reason, the term **urothelial carcinoma** can refer to cancer that begins in the urinary bladder or in the transitional cells of the renal pelvis, ureters, or urethra. Urothelial carcinoma is by far the most common form of bladder cancer seen in the United States, and is the main focus of this discussion.

Bladder cancer is the sixth most common cancer in the United States, diagnosed in over 70,000 people each year, and causing about 15,000 deaths. It is usually a disease of mature people; the median age at diagnosis is 68 years.

Etiology: What Happens?

Like most types of cancer, bladder cancer usually involves epithelial cells, in this case, the transitional epithelium that lines the urinary bladder. Because the kidneys filter environmental irritants out of the blood and into the urine, this delicate tissue is often bathed in toxic chemicals. Constant repetitive damage causes the mature cells to die. This stimulates rapid replication in the basal layer, and colonies of immature cells then migrate to the surface. These new cells are easily disrupted by genetic mutations and may become malignant growths that cause bleeding into the bladder. Papillary bladder cell tumors are wart like, and attached to a stalk. Nonpapillary tumors are embedded in the bladder wall. They are less common, but more likely to become invasive.

Causes of bladder cancer vary according to medical history and geographic region. Persons who have undergone pelvic radiation for other problems are at an increased risk for developing bladder cancer, as are people who have had chronic infections, bladder stones, or catheter use. One type of chemotherapy used for lymphoma has been identified as a possible cause. In some developing countries, bladder cancer is associated with a parasitic infestation, **Schistosoma haematobium**.

Several genetic mutations that limit the body's ability to inhibit tumor growth or invasion have been linked to bladder cancer. These mutations are frequently triggered by exposure to carcinogenic substances. In the United States and Europe, approximately half of bladder cancer cases are believed to be related to cigarette smoking. Other triggers include exposure to aromatic amines (chemicals used in dry cleaning fluid, hairdressing chemicals, and textile and rubber industries).

Most bladder cancer diagnoses are made when the cells affect only superficial layers of tissue. This is excellent news, because the survival rate for cancers caught early is much better than for cancers caught in stage III or later. Nevertheless, bladder cancer has an unusual habit of growing in several places at the same time, so although it may be possible to catch one or two tumors, the invisible third, fourth, and fifth tumors may not become symptomatic for another several months. This means that the recurrence rate for bladder cancer is high: up to 80% of patients have at least one recurrence.

Types of Bladder Cancer

- *Transitional cell carcinoma*. This accounts for about 90% of all bladder cancer diagnoses in the United States.
- *Squamous cell carcinoma*. This accounts for about 8% of diagnoses in the United States, but in developing countries, it is the most common type of bladder cancer. It can be caused by infection with Schistosoma.
- *Other types of bladder cancer*: Small cell carcinoma and adenocarcinoma of the bladder account for 1% to 2% of bladder cancer cases in the United States.

Signs and Symptoms

The earliest and most dependable sign of bladder cancer is hematuria, or blood in the urine. The urine of a bladder cancer patient is often visibly reddened or rust colored, although the patient has no particular pain in the early stages of the disease. If the tumors continue to grow and invade deeper layers of the bladder, secondary symptoms may develop. These are the result of mechanical pressure, including bladder irritability (painful urination, increased urinary frequency, reduced urine output) and compression on the rectum, pelvic lymph nodes, and any other structures that happen to be in the way.

Treatment

Bladder cancer treatment depends on the stage at diagnosis. See Sidebar 10.3 for bladder cancer staging protocols.

Surgeons can use a cystoscope and a variety of tools to remove abnormal tissue. More invasive surgeries may remove part or all of the bladder, and if signs of pelvic metastasis are present, other tissues as well. Men may lose the prostate gland; women may lose the uterus, ovaries, and parts of the vaginal wall. Pelvic lymph nodes are also removed, leading to the risk of lymphedema in the legs. Urine flow may be routed out of the body through a stoma, or a variety of surgeries have been developed to form artificial bladders from parts of the large or small intestines.

In addition to surgery, radiation therapy and chemotherapy may be used to battle bladder cancer. Chemotherapy may be administered intravenously, orally with pills, or through a site-specific bladder wash to distribute the medication directly to the target tissues.

Biologic therapies involve introducing substances into the bladder that stimulate immune system responses. The Bacille Calmett-Guerin vaccine (sometimes used for tuberculosis) is successful in many cases. In other situations, interferon or other substances may be used.

Administering medication by bladder wash is most effective in combination with surgery to remove cancerous cells. After bladder cancer treatment is completed, it is especially important to be diligent about follow-up care because this cancer recurs in most patients.

Medications

- Chemotherapeutic agents orally or by bladder wash
- Biologic therapy by bladder wash to trigger immune system activity against cancer cells

Massage?

RISKS Because bladder cancer has a high rate of recurrence, patients often undergo surgery in early stages. This may leave them with stomas, catheters, or other medical devices that must be accommodated for.

BENEFITS The benefits of massage for bladder cancer patients are the same as those for any kind of cancer patients. While bodywork can promote pain reduction, anxiety reduction, and general support, massage therapists must work as part of a team, sharing information and concerns with the rest of the client's health care staff. A client who has successfully treated his bladder cancer can enjoy the benefits of any type of bodywork that is within his capacity for adaptation. More information on massage in the context of cancer can be found in Chapter 12.

SIDEBAR 10.3 Staging Bladder Cancer

Bladder cancer is staged with the traditional TNM classifications. Here is a simplified version:

Tumor (T)	Node (N)	Metastasis (M)
Ta: noninvasive papillary tumor	Nx: nodes cannot be assessed	Mx: metastasis cannot be assessed
TIS (cancer in situ): noninvasive flat, nonpapillary cells	N0: no nodes involved	M0: no metastasis found
T1: cancer cells invade urothelium but not muscle tissue	N1: one pelvic node involved; cells <2 cm	M1: distant metastasis to organs or bones
T2: cancer cells invade muscle tissue	N2: 2 or more pelvic nodes are involved.	
T3: cancer cells invade through muscular wall into connective tissue and exterior fat	N3: Nodes along the iliac artery are involved	
T4: cancer cells invade other tissues, including the prostate, uterus, pelvic wall, or abdominal wall		

These delineations are translated to Stages 0 to IV in this way:

Stage 0a	Ta, N0, M0
Stage 0 IS	TIS, N0, M0
Stage I	T1, N0, M0
Stage II	T2, N0, M0
Stage III	T3 or T4, N0, M0
Stage IV	T4, N0, M0; or any T, N3, M0; or any T, any N, M1

Interstitial Cystitis

Definition: What Is It?

Interstitial cystitis (IC) is a condition in which the urinary bladder becomes irritated and inelastic. Because the diagnostic criteria for IC are still in development, it is sometimes referred to as IC/PBS (interstitial cystitis/painful bladder syndrome).

Etiology: What Happens?

The bladder, a hollow organ, shrinks when it is empty and expands when it is full. A healthy bladder can hold 8 to 12 oz of urine. Normal urine is composed of water, excess salts and hormones extracted from the blood, nitrogenous wastes such as urea and uric acid, and other debris. It should not contain significant numbers of microorganisms. Protective mucous membranes shield the bladder from the acidity of urine.

IC occurs when the inner lining of the bladder no longer protects the organ from acidity. Many IC patients develop tiny bleeding areas called pinpoint hemorrhages or **glomerulations** in the bladder wall. About 10% of patients develop a deeper lesion called a **Hunner ulcer** inside the bladder. As the problem progresses, the muscular walls of the bladder become fibrotic and inelastic; this is true especially for people with Hunner ulcers. Patients find that they have little capacity for storing urine, even if their bladder is a normal size. It is common for IC patients to have to use the bathroom dozens of times each day.

The cause of IC is a mystery. One hypothesis is that this may be an autoimmune disease or allergy that weakens the protective mucous membrane in the bladder's epithelium. In this way, irritating chemicals from urine can infiltrate and damage the bladder wall. The presence of abnormal numbers of mast cells in some IC patients supports this idea. A pathologic thinning of

Interstitial Cystitis (IC) in Brief

Pronunciation: in-ter-STIH-shul sis-TY-tis

What is it?
IC is a chronic inflammation of the bladder involving pain, scar tissue, stiffening, decreased capacity, pinpoint hemorrhages, and sometimes ulcers in the bladder walls.

How is it recognized?
Symptoms of IC are very much like those of urinary tract infections: burning, increased frequency, and urgency of urination; decreased capacity of the bladder; and pain, pressure, and tenderness.

Massage risks and benefits
Risks: Patients with IC may not be comfortable on a table for a full massage session; appropriate adjustments must be made so they can empty their bladder if necessary.
Benefits: IC may be exacerbated by stress, and if massage is comfortable to receive, it may be a helping strategy for a frustrating condition.

the mucous membrane on the bladder wall is another factor to consider. IC does not respond to antibiotic therapy, so it is clear that no known strain of bacteria causes this problem. Other hypotheses suggest a neurological hypersensitivity to bladder fullness, or problems with the perineum muscle that may refer pain into the pelvis. This is likely if the symptoms don't interfere with sleep.

Signs and Symptoms

Symptoms of IC include chronic pelvic pain, pain and burning on urination, increased urinary frequency and urgency, and painful intercourse. Symptoms are worst when the bladder is full, and they abate somewhat when the bladder is empty. Menstruation can exacerbate symptoms. Some patients find that symptoms occur in periods of flare and remission; others find that their daily experiences are all about the same.

Treatment

Because IC is a disease without a known cause, it is also without a known cure. IC treatment is generally aimed at symptomatic relief and the development of coping skills. Often the diagnostic tool of bladder distension can give temporary relief, as can an instillation, or bladder wash. This is sometimes done with dimethyl sulfoxide (DMSO), which can pass into the bladder wall to act as an anti-inflammatory and to block pain sensation. Lesions on the bladder wall may be removed with lasers or electrical wires. An oral medication to help repair the mucous lining has been approved, but it may take several months to be effective and some patients don't respond to this intervention. Aspirin and other painkillers may be recommended, as are exercise, smoking cessation, and dietary changes to avoid highly acidic foods and drinks. Antidepressants can be effective pain modulators. Various nerve stimulating devices may provide symptomatic relief. No single intervention is successful for all patients, and nothing has yet provided a permanent solution. IC may recur after months or even years of remission.

Some patients have such severe problems that surgery becomes an option. They may have a new bladder constructed from a segment of the colon, or they may have the bladder removed altogether and replaced with a stoma and external bag.

Medications

- Pentoson polysulfate sodium to help rebuild the bladder lining
- Bladder instillation with DMSO
- Analgesics, antidepressants or antiseizure drugs for pain management

Massage?

RISKS The primary challenge for interstitial cystitis (IC) or irritable bladder patients who want to receive a massage is that they may need to interrupt the session to use the bathroom. If accommodations can be made for this, massage holds little risk for this clientele.

BENEFITS Massage may be a useful intervention for the goal of relieving stress and anxiety, although it will probably have little direct effect on bladder irritation.

A person in remission from IC can enjoy all the benefits of massage as the rest of the population.

OPTIONS A client with an external bag to act as a urine reservoir requires special positioning and care not to disrupt the stoma or the device. Consult with the client for best options.

Urinary Tract Infection

Definition: What Is It?

A urinary tract infection (UTI) is an infection that may occur anywhere in the lower urinary system. This discussion focuses on infections of the lower urinary tract, that is, the urethra (urethritis) and the bladder (cystitis).

UTIs are almost always women's disorder, because the female urethra is short and close to the anus, where bacteria that are harmless in the digestive tract can wreak havoc if they gain access to the urinary tract. People who must drain their bladder with a catheter are also at increased risk for UTI. When men have a UTI, it may be the warning sign of a prostate problem or a sexually transmitted infection.

Etiology: What Happens?

Under normal circumstances, the environment in the bladder is essentially sterile. The urine contains waste products to be expelled from the body, but few or no living microorganisms should be present. Furthermore, the bladder is lined with a protective mucus-producing layer of cells that works to prevent infectious or noxious agents from harming the bladder walls.

Sometimes foreign microorganisms are introduced into the urethra. *E. coli* are the causative agent behind close to 90% of UTIs. These strains of bacteria live normally and harmlessly in the digestive tract, but they can damage the urinary tract. Other pathogens can invade as well, but they are not typical. It is important to identify the correct causative agent, because not all of them respond to the same antibiotics.

Chronic irritation can also contribute to the development of UTIs. "Honeymoon cystitis" is inflammation and subsequent infection brought about by repeated irritation of the urethra from sexual activity.

Some women are more susceptible to UTIs than others, although the reasons for this are not completely clear; they may have to do with immune system differences and shortages of certain types of antibodies. Some factors, however, are reliable predictors of who is at risk for developing a UTI:

- Spermicide use. Spermicide foams and jellies used with a diaphragm or alone have been shown to raise the risk of UTIs in some women.
- Diaphragm use. Women who use a diaphragm show statistically higher rates of UTIs than women who do not.
- Pregnancy. Pregnant women do not necessarily get more UTIs than women who are not pregnant, but the risk of having a simple infection complicate into a more dangerous one is higher for these patients.
- Diabetes. Elevated sugar levels in the urine make a hospitable environment for bacteria to grow in the bladder.
- Neurogenic bladder. A **neurogenic bladder** has lost motor function and does not empty as completely as a normal one. This raises the potential for infection, as does the presence of catheter tubes, which are used for people with limited bladder function.

If the bacteria that invade the urethra and bladder are able to travel up the ureters, they may complicate into a kidney infection. Chronic UTIs with progressive damage to the kidneys may contribute to chronic renal failure. Untreated kidney infections can also lead to the release of infectious bacteria in the blood and life-threatening septicemia.

Urinary Tract Infection (UTI) in Brief

What is it?
A UTI is an infection usually caused by bacteria that live harmlessly in the digestive tract finding their way into the urinary tract.

How is it recognized?
Symptoms of UTIs include pain and burning sensations during urination, increased urinary frequency and urgency, and cloudy or blood-tinged urine. Abdominal, pelvic, or low back pain may occur. In the acute stage, fever and general malaise may be present.

Massage risks and benefits
Risks: Acute UTIs are painful and may involve fever and malaise. Left untreated they carry a risk for complicating to pyelonephritis. For these reasons, it is best to delay any rigorous bodywork until after the infection has been resolved.
Benefits: Very gentle noninvasive bodywork may be soothing during a UTI. A client who has fully recovered from this condition can enjoy the same benefits from bodywork as the rest of the population.

10 Urinary System Conditions

Unfortunately, not all UTIs show symptoms, so they may be neglected, especially in children. It is possible for some people to have complications of this type of infection that can easily lead to permanent kidney damage or even to death.

Some basic precautions can help prevent UTIs, especially for women who are especially vulnerable to them. These include drinking lots of water and acidic juices; urinating whenever necessary rather than holding it for a more convenient time; wiping from front to back after a bowel movement to prevent the introduction of digestive bacteria into the urethra; taking showers rather than baths; emptying the bladder after sex; and avoiding feminine hygiene sprays and douches, which can aggravate the urethra.

Signs and Symptoms

The symptoms of UTIs are painful, burning urination; a frequent need to urinate; reduced bladder capacity; urinary urgency; and blood-tinged or cloudy urine. Pelvic, abdominal, or low back pain may also occur. Men with UTIs may have pain in the penis or scrotum. If severe flank or back pain and high fever develop, a kidney infection should be suspected.

Treatment

The first step in self-treatment of a UTI is to drown it: radically increasing fluid intake gives the body the much needed opportunity to fully and frequently empty the bladder—not only of urine but of bacteria as well. Drinking blueberry or cranberry juice is helpful for many women. These berries contain chemicals that limit the ability of bacteria to cling to bladder walls. It is important, however, to avoid sweetened juice; the amount of sugar it takes to make cranberry juice sweet may actually make the bladder a more hospitable environment for infection. In subacute infection, hydrotherapy in the form of hot and cold sitz baths may be recommended.

UTIs usually respond well to antibiotics. With bladder infections, as with all types of bacterial infections, it is important to take the full prescription. Stopping too soon may result in recurrent infections with more highly resistant bacteria.

People who have low-grade, chronic UTIs that do not clear up with normal treatments are sometimes successfully treated with long-term low doses of antibiotics. Structural problems with the way urine drains from the bladder may contribute to chronic infections; surgery may be recommended to correct these problems.

Medications

- Antibiotics for bacterial infection
- Analgesics for pain management

Massage?

RISKS Urinary tract infections (UTIs) are uncomfortable and, when acute, may involve fever and malaise. Clients may not be comfortable on a table for a full session in this state. Further, any but the most gentle bodywork is probably not welcome at this time.

BENEFITS Noninvasive bodywork may be soothing during an infection, and any client who has fully recovered from a UTI can enjoy the same benefits from massage as the rest of the population.

CHAPTER REVIEW QUESTIONS: URINARY SYSTEM CONDITIONS

1. What pushes fluid from the glomerulus into the Bowman capsule?
2. What happens to kidney function if blood pressure suddenly drops as a result of circulatory shock or loss of blood volume?
3. What condition is staged according to declining GFR?
4. When do kidney stones cause pain?
5. What is the most common cause of bladder cancer in the United States?
6. What is the difference between a UTI and IC?
7. How can kidney dysfunction lead to anemia?
8. A client has IC and would like to receive massage. What are the potential benefits and risks? How might the practitioner need to adjust bodywork to meet this client's needs?

9. A client with chronic renal failure is on the waiting list for a kidney transplant. He undergoes dialysis regularly. He would like to receive a massage for stress and pain relief. What are the potential benefits and risks? How might the practitioner need to adjust bodywork to meet this client's needs?

10. A client received a donated kidney 2 years ago. He would like to receive a massage for stress and pain relief. What are the potential benefits and risks? How might the practitioner need to adjust bodywork to meet this client's needs?

11

Reproductive System Conditions

Chapter Objectives

After reading this chapter, you should be able to . . .

- Name a causative agent of cervical cancer.
- Identify the difference between primary and secondary dysmenorrhea; name three contributors for secondary dysmenorrhea.
- Identify an important trigger for the genetic mutation that leads to uterine cancer.
- Explain why endometrial growths change with a menstrual cycle.
- Name the two most common varieties of breast cancer.
- Explain why ovarian cancer has a high death rate.
- Describe how prostate cancer and benign prostatic hyperplasia are similar.
- Explain why the term prostatitis is often a misnomer.
- List two classes of testicular cancer.
- List four pregnancy-related complications.
- List three bacterial or viral sexually transmitted diseases.

Introduction

Massage therapists are often shortchanged in their education about the reproductive system. This may be because of time constraints in the classroom or because of a tendency to skip over this system because of a lingering stigma that confuses massage therapy with the sex industry. While massage is not a treatment of choice for most reproductive system diseases, many clients live with them, and the conditions themselves or their treatment options may have repercussions for bodywork choices.

Another stumbling block in the topic of reproductive system conditions is the perception that two perfectly normal, nonpathological states are often addressed as diseases: pregnancy and menopause. It is important for massage therapists (and other people too!) to understand that these conditions are not diseases, but simply conditions that change the way the body functions; for that reason, we should know about them.

Terminology for structures in the reproductive system can sometimes be confusing. Many resources have moved toward labeling structures by their location or function rather than by their traditional names, which commonly refer to the physicians or anatomists who first recorded them. Thus, fallopian tubes, named for 16th-century anatomist Gabriele Falloppio, may now be called oviducts or uterine tubes, which is more descriptive. Traditional names are still in common use, however. In this chapter, structures will be referred to by both traditional and functional or locational names, so that practitioners educated in either terminology may feel at home.

To hear the author's thoughts on reproductive system conditions and massage, go to http://thePoint.lww.com/Werner5e.

Structure and Function of the Female Reproductive System

Most of the female reproductive structures are low in the pelvis. In a healthy, nonpregnant woman with no scar tissue or other anomalies, the ovaries are typically behind the upper corners where the pubic hair starts to grow. They are attached via the ovarian ligament to the uterus. The ovaries produce hormones, which are released into the bloodstream, and they release eggs, usually one each month during ovulation, which are released into the peritoneal space.

Mittelschmerz is a term derived from German for "middle pain." It refers to the sensation some women have when the dominant follicle on an ovary ruptures and the egg is released into the pelvic cavity. It is called "middle" because it occurs precisely in the middle (about day 14) of the menstrual cycle.

The fimbriae of the fallopian (uterine) tubes gently caress the ovaries, coaxing the released egg toward them. Once inside the tubes, the eggs make the 5-day journey to the uterus itself. If an egg is fertilized, it generally happens inside the uterine tube.

When the egg reaches the uterus, it finds a hollow organ that is built of criss-crossed layers of muscle. The inside surface of the uterus, the **endometrium**, is made of delicate epithelial tissue that holds vast billowy supplies of specialized capillaries to provide a nest for that fertilized egg (Figure 11.1). If the egg is not fertilized, the uterus sheds the tissue and egg with it in the **menses**. Then it begins to build a new nest for next month's candidate.

The timing of the ripening and release of eggs from the ovaries and the building and shedding of the endometrial nest is under the control of the endocrine system. Hormones secreted from the ovaries themselves and from the pituitary gland determine when and how these various events will happen. Birth control pills and other hormonal applications work by

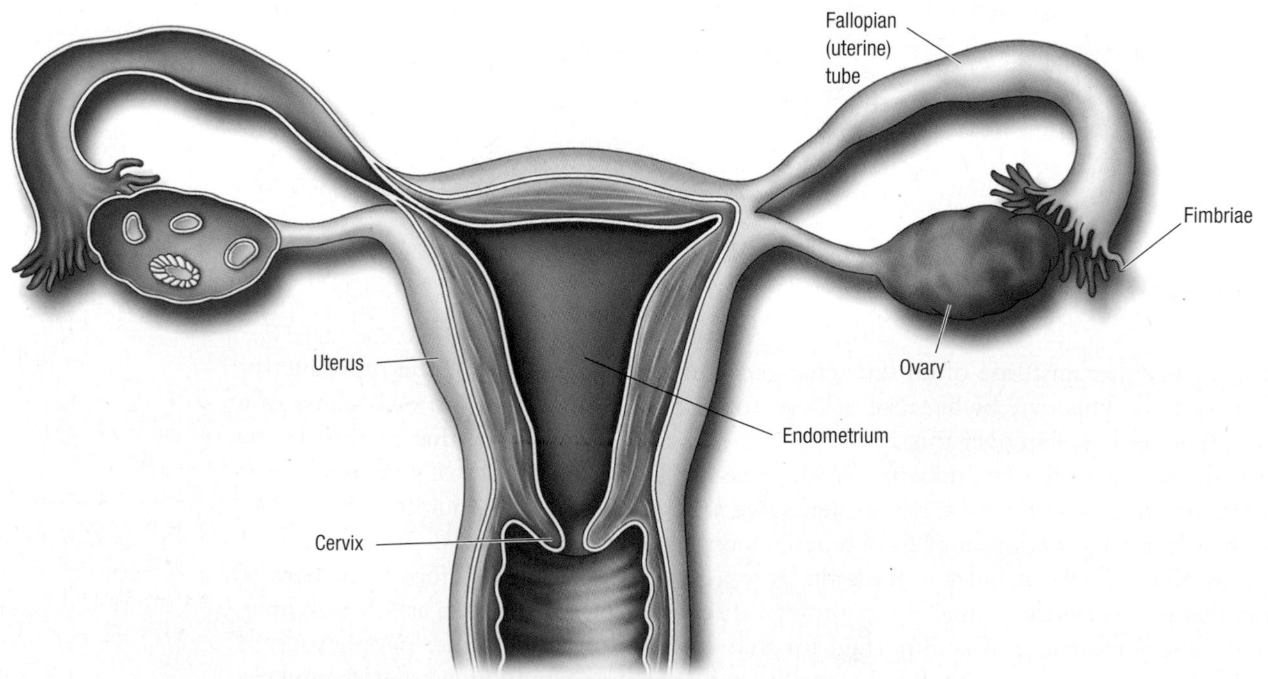

Figure 11.1. Female reproductive organs

introducing artificial hormones into the blood. These trick the pituitary into believing that the woman is always pregnant, so she never ovulates.

The relation between the reproductive system and the endocrine system is extremely tight; the female reproductive cycle is under the control of hormone secretions. Several of the conditions discussed in this chapter could be considered endocrine system disorders, but the tissue changes occur in reproductive system organs, so they are discussed here (Sidebar 11.1).

Female reproductive conditions that have significance for massage therapists generally have to do with growths or local tenderness deep in the abdomen. Although intrusive work in the vicinity of the uterus or ovaries is not generally done, sometimes these conditions can displace internal organs, making them vulnerable in places they wouldn't ordinarily be found.

Structure and Function of the Male Reproductive System

The male reproductive system consists of the testes, the **epididymis**, the spermatic cord, other glands that contribute to the production of semen, and the urethra, which expels semen through the penis (Figure 11.2).

Sperm cells are among the smallest of human cells and the only ones equipped with flagella for locomotion. They are manufactured in specialized tubes in the testes, the **seminiferous tubules**. Sperm cells grow and mature in the testes. The testes are suspended from the body in the scrotal sac, because sperm cells flourish best when the temperature is slightly lower than internal body temperature. Mature sperm cells are stored in the epididymis, a long tube that is coiled up behind the testes in the scrotum. Sperm cells leave

SIDEBAR 11.1 What Is This Thing Called Estrogen?

Estrogen is not a single hormone but a group of closely related chemicals that includes estradiol, estriol, and estrone. These chemicals are synthesized from cholesterol primarily in the ovaries during a woman's fertile years. After menopause, they continue to be manufactured in peripheral tissues in much smaller amounts, using root chemicals secreted by the adrenal cortex.

Estrogens are received by target tissues all over the body. They not only are associated with sex organ function but also influence the growth, health, and activity of many organs, including the bones and heart. They influence cell production and differentiation. Estrogens are also associated with mood swings and emotional responsiveness.

The liver makes estrogens chemically able to stimulate biological activity in their target cells. This metabolism can occur in a variety of ways, with great implications for long-term health. Some "bad" estrogen metabolites are associated with tissue proliferation (i.e., cancer) of the breast, uterus, cervix, ovaries, and thyroid. "Good" estrogen metabolites are associated with healthy bone maintenance and cardiovascular protection.

What determines which estrogen metabolites are present in a woman's body? Two main factors are at work here: diet and estrogen exposure.

Diet

High-fat, low-fiber diets provide excessive cholesterol, thereby allowing the body to manufacture more estrogens than it otherwise would. With a minimum of fiber, they prevent the binding of excessive estrogens to the molecules that would inactivate them. And by disrupting the healthy balance of bacteria in the intestines, poor diets allow some estrogens to reenter the circulation.

Estrogen Exposure

People are exposed to estrogen from internal production (endogenous estrogens) and external sources (exogenous estrogens). Endogenous estrogens have already been discussed as a function of diet and estrogen metabolism. Endogenous estrogen exposure is also increased by obesity, as fat cells can contribute to estrogen production. Exogenous estrogen exposure is a topic that has only recently begun to be discussed. Oral birth control pills, hormone replacement therapy, and supplements in meat and dairy products, along with environmental chemicals such as pesticides, herbicides, plastics, and industrial solvents all contribute to cumulative endogenous estrogen exposure.

Excessive estrogen exposure and the metabolism of "bad" estrogens have been identified as contributing factors in several cancers of hormone-dependent tissues. In addition, **estrogen dominance** is being investigated as a factor in other reproductive system disorders, including premenstrual syndrome, endometriosis, uterine fibroids, and menopause. The good news is that estrogen exposure and metabolism can be influenced by diet and nutrition. Estrogen receptor sites in target tissues can bind with several estrogen-like substances (phytoestrogens, including soy, legumes, and other sources), and some nutritional supplements can help disable free estrogen metabolites before they influence cell proliferation or differentiation. Ultimately, these reproductive system disorders may be treated or even prevented by having patients take greater control over how much estrogen they are exposed to and how their bodies put that estrogen to use.

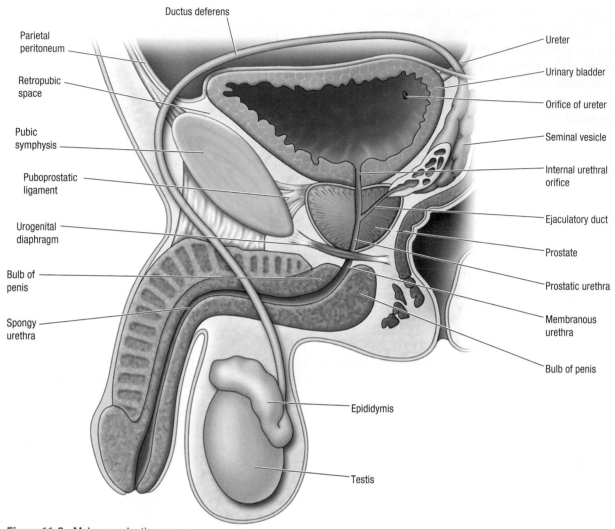

Figure 11.2. Male reproductive organs

the epididymis through the left and right **vas deferens**, which carries them through the inguinal ring into the abdomen. Along the way, other glands, including the seminal vesicles and prostate, contribute to the fluid that suspends and nourishes the sperm on their long journey toward the ovum. The left and right vas deferens join together at the urethra, and sperm leaves the penis during ejaculation.

The most common disorders of the male reproductive system have to do with the prostate gland, which is in a position to obstruct the urethra during ejaculation or urination. While prostate massage is typically conducted by a urologist through the wall of the rectum during an examination (and is therefore outside the scope of practice of most massage therapists), prostate problems can seriously diminish a person's quality of life. Consequently, some clients seek bodywork as a coping mechanism while managing prostate problems. Massage conducted to maximize the benefits of parasympathetic effect and improved immune system function can be a safe and appropriate choice.

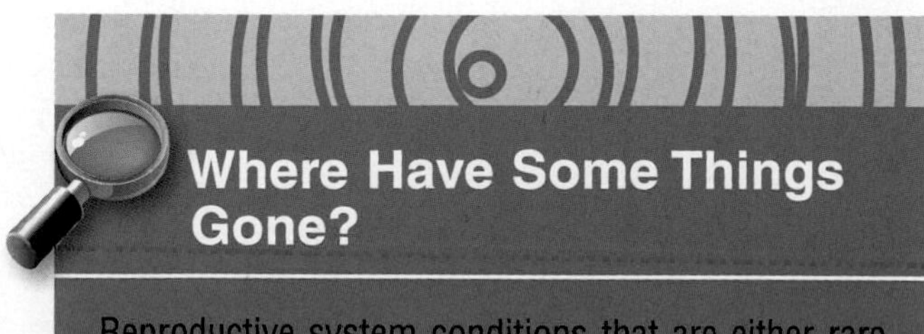

Where Have Some Things Gone?

Reproductive system conditions that are either rare or seldom seen in a stage that presents problems for massage have been relocated. For this chapter, that means spontaneous and elective abortion, pelvic inflammatory disease, and uterine prolapse can be found in Appendix C, Extra Conditions at a Glance.

Reproductive System Conditions

Disorders of the Uterus

- Cervical cancer
  - Squamous cell carcinoma of the cervix
  - Adenocarcinoma of the cervix
  - Other types of cervical cancer
- Dysmenorrhea
  - Primary dysmenorrhea
  - Secondary dysmenorrhea
- Endometriosis
- Fibroid tumors
- Uterine cancer
  - Endometrial cancer
  - Uterine sarcoma

Disorders of Other Female Reproductive Structures

- Breast cancer
  - Ductal carcinoma
  - Lobular carcinoma
  - Inflammatory breast disease
  - Other types of breast cancer
- Ovarian cancer
  - Adenocarcinoma of the ovary
  - Germ cell ovarian cancer
  - Stromal cell ovarian cancer
- Ovarian cysts
  - Follicular cysts
  - Corpus luteum cysts
  - Polycystic ovaries
  - Endometriomas
  - Dermoid cysts
  - Cystadenomas

Disorders of the Male Reproductive System

- Benign prostatic hyperplasia
- Prostate cancer
- Prostatitis
  - Acute bacterial prostatitis
  - Chronic bacterial prostatitis
  - Chronic nonbacterial prostatitis/chronic pelvic pain syndrome
  - Asymptomatic inflammatory prostatitis
- Testicular cancer
  - Germ cell tumors
  - Stromal cell tumors

Other Reproductive System Conditions

- Menopause
- Pregnancy
- Premenstrual syndrome
- Sexually transmitted infections
  - Bacterial vaginosis
  - Chlamydia
  - Gonorrhea
  - Syphilis
  - Nongonococcal urethritis
  - Trichomoniasis
  - Molluscum contagiosum
  - Genital warts

Disorders of the Uterus

Cervical Cancer

Definition: What Is It?

Cervical cancer is the growth of malignant cells in the lining of the cervix. While some types of abnormal cells grow slowly and don't present a serious threat, other types are aggressive and invasive.

Although rates of cervical cancer diagnosis and death have been falling, it is still responsible for about 12,700 diagnoses and 4,300 deaths each year in the United States. For more information on the history of cervical cancer, see Sidebar 11.2.

Etiology: What Happens?

Cervical cancer is a malignancy brought about directly by a viral infection, in this case with some of the 100 varieties of the human papilloma virus (HPV) family. Being infected with HPV is not a dependable indicator of cervical cancer, however: most of the viruses in this family are not associated with aggressive or invasive cancers.

When a woman is infected with HPV, the virus may trigger cellular changes in the lining of her cervix. Precancerous changes called **dysplasia** can be stimulated by both low-risk and high-risk types of HPV.

If a woman is infected with a low-risk type of virus, her abnormal cells may spontaneously resolve, and she may never know anything had happened. But if she is infected with an aggressive form of HPV, cancerous cells may grow in the lining of the cervix and then may spread throughout the uterus, the vagina, and into the pelvic cavity, affecting the bladder, colon, and inguinal lymph nodes. Ultimately, the cancer may travel to distant parts of the body.

Cervical Cancer in Brief

Pronunciation: SER-vih-kal KAN-ser

What is it?
Cervical cancer is the development of cancerous cells in the lining of the cervix. These may spread to affect the whole cervix, the rest of the uterus, and other pelvic organs.

How is it recognized?
Early stages of cervical cancer are virtually silent; this disease is detected by Pap (Papanicolaou) tests before symptoms develop. Later signs and symptoms include bleeding or spotting outside a normal menstrual period, vaginal discharge, and pelvic pain.

Massage risks and benefits
Risks: A woman with advanced cervical cancer must handle the challenges of both the disease and its treatments. Any massage in this context must respect those challenges.
Benefits: Most cases of cervical cancer are found before significant risks develop. Women in this situation who are receiving care, and those who have successfully treated cervical cancer in the past, can enjoy the same benefits from massage as the rest of the population.

HPV is a sexually transmitted disease, transferred by direct skin-to-skin touching. While condoms have been seen to reduce the risk of developing cervical cancer, they do not prevent the spread of all HPV, because skin still comes in contact during sexual activity.

NOTABLE CASES Argentinean political leader Eva Peron died of complications due to cervical cancer at age 33. Rumors suggest that it was purposely misdiagnosed as appendicitis when it could have been stopped earlier. The prolific, award-winning comedian, writer and actress Julia Sweeney is a cervical cancer survivor.

Exposure to HPV is the central risk factor for developing cervical cancer. However, other factors may contribute to the likelihood of those abnormal cells becoming malignant. Sexual activity at an early age may increase the transmission rate of HPV, especially if a woman has multiple partners. Alternatively, if a woman has only one sexual partner but that person has a history of multiple partners, her risk of cervical cancer is increased. Smoking raises the risk of cervical cancer by roughly 100%. Increased risk is also seen with women who are overweight and whose diet is low in fruits and vegetables.

SIDEBAR 11.2 Cervical Cancer: History of a Disease

In the early part of the 20th century, cervical cancer was one of the leading causes of death by cancer for women in this country. This disease is virtually silent, causing no signs or symptoms until it has spread throughout the pelvic cavity and into the lymph system—by which time survival rates are very low.

Then from 1955 to 1992 a remarkable phenomenon occurred: rates of death by cervical cancer dropped by 74%.

What made the difference? A simple examination: the **Papanicolaou test**, which makes it possible to detect precancerous cells in the cervix before they spread. Because of the Pap test, women could have abnormal cells detected and removed before they had a chance to become malignant, and women could find and remove malignancies before they had a chance to spread throughout the pelvic cavity.

Today the recommended protocol for cervical cancer detection is to receive a traditional Pap test once a year or a liquid Pap test (a more complicated version that can yield more accurate results) every 2 years. If a woman over 30 years old has three consecutive years without any sign of dysplasia, her doctor may recommend that she can have Pap tests less frequently. If a test is positive for abnormal cells, tests for HPV DNA may be conducted. These tests are most accurate for women over 40, but they can give very specific information about what type of virus may be present, which then dictates the best treatment options.

Higher mortality rates in women of low socioeconomic status in the United States and around the world point out the fact that many at-risk women still do not have access to this inexpensive and highly useful test.

Being the daughter of a woman who took **diethylstilbestrol**, a drug prescribed to prevent miscarriage from 1940 to 1971, increases the possibility of cervical cancer, as does immune system suppression through HIV infection or immunosuppressant drugs. Coinfection with chlamydia also raises the risk. Finally, socioeconomic standing is a major factor, as this often determines whether a woman has adequate access to early detection and care.

A vaccine for certain types of HPV now provides some protection from transmission of HPV types 6 and 11 (the cause of some 90% of genital warts) and of HPV types 16 and 18 (the cause of about two-thirds of all cervical cancers). This vaccine does not prevent cervical cancer in a woman who has already been exposed to the virus. Furthermore, while it prevents most cervical cancers, it does not protect against all aggressive forms of HPV. For this reason, a woman who has had the vaccine series still must undergo routine cervical cancer screening.

Types of Cervical Cancer

- *Squamous cell carcinoma of the cervix*: This accounts for 80% to 90% of all diagnoses, and it tends to affect cells on the inferior part of the cervix.
- *Adenocarcinoma of the cervix*: This is more rare, and typically begins in the mucus-producing cells at the superior aspect of the cervix.
- *Other types of cervical cancer*: In very rare cases, melanoma, lymphoma, or sarcoma can develop at the cervix.

Signs and Symptoms

Early stages of cervical cancer have no symptoms to speak of. The cancer must be significantly advanced before any signs appear. These usually include bleeding or spotting between menstrual periods or after menopause, vaginal discharge, and pelvic or abdominal pain.

Treatment

Treatment for cervical cancer depends on the stage at which it is diagnosed (see Sidebar 11.3 for staging protocols). Most cases are found in stage 0 or I, which means treatment can be limited to removing the abnormal cells and watching carefully for further changes. Surgical interventions to remove cervical dysplasia include cryotherapy, in which cells are frozen off; loop electrosurgical excision procedure, in which electricity is passed through a loop of thin wire to slice off the suspicious tissue; laser surgery; and cone biopsy.

Surgical procedures for cancer caught in later stages may range from full or partial hysterectomy (including a procedure that may preserve most of the uterus for the possibility of future childbearing) to full pelvic **exenteration**, in which virtually all of the pelvic organs are removed.

Radiation therapy and chemotherapy may also be employed with advanced cases of cervical cancer.

SIDEBAR 11.3 Staging Cervical Cancer

The staging protocols for cervical cancer can be confusing, and as they are constantly under review, they change frequently. At this writing, the recommendations for cervical cancer divide this disease into precancerous and cancerous stages.

Precancer Staging

When abnormal cells are found in cervical cancer screening, they are classified into these four subgroups:

- *Atypical squamous cells.* Cells look abnormal, but infection or irritation may be the cause.
  - *Atypical squamous cells of unknown significance.* The patient may be told to repeat the test in several weeks or months.
  - *High-grade atypical squamous cells.* They look dangerous and should be removed for further study.
- *Squamous intraepithelial lesions.* These lesions may be classified as low grade or high grade, but they all need further study
- *Squamous cell carcinoma.* These cancerous cells must be staged and removed
- *Atypical glandular cells.* Mucus-producing cells are affected.

Cancer Staging

The staging protocol for invasive cervical cancer was developed by the Fédération Internationale de Gynécologie et d' Obstétrique, so it is sometimes called the FIGO system. A simplified version is included here:

- Stage 0. Cancer cells are found only in the superficial layer of the cervix.
- Stage I. Cancer cells are found only in the cervix. Lesions can range from microscopic to 4 cm in width.
- Stage II. Cancer cells have moved from the cervix into the surrounding area, involving the upper vagina or tissue surrounding the uterus.
- Stage III. Cancer cells are found in the lower vagina and/or the pelvic wall. A growth may be big enough to block the flow of urine through the ureters. Pelvic lymph nodes may also be involved.
- Stage IV. Cancer cells are found in the bladder, rectum, or distant organs.

Medications

- Chemotherapeutic agents, if necessary

Massage?

RISKS Massage has many benefits for women with advanced cervical cancer, as long as appropriate adjustments for the cancer and treatments, which can include surgery, radiation, and chemotherapy, are respected. For more information on working with cancer patients, see Chapter 12.

BENEFITS Massage has no risks for a woman with cervical dysplasia or early cervical cancer that is successfully treated.

Dysmenorrhea

Definition: What Is It?

Dysmenorrhea is a technical term for painful menstrual periods. Generally a woman is said to have dysmenorrhea if she has to limit her regular activities or requires medication to function for 1 day or more every cycle.

Dysmenorrhea is a leading cause of lost time from school or work for women of childbearing age.

Dysmenorrhea in Brief

Pronunciation: dis-men-o-RE-ah

What is it?
Dysmenorrhea is the technical term for menstrual pain that is severe enough to limit the activities of women of childbearing age. It may be a primary problem or secondary to some other pelvic pathology.

How is it recognized?
The symptoms of dysmenorrhea are dull aching or sharp severe lower abdominal pain preceding and/or during menstruation. Nausea and vomiting may accompany very severe symptoms. Secondary dysmenorrhea may cause pelvic pain outside normal periods as well.

Massage risks and benefits
Risks: If extreme menstrual pain is being generated by an underlying problem, that must be identified before doing any intrusive abdominal massage. Most women would probably also rather avoid deep abdominal work during their period.
Benefits: Massage can have a profoundly positive affect for primary dysmenorrhea, and it can be a helpful coping strategy for pain caused by underlying problems.

Etiology: What Happens?

Painful menstrual cramps can be free standing (primary dysmenorrhea) or a symptom of an underlying disorder (secondary dysmenorrhea). Ultimately the result is the same: pain that is severe enough to limit activity every month.

In addition to pain being generated at the uterus, many women find that emotional stress—sometimes simply the stress of anticipating menstrual pain—can exacerbate that pain. Add to this the problem of ligament laxity and subsequent muscle tightening that many women experience during their cycle, and pain associated with menstruation becomes a very complicated problem.

Types of Dysmenorrhea

- *Primary dysmenorrhea*: This usually starts within 3 months of **menarche**. Several factors can contribute, including excessive prostaglandin and vasopressin release (prostaglandins and vasopressin promote pain, inflammation, and smooth muscle contraction), the pain-spasm cycle created when the uterus contracts to expel its contents, and irritation as the uterine ligament that anchors the uterus is tugged.

Secondary dysmenorrhea: This is a complication of some other pelvic disorder. Some of the most common problems that cause menstrual pain include pelvic inflammatory disease (PID), fibroid tumors, intrauterine devices (IUDs), sexually transmitted infections (STIs), and endometriosis. Torsion or cysts that affect the ovaries can cause extreme menstrual pain, and pelvic adhesions, deposits of scar tissue from previous surgeries, or trauma may also contribute.

Signs and Symptoms

Signs and symptoms of dysmenorrhea vary. They can include dull aches in the abdomen and low back or sharp pains and cramping in the pelvis and abdomen.

These usually happen early in menstruation, but some women have symptoms during their whole period. Headaches, nausea, vomiting, diarrhea, and constipation are all possibilities, along with a frequent need to urinate.

Secondary dysmenorrhea typically begins after some years of relatively pain-free menstruation. Symptoms may not be limited to the menstrual period; menstrual flow may be irregular or abnormally heavy; pain medication is often not effective; and this condition is often accompanied by infertility.

Treatment

For most cases of dysmenorrhea, painkillers such as ibuprofen or naproxen provide some relief by inhibiting the secretion of prostaglandins. These are recommended along with warm or hot packs to the abdomen and increased exercise and stretching of the low back.

If painkillers, heat, and stretching are inadequate, more aggressive interventions may be considered. Narcotic painkillers may be prescribed. High-frequency TENS units have shown some success to manage symptoms. Low-dose birth control pills suppress ovulation, which in turn prohibits the secretion of prostaglandins in the uterus. If a structural condition, such as fibroid tumors, is at the root of the problem, surgery may be an option. And laparoscopic surgery for endometriosis may alleviate symptoms if that is the source of the problem.

Dysmenorrhea is often responsive to many alternative treatment options. A thorough nutritional analysis may reveal strategies for dealing with menstrual pain. Vitamin B_1, vitamin E, fish oil, magnesium, and thiamine have all shown improvement in small-scale trials. Dietary changes to reduce fats and animal proteins while increasing fiber and calcium are often recommended. Exercise and stretches can also relieve the pain in the uterine ligament, which may be irritated by a uterus in spasm.

Medications

- Anti-inflammatories to manage inflammation and pain
- Narcotic analgesics if necessary (especially for secondary dysmenorrhea)
- Low-dose birth control pills to suppress ovulation

Massage?

RISKS Deep or intrusive work for an undiagnosed problem that causes menstrual pain or during a menstrual period should be avoided.

BENEFITS Massage can be very helpful for primary dysmenorrhea by relieving stress, indirectly addressing the uterine pain-spasm cycle, and helping any muscle tightness brought about by ligament laxity that accompanies the menstrual cycle.

OPTIONS Unlike most referred pain patterns, the tendency for the uterus to refer pain the sacral area of the low back appears for many women to be reversible. In other words, gentle work around the skin of the sacrum can cause a reflexive relief of pain in the pelvic cavity.

Massage to the abdomen when the client is not menstruating may improve tissue quality and help to minimize abdominal adhesions that contribute to pain.

Endometriosis

Definition: What Is It?

Endometriosis is a condition in which cells from the endometrium implant elsewhere in the body. Growths usually begin in the pelvic cavity but may spread further into the abdomen and in rare cases above the diaphragm.

It is estimated that anywhere from 5% to 20% of women of childbearing age have this disorder, although not all have symptoms.

Etiology: What Happens?

Endometriosis is implantation and growth of endometrial cells anywhere outside the uterus. It was first described in 1921 by American gynecologist James Sampson, who noticed these growths in the peritoneal cavities of women undergoing abdominal surgery. He hypothesized that the endometrial cells got out of the uterus via retrograde backflow through the uterine tubes.

Retrograde backflow is still a leading theory about the pathophysiology of this disorder, but since it has been found that most women have some endometrial cells in the pelvis during menstruation, clearly other factors are involved. These include

Endometriosis in Brief

Pronunciation: en-do-me-tre-O-sis

What is it?
Endometriosis is the implantation and growth of endometrial cells in the peritoneal cavity (and possibly elsewhere) that grow and then decay with the menstrual cycle.

How is it recognized?
Endometriosis may have no symptoms. When it does, they generally include heavy, painful menstruation; pelvic and abdominal pain; difficulties with urination or defecation; painful intercourse; and other problems, depending on which tissues are affected. Symptoms are worst just before and during menstruation. Infertility is a frequent complication of endometriosis.

Massage risks and benefits
Risks: If a client knows she has endometriosis, invasive abdominal work must be done with extra care. Otherwise, massage carries no specific risks for clients with this condition.
Benefits: Massage is unlikely to change the course of endometriosis but its generally soothing and calming effects can improve the quality of life for a woman who struggles with a very frustrating condition.

coelomic metaplasia (the metamorphosis of some cells into endometrial cells, possibly triggered by inflammation), endometrial cells spread via surgical procedures (deposits located in the scar tissue from C-sections and laparoscopic procedures support this theory), metastasis via blood or lymph (endometrial deposits are rarely found outside the abdominopelvic cavity, but this would be the mechanism), or immune system anomalies that promote inflammation but suppress activity against cells that are notably out of place.

Wherever the cells land, if they are able to colonize the tissue, they stimulate the growth of supplying blood vessels, and they proliferate in accordance with the hormonal commands in the body. But these growths cannot be shed with normal menstruation. Instead, they decay and accumulate in local areas, stimulating an inflammatory response. The body attempts to isolate them by surrounding the deposits with fibrous connective tissue. Eventually multitudes of fibrous "blood blisters" called endometriomas accumulate (Figure 11.3).

Endometrial growths that are found early look like clear vesicles on the structures they have colonized. Later these vesicles become bright red. Over a course of 10 or more years, they become thick, black, and scarred. Growths on ovaries that have darkened over time are sometimes called "chocolate cysts."

Accumulations of deposits and fibrous connective tissue can create adhesions in or on the uterine tubes and ovaries, which raise the risk of infertility or ectopic pregnancy. The collecting of blood in these deposits routes blood away from where it can be useful, resulting in anemia. Uterine hyperplasia is a condition that occasionally accompanies endometriosis; the normal endometrial lining becomes pathologically thickened, leading to excessive bleeding and further difficulties with fertility.

Signs and Symptoms

Very often infertility is the complaint that brings a woman with endometriosis to a doctor for a first diagnosis. Other signs and symptoms of endometriosis are often nonexistent, at least in the early stages, but premenstrual spotting, a sensation of urinary urgency with painful urination, and diarrhea and rectal bleeding during menstruation may occur. Some cases include severe dysmenorrhea before, during, and after periods. Interestingly, the amount of pain does not correlate with the size of the endometrial growths.

Symptoms of endometriosis are cyclical, reaching a peak during menstruation. This feature has probably prevented a lot of women from seeking medical help, since traditionally it has been assumed that painful menstruation is a normal and expected part of having "the curse." As women have become more proactive about health care, they have discovered that painful menstruation is not a given and have become more willing to explore the causes and possible solutions to their pain.

Treatment

Treatment for endometriosis depends on what outcome the woman desires. No permanent solution for this disorder exists; even a complete hysterectomy won't protect a patient from endometriosis if any remaining microscopic deposits are stimulated with hormone replacement therapy (HRT).

Because many women wish to treat endometriosis to become pregnant, treatment options are often geared toward limiting symptoms and progression

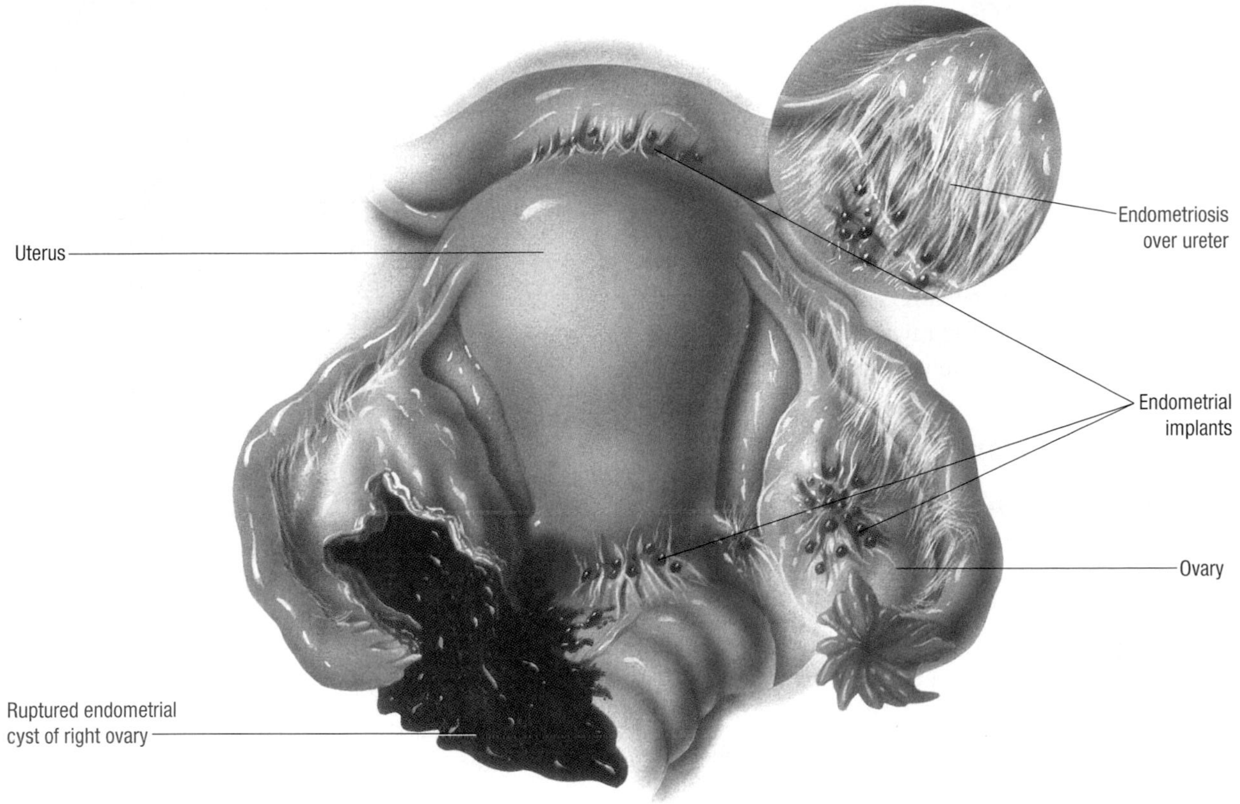

Figure 11.3. Sites of endometriosis.

long enough to allow fertilization to take place. Symptoms disappear during pregnancy, but they usually recur after a baby is born.

Four main goals are at the center of medical intervention for endometriosis. These are to relieve pain, to stop the progression of established growths, to prevent the establishment of any new growths, and to maintain or restore fertility if that is the patient's wish. Nonsteroidal anti-inflammatory drugs or other analgesics may be adequate for pain relief. Hormone therapy that disrupts the secretion of estrogen may be employed to limit growths. These may be used alone or as a preparation for surgery. Surgical intervention may include the use of lasers or electrocauterization to ablate (remove the top layer of tissue) or cut out visible growths and to reduce adhesions between pelvic organs.

Medications

- Nonsteroidal anti-inflammatory drugs for pain and inflammation
- Narcotic analgesics if necessary for pain management
- Oral contraception to suppress estrogen and ovulation
- Other hormonal analogs (by nasal spray, orally, or by injection) to suppress ovulation

Massage?

RISKS Endometriosis can cause scarring and adhesions in the pelvic cavity. This possibility requires special caution and care when doing anything more than superficial work on the abdomen.

BENEFITS Many women with endometriosis live in a state of anxiety and frustration with their own body that may exacerbate their most painful symptoms. Massage therapy along with other relaxation techniques is frequently recommended for women who must learn to cope with the long-term consequences of a disorder that has no permanent cure.

OPTIONS Special training in abdominal and pelvic bodywork may help to relieve pain and some other symptoms (including infertility) for women with endometriosis.

Fibroid Tumors

Definition: What Are They?

Fibroid tumors, or leiomyomas, are benign tumors that grow in or around the uterus. They can grow within the smooth muscle walls, or, more rarely, they can be suspended from a stalk into the pelvic cavity or uterus (Figure 11.4). Some even hang down into the vagina. Fibroids can grow singly or in clusters, and they vary in size from being microscopic to weighing several pounds and completely filling the uterus.

Etiology: What Happens?

The pathophysiology of uterine fibroids is not well understood. While they sometimes run in families, they are not strictly genetically linked. They seem to be stimulated by estrogen; after menopause, many shrink and ultimately disappear. Many experts believe that fibroid tumors arise as a combination of genetic, environmental, and hormonal factors.

Histological studies show that the extracellular matrix of fibroid tumors lacks a key protein, and the collagen filaments are disorganized and not discretely formed. This is especially interesting because the same growth pattern has been observed in keloid scars. Both fibroids and keloids are about three times more common in African Americans than in the rest of the population.

Fibroid Tumors in Brief

Pronunciation: FY-broyd TU-morz

What are they?
Fibroid tumors are benign growths in the muscle or connective tissue of the uterus.

How are they recognized?
Fibroid tumors are often asymptomatic. They may cause heavy menstrual bleeding or put mechanical pressure on other structures in the pelvis.

Massage risks and benefits
Risks: Massage carries little risk for a client with fibroid tumors unless a tumor is very large and massage is deep, intrusive, and low in the pelvis.
Benefits: Massage is unlikely to have any effect on fibroid tumors. Clients with this condition can enjoy the same benefits from bodywork as the rest of the population.

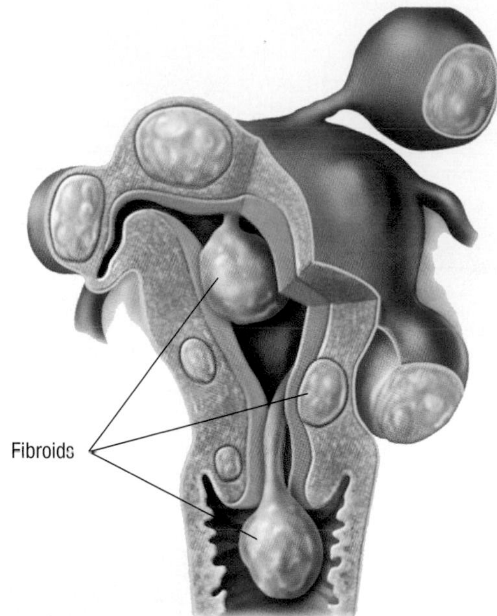

Figure 11.4. Uterine fibroids

Fibroids are typically classified by their location. Submucosal fibroids grow under the mucous lining of the uterus; they are the deepest type. Intramural fibroids grow within layers of the muscular wall of the uterus. Subserosal fibroids grow on the superficial aspect of the uterus but deep to the peritoneum.

Fibroids are very seldom serious, but they can lead to some troubling consequences. The heavy periods they cause sometimes lead to anemia. They can cause infertility by obstructing fallopian tubes or interfering with the implantation of a fertilized ovum. They can also interfere in pregnancies brought to term: if a fibroid is large enough, it can crowd the growing fetus or block the exit through the cervix. These problems can lead to premature births and cesarean sections.

Pedunculate fibroids, the type that dangle into the uterus or vagina, can twist on their stalk. This causes extreme pain and requires surgery for removal. It is also possible for very large fibroids to outgrow their blood supply. This leads to degeneration, in which tissue that is deprived of oxygen dies. The body slowly reabsorbs the necrotic mass, but it can be a long and painful process; more often, surgery is performed to remove the fibroid.

Signs and Symptoms

Usually fibroids produce no symptoms at all. In extreme cases, the tumor may grow large enough to press on the sensory nerves inside the uterus. If they press on the bladder, they can cause urinary frequency; if on the rectum, they can cause difficulties with defecation. If they press on the fallopian (uterine) tubes, they may interfere with pregnancy. They can also cause heavy menstrual bleeding and occasionally bleeding between menstrual periods.

Fibroids typically grow slowly, but occasionally they grow fast, doubling their size within a few months. In this situation, a biopsy is recommended to rule out uterine malignancy.

Treatment

Fibroids seldom require treatment unless they cause pain and excessive bleeding, or if they interfere with pregnancy.

Hormone therapy can shrink them, but they grow back when medication is stopped. Other options include minimally invasive procedures to shrink the growths with hormone therapy or minimally invasive procedures that remove parts of the tumors, or blocking off the supplying arteries (uterine artery embolization). Surgical possibilities include laser ablation, myomectomy (the removal of the tumor while preserving the rest of the uterus), or full hysterectomy.

Medications

- Gonadotropin releasing hormone inhibitors to help shrink the tumors before surgery
- Progesterone or progestin to counter the effects of estrogen

Massage?

RISKS If a client knows she has large fibroid tumors, it is best not to disrupt them with intrusive massage low in the abdomen. Bodywork holds no other specific risks for a person with this condition.

BENEFITS Massage has no direct impact on the presence of fibroid tumors. Most clients with this condition can enjoy all the same benefits of bodywork as the rest of the population.

Uterine Cancer

Definition: What Is It?

Uterine cancer is the development of cancerous cells in the uterus. It is classified as endometrial cancer or uterine sarcoma. It is diagnosed in about 43,000 American women each year, and leads to about 8,000 deaths.

Uterine Cancer in Brief

Pronunciation: YU-tah-rin KAN-ser

What is it?
Uterine cancer is the development of cancerous cells in the endometrium or other tissues of the uterus.

How is it recognized?
The most dependable symptom of uterine cancer is postmenopausal spotting or bleeding. Other signs can include spotting between periods for premenopausal women, vaginal discharge, pelvic pain, pain with sex, and unexplained weight loss.

Massage risks and benefits
Risks: The risks for uterine cancer patients who wish to receive massage or bodywork are the same as those for other cancer patients: both the challenges of the disease and of its treatments must be respected. For uterine cancer, this can involve chemotherapy, radiation, and surgery.
Benefits: If bodywork accommodates for the limitations brought about by uterine cancer and its treatments, the benefits it can offer include decreased pain and anxiety, increased appetite and energy, improved sleep and less depression.

Etiology: What Happens?

Uterine cancer begins with a mutation in the DNA of the affected cells. Most often these are cells in the endometrium, but uterine cancer can also develop in the connective tissue or muscle tissue of the uterus.

The primary trigger for many cases of uterine cancer appears to be exposure to excessive estrogen. That source can be endogenous (for instance if the ovaries or fat cells produce more estrogen than can be tolerated) or exogenous (with HRT or other sources). Other factors, including race, age, and history of other cancers, also influence a woman's chance of developing uterine cancer.

When a new growth develops in the uterus, it tends to be fragile and easily disrupted. This leads to vaginal bleeding or spotting, especially in postmenopausal women; this is the most dependable early symptom of the disease.

Uterine cancer is often slow growing and not aggressive. When it does spread, however, it can use any of four mechanisms. Direct contact can allow cells on the exterior of the uterus to become established on nearby organs, such as the bladder or the colon. Cells from the uterus can also float through peritoneal fluid to land elsewhere in the region and set up new growth sites. Finally, both the lymphatic and circulatory systems can be recruited to carry cancerous cells outside the pelvis to the lungs, bones, or other areas.

Risk factors for uterine cancer have been extensively studied, and the most potent triggers all have to do with estrogen exposure. Uterine hyperplasia is a condition that develops in some perimenopausal women, especially when they supplement estrogen. This enlargement of the uterus can sometimes develop into cancer. Estrogen replacement therapy that is unopposed with progestin; obesity (abdominal fat cells can produce estrogen); a high-fat, low-fiber diet; never having had children; early menarche combined with late menopause; polycystic ovarian disease; and taking tamoxifen to reduce the risk of breast cancer recurrence can all increase the risk of uterine cancer.

NOTABLE CASES Actress ("Mrs. Robinson") Anne Bancroft succumbed to uterine cancer at age 73 in 2005. Actress and author (*Cancer, Schmancer*) Fran Drescher is a uterine cancer survivor and outspoken advocate for uterine cancer patients.

Other risk factors for uterine cancer include age, race, and the genetic anomaly associated with a high risk of colorectal cancer. Type 2 diabetes is associated with uterine cancer; this is probably due to a tendency toward obesity, but the metabolic problems of diabetes itself may also have something to do with an increased risk of this disease.

Types of Uterine Cancer

- *Endometrial cancer*: This accounts for the vast majority of uterine cancer diagnoses. Its subtypes include the following:
    - Adenocarcinoma: This is the most common form of endometrial cancer. It involves cells that resemble normal endometrial cells. It tends not to be aggressive.
    - Adenosquamous carcinoma: This involves squamous epithelial cells along with typical endothelial cells.
    - Papillary serous adenocarcinoma: this is rare and potentially aggressive.
    - Clear cell adenocarcinoma: This is the rarest form of endometrial cancer, and it has a high risk of being aggressive.
- Uterine sarcoma: This cancer originates from nonglandular tissues. While it progresses with essentially the same pattern as endometrial cancer, uterine sarcoma tends to be much more aggressive and has a poorer survival rate. Subtypes include the following:
- Stromal cell cancer: This affects the connective tissue of the uterus.
- Leiomyosarcoma: This starts in the smooth muscle cells of the uterus.
- Mixed Müllerian sarcoma: This combines features of adenocarcinomas and sarcomas.

Signs and Symptoms

Most women with uterine cancer are postmenopausal, so the most common early sign of this disease, vaginal spotting or bleeding, is easy to identify. While most women who have postmenopausal bleeding do not have uterine cancer, this early sign contributes to the excellent survival rates for this disease: it is often found in Stage I or II.

For women who still have a menstrual cycle, uterine cancer can be harder to identify early, but spotting between periods should be investigated.

Other signs and symptoms include vaginal discharge, pelvic pain, a pelvic mass, pain with sex, a change in bladder or bowel habits, and unintended weight loss.

Staging protocols for uterine cancer can be found in Sidebar 11.4.

Treatment

The mainstay of uterine cancer treatment is a hysterectomy, which is usually accompanied by the removal of the ovaries and uterine tubes as well. This may be followed by radiation and/or hormone therapy, depending on findings. Lymph nodes near the aorta and in the groin are often dissected for signs of metastasis. Chemotherapy is used most often for uterine sarcomas or for women who are not good candidates for open surgery because of age or other health problems.

If a young woman is diagnosed with uterine cancer and wants to preserve her uterus for the possibility of childbearing, she may choose to have a dilatation and curettage procedure with progestin supplements instead of surgery. This option carries a high risk of recurrence, however, so it must be followed by careful surveillance.

SIDEBAR 11.4 Staging Uterine Cancer

As with cervical cancer, the staging protocol for uterine cancer was developed by the Fédération Internationale de Gynécologie et d' Obstétrique, so it is sometimes called the FIGO system.

A simplified version of the TNM system for staging uterine cancer looks like this:

Tumor	Node	Metastasis
T0: No signs of a tumor in the uterus.	N0: No spread to nearby nodes.	M0: No spread to distant nodes or tissues.
Tis: Preinvasive cancer (in situ); cells are limited to the endometrium.	N1: Lymph nodes in the pelvis are involved.	M1: Spread to distant organs and lymph nodes.
T1: Tumor is growing in the body of the uterus but not beyond.	N2: Lymph nodes along the aorta are involved.	
T2: The tumor has spread into supporting connective tissue of the cervix.		
T3: The cancer has spread from the uterus into nearby tissues, including superficial layers of the rectum and bladder.		
T4: The cancer has fully invaded other nearby organs or spread to distant organs.		

These are then translated into stages in this way:

Stage I	T1, N0, M0
Stage II	T2, N0, M0
Stage III	T3, N0, M0
Stage IV	T4, any N, M0, *or* any T, any N, M1

Medications

- Chemotherapeutic agents
- Hormone therapy, including progesterone and progestin; tamoxifen; aromatase inhibitors (to reduce estrogen production at fat cells); and gonadotropin-releasing hormone inhibitors

Massage?

RISKS Uterine cancer may be treated with any combination of surgery, chemotherapy, hormone therapy, or radiation. Any bodywork delivered in this setting must accommodate for the challenges of the disease as well as the challenges of its treatments.

BENEFITS Bodywork has many demonstrated benefits for cancer patients, as long as appropriate adjustments are made. For more information on massage in the context of cancer, see Chapter 12.

Disorders of Other Female Reproductive Structures

Breast Cancer

Definition: What Is It?

Breast cancer is the development of tumors in the epithelial or connective tissue of the breast. These growths may start out as nonmalignant, but may become invasive if neglected for a long period.

About 230,000 new cases of invasive breast cancer are diagnosed in women (this does not include diagnoses found in situ), and about 1,900 cases in men each year in the United States. About 39,000 women and about 500 men die of this disease each year. It is estimated that 2.5 million breast cancer survivors are alive in the United States today.

Breast Cancer in Brief

What is it?
Breast cancer is the growth of malignant tumor cells in breast tissue. These cells can invade skin and nearby muscles and bones. If they invade lymph nodes, they can metastasize to the rest of the body.

How is it recognized?
The first sign of breast cancer is a small painless lump or thickening in the breast tissue or near the axilla. The lump may be too small to palpate, but may show on a mammogram. Later the skin may change texture, the nipple may change shape, and discharge may occur.

Massage risks and benefits
Risks: Breast cancer patients undergo treatments that are extremely taxing on general health as well as on physical and emotional well-being. Ports or other surgical equipment may be present. Further, this cancer can invade the skeleton, leading to unstable and easily fractured bones. Any bodywork in this context must respect all these challenges.
Benefits: As long as the challenges of both breast cancer and its treatments are accommodated, massage can be a wonderful, supportive, important coping mechanism for many patients.

Etiology: What Happens?

Breasts are constructed of 15 to 20 lobes where milk is produced in lactating women; ducts that deliver milk to the nipple; and the stroma, or collagen, elastin, and fat cells that provide support and the bulk of breast tissue. The lobes and ducts are made of epithelial cells; the stroma is connective tissue and lipid cells. Although cancer may grow in any of these tissues, malignant cells are most likely to grow in the lobes and ducts.

NOTABLE CASES The list of well-known people with breast cancer is long and varied. It includes activist Gloria Steinem, singer Olivia Newton-John, journalist Linda Ellerbee, and—as a demonstration that breast cancer is not just a woman's disease—"Shaft" actor Richard Rountree. Perhaps the most eloquent breast cancer patient in recent years was columnist Molly Ivins, who declared, "Having breast cancer is massive amounts of no fun. First they mutilate you; then they poison you; then they burn you. I have been on blind dates better than that." Molly Ivins died from inflammatory breast disease in 2007.

Many types of breast cancer begin as in situ growths that eventually develop malignant characteristics. It can take a long time for a tumor to become large enough to notice; it is estimated that it takes several years for a growth to reach a diameter of 1 cm.

As tumors grow, cells may invade the circulatory or lymphatic system. The proximity of the axillary lymph nodes makes these a common site for the spread of malignant cells (Figure 11.5).

Breast cancer usually metastasizes to nearby lymph nodes in the axilla and thoracic cavity first; invasion of chest muscles, bones, and skin follows. Finally, distant metastatic sites include the liver, lung, and brain. If the cancer is not successfully treated, complications may include spinal cord pressure, bone fractures, pleural effusion, and bronchial obstruction.

One of the most frustrating things about breast cancer is that no dependable profile of the women most likely to get it has ever been developed. Some cancers, such as lung, colon, and skin cancer, can be directly linked to diet or environmental factors; breast cancer cannot. Although some risk factors have been identified as increasing the chance that a woman may develop breast cancer, most women with these risk factors (outside of genetic predisposition) never develop the disease, and most breast cancer patients don't carry most of these risk factors (outside of age).

Age is the leading risk factor for breast cancer: most patients are diagnosed when they are over 50 years old. Prolonged estrogen exposure is another factor: women with early menarche and late menopause; who had children after age 30 or not at all; who are obese, especially after menopause; or who use HRT are at greater risk than the general population. Women who have more than one alcoholic drink every day, who have a history of radiation treatments to the chest, or who have a history of lobular carcinoma in situ (LCIS) are more likely than the rest of the population to develop breast cancer.

One reliable risk factor is the presence of two abnormal breast cancer genes, BRCA 1 and BRCA 2. About 80% of women carrying these genes will develop breast cancer, but they account for only 5% to 10% of diagnosed patients. For the other 90% of breast cancer patients, the only dependable risk factor is age.

Breast cancer is not a preventable disease. Therefore, efforts for prevention are targeted at early detection,

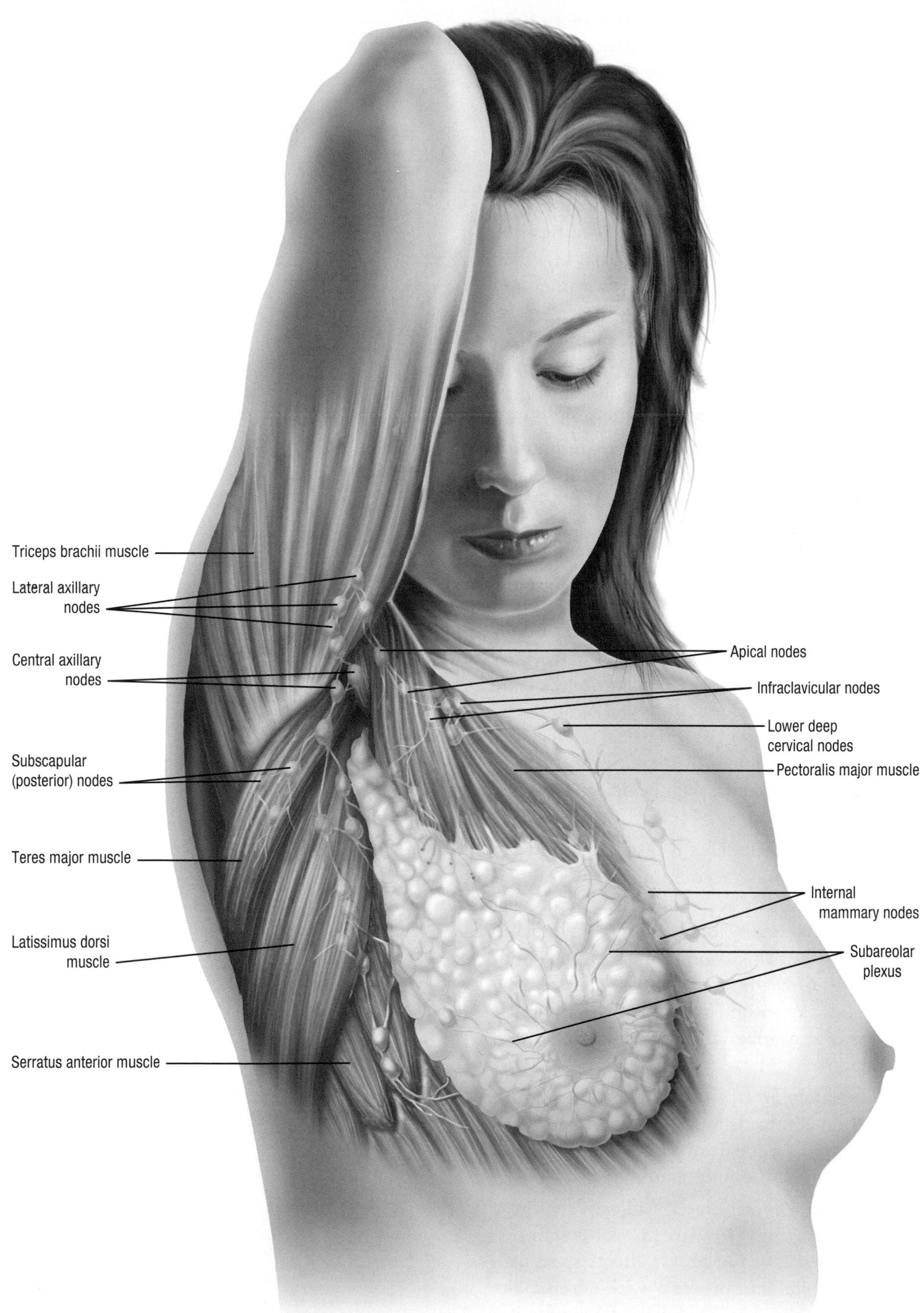

Figure 11.5. Breast cancer: proximity of lymph nodes

which significantly increases the life expectancy of the breast cancer patient. The three main courses for early detection are self-examination, breast examination by a professional, and mammograms, which use radiation to look for unusually dense masses in the breast tissue. MRI or ultrasound imaging is typically saved for high-risk women who are under 40 years old.

Women who have a personal or family history of breast cancer, who are positive for the breast cancer genes, or who are otherwise considered at high risk for this disease may be counseled to test earlier and more often than the general public.

It is important to emphasize that a mammogram is not a definitive test for breast cancer. Mammogram interpretations vary widely, and mammograms may miss the subtle changes in breast tissue that only women who perform monthly self-examinations may notice. Therefore, an "all-clear" from a mammogram does not rule out breast cancer.

Types of Breast Cancer

- *Ductal carcinoma*: This is the most common type of breast cancer, accounting for 70% to 80% of diagnoses. It can occur in situ, in which case cells affect only the epithelial lining of the ducts, or it can become invasive (Figure 11.6). Ductal carcinoma in situ (DCIS) is associated with the development of small calcified deposits in the breasts and a slightly increased risk for invasive breast cancer.
- *Lobular carcinoma*: This is less common than ductal carcinoma, accounting for 5% to 10% of tumors. It can be limited to the epithelial lining of the lobes (lobular carcinoma in situ, or LCIS), but this condition carries a significant risk of becoming invasive (Figure 11.7). Lobular carcinoma also has a higher incidence of appearing in both breasts than ductal carcinoma.
- *Inflammatory breast disease*: This is a form of breast cancer that is relatively rare in the West. It resembles a local infection or insect bite, with warm, red, itching skin.
- *Other types of breast cancer*: Collectively, these account for only 10% to 15% of diagnoses. Paget disease of the breast affects specifically the nipple, and presents with eczema-like changes in the skin. Medullary carcinoma is a rare malignancy of the connective tissues in

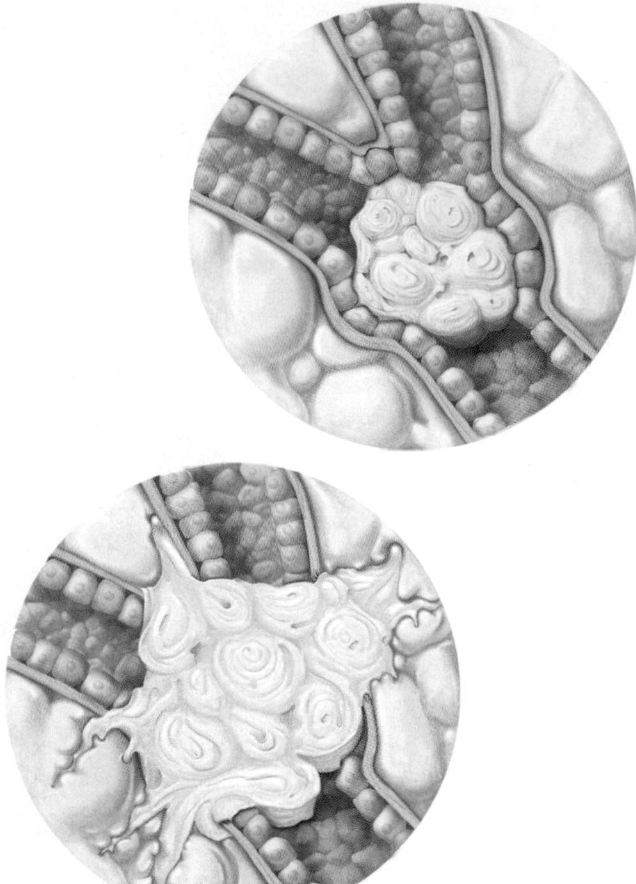

Figure 11.6. Ductal breast cancer

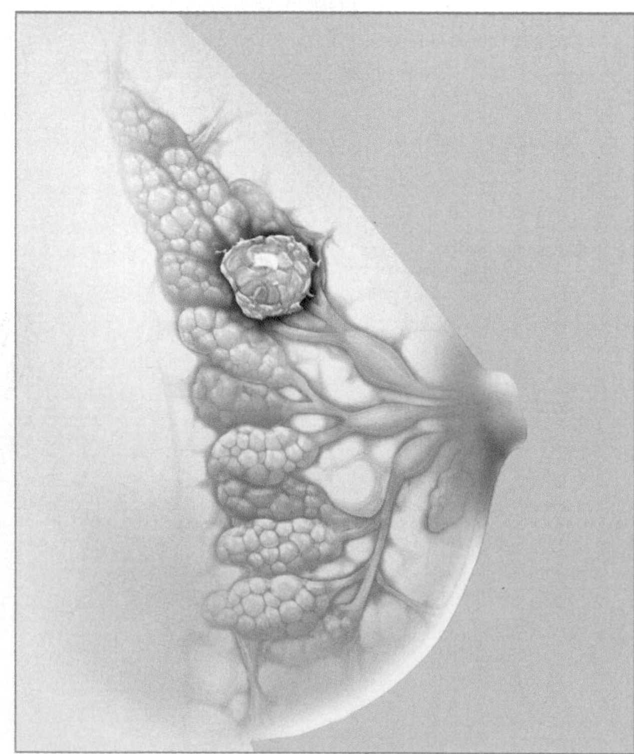

Figure 11.7. Lobular breast cancer

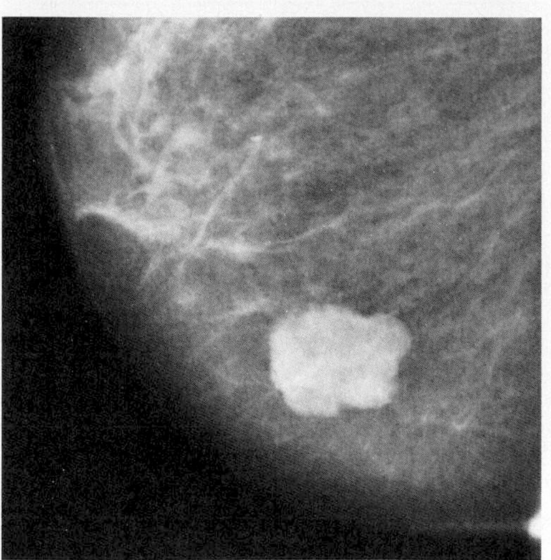

Figure 11.8. Mammogram showing a breast cancer tumor: note the irregular shape and borders of growth

the breast. Tubular carcinoma refers to the shape of the mutated cells. And mucinous carcinoma is a rare type with a good prognosis.

Signs and Symptoms

Early symptoms of breast cancer are subtle. Breast tissue is soft and loose, so tumors have ample room to grow without causing pain. Sometimes self-examination can find changing textures or lumps before a mammogram can show them, and sometimes a mammogram reveals thickenings or minute calcifications that are too subtle to feel (Figure 11.8). Self-exams may also find nonmalignant breast changes that can easily be mistaken for breast cancer (see Sidebar 11.5).

Advanced cases of breast cancer show asymmetrical breast growth, inverted nipples that may have discharge, and sometimes a characteristic "orange peel" texture of the skin on the breast. Advanced cases may also cause symptoms in other parts of the body that are damaged by the growth of invasive tumors: bone pain, weight loss, spinal cord compression, and swelling in the arms may be the result of tumors far from the original site of the cancer.

SIDEBAR 11.5 Nonmalignant Breast Changes

Not all breast growths are malignant. Most growths in breast tissue are cysts or benign tumors; many fall into the classification of fibrocystic breast changes. Some of these growths carry a risk of eventually becoming malignant, but for the most part they are not serious conditions and can easily be distinguished from malignancies with testing procedures that include mammograms, fine-needle aspiration, ultrasound, or biopsy.

Breasts can also be affected by infection (called **mastitis** if a woman is lactating or **ductal ectasia** if she is not). Injury from trauma, surgery, or radiation may cause fat necrosis, a condition in which the fat cells that make up the bulk of breast tissue degenerate and die. Breast infections and fat necrosis can be serious, requiring medical intervention for the best outcomes.

Treatment

Treatment for breast cancer depends on the stage of the disease when it is found; staging protocols are discussed in Sidebar 11.6. Several options for treatment are often used in combination for best results:

- *Surgery*. Lumpectomies, partial mastectomies, total mastectomies, and modified mastectomies are surgical options for removing tumors and nearby lymph nodes. Lymph nodes are examined for signs of further metastasis. Lymphedema and postmastectomy pain syndrome from damaged nerves are possible negative side effects.
- *Radiation therapy*. Radiation is aimed at tumors to slow or stop growth or to shrink tumors to make them easier to remove surgically. Radiation may be applied externally or internally, with radioactive pellets that are surgically placed around the tumors and removed later.
- *Chemotherapy*. Chemotherapy may be used before surgery to reduce the size of a growth for a better chance of full removal, after surgery as a protective measure, or instead of surgery when tumors are determined to be inoperable.
- *Hormone therapy*. Some breast cancer tumors have been found to be sensitive to estrogen levels; they need access to this hormone to grow. Medications called selective estrogen receptor modulators can block estrogen receptor sites or inhibit estrogen production to limit these growths.
- *Biologic therapy*. Monoclonal antibodies may be used to attack potential cancer cells and reduce the risk of recurrence.

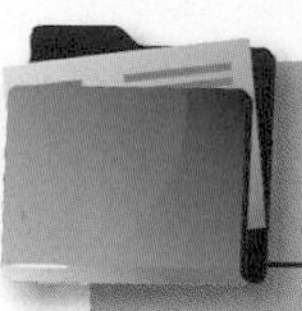

CASE HISTORY 11.1 Breast Cancer

Right before my 57th birthday, I found a lump in my left breast while doing a breast examination in the shower. When I went in for my mammogram, the doctor said he couldn't feel it, and the mammogram was normal. A subsequent ultrasound did not reveal anything, and the technician also could not feel what I felt. So, even though I knew better, this gave me a sense of security that all was well.

Until January. I could still feel the lump and by now my husband could also, so I was not imagining it. I made an appointment with a surgeon. He not only felt what I had felt (which was a thickening, more than a lump), but in checking my previous mammogram, he found pinpoints of calcium in the right breast, which are sometimes indicators of cancer. Three days later I had bilateral biopsies.

During the biopsies, a frozen section was done on the thickening on the left side, which meant the pathologist could tell right away whether the tissue was malignant. (The tissue from the right breast biopsy went through routine pathology, and I had to wait for several days for those results.) So there I was, in the recovery room, when the doctor came in and told me that the left breast biopsy revealed a malignancy. Then he left to talk to my husband, and I was by myself. The greatest feeling I had was just incredible sadness. I don't know why I wasn't angry or anything else; I was just so sad. After a few minutes, I was able to join my husband and we both cried.

After 3 days, the call came saying the second biopsy showed no malignancy. By that time, I was thankful that only one breast had a malignancy. Strange thing for which to be thankful.

My diagnosis was a stage I infiltrated ductal carcinoma, upper medial quadrant, left breast. After I got a second opinion, surgery was scheduled for the following Monday. Before that, I had to have chest x-rays, a bone scan, and a radiation oncology consult, as I had opted to have conservative surgery (a lumpectomy followed by 6 weeks of radiation).

CAROL E., 60 YEARS OLD
"When you have had breast cancer, the thought of possible recurrence is always with you. It makes you look at what is really important in life."

The surgeon performed a lumpectomy and also did an axillary dissection—removal of some lymph nodes in the armpit. It is during this surgery that a nerve in my armpit was either severed or damaged. This produces numbness in the underarm and inner upper arm that can be permanent. The lymph nodes removed (16 in my case) were tested for malignancy, and later I learned that they showed no cancer. Chances were that the cancer had been confined to the breast tissue. Good news indeed!

But then the surgeon called and said that the margins of the tissue removed were not clean—meaning that there were still some cancer cells in the breast. So back to surgery for another resection of the breast. My surgeon did not usually do this, but he felt that there was very little cancer left, and a mastectomy could still be avoided. Unfortunately, the margins on that sample weren't clean either. The following week again found me in surgery having a total mastectomy. Three major surgeries in 3 weeks with general anesthetic each time are a lot to cope with, but you do what you have to do.

Because I had a mastectomy, I did not have to have any radiation, and because my lymph nodes were negative for cancer cells, I also did not have to have chemotherapy. A big relief!

I do take tamoxifen, and amitriptyline, a mild antidepressant, to help break the cycle of chronic nerve pain that I have had in my left arm—an unusual and difficult complication. About 8 months ago I also started on Neurontin, an antiseizure drug that can also work on nerve pain, and in my case it has really helped. So after almost 2 years, the pain in my arm is under control. I have no lymphedema (swelling of the arm due to a compromised lymph system). However, this could happen at any time.

I do not feel that the doctors emphasize enough how vulnerable the affected arm is. Infections can develop very easily, and I have to be really careful, especially working in the garden. It seems that little burns and scratches take forever to heal. I should not lift more than 10 lb with the affected arm and should not have any needle sticks or have blood pressure taken on that arm. Once I awoke after minor surgery to find a blood pressure cuff on my left arm, and was I upset! I thought that I had taken enough precautions that this should not have happened. The prescription for medication post surgery had been clipped over the warning note! The next time I had an anesthetic, I wrote on my left arm with a surgical pen, and that did not come off!

When you have had breast cancer, the thought of recurrence is always with you. Breast cancer does not follow the 5-year rule; it can come back at any time. It is a lifelong commitment always to be on the watch and take really good care of yourself. This makes you look at what is really important in life. You try not to put off things that you want to say or do. Life is precious and I am glad to still have it!■

SIDEBAR 11.6 Staging Breast Cancer

Although the progression of cancer from stage to stage has been categorized for the sake of convenience, it is impossible to predict exactly how this disease will progress in each patient. Every person who develops breast cancer will undergo a unique disease process, unlike anybody else's.

Here is a simplified version of TNM classifications for breast cancer:

Tumor	Node	Metastasis
T0: no tumors found	N0: no nodes involved	M0: no metastasis
T-IS: cancer in situ; first layer of tissue involved; could be DCIS or LCIS	N1: 1–3 lymph nodes involved on affected side; not attached to each other or to other tissues	M1: distant metastasis
T1: ≥1 tumors, <2 cm in diameter	N2: 4–9 nodes on same side as tumor involved; nodes attached to each other or to surrounding tissues	
T2: ≥1 tumors 2–5 cm in diameter	N3: ≥10 axillary nodes involved, or nodes from other groups (e.g., infraclavicular, supraclavicular, internal mammary nodes)	
T3: ≥1 tumors >5 cm in diameter		
T4: Tumors invade chest wall or skin		

These are translated into stages I–IV in this way:

Stage 0	T IS, N0, M0
Stage I	T 1, N0, M0
Stage IIA	T0-T2, N0-N1, M0
Stage IIB	T2-T3, N0-N1, M0
Stage IIIA	T0-T3, N1–2, M0
Stage IIIB	T4, N0–2, M0
Stage IIIC	Any T, N3, M0
Stage IV	Any T, Any N, M1

All of these treatment options have serious potential side effects that may influence choices about massage and bodywork. These are discussed in detail in Chapter 12.

Medications

- Chemotherapeutic drugs
- Hormone therapy to block receptor sites on cells and to disable growth-promoting proteins
- Biologic therapy: monoclonal antibodies to reduce the risk of recurrence
- Bisphosphonates to promote bone density
- Antiemetics to limit chemotherapy-induced vomiting

Massage?

RISKS The risks of massage and bodywork in the context of breast cancer are the same as those for all other cancers: accessible tumors, unstable bones, compromised organs, challenges of treatment, and surgical equipment must all be accommodated. For more information about working with clients who have cancer, see Chapter 12.

BENEFITS Breast cancer was one of the first types of cancer studied for possible benefits offered by massage therapy. Among these patients it was found that massage can improve sleep, soothe anxiety, reduce depression, and help to manage pain. As long as basic precautions are taken, it is clear that massage and bodywork have much to offer this population.

Ovarian cancer

Definition: What Is It?

Ovarian cancer is the growth of malignant tumors on the ovaries. Several varieties of ovarian cancer have been identified, but most of them begin in the epithelial cells of these organs. The tumors may take a long time to become established, but once they do, some types may grow quickly and metastasize readily through the peritoneal cavity to the pelvic wall and other organs.

Ovarian cancer is diagnosed in about 22,000 women in this country each year. Although the numbers of women with this disease is low compared to those of other cancers, its mortality rate is high: ovarian cancer kills about 15,000 women every year.

Etiology: What Happens?

The ovaries, by definition, are made primarily of cells that are primed for reproduction; this makes it vulnerable to the DNA mutations that can lead to malignancy and metastasis. Furthermore, they are located in close contact with several other organs, so the seeding of malignant cells via direct extension, through the peritoneal cavity, or through the circulatory or lymph systems happens easily. This all develops without major symptoms, which is why most diagnoses of ovarian cancer are made at Stage III or IV (Figure 11.9).

Although the specific triggers for the growth of tumors on the ovaries are unknown, some of the most important risk factors for developing the disease have been identified:

- *Familial history.* A significant risk factor for ovarian cancer is having it in the family. Women who have a first-degree relative (mother, sister, or daughter) with ovarian cancer have a roughly 1 in 3 chance of developing the cancer themselves. Having a second-degree relative (grandmother, aunt, half-sister) with ovarian cancer also increases the chance of developing the disease. Families with a history of breast or colorectal cancer have statistically higher rates of ovarian cancer than the general population. This is true especially if identified breast or colorectal cancer genes are present.
- *Reproductive history.* Women who never have a break in their menstrual cycle (i.e., never been pregnant or taken birth control pills) are at significantly increased risk for this disease. This supports a theory that ovarian cancer may be related to ovulation trauma: the ovaries must heal every time an egg is released, and this wear and tear may trigger genetic mutations in ovary cells. In addition, women who have taken fertility drugs without conceiving and bearing a child may also be at increased risk, although the statistics for these women have been inconsistent.
- *Hormone replacement therapy.* Women who have employed HRT have a higher chance of developing ovarian cancer than others. This is most likely when a woman who had a hysterectomy used estrogen alone for more than 10 years.
- *Other.* Other risks include exposure to radiation or asbestos, the use of talcum powder on the genitals, a high-fat diet, and age; the chance of developing ovarian cancer goes up considerably between age 40 and 60.

Ovarian Cancer in Brief

Pronunciation: o-VARE-e-an KAN-ser

What is it?
Ovarian cancer is the development of malignant tumors on the ovaries that may metastasize to other structures in the pelvic or abdominal cavity.

How is it recognized?
Symptoms of ovarian cancer are generally subtle until the disease has progressed to life-threatening levels. Early symptoms include a feeling of heaviness in the pelvis, vague abdominal discomfort, occasional vaginal bleeding, and weight gain or loss.

Massage risks and benefits

Risks: As with all cancers, the risks of massage for ovarian cancer patients depend on both the cancer and the treatments the patient is using. Ovarian cancer patients usually undergo aggressive therapies, so their overall resilience is often extremely challenged.

Benefits: As long as accommodations are made for surgery, chemotherapy and other interventions, bodywork can be a useful intervention for anxiety, insomnia, pain and depression during an extremely trying, and often life-threatening process.

Types of Ovarian Cancer

- *Adenocarcinoma of the ovary*: These epithelial cell tumors comprise about 90% of all ovarian cancer diagnoses. Several subcategories have been identified with varying growth patterns. Some are entirely benign; some are not threatening, but others aggressively invade other abdominal and pelvic organs, often without major symptoms.
- *Germ cell ovarian cancer*: These rare tumors occur most often in women under 30 years old. Several subtypes have been identified, but the prognosis is generally positive.
- *Stromal cell ovarian cancer*: These rare tumors can be benign or malignant. They grow in the connective tissue and hormone-producing cells of the ovaries, so symptoms often have to do with excessive estrogen or testosterone. The prognosis for stromal cell ovarian cancer is usually good.

Signs and Symptoms

The feature that makes ovarian cancer an especially dangerous disease is that early symptoms are practically silent, or so subtle that they are easily passed over. When the cancer is finally identified, often it has already metastasized.

Symptoms of ovarian cancer include a feeling of heaviness in the pelvis; vague abdominal discomfort, including bloating, nausea, diarrhea, and constipation; urinary frequency or urgency; vaginal bleeding; a change in menstrual cycles; and weight gain or loss. Because the most common age for women to be affected by ovarian cancer is also the time when symptoms of perimenopause develop, these signals are easily ignored. Later symptoms can include a palpable abdominal mass, increased girth around the abdomen, and ascites—the accumulation of fluid in the peritoneum.

NOTABLE CASES Mary Tudor, also known as "Bloody Mary" for her relentless persecution of Protestants during her time as Queen of England, is believed to have died of uterine or ovarian cancer at age 42. More recently, civil rights activist Coretta Scott King and actors Madeline Kahn and Gilda Radner succumbed to ovarian cancer. Oscar-winning actor Kathy Bates and US Congresswoman Rosa de Lauro are both long-term ovarian cancer survivors.

Ovarian cancer survivor, triathlete, and Licensed Massage Therapist Jenn Sommerman's response to her experience is this: "I am doing 50 triathlons in all 50 states by the time I am 50 years old to raise $100,000 for ovarian cancer research. As a survivor, I am passionate about finding a method of early detection for this deadly 'silent killer.'"

Treatment

Ovarian cancer is generally treated according to stage (see Sidebar 11.7 for staging protocols). Surgery and chemotherapy are the usual first-line strategies. Surgery removes the ovaries (**oophorectomy**) and often the uterine tubes and uterus as well. Surgical "debulking" removes of as

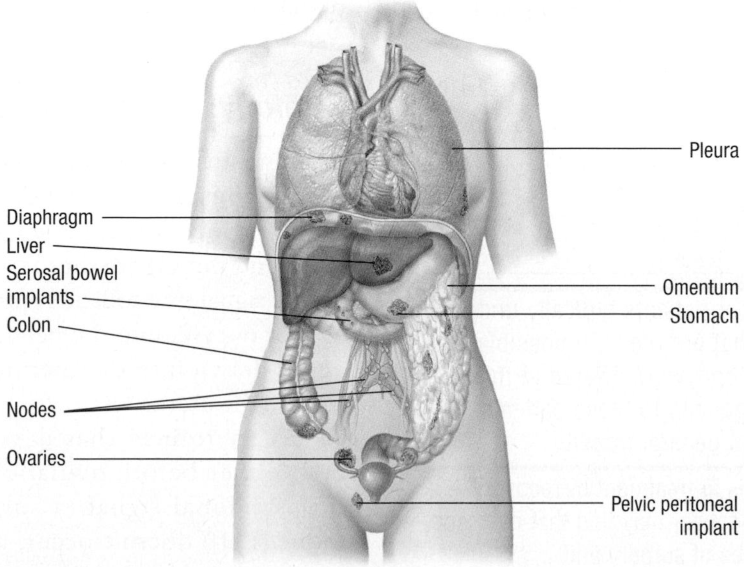

Figure 11.9. Metastasis of ovarian cancer

SIDEBAR 11.7 Staging Ovarian Cancer

The Fédération Internationale de Gynécologie et d' Obstétrique (FIGO) has developed the most commonly used staging system for ovarian cancer. The tumors are described as being superficial or deep, and the capsule around the tumor is either intact or ruptured. Here is a simplified version of the FIGO system for ovarian cancer staging:

Stage	Subdivisions of Stages
I: Growth limited to ovaries	IA: One ovary affected; tumor deep; capsule intact; no ascites IB: Two ovaries affected; tumors deep; capsules intact IC: Tumor(s) superficial; capsule(s) ruptured; cancer cells in peritoneal fluid
II: One or both ovaries involved; extensions into pelvis	IIA: Metastases to uterus and/or uterine tubes IIB: Metastases to other pelvic organs IIC: Metastases to uterus, tubes, other pelvic organs
III: One or both ovaries involved; cells in peritoneal fluid; possible metastases in abdomen	IIIA: Metastases limited to pelvis; no lymph nodes involved IIIB: Tumors <2 cm outside pelvis; no lymph nodes involved IIIC: Tumors >2 cm outside pelvis; lymph nodes may be involved
IV: Distant metastases	Metastases in liver or lungs

much cancerous tissue as possible. This may involve taking out parts of the large or small intestines or other structures. Chemotherapy can be administered orally at home, intravenously, or directly into the peritoneum, where it can have immediate access to malignant tumors. Radiation is seldom used for ovarian cancer itself, but may sometime be employed as adjunctive therapy.

Medications

- Chemotherapeutic agents by mouth, IV, or directly into the peritoneum
- Biologic therapies are sometimes used but have not been approved for ovarian cancer treatment

Massage?

RISKS Ovarian cancer patients typically undergo treatments that are rife with possible negative side effects. Any bodywork offered in this setting must be carefully gauged to these patients' capacity for adaptation and general fragility.

BENEFITS A client who is in treatment or recovery from ovarian cancer may find that massage can ameliorate the challenges of surgery and chemotherapy.

Ovarian Cysts

Definition: What Are They?

A variety of cysts may grow on the ovaries. They may be related to endometriosis, or they may be types of precancerous growths that eventually develop into ovarian cancer. Most cysts however arise from normal ovaries, either just before or just after ovulation. For this reason they are often called functional cysts.

Etiology: What Happens?

Each month a fertile woman develops several follicles (pockets where eggs are held) on one of her ovaries. As her cycle progresses, a single follicle becomes dominant and the others recede. At the appropriate hormonal signal, the follicle ruptures, releasing a mature egg, or oocyte, into the pelvic cavity. From there the egg is drawn into the uterine tubes for the journey toward the uterus.

Every follicle that develops could become a cyst, either before ovulation or after. Sometimes the hormonal signal (a surge in luteinizing hormone [LH]) doesn't occur, and the follicle doesn't rupture completely. Consequently, a blister forms on the ovary, locking the egg inside. Sometimes

Ovarian Cysts in Brief

Pronunciation: o-VARE-e-an SISTS

What are they?
Most ovarian cysts are fluid-filled growths on the ovaries. Some types of cysts are associated with ovarian cancer, but the cysts considered in this discussion are benign.

How are they recognized?
Ovarian cysts may have no signs or symptoms, or they may cause a disruption in the menstrual cycle. Constant or intermittent pain in the pelvis, pain with intercourse, or symptoms similar to early pregnancy may arise from some ovarian cysts.

Massage risks and benefits
Risks: Diagnosed ovarian cysts contraindicate intrusive abdominal massage, which could cause them to rupture and bleed. A client with painful symptoms of ovarian cysts that persist for more than a few days would be well-advised to get a formal diagnosis.
Benefits: Massage has no specific benefits for ovarian cysts. A client with this condition can enjoy the benefits of any bodywork that does not threaten to mechanically disrupt a cyst, and clients who have had cysts in the past with no current symptoms can receive massage or bodywork without restrictions.

the ruptured follicle (now called the corpus luteum) seals up behind the discharged ovum, trapping the hormones that should flow freely from it. This kind of blister may eventually break and bleed into the pelvic cavity.

The reasons some women develop cysts and others do not are complex and multifactoral. Estrogen dominance may play a role, as well as hypersensitivity to gonadotropin-stimulating hormone. Infertility treatments (which drastically alter hormone levels) can also cause ovarian cysts to develop.

Size is the major factor that determines whether or not ovarian cysts cause any trouble. They can grow big enough to interfere with blood flow; they may also rest on the bladder. In rare cases they grow to incredible dimensions. An ovarian cyst that hangs from a stalk sometimes gets twisted; this is called torsion. Large cysts can also cause the whole ovary to twist. If a torsion develops, acute abdominal pain, nausea, and fever develop; medical intervention is necessary, as the tissue may become necrotic. The risk of peritonitis is high in this situation.

Perhaps the most serious complicating factor of ovarian cysts is that their early symptoms, subtle as they may be, mimic an advanced case of ovarian cancer. This is a threatening cancer that has few early symptoms. By the time a person can feel a firm, painless swelling in her pelvis, the disease is dangerously advanced. Therefore, if a client displays any of these symptoms but has not been examined, it is important for her to get more information as soon as possible.

Types of Ovarian Cysts

- *Follicular cysts.* When a follicle that holds a mature egg doesn't rupture completely, a blister forms at the site; this occurs before ovulation. Follicular cysts rarely get bigger than 2 to 3 inches across, and they usually spontaneously recede within two menstrual cycles (Figure 11.10). Follicular cysts are the most common ovarian cysts.
- *Corpus luteum cysts.* Blisters can form over the corpus luteum, which blocks the hormones that should be secreted from the ovaries. This happens after ovulation. Corpus luteum cysts delay subsequent ovulations and produce symptoms mimicking pregnancy (nausea, vomiting, breast tenderness) until they spontaneously resolve, usually within a month or two. Corpus luteum cysts are less common than follicular cysts, but they can be more serious, as they may rupture and bleed.

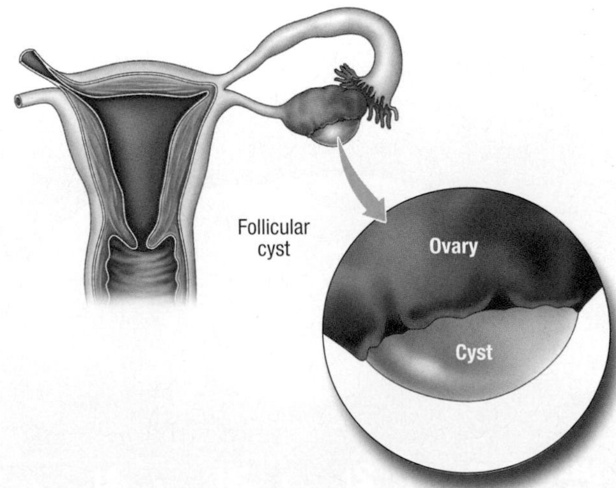

Figure 11.10. Follilcular cyst

- *Polycystic ovary syndrome*. Also called Stein-Leventhal syndrome, this condition is characterized by enlarged ovaries with multiple small cysts that are immature follicles with no ovulation (Figure 11.11). The changes in hormone secretion that this condition produces may lead to loss of menstrual cycle, acne, and **hirsutism** (thickened body hair, especially on the face and legs). Polycystic ovary syndrome (PCOS) is also closely linked to poor insulin sensitivity, high triglycerides, low high-density lipoproteins, and other signs associated with metabolic syndrome, diabetes, and heart disease.
- *Endometriomas*: These are pockets of endometrial cells on the ovaries as a part of endometriosis. They are sometimes called chocolate cysts.
- *Dermoid cysts*: In dermoid cysts, also called **teratomas**, some primitive cells have been isolated from the rest of the body, and these develop into various types of tissues. Dermoid cysts may contain teeth, hairs, bone fragments, and other types of tissue. They are usually harmless in women, although they can limit ovarian function. Men can develop them too, but for males teratomas are a much more serious condition that may lead to testicular cancer
- *Cystadenomas*: These are usually benign fluid-filled cysts on the surface of the ovary, but they bear watching, because they can develop malignant characteristics.

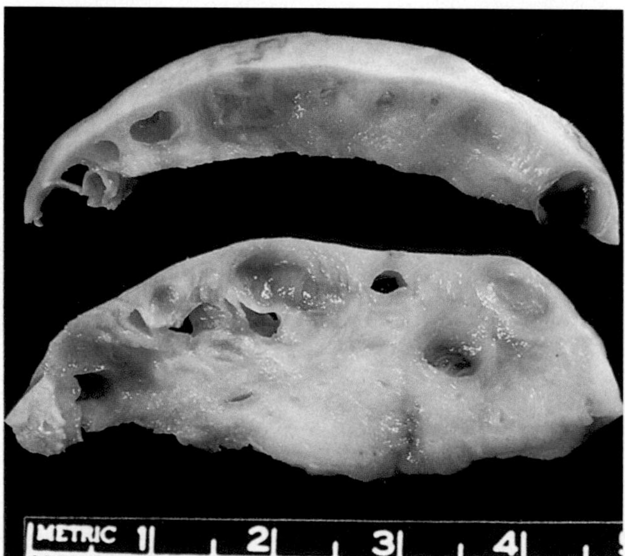

Figure 11.11. Polycystic ovary

Signs and Symptoms

Most ovarian cysts have no symptoms until the cyst is injured in some way. Some women however, have a dull ache in the lower abdomen on the affected side. A firm, painless swelling may develop in the pelvis, and occasionally an ovarian cyst causes pain with intercourse. Large cysts may cause low back pain or, through pressure on the lumbar plexus, pain in the legs.

In the absence of these signs, a person might never know a cyst is there unless it grows big enough to interfere with other functions, or if it twists or ruptures.

Treatment

Follicular and corpus luteum cysts are often treated with watchful waiting to make sure they resolve. Oral contraceptives alter hormonal secretions and prevent new cysts from forming.

Surgery may be recommended if hormone treatment is not successful. This can be in the form a closed laparoscopy or an open laparotomy, depending on the type of cyst and the risks involved. In some cases, complete removal of the ovaries and uterus is recommended because some types of cysts tend to recur and can develop into cancer.

Medications

- Oral birth control pills
- Luteinizing hormone analogs for PCOS
- Anti-androgenizing hormones if birth control pills are unsuccessful

Massage?

RISKS Ovarian cysts locally contraindicate intrusive abdominal massage. Cysts can be quite large, and they can cause the pelvic contents to shift so that structures are vulnerable outside of their usual locations. Pressure may cause them to rupture and bleed, which can be a medical emergency. Clients with polycystic ovary syndrome are at increased risk for diabetes and metabolic syndrome, each of which has its own set of cautions for bodywork.

BENEFITS While massage is unlikely to change the course of ovarian cysts for the better, simple precautions can allow clients with this condition to receive many benefits from bodywork. A history of ovarian cysts with no current symptoms carries no cautions for massage.

Disorders of the Male Reproductive System

Benign Prostatic Hyperplasia

Definition: What Is It?

Benign prostatic hyperplasia (BPH) is a condition in which the prostate gland of mature men grows new cells and becomes enlarged. This growth late in life is not related to prostate cancer, hence the name "benign." For more information on BPH vocabulary, see Sidebar 11.8.

Nearly 50% of men over 60 years old have some level of BPH; 70% of men over 70 have it; 80% of men over 80 have it, and so on. Approximately 14 million men in the United States have been diagnosed with this condition, although many of them do not experience significant symptoms.

SIDEBAR 11.8 Vocabulary Check: Hypertrophy v. Hyperplasia: A Small but Important Difference

In discussions of prostate enlargement, the terms *hypertrophy* and *hyperplasia* are sometimes used interchangeably. This is understandable, because both of them suggest an increase in size. But they mean two different things, and it is important to be accurate.

Hypertrophy means each cell in the tissue under discussion gets larger, but the structure does not grow new cells. For instance, when we exercise and our muscles get bigger, it is because each muscle cell is expanding—we are not adding to our total number of muscle cells.

Hyperplasia means the cells stay the same size, but the structure grows more of them. This is the case with tumors, for instance. Benign prostastic hyperplasia then describes a prostate that grows new cells—not cancerous ones, but because its symptoms are so similar to those of prostate cancer, it is wise to track this process carefully.

Benign Prostatic Hyperplasia (BPH) in Brief

Pronunciation: be-NINE pros-TAT-ik hi-per-PLA-zhah

What is it?
BPH is a condition in which the prostate gland of a mature man begins to grow for the first time since the end of puberty. It is not related to cancer, which is why this condition is called "benign."

How is it recognized?
The primary symptoms of BPH have to do with mechanical obstruction of the urethra. This leads to problems with urination, including a feeling of urgency, difficulties with initiating flow, leaking, and the sensation that the bladder is never emptied. Obstructions may also raise the risk of urinary tract infection or kidney irritation. For many men however, BPH is a silent condition.

Massage risks and benefits
Risks: Bodywork has no particular risks for men with BPH as long as they are free from urinary tract infection or kidney disorders.
Benefits: Bodywork is unlikely to have a directly positive effect on BPH, but as long as they are comfortable on the table, clients with this condition can enjoy the same benefits from massage as the rest of the population.

Etiology: What Happens?

The prostate gland of a preadolescent male is very small. As a boy enters puberty, this pea-sized gland that wraps around the urethra just below the bladder grows approximately to the size of a walnut. It stays that size until a man is 25 to 40 years old, and then some prostates begin to grow again.

It is unclear why some prostate glands grow and others do not. Theories about triggers for late prostate growth involve hormonal changes with maturity. One possible factor may be the formation of dihydrotestosterone (DHT). This hormone is a form of testosterone that has been seen to increase prostate size. Another theory is that as men age, they produce less testosterone to balance out their normal levels of estrogen plus estrogen from outside sources; this may lead to hyperplasia, as estrogen is also associated with prostate growth.

Regardless of the cause of prostate growth, BPH may lead to mechanical pressure on the urethra (Figure 11.12). This occurs for two reasons: the prostate is surrounded by a tough fascial capsule that does not allow it to expand outward, and the tissue usually affected by BPH is in the periurethral and transitional sections of the gland. (This helps to distinguish BPH

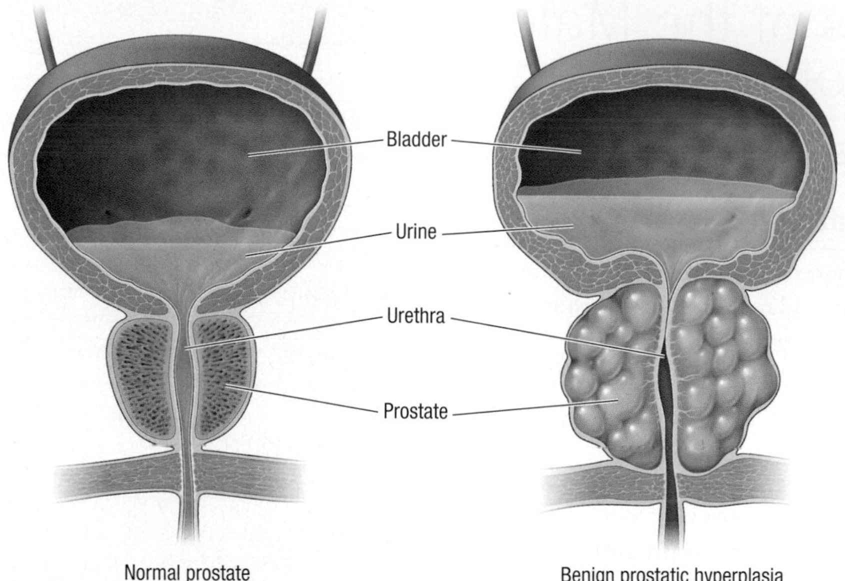

Figure 11.12. Benign prostatic hyperplasia

from prostate cancer, which typically begins on the outer borders of the prostate.)

The extent of growth does not always correspond with the amount of pressure on the urethra; some men have advanced BPH with no urinary symptoms at all, while others have minimal amounts of prostate growth and severe urethral constriction.

Mechanical pressure on the urethra makes it difficult to expel urine from the body. Long-term consequences can include pathological changes in the bladder, which can become stiff, inelastic, and irritable. The risk of urinary tract infections, pyelonephritis, and bladder stones is much higher in men who cannot urinate easily; these are common complications of BPH.

Signs and Symptoms

Signs and symptoms of BPH, when any develop at all, involve difficulties with urination. Weak flow, interrupted flow, frequency, and a feeling that the bladder is never completely emptied are often reported. Leaking or dribbling urine between visits to the bathroom is common. Some men find it difficult to initiate urination, and they must strain or push to start their flow. Other men find that they need to urinate more frequently, especially at night. BPH does not typically cause pelvic pain, which distinguishes it from prostatitis.

One rare but serious sign of BPH is an abrupt obstruction of the urethra, called acute urinary retention. In this situation the urethra is suddenly completely obstructed and urine has no way to get out of the body. This situation is often associated with the use of over-the-counter cold or allergy medications. It is a medical emergency, and must be treated in a hospital.

Treatment

BPH is treated according to severity. If it does not seriously affect a man's ability to urinate, it may be left untreated but closely monitored for signs of further growth. A number of options have been developed to limit prostate growth, including medications and a variety of minimally invasive surgeries.

Medications for BPH include drugs designed to lower levels of DHT, the testosterone derivative believed to stimulate prostate growth, and alpha-blockers. These are a group of medications originally developed to treat high blood pressure that help the prostate and bladder neck to relax. The side effects of these medications can be significant, however, including inability to achieve erection, lowered sex drive, lowered sperm counts, dizziness, fatigue, and others.

Surgical options for BPH include a variety of techniques that cut away, vaporize, burn, microwave, or otherwise remove small sections of the prostate gland to relieve pressure on the urethra.

Medications

- Hormones to alter prostate cell behavior
- Alpha-blockers to relax smooth muscle tissue and improve urinary symptoms

Massage?

RISKS If a client with benign prostatic hyperplasia (BPH) reports any symptoms of a urinary tract or kidney infection, it is important that he get appropriate care as soon as possible. Otherwise massage carries no specific risks for a client with BPH.

BENEFITS Most bodywork is safe and appropriate for clients who have BPH, as long as they are comfortable receiving it, but massage is unlikely to have a direct effect on prostate size.

OPTIONS Practitioners trained in visceral manipulation report that clients with BPH may experience some symptomatic relief with careful abdominopelvic bodywork. It is important to work knowledgeably in this area, and to rule out the risk of prostate cancer.

Prostate Cancer

Definition: What Is It?

Prostate cancer is the growth of malignant tumor cells in the prostate gland. This cancer often grows slowly, but some versions of it can be aggressive. Prostate cancer can metastasize to other parts of the body, most often the bladder, rectum, and bones of the pelvis.

Each year about 241,000 cases of prostate cancer are diagnosed in this country, and about 34,000 men die of the disease. Most patients are men over 65; prostate cancer is rare in men under 40.

NOTABLE CASES Prostate cancer is often so treatable that many of the first people who were willing to publicize their disease are still living. Politicians Bob Dole, Rudolf Giuliani and John Kerry are all prostate cancer survivors. This puts them in company with former President of South Africa Nelson Mandela, former Secretary of State Colin Powell, and musician, artist and activist Harry Belafonte.

Sadly, the diagnosis of prostate cancer came too late for actor Telly Savalas, musician Frank Zappa, and two-time Nobel Prize winner Linus Pauling, PhD.

Prostate Cancer in Brief

Pronunciation: PROS-tate KAN-ser

What is it?

Prostate cancer is the growth of malignant cells in the prostate gland, which may metastasize, usually to nearby bones or into pelvic or inguinal lymph nodes.

How is it recognized?

The symptoms of prostate cancer include problems with urination: weak stream, frequency, urgency, nocturia, all arising from constriction of the urethra. Later symptoms include blood in the urine, painful ejaculation, and persistent bone pain.

Massage risks and benefits

Risks: Massage for prostate cancer patients, as with all cancer patients, must be gauged to the constitutional health and resilience of the client. Accommodations for both the disease, which may lead to bone damage, and for the treatments, which can involve anything from chemotherapy to radiation to surgery, must be individualized for each client.

Benefits: As with all cancer patients, massage that respects both the disease and the challenges presented by treatment can be an effective strategy for managing pain, insomnia, depression, anxiety, and many other complications related to this challenging disorder.

Etiology: What Happens?

The prostate is a doughnut-shaped gland that lies inferior to the bladder and encircles the male urethra. It produces the fluid that allows for the motility and viability of sperm. The prostate also controls the release of urine from the bladder. Some enlargement of the prostate in later years is a guarantee for most men. Simple enlargement with no malignant cells is benign prostatic hyperplasia (BPH). But sometimes the growth and thickening of the prostate gland is not benign; it indicates prostate cancer.

When cancerous cells begin to form a tumor in the prostate, they can exert direct pressure on the urethra. This can lead to a number of different problems, from difficulty in urinating to urgency, frequency, **nocturia**, painful ejaculation, and bladder infections. Because the symptoms of prostate cancer are so similar to those of BPH, these signs may be ignored until the urethra is seriously restricted. (Compare & Contrast 11.1.) Prostate cancer often grows slowly, and it can stay silent long enough for cells to metastasize before it is detected.

Three main red flags for prostate cancer risk have been identified from biopsied tissues. **Prostatic intrathelial neoplasia** can be rated as low grade or high grade, **atypical small acinar proliferation** is associated with a significant risk of prostate cancer, and **proliferative inflammatory atrophy** has also been associated with an increased risk. Men whose biopsies return these findings don't have prostate cancer per se, but they need to be more diligent than others about tracking their prostate health.

COMPARE & CONTRAST 11.1 Prostate Dysfunction

When the prostate gland becomes enlarged or irritated, symptoms are predictable: restriction of urinary flow, bladder irritation, and a risk of urinary tract infection that can complicate to pyelonephritis. The causes of prostate enlargement, however, are not so consistent. Benign prostatic hyperplasia (BPH) can be hard to distinguish from prostate cancer, and prostatitis adds to the general confusion. Here are some general guidelines about similarities and differences with these conditions.

CHARACTERISTICS	PROSTATE CANCER	BENIGN PROSTATIC HYPERPLASIA	PROSTATITIS
Who gets it?	Usually affects men older than 50 but can occur in younger men with certain risk factors.	Very common in mature men; incidence increases with age.	Can occur in males of any age; leading cause of visits to urologist for young men.
Signs and symptoms	Restricted urinary flow; pain with pressure on other structures or bone damage; blood in urine possible.	Restricted urinary flow, bladder irritation.	Symptoms vary with causes, but usually significant pelvic pain.
Diagnosis	DRE, PSA tests, ultrasound to evaluate risk of prostate cancer; findings confirmed with biopsy.	DRE, PSA tests, tests to measure urinary flow usually confirm BPH.	DRE, examinations of urine, semen, prostate secretions to evaluate type of prostatitis.
Treatment	Determined by age of patient, stage of cancer. Options include surgery, chemotherapy, radiation, watchful waiting.	Medications to limit prostate growth may be prescribed; surgery to enlarge passageway for urethra may be performed.	Antibiotics for infections; otherwise treated symptomatically.
Implications for massage	Therapists must adapt to chosen treatment options (see Chapter 12).	Massage has no direct effect on BPH, is safe as long as no infection is present and client is comfortable on table.	After any infection is treated massage is safe. Some pelvic pain may be referred from trigger points.

DRE, digital rectal exam; PSA, prostate-specific antigen.

The triggers for prostate cancer are unknown. However, for tumors to grow, they must have access to testosterone from fully functional testes. This disease is not seen in men who have been physically or chemically castrated, and removal of the testes shrinks cancerous tumors.

Men with prostate cancer in their immediate family are more likely than others to develop this disease. Likewise, men from families whose women have breast cancer have a higher risk. Heredity is estimated to account for about 5% to 10% of prostate cancer cases.

Signs and Symptoms

Signs of prostate cancer are similar to those for BPH: an enlarged, hard prostate; obstruction of the urethra with resulting difficulty in urination; and susceptibility to urinary tract and kidney infections. In addition, men with prostate cancer may also have pain while urinating or ejaculating, blood in the urine, and an inability to maintain an erection. Low back pain and pain that refers into the upper thighs may follow as the growths become large enough to put mechanical pressure on pelvic nerves or erode into bone tissue.

One possible sign of prostate cancer is a positive PSA (prostate-specific antigen) blood test. Its usefulness is somewhat debatable, since many variables may cause PSA levels to rise or fall, but when levels are higher than normal, this blood test can serve as a warning sign to consider the possibility of prostate cancer. For more information on PSA tests, see Sidebar 11.9.

SIDEBAR 11.9 What Does a PSA Test Tell?

One of the diagnostic procedures for prostate cancer is a blood test to measure levels of a substance called prostate specific antigen (PSA). PSA is a protein secreted by the prostate gland. Under certain circumstances levels of this protein can rise; one of those circumstances is the growth of malignant tumors in the prostate gland.

PSA tests can be used to predict the possibility of prostate cancer, to monitor the effectiveness of prostate cancer treatment, and to detect the recurrence of prostate cancer. However, lots of things can elevate PSA levels, including infection or inflammation, ejaculation within the past 24 hours, riding a bicycle, and some herbs and medications. Any of these can falsely elevate PSA levels in a blood test.

A "normal" PSA test shows fewer than 4 nanograms of this protein per milliliter of blood (ng/mL). Even at this level. Up to 15% of men tested still have prostate cancer, so this rating system may be recalibrated. PSA readings show the following for the risk of prostate cancer:

PSA levels	% Diagnosed with prostate cancer
<4 ng/mL	15%
4–10 ng/mL	25%
>10 ng/mL	>50%

A PSA test is just the beginning of gathering information about the risk of prostate cancer. Other variables include whether the PSA is free or attached to other blood proteins: higher ratios of free PSA indicate a higher chance for a nonmalignant situation, while higher ratios of attached PSA are associated with an increased risk of prostate cancer. PSA velocity (how the levels change over time), and PSA density (the relationship between PSA and the size of the prostate), and other factors can yield information about the risk of prostate cancer.

As our ability to interpret PSA tests improves, we are becoming more skilled at finding the balance between careful vigilance and the risks of overdiagnosis that is followed by invasive and unnecessary procedures.

Treatment

Treatment options for prostate cancer depend on the stage at which it is diagnosed. For information on staging prostate cancer, see Sidebar 11.10. Treatments include watchful waiting; radiation from surgically implanted pellets (this is called **brachytherapy**) or external beams or precisely aimed protons; surgery to remove part or all of the prostate, seminal vesicles, or testes; and hormone therapy to counteract elevated levels of testosterone. Chemotherapy is generally reserved for very advanced cases. The "training" of white blood cells to attack cancer cells is a form of vaccine that is also used in advanced cases.

Most treatment options for prostate cancer have daunting side effects, including temporary or permanent incontinence, erectile dysfunction, sterility, and the development of feminine characteristics. For these reasons, elderly men or men with other health problem who have slow-growing tumors may opt not to treat their disease because their quality of life would be so seriously affected.

Medications

- Hormone therapy to interfere with cancer cell receptors or suppress testosterone production
- Analgesics for pain management
- Bisphosphonates to maintain or recover bone density
- Chemotherapeutic agents for advanced disease
- Biologic therapy to sensitize white blood cells to attack cancer cells

Massage?

RISKS Any massage therapists who number elderly men among their clientele will have some clients living with the threat of prostate cancer. This condition can be slow-growing and relatively nonthreatening, but it can also be aggressive. Any bodywork must accommodate not only prostate cancer but also whatever treatment options the client has chosen to pursue. Clients who have chosen brachytherapy are best delaying massage until the radioactive pellets have been removed.

BENEFITS Massage is a wonderful option deal with the often under-addressed issues related to cancer: depression, anxiety, insomnia, and general pain. For more information on massage in the context of cancer, see Chapter 12.

SIDEBAR 11.10 Staging Prostate Cancer

Most specialists in the United States use the tumor, node, metastasis (TNM) staging system for prostate cancer, in combination with a cancer cell rating system, the Gleason scale. This rates cells according to their appearance and aggressiveness; a low score suggests a less threatening problem, and a higher score means a more threatening problem. The Gleason ratings range from 2 to 10, but may be doubled if multiple neoplasms are found in the prostate.

Prostate cancer, like some other cancers, sometimes cannot be fully staged until surgery is conducted and tissue is examined. The following is a combination of clinical staging (based on best estimates without surgery) and pathological staging (based on findings during or after surgery).

Tumor	Tumor Substage	Node	Metastasis
T1: tumor cannot be palpated or found with transrectal ultrasound	T1A: tumor found with treatment for BPH; affects <5% of tissue T1B: tumor found with treatment for BPH; affects >5% of tissue T1C: tumor found with needle biopsy, elevated PSA levels	N0: no nodes involved N1: ≥1 regional nodes involved	M0: no metastasis M1: Distant metastasis
T2: tumor palpable with DRE; confined to the prostate	T2A: <50% of one side is affected T2B: >50% of one side is affected T2C: both sides affected		
T3: tumors outside prostate and/or on seminal vesicles	T3A: tumors outside prostate but not on seminal vesicles T3B: tumors on seminal vesicles		
T4: tumors on other tissues, including bladder and wall of pelvis			

The TNM ratings are then combined with Gleason scores to stage prostate cancer from stage I to IV in this way:

Stage	Tumor	Node	Metastasis	PSA	Gleason score
I	T1A or 2A	N0	M0	<10	<6
II	T1–2	N0–1	M0	10–20	2–10
III	T3	N0	M0	any	Any
IV	Any	N0	M0	any	Any
IV	Any	Any	M1	any	Any

Prostatitis

Definition: What Is It?

Prostatitis is a condition in which the prostate becomes painful and possibly inflamed. Unlike benign prostatic hyperplasia, prostatitis usually involves significant pain throughout the pelvis and groin. While occasionally connected to a specific infection, it is often difficult to identify and treat the causes of prostatitis.

Etiology: What Happens?

The prostate is a walnut-sized gland that surrounds the urethra just distal to the urinary bladder of males. It is composed of ducts and channels into which epithelial cells secrete seminal fluid, a constituent of semen. The seminal fluid is expressed into the urethra during ejaculation.

The draining channels in the prostate are arranged in a basically horizontal plane around the periphery of the organ. This allows material to become stagnant within the gland if it is not frequently expelled. Furthermore, bladder reflux, in which urine collects in the prostate, can cause irritation or even direct bacterial exposure to these delicate epithelial tissues, leading to a risk of prostate stones and acute or chronic infection that may be difficult to treat.

Prostatitis in Brief

Pronunciation: pros-tah-TY-tis

What is it?
Prostatitis is inflammation or irritation of the prostate gland, either from pathogenic or nonpathogenic causes.

How is it recognized?
Symptoms of prostatitis vary according to their cause. Acute prostatitis involves fever, extremely painful urination, urinary frequency and urgency, and pain in the penis, testicles, perineum, and low back. Chronic prostatitis has similar signs and symptoms, but they tend to be less severe, and they may not include fever.

Massage risks and benefits
Risks: A person with an acute bacterial infection of the prostate is unlikely to seek massage before other types of care, so it is unlikely that a massage therapist or bodywork practitioner will have a client with fever, malaise and debilitating pelvic pain. If that does occur, gentle noninvasive work and a recommendation to consult a primary care provider are the best options.
Benefits: A person who has a chronic condition with no acute signs of infection may receive massage without risk, as long as he is comfortable on the table.

Prostatitis is an umbrella term for four basic types of problems. These classes of prostatitis were outlined by the National Institute of Health in 1995 to create a framework for more efficient study of this often mysterious and difficult problem.

Types of Prostatitis

- *Type 1, Acute bacterial prostatitis*: This is an acute infection of the prostate. This may be accompanied by an abscess, which requires surgical removal.
- *Type 2, Chronic bacterial prostatitis*: This is a recurrent infection of the prostate. The most common infectious agent for types 1 and 2 is *E. Coli*.
- *Type 3, Chronic nonbacterial prostatitis/chronic pelvic pain syndrome (CPPS)*: This is prostate irritation with no demonstrable infection. Subgroups of this class include these:
    - *Type 3a, Inflammatory CPPS*: White blood cells are found in the semen, expressed prostatic secretions, or urine.
    - *Type 3b, Noninflammatory CPPS*: White blood cells are not found in semen, expressed prostatic secretions, or urine. This is by far the most commonly reported version of prostatitis. It is not well understood, because no specific causative factors have been identified. Some experts suggest that CPPS may be due to bacteria that are difficult to culture and treat; others think that chronic hypertonicity or trigger points are referring pain from the perineal muscle; this suggests that some cases may be related to myofascial pain.
- Type *4, Asymptomatic inflammatory prostatitis*: This has no subjective symptoms, but white blood cells are found in prostate secretions or in prostate tissue during an evaluation for other disorders.

Signs and Symptoms

Acute bacterial prostatitis has all of the signs and symptoms of a urinary tract infection: pain and burning with urination along with urinary frequency and urgency. In addition, pain in the pelvis, perineum, testicles, and penis may be present, along with penile discharge, painful ejaculation, possible erectile dysfunction, low back pain, and fever. The prostate, palpated through the wall of the rectum, is exquisitely painful and palpably hot.

Chronic bacterial prostatitis, which indicates recurrent low-grade infection, produces the same symptoms, but with less severity.

CPPS has the same profile without the element of fever, and palpation of the prostate often shows no inflammation.

Treatment

Acute bacterial prostatitis responds well to antibiotics, but chronic bacterial prostatitis does not. It may take 6 weeks or more of antibiotic therapy, and it frequently recurs.

If prostate stones are discovered, they are surgically removed, typically with laser surgery through the urethra.

Chronic pelvic pain is often treated with a short or long course of antibiotics just in case some bacteria were missed, and then dealt with symptomatically. Alpha-blockers relax the smooth muscle tissue in the bladder for easier urination; anti-inflammatories, frequent ejaculations, and sitz baths (a bath just for the pelvic area) to help relax the perineal muscle are also recommended. Antianxiety medications are sometimes prescribed. Biofeedback techniques to increase awareness of tightness in the perineal muscle have some success, as do some dietary supplements and some forms of acupuncture. For many men, however, CPPS is a stubborn disorder with no simple answers; it can have a long-term and severe impact on their quality of life.

Medications

- Antibiotics for bacterial infection
- Anti-inflammatories and analgesics for chronic pain
- Alpha blockers to improve urine flow
- Antianxiety medication for chronic pain

Massage?

RISKS When acute infection with fever and inflammation is present, invasive or rigorous massage is inappropriate.

BENEFITS Massage is unlikely to have a direct impact on prostate irritation, but anything that can improve the quality of life for a patient with a chronic, non-acute problem can be helpful.

OPTIONS It is possible that some pelvic pain is related to trigger points in the perineal muscle that refer to the pelvic cavity. That makes this a musculoskeletal condition. In most massage laws, however, work on the perineal muscle is not within the scope of practice for massage therapists.

Testicular Cancer

Definition: What Is It?

Testicular cancer is growth of malignant cells in the testicles. These cells usually grow slowly, but they may metastasize through the lymph or blood systems to the bones, liver, lungs and brain.

Testicular cancer is diagnosed about 8,000 times per year and causes about 400 deaths per year in this country. It is most often found in white men between 20 and 55 years old, but it has been found in males of any age and race.

> **Testicular Cancer in Brief**
>
> Pronunciation: tes-TIK-yu-lar KAN-ser
>
> **What is it?**
> Testicular cancer is the growth of malignant cells in the testicles, which may metastasize to the rest of the body.
>
> **How is it recognized?**
> Early signs of testicular cancer include a painless lump in the scrotum, a dull ache in the low abdomen or groin, a sense of heaviness in the scrotum, and enlarged or tender breasts.
>
> **Massage risks and benefits**
> ***Risks:*** The risks of bodywork for a client with testicular cancer are the same as those for other cancers: the challenges presented by both the disease and its treatments must be accommodated. Because this type of cancer is often very treatable, patients may be more resilient and less fragile than some other cancer patients.
> ***Benefits:*** As long as bodywork is within a client's tolerance for adaptation, massage for testicular cancer patients can be a helpful tool to deal with some of the common complications of cancer in general: anxiety, pain, depression, insomnia, and poor appetite.

Etiology: What Happens?

As with many other cancers, testicular cancer begins with a mutation to fast-growing cells that causes them to pile up into tumors that can invade healthy tissue. The causes or contributing factors of testicular cancer are not well understood. The only consistent risk factor is that males who were born with an undescended testicle (**cryptorchidism**) have a slightly higher risk of developing this disease. Other risk factors include other congenital abnormalities, age, race, personal or family history of testicular cancer, and HIV status: men who are HIV positive have a slightly higher risk of testicular cancer than others.

Types of Testicular Cancer

- *Germ cell tumors*: These are tumors that arise within the sperm and hormone-producing cells

SIDEBAR 11.11 Staging Testicular Cancer

Testicular cancer is staged differently from most other cancers; instead of progressing from Stage 0 to Stage IV, it is usually discussed as Stages 0 to III. Specialists use highly defined and detailed staging protocols to make appropriate treatment plans and prognoses. These often include measurements of cancer markers in the blood along with tumor, node, and metastatic progress. The following is a simplified version of testicular cancer staging:

- Stage 0. This is cancer in situ: preinvasive germ cell cancer.
- Stage I. The testicle and spermatic cord are affected; no spread to lymph nodes; blood tests are normal.
- Stage II. Nearby lymph nodes are invaded.
- Stage IIA. The nodes show signs of microscopic invasion. This is sometimes called "nonbulky stage II."
- Stage IIB. The nodes are larger than 5 cm; this can be called "bulky stage II."
- Stage III. Distant lymph nodes and other tissues are invaded.
- Stage IIIA. Only lymph nodes are invaded, but growths are smaller than 2 cm (nonbulky stage III).
- Stage IIIB. Other tissues are invaded, usually the central nervous system and/or lungs. Lymph node metastases are larger than 2 cm (bulky stage III).

of the testicle. Germ cell tumors are further classified into seminomas and nonseminomas.

- *Seminomas*: These are the most common variety of testicular cancer, accounting for 40% to 45% of diagnoses. They tend to grow slowly and are highly sensitive to radiation.
- *Nonseminomas*: These are several different types of testicular tumors, some of which are more aggressive than others. Embryonic carcinomas, yolk sac tumors, and teratomas are growths that resemble the growth pattern of embryos. Choriocarcinoma is the most aggressive form of testicular cancer, and has the poorest prognosis.

- *Stromal cell tumors*: These are growths within the supportive tissue for the testicle. They are quite rare and account for only 5% or less of testicular cancers.

Signs and Symptoms

Testicular cancer usually begins with a painless lump on the testicle. It may be accompanied by a feeling of fullness or heaviness or fluid in the scrotum. A dull ache in the low abdomen or groin may develop, along with enlargement and tenderness at the breasts. If any of these symptoms persist for more than 2 weeks, the person should consult his physician as soon as possible.

Later signs of testicular cancer indicate metastasis: coughing and shortness of breath if tumors have invaded the lungs, painless lumps in the neck if the cervical lymph nodes are affected, and so on.

NOTABLE CASES Perhaps the most famous public figure with testicular cancer is multiple Tour de France winner bicyclist Lance Armstrong, who was diagnosed with a combination of non-seminoma growths that had metastasized to his lungs and brain. Other familiar names include Olympic figure skater Scott Hamilton, the subject of the movie "Brian's Song" football player Brian Piccolo, and actor and comedian Richard Belzer, who, coincidentally, produced a CD titled, "Another Lone Nut."

Treatment

The treatment options for testicular cancer depend on the stage at diagnosis (see Sidebar 11.11), but they usually begin with surgery to remove the affected testicle and any secondary tumors that are found. If the cancer is identified as a seminoma, radiation therapy follows surgery; these cancer cells are extremely sensitive to radiation, and this protocol is usually completely successful. If the cancer was a mixed tumor or a nonseminoma, chemotherapy may be used following surgery.

Depending on the findings in the removed tissue, a second surgery may be conducted to take lymph nodes from the pelvis or abdomen. This is a more invasive procedure that has a higher risk of complications, including damage to the nerves that control ejaculation which can be permanent.

Follow-up care after testicular cancer treatment is critical to make sure no metastases were missed. Furthermore, testicular cancer survivors have a small but significant risk of developing cancer in the other testicle.

The survival rate for testicular cancer is so high and the treatments available are so effective that no invasive early screening protocols for this disease have been demonstrated to improve life expectancy. Nonetheless, many men are taught to conduct testicular self-examinations, just as women are taught to do breast self-examinations. In this way any changes in the tissue may be identified and investigated as quickly as possible.

Medications

- Chemotherapeutic agents

Massage?

RISKS Most testicular cancer patients undergo cycles of radiation or chemotherapy. Any bodywork must be adjusted for these challenges.

BENEFITS Many testicular cancer patients are encouraged to exercise; this is a good sign that massage is also appropriate. Any bodywork that supports, rather than challenges, a client's capacity for adaptation is safe and appropriate in this setting, as it can help with pain, anxiety, depression, and other common cancer complications. For more information on massage in the context of cancer, see Chapter 12.

Other Reproductive System Conditions

Menopause

Definition: What Is It?

Menopause is a specific event: it describes the moment the ovaries permanently stop secreting enough hormones to initiate a menstrual cycle. The time leading up to this event and for a year after the last menstrual period is called perimenopause, and many of the symptoms associated with declining hormone secretion occur during this period. Menopause itself is not conclusively identified until a full year after the last menstrual period.

It is important to point out that menopause is not a disease: it is a normal part of aging that every woman, if she lives long enough, will experience. Nevertheless, it can cause significant symptoms that can impact function and quality of life. For more information on women's "men-" vocabulary, see Sidebar 11.12.

The average age for the onset of perimenopausal symptoms is 47.5 years; the average age at which

Menopause in Brief

Pronunciation: MEN-o-pawz

What is it?
Menopause refers to the moment when ovaries no longer respond to chemical signals to establish a reproductive cycle. Although this usually happens as a normal part of aging, menopause can be induced through surgery, radiation, or medication.

How is it recognized?
The symptoms associated with a decline in ovarian function (perimenopause) include night sweats, hot flashes, insomnia, mood swings, decreased sex drive, vaginal itchiness or dryness, urinary incontinence, and poor concentration and memory. Longer-term changes include an increased risk of osteoporosis and cardiovascular disease.

Massage risks and benefits
Risks: Massage has no particular risks for a healthy woman who is going through the changes leading up to menopause.
Benefits: Massage is unlikely to alter the course of perimenopause, but it can be a powerfully positive experience for a woman undergoing fundamental changes in her self-identity and physical processes.

SIDEBAR 11.12 Menarche, Menstruation, Menses, Menopause: What Are All These *Men* Doing In Women's Health Vocabulary?

The root word is mēn, which is Greek for "month."

- Menarche is mēn plus arche, or beginning.
- Menstruation is mēn plus atus, meaning to be menstruant.
- Menses is the plural for mēn, meaning many months.
- Menopause is mēn plus pausis, or cessation.

Another anatomic application of the moon analogy is "meniscus": this describes crescent-moon shaped cartilaginous structures found in the knee and the jaw.

the transition is final is 51.4 years. It is estimated that about 46 million women in the United States are postmenopausal, and with the increasing number of mature Americans, about 50 million women will be postmenopausal by 2020.

Etiology: What Happens?

In addition to ripening several eggs each month and releasing at least one for the possibility of fertilization, the ovaries secrete a variety of chemicals (mostly estrogen and progesterone) into the bloodstream. They do this under the control of hypothalamus and pituitary secretions of follicle-stimulating hormone (FHS) and luteinizing hormone (LH).

As ovaries age, they become less sensitive to these hormones. Consequently, FHS levels go up, but estrogen and progesterone levels go down. It is somewhat misleading to refer to estrogen and progesterone as only two hormones, as both of these substances are produced in various chemical forms, each of which is metabolized and used in different ways.

Estrogens and progesterones influence sex organs either to support a pregnancy or to shed the endometrial lining of the uterus. When the ovaries lose function, either as a normal part of aging or because their function has been interrupted by surgery, irradiation, or drugs (this is called "induced menopause"), these processes come to a stop. When a woman no longer ovulates, she no longer grows an endometrial lining in her uterus, and she no longer sheds that lining during menstruation. But these ovarian hormones also work on many other tissues in the body in ways that are only just beginning to be explored.

- *Bone density.* The role of estrogens and progesterones in maintaining bone density is complex. Estrogen inhibits osteoclast activity, that is, it helps to prevent the thinning of bone tissue. But some forms of progesterone are involved in maintaining bone density as well, stimulating osteoblast activity. In other words, estrogen prevents bone from being dissolved, while progesterone helps it to build up. When both of these are in short supply, women can lose up to 20% of their bone mass during the first years of hormonal fluctuation.
- *Cardiovascular health.* As women age, the types of cholesterol in their blood change. Premenopausal women have a higher proportion of HDLs (the "good" cholesterols), and postmenopausal women have higher levels of low-density lipoproteins and triglycerides (the "bad" types of cholesterol). In other words, the blood lipids of post-menopausal women resemble that of men, which contributes to why heart disease is the number one killer of both men and women. Further, estrogens appear to have a role in healthy endothelial growth, which influences the inner layer of blood vessels.
- *Protection from some types of cancer.* This is an extremely complex issue that reflects just how little is understood about the effects of different types of estrogens and progesterones on different types of tissues. High levels of some types of estrogen have a statistical link with lower rates of colon cancer but with higher rates of some other types of cancer, including breast and ovarian cancers. Ultimately it may be found that whether hormone levels are dangerous or protective depends on the chemical variation of the hormone, where it comes from, how it is metabolized, where it is used, and other variables that haven't even been considered yet.
- *Central nervous system functions.* Estrogen seems linked to mood, depression, and basic cognitive function. Supplementing low doses of estrogen has been seen to be effective for dealing with the mild depression, insomnia, and short-term memory loss that may accompany perimenopause, but it is not effective for more severe depressive disorders.

When the ovaries decrease hormonal production, a woman becomes dependent on other tissues to secrete enough hormones to provide for her daily function. Some fat cells and other tissues continue to produce estrogen after the ovaries atrophy, but at a fraction of previous levels. Further, while some estrogen production continues after menopause, most progesterone production does not. Combine this with exposure to excessive exogenous estrogens, and it is clear to see how the correct ratio between estrogens and progesterones is lost.

Signs and Symptoms

The symptoms of perimenopause are related to changes in hormone secretion. Symptoms generally subside when hormone levels stabilize, but this may not happen until a year or more after a final menstrual period.

SIDEBAR 11.13 Hormone Replacement Therapy (HRT)

The Women's Health Initiative was a study of 161,809 postmenopausal American women between 50 and 79 years of age. The goal was to track these participants over 8 years to gather information about health trends for older women. One question they pursued concerned the benefits and risks of the most common version of hormone replacement therapy: concentrated equine estrogens (Premarin) plus medroxyprogesterone acetate (progestin) for women who had not had a hysterectomy. This hormone supplement regimen has traditionally been prescribed to reduce perimenopausal symptoms like hot flashes and vaginal dryness, and to reduce the risk of heart disease and osteoporosis.

After 5 years of following the study participants, researchers found some surprising results. While the relative risk of osteoporosis and colorectal cancer went down as expected, all other health concerns being tracked actually increased, as follows:

Heart attack	Increased	29%
Breast cancer	Increased	26%
Stroke	Increased	41%
Blood clot in leg or lung	Increased	111%
Dementia	Increased	105%
Hip fractures (as measure of osteoporosis)	Decreased	33%
Colorectal cancer	Decreased	37%

The cardiovascular risks rose within 2 years of beginning HRT, and the increase in breast cancer risk was found after 4 years. Protection against osteoporosis was lost within 2 years of stopping therapy. These findings were so significant that it was considered unethical to keep women on HRT without informed consent, and this branch of the study was concluded in July 2002.

When the results of the WHI became public, thousands of women stopped using HRT. Interestingly, within a year the per capita diagnosis rate of breast cancer began to go down. That trend continued over several years, and statistical analysis suggests that the two phenomena are related.

Researchers have continued to look at this issue, and current findings suggest that HRT for women at the onset of perimenopause does help to manage symptoms and to reduce the risk of colorectal cancer and osteoporosis. However, the general recommendation is to encourage women to use the lowest possible dosage of hormones for the shortest period possible.

The signs and symptoms of menopause vary with each individual, but some of the most common ones are hot flashes (some women call them power surges), night sweats, insomnia, mood swings, urinary urgency, loss of urinary continence, decreased sex drive, vaginal dryness or itchiness, confusion, short-term memory loss, and poor concentration. Some of these symptoms may be interrelated: for instance, insomnia may have to do with night sweats and hot flashes; depression and decreased sex drive may have to do with a change in self-perception as a woman becomes no longer fertile. But for some women, the symptoms of perimenopause are directly linked to hormonal disruption, and taking steps to smooth out the hormonal shifts can alleviate a lot of discomfort.

The long-term consequences of menopause include pathological thinning of bones and decreased resistance to heart disease, although these phenomena are certainly controllable.

Treatment

Treatment options for the symptoms of perimenopause and the long-term consequences of reduced estrogen and progesterone secretion are many and varied. Estrogen replacement therapy provides supplements of various types of estrogens. This seems to be adequate for some women, but it doesn't address the lost balance between estrogens and progesterones that are implicated in many health issues. Further, it is appropriate only for women who have had a hysterectomy, because unopposed estrogen stimulates potentially dangerous endometrial growth.

While hormone replacement therapy (HRT) can address some symptoms of perimenopause and it can reduce the risk of osteoporosis and colorectal cancer, it is also associated with some increased risk of other problems. This is especially true for women who have supplemented hormones for prolonged periods. See Sidebar 11.13 for more information on HRT risks and benefits. Some specialists suggest that the benefits of HRT can be experienced with fewer risks if they are administered by a non-oral route, that is, by patch, cream, or vaginal suppository.

If a woman decides not to supplement hormones to treat her menopausal symptoms, she may consider other options. Medications to support bone density and decrease the risk of heart disease are possibilities, as are a variety of herbal preparations. Options include black cohosh (which should be avoided when other estrogen supplements are used), red clover, dong quai (which should not be used along with blood thinners), ginseng, wild yam, and kava (which has been associated with a risk of liver problems).

Medications

- HRT (estrogen only for women with no uterus; estrogen and progesterone for women with a uterus)
- Herbal preparations (these are not risk free; they may cause problematic interactions with other medications)
- Statins and other cardiovascular disease treatments if necessary
- Bisphosphonates for osteoporosis if necessary

Massage?

RISKS Massage and bodywork have no risks for women who are fundamentally healthy while they go through perimenopause.

BENEFITS While massage is unlikely to have a direct impact on perimenopausal processes, it may help to mitigate some of its symptoms, including mood disruptions, insomnia, and fatigue.

OPTIONS Menopause can be both tremendously challenging as a basic part of a woman's self-definition changes, and wonderfully fulfilling, as her commitments to children and parents are often tapering off, and she may be able to devote more of her time, energy, creative drive and focus to her own purposes. Massage can be a way to reinforce a sense of physical joy and wholeness during a time of great transition.

Pregnancy

Definition: What Is It?

Pregnancy, obviously, is the condition in which a woman carries a fetus.

Etiology: What Happens?

The physiologic changes that occur when a woman is pregnant are wide-ranging and complex, and this text will not pursue them fully. Instead, the most common or dangerous complications of pregnancy will be discussed, and several symptoms that many pregnant women experience that are especially pertinent to massage and bodywork will be examined.

Pregnancy in Brief

Pronunciation: PREG-nan-se

What is it?
Pregnancy is the state of carrying a fetus.

How is it recognized?
The signs and symptoms of advanced pregnancy are obvious, but symptoms that specifically pertain to massage include loose ligaments, muscle spasms, clumsiness, and fatigue.

Massage risks and benefits
Risks: The risks of bodywork for a pregnant client vary by trimester, and they may also be connected to any complications the woman experiences.
Benefits: Bodywork can be adapted for every trimester to help the mother with some of pregnancy's most common problems, including fatigue, muscle and joint pain, and clumsiness.

Types of Pregnancy Complications

- *Asthma*: Many pregnant women have asthma, and incomplete control of this condition has serious repercussions for both mother and baby. It has been linked to low birth weight and prematurity, an increased risk of cerebral palsy and mental disability, and preeclampsia. Well-controlled asthma, by contrast, is not associated with significant risks.
- *Thromboembolism*: This is a combination of deep vein thrombosis and pulmonary embolism, both of which are discussed in Chapter 6. Pregnant and newly postpartum women have approximately ten times more risk of blood clots as the nonpregnant population. The risk increases as the pregnancy develops, and is highest in the first few days after the baby is delivered. Identifying risk factors for thromboembolism may eventually lead to the use of prophylactic blood thinners during the postpartum period.
- *Gestational diabetes*: Pregnancy-related diabetes is diagnosed with a glucose tolerance test, in which the woman drinks a sweet beverage, and then her urine is examined for elevated levels of glucose. Gestational diabetes is usually identified in the fifth or sixth month of pregnancy (between 24 and 26 weeks of gestation).

If diabetes develops during pregnancy, risks to the baby and mother are significant. The rerouting of nutrients in the blood can cause babies to grow abnormally large in a condition called **macrosomia**, which may require a cesarean section. Babies born to women with gestational diabetes also have a high risk of respiratory distress syndrome, early hypoglycemia, and later obesity and type 2 diabetes.

A woman who develops gestational diabetes has a high risk of doing so again with subsequent pregnancies, and of developing type 2 diabetes later in life.

- *Pregnancy-induced hypertension*: This is a condition that generally starts mildly but can quickly become life-threatening both for the baby and the mother. It occurs in three categories: hypertension alone; **preeclampsia**, which is hypertension along with elevated proteins in the urine and possible systemic edema; and **eclampsia**, which is the same condition along with convulsions or coma.

  Most cases of pregnancy-induced hypertension occur during the first pregnancy, in teens, or in women over 40. Other women at risk include those who are obese prior to pregnancy, those who have a personal or family history of chronic high blood pressure, women carrying multiple babies, and women who have an underlying disease that can affect the circulatory system, including diabetes, lupus, and scleroderma. Treatment includes medication to bring down the blood pressure, strict bed rest, and, where appropriate, early delivery of the baby.

  A complication of pregnancy-induced hypertension is **HELLP syndrome**: hemolysis with elevated liver enzymes and low platelet count. This disorder of damaged blood cells and impaired liver function can result in bleeding and severe liver damage. Other complications of pregnancy-induced hypertension for mothers include renal failure, cerebral hemorrhage, liver damage, and retinal detachment leading to blindness. Risks to the baby include reduced growth from circulatory impairment and **placenta abruptio**, a condition in which the placenta prematurely separates from the uterus.

- *Ectopic pregnancy*: An ectopic pregnancy is a fertilized egg that implants outside of the uterus. Most ectopic pregnancies develop in the fallopian tubes; some implant in the peritoneum, on the ovaries, or on the cervix.

  Risk factors for ectopic pregnancy include IUD use; a history of PID, endometriosis, or sexually transmitted disease; and adhesions from previous abdominal surgeries. Ectopic pregnancies cannot come to term; the fallopian tube inevitably ruptures, killing the fetus and endangering the life of the mother. Ectopic pregnancies that are recognized early (usually by ultrasound and testing for hormone levels) may be terminated by medication or laparoscopic surgery, preserving the ovary and oviduct for the chance of a future successful pregnancy.

Signs and Symptoms

Pregnancy creates a wide array of signs and symptoms, and some of them have specific implications for massage. Here are some of the complaints of pregnant women that bodywork practitioners can influence:

- *Loose ligaments*: Pregnant women often experience ligament laxity, even early in fetal growth. This can lead to joint instability, including subluxations of the vertebrae and the sacroiliac joints. Muscles then work hard to stabilize the joints, causing spasm and pain.
- *Fatigue*: Pregnant women carry a lot of extra weight. The baby itself is only a fraction of the whole load, which includes the placenta, amniotic fluid, 40% more blood, and any extra fat she may accumulate during her pregnancy. In addition to carrying extra weight, a pregnant woman tends to have low blood pressure and low blood sugar, and she secretes hormones that signal her to get a lot of rest. This is a command that many pregnant women don't have the luxury of obeying, at least if they're trying to hold a job until the baby is born.
- *Shifting proprioception*: Pregnant women change their size every day. This is true especially in the last trimester, when the baby grows at an astounding rate. The result is that a pregnant woman never knows exactly how much room she takes up. Her sense of where in space her body ends and the rest of the world begins is very shaky. This, along with newly loose ligaments and a shifted center of gravity, tends to make a pregnant woman clumsy and prone to injury. Massage provides an extraordinary sense of where bodies are in space. It can improve

proprioceptive senses by giving continuous and accurate feedback about boundaries.

- *Depression*: Many women experience anxiety and depression in a new pattern when they are pregnant. This condition can significantly alter her quality of life and interfere with her ability to bond with and enjoy her child.

Treatment

No medical treatment for an uncomplicated pregnancy is necessary.

Treatment for pregnancy complications obviously depends on the situation. They may include anticoagulants, antihypertensive drugs, steroids and other anti-inflammatories for asthma, antidepressants, and others.

Massage?

RISKS First trimester: from the time a woman knows she is pregnant until she delivers, intrusive work in the abdomen is contraindicated. Practitioners of acupressure or shiatsu may also suggest against specific points that are believed to trigger uterine contractions.

Second trimester: this is the most stable, least risky phase of pregnancy. At some point during this time, it will no longer be comfortable for a client to lay prone without special accommodations in the way of support cushions, extensive bolstering, or a specially designed pregnancy table.

Third trimester: during this time, a woman may not be able to lay prone or supine, as reclining allows the fetus to compress major blood vessels which can lead to dizziness and/or muscle cramps (Figure 11.13). In addition, the risk of blood clots causing deep vein thrombosis and the possibility of pulmonary embolism is high at this time, and through the first few weeks post-partum. Any fever, edema, dizziness, headache or nausea during this time requires immediate medical attention.

BENEFITS As long as a pregnancy is not complicated by diabetes, hypertension, or other disorders, massage is a wonderful gift for a person whose body doesn't quite belong to herself for a while. Particularly for issues of anxiety, fatigue and shifting proprioception, massage can be a powerful intervention.

OPTIONS Specific guidelines for positioning pregnant clients are discussed in the *risks* section. Some experts suggest having the mother lay only on her left side in late stage pregnancy. Special training for working with pregnant and post-partum women is widely available and highly recommended. This is a precious group of clients who require some specific skills for the safest and most effective bodywork.

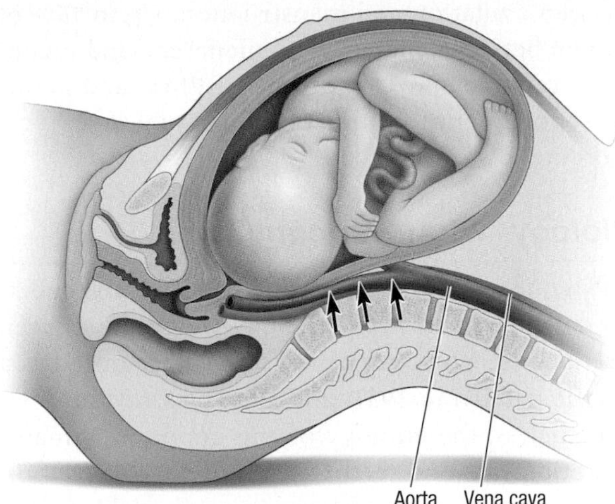

Figure 11.13. Pregnancy: a late-term fetus can obstruct blood flow through the iliac arteries or the vena cava

Premenstrual Syndrome

Definition: What Is It?

Premenstrual syndrome (PMS) is a collection of signs and symptoms that combine to interfere with a woman's ability to function normally during the luteal phase of the menstrual cycle: the time

Premenstrual Syndrome in Brief

Pronunciation: pre-MEN-stru-al SIN-drome

What is it?
Premenstrual syndrome (PMS) is a collection of many signs and symptoms that occur in the time between ovulation and menstruation, and then subside after menstruation begins. It may have several causes and triggers.

How is it recognized?
Signs and symptoms of PMS are often divided into physical and emotional features. Physical symptoms include breast tenderness, bloating, digestive upset, fatigue, changes in appetite, backache, and many others. Emotional signs include irritability, anxiety, depression, mood swings, and other possible problems.

Massage risks and benefits
Risks: Massage has no specific risks for women with PMS.
Benefits: Massage and bodywork may offer wonderful support for a woman whose negative physical experience is predictable, potentially debilitating, and tremendously frustrating.

between ovulation and menstruation. Up to 75% of women between the onset of menarche and menopause report some symptoms of PMS, and about 5% report symptoms of premenstrual dysphoric disorder.

Etiology: What Happens?

PMS is one of the most common and least well understood conditions that women experience. It has been described since ancient times; it was recognized as a specific pattern in 1931, and finally named in 1953. Nonetheless, the etiology of this condition remains mysterious. Several factors seem to contribute to it, and each woman's experience is unique. This makes it difficult to predict or treat, as no single approach is universally successful.

Some of the hypotheses for the causes or triggers of PMS include the following:

- *Hormonal hypersensitivity*. The precipitous drop in hormones just before a period occurs in every menstruating woman, but some appear to be especially sensitive to the change. In addition, exposure to environmental estrogens in animal fats and other sources may cause the endometrial lining to become overactive, leading to an even more extreme fluctuation in hormonal levels.
- *Nutritional deficiencies*. Some women with PMS are deficient in specific nutrients, notably calcium, magnesium, folic acid, vitamin B_6, and some essential fatty acids.
- *Neurotransmitter imbalance*. Plunging estrogen and progesterone levels have been seen to suppress the secretion of serotonin, a neurotransmitter that is strongly related to mood swings and depression. Opioid peptides are other brain chemicals that appear to be adversely affected by hormone disruption. These chemicals also help to determine mood.
- *Other factors*. Some factors that may contribute to PMS are more vague but definitely a part of the picture for many women. Genetic predisposition may be a factor, but it is unclear whether it is passed on through heredity or the likelihood to seek help for it is passed on through environmental influence. Cultural expectations, general stress, and a number of unrelated disorders may also contribute to PMS.

Signs and Symptoms

PMS is identified when symptoms are present in the 10 days leading up to a period, and disappear within the first 4 days after a period begins.

More than 150 signs and symptoms have been documented among PMS patients. These have been loosely categorized into physical and emotional indicators of this disorder.

- *Physical manifestations*. The most common physical signs and symptoms associated with PMS include bloating, breast tenderness, acne, salt and sugar cravings (along with binge eating), headaches (including migraines), backaches, insomnia, and digestive upset, that is, diarrhea and/or constipation. Less common physical manifestations include sinus problems, heart palpitations, and dizziness. Asthma, hay fever, migraines and seizures all tend to get worse during the luteal phase for women who live with these challenges.
- *Emotional manifestations*. These include confusion, poor concentration, depression, anxiety, panic attacks, mood swings, and general irritability.

Another disorder, called premenstrual dysphoric disorder (PMDD), is essentially like PMS but with the added factor of extremely depressed mood and/or anxiety. It occurs cyclically, just as PMS does, but it is typically treated with antidepressants and antianxiety medications rather than with birth control pills.

It is important to point out that PMS or PMDD symptoms are restricted to the luteal phase of the menstrual cycle. If they occur outside of this pattern, other causes must be pursued.

Treatment

PMS is typically treated symptomatically. Conventional physicians often prescribe low-dose birth control in the form of pills or other delivery systems to control estrogen and progesterone levels; diuretics to control water retention; or antidepressants to address serotonin levels. Most women are also strongly advised to make sure that they get the best sleep they can muster during their difficult time, and to exercise regularly.

Health professionals who focus on nutritional aspects of PMS often recommend that patients follow a low-fat vegetarian diet to avoid excessive estrogen exposure, and that they avoid salt, sugar, caffeine, and alcohol. Many herbal remedies have been reputed to help PMS; some of the more common herbal recommendations include borage or evening primrose (for essential fatty acids), Crocus sativus (saffron), black cohosh, and chasteberry. Homeopathic remedies are successful for many women with this condition.

Ultimately PMS usually can be successfully managed so that a woman doesn't have to lose function for 10 days every month, but it is unlikely to spontaneously disappear until the onset of menopause.

Medications

- Hormone supplements that suppress ovulation
- Diuretics to manage water retention
- Antidepressants or antianxiety medications to manage mood swings or PMDD (these come with special cautions for adolescent patients)
- Herbal remedies

Massage?

RISKS Because premenstrual syndrome (PMS) is not related to underlying infection, structural problems, neoplasm, or other dysfunctions, massage and bodywork carry no specific risks for clients with this condition.

BENEFITS Massage and other types of bodywork have been seen to be able to reduce depression and anxiety, and to help with some other physical symptoms that make PMS so uncomfortable.

Sexually Transmitted Infections

Definition: What Are They?

STIs are infections that spread through intimate contact. The primary mode of transmission is through vaginal, oral, or anal sex, although a mother carries a risk of infecting her baby either through the blood or through direct contact during birth.

More than 20 infectious diseases are spread through intimate contact. Several have been discussed elsewhere in this book; they include herpes simplex, HIV/AIDS, pubic lice, and hepatitis B. This discussion has been reserved for some common bacterial STIs, followed by a brief look at some viral and protozoan infections.

Sexually Transmitted Infections in Brief

Pronunciation: SEKS-u-ah-le tranz-MIH-ted

What are they?
Sexually transmitted infections (STIs) are contagious conditions that are spread through intimate contact. Pathogens can be bacteria, viruses, or protozoa.

How are they recognized?
The major STIs all share some signs when any signs are present at all. These include penile or vaginal discharge, painful urination, and painful intercourse. Other more specific symptoms vary by causative agent.

Massage risks and benefits
Risks: Massage is unlikely to have a directly negative impact on an STI, but undiagnosed conditions can continue to spread and damage more tissue until they are treated. People with very advanced infections may have cautions for massage related to having other tissues affected.
Benefits: Once an infection has been identified and controlled, massage within a client's capacity for adaptation is appropriate. People who have fully recovered from STIs can enjoy the same benefits from bodywork as the rest of the population.

Etiology: What Happens?

The pathophysiology of each STI discussed here is covered in the discussion of the infectious agents. Most are spread through sexual activity with an infected partner, but some may also be shared from mother to fetus.

The transmission of STIs can be prevented, but the only completely successful method is to practice abstinence or to have sex with one partner who is known to be uninfected. Barrier methods of birth control (male or female condoms) provide protection from some but not all STIs: molluscum contagiosum, genital warts, and syphilis may spread to areas not covered by condoms. And of course, other methods of birth control (spermicidal cream, birth control pills, IUDs, and other hormonal applications) provide no protection from STIs.

Types of Sexually Transmitted Infections

- *Bacterial Vaginosis*: This condition is exclusive to women. It involves an imbalance in the normal bacterial environment of the vagina with the result of malodorous discharge, irritation, and an increased risk of catching and transmitting other STIs, pelvic inflammatory disease (PID) and complicated pregnancy. The triggers for bacterial vaginosis are not well understood, but having multiple partners and frequent douching are seen to increase the incidence of this condition. It is treated with antibiotics.

NOTABLE CASES Of the conditions discussed here, only syphilis (sometimes called "Cupid's disease") is potentially life-threatening. Before penicillin was available, it was treated with near-lethal doses of mercury or arsenic. One theory behind the death of Napoleon Bonaparte is that he died of poisoning in an attempt to cure syphilis. Other notable figures whose lives were shortened by this infection include Franz Schubert, Christopher Columbus, Scott Joplin, and Al Capone.

- *Chlamydia*: This is a bacterial infection with *Chlamydia trachomatis*. These bacteria have an affinity for columnar mucus-producing cells. These infections can develop at any site of sexual contact: the reproductive tract, the mouth and throat, and the anus.

While chlamydia silently attacks columnar mucus cells in the reproductive tract, it also invades the uterus and uterine tubes, where a chronic low-grade infection and inflammatory response may lead to permanent scarring and infertility. This is one variety of PID.

Chlamydia is often silent; three-quarters of infected women and about half of infected men report no symptoms. When symptoms are present, they include vaginal or penile discharge, pain and burning during urination, and painful intercourse.

The primary complication of a chlamydia infection for a woman is PID and the risk of ectopic pregnancy or lifelong infertility. An infection in a man may cause **epididymitis**, swelling of the testicles, and a risk of infertility for him too. A baby born to a woman with undiagnosed chlamydia has a risk of exposure in the birth canal that may lead to conjunctivitis or life-threatening pneumonia. A chlamydia infection also increases the risk of HIV transmission.

Chlamydia is treatable with appropriate antibiotics, as long as sexual partners are treated too. It often appears with gonorrhea, which requires a different antibiotic treatment, so it is important to get a thorough diagnosis. Exposure and treatment for chlamydia does not impart immunity, so any future exposure to this pathogen can lead to a new infection that requires treatment.

- *Gonorrhea*: This is an infection with *Neisseria gonorrhoeae*: a diplococcal bacterium. It is spread through intimate contact, affecting mucous membranes of the throat, vagina, and rectum. It is rarely transmitted by any contact other than sex; it is unusual for a pregnant mother with gonorrhea to pass it to her child. Once inside the body, gonorrhea may infect tissues other than mucous membranes; **gonococcal arthritis** is an infection of joints that can lead to permanent damage.

Gonorrhea is often silent, especially in women. If symptoms do appear in a woman, they typically include vaginal discharge, urinary discomfort, and painful intercourse. An infection from oral sex may lead to sores in the mouth and a sore throat.

Male symptoms of gonorrhea include burning on urination, a yellow-white discharge from the penis, and **orchitis**, or swelling of the testicles.

This infection is responsive to antibiotics, although it has developed resistance to a number of them. It frequently appears with chlamydia, which requires concurrent treatment with a different antibiotic.

- *Syphilis*: This infection with the bacterial spirochete *Treponema pallidum* spreads through sexual contact and from mother to unborn child. It travels through the blood and may affect joints, bones, blood vessels, and the central nervous system if it is untreated. This bacterium is very fragile outside a host, and does not survive when exposed to air or sunlight.

Syphilis moves through the system in predictable stages. It is communicable only in the first two stages of infection. In the late stage, although it may cause very serious problems in the infected person, it is no longer contagious.

- Primary syphilis is detectable 10 days to 3 months after exposure, when a characteristic **chancre**, or open ulcer, appears. A chancre is usually not acutely painful, and if it appears inside the vaginal canal, a woman may not be aware of it. The tissue in chancres is very contagious. A typical chancre heals in 3 to 6 weeks.

- Secondary syphilis takes the form of a rash of open brownish sores that appear several weeks after the chancre heals. This rash is often on the soles of the feet or palms of the hands, but it may be anywhere. These lesions are also highly infectious. The rash associated with secondary syphilis may come and go for 1 to 2 years before the infection becomes latent.
- In some people syphilis becomes a silent infection after the secondary stage and may produce no further symptoms. No skin lesions appear, and the infection is no longer contagious. However, about one-third of people with secondary syphilis develop tertiary syphilis, a condition in which the bacteria invade other body systems. At this point the infection may attack the bones and joints, causing rheumatic pain, or the blood vessels, causing a risk of aneurysm. Most significantly, syphilis may attack the central nervous system, leading to a range of problems including blindness, loss of hearing, stroke, meningitis, or psychosis.

Like other bacterial STIs, syphilis significantly increases the transmission rate of HIV. A pregnant woman with syphilis, if she doesn't miscarry, has a nearly 100% chance of spreading the disease to her newborn through the bloodstream. Babies born with syphilis may not have symptoms immediately, but may develop vision or central nervous system problems along with syphilitic rhinitis; their mucus secretions are highly contagious.

Syphilis is sensitive to penicillin, and a single dose is typically adequate. Treatment must be administered before organ damage takes place, however. Syphilitic damage to the central nervous system, blood vessels, and other structures is irreversible.

- *Nongonococcal urethritis*: This is a bacterial infection of the urinary tract by an agent other than gonorrhea. It is often related to chlamydia, *Ureaplasma urealyticum*, or *Mycoplasm genitalium*. It is usually an STI but can also be related to prostatitis, urinary tract infection, or catheterization. If it is identified as a bacterial infection, it can be successfully treated with antibiotics.
- *Trichomoniasis*: This infectious agent is a protozoan parasite that causes vaginal discharge, pain, itching, and an increased risk of HIV transmission. **Trichomoniasis** is treatable with antibiotics.
- *Molluscum contagiosum virus* (MCV): This is a generally benign condition that is commonly seen among children, in whom it is not an STI. When MCV appears as an STI, it appears on the thighs, buttocks, groin, external genitalia, and anus. It is treated by removing the growths with topical chemicals or cryotherapy.
- *Genital warts*: These are also called **Condylomata acuminata**. They can grow on the vulva, the walls of the vagina, the perineum, or cervix of a woman or on the penis, scrotum, or anus of a man. Oral infections may grow in the mouth or throat. They have a high transmission rate; exposure leads to infection about two-thirds of the time. Genital warts are typically small, but they can grow in clusters large enough to interfere with a pregnancy. Many types of HPV can cause genital warts, and some of them are associated with cervical, penile, or vulvar cancer. Genital warts can be removed, but over-the-counter medications that treat common warts are inappropriate for these lesions, which grow on sensitive, delicate tissues.

Medications

- Antibiotics for bacterial and protozoan infections
- Antiviral medications for viral infections
- Topical application for genital warts and molluscum contagiosum

Massage?

RISKS Most sexually transmitted infections (STIs) are only spread through sexual contact, which makes communicability for massage therapists a nonissue. Exceptions to this rule include herpes simplex, molluscum contagiosum, genital warts, and open syphilis lesions. These can travel by skin-to-skin contact, and lesions may not be confined to genitalia.

BENEFITS Clients who are under treatment for STIs, or who have fully recovered from an infection, can enjoy all the benefits from bodywork as the rest of the population.

CHAPTER REVIEW QUESTIONS: REPRODUCTIVE SYSTEM CONDITIONS

1. Why have death rates from cervical cancer decreased in the past century? Why will they probably continue to decline?
2. A client in her 30s reports severe menstrual pain in a new pattern. What information should be conveyed before a massage?
3. How can endometriosis lead to infertility?
4. What is the most common symptom of uterine fibroids?
5. Is breast cancer a preventable disease? Why or why not?
6. Your client is a 76 year old man who complains that he has to get up to urinate frequently at night, and he often feels that he cannot fully empty his bladder. What two conditions should he have checked out?
7. Why is a man more likely to die *with* prostate cancer than *of* prostate cancer?
8. Your client is a 35 year old man who complains of chronic pain low in his abdomen. He does not have an infection. What condition is probably present?
9. What is the difference between perimenopause and menopause?
10. Your 25 year old client has PMS. She is in the luteal phase of her cycle and would like to receive massage. What are the potential risks and benefits?

12

Principles of Cancer

Chapter Objectives

After reading this chapter you should be able to . . .

- Describe the difference between a carcinoma and a sarcoma.
- Identify the difference between external and internal factors for cancer development.
- Name five infectious agents associated with cancer risk.
- Name six early signs of cancer.
- Name five habits that reduce the risk of cancer.
- Identify what TNM stands for.
- Name five treatment options for cancer.
- Name three complications or side effects of cancer treatment.
- Name three cautions for massage and cancer.
- Name three cautions for massage and cancer treatments.

Principles of Cancer

Cancer is not a single disorder. It comprises more than 100 diseases that have one thing in common: normal body cells mutate slightly and begin to replicate uncontrollably. When the malignant cells begin in epithelial cells, the cancer is called **carcinoma**. When the original cells are muscle or connective tissue, the cancer is a type of **sarcoma**. Carcinomas and sarcomas typically involve solid tumors. Cancers of the blood and lymph (leukemia, myeloma, lymphoma) usually do not; these are called **hematologic** cancers.

The principles laid out here are designed to provide background information for the discussions that appear throughout this book, which include skin cancer (Chapter 2); osteosarcoma (Chapter 3); leukemia and myeloma (Chapter 5); lymphoma (Chapter 6); laryngeal and lung cancer (Chapter 7); esophageal, stomach, colorectal, liver, and pancreatic cancer (Chapter 8); thyroid cancer (Chapter 9); kidney and bladder cancer (Chapter 10); and cervical, uterine, breast, ovarian, prostate, and testicular cancer (Chapter 11).

It is important to point out that massage therapy education has a history of overstating the risks of receiving bodywork if a client has cancer. While it is appropriate to be conservative and to "do no harm," it is also appropriate to use massage to provide many benefits to people who are going through a difficult time. To quote Tracy Walton's *Massage Contraindication and Cancer Principle*, "Skilled massage therapy is safe for people with cancer and will not spread the disease. Specific massage adjustments are based on *clinical presentations* of cancer, not the presence of a cancer diagnosis*." In other words, the guidelines for massage and bodywork for clients with cancer are determined by the circumstances presented in each case and not by the fact that cancer is an issue.

To see the author's video on massage therapy and cancer, visit http://thePoint.lww.com/Werner5e.

Cancer Statistics

About 40% of all men and women in the United States will develop some sort of cancer in their lifetime. Cancer is diagnosed in about 1.5 million people and leads to the death of about 570,000 in the United States every year. It is the second leading cause of death in the United States (heart disease is the first). Approximately 12 million people alive in the United States have had cancer.

Skin cancer is the most common variety reported (and these statistics do not reflect the countless moles that are removed as a safeguard against melanoma development), but lung cancer is the leading cause of death by cancer for both men and women. Other leading causes of death in the United States include breast and ovarian cancer for women, prostate cancer for men, and cancer of the colon, rectum, and pancreas for both genders. In other countries, most cancer deaths are due to lung cancer as a result of smoking, and liver and cervical cancers as a result of infection with hepatitis B or C and human papilloma virus, respectively.

Steps in Metastasis

It is still unclear exactly why or how a healthy cell changes into a malignant cell. One thing that all cancers have in common is that the DNA of a cell mutates so that the cell acquires certain growth properties. As researchers learn more about metastasis, new ways to interrupt the process and limit the ability of cancer cells to invade and destroy healthy tissue are being discovered.

The following is a simplified version of metastasis as it is currently understood:

- *Oncogene activation*. An **oncogene** is a gene that initiates malignant characteristics within a cell. Oncogene activation is the beginning of the changes that cause certain cells to become malignant. The trigger for activation may be toxic environmental exposures, diet, genetic predisposition, or some combination of factors, but it is often not clear. Oncogenes are typically inhibited by the activity of tumor suppressor genes. Eventually, it may be found that a lack of tumor suppressor genes (instead of or in addition to a surfeit of oncogenes) may be a significant factor in cancer risk.
- *Local invasion*. Mutated cells invade healthy tissue. They often do this without creating an inflammatory response because they secrete chemicals that suppress immune system reactions against them.
- *Proliferation*. The mutated cells proliferate without control, often piling up into distinct masses called tumors. As masses of cells accumulate, they begin to lose the characteristics that define their tissue type. This lack of differentiation is associated with aggressiveness of the tumor.
- *Angiogenesis*. **Angiogenesis** is the growth of blood vessels to supply a tumor. Any growth of more than 1 or 2 cm^3 requires a dedicated blood supply. Some cancer cells seem well supplied with the chemical messengers that command the body to build new capillaries. The more highly invested a tumor is with blood vessels, the more likely it is to have metastasized.
- *Migration*. Cancer cells break off the primary tumor and travel to new areas. The circulatory or lymphatic system may be used as a transfer medium, but cancer cells can also spread through direct contact with other organs or in peritoneal fluid.
- *Colonization*. When cancer cells land in a new target tissue, they must begin the process over again, starting with proliferation. This requires that the cells be able to adhere to the new tissue and that they secrete the correct enzymes to suppress an immune system attack, create new blood vessels, and erode the new extracellular matrix. The first tumor that grows in the

*Walton T. Medical Conditions and Massage Therapy a Decision Tree Approach. p. 376. (c) 2011, Lippincott Williams & Wilkins.

disease process is called the primary tumor; other tumors that grow from metastasis of the primary tumor are called secondary tumors. In other words, a tumor in the bladder that metastasized from the ovary is not bladder cancer. It is secondary ovarian cancer in the bladder.

Causes of Cancer

Triggers for oncogene activation vary by tissue type and individual case. Causes of cancer are slowly being narrowed to some identifiable factors. These are generally discussed as *internal* or *external* factors.

Internal Factors

Every cell in the body has a built-in capacity for self-destruction. This is a natural and healthy process called **apoptosis**, or programmed cell death. A specific gene in some cancer cells has been found to inhibit apoptosis. Therefore, some cancers may be as much related to cells that refuse to die as it is to new cells coming to life.

Some cancers are brought about by or connected to inherited characteristics. This means an inherited gene is likely to cause cellular mutations sometime in the future. Such genes have been identified for a small percentage of breast and colorectal cancers. It may also mean that a person has a genetic susceptibility to environmental factors that might not be a threat to someone else.

Other internal factors may include hormonal activity (some hormones appear to stimulate malignant cell division; others may suppress it) and immune system problems in recognizing and fighting off cancer cells.

External Factors

Carcinogens are chemical or environmental agents that have been identified as cancer causers. The National Toxicology Program is a consortium of several government entities including the National Institutes of Health, the Centers for Disease Control and Prevention, and the Food and Drug Administration. This organization lists 243 substances as known or highly probable carcinogens. This list includes the hydrocarbons in cigarette smoke; compounds created when meats are grilled over high heat; and several substances found in dyes, inks, and paint. Radiation from the sun, radon gas, gamma rays, or x-rays and CT scans can cause cancer, as can exposure to asbestos, benzene, nickel, cadmium, uranium, and vinyl chloride.

In addition to environmental irritants and pollutants, some pathogens have been determined to cause certain types of cancer. Others simply have a strong statistical link with the development of various cancers, but the cause-and-effect relationship has not been defined. Cancer-related pathogens include viruses, bacteria, and animal parasites.

Viruses

- *HTLV-1* (human T-lymphotrophic virus) resembles HIV; it is a retrovirus that is spread through intimate fluids. It can cause lymphocytic leukemia and non-Hodgkin lymphoma.
- *HPV* (human papillomavirus) is a large group of viruses associated with various types of warts. A few viruses in this group can cause cancer of the cervix, penis, anus, vagina, vulva, mouth, and throat. At this point, it is not possible to tell from early cellular changes whether the HPV involved is dangerous, so all dysplastic cells are removed. Vaccines against some forms of HPV are available.
- *HHV-8* (human herpesvirus 8) can cause Kaposi sarcoma, a type of skin cancer. HHV-8 is active only when the immune system is suppressed. Consequently, Kaposi sarcoma is an indicator disease for HIV infection or other immune-suppressing conditions.
- *HIV* is indirectly associated with cancer via suppressed immune system function that would otherwise protect against both HPV and HHV-8.
- *EBV* (Epstein-Barr virus) is another herpesvirus. It resides in B cells and usually causes mononucleosis in its first infection. EBV is associated with an increased risk of nasopharyngeal cancer, Burkitt lymphoma, Hodgkin lymphoma, and stomach cancer.
- *HBV* and *HCV* (hepatitis B and C viruses) open the door to liver cancer through chronic long-term inflammation that interrupts function in epithelial cells.

Bacteria

- *Helicobacter pylori,* which is also associated with peptic ulcers, has been seen to convert nitrites in foods to potential carcinogens. It is implicated in stomach cancer and lymphoma.
- *Others* include *Borrelia burgdorferi* (the spirochete that causes Lyme disease) and *Campylobacter jejuni*, which have both been associated with digestive tract lymphomas.

Animal parasites

- *Liver flukes* are associated with cancer in bile ducts. They are spread through the consumption of raw or undercooked fish.
- *Schistosoma haematobium* can cause cancer of the urinary bladder. They are spread through contaminated water. They are not found in the United States but may be carried by those who travel to areas where the parasites are common.

It is often a combination of external and internal factors that tips the scales in favor of developing cancer. Exposure to carcinogens in certain combinations can also be dangerous. For example, heavy smoking combined with excessive alcohol consumption is an especially potent combination for developing cancers of the mouth or upper gastrointestinal tract. Very often, many years or even decades may pass between the initial exposure to a carcinogen and the development of distinguishable tumors. This makes it difficult to pin down precise causes of cancer that are consistent from person to person.

Signs and Symptoms

Signs and symptoms of cancer vary widely, depending on the site. One of the most insidious features of this disease is that it is often painless until it is far advanced. Tumors begin to cause pain when they press on nerve endings or when they cause a blockage in a tube or duct that in turn presses on nerve endings. A list of common signs that are red flags for the possibility of cancer includes the following:

- A change in bowel or bladder habits; blood in the stool or urine
- A sore that does not heal, or that comes and goes in the same place; a change in a wart or a mole
- Uterine bleeding between periods or postmenopause
- Thickening or lump in the breast or elsewhere
- A prostate exam that shows enlargement
- Indigestion or swallowing difficulty
- Persistent cough or hoarseness; coughing up blood
- Unexplained weight loss
- Fatigue, anemia
- Unexplained fever

Cancer screening recommendations vary for types of cancer, risk factors, genetic history, and other issues. The most successful screening protocols aim to do two things: to find cancerous cells while treatment is most likely to be completely successful, and to lead to an increased survival rate. Not all screening protocols accomplish these goals equally well, and some procedures carry risks themselves, including exposure to radiation, perforation of hollow organs, false-negative results, false-positive results, and overdiagnosis that may lead to anxiety and unnecessary interventions, even surgery, for the patient. For more details on cancer screening recommendations, see Sidebar 12.1.

If suspicious changes are noted during screening, tissue samples are taken and analyzed for the presence of malignant cells; this is called a **biopsy**. If these tests are positive, further examinations of the patient follow to determine how far the cancer has developed.

Staging

Most types of cancer develop in predictable enough patterns that they can be staged, or given a label that indicates how far the cancer has advanced. Staging is based on collected knowledge about how cancer grows and how readily various types of cancer may metastasize. Some variables include the location of the primary tumor, the size and number of tumors, lymph node involvement, the characteristics of cells in the examined tissue, and the presence or absence of distant growths. Some cancers can be staged with typical screening mechanisms; others cannot be accurately staged until surgery is performed. Staging may be further qualified

SIDEBAR 12.1 Cancer Screening: Who, What, Where, When, Why?

The science of early cancer detection is far from fully developed or universally accepted. A survey of several medical agencies yields significantly different guidelines for individuals to follow in the attempt to be vigilant against early signs of cancer. One of the concerns with making screening recommendations is the risk of false positives, or the identification as cancerous of nonthreatening growths. These findings may lead to unnecessary interventions and even dangerous surgeries. Screening recommendations are further complicated by differences for low-risk and high-risk populations.

The following is a brief synopsis of the leading recommendations for early cancer detection.

Cancer type	Low-risk population recommendations	High-risk population recommendations
Breast cancer	Self-exam, monthly after age 20 onward. Clinical exam, every 3 years from ages 20 to 39; annually from 40 onward. Mammogram, opinions vary; most suggest exams every 1 to 3 years starting at age 40 or 50.	This includes women with the identified breast cancer genes, women who have first-degree relatives with breast cancer, or women who have had breast or other types of cancer before. Screening schedules are matched to individual cases.
Cervical cancer	When a woman becomes sexually active or reaches age 21 (whichever comes first), she should have an annual pelvic exam and Pap test; with three normal tests in a row, she can cut back to once every 3 years, or by her doctor's recommendation, for as long as she has a cervix. Testing can be suspended after age 70 if she has had 3 normal tests in a row.	This includes women who have shown signs of cervical dysplasia in pelvic exams or Pap tests. Screening should continue on a yearly basis until patients have three normal tests in a row. Screening can be discontinued if a patient has had a hysterectomy, **unless** the surgery was related to surgical cancer.
Skin cancer	Several agencies recommend a monthly self-exam for changes in skin, with a clinical visual exam every 3 years from age 20 to 40, and annually from age 40 onward.	This includes fair-skinned people, and anyone previously diagnosed with any type of skin cancer or precancerous condition; clinical exams should be scheduled on an as-needed basis.
Prostate cancer	A PSA test and DRE are recommended yearly for men over 50 years old with high PSA readings, and every 2 years for men with low PSA tests. Early screening for prostate cancer carries a high risk of false-positive results or overdiagnosis.	This includes African American men, and men with a father, brother, or son who have prostate cancer; testing should begin at age 40 to 45.
Colorectal cancer	Beginning at age 50, patients should choose one of the following: • A FOBT or FIT every year • A flexible sigmoidoscopy every 5 years • A double-contrast barium enema every 5 years • A colonoscopy every 10 years	This includes people with a history of colon polyps, inflammatory bowel disease, or a family history of hereditary colorectal cancer; screening should begin before age 50.
Lung, ovarian, and endometrial cancer	No effective noninvasive screening measures have been developed to detect these cancers in early stages. Postmenopausal women with any vaginal bleeding or spotting should consult with their doctor.	Some screening techniques may find these cancers, but they tend to be invasive procedures that are reserved for patients with a high risk for developing them.

DRE, digital rectal examination; FOBT, fecal occult blood test; FIT, fecal immunochemical test.

by the use of A and B designations to allow for differences in patterns of progression. Accurate cancer staging allows care providers to choose treatment strategies with the best chances for success.

Several staging protocols have been developed, but most cancers are rated by the TNM system, which may be translated into the stage 0 to IV system. In addition, cancer cells may be rated by grade, which describes their appearance and potential aggressiveness.

- *TNM system.* The TNM system rates cancer progression by evaluations of tumors, nodes, and metastasis. These are further explained in Tables 12.1 to 12.3.

TABLE 12.1 T: Tumor

Tumor	Definition
Tx	Tumor cannot be evaluated.
T0	No evidence of primary tumor.
Tis	In situ: tumor has not spread to nearby tissue.
T1, T2, T3, T4	These refer to the size and extent of primary tumor(s).

- *Stages 0 to IV system.* TNM ratings are often translated to the more familiar stages 0 to IV. Cancers have varying growth patterns, though, so the exact translation from TNM to stages 0 to IV varies by type. Stage 0 typically means that malignant cells are restricted to the first layer of affected tissue; stage IV means that distant metastasis has occurred. The 0 to IV staging system is explained in more detail in Table 12.4.
- *Grade.* Another predictor for how cancer grows is the grade of tumor cells. This refers to two issues: how well differentiated the cells are (the higher the differentiation, the better the prognosis), and the propensity for proliferation, or aggressiveness. Cancer grading is explained further in Table 12.5.

TABLE 12.2 N: Node

Node	Definition
Nx	Node involvement cannot be evaluated.
N0	No cancer is found in nearby nodes.
N1, N2, N3	These refer to the number and extent of regional lymph nodes invaded by cancer cells.

TABLE 12.3 M: Metastasis

Metastasis	Definition
Mx	Metastasis cannot be evaluated.
M0	No distant metastasis can be found.
M1	Distant metastasis is found.

Not all cancers lend themselves to the TNM or 0 to IV staging systems. Leukemia and lymphoma do not involve primary tumors, so their staging systems refer to blood counts, symptoms, and grade of cancer cells. Some cancers may be discussed in other terms, such as whether the lesion is operable or whether it has reached nearby organs.

Treatment

Decisions on how to treat cancer depend on the stage, the age, general health, and wishes of the patient, and

TABLE 12.4 Numerical Staging

Stage	Definition
0	Cancer in situ: cells have not penetrated tissue beyond original layers of affected tissue.
I, II, III	These refer to the size and extent of tumors, nodal involvement, and invasion of adjacent tissues.
IV	Cancer has spread to another organ. By convention, stage IV often means metastasis to other side of diaphragm or into central nervous system.

CNS, central nervous system.

TABLE 12.5 Grading Cancer

Grade	Definition
Gx	Grade cannot be assessed.
G1	Cells are well differentiated (low grade).
G2	Cells are moderately well differentiated (intermediate grade).
G3	Cells are poorly differentiated (high grade).
G4	Cells are undifferentiated (high grade).

what kind of cancer is present. Within each tumor, different kinds of cells may require different modes of attack. This makes successful treatment of cancer a matter of finding the correct combination of therapies.

Neoadjuvant therapy is the use of an intervention before main treatment begins, to increase the chances for success. Radiation to shrink tumors before surgery is an example of neoadjuvant therapy. **Adjuvant** therapy is the use of an intervention after the main treatment is completed to increase the chance for complete success, or to reduce the risk of future recurrence. Using Tamoxifen after breast cancer is an example of adjuvant therapy. **Palliative** therapy is given to a patient who is not likely to survive. For example, surgery to reduce tumor size and take pressure off of tissues might be conducted, not to cure the cancer, but to relieve pain and improve quality of life.

- *Surgery.* Cancer surgeries are performed to remove malignant tumors with a layer of healthy tissue around them when possible: this is called a "clean margin." A sample of nearby lymph nodes is often taken as well to examine them for signs of metastasis. If a **sentinel lymph node** can be identified (this is a node through which most or all of the lymph entering an area passes before going on to other nodes), it can be taken alone for examination.
- *Radiofrequency thermal ablation.* This is a procedure in which instruments are inserted through the skin to the depth of a targeted tumor, and an electrical current essentially "microwaves" cancerous material. It is used for tumors that are not easily accessible for traditional surgery, especially in liver cancer. It may find applications in treatment for kidney and prostate cancer as well.
- *Chemotherapy.* A variety of **cytotoxic** drugs have been developed for use in cancer treatment. These drugs specifically target any fast-growing cells in the body. Therefore, in addition to killing cancer cells, they may cause several side effects.
- *Autologous bone marrow transplant.* **Autologous bone marrow transplant** is a procedure in which some healthy bone marrow is harvested from the patient and stored. Then a very extreme course of cytotoxic drugs is administered. This kills the cancer cells, but kills most white blood cells too. After chemotherapy, the stored bone marrow is replanted in the patient, where it replaces the immune system cells killed by chemotherapy. This procedure is for use only in very extreme cases; it has a number of dangerous side effects and serious complications, but it can be a lifesaver if nothing else works. **Allogenic bone marrow transplantation** is a similar procedure with use of the marrow of a closely matched donor.
- *Radiation therapy.* Radiation therapy involves high-energy rays that are focused on tumors to kill them or slow their growth. The radiation may be applied from an external machine, which requires daily outpatient visits for several weeks, or it may come from small radioactive pellets that are temporarily implanted close to the tumor. **Stereotactic radiotherapy** involves doses of rays from several directions at once.
- *Hormone therapy.* Some tumors both depend on certain hormones to grow. Therapies to limit the secretion of these hormones or to change the way they affect the body are used in the treatment of these cancers.
- *Hypothermia.* In some cases, specifically with precancerous cells on the skin or cervix, potentially malignant cells may be killed by freezing them off the affected structure.

- *Hyperthermia.* Raising the body's temperature has been seen to make some cancer cells more vulnerable to the effects of chemotherapy. Drugs are sometimes administered through warmed intravenous fluids or when the core temperature has been raised.
- *Biologic (targeted) therapy.* These strategies work to support the immune system in various ways to identify and fight cancer more aggressively. They may involve injecting antigens that trigger an immune system attack, along with other substances that make the immune system more powerful as it hunts down cancer cells.
- *Stem cell implantation.* The implantation of stem cells specifically for leukemia patients carries promise as an effective treatment. These cellular blanks have the potential to grow into whatever kinds of cells the body needs to replace.

Prevention

Most resources that study cancer publish a list of simple lifestyle choices that can reduce the risk of developing this disease. While different aspects are emphasized for different types of cancer, a basic approach includes these recommendations:

- Stop smoking and other tobacco use.
- Avoid known carcinogens like radon and hazardous materials.
- Use sunscreen or clothing to protect the skin from ultraviolet radiation.
- Eat more fruit, vegetables, and whole grains, controlling dietary fat.
- Exercise regularly and control weight.
- Use alcohol moderately.
- Practice safe sex. (This is as a precaution against contracting HPV, which is associated with cervical cancer. However, barrier methods such as condoms do *not* reliably protect against the spread of this virus. Therefore, "safe sex" in this context means to have relations only with an uninfected partner.)
- Vaccinate against cancer-causing pathogens when possible.
- Use early cancer screening methods.

Massage?

Although it has traditionally been believed that circulatory types of massage carry the risk of aiding metastasis by boosting blood and lymph flow, research shows that cancerous growths can take years to become established before they are detectable by palpation. It seems far-fetched to suppose that a 60-minute massage could contribute to that process any more significantly than a brisk walk around the block or a long hot shower. Nonetheless, it is obviously inappropriate to rub on a tumor or any undiagnosed swelling or thickening of tissue.

Massage for persons undergoing cancer treatment, however, has a vital and useful role. Five symptoms of cancer and cancer treatment that are common in most patients include pain, anxiety, nausea, fatigue, and depression: all of these can be addressed with massage. In addition, constipation, altered body image, and poor sleep are problems that massage and bodywork can help with. Massage in various forms is being researched in all of these contexts. Perhaps most of all, massage provides for a basic human need: nurturing, caring, and informed touch at a time when many cancer patients feel isolated and dehumanized. The benefits massage has to offer are so well accepted as helpful, and so consistently requested by patients, that many hospitals are now including massage treatments for cancer patients and their families.

It is important to bear in mind that the complications associated with cancer and various cancer treatments can have serious implications for the choice of bodywork modalities, especially when multiple treatments are employed. One way to clarify choices about massage for cancer patients is to determine whether certain risks are brought about by the cancer itself, or by cancer treatment.

Massage Risks for Cancer

- *Tumor sites.* Massage should not disrupt any site where tumors or undiagnosed lesions are located close to the surface of the body. Further, a person with any kind of abdominal cancer is not a good candidate for intrusive abdominal work.
- *Bone involvement.* When cancer metastasizes to bones, they can become brittle and unstable.

This can make a person extremely vulnerable to fractures. Cancers of the breast, thyroid, kidney, lungs, and pancreas are most likely to metastasize to the bones.

- *Vital organ involvement.* A client who has cancer or metastasis in a vital organ (this includes the lungs, liver, brain, kidneys, and heart) may have compromised function of any of those organs. This risk should be evaluated to see how well the patient can adapt to bodywork.
- *Deep vein thrombosis.* A potential complication of both cancer and cancer treatment, the risk of deep vein thrombosis is a red flag for massage.

Massage Risks for Cancer Treatment

- *Surgery.* Several complications of cancer surgery can have implications for massage. Infection obviously contraindicates massage until the client is out of danger. Constipation is a frequent postsurgical complaint, but intrusive abdominal massage may be inappropriate, depending on the cancer site; lighter work can be helpful here.

  Medical devices may be present after surgery, including ports, catheters, drains, or ostomies. These should be locally avoided, and the client must be positioned in ways that minimize the risk of their disruption.

  When regional lymph nodes are surgically removed for staging purposes, **lymphedema** may develop; see Sidebar 12.2 for details on this complication. (Figures 12.1 and 12.2)
- *Radiation therapy.* Radiation can create several problems. When it is applied by an external machine, the skin at the entry and exit sites may become thin, red, and irritated. If radioactive pellets have been implanted, the patient may have to avoid contact with others until they have been removed. The gastrointestinal tract may be irritated, leading to nausea, vomiting, and diarrhea. Bone marrow suppression can lead to anemia, fatigue, poor clotting, and susceptibility to infection. Irradiated lymph nodes can be damaged, leading to a risk of lymphedema. Finally, externally or internally applied radiation can cause debilitating fatigue.

SIDEBAR 12.2 Lymphedema

The removal and examination of local lymph nodes for signs of metastasis is an important part of cancer staging. If cancer cells are found, the remaining nodes may be treated with radiation therapy. Both the surgery to remove sample nodes and the treatment to kill cancer that might be growing in remaining nodes can lead to a serious complication called lymphedema.

Lymphedema describes the accumulation of protein-rich fluid in interstitial spaces as a result of lymph system dysfunction. (This distinguishes it from simple edema, which is typically related to venous insufficiency or local trauma.) The chemistry of interstitial fluid is such that when it doesn't flow freely into nearby lymph vessels, it attracts water. That is, a small amount of fluid retention can become a significant problem in a short period.

Lymphedema can develop in the days or weeks after cancer surgery or radiation therapy, or it can suddenly appear decades later; all that is required is an insufficiency in lymph node function. Patients most at risk for this problem are those who have had nodes removed, had radiation therapy following surgery, who are overweight, and who are sedentary. Once the shift in tissue proteins occurs, the symptoms may subside, but the risk of recurrence is always high.

Signs and symptoms of lymphedema can include redness, heat, and pain; these signs indicate infection along with fluid retention. Often, however, it is simply the deep ache and loss of function of a limb that grows to huge proportions. Pitting edema is another indicator. Lymphedematous limbs are particularly vulnerable to bacterial and fungal infections and must be cared for very carefully.

Long-standing lymphedema can lead to fibrosclerotic changes in the interstitial spaces of the superficial fascia. As a result, the tissue and skin on the affected limb become indurated, or hardened. Once this stage is reached, it is very difficult to reverse.

Standard treatment options for lymphedema are limited. Compression machines, bandages, and supportive clothing are often unsatisfactory. Lymphedema is of particular relevance for massage therapists, because it would seem tempting to use Swedish massage, reputed to influence fluid flow, to help resolve it. However, because of the chemical imbalance in the interstitial spaces, any kind of work that compresses blood vessels may make lymphedema worse. Various kinds of bodywork techniques have been developed to address lymphedema, but they employ extensive knowledge of the anatomy and physiology of the lymph system to maximize benefits while minimizing risks. Practitioners who learn these techniques, however, are likely to find an eager group of clients hoping to benefit from their work and acceptance in the medical community.

Clients with a history of lymphedema live with a lifetime risk of repeated episodes. While massage to the rest of the body may be safe, massage to the affected extremity must be conducted very conservatively.

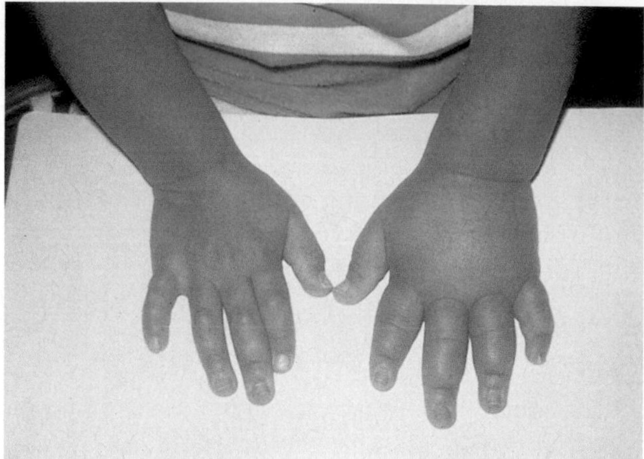
Figure 12.1. Lymphedema

- *Chemotherapy.* Chemotherapeutic drugs may be administered orally or through intravenous drips. They often suppress bone marrow activity, leading to anemia, a risk of infection, and clotting problems. Gastrointestinal tract irritation, mouth sores, **hand-foot syndrome,** and hair loss are other side effects of drugs that kill fast-growing cells. Other complications of chemotherapy include neuropathy, constipation, skin rashes, and mood changes.

  Some varieties of chemotherapy are expressed through the skin. It may not be appropriate for a patient to be extensively touched skin-to-skin during this process, but gloves can be used. In some care centers, the risk of infection among immune-compromised patients is so high that using gloves is a standard protocol regardless of chemotherapy type.

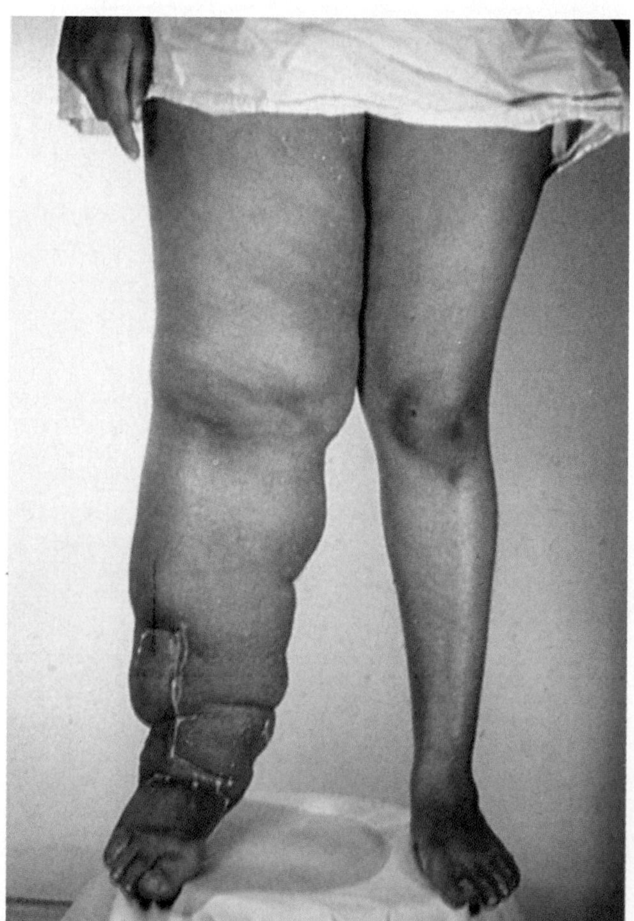
Figure 12.2. Extreme lymphedema

- *Other therapies.* Other cancer treatments may also hold cautions for massage. Hormone treatments may increase the risk of blood clots, biologic therapies may cause fatigue and flulike symptoms, cryotherapy can leave irritated areas on the skin, and so on.

  No matter what kind of cancer or cancer treatments a person is going through, it is vital for his or her massage therapist to communicate with the rest of the health care team to provide the best benefits that bodywork has to offer with minimal risks. For more information on the role of massage and bodywork for cancer patients, please consult the works cited in the bibliography.

Massage Benefits for Cancer Patients

Cancer has been a focal point of massage therapy research since the early 1990s when some brave people challenged the concept that massage had no safe role for cancer patients. While the results of the research have some variations, the general themes are these: expertly performed massage for cancer patients can

- Improve sleep
- Increase appetite
- Relieve constipation
- Improve mood
- Reduce anxiety
- Decrease depression
- Alleviate pain

These benefits can be applied to both cancer and cancer treatments, as long as appropriate adjustments for the risks listed above are employed. Further, massage must of course be gauged to fit within a client's typical activity levels and capacity for adaptation, which may vary greatly from one person to another. Even though massage alone is unlikely to reverse the course of cancer, by interfering with some of the most common and debilitating side effects of the disease and its treatments, bodywork can without doubt improve the quality of life for people who face this challenge.

CHAPTER REVIEW QUESTIONS: PRINCIPLES OF CANCER

1. Briefly define cancer.
2. Briefly define metastasis.
3. What is the purpose of removing lymph nodes from cancer patients?
4. What is a "sentinel node"?
5. When cancer cells have been found but are limited to only one layer of tissue, what stage is it?
6. When cancer cells have been found in the central nervous system or on the other side of the diaphragm from the original growth, what stage is it?
7. What is the most commonly diagnosed form of cancer?
8. Which is the leading cause of death by cancer for both men and women?
9. Your client is between cycles of chemotherapy for stage III breast cancer. She has undergone an initial surgery and the chemo is an adjunctive therapy to follow up. What are some questions you need to ask in order to work with her safely?
10. Describe the benefits massage has to offer cancer patients undergoing treatment.

Appendix A
Medications

Massage therapists are always encouraged to ask about what medications, prescription or otherwise, their clients might be taking. Traditionally, this has been to help discover what conditions a client might have that could influence the way massage needs to be conducted. But the possible interactions between bodywork and medications themselves are a related but separate topic.

The following is a *very* short collection of classes of medications that are commonly prescribed for chronic conditions. Massage therapists must balance the effects of medications, medical interactions, all possible side effects, and the potential for bodywork to tip the scales in one direction or another. In many cases, a conversation with the primary care provider is in order—not so much to ask permission to do massage as to investigate whether the generally parasympathetic changes massage brings about carry any concern or risk in the presence of prescription drugs.

Recently, some excellent resources about bodywork in the context of pharmaceuticals have been developed. I recommend these resources:

- Wible J. Pharmacology for Massage Therapy. Philadelphia, PA: Lippincott Williams & Wilkins, 2005.
- Persad R. Massage Therapy and Medications. Toronto, ON: Curties-Overzet Publications, 2001.

In addition, massage offices would do well to have a general reference about medications on hand. In this way, when a client enters "doxercalciferol" on her intake form and neither one of you are sure what it's for, you'll have a way to find out.

Two good options are

- Springhouse Nurse's Drug Guide 2006.
- Wible J. Portable Pharmacology for Massage Therapists. Philadelphia, PA: Lippincott Williams & Wilkins, 2008.

The short list of medication classes under discussion here includes the following:

- Antianxiety drugs
- Antidepressant drugs
- Anti-inflammatory/analgesic drugs
- Autonomic nervous system (ANS) drugs
- Cardiovascular drugs
- Cancer drugs
- Clotting management drugs
- Diabetic drugs
- Muscle relaxant drugs
- Thyroid supplemental drugs

Within each description, the following information is provided:

- Examples of common name brands and some generic names: please be aware that this information is perhaps the most changeable of all and requires that every therapist get accurate and current information from every client. Generic names are in lowercase.
- Basic mechanism of the drug
- Massage cautions and implications associated with the medication or the condition it treats

Antianxiety Drugs

These medications are used to alter the sympathetic "flight or fight" response that is so prevalent for many people with anxiety disorders. They act on the central nervous system (CNS), but their effects may be far-reaching. Common side effects of antianxiety medications include CNS depression, poor reflexes, dry mouth, and feeling unusually exhausted. All of these side effects impact decisions about bodywork. While most of the time side effects are mild and easily tolerated, they can become a medical emergency. Clients should be encouraged to report any troubling symptoms to their primary physician.

Classes of antianxiety drugs:

- Benzodiazepines
- Buspirone HCl

Benzodiazepines

Common Examples

Valium, Ativan, Xanax, Loftran, Halcion, Dalmane, Restoril, Librium, Tranxene, Paxipam, Serax

Basic Mechanism

It is believed that these medications mimic the inhibitory action of the neurotransmitter gamma aminobutyric acid, making neurons harder to activate and suppressing the emotional component of anxiety in the limbic system. Benzodiazepines are used for short-term anxiety, seizures, insomnia, and convulsions. They are potentially addictive.

Implications for Massage

When a person's sympathetic response is suppressed, she is more prone to slide into a deep parasympathetic state. This is fine, until she tries to sit up, and falls off the table because of orthostatic hypotension. Massage in the presence of these drugs must be conducted conservatively to respect the client's reduced ability to adapt to external changes. Using more stimulation throughout the massage may help the client to avoid dizziness and fatigue at the end of the massage.

Buspirone HCl

Common Example

BuSpar

Basic Mechanism

The mechanism of this medication is not well understood. It appears to bind up serotonin and dopamine receptors in the brain, leading to calmer effect without the CNS side effects seen with benzodiazepines. It is less addictive as well. BuSpar is used for short-term anxiety and for chronic problems like general anxiety disorder.

Implications for Massage

The systemic side effects with BuSpar are less than those with other antianxiety medications, but the rules are the same: clients need to move carefully after a session because of sympathetic suppression and more stimulating massage throughout the session will aid in avoiding dizziness and fatigue.

Antidepressant Drugs

The exact causes of depression remain under dispute, and so do the exact working mechanisms of antidepressant medications. Three main classes have been developed: tricyclic antidepressants (TCAs), monamine oxidase inhibitors (MAOIs), selective serotonin reuptake inhibitors (SSRIs)/ serotonin norepinephrine reuptake inhibitors (SNRIs), and some miscellaneous drugs. and some miscellaneous drugs. As a whole, these drugs prolong the availability of various types of neurotransmitters in synapses in the brain, although why exactly this makes a difference is still an issue of some contention. It takes time for the body to adapt to these changes however; 4 weeks or more are often needed for the drugs to take effect.

Antidepressants all have some side effects, although these are usually temporary and mild. Agitation at the beginning of treatment is common, along with increased anxiety, headaches, and insomnia; these often fade quickly. Other side effects include dry mouth, constipation, reduced sexual function, bladder problems, increased heart rate, and dizziness. If these symptoms don't subside, or if they become a significant issue, patients should consult with their prescribing doctors as soon as possible.

Two types of antidepressants are associated with significant health risks: MAOIs have dangerous interactions with decongestants and some food groups that lead to dangerously high blood pressure and a risk of stroke, and Serzone has been associated with liver toxicity.

Dizziness, drowsiness, and lightheadedness are common side effects to many antidepressants. Massage may exacerbate these symptoms, so the therapist should take care not to overtreat, especially when a client is just starting new course of drugs.
Classes of antidepressant medications:

- Tricyclics
- Monamine oxidase inhibitors
- Selective serotonin reuptake inhibitors/ serotonin norepinephrine reuptake inhibitors
- Other antidepressants

Tricyclics

Common Examples

Imipramine / Tofranil, amitriptyline / Elavil, nortriptyline / Pamelor, desipramine / Norpramin, clomipramine / Anafranil, doxepin / Sinequan, protriptyline / Vivactil

Basic Mechanism

Tricyclics block the reuptake of norepinephrine and serotonin at synapses; this leads to "down regulation" and more normal function of the postsynaptic receptors, but it may take 4 weeks or more before improvement is noticed.

Implications for Massage

Like other antidepressants, tricyclics may have dizziness as a side effect. Clients may need some gently stimulating strokes at the end of the session to come back to full alertness. Of all the antidepressants, tricyclics tend to have the most extreme side effects.

Monoamine Oxidase Inhibitors

Common Examples

Nardil, Parnate, Marplan

Basic Mechanism

MAOIs work by inhibiting monamine oxidase, an enzyme that breaks down the neurotransmitters, but are used less often than other antidepressants because of the risk of dangerous interactions with some substances, notably decongestants, and aged cheeses, red wine, pickles, and other foods with tyramine.

Implications for Massage

MAOIs and other antidepressants have the tendency to cause excessive drowsiness and dizziness; massage must be performed and concluded appropriately.

Selective Serotonin Reuptake Inhibitors/ Serotonin Norepinephrine Reuptake Inhibitors

Common Examples

Prozac, Zoloft, Luvox, Paxil, Celexa, Lexapro, Effexor, Pristiq, Cymbalta..

Basic Mechanism

These drugs all work to keep serotonin and norepinephrine present in CNS synapses for a longer period of time. The theory is that this will lead to a more normalized uptake of neurotransmitters from presynaptic neurons and a decrease in symptoms. SSRIs and SNRIs are used to treat various types of anxiety disorders and eating disorders as well as depression.

Implications for Massage

SSRIs and SNRIs often have fewer side effects than other antidepressants, but therapists should be alert for signs of excessive dizziness or drowsiness and compensate appropriately.

Other Antidepressants

Common Examples

Serzone, Wellbutrin, Remeron, Ludiomil, Desyrel, Symbyax

Basic Mechanism

These drugs are similar to other antidepressants, although they focus on serotonin, norepinephrine, or dopamine uptake.

Implications for Massage

In addition to the general guidelines about massage and antidepressants, Serzone, in particular, is associated with a risk of liver toxicity. Clients with signs of jaundice, chronic nausea, or other abdominal discomfort, should immediately consult their primary caregiver.

Anti-Inflammatory and Analgesic Drugs

Inflammation is frequently a source of nerve irritation at acute or chronic sites of tissue damage. Consequently, many analgesics work to reduce pain sensation by reducing or inhibiting the inflammatory process. Other analgesics alter pain perception in the CNS, and do not affect inflammation.

Regardless of the site of drug activity, analgesics and anti-inflammatories change tissue response. It is important to work extremely conservatively with clients who take these medications, because information therapists gather about temperature, muscle guarding, local blood flow, and other signs will be altered, and overtreatment is a significant risk. Although it is inappropriate to suggest that clients skip or change their medication for massage, it is important to be aware of when these drugs are at their peak of activity so that therapists may be prepared for the changes in tissue and the effects on clients.

Classes of drugs

- Salicylates
- Acetaminophen
- Nonsteroidal anti-inflammatory drugs (NSAIDs)
- Steroidal anti-inflammatories
- Narcotics and mixed narcotics

Salicylates

Common Examples

Aspirin, Bayer, Empirin, Doan's Pills, Trilisate, Dolobid

Basic Mechanism

Salicylates inhibit prostaglandin synthesis, which then reduces pain sensitivity and inflammatory response. They also reduce fever by acting on the hypothalamus and promoting peripheral vasodilation. (They do not reduce a normal temperature.) In addition, aspirin works to inhibit platelet aggregation (see *anticoagulants*).

Implications for Massage

Reduced pain perception and inhibited inflammation means that compromised tissue may not send a strong signal about pain; bodywork needs to be conducted conservatively to avoid overtreatment and deep tissue massage used with caution. Also the tendency for peripheral vasodilation raises the risk for hypotension (dizziness and lethargy) and chilling during and after a massage.

Acetaminophen

Common Examples

Tylenol, Anacin

Basic Mechanism

The mechanism for acetaminophen is not thoroughly understood. It is clear that these medications act on the heat-regulating center of the hypothalamus to reduce fever. These drugs reduce pain sensation, possibly in both the CNS and in the peripheral tissues, but do *not* influence inflammation.

Implications for Massage

As with other pain medications, caution must be used to avoid overtreatment.

Nonsteroidal Antiinflammatory Drugs

Common Examples

Celebrex, Lodine, Advil, Excedrin, Nuprin, Relafen, Indomethacin/Indocin, Aleve, Ansaid, Ketoprofen, Mobic, Clinoril

Basic Mechanism

All of these medications work to inhibit prostaglandin synthesis at sites of tissue damage to reduce inflammation and the pain associated with it.

Implications for Massage

NSAIDs are effective for pain and inflammation, but they are also associated with stomach and kidney damage; clients need to consult their doctor if they have any discomfort (bear in mind that kidney pain may present as low back pain). Regular use of Vioxx and Celebrex has been shown in some studies to increase the risk of cardiovascular disease, including heart attack and stroke.

Massage therapists carry the responsibility to avoid overtreatment, even if the client doesn't report feeling pain.

Steroidal Anti-Inflammatories

Common Examples

Cortisone, Compound E, Beconase, Propaderm, H-Hydrocort, Hydrocortisone, Depo-Medrol, Prednisol, Prednisone, Decadron, and Methotrexate

Basic Mechanism

These synthetic analogs to glucocorticoids produced in the adrenal cortex all work to undo the main symptoms of inflammation: they reduce pain, heat, redness, and edema in the short run. The mechanism by which they do this is not well understood, although some researchers suggest that they change local cellular activity leading to suppressed production of prostaglandins, histamine, and other inflammatory substances.

Implications for Massage

Steroidal anti-inflammatories are powerful, but have several serious side effects. In addition to altering tissue response (which requires extra caution with massage), they suppress immune system activity. Long-term use is associated with weakened connective tissues, fat deposition, muscle wasting, reduced bone density, fluid retention, hypertension, and easy bruising. Topical applications of steroid creams can lead to thinning skin. All of these features influence bodywork choices. Deep tissue massage should not be used when these drugs are used long-term, and myofascial techniques should be used with great caution.

Steroidal anti-inflammatories may also be prescribed in inhalant form for the treatment of asthma. While these medications specifically target the lung, long-term use may have negative impact on other tissues.

Narcotics and Mixed Narcotics

Common Examples

Codeine, Demerol, Oxycontin, Darvon, Percocet, Lortab, Vicodin, fentanyl/Duragesic, Dilaudid, MS Contin, Morphine

Basic Mechanism

Narcotics bind to opiate receptors in the brain to mimic the action of pain-killing endorphins. This leads to a reduced sensation of pain without loss of consciousness, along with suppression of the cough reflex, and gastrointestinal (GI) tract sluggishness. Narcotics are potentially addictive; mixed narcotics were developed to minimize the risk of dependence, but have proven to be addictive also.

Implications for Massage

A client taking these medications has a problem that is too extreme to be managed with less intrusive analgesics. Interference with pain perception is more complete, and appropriate caution is called for. Furthermore, clients taking narcotic analgesics may be prone to mood swings and difficulties with accurate communication. Deep tissue massage should not be used and stimulation during or at the end of the session is needed to prevent side effects of dizziness and fatigue. Avoid massaging around the area of transdermal patches.

Autonomic Nervous System Drugs

ANS drugs work to stimulate or block the action of the sympathetic or parasympathetic nervous systems. They are used for a wide variety of diseases including gastrointestinal, urinary, cardiac, and respiratory conditions. They can work directly on the receptors to stimulate or block them, or they can work to increase or decrease the associated neurotransmitters.

Classes of ANS drugs:

- Cholinergic (increase parasympathetic nervous system actions)
- Anticholinergic (block the actions of the parasympathetic nervous system)
- Adrenergic (increase sympathetic nervous system actions)
- Adrenergic blockers (block sympathetic nervous system actions)

Cholinergics

Common Examples

Urecholine, Carbastat, pilocarpine, Aricept

Basic Mechanism

These drugs mimic the action of the parasympathetic system.

Implications for Massage

Since these drugs do the exact thing that massage is usually meant to do (activate the parasympathetic nervous system), care should be taken not to overtreat. Stimulating forms of massage should be used throughout the session so the client is alert at the end, rather than dizzy and in a deep parasympathetic lethargy.

Anticholinergic Drugs

Common Examples

Atropine, Transderm Scop, Scopolamine, Anaspaz, Librax, Cogentin, Bentyl, Ditropan, Detrol, Artane

Basic Mechanism

The actions of these drugs can vary. They are often organ specific and may suppress or stimulate parasympathetic nervous system receptors.

Implications for Massage

These drugs affect the parasympathetic response of the client, and therefore the effects of massage. Looking up the drug, target organ, and side effects, as well as talking with the client about how the drug affects them will help determine if the parasympathetic response is stimulated or blocked. Massage can then be given with these individual effects in mind.

Adrenergic Drugs

Common Examples

Dopamine, Epinephrine, Isuprel, albuterol, terbutaline, Serevent, Neo-Synephrine.

Basic Mechanism

These drugs stimulate the sympathetic nervous system.

Implications for Massage

The goal of massage to induce a parasympathetic response is more difficult to achieve with the actions of these drugs. Longer, slower massages may be needed. Be cautious with strokes that stimulate, such as tapotement and friction.

Adrenergic Blockers

Common Examples

Cardura, Minipress, Flomax, Migranal, Coreg, Normodyne, Betagan, Corgard, Inderal, Betapace.

Basic Mechanism

These drugs block the action of the sympathetic nervous system at various receptor sites, and include alpha and beta blockers. They can be very specific to the target organ, but may have side effects that are systemic.

Implications for Massage

Blocking the sympathetic nervous system means the client may be susceptible to going into a deep parasympathetic state with massage. Caution should be used to be certain the client is awake and not experiencing dizziness or other effects.

Cardiovascular Drugs

Most of the drugs used to treat cardiovascular disease work in some way to minimize a sympathetic response or to dilate peripheral blood vessels. The overriding rule when a client uses these substances is that their slide into a parasympathetic state may be intensified by massage, leaving the client dizzy, fatigued, and lethargic. Ending a session with strokes that are more stimulating may help to ameliorate these effects, as long as they fit into a protocol that is suitable for a person with compromised cardiovascular health. Clients should be instructed to sit up and move slowly after their massage, in order to minimize dizziness or discomfort.

Hydrotherapeutic techniques can present a greater challenge to maintain homeostasis than many other modalities. Many clients with cardiovascular diseases should avoid total immersions in favor of smaller, localized hydrotherapy applications.

Classes of cardiovascular drugs:

- Beta blockers
- Calcium channel blockers
- Angiotensin converting enzyme inhibitors
- Digitalis
- Antiangina drugs
- Antilipemic drugs
- Diuretics

Beta Blockers

Common Examples

Inderal, Normodyne, Levatol, Corgard, Tenormin, metoprolol/Lopressor, Toprol, Sotalol, Coreg, Betagan.

Basic Mechanism

These affect beta receptors at the heart, bronchi, blood vessels, and the uterus. They lower blood pressure and cardiac output. They are used to treat angina, hypertension, anxiety, and some other disorders. Beta blockers may be selective for action on the heart only, or nonselective for a more general effect.

Implications for Massage

Beta blockers can lead to excessively low blood pressure, especially when the client is in a relaxed state. Hydrotherapy is generally safer with local applications than systemic immersions in hot tubs, saunas, or other facilities.

Calcium channel blockers

Common Examples

Norvasc, ardene, Isoptin, Procardia, Plendil, Verapamil.

Basic Mechanism

These drugs block the movement of calcium ions in smooth and cardiac muscle tissue. The result is vasodilation and more efficient myocardial function. They are used for hypertension and long-term (not acute) angina.

Implications for Massage

Side effects of these drugs include flushing, dizziness, and hypotension. Massage should be conducted to minimize the risk of exacerbating these: less emphasis on big, draining strokes and more emphasis on smaller, less circulatory strokes is appropriate.

Angiotensin Converting Enzyme Inhibitors

Common Examples

Lotensin, Captopril, Vasotec, Monopril, Accupril, Altace, Zestril

Basic Mechanism

ACE inhibitors work by limiting the action of an enzyme that is employed in the renin-angiotensin system: the loop between blood pressure and kidney function. They promote the excretion of sodium and water, reducing load on the heart. They are used to control hypertension and heart failure.

Implications for Massage

As with other drugs for cardiovascular disease, excessive hypotension is a possible side effect. Clients may experience fatigue, dizziness, and lethargy if gently invigorating strokes are not administered toward the end of the session.

Digitalis

Common Examples

Digitek, digoxin, Lanoxicaps, Lanoxin.

Basic Mechanism

Digitalis increases the force of the heartbeat by boosting calcium in cardiac muscle cells; it also slows the heartbeat through action in the CNS. It is used to treat arrhythmia and heart failure.

Implications for Massage

Clients who take any form of digitalis to control heart failure are not good candidates for rigorous circulatory massage. Invigorating strokes to conclude a session must be chosen to support alertness rather than circulatory flow.

Antilipemic Drugs

Common Examples

LoCholest, Lopid, Prevalite, Questran, Lipitor, Lescol, Zocor, Crestor, Mevacor, Pravachol, Zetia, Lopid, Tricor, Niaspan, Vytorin.

Basic Mechanism

Cholesterol-lowering drugs work by sequestering bile or by inhibiting cholesterol synthesis. Bile-sequestering drugs promote the excretion of bile in stool, requiring the liver to use more cholesterol in bile manufacturing; this lowers blood cholesterol. Cholesterol synthesis inhibitors interfere with enzyme activity in the liver that leads to cholesterol synthesis. Both approaches lead to lower low-density lipoprotein levels.

Implications for Massage

A common side effect for all these drugs is constipation as they influence the GI tract. Massage may help to relieve this symptom, but if a client has abdominal pain and has had no bowel movement for several days, an acute bowel impaction is possible; this is a medical emergency.

Other side effects (which are not always listed) may include muscle soreness, cramping, and weakness. If a client taking an antilipemic drug has these problems, the prescribing doctor should be consulted before the massage therapist works to resolve them.

On rare occasions, these drugs can cause a life-threatening muscle-wasting disease called rhabdomyolysis. Symptoms include worsening muscle pain and weakness. If your client has these symptoms, refer them to the physician immediately.

Diuretics

Common Examples

Thalidone, Kaluril, Lasix, Bumex, Lozide, Lozol, spironolactone/Aldactone, Chlorthalidone, Demadex, Zaroxolyn, Dyazide, Maxzide, hydrochlorothiazide

Basic Mechanism

Some diuretics prevent sodium from being reabsorbed in the kidney. As it is processed into urine, sodium then pulls water along with it. Other medications target specific parts of the nephron to prevent water and salt reabsorption, but can control the loss of other electrolytes more carefully.

Implications for Massage

Rigorously applied massage may put an extra load on the kidneys. Resting hypotension may also be a problem for people taking these medications. General diuretics may cause a loss of potassium that can contribute to muscle cramps. This needs to be addressed by a doctor rather than by a massage therapist.

Antiangina Medication

Common Examples

Apo-ISDN, Cedocard, IMDUR, Monoket, Nitrodisc, Nitrostat, Transderm-Nitro, nitroglycerin

Basic Mechanism

Antiangina drugs reduce myocardial oxygen demand, or they increase the supply of oxygen to the heart, or both. Chronic angina is treated with beta blockers or calcium channel blockers, discussed elsewhere. Acute angina is typically treated with various nitrates. These cause vasodilation, especially of veins, leading to decreased load on the heart. They are typically dissolved under the tongue for fast action, or applied with a skin patch or ointment for longer-lasting effect.

Implications for Massage

If a client has a transdermal patch for antiangina medication, that area and the adjacent tissue must be avoided so that dosage is not influenced. Clients taking these medications have the same risk of hypotension, flushing, and dizziness seen with other cardiovascular drugs.

Cancer Drugs

Cancer drugs or chemotherapy drugs are a large group that act in a wide variety of ways on the body. While the goal is to attack the cancer cells, cancer drugs are generally toxic to the whole body. Newer drugs can target cancer cells more carefully, but still tax the body as a whole. Massage should be applied very conservatively, and circulatory massage minimized. Timing of the session should be related to excretion rates of the drug and discussed with the client's physician in detail.

Classes of drugs:

- Alkylating drugs
- Antimetabolite drugs
- Antibiotic antineoplastics
- Hormonal antineoplastics
- Natural antineoplastics
- Other antineoplastic drugs

Common Cancer Drugs

Common Examples

This is a limited list of the most commonly seen drugs: Cytoxan, dacarbazine/DIC, CCNU, TSPA, cisplatin, methotrexate, 5-FU, actinomycin, Tamofen, Teslac, vinblastine, vincristine, interleukin-2, interferon.

Basic Mechanism

These drugs target the cancer cells and kill them, block the growth of the cells, or block the vascular feeding of the cells.

Implications for Massage

Always consult with the physician. Massage application should be very conservative. Be aware of methods of excretions (some excrete through the skin) and take appropriate precautions. If radioactive elements are implanted in the body, check with the physician on any limits to the time that should be spent in close proximity to the client.

Clotting Management Drugs

Medications to manage blood clots come in three basic forms: anticoagulants to prevent the formation of new clots by acting on clotting factors; antiplatelet medications prevent the clumping of platelets to form new clots; and thrombolytics, which are used to dissolve preexisting clots. Thrombolytics are used only in emergency situations (i.e., in early treatment for heart attack or ischemic stroke), and so won't be discussed here. Other clot management drugs are used for chronic problems or to lower the risk of future clots.

Classes of drugs:

- Anticoagulants
- Antiplatelet drugs

Anticoagulants

Common Examples

Heparin, Lovenox, Coumadin

Basic Mechanism

Heparin and Lovenox are injected anticoagulants; Coumadin is an oral medication. All of them alter the formation of clotting factors in the liver to prevent the formation of new clots, although they do not help to dissolve preexisting clots. These medications are used for people with atrial fibrillation, a high risk of deep vein thrombosis (DVT), or for people using hemodialysis. Heparin may also be used in orthopedic surgery to reduce the risk of postsurgical DVT.

Implications for Massage

All blood-clotting medications carry a risk for bruising, even with relatively light massage. Furthermore, the need for these medications indicates a tendency to form blood clots that may contraindicate all but the lightest forms of bodywork. If a blood clot is present, massage should not be given.

Antiplatelet Drugs

Common Examples

Aspirin, Empirin, Pletal, Plavix

Basic Mechanism

These drugs prevent platelets from clumping at the site where a clot might otherwise form.

Implications for Massage

Although these are typically less powerful than anticoagulants, the risk of bruising must still be respected for clients who take antiplatelet drugs.

Diabetes Management Drugs

Because type 2 diabetes is so prevalent in the United States, the chances that a massage therapist might have diabetic clients are excellent. When type 2 diabetes cannot be managed by diet and exercise alone, other interventions are used. They often start with diabetes management drugs, and may eventually culminate with the supplementation of insulin in various forms. Type 1 diabetes is also fairly common, and is managed with the use of insulin injections in various forms.

The implications for diabetes and massage therapists are many and complicated. While many diabetics manage their disease well and minimize their risk for secondary complications, others are prone to several problems that pose serious cautions for massage: systemic atherosclerosis, an increased risk of stroke, diabetic ulcers, and peripheral neuritis to name a few.

Furthermore, massage lowers blood glucose. While this is an advantage to diabetic clients, this challenge to homeostasis may sometimes be overwhelming enough to trigger a hypoglycemic episode. Massage therapists with diabetic clients should be aware of signs of hypo- and hyperglycemia, and should consult with those clients about how best to address their needs in an emergency.

Classes of drugs

- Insulin
- Oral glucose management drugs

Insulin

Common Examples

Humulin, Humalog, Lantus, Novolog, Novolin

Basic Mechanism

Insulin is a protein-based hormone that would be destroyed by digestive juices if taken orally. Consequently, it is administered by injection, either through multiple daily injections or through an insulin pump. It decreases blood glucose by helping to deliver glucose to cells that need this clean-burning fuel to do their jobs.

Implications for Massage

Clients who supplement insulin vary their injection sites; these areas need to be locally avoided in order not to interfere with normal uptake of the drug. Length of time for peak effect of the drug varies with the type of insulin; it is best to avoid the injection area for at least that amount of time. If uncertain, avoid it for 24 hours.

Because blood glucose stability is an issue for diabetic clients, it is best for them to receive massage in the middle of their insulin cycle, rather than at the end or at the beginning.

It might also be useful for a new client to check blood glucose before and after the session, so that if he or she needs to take in sugar in an easily accessible form, the therapist can plan ahead and have some juice, milk, or candy available.

Oral Glucose Management Drugs

Common Examples

Diabinase, Glucotrol, Glyburide, Glucophage, Precose

Basic Mechanism

These drugs work in a variety of ways to inhibit the production of sugar in the liver, to improve the output of insulin in the pancreas, and to increase the sensitivity of insulin receptors on target cells.

Implications for Massage

Of these drugs, Glucophage may have the least risk for setting up a hypoglycemic episode. Nonetheless, any clients who manage their diabetes with any combination of drugs and insulin must be monitored carefully for blood glucose stability. As with insulin, it is safest to work with these clients *after* the peak of drug activity.

Muscle relaxant drugs

Muscle relaxants are prescribed to deal with acute spasms related to trauma or anxiety, or to help with chronic spasticity from central nervous system damage as seen with multiple sclerosis, stroke, spinal cord injury, or cerebral palsy. They can act on the brain, the spinal cord, or in the muscle tissue itself.

A client who takes muscle relaxants is *not* inherently relaxed, although his or her tissues may seem that way. These drugs interfere with muscle protection reflexes, and so the risk of overtreatment with deep tissue work, range of motion exercises, or stretching is significant.

Classes of muscle relaxant drugs:

- Centrally acting skeletal muscle relaxants
- Peripherally acting skeletal muscle relaxants

Centrally acting skeletal muscle relaxants

Common Examples

Soma, Paraflex, Flexeril, Skelaxin, Norflex, Baclofen, Valium, Robaxin, Zanaflex

Basic Mechanism

These medications are central nervous system depressants. They suppress reflexes that would tighten muscles in response to stretching or damage. They are used to control painful acute spasms related to trauma or anxiety.

Implications for Massage

These drugs enforce a parasympathetic state, which may then be intensified by massage. Therapists should take care that clients are not overly exhausted at the end of a session. In addition, the protective stretch reflex is inhibited under these medications; therapists should not try to create an increased range of motion while the client is in this altered state.

Peripherally Acting Skeletal Muscle Relaxants

Common Examples

Dantrium

Basic Mechanism

This drug interferes with calcium release at the sarcoplasmic reticulum of muscle cells, leading to weaker contractions. It is used to treat chronic spasticity associated with central nervous system damage, but the overall weakness that ensues makes it a questionable choice for patients whose strength is borderline.

Implications for Massage

A client taking Dantrium will have a compromised stretch reflex and falsely hypotonic muscles; massage must be conducted conservatively.

Thyroid Supplement Drugs

Hypothyroidism is typically treated with supplements to replace thyroid secretions T3 and T4. Levothyroxine sodium is chemically identical to the thyroid secretion T4, and is meant to be converted to bioactive T3. While many hypothyroidism patients successfully treat their disease with levothyroxine sodium, some supplement T3 instead of or in addition to T4. This substance has traditionally been available in the form of desiccated animal glands, but a synthetic form of T3 has recently become available.

Classes of drugs:

- Levothyroxine sodium
- Desiccated extract
- Liothyronine sodium

Levothyroxine Sodium

Common Examples

Synthroid, Eltroxin, Levo-T, Levothroid, Levoxyl

Basic Mechanism

Synthetic thyroid hormones mimic the action of naturally occurring thyroid hormones to boost protein synthesis in cells, promote the use of glycogen stores, increase heart rate and cardiac output, and increase urine output.

Implications for Massage

New users of synthetic thyroid supplements may go through a period of nervousness, agitation, and insomnia, which massage may help to improve. If these symptoms persist, the dosage may not be correct, and the person should consult with the prescribing physician.

Someone who has been taking synthetic thyroid supplements for a long time probably has no significant side effects, and no implications for massage therapy.

Desiccated Extract

Common Examples

Armour Thyroid, Nature-Throid, Thyroid USP, Westhroid.

Basic Mechanism

These forms of thyroid hormone have the same action as synthetic supplements: they mimic the action of naturally occurring thyroid hormones to boost protein synthesis in cells, promote the use of glycogen stores, increase heart rate and cardiac output, and increase urine output. The difference is that the potency of these dosages is more difficult to predict, so users may experience significant fluctuation of symptoms.

Implications for Massage

As with synthetic hormones, a new user may experience increased anxiety, insomnia, or agitation, all of which indicate massage. If symptoms persist, the person needs to consult with the physician. Otherwise, massage is perfectly appropriate for clients who supplement thyroid hormones.

Liothyronine Sodium

Common Examples

Cytomel, Triostat.

Basic Mechanism

These synthetic forms of T3 are prescribed for patients who don't have success with levothyroxine sodium. They are meant to mimic the action of naturally occurring thyroid hormones to boost protein synthesis in cells, promote the use of glycogen stores, increase heart rate and cardiac output, and increase urine output.

Implications for Massage

As with other hormone supplements, anxiety, insomnia, or agitation may occur until dosage is correctly gauged. If symptoms persist, the person needs to consult with the physician. Otherwise, massage is perfectly appropriate for clients who supplement thyroid hormones.

Appendix B
Research Literacy, Research Capacity

"But We've Always Done It This Way"

Many people who were educated in massage therapy more than a few years ago learned about its physiological effects through revered but seldom-questioned lore, common sense, and educated guesses. Based on this tradition, massage therapists have been taught that "massage boosts circulation," without guidance for what kind of massage, for how long, and for whom. Many were taught that "massage spreads cancer" based on guesses about massage and fluid flow, but this claim turns out to be probably overstated. We have traditionally assumed that massage has its best applications for musculoskeletal issues, but our impact on the nervous and endocrine systems may be even more profound. What other traditions have we clung to out of loyalty rather than knowledge?

Every health care profession must go through the process of having its beloved mythologies tested and analyzed. The justification of the traditional "we've always done it this way" approach doesn't always hold up under scrutiny. The process of testing and analysis is a reflection of a basic aspect of human nature: the drive to know the best possible way to go about achieving certain goals. Massage therapy is finally entering this world, and massage therapists must become capable of reading and interpreting results: this is *research literacy*. Some practitioners must also become capable of conducting research projects—otherwise, clinical trials will not accurately reflect what happens in a realistic massage setting. The ability to conduct credible research is *research capacity*.

Good research creates amazing opportunities: it can supply information to massage therapists and educators; it can offer informed guidance to licensing and regulatory bodies; it provides a bridge to other health care practitioners. But, as Benjamin Disraeli wrote (and Mark Twain famously quoted), "*There are three kinds of lies: lies, damned lies, and statistics.*" This can be especially true when highly individualized modalities, such as massage therapy, are studied with the intent to quantify the unquantifiable, and where the practice of massage is often unique to each client-therapist relationship. This presents challenges to many traditional kinds of research design.

Fortunately, a number of invaluable resources have emerged to help massage therapists work their way through this jungle of observational studies, experimental studies, randomizing, blinding, confounds, and controls. This document is a grateful nod toward the pioneers who are working to make research literacy an attainable goal for massage therapists everywhere. These sources are listed with great appreciation and respect in the references section of this appendix.

Some vocabulary for research issues may be new to many readers. A brief definition of **bolded terms** is provided in Table B.1.

Traditionally, **quantitative** research has been held in higher regard than research on those processes that cannot be quantified. For example, if a patient with high blood pressure gets a massage, her blood pressure may go from 145/95 to 130/85, a quantitatively measurable change. However, recent innovations have strengthened the acceptability of **qualitative** research, which focuses on describing process and experience, rather than on numbers. For example, **Likert scales** (Figures B.1 and B.2) or **visual analog scales** (Figure B.3) are validated methods by which measurement can be carried out qualitatively. In many ways, these methods are better suited to track benefits of massage and bodywork, and as the results come in, we are discovering exciting, unexpected, and sometimes paradigm-shifting pieces of information.

Research in massage therapy is happening at an astonishing pace. As of this writing, a search for massage therapy that is limited to humans and the

TABLE B.1 Research Literacy Vocabulary List: Definition of Terms

Term	Definition
Anecdotes	Informal stories, which are not rigorously analyzed.
Best practices	An example or guideline of a standard which a profession recognizes as embodying the highest knowledge available.
Bias	To be influenced or to make errors in a particular direction, rather than to objectively evaluate the evidence.
Case series	Multiple case studies for a particular condition or treatment.
Case study	A detailed rigorous observation and analysis of the effects of a treatment or a condition in one patient.
Confound	A factor in a study that can interfere with, or confuse, the connection between treatment and outcome.
Control group	A group of subjects in an experiment/study that does not receive the treatment being studied. Sometimes the control group receives a placebo treatment; other times it simply receives a different treatment from the one being studied.
Crossover study	A form of research studies where each subject receives, in random order, both the control treatment and the experimental treatment. In this way, each subject serves as his own control.
Descriptive studies	A form of research studies that simply describes the observed effects of treatments without forming a hypothesis or trying to find a cause for whatever effects were observed.
Double-blinded	A form of research studies where neither the persons carrying out the experiment nor the subjects know which treatment the subjects are getting (the treatment being tested, or a placebo in its place). In other words, **both** the researchers and the study subjects are **blinded** to that information.
Empirical	Based on practical experimentation and observation
Evidence-informed medicine	Attaining to the highest standard of clinical care of patients by combining the best scientific evidence available with the practitioner's clinical judgment and experience, as well as with respect for the patient's preferences.
Experimental/ explanatory studies	A form of research studies concerned with not only describing the effects of a treatment, but also with discovering **how** and **why** it works or not—the relationship between cause (treatment) and effect (outcome).
Likert scale	A scale in which a patient or a subject in a study indicates a level of agreement with statements that are arranged in order from more to less strongly (or vice versa).
Power	A measurement of the number of study participants or subjects are necessary to ensure that the study will be able to reliably detect treatment effects.
Qualitative	Observations that are measured by "qualities" or descriptive properties of the experience, rather than with numbers ("soft," "hard," "easy," "difficult," "feels good," "hurts," "big," "small," "sad," "happy," etc. are all qualitative descriptions of outcomes).
Quantitative	Observations that are measured by numbers, such as 98.6°F temperature, 120/80 blood pressure, etc.
Randomization	A technique for lowering the opportunity for bias in a study, by using chance to decide which group (treatment or control) the subjects of a study are assigned to.

continues

TABLE B.1 Research Literacy Vocabulary List: Definition of Terms *continued*

Randomized control trial (RCT)	A form of research studies where outcomes for a treatment group are compared to outcomes for a control group, and the assignment of study subjects to one of the two groups is carried out through randomization.
Sham	A fake treatment, used to blind study subjects as to whether or not they are receiving the real treatment, so that their expectations cannot unconsciously bias the outcomes.
Single-blinded	A form of research studies where the persons carrying out the experiment know which treatment the subjects are getting (the treatment being tested, or a placebo in its place), but the subjects do not know which treatment they are receiving. In other words, **only** the study subjects are **blinded** to that information.
Validity	A measure of how well a study or experiment actually tests what it is intended to test.
Visual analog scale	A scale in which a patient or a subject in a study reports a subjective opinion of the intensity of a sensation. The visual analog scale is often used, for example, to report the degree of pain (i.e., from tolerable/less intense to intolerable/very intense).

English language in the PubMed database of health sciences research articles (http://www.pubmed.com) yields over 5,000 entries: each one an article describing some kind of research project in which massage was studied. The amount of information that is being generated today is dizzying—but how do we make sense of it, and put it to use?

Science and the Scientific Method

Reading technical research reports on massage can feel intimidating at first, but a few basic principles make the process much more straightforward. Most research articles follow a basic framework, and all credible studies are grounded in science and the scientific method. This is simply a formalized way of observing and describing something about the natural world in a way that others can repeat.

Evidence from scientific studies is often referred to as **empirical**, meaning it is derived from experiments. People frequently assume that "doing science" requires lots of fancy machines or special training, but all it really means is that we are making observations about the world that are organized, unbiased, well documented, reproducible, and understandable to others.

The scientific method is a widely applicable set of steps that can be adjusted for any scientific study, from physics to biology. For the context of massage, it can be described in the following steps:

1. Make an observation about the natural world.
2. Develop a testable theory about how massage or bodywork might influence that observation.
3. Make a prediction or hypothesis for what you expect to happen when you test your theory.
4. Carry out an experiment that tests your theory. Try to control the circumstances around your test so that you can accurately connect the experiment to the outcomes.

How interested are you in the topic of research literacy? (Circle one)				
Very interested	Somewhat interested	Neutral	Not very interested	Not at all interested

Figure B.1. Likert scale

Research literacy is...

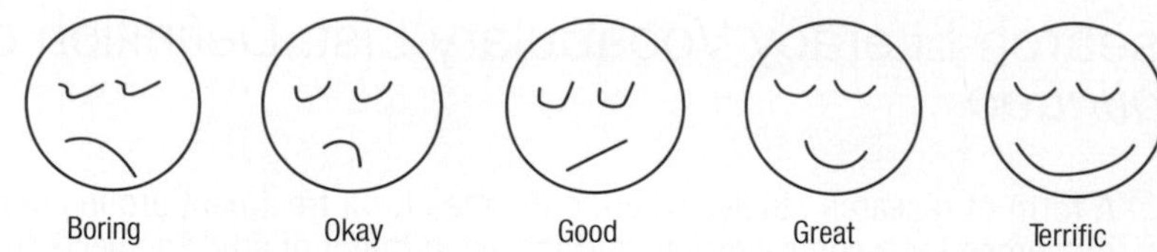

Figure B.2. Likert scale alternate

5. Observe and document your results. Did the test go as you expected, or not?
6. Based on your results, decide whether your theory needs to be modified, or if it really did successfully predict what happened.

It is important to point out that the scientific method can be much broader than what is presented here, but this model provides a good starting point for this discussion.

Structure of a Journal Article: IMRAD

In keeping with the scientific method explained above, most research articles follow a standard format, which describes a project in an organized way. This allows other researchers to repeat the study to see if they get similar results. The format is sometimes called IMRAD, an acronym that stands for *introduction, methods, results, and discussion*. We'll use a study that tested whether massage could benefit the health of infants in an orphanage[1] to see how the parts of an article correspond to the scientific method.

I = *Introduction*

The "I" in IMRAD stands for "introduction," which is the first part of the body of an article. The author uses the introduction to explain the importance of the research, to share an observation, and to offer a testable explanation and prediction for what is expected to happen in the study. In other words, the introduction covers steps 1 to 3 of the scientific process.

Step 1: Make an observation about the natural world

> According to a recent World Health Organization report, during the 2000-2003 period, diarrhea remained the second most common factor responsible for mortality of children younger than 5 years in the world...Diarrhea is quite common in institutions such as orphanages where infants come in close contact with each other for prolonged periods of time.[1, p. 314]

Step 2: Develop a testable theory about how massage or bodywork might influence that observation

> It is imperative that interventions with the potential to decrease the incidence of diarrhea be developed and tested to decrease the likelihood of diarrhea in infants and young children. Massage therapy is one intervention with such potential as it has been linked to positive health outcomes in a variety of populations.[1, p. 315]

Step 3: Make a prediction or hypothesis for what you expect to happen when you test your theory

> The purpose of this study was to determine whether infant massage would decrease the incidence of diarrhea and overall illness in infants living in orphanage settings.[1, p. 315]

M = *Methods*

The "M" in IMRAD stands for the "methods" section of the article. This segment describes exactly how the experiment is conducted. It needs to be especially

How much of an impact on your work has learning about research literacy had?

No effect ——————————————————— Huge effect

Figure B.3. Visual analog scale

clear, because the **validity** of the results depends mostly on the integrity of the methods.

Step 4: Carry out an experiment that tests your theory. Try to control the circumstances around your test so that you can accurately connect the experiment to the outcomes

> Infants in the experimental group received a 15-minute full-body (including the legs, stomach, chest, arms, face, and back) massage daily, usually in the morning, delivered by orphanage volunteers or staff, all of whom were trained in infant massage by a PhD-level, certified instructor using techniques endorsed by Infant Massage USA.[1, p. 316]

R = Results

The "R" in IMRAD stands for the "results" section of the article. This is where the researcher reports what happens, without interpretation. This may be done as a verbal description, and/or with charts or graphs to display data.

Step 5: Observe and document the results—did your prediction occur as expected, or not?

> The prevented fraction for the target population was estimated to be 16%, indicating that by participating in the massage intervention, the incidence of diarrhea could possibly be reduced by 16% among similar populations of infants.[1, p. 317]

AD = *and Discussion*

"A" stands for "and", and "D" stands for the "discussion" section of the article. In this segment, the researcher discusses the meaning of the results; whether the hypothesis was confirmed or not, and why; and what this means both for future research and in current applications.

Step 6: Based on your results, decide whether your theory needs to be modified, or if it really did successfully predict what happened

> Results of this experimental pilot project were promising in that infants who were massaged daily had significantly fewer days of diarrhea and slightly lower rates of overall illness than infants in the control group. As noted above, other studies have indicated that massage improves immune functioning, and there may have been increased immunity in the infants in the experimental group in this project. Another possibility is that massage improved infants' gastrointestinal functioning through stimulation of the vagus nerve. If massage can indeed decrease the incidence of diarrhea among orphaned infants, this avenue of intervention should be pursued, particularly given the high risk of mortality associated with this condition in developing countries.[1, p. 317]

Understanding the structure of the scientific method and of research articles can help you to navigate the literature and decide what specific studies mean for you and your practice. But life is wonderfully complex, and the approach described above cannot be applied to all types of questions. Consequently, researchers have developed a wide array of designs to apply the scientific method to real-life circumstances that occur whenever we work with people. We'll discuss some of those approaches below, relating them to the steps we just went over, in order to keep them understandable in context.

The Scientific Method and Massage: Strengths and Weaknesses

The scientific method often derives information about the natural world by separating components of a process, and studying each piece independently of the others. Then that knowledge is reintegrated into a larger context. This is analysis (looking at individual pieces), followed by synthesis (putting ideas together).

An effective way to study how massage works is to isolate various aspects of the practice, which can later be reintegrated into larger pictures. This control of variables allows us to be more precise about how we link exposure to outcome, or cause to effect. For example, look at the following questions and identify which one is likely to yield the most reliable information about how massage affects human function?

> Example A: What is the effect of massage therapy administered by parents on sleep disturbances in autistic children?

Example B: What is the effect of pétrissage administered by sports massage practitioners to marathon runners on postevent soreness in the gastrocnemius (calf) muscle?

Example B is the correct answer for several reasons: the scope of the research question is much narrower (one muscle versus the whole process of sleep). The population is much more similar to each other (highly trained athletes have more in common than does a diverse group of children with a poorly understood condition). The amount of time being studied is much shorter for the athletes (postevent versus all night). There is much less variation in the one stroke (pétrissage) than in all of massage therapy, and finally sports massage practitioners have more standardized training than do parents. All of these factors make a study of the effect of massage therapy administered by parents on sleep disturbances in autistic children much more challenging than a study of the effect of pétrissage administered by sports massage practitioners to marathon runners on postevent soreness in the gastrocnemius muscle. This does not mean that we can't study how massage affects the sleep patterns of autistic children, but we have to make some adjustments to the research design in order to do so.

The Randomized Control Trial

A **randomized controlled trial** (RCT) is considered the gold standard of research study design, because it adheres as closely as possible to the ideal scientific method. A treatment group and a **control group** are studied, so that outcomes can be compared between them; this helps to isolate cause and effect, and helps to eliminate **bias**. Participants are **randomized** into the two groups, so that any differences among the groups average out as much as possible, and don't confuse or **confound** the outcome.

Other steps to reduce bias include blinding. The trial may be **single-blinded**, in which case the participants don't know whether they are receiving the treatment or not: in this way, preconceived notions about effectiveness won't taint the outcomes. In blinded tests, some participants receive a **sham** treatment, or participants could receive some different kind of intervention: a friendly visit, or a relaxation tape for instance, but not know which intervention is truly being studied. If the people analyzing the data don't know which participants received the real treatment, they work with the data exactly as it is created, and expectations cannot creep in and taint their analysis. When analysts are blinded in this way as well, we say the trial is **double-blinded.**

You probably see some design challenges with this for massage already: if you're studying a drug, you can give the control group a sugar pill, and if you're studying acupressure, you can use a sham point instead of the real one as a placebo. But how do you give someone a placebo massage? That is one of the difficulties with carrying out RCTs in this context.

Another challenge is ethical. In order to carry out a full-fledged RCT, the study needs a large enough number of participants (sufficient **power**) in order to determine what is a real treatment effect, and what is not. But it can be difficult and expensive to round up a significant number of participants and qualified therapists and analysts to conduct a large-scale study. In this case, two ethical imperatives compete against each other. On one hand, it is unethical to claim knowledge about massage that cannot be backed up with reliable evidence. On the other hand, if logistical problems interfere with the collection of information, is it right to deny patients the relief that massage may provide? In this situation, **evidence-informed medicine** advises that we follow the **best practices** standard in the profession. It is our responsibility then to evaluate the effectiveness of massage to the best of our abilities, and to neither overpromise what massage can do, nor deny patients the benefits of massage, simply because it cannot meet the standards of an RCT.

Beyond the Randomized Control Trial

The RCT can be difficult or impossible to apply to some aspects of massage research, but other research designs may be a better fit. They can help identify best practices for massage, and they can provide research questions for later, methodologically stronger, studies. For example, practitioners who work with someone with catastrophic burn injuries, or brain damage from oxygen deprivation, can write up their work as case studies. Other practitioners with similar clients can use that work, and write up their case studies in turn. And a university researcher can decide that several case studies indicate a trend that deserves further investigation, and marshal the resources of the university and medical communities to design a larger RCT on the same research questions.

Researchers have created a hierarchy of evidence, ranging from the RCT at the strongest end, to the **case study** and **anecdotes** (stories) at the weakest end. A **case series** is a collection of case studies that all address a similar question or make a similar observation. **Experimental** or **explanatory studies** allow the investigators to control the variables, and to look for mechanisms or causes to explain results. **Descriptive** studies observe phenomena without attempting to explain cause and effect. In a **crossover study**, each participant serves as his or her own control, and the results of an intervention are measured twice: once when the subject gets no treatment, and again when the subject receives the treatment. Each type of study is valuable in different situations.

What Can One Massage Therapist Do?

The easiest and fastest way to begin moving from research literacy into research capacity is by conducting a case study. If you want to be part of a research team that is funded to carry out studies on massage, a long journey of learning is probably ahead. But you can start to along that path, and you can give back to others who would benefit from your experience, by writing up interesting or unusual case reports from your practice. Most trade journals for massage dedicate space to research issues; consider submitting your report for publication. You may also consider participating in the Massage Therapy Foundation's student or practitioner case report contests. Visit *http://www.massagetherapyfoundation.org/* for more information.

Remember the IMRAD structure as you document your experience.

- **I:** Write the introduction first. What is this patient's need? What is the larger context? What does the literature say about it? You can learn how to find articles related to your topic from databases such as PubMed, the Massage Therapy Foundation, and other sources. Explain your basis for thinking that massage would be a good treatment. The literature you refer to here will become your References/Bibliography section.
- **M:** Next comes the methods section: describe what you did to treat the patient. Be careful, clear, and detailed, so that an interested reader could reproduce your study if he or she wanted to.
- **R:** Report the outcome in your results section. This is a place just for the facts you have gathered; interpretation comes next.
- **D:** The discussion or conclusions section is the place to interpret or relate the meaning of your results to the larger context from your introduction, and where you recommend what you consider is the next step for other people to take.

Finally, write the abstract. An abstract is a very short summary that sketches out the entire article. Readers use it to decide whether your report is pertinent to their practice. If you have addressed an issue interesting to them, they can read the full text.

As a practicing massage therapist, you have a lot of knowledge to offer. Developing your research literacy and research capacity is a way of making an important contribution, both to other massage therapists, and to the profession as a whole.

It is not an easy journey, but it is a wonderful one.

Reference

1. Jump VK, Fargo JD, Akers JF. Impact of massage therapy on health outcomes among orphaned infants in Ecuador: results of a randomized clinical trial. Family Community Health. 2006;29(4):314–319.

Suggested Readings

1. Dryden T, Achilles R. The Massage Therapy Research Curriculum Kit. Evanston, IL: Massage Therapy Foundation, 2004.
2. Hymel G. Research Methods for Massage and Holistic Therapies. Philadelphia, PA: Mosby, 2005.
3. Menard MB. Making Sense of Research. 2nd edition Toronto, ON: Curties-Overzet Publications Inc., 2010.
4. Jump VK, Fargo JD, Akers JF. Impact of massage therapy on health outcomes among orphaned infants in Ecuador: results of a randomized clinical trial. Family and Community Health. 2006 Oct-Dec;29(4):314–9.

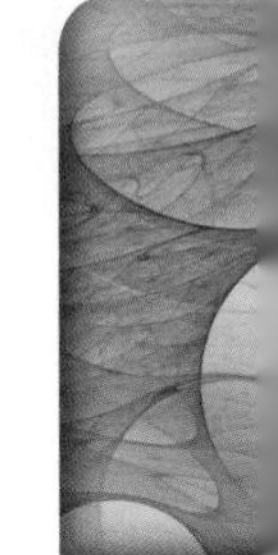

Appendix C
Extra Conditions—At a Glance

Abortion, Spontaneous and Elective

Definition: What Is It?

An elective abortion is the intentional termination of a pregnancy; a spontaneous abortion is an unintentional termination. In either case, the fetus and placenta are detached from the uterine wall and cannot continue to develop.

Etiology: What Happens?

A pregnancy can be electively terminated in different ways, depending on the stage. If it happens within the first 12 weeks, an elective abortion is usually conducted with medication or vacuum suction. In the thirteenth to fifteenth weeks, a D&C (dilation and curettage) may be performed. Later terminations are brought about by inducing premature labor. They can be very difficult and requires hospitalization.

Spontaneous abortion is called miscarriage if it happens in the first 14 weeks of pregnancy, and stillbirth if it happens late in gestation. Several factors may contribute to the spontaneous disruption of a pregnancy. Some of these are controllable, but many of them are not.

Controllable factors that may raise the risk of miscarriage include smoking, untreated infections of the reproductive tract, untreated diabetes or thyroid disorders, exposure to toxic chemicals, especially solvents, and progesterone deficiency in the early weeks of pregnancy. An immune system response that causes blood in fetal vessels to clot can be controlled with low doses of aspirin or other blood thinners.

Uncontrollable factors include structural problems in the uterus (fibroid tumors or a weak cervix), the fertilization of multiple eggs, age, autoimmune disease, an immune system rejection of fetal tissue, failure of the fetus to implant into the endometrium, or what is perhaps the most common cause of miscarriage: the fetus is simply missing key genetic information that would allow it to continue to develop. When the moment comes that the needed genes are missing, the fetus dies.

Signs and Symptoms

When the endometrial lining of the uterus is disrupted in any way but a normal menses, the endometrium is traumatized. This is true for elective and spontaneous abortions and also for childbirth. Symptoms of this trauma can include pain (local and referred), bleeding, and cramping. These are generally self-limiting; that is, the symptoms resolve themselves with time, unless complications develop.

Complications

Complications of elective abortions or miscarriages can include infection from incomplete shedding of the uterine lining; damage to the uterus, bladder, or colon from surgical instruments; and possible hemorrhaging. Depression or anxiety disorders are other frequent complications. The later the gestational age of the fetus, the higher the risk of complications from elective or spontaneous abortion.

Treatment

Spontaneous abortions that are complete require no treatment. Elective abortions, or spontaneous abortions that are incomplete or complicated, may require procedures ranging from medication to stimulate uterine contraction, to dilation and curettage, and to open surgery. Other treatments are determined by the needs of the woman, and may include antibiotics for infection, analgesics, counseling, or other interventions.

Medications

- For medical abortion: drugs that mimic hormonal activity, administered orally, by injection, or via the vagina
- Analgesics, including NSAIDs or codeine
- Ergot alkaloids to promote uterine contraction
- Prostaglandins, oxytocin, or other medication to control bleeding

Massage?

RISKS	Intrusive abdominal work is not indicated for a woman recovering from a recent pregnancy loss until the bleeding has stopped and she is free from any signs of complications.
BENEFITS	Gentle bodywork can be supportive and helpful during an extremely stressful time.

Acromegaly

Definition: What Is It?

Acromegaly ("acro-" means extremities, "megaly" means enlargement) is a disorder involving the production of too much growth hormone in adults. It is usually related to the development of a slow-growing benign tumor on the pituitary gland, although it can occasionally be connected to tumors elsewhere.

Etiology: What Happens?

The pituitary gland secretes growth hormone (GH), under the command of the hypothalamus. The secretion of GH stimulates in turn the release of a chemical from the liver: insulin-like growth factor I (IGF-I). GH and IGF-I stimulate the metabolism of fuel into new cells for growth (in young people) and for repair (in older people).

A tumor on the pituitary gland leads to the release of excessive amounts of GH and IGF-I. This stimulates the production of masses of new tissues, resulting in bone enlargement, which can cause joint distortion and pain, and enlargement and weakening of the heart. In addition, the tumor itself can exert mechanical pressure on the pituitary and other brain structures, causing a variety of problems. The type of tumor associated with acromegaly is benign, but dangerous for the symptoms it causes.

Signs and Symptoms

Often, the earliest symptoms of acromegaly are headaches and vision problems brought about by pressure inside the cranium. The hands and feet may grow, along with facial changes including enlarged mandibles and spaces between teeth. Joint pain, fatigue, hyperhydrosis (excessive sweatiness) with body odor, and sleep apnea (probably related to an enlarged tongue) are frequent problems. Skin tags are common, along with a deeper voice. If a tumor grows to a significant size, other central nervous system symptoms may occur, including cranial nerve damage.

Complications

Midlife changes in bone size and shape put acromegaly patients at risk for painful arthritis. If the tumor interferes with other pituitary functions, other endocrine-related dysfunctions might include thickened, oily skin, heavy menstrual periods, growth of body hair, and breast discharge. Because the sudden growth of new tissues can stress the heart, some of the most serious complications of acromegaly have to do with cardiovascular challenge. High blood pressure is common, along with a pathologic enlargement of the heart: cardiomegaly. Eventually, untreated acromegaly patients may experience congestive heart failure.

Some acromegaly patients develop insulin resistance or diabetes mellitus. A higher-than-average risk of colorectal cancer has also been observed among this population. Women are more prone to uterine fibroid tumors as well.

Treatment

Surgery for acromegaly is most successful when the pituitary tumor is small. This transsphenoidal surgery is conducted through the nose or upper lip. Postsurgical radiation may be recommended. Other therapies focus on attempts to balance the GH/IGF-I balance that is lost when the pituitary gland becomes hyperactive.

Medications

- Somatostatin analogs to suppress GH production and shrink the tumor
- GH receptor antagonists to interfere with GH activity and normalize IGF-I secretion
- Dopamine agonists to lower GH and IGF-I secretion

Massage?

RISKS	Serious or extreme cases of acromegaly carry a risk of heart failure; this requires adaptation of bodywork choices. Acromegaly patients also have higher-than-average rates of colorectal cancer and diabetes: these must be investigated for safety.
BENEFITS	Massage is unlikely to change the course of acromegaly, but within safety limits it can certainly improve a patient's quality of life. Clients who have successfully treated their pituitary tumor with no long-term damage can enjoy the same benefits from massage as the rest of the population.

Addison Disease

Definition: What Is It?

Addison disease involves the destruction of the adrenal cortex, limiting the secretion of any combination of cortisol, aldosterone, or androgenic hormones. It can be related to an infection, but it is usually an autoimmune condition.

Etiology: What Happens?

The adrenal glands are composed of two main regions: the medulla and the cortex. The adrenal cortex produces hormones in three main classes: glucocorticoids, mineralocorticoids, and androgens. Glucocorticoids, of which cortisol is the most well known, create appropriate stress responses; influence the metabolism of proteins, fats, and sugars; suppress immune system activity; and do several other important jobs. Mineralocorticoids help to maintain blood pressure by affecting water and salt retention at the kidneys; aldosterone is the primary mineralocorticoid. Androgens are male sex hormones; women secrete much of their androgens from the adrenal cortex, while men secrete most of theirs from the testes.

Addison disease develops when autoimmune disease or infection destroys much of the adrenal cortex and interferes with the secretion of adrenal cortex hormones. Pituitary disruption can also suppress adrenal cortex secretion.

Signs and Symptoms

Signs and symptoms of adrenal cortex insufficiency include muscle weakness and fatigue, low blood pressure, hypoglycemia, irritability, and depression. When aldosterone levels are low, salt craving and dehydration develop. Low androgen levels in women result in the loss of pubic and axillary hair; men, who secrete most of their androgens from the testes, are not affected in this way.

A link between corticotrophin-releasing hormone (which increases when the adrenals are low functioning) and melanocyte-stimulating hormone means that Addison disease often involves patches of darkened skin and mucous membranes where melanocytes become overactive.

Types of Addison Disease

- Primary Addison disease: This is usually an autoimmune attack on the adrenal glands, called idiopathic adrenal insufficiency. If other glands are affected, it is called polyendocrine deficiency syndrome. About 20% of primary Addison disease in the United States is related to tuberculosis, but in countries where TB is more common this percentage is much higher. Adrenal damage can also occur because of cancer metastasis, chronic fungal infections, local hemorrhage, and other more obscure reasons.
- Secondary Addison disease: This occurs when pituitary secretions of adrenocorticotropic hormone (ACTH) are abnormally low. If ACTH levels drop, then cortisol secretion also drops. This can happen when a person who supplements steroidal hormones suddenly stops taking his or her medication, or when the pituitary is affected by a tumor or surgery.

Complications

An addisonian crisis involves a sudden onset of sharp abdominal pain, severe nausea, vomiting, and diarrhea. Low back pain and pain in the arms and legs may occur, along with dangerously low blood pressure, high potassium levels, and loss of consciousness. An addisonian crisis is a medical emergency.

Treatment

Addison disease is highly treatable with oral or injected doses of steroids to replace the missing hormones. Salt supplementation is recommended for patients low on aldosterone, especially during hot weather or with excessive physical work that involves sweating.

Medications

- Oral or injected corticosteroids to replace depleted cortisol
- Synthetic mineralocorticoid (fludrocortisone acetate) to replace depleted aldosterone
- Androgen replacement therapy for women with Addison disease

Massage?

RISKS	Addison disease often involves weakness and low blood pressure, and the treatment involves taking steroids that carry important side effects. Massage therapists and other bodywork practitioners must make adjustments accordingly.
BENEFITS	While massage is unlikely to change the prognosis of Addison disease, within the limits of client adaptation it can certainly add to a client's quality of life.

Avascular Necrosis

Definition: What Is It?

Avascular necrosis (AVN) is a condition in which blood supply to a bone is impeded by some combination of factors. Bone tissue and blood vessels disintegrate and are never fully replaced. The resulting weakness leads to a high risk of fractures, arthritis, and joint collapse.

Etiology: What Happens?

Several factors may work together to interrupt blood flow to a bone, including trauma or tiny emboli made of blood clots, fat cells, or nitrogen bubbles: this can be a complication of decompression sickness, or "the bends."

Other conditions that can lead to AVN include excessive alcohol consumption, steroids for autoimmune disease or organ transplant patients, hemophilia, sickle-cell disease, HIV, and pancreatitis.

Because it relies on only one major blood source, the head of the femur is particularly vulnerable to interruptions in blood flow. The end result of AVN often involves serious damage to this important structure. Damage is usually unilateral.

Signs and Symptoms

AVN often has a slow onset. It may begin with loss of range of motion, limping and joint pain just during movement, but the pain worsens and becomes prevalent even during rest. Pain may refer to the lateral thigh or knee. In later stages, AVN shows all the signs of osteoarthritis. Eventually, it may lead to total collapse of the joint.

Types of Avascular Necrosis

- **Legg-Calve-Perthes disease:** This is a type of AVN that is almost exclusive to young children. This rare condition affects boys about four times more often than girls, and is typically diagnosed between age 3 and 10. Most cases of LCPD have an excellent prognosis, but children may temporarily need braces, crutches, and surgery to reshape the head of the femur.
- **Osteonecrosis of the jaw:** This is a rare form of AVN that affects the mandible. It is related to the use of bisphosphonate drugs used to treat osteoporosis or the bone loss that sometimes develops with cancer or cancer treatments.

Treatment

Treatment options for AVN are determined by several variables, including age, cause, and severity. Nonsurgical treatments include the use of physical therapy, braces or crutches to temporarily relieve weight-bearing stress. Electrical stimulation of the bone may be recommended to stimulate healthy new growth.

Many AVN patients eventually undergo some kind of surgery to decompress the medullary canal, to remove dead tissue, to reshape the bone for better strength, or to replace a ruined joint.

Medications

- Anti-inflammatories to control inflammation and pain (this does not include aspirin for young children)
- Anticholesterol drugs to limit the risk of fat emboli

Massage?

RISKS	Avascular necrosis involves severely damaged bone with loss of range of motion and the risk of fracture. Any massage needs to be adjusted for this vulnerability at and around the affected area. AVN is often a complication of an underlying disorder: this must be pursued in case other cautions for massage exist.
BENEFITS	As long as the rest of circulation is healthy, massage anywhere away from the affected area may help to manage some of the compensatory postural and movement patterns that develop when walking is painful.

Bronchiectasis

Definition: What Is It?

Bronchiectasis is a condition in which the bronchi and bronchioles of the lungs become permanently dilated, thickened, and unable to clear mucus. It is related to a wide variety of underlying disorders.

Etiology: What Happens?

In this condition, chronic or repeated irritation to the proximal and medium-sized bronchi causes the smooth muscle and elastin in these tubes to degenerate. The structures become rigidly open and thickened, and the ability to clear mucus is seriously impaired. This allows the lungs to become a veritable growth medium for bacteria or other pathogens, leading to more mucus production, and a vicious circle of lung dysfunction.

Bronchiectasis is part of the process of a wide variety of disorders. It is considered part of the chronic obstructive pulmonary disease (COPD) group, along with chronic bronchitis and emphysema, but instead of being related closely to cigarette smoking, it is most often connected to repeated infections (especially pneumonia or pertussis), congenital disorders (especially cystic fibrosis), autoimmune disease, gastroesophageal reflux disease, or other conditions.

Signs and Symptoms

Signs and symptoms of bronchiectasis typically begin with a productive cough. Shortness of breath and chest pain are frequently present. During an infective flare, mucus may be thick, opaque, and foul smelling. Lung sounds called crackles may be audible with a stethoscope.

Complications

Bronchiectasis has several serious possible complications. Increased vulnerability to infection raises the risk of lung abscesses or life-threatening pneumonia. Rarely, extreme coughing can damage an artery in the lung leading to excessive bleeding into the sputum; this is called hemoptysis. Progressive respiratory failure can develop as the lungs lose function. And resistance in the pulmonary circuit can put an excessive load on the right side of the heart, leading to cor pulmonale, or right sided heart failure.

Treatment

Treatment for bronchiectasis is directed at improving lung clearance, controlling infection, addressing underlying conditions, and improving the strength of breathing muscles. Patients are counseled to avoid smoking and secondhand smoke, and to keep current on immunizations for flu and pneumonia. Physical therapy often includes aggressive manual clapping over the thorax; this may also be accomplished with devices that range from an inflatable percussive vest to a handheld inhaling instrument that sends vibrations into the chest. If the bronchiectasis is limited to a focal area of the lung and other interventions are not successful, resection surgery may be recommended. Patients at risk for cor pulmonale may supplement oxygen.

Medications

Medications may vary according to other conditions that contribute to lung damage.

- Antibiotics to treat and prevent bacterial and mycoplasma infections
- Expectorants to assist lung clearing
- Inhaled medications
  - Bronchodilators
  - Corticosteroids
  - Beta-agonists for smooth muscle relaxation
- Immuno-suppressant drugs to treat autoimmune diseases
- Medications to treat gastroesophageal reflux disease

Massage?

RISKS	A person with bronchiectasis may be at significantly increased risk for developing respiratory infections; massage should be rescheduled if either the client or the therapist shows any signs of respiratory infection. Patients may also have a variety of underlying disorders, any of which may require adaptation for massage.
BENEFITS	Pulmonary physical therapy is a mainstay of bronchiectasis treatment, and massage may be adapted to fit into this context as well. Any bodywork that improves resilience, immune system activity, and fatigue will be welcomed, as long as it respects other challenges that the patient faces.

Carditis

Definition: What Is It?

Technically, carditis is inflammation of the heart. In reality, this term refers to any of three sites of inflammation: the pericardium, the myocardium, or the endocardium, especially where it covers the heart valves.

Etiology: What Happens?

Carditis is often related to an infection. Many viruses, bacteria, and fungi can colonize the layers of the heart, and each pathogen has its own pattern of symptoms, damage, and response to treatment. Other causes of inflammation in and around the heart include autoimmune activity (especially with systemic lupus erythematosus, scleroderma, and sarcoidosis), trauma, or reactions to medications.

Signs and Symptoms

Signs and symptoms of carditis vary according to the causative factors and the part of the heart that is affected. Some forms of myocarditis are practically silent in early stages, but most acute viral and bacterial infections cause a predictable set of symptoms including fever, malaise, dyspnea, and stabbing chest pain. Pain often refers to the left arm, shoulder, and scapula. Many patients find that inhalation becomes painful, but sitting with the trunk in flexion relieves pain: this is a characteristic sign of carditis. Heart rhythms may become abnormal, and sounds from the friction of scarred layers of pericardium rubbing together may be audible through a stethoscope.

Types of Carditis

- **Pericarditis:** This is inflammation of the pericardial sac, but it may penetrate to the myocardial cells as well. It is usually due to a viral or bacterial infection. Damage to healthy cells comes about both through pathogenic activities and through immune system responses. While most cases of pericarditis are short-lived, two serious complications can develop: cardiac tamponade, where the pericardial sac fills with fluid that puts mechanical pressure on the heart and can lead to circulatory failure, and constrictive pericarditis, where enough scar tissue builds between the visceral and parietal layers of the pericardium that a normal heartbeat is inhibited.
- **Myocarditis:** This is inflammation of the myocardium. It is often related to a viral attack, but autoimmune diseases can cause it as well. The net result is that myofibers are destroyed and replaced with noncontractile connective tissue. The prognosis of myocarditis is unpredictable: it can go to full recovery with no long-term ill effects, or it can lead to heart failure.
- **Endocarditis:** This is inflammation of the endocardium, especially where it covers the valves of the heart. People with a history of heart or valve problems are at heightened risk for developing an infection here, so they are often counseled to use prophylactic antibiotics before undergoing any dental procedures or other types of surgery. Pathogens tend to colonize the heart valves downstream from blood flow, where they trigger the growth of structures called vegetations. These are formed of platelets, fibrin, pathogens, and immune system cells. Vegetations can be large enough to occlude a valve opening, but they tend to be delicate and easily breakable.

Fragments that enter the bloodstream become arterial emboli and can have serious repercussions.

Treatment

Most forms of carditis are treated with bed rest, good nutrition, and drugs to address infection, autoimmune activity, or the risk of heart failure. Pericardiocentesis is a procedure using a long thin needle to extract excess fluid from the pericardial sac: this is used to treat cardiac tamponade. Surgery to replace damaged valves or to repair or remove a seriously scarred pericardium is sometimes recommended.

Medications

- NSAIDs to manage pain and inflammation
- Antibiotics for bacterial infection (note: these may be given intravenously for several weeks)
- Narcotic analgesics if necessary
- Steroidal anti-inflammatories to manage autoimmune disease (note: these must be avoided in the presence of infection)
- Beta-blockers, ACE inhibitors, diuretics, and other hypertension management drugs in the presence of heart failure

Massage?

RISKS	Whichever type of carditis is present, it is an indication that the homeostatic processes of the body are severely impaired. Any kind of bodywork that requires significant adaptation should be postponed until the inflammation has subsided and the patient is restored to health.
BENEFITS	Bodywork that does not present a challenge to homeostasis may be soothing and welcome during a time of significant fear and stress. Clients who have fully recovered from carditis and are cleared for physical activity can enjoy the same benefits from massage as the rest of the population.

Charcot-Marie-Tooth Syndrome

Definition: What Is It?

Charcot-Marie-Tooth syndrome (CMT) is a collection of genetic neurologic conditions that affect the myelin or long axons of the peripheral nervous system. It affects about 125,000 people in the United States.

Etiology: What Happens?

The inherited genetic mutations that cause CMT can be dominant, recessive, X linked, or spontaneous. Each type of CMT involves a different mutation, but the ultimate results on the body are the same. Most versions lead to problems with the production of the myelin sheath by Schwann cells in the peripheral nervous system. Areas of unstable myelin develop; the myelin breaks down; and then Schwann cells proliferate, make extra myelin that may be defective, and the cycle begins again. Ultimately, poorly myelinated axons have slowed conduction, and sensation is impaired. In a slightly different form of CMT, the damage occurs not to the myelin but to the nerve fibers themselves. All forms of CMT lead to poor conduction of motor impulses and some sensory messages.

Interestingly, the sensory deficit brought about by the most common type of CMT is restricted to texture and pressure sensation. Pain and temperature-sensitive neurons are not myelinated, and so are usually unaffected by this disease.

Signs and Symptoms

CMT symptoms usually develop by adolescence or early adulthood. Weakness and muscle wasting in the feet and lower legs are common early signs. Clumsiness, frequent tripping, and falls may be the first things parents notice. As the muscles of the foot atrophy, the flexor tendons may distort the foot into an extremely high arch (pes cavus) with hammertoes, along with a risk of sores and infections at the foot. Foot drop and an exaggerated gait to accommodate for this weakness may develop.

Many CMT patients don't report numbness or loss of sensation, but this may be because pain and temperature sensation are usually intact, and the other sensations (texture and pressure) had never fully developed. Some patients experience pain with nerve degeneration and severe muscle cramps.

CMT is often slowly progressive, and may eventually affect the muscles of the hand and arm. In rare cases, it impairs the action of the phrenic nerve, leading to problems with breathing.

Treatment

As a genetic disorder, CMT has no specific treatment. Instead, symptoms and complications are addressed with orthotics; crutches, canes, or braces; medication to manage pain; and therapy to enhance strength and stability.

Medications

- NSAIDs for pain and inflammation
- Tricyclic antidepressants for neuropathic pain and depression
- Anticonvulsant medications for pain and sedation

Massage?

RISKS	CMT patients have some reduced sensation in the affected limbs. Fortunately, pain and temperature sensation tend to remain intact, but care must be taken to respect the fact that pressure and texture sensation may be impaired. The pain related to CMT is mainly related to nerve damage and muscle spasm. Carelessly applied massage may make either of these situations worse.
BENEFITS	CMT patients are often engaged in extensive physical and occupational therapy to counteract progressive muscle weakness, contracture of tendons, and postural instability. Massage, with respect for cramping, nerve pain, and loss of sensation, could have a useful place here as well.

Cushing Syndrome

Definition: What Is It?

Cushing syndrome is a condition in which cortisol levels in the blood are excessively high for a prolonged period, leading to tissue changes and possible death. It is also called hypercortisolism.

Etiology: What Happens?

Cortisol, the principal glucocorticoid hormone, is secreted by the adrenal cortex. It has many functions, including working with the stress response, immune system activity, fluid retention, metabolism of food into energy, and balancing insulin activity. Cortisol production is controlled by a chain that begins in the hypothalamus, which signals the pituitary gland to release adrenocorticotrophic hormone, or ACTH. ACTH stimulates the adrenal glands to release cortisol. When cortisol levels are dangerously high for a prolonged period, many tissues throughout the body are affected.

The most common forms of Cushing syndrome occur when ACTH levels are abnormally high (endogenous hypercortisolism), or as a reaction to cortisol-based medication (exogenous hypercortisolism).

Signs and Symptoms

Perhaps the most well-recognized sign of Cushing syndrome is the development of fatty deposits around the neck and face (giving rise to a "moonface" presentation), and around the abdomen and upper back. Arms and legs typically become thin and weak.

High levels of cortisol can damage supportive collagen. This is reflected in bone thinning, and in the development of very thin, delicate skin, often with purple stretch marks.

Other effects of hypercortisolism include high blood pressure; high blood glucose with an increased risk of developing diabetes; mood changes that involve irritability, anxiety, and depression; severe acne; slowed healing with suppressed immune system activity; the development of excessive body hair (hirsutism) and disrupted menstrual cycles for women; and decreased fertility, decreased sex drive, and erectile dysfunction for men.

Types of Cushing Syndrome

- **Endogenous Hypercortisolism:** This develops when too much ACTH is secreted by the pituitary gland or other tissues, or when the adrenal glands themselves secrete too much cortisol. It can come about because of a benign tumor on the pituitary gland (this is called Cushing disease), or because tumor cells in other tissues produce abnormal levels of ACTH. Rarely, Cushing syndrome is related to tumors on the adrenal glands themselves.
- **Exogenous Hypercortisolism:** Patients who have autoimmune diseases or who are organ transplant recipients may take cortisol-based steroid medications to control their disease or to prevent tissue rejection. These medications have serious side effects, including bone thinning, diabetes, mood swings, and high blood pressure: this is exogenous hypercortisolim, and it is the most common form of Cushing syndrome.

Treatment

Cushing syndrome is treated according to its cause. Exogenous Cushing syndrome is treated by reevaluating the correct dose of corticosteroid drugs to achieve the best benefits with the least risk. Pituitary adenomas are usually surgically removed; radiation therapy may be part of this treatment course. Cushing syndrome brought about by tumor cells secreting ACTH is treated by dealing with the tumors, but drugs that inhibit cortisol may also be used.

Medications

- Adrenal steroid inhibitors to limit cortisol production
- Supplements of hydrocortisone (postsurgery for pituitary tumor)
- Chemotherapeutic agents for adrenal carcinoma

Massage?

RISKS	Hypercortisolism affects the body in many ways that influence decisions about bodywork: hypertension, brittle bones, a risk of diabetes, and immune system suppression are just a few examples. The cause and treatment options for a client with Cushing syndrome may require significant adaptations to design a safe bodywork session.
BENEFITS	As long as massage stays within the average physical challenges of a person with Cushing syndrome, it can be a useful treatment option. Clients who have successfully treated their Cushing syndrome can enjoy the same benefits from massage as the rest of the population.

Diabetes Insipidus

Definition: What Is It?

Diabetes insipidus (DI) is a problem in the brain or in the kidneys, leading to a failure to concentrate urine appropriately. It is a relatively rare condition that is often linked to underlying trauma or disorders. It is unrelated to diabetes mellitus.

Etiology: What Happens?

Fluid levels in the body are controlled through a feedback loop that employs the thirst mechanism; a hormone made in the hypothalamus and stored in the pituitary gland called antidiuretic hormone, or ADH; and the kidneys. When a person takes in more fluid than he or she needs, the kidneys extract it from the blood to excrete it as urine. ADH limits urine production and increases concentration. Without adequate ADH, or without sensitivity to ADH in the kidneys, the urine is not adequately concentrated.

Whether DI begins in the kidneys or in the brain, the result is the same: urine is too diluted. This means that the patient expels anywhere from 2.5 to 15 liters of urine every day, and must replace that fluid by drinking.

Signs and Symptoms

Polyuria (frequent urination) and polydipsia (frequent thirst) are the two leading indicators for this disease. Nocturia (needing to urinate in the nighttime) is frequent, and even adults may experience bedwetting. Many patients develop an enlarged bladder to accommodate excessive urine flow. Signs of dehydration may also develop, including sunken eyes, muscle weakness, hypotension, rapid heartbeat, and headache.

Types of Diabetes Insipidus

- **Central diabetes insipidus:** This is the most common form of DI, and it is the result of a reduction of ADH production in the hypothalamus, or a reduction of ADH release from the pituitary. It can be the result of brain tumors, traumatic brain injury, or a postsurgical complication of brain surgery.

- **Nephrogenic diabetes insipidus:** This is a problem with ADH sensitivity at the collecting tubules in the kidney. It can be idiopathic, but it may be related to lithium toxicity, too much calcium in the blood (hypercalcemia), too much potassium in the blood (hyperkalemia), or rare diseases of the kidneys.
- **Gestational diabetes insipidus:** This condition develops during pregnancy, when placental enzymes destroy ADH in the mother. It resolves after the birth of the infant.
- **Dipsogenic diabetes insipidus:** This is the result of too much fluid intake, which can alter the activity of ADH. It may be related to a psychiatric disorder that causes a person to drink too much water or other liquids.

Treatment

DI is treated according to its type and cause. If it is related to a tumor, surgery may be recommended. Central DI is treated with a synthetic form of ADH. Nephrogenic DI is treated with drugs that change the way the kidneys respond to ADH. Dipsogenic DI may be treated with counseling or other psychiatric interventions.

Medications

- Desmopressin (synthetic ADH) to activate urinary concentration in kidneys
- Hydrochlorothiazide to decrease urinary volume
- Ibuprofen and indomethacin to reduce the delivery of urinary solute to the tubules of the kidney

Massage?

RISKS	Massage has no particular risks for a person with treated diabetes insipidus, as long as he or she is comfortable on a table or chair.
BENEFITS	A client under treatment for diabetes insipidus can enjoy the same benefits from massage as the rest of the population.

Ehlers-Danlos Syndrome

Definition: What Is It?

Ehlers-Danlos syndrome (EDS) is a group of genetic disorders that lead to problems in the production of various types of connective tissue proteins. It affects about 50,000 people in the United States, but it is very mild and not easily recognized in many cases.

Etiology: What Happens?

EDS is the result of genetic mutations that affect the production of collagen, elastin, and some other parts of the extracellular matrix that forms the bulk of connective tissues. Most people with this disorder experience hypermobility of the joints, along with chronic joint pain, delicate skin, and poor wound healing.

EDS is an inherited disorder, but that inheritance may be through autosomal-dominant, autosomal-recessive, or X-linked chromosomes. The most common versions are autosomal dominant, which means a child needs to inherit only one chromosome from a parent to develop this disorder.

Signs and Symptoms

The signs and symptoms of EDS are determined by the type of genetic mutation that is present. Most symptoms are related to extremely delicate skin, hypermobile joints, and chronic joint pain. Common signs include easy bruising, poor wound healing, frequent joint dislocations, and eye problems, including myopia, detached retina, and damage to the connective tissue that maintains the globular shape of the eyeball. The risk of mitral valve prolapse is higher for EDS patients than for the rest of the population. Rarer signs of EDS include extreme postural deviations and slack, baggy skin.

Types of Ehlers-Danlos Syndrome

- **Classic EDS:** This involves delicate skin that is fragile and prone to bruising, slow wound healing, and joints that are loose and vulnerable to injury.
- **Hypermobility EDS:** Patients with this disorder are prone to multiple dislocations, joint pain, and early-onset osteoarthritis
- **Arthrochalasia EDS:** This is a different genetic anomaly than hypermobility EDS, but the result is the same: easy joint disruptions, including hip dysplasia and frequent subluxations.
- **Dermatosparaxis EDS:** This involves involves very loose and baggy skin that sags and wrinkles, even in childhood.
- **Kyphoscoliosis EDS:** This leads leads to a severe, progressive curvature of the spine.
- **Vascular EDS:** This affects affects the connective tissues in blood vessels and other tubes with serious repercussions: midsized blood vessels and the gastrointestinal tract are vulnerable to damage or even rupture. This is a life-shortening version of the disease.

Treatment

EDS is treated according to symptoms or related problems. People with hypermobile joints are taught how to preserve joint function and are discouraged from stretching joints beyond a healthy range of motion. Skin wounds are typically treated with bandages or wound glue rather than sutures, because the skin is so delicate. Any surgery or dental work is conducted with extreme care because of poor wound healing and because people with a risk of mitral valve prolapse are also at risk for endocardial bacterial infections.

Massage?

RISKS	Most EDS patients have hypermobile joints; bodywork that challenges range of motion must be done with respect for this problem. Skin and cardiovascular health may inform modality choices.
BENEFITS	Because joints tend to be loose, EDS patients may experience muscle tightness, pain, and inefficient movement. Massage that can reduce pain and increase ease of movement—without compromising joint integrity or other tissue weaknesses—is helpful and appropriate.

Fractures

Definition: What Are They?

Fractures are any variety of broken bone, from a hairline crack to a complete break with protrusion through the skin.

The three basic classes are simple fracture (the bone is completely broken but little or no damage has occurred to the surrounding soft tissues); incomplete fractures (the bone is cracked but not completely broken); and compound fractures (the bone is completely broken and a great deal of soft tissue damage has occurred). Beyond that, fractures are named for the type or shape of the lesion.

Etiology: What Happens?

When a bone undergoes more mechanical stress than it can accommodate, it cracks or breaks altogether. This typically occurs as a trauma, a result of osteoporosis, or because of overuse. If a bone is appropriately stabilized during the healing process, osteocytes can lay down a thickened area of new growth over the break site, leading to a structure that is actually denser than before it was broken. Fractures become problematic when they affect the growth plate in children, or when the healing process is slowed due to age, nutrition, unrelenting stress, or other factors.

Signs and Symptoms

Big bone breaks are usually obvious: they are painful, they usually follow a specific traumatic event, and they severely limit the function of the adjacent joints. But some fractures can be difficult to identify, particularly if they are accompanied by a lot of soft tissue trauma. Sprained ankles and shin splints are two conditions that frequently hide minor bone fractures.

Types of Fractures

- **Avulsion fractures:** These occur when a bone fragment of bone is pulled away. This is an occasional complication of Osgood-Schlatter disease, for example.
- **Comminuted fractures:** These involve a bone that shatters into multiple pieces.
- **Compression fractures:** These involve collapsed vertebral bodies. They are often associated with low bone density, as seen with osteoporosis and osteogenesis imperfecta.
- **Greenstick fractures:** These involve bending and partial breakage of the bone.
- **Malunion fractures:** These occur when the bone fragments heal in a nonanatomic position.
- **Stress fractures:** These are common minor cracks that occur with chronic overuse. They can be difficult to identify without tests.

Treatment

Most fractures heal well if the bones are immobilized with a cast or other device. More complicated situations may call for pins, plates, screws, or reparative surgery. Grafts of bone tissue or bone paste along with electrical stimulation to the site may help to speed healing when recovery is impaired.

Medications

- NSAIDs for pain and inflammation

Massage?

RISKS	Acute fractures locally contraindicate massage, until the bones are stabilized and other soft tissue damage is addressed.
BENEFITS	Swelling is a frequent complication of casting. Any lymphatic work to decrease fluid retention can help with both comfort and speed of circulatory turnover in the compromised area. Massage elsewhere to the body while a fracture is healing can help address the challenge of having impaired movement, as well as any limping or other compensations that may occur. A person who has fully recovered from a fracture can enjoy the same benefits from massage as the rest of the population.

Guillain-Barré Syndrome

Definition: What Is It?

Guillain-Barré syndrome (GBS) is a condition involving acute inflammation and destruction of the myelin layer of peripheral nerves. It usually starts in the extremities and moves toward the trunk, but some variants of this syndrome affect only cranial nerves or have other patterns. It is the most frequently seen form of acute neuromuscular paralysis in the Western Hemisphere.

Etiology: What Happens?

GBS is not fully understood, but it is believed that for many patients a triggering infection stimulates an immune system attack mistakenly directed against the myelin sheaths of peripheral nerves. This disorder has also been seen in conjunction with pregnancy, surgery, and administration of certain vaccines, specifically the swine flu vaccine that was distributed in 1976.

Regardless of what initiates the disease process, the result is that the myelin sheaths on peripheral nerves are attacked and destroyed by macrophages and lymphocytes. It can affect primarily motor or sensory neurons, or both. The damage progresses proximally and may also affect cranial nerves. This can be life threatening if the nerves that control breathing are damaged; many GBS patients spend time on a ventilator before they recover.

Signs and Symptoms

When GBS first appears, it often involves symmetrical weakness or tingling in the affected limbs. Reflexes become dull or disappear altogether. Loss of sensation progresses proximally, although pain frequently develops in the hips and pelvis. If the GBS affects cranial nerves of the face, facial weakness, pain, and difficulty with speech and swallowing may develop. If GBS attacks cranial nerves, then autonomic symptoms may develop. These can include variable heart rate and blood pressure, flushing, excessive sweating, or lack of sweating. As the disease progresses, the nerves that supply respiratory muscles are affected, and dangerous problems with breathing develop.

GBS symptoms usually peak 2 or 3 weeks after onset, and they may persist for several weeks before they begin to subside. Full recovery can take 18 months or more. Some patients experience permanent weakness after GBS, and a small number of patients don't survive.

Types of Guillain-Barré syndrome

- **Acute inflammatory demyelinating polyradiculoneuropathy:** This is the most common form, accounting for 90% of GBS diagnoses.
- **Acute motor axonal neuropathy:** This affects motor neurons only. It is most common in children and has a good prognosis.
- **Acute motor-sensory axonal neuropathy:** This affects motor and sensory function. It is most common in adults and has a poorer recovery rate than other forms of GBS.
- **Miller-Fisher syndrome:** This is a rare variant of GBS that involves only the cranial nerves. It leads to poor control of the eyes and other facial muscles.

Treatment

Two treatment options have been successfully used to shorten recovery time for GBS patients: plasmapheresis and injections of high concentrations of immunoglobulin (donated antibodies).

Other interventions for GBS patients are dictated by their individual needs. About one-third of patients require the use of a ventilator until the respiratory nerves regain full function. Pain management is problematic because powerful pain medications can depress the nervous system; massage and other nondrug options are often recommended for this purpose. Once the acute inflammation has passed, occupational and physical therapy is used to help the patient regain as much muscle function as possible.

Medications

- Immunomodulators to inhibit antibody production
- Anticoagulants to reduce risk of deep vein thrombosis and pulmonary embolism
- NSAIDs for pain management
- Narcotics for pain management if NSAIDs are insufficient

Massage?

RISKS	A GBS patient may have weakness, pain, and numbness that progressively move from the extremities toward the trunk. Any massage must respect the many challenges that this person is undergoing, including the disease process and any medical efforts to control it. This includes medications, assisted ventilation, and other interventions.
BENEFITS	When a person has begun to recover from a GBS attack, physical and occupational therapy are often employed to speed recovery and prevent muscle atrophy. Massage at this stage may be useful to limit pain, improve circulation, and reduce fatigue and anxiety.

Glomerulonephritis

Definition: What Is It?

Glomerulonephritis is a relatively rare but serious situation involving inflammation and scarring of the glomeruli in the kidneys. This can occur as a result of toxic exposure, as a complication of a bacterial infection, or related to autoimmune disease. Some cases are idiopathic.

Etiology: What Happens?

"Glomerulus" is the diminutive form of the Latin word glomus, for "ball of yarn," which is an excellent description of the tufts of capillary loops that allow for diffusion and filtration in the kidneys. These points of interface between circulatory capillaries and nephrons act as filters to keep vital blood components in the bloodstream while allowing water and wastes to exit into the urinary system.

When the body launches an immune system attack against an invader, one consequence can be the formation of "immune complexes": sticky clumps of antigens and antibodies. Ordinarily, these would be consumed by macrophages, but occasionally they can develop in or get caught by the glomeruli, leading to a localized inflammatory reaction: glomerulonephritis. Triggers for this process can include bacterial infections (especially with Streptococcus), toxic exposures, or autoimmune disorders.

Acute or chronic inflammation in the glomeruli can compromise their effectiveness and allow important substances to leave the body through the urine, while allowing toxins to accumulate in the bloodstream. Inflammation in the kidneys leads to an accumulation of scar tissue where only soft, pliable epithelium should be; consequently the kidneys become progressively less able to manage fluids in the body, which may lead to chronic renal failure.

Signs and Symptoms

Early symptoms of glomerulonephritis include abnormalities in the urine such as high protein levels or red blood cells. Hematuria, or blood in the urine, can be observed as dark or rust-colored urine. Protein in the urine makes it look foamy. Occasionally, no observable signs develop, and glomerulonephritis is found only when a routine analysis reveals higher-than-normal levels of protein or blood in the urine.

Hypertension that does not respond to normal interventions is both a symptom and a complication of glomerulonephritis. Later symptoms are indicators of renal failure, including general malaise, skin discoloration, itching, fatigue, anemia, low urine output, systemic edema, and, in very severe cases, lethargy, confusion, and coma.

Treatment

The treatment for glomerulonephritis depends entirely on the cause, and is generally geared toward symptom abatement and improved kidney function. Controlling high blood pressure is the first priority; this may be done antihypertensive drugs as well as restricting salt and protein intake. If glomerulonephritis is a complication of a general infection, antibiotics may lead to a complete recovery. If it is an autoimmune or other inflammatory problem, steroids or other immunosuppressant drugs may be used to limit damage to the nephrons. In some cases plasmapheresis is recommended to remove inflammatory immune complexes.

Medications

- Diuretics to promote urine production
- ACE inhibitors or angiotensin II receptor antagonists to control hypertension
- Antibiotics in the presence of bacterial infection
- Steroidal anti-inflammatories or immunosuppressants for autoimmune diseases

Massage?

RISKS	Glomerulonephritis is an inflammatory condition that impairs the body's ability to manage circulatory turnover in the kidneys. Any bodywork that targets fluid flow may exceed a client's ability to adapt.
BENEFITS	Noncirculatory types of massage or bodywork may be appropriate for glomerulonephritis patients to receive, as long as the contributing factors and medications are identified and accommodated.

Heterotopic Ossification

Definition: What Is It?

Heterotopic ossification describes a condition in which calcifications form in soft tissue. The most common form is seen most often in adolescents and young adults, and usually affects the quadriceps and brachialis muscles.

Etiology: What Happens?

The most common variety of heterotopic ossification follows an injury with bleeding into the muscle belly or between fascial sheets. Eventually, a formation develops at the site of the contusion that looks and feels like a bone embedded in soft tissue. Bone-like growths can be suspended within muscle or other soft tissue, but in many cases they are attached continuously or by a stalk to nearby periosteum.

Other forms of heterotopic ossification are associated with disorders that either limit mobility or promote excessive growth of bone tissue. Spinal cord injury, traumatic brain injury, ankylosing spondylitis, Paget disease, and some autoimmune disorders carry an increased risk for developing this condition. Hip replacement surgery also carries a significant risk of developing bony deposits in surrounding soft tissues.

Signs and Symptoms

In the acute stage of trauma-based heterotopic ossification, the area feels bruised; within a few days it may feel hard and locally very tender. The range of motion in the nearby joint is limited: if it occurs in the brachialis, the elbow doesn't fully extend, and when it occurs in the quadriceps, the knee can't fully flex. Eventually, little or no local pain may be present, but a dense, unyielding mass develops where nothing hard should be.

Treatment

Treatment for heterotopic ossification tends to be conservative. Patients are recommended to rest and isolate the injured area in the acute stage to limit further bleeding. Later passive stretching is employed for range of motion, followed by exercises to restore normal muscle strength.

If a fully mature and calcified mass interferes with muscle or tendon function, it can be surgically removed. This kind of surgery is avoided if possible, however, because many patients have a postsurgical recurrence of the growth.

Medications

- NSAIDs against pain and blood clotting to prevent heterotopic ossification from developing or recurring

Massage?

RISKS	Heterotopic ossification locally contraindicates rigorous massage because of the risk of increased internal bleeding: this is true for both a new and mature injury.
BENEFITS	Gentle massage around the edges of a calcium deposit may stimulate bony resorption. Massage elsewhere is safe and appropriate.

Hyperparathyroidism

Definition: What Is It?

Hyperparathyroidism is a condition in which the parathyroid glands produce too much hormone. It affects about 100,000 people in this country each year. Women are affected about twice as often as men, and it is most common in people over 60 years old.

Etiology: What Happens?

The parathyroid glands are tiny glands located behind or close to the thyroid gland. They secrete parathyroid hormone (PTH). Unlike many endocrine glands that operate under control of the hypothalamus and pituitary, the parathyroids are essentially self-regulating: they release PTH when plasma calcium is low, and stop when plasma calcium is high.

PTH has several functions in blood calcium maintenance. It causes the demineralization of cortical bone to increase plasma calcium and phosphate; it increases the absorption of calcium in the intestines, and the reabsorption of calcium in the kidneys; and it promotes the conversion of vitamin D into a usable form.

The etiology of hyperparathyroidism depends on the type; these are described below. Regardless of the version, this disorder causes the secretion of excessive amounts of PTH, leading to elevated blood calcium. This can be a minor abnormality that produces no symptoms and requires no treatment, or it can be severe and potentially life threatening.

Signs and Symptoms

Signs and symptoms of hyperparathyroidism are related to elevated plasma calcium levels. They include muscle weakness and fatigue at the mild end of the scale, and nausea, vomiting, diarrhea, depression, and confusion at the more severe end.

Types of Hyperparathyroidism

- **Primary hyperparathyroidism:** This is the most common form, and is usually related to the growth of one or more adenomas (benign epithelial tumors) on the parathyroid glands. Very rarely it may be related to parathyroid cancer.
- **Secondary hyperparathyroidism:** This form of the disease is usually related to kidney dysfunction. It is almost always seen with end-stage renal failure, but may also develop because of an extreme deficiency in calcium or vitamin D.
- **Tertiary hyperparathyroidism:** This is a situation where long-term dysfunction becomes self-sustaining, and the parathyroids continue to produce too much hormones after other contributing factors, especially renal failure, have been resolved.

Complications

The complications of hyperparathyroidism may be among the first indicators of the disease. They include hypertension, bradycardia, osteopenia that affects cortical bone (this distinguishes it from osteoporosis which affects mainly trabecular bone), kidney stones, and pseudogout.

Treatment

Surgery to remove the affected parathyroid gland or glands is the most common treatment option for hyperparathyroidism that requires treatment. Patients may need to supplement calcium and vitamin D after surgery, especially as the bones quickly pull calcium from the blood to add density in a condition called "hungry bone syndrome." In addition, patients are advised to hydrate well, to exercise within tolerance, and to avoid any diuretics if possible.

Medications

- Hormone replacement therapy if surgery is not an option
- Bisphosphonates to improve bone density
- Calcimimetic drugs for secondary hyperparathyroidism

Massage?

RISKS	A person with hyperparathyroidism may have kidney problems as well: these must be addressed for best safety. Patients may also have significant bone thinning in cortical bone, which requires adjustments in depth of bodywork.
BENEFITS	Massage won't change the course of hyperparathyroidism, but it can improve the quality of life for people with this condition. A client who has a mild case that is under observation, or who has fully recovered from surgery, can enjoy the same benefits from massage as the rest of the population.

Hypoparathyroidism

Definition: What Is It?

Hypoparathyroidism is a rare condition in which the parathyroid glands don't produce an adequate amount of parathyroid hormone.

Etiology: What Happens?

Calcium in plasma and extracellular fluid is extremely important for many body functions, including regulating muscle contraction, blood clotting, nerve transmission, and kidney function. Normal levels of circulating calcium are usually extremely stable. Special cells in the parathyroid glands (as well as a few other areas) are sensitive to calcium, and when these levels drop, parathyroid hormone (PTH) is released.

Parathyroid hormone has several jobs: it activates osteoclasts to pull calcium off bone and add it to plasma; it influences kidney function to retain calcium and eliminate phosphorus; and it stimulates the kidneys to metabolize vitamin D for calcium absorption. When PTH is in short supply, these functions are lost. Consequently, the kidneys pull excessive calcium out of the blood, leading to high urinary calcium and a risk of kidney stones. Circulating calcium levels drop, along with the ability to absorb this important mineral from the diet, while phosphorus levels go up. Lack of plasma calcium prevents bones from increasing their density, changes muscle contractions, and ultimately affects the central nervous system.

Hypoparathyroidism can be the result of a congenital birth defect, or a complication of an autoimmune attack against several endocrine glands. The most common form, however, is related to a history of neck surgery or radiation that damages the parathyroid glands. This condition is permanent; while it is treatable, it never resolves.

Signs and Symptoms

Signs and symptoms of hypoparathyroidism often begin with tingling and parasthesia in the lips, fingers, and toes. Skin and hair become dry, and severe and long-lasting muscle cramps called tetany may occur. Severe muscle cramping at the larynx and bronchi is rare, but may be life threatening. Excessive calcium processing in the kidneys raises the risk for kidney stones. Headache, fatigue, mood swings, and irritability are common. Children born with this condition may have abnormal calcification of teeth and bones, and delayed growth patterns.

Treatment

Hypoparathyroidism is typically treated with calcium and vitamin D supplements. Surgical implant of parathyroid tissue has been used, but the results are inconsistent compared with the simpler strategy of supplementation.

Medications

- Supplements of calcium and vitamin D
- Synthetic parathyroid hormone is under investigation

Massage?

RISKS	Hypoparathyroidism is easily treatable and not usually life threatening; it carries no specific risks for massage as long as the bodywork does not trigger painful muscle cramps.
BENEFITS	Massage is unlikely to improve the course of this condition, but it can certainly add to the quality of life of the person who lives with hypoparathyroidism.

Ichthyosis

Definition: What Is It?

Ichthyosis vulgaris or common ichthyosis (from the Greek for "fish condition") is a group of problems that lead to the formation of dried, scaly skin. It is usually an inherited genetic anomaly; it can develop as a symptom or complication of another underlying disorder.

Etiology: What Happens?

Ichthyosis develops when a normal water-proofing protein in the skin is impaired, usually because of a genetic anomaly. The normal balance between new skin cell production and old skin cell exfoliation is upset, and the result is the development of small scales of dead cells. The scales are firmly attached to new cells underneath, so the risk of skin cracking and bleeding is high.

This is usually a genetic disorder, but acquired ichthyosis can develop as a symptom or a complication of other diseases, including cancer (especially lymphoma), Hansen disease (also called leprosy), lupus, sarcoidosis, thyroid dysregulation, and some other conditions.

Signs and Symptoms

The hallmark of ichthyosis is dry skin with irregular polyhedronal scales. It is most common on the extensor side of the extremities and the abdomen, but it can develop elsewhere. Ichthyosis symptoms tend to be worst during cold, dry weather.

Types of Ichthyosis

- **Ichthyosis vulgaris:** This is a mild form, and accounts for the majority of ichthyosis diagnoses.
- **Lamellar ichthyosis:** This is a severe, potentially disfiguring variety with deep painful cracks, especially on the palms or soles.
- **X-linked ichthyosis:** This is mild, and seen only in males.
- **Epidermolytic hyperkeratosis:** This rare version affects babies with massive blistering and peeling of superficial skin.

Treatment

Soothing lotions and moisturizers along with mild applications of salicylic acid to remove loosened scales are often recommended.

Medications

- Hypoallergenic moisturizers to manage ichthyosis vulgaris.
- Retinoins to slow the production of new skin cells.
- Steroidal anti-inflammatories to manage itchiness.

Massage?

RISKS	Skin that is bleeding or oozing locally contraindicates massage.
BENEFITS	If the skin is intact, a client with ichthyosis can enjoy the extra moisturizing that massage may offer, along with the wonderful experience of having their skin be carefully tended. Be sure to use a hypoallergenic lubricant.

Impetigo

Definition: What Is It?

Impetigo is a staphylococcal or streptococcal infection of the skin. It occurs mostly among infants and young children, although adults can get it too.

Etiology: What Happens?

Most cases of impetigo in the United States are caused by *Staphylococcus aureus.* In a typical infection, the bacteria gains access through a minor skin injury. Lesions are usually restricted to the epidermis and don't cause permanent scarring, but one type of impetigo can penetrate to deeper layers of the skin. Scratching the infected areas allows the bacteria to spread over large areas.

Impetigo can lead to serious complications including renal failure, meningitis, cellulitis, and blood poisoning. For this reason, it is usually treated quickly and aggressively.

Signs and Symptoms

Impetigo lesions usually occur around the nose and mouth, but it can infect the skin anywhere on the body. The characteristic presentation is a cluster of small red sores that blister, then rupture, and form yellow or honey-colored crusts. Left untreated, these sores heal in 2 to 3 weeks, leaving no scars (Figure 2.20).

Types of Impetigo

- **Impetigo contagiosa:** This is the most common version; sores are itchy but not painful.
- **Bullous impetigo:** This involves large, painless, delicate blisters on the trunk, arms, and legs; it may be accompanied by fever, diarrhea, and general weakness.
- **Ecthyma:** This penetrates to deep layers of the skin, and causes permanent scarring.

Treatment

For prevention of impetigo, chapped skin should be treated with lubricant to prevent damage, and all other wounds should be cleaned thoroughly, treated with antibacterial ointment, and covered.

Patients are counseled to keep lesions clean and dry, and to remove crusts as soon as possible. The patient's bedding and towels must be strictly isolated during the infection. Children should avoid contact with others for at least 24 hours after they begin treatment.

Antibiotics are the mainstay of medical treatment for impetigo, but the increasing incidence of methicillin-resistant *Staphylococcus aureus* (MRSA) in these infections has made antibiotic choice more challenging.

Medications

- Topical over-the-counter or prescription antibiotic ointment
- Oral or parenteral antibiotics for severe cases

Massage?

RISKS	Because of the risk of communicability, impetigo systemically contraindicates massage until the lesions have healed completely. If a client reports that someone in his or her house has impetigo, it is best to reschedule the appointment for after the infection is over.
BENEFITS	A client who has fully recovered from impetigo can enjoy the same benefits of bodywork as the rest of the population.

Jaundice

Definition: What Is It?

Jaundice, from the French jaune (yellow), is also called icterus. It is a condition involving a yellowish tinge to skin, mucous membranes and the sclera of the eyes, brought about by liver dysfunction.

Etiology: What Happens?

Bilirubin is dark-pigmented material recovered by the spleen from dead erythrocytes. The spleen sends bilirubin to the liver via the portal vein. One of the many functions of the liver is to change bilirubin into bile. Bile drips from the liver to the gallbladder, which squirts it into the duodenum when fatty food is present. Bile helps hold particles of fat in suspension, so that fat-dissolving enzymes from the pancreas can break them down effectively. Eventually all the bilirubin gets into the digestive tract, where it is a coloring agent for feces.

If dark reddish-brown bilirubin can't leave the liver, it accumulates in the bloodstream and the tissues. Eventually, it can visibly stain the skin, mucous membranes, and the sclera of the eyes.

Signs and Symptoms

Yellow-tinted skin, mucous membranes, and sclera of the eye are the main signs of jaundice. Urine often becomes dark, as the kidneys pull bilirubin out of the bloodstream. In contrast, stools tend to become light or clay-colored because the bilirubin doesn't enter the GI tract.

Other signs and symptoms are related to underlying liver disease, which may involve infection, cirrhosis, or other problems.

Types of Jaundice

- **Neonatal jaundice:** Also called kernicterus, this occurs in newborn babies if their livers are not mature enough to keep up with the turnover of fetal red blood cells. It takes a few days to catch up with this extra workload. Treatment is usually exposure to sunlight or full-spectrum "bili lights," which stimulate liver activity.
- **Hemolytic jaundice:** In this situation, red blood cells break down too fast, overwhelming the spleen and liver with too much material: this is seen with sickle-cell disease, mismatched blood transtusions, and some infections.
- **Hepatic jaundice:** This describes internal liver dysfunction due to scar tissue, hepatic carcinoma, infection, or a congenital malfunction of enzyme systems.
- **Extrahepatic jaundice:** This is related to a mechanical obstruction outside the liver. Gallstones, pancreatic tumors, or tumors in the GI tract are usually responsible.

Complications

Jaundice is a sign of liver dysfunction, which is often slowly progressive. Left untreated, it can lead to liver failure and the need for a liver transplant. Untreated neonatal jaundice can lead to brain damage as toxins accumulate in the bloodstream.

Treatment

Jaundice is treated according to the cause. Antiviral medications can reduce the impact of viral hepatitis; gallbladder surgery can correct an obstructed bile duct; other interventions are also tied to underlying causes.

Massage?

RISKS	A person with jaundice predictably has some liver dysfunction. Problems may be mild or severe, but they must be addressed before any rigorous or challenging bodywork can be done. If the condition is due to hepatitis B or C, hygienic precautions must be especially scrupulously observed.
BENEFITS	Gentle or energetic bodywork may be well received by a person dealing with a liver problem. A person who has fully recovered from jaundice can enjoy the same benefits from massage as the rest of the population.

Lichen Planus

Definition: What Is It?

Lichen planus is a noncontagious inflammatory condition involving small, flat, hard lesions on the skin. It may also affect some mucous membranes.

Etiology: What Happens?

Lichen planus is an idiopathic disease that most often affects middle-aged people. It often appears with autoimmune conditions or in conjunction with allergic reactions to medications, leading experts to theorize that it is somehow connected to immune system dysfunction.

Signs and Symptoms

Lichen planus lesions are small, purplish, flat-topped, angular bumps that usually appear on the wrists, ankles, shins, and in the mouth, but they are also found on the low back, neck, and genitals. The bumps may be intensely itchy. They may form where the skin has been damaged, so people prone to this condition are advised to be careful about skin injuries. Skin lesions may be covered with fine lacey white lines; this is called Wickham striae. This form of the disease usually disappears in 6 to 18 months.

When lichen planus occurs in the mouth, it looks like patches of white dots or lines on the tongue, gums, or cheeks. Larger lesions may become painful ulcerations. Oral lichen planus is associated with an increased risk of squamous cell carcinoma, so it is useful to be aware of this condition. Mouth lesions tend to last longer than the skin form: it persists here for up to five years.

Treatment

Lichen planus is typically treated with steroids or antihistamines to address itching. Severe cases may call for systemic steroids or medication in combination with UV radiation.

Medications

- Topical or oral corticosteroids for itching on the skin and in the mouth
- Antihistamines for itching
- PUVA: psoralen with UV radiation

Massage?

RISKS	The only risk for a client with lichen planus is that massage may exacerbate itching.
BENEFITS	Massage probably won't improve the prognosis for lichen planus, but clients can enjoy the same general benefits from bodywork as the rest of the population.

Malaria

Definition: What Is It?

Malaria is a vector-borne infection of blood cells. The causative agent comes from a group of single-celled parasites from the genus of protozoa called *Plasmodium*, and the vector is the bite of an infected female mosquito from the Anopheles species. Globally, malaria infects about 500 million people each year, and causes about a million deaths. In North America, it is relatively rare, but not unheard of.

Etiology: What Happens?

When a human is bitten by a mosquito infected with malaria-causing protozoa, an immature form of the parasite is introduced into the bloodstream. It travels to the liver, where it grows for six to nine days. At that time it goes back into the bloodstream, where it begins to invade healthy red blood cells.

The protozoa feed on hemoglobin, and replicate inside the RBCs. The infected cells rupture, releasing toxic wastes and more protozoa. These go back to the liver to grow and then newly released protozoa invade more erythrocytes. Each cycle damages more liver cells and destroys more erythrocytes. When an uninfected mosquito bites this person, immature parasites enter the insect to begin the cycle again.

Signs and Symptoms

The signs and symptoms of malaria include extreme fluctuations between fever and chills (these reflect whether red blood cells are being invaded or rupturing), in cycles that may recur over several days.

When enough red blood cells have been invaded, anemia develops. Malaria is a type of hemolytic anemia: a situation in which red blood cells are destroyed faster than they can be replaced. Jaundice is another complication: this is related to the rapid destruction of erythrocytes that allows bilirubin to accumulate in the skin and mucous membranes. In some forms of the infection, the central nervous system, lungs, and kidneys may also be damaged.

A typical infection with the less virulent protozoa lasts about two weeks and then subsides, but some parasites may remain in the liver to launch a new episode months or years later.

Treatment

The treatment options for malaria are limited, and the most common and aggressive parasites are developing resistance to chloroquine, the most frequently used and cost-effective treatment option. Most malaria patients can be treated successfully if they have full access to all the drugs necessary, and if they take the drugs according to prescription.

Medications

- Topical applications of DEET to prevent mosquito bites
- Antimalarial medications, including
  - Chloroquine, hydroxychloroquine, and doxycycline to prevent or treat some types of malaria
  - Quinine to treat but not prevent new infection

Massage?

RISKS	Malaria carries a risk of brain, liver, and kidney damage. For this reason, any client who may be dealing with this disease must be fully treated before receiving any kind of rigorous bodywork.
BENEFITS	People who have had malaria may have long-term organ damage. Any bodywork that is conducted within these parameters may be safe and supportive. People who successfully treated malaria with no long-term repercussions may enjoy the same benefits from massage as the rest of the population.

Marfan Syndrome

Definition: What Is It?

Marfan syndrome is the result of a genetic mutation that leads to the production of dysfunctional fibrillin, a key connective tissue fiber.

Etiology: What Happens?

Marfan syndrome is a result of the production of faulty protein fibers with the consequence that certain connective tissues throughout the body may be weak or otherwise dysfunctional. The musculoskeletal system, the meninges, the heart and aorta, and the eyes are most at risk for problems related to Marfan syndrome.

Signs and Symptoms

Marfan syndrome affects several body systems. In the musculoskeletal system, it can lead to abnormally long extremities and digits. One sign of this disorder is the wrist test: persons with Marfan syndrome can overlap the thumb and fifth digit (little finger) of one hand while encircling the opposite wrist. Ligament laxity, joint hypermobility, and anomalies in the shape of the thorax are also common. A protruding sternum is called pectus carinatum; a sunken sternum is called pectus excavatum. Scoliosis and hyperkyphosis are also possible indicators of Marfan syndrome. These bony anomalies can be severe enough to interfere with breathing and raise the risk of pneumonia.

In the cardiovascular system, Marfan syndrome can weaken the aortic and mitral valves of the heart. Prolapsed valves lead to the regurgitation of blood and an irregular heartbeat. An enlarged aorta with a risk of a dissecting aneurysm is a potential cause of death for Marfan syndrome patients.

In the nervous system, patients may experience dural ectasia: a situation in which the dura mater stretches and weakens with age.

Other symptoms include stretch marks on the skin; hernias; and eye problems that range from myopia to dislocated lens, detached retina, and possible blindness.

Treatment

Marfan syndrome is treated according to the symptoms. Surgery may be needed for heart valves to correct an aortic aneurysm, to deal with postural deviation, or to repair a deformed thorax.

Medications

- Beta-blockers to reduce cardiac load
- Prophylactic antibiotics to prevent infection of the valves of the heart

Massage?

RISKS	Marfan syndrome patients have fragile connective tissues. Hypermobility in the joints and a risk of blood vessel weakness require accommodations in bodywork.
BENEFITS	As long as the challenges of massage are kept within the client's ability to adapt, a person with Marfan syndrome can enjoy the same benefits from massage as the rest of the population.

Myasthenia Gravis

Definition: What Is It?

First described by Wilhelm Erb in 1890, MG is an autoimmune disease that involves destruction of receptor sites at neuromuscular junctions. It is a progressive disease, but it is usually manageable with medical and surgical intervention. It diagnosed most often in women under 40 and men over 60, and it affects about 36,000 people in the United States.

Etiology: What Happens?

Acetylcholine (ACh), a neurotransmitter associated with increased excitability, is a key player in the lightning-fast cascade of events that translates electrical stimulation from the brain into chemical reactions in the muscles. In myasthenia gravis, the ACh receptor sites are attacked by antibodies. They don't function correctly and the muscle loses the ability to respond and ultimately to contract. Symptoms develop when about 70% of receptors have been lost.

It is not clear why antibodies attack the neuromuscular junction, but many experts believe the thymus may be involved in some way because the vast majority of MG patients show signs of thymus disruption.

Signs and Symptoms

Most people with MG report weakness and fatigability in affected muscles. The process begins most often around the eyes, face, and throat. Early signs include a flattened smile, droopy eyelids (ptosis), blurred vision, and difficulty with eating, swallowing, and speech.

Symptoms tend to fluctuate during the day and are worst early in the morning and late at night. Repetitive activity, emotional stress, overexertion, exposure to heat, and some medications can make symptoms much worse.

One very serious consequence of MG is called a myasthenic crisis. In this situation, an event like a respiratory infection or a reaction to medication triggers a sudden and rapid loss of strength in the muscles that control respiration. Patients need assisted ventilation until the crisis passes.

Treatment

Treatment of MG is intended to boost nerve transmission and to suppress immune system activity at neuromuscular junctions. Surgery is occasionally recommended to remove an abnormal thymus gland. In extreme situations, plasmapheresis may be conducted to remove faulty antibodies from the blood.

Medications

- Cholinesterase inhibitors to increase the availability of ACh at neuromuscular junctions
- Corticosteroids to suppress immune system activity

Massage?

RISKS	Excessive heat may aggravate MG symptoms, so this must be avoided. People with MG may treat it with immunosuppressant drugs, so they are at higher risk than the general population for picking up infections.
BENEFITS	Because MG involves motor paralysis but not sensory deprivation, carefully applied massage can be safe and supportive.

Multiple System Atrophy

Definition: What Is It?

Multiple system atrophy (MSA) is a fairly rare progressive disease that involves degeneration of neurons in the brain that control several autonomic functions. It usually affects adults in their 50s, and typically progresses from onset of symptoms to death over the course of about ten years.

Etiology: What Happens?

MSA occurs when oligodendrocytes (insulating cells in the central nervous system) accumulate an abnormal amount of a protein called alpha-synuclein. This interferes with several functions, including the production of dopamine, which is why MSA can sometimes be difficult to distinguish from Parkinson disease. The cause of the buildup of alpha-synuclein is not clear. Neither heredity nor toxic exposure appears to be factors.

Until recently, MSA was discussed as three different phenomena: Shy-Drager syndrome (involving a whole-body autonomic system degeneration), striatonigral degeneration, and olivopontocerebellar degeneration. Now neurologists recognize that these three problems are all the same process, each happening in a different location in the brain.

Signs and Symptoms

Signs and symptoms of MSA vary according to the location of the damage. And because this disease is progressive, symptoms can evolve and encompass more and more of autonomic function. This includes difficulty with maintaining appropriate blood pressure: it tends to be too high when a person is laying down, and too low when a person is standing—leading to syncope, or fainting spells. Heart rate may be extremely variable. The digestive system may be impaired from swallowing to peristalsis to continence. Bladder control is likewise vulnerable. Loss of muscle control of the limbs, along with rigidity, tremor, and flexion of the trunk raise the risk of falls.

Types of Multiple System Atrophy

Specialists sometimes discuss MSA as two types. It is possible to begin with one version and progress to have symptoms of another version.

- **MSA-P:** This is a version that resembles Parkinson disease in many ways. Its primary symptoms are rigidity, bradykinesia, and tremor.
- **MSA-C:** This is named for its focus on cerebellar damage. Leading symptoms of this type of MSA include loss of motor control for gait and limb movement, slurred speech, and difficulties swallowing.

Treatment

MSA has no cure and does not enter remission. Treatment is aimed solely at managing symptoms. Patients who have difficulty with regulating their heart rate may have a pacemaker surgically implanted. A speech pathologist may be employed to help with speech and swallowing skills.

Medications

- Blood pressure medication to either raise or lower blood pressure
- Parkinsonism drugs to improve dopamine uptake and muscle control
- Dietary fiber or laxatives for constipation
- Drugs to manage bladder control

Massage?

RISKS	A client with MSA may have any number of problems that massage might exacerbate, including low blood pressure, high blood pressure, incontinence, balance and coordination problems, and others.
BENEFITS	Using a massage chair rather than a table and aiming for short sessions to track the client's tolerance are probably good strategies for working with people who have MSA. The relaxation provided by massage may help to mitigate some stress-related symptoms, as long as the work is within the client's ability to adapt.

Osteogenesis Imperfecta

Definition: What Is It?

Osteogenesis imperfecta (OI) is a group of genetic disorders that change the quality or the quantity of certain collagen fibers, leading to bones that are pathologically thin and possibly brittle. About 50,000 people in the United States have OI; men and women are affected equally.

Etiology: What Happens?

Type I collagen provides the scaffolding for bones and invests connective tissues of organ capsules, fascia, the cornea and sclera, tendons, meninges, and skin. Osteogenesis imperfecta is the result of a genetic mutation that alters the quality or quantity of type I collagen fibers. Consequently, the creation of healthy bone tissue is impaired.

This mutation is autosomal dominant (a person can inherit the trait from just one parent), but about a third of all cases seem to be spontaneous mutations.

Signs and Symptoms

The primary feature of OI is having bones that fracture extremely easily, especially in infancy and early childhood. Children with OI are sometimes mistaken for victims of child abuse because their radiographs show a history of multiple broken bones. Other possible signs include brittle teeth, ligament laxity, easy bruising, short stature, bowed long bones, extreme postural deviations (especially hyperkyphosis with scoliosis), hearing loss, and low muscle mass.

Having poorly formed or inadequate type 1 collagen can lead several problems outside of the musculoskeletal system, including heart valve weakness, dilation of the aorta, distortions of the sclera with vision loss, and muscle weakness. An especially serious complication occurs when ligament laxity allows the skull to press on the spinal column; this is called basilar invagination.

Treatment

The main goals of OI treatment are to maintain health and independence, to preserve bone density, and to minimize cardiovascular problems. Children and adults are encouraged to be physically active within safety parameters. A healthy diet is strongly promoted to control weight and assist with bone density.

Surgery to straighten and support bowed long bones may be conducted, and other assistive devices, from crutches to braces to wheelchairs, may be used to improve mobility. TENS units or nerve blocks may be used for pain if other drugs are not sufficient.

Medications

- NSAIDs for pain management
- Bisphosphonates to promote bone density
  - This is an off-label use for these medications, and is still being investigated

Massage?

RISKS	OI involves bones that are abnormally brittle. Very severe versions of the disease can lead to fractures with little or no trauma. It is imperative that any massage therapist working with an OI patient be fully informed about this risk.
BENEFITS	People with OI are directed to manage stress and to exercise to maintain muscle mass and control weight. Carefully conducted massage that stays within the client's ability to adapt may have a role here, as long as the fragility of the bones and other tissues is respected.

Osteomalacia

Definition: What Is It?

Osteomalacia, which technically means "bone softening," is a condition in which bone tissue breaks down faster than it can rebuild. It is distinguished from osteoporosis by the fact that it involves problems with the bone-building process, rather than the dismantling of previously healthy bones. When osteomalacia is seen in children, it is often called by its traditional name, rickets.

Etiology: What Happens?

Healthy bone tissue is formed within units called osteoids. Type 1 collagen forms the scaffolding of the osteoids, and minerals collect around the fibers to become typical bone tissue. In osteomalacia, some osteoids don't mineralize completely or correctly, leading to gaps within healthy bone tissue, bone weakness, a high risk of fractures, and bowing in the weight-bearing long bones of the leg.

Osteomalacia has several contributing factors, but they all lead to problems with building bone density. The nutrients that are deficient in some cases of osteomalacia include calcium, vitamin D, and phosphate. Some people with celiac disease or a history of stomach or small intestine surgeries are incapable of absorbing these important nutrients from their diet. Certain thyroid, kidney, and liver diseases can interfere with bone development. Long-term exposure to toxins, use of some antiseizure drugs, and overuse of over-the-counter antacids have also been seen to trigger osteomalacia.

Signs and Symptoms

The leading symptom of osteomalacia in adults is progressive deep, achy bone pain, especially in the legs, pelvis, and low back. Muscle weakness and general fatigue are often present as well. A waddling gait may develop as the leg bones begin to bow.

X-rays of people with osteomalacia may show characteristic zones where the bone tissue forms abnormally. These seams of low-density bone often resemble stress fractures. In children, this is especially visible at the growth plates, which stay wide and irregular. Eventually, the long bones of the leg weaken and bow outward.

Treatment

Osteomalacia is treated according to its cause. Vitamin and mineral supplements and treating other underlying conditions that contribute to the problem are the highest priorities.

Medications

- Vitamin or mineral supplements

Massage?

RISKS	In adults, osteomalacia is frequently associated with underlying disorders that must be addressed to work safely. This condition involves weak bones with a high risk of fracture, so any bodywork or massage must be adapted for that vulnerability.
BENEFITS	As long as the pressure is appropriate for the client and other underlying problems have been addressed, massage may be a useful strategy to deal with the deep pain and muscle weakness that frequently accompany this condition.

Osteomyelitis

Definition: What Is It?

Osteomyelitis is an acute or chronic bone infection.

Etiology: What Happens?

The infectious agents that cause osteomyelitis are usually varieties of staphylococcus including MRSA (methicillin-resistant *Staphylococcus aureus*), streptococcus, enterobacter, and some others. The pathogens access the bones through a variety of routes. Compound fractures allow environmental agents to directly access bones. Osteomyelitis is an occasional surgical complication as well. Sometimes a relatively minor skin wound becomes a portal of entry for pathogens to gain deep access. And in some cases, a condition like pneumonia or a urinary tract infection can allow pathogens to travel elsewhere in the body, leading to bone infections.

Some populations are particularly vulnerable to osteomyelitis. Long-term users of any surgical tubing such as central lines or dialysis are at risk, as are people who are HIV positive or otherwise immune-suppressed, sickle-cell disease patients, people with advanced diabetes, those with peripheral artery disease, intravenous drug users, and those who have undergone joint replacement surgeries.

Signs and Symptoms

Osteomyelitis can be acute or chronic. A chronic situation generally involves a stubborn infection that persistently recurs despite aggressive treatment.

Acute bone infections typically show a slow onset. When they occur in children, the long bones of the extremities are usually the target. In adults, the vertebrae or pelvic bones are the most common infection sites. In either case, fever, lethargy, irritability, edema, and limited movement of the affected area are seen in conjunction with redness and swelling at the affected bone.

Treatment

Intravenous antibiotics are the first recourse to treat osteomyelitis, but surgery to remove necrotic tissue may follow.

If this condition becomes a chronic situation that is resistant to treatment, chronic skin ulcers or sinuses may develop where the internal infection seeps to the surface. Inadequately treated osteomyelitis may lead to extensive loss of bone and soft tissue, raising the risk for fractures, loosening of implanted joint prostheses, spinal cord compression, deep vein thrombosis, and other serious complications.

Medications

- Antibiotics for bacterial infection; these are typically administered intravenously for several weeks

Massage?

RISKS	A person with osteomyelitis has an active and potentially dangerous infection. Massage that intends to mechanically influence fluid flow is inappropriate until this situation has been resolved. A person who has recently had surgery to treat osteomyelitis may need special considerations during recovery.
BENEFITS	Bodywork that focuses on soothing, parasympathetic support during recovery from infection may be safe and appropriate, as long as local skin problems are avoided. Clients who have fully recovered from osteomyelitis can enjoy the same benefits from massage as the rest of the population.

Paget Disease

Definition: What Is It?

Paget disease, also called osteitis deformans, is a condition in which bone is reabsorbed much faster than normal. It is replaced with disorganized fibrous connective tissue, which never completely matures, leaving the affected bones weakened and distorted. Paget disease is most common in people over age 50 of Northern European descent.

Etiology: What Happens?

Normal bone activity involves osteoclasts and osteoblasts that keep each other in balance. In Paget disease, the osteoclasts become huge and hyperactive. Osteoblasts also increase activity, but they don't change in size or form. The result is that bony tissue is broken down and replaced at an accelerated pace, but the new tissue is extremely brittle and disorganized. The cause or trigger for this change in cellular behavior is not fully understood. A genetic component seems clear because it runs in families, but the precise mutation has not been found.

Paget disease can occur in one bone or several. The vertebrae, pelvis, leg, and skull bones are affected most often. Once established, the lesions may grow, but they do not appear to spread to other bones.

Signs and Symptoms

Paget disease usually has no symptoms until it is advanced enough to cause visible changes to the affected bones. Later signs and symptoms include deep bone pain, palpable heat where the bone is affected, and problems related to a change in bone shape in the affected area. These can include a loss of hearing and chronic headaches if the skull is affected, pinched nerves and vertebral fractures if the disease is in the spine, and a visible change in the shape of long bones, which may become bowed and distorted.

Complications

The most common complications of Paget disease are arthritis and fractures in the affected bones. If the cranial bones press on parts of the central nervous system, deafness, headaches, or vision problems could develop. Teeth can loosen if the disease distorts the mandible. Congestive heart failure may occur because the heart must pump blood through whole massive networks of vessels in the new, useless fibrous tissue. A small number of Paget disease patients may develop a rare but aggressive form of bone cancer.

Treatment

Treatment for Paget disease includes recommendations for exercise and physical therapy to maintain function and healthy bone mass. Medications can address symptoms of the disease, but may not interrupt the progress. Surgery may become necessary to repair fractures or replace joint surfaces when the bones become badly distorted.

Medications

- NSAIDs for pain and inflammation
- Bisphosphonates to inhibit osteoclast activity
- Calcitonin, if bisphosphonates aren't successful

Massage?

RISKS	People with Paget disease have bones that are severely compromised. This fragility must be accommodated with modality and positioning choices.
BENEFITS	Early-stage Paget disease may be treated with physical therapy to maintain flexibility and bone density. Massage in this context, and in concert with the rest of the health care team, may be safe and appropriate.

Pelvic Inflammatory Disease

Definition: What Is It?

Pelvic inflammatory disease (PID) can involve infection of the uterus (endometritis), infection of the uterine tubes (salpingitis), or abscesses on the ovaries (oophoritis).

Etiology: What Happens?

PID is usually the result of a bacterial infection that begins in the vagina. The infectious agent is often chlamydia or gonorrhea or both, but possible causes also include irritation from an IUD or incomplete elective or spontaneous abortion.

Common complications of PID include infertility, ectopic pregnancy, and chronic pelvic pain. PID becomes dangerous when the infection backs up from the vagina to the uterus and into the fallopian tubes, where it can start growing in the open pelvic cavity. Occasionally, PID causes the growth of tubo-ovarian abscesses. If an abscess ruptures, it releases infectious material into the pelvis. In either case, life-threatening peritonitis is the result.

Types of Pelvic Inflammatory Disease

- **Acute PID:** This is a high-grade infection with symptoms that include fever, low back pain, nausea, vomiting, lethargy, painful intercourse, and heavy vaginal discharge.
- **Chronic PID:** This condition involves long-term low-grade inflammation that can cause subtle symptoms, but can also lead to extensive scarring of the uterine tubes and a high risk of infertility or ectopic pregnancy.

Signs and Symptoms

The signs and symptoms of PID depend on whether the infection is acute or chronic. They are described above under types of pelvic inflammatory disorder.

Treatment

PID is usually a fairly simple bacterial infection. Caught early, it responds well to antibiotics and bed rest, although some women need hospitalization and intravenous antibiotics. Sexual activity must be curtailed for several weeks, and the woman's sexual partner or partners should also be treated for gonorrhea or chlamydia if either of those is causing the infection.

Medications

- Antibiotics for bacterial infection

Massage?

RISKS	Acute PID contraindicates any but the most gentle, noninvasive bodywork until the infection has been resolved. Chronic PID (if it is identified at all) calls for special caution for abdominal work, and of course any other massage must fit within the client's capacity for adaption.
BENEFITS	Massage is unlikely to have a direct positive impact on PID, but it may be a helpful and soothing coping mechanism for a woman going through a difficult time. Clients who have fully recovered from PID can enjoy all the same benefits from massage as the rest of the population.

Peritonitis

Definition: What Is It?

Peritonitis is usually an infection that has become established in the peritoneal space, where infectious agents can grow easily. Other irritants may also cause inflammation of the peritoneum, including gastric juice from a perforated peptic ulcer, or bile from the gallbladder or injured liver.

Etiology: What Happens?

Peritonitis that is related to infection can begin when pathogenic agents gain access to the peritoneal space. This can happen in a variety of ways: mechanical perforation (as in a knife wound or a complication of surgery); with the rupture of an abdominal or pelvic abscess (pelvic inflammatory disease); or with organ damage related to underlying disease (perforating ulcers, acute appendicitis, Crohn disease, ulcerative colitis, or diverticulitis). Peritonitis can also happen spontaneously; this is an occasional complication of ascites: massive abdominal fluid retention that is seen with cirrhosis and some other disorders. Experts theorize that in this case bacteria seep into the abdominal fluid through the gut wall or mesenteric lymph nodes.

One form of peritonitis is related to peritoneal dialysis. This is a procedure that uses the peritoneum as a filter for blood dialysis, but it carries a significant risk of contamination and infection.

Once bacteria establish residence in the peritoneal space, they promote the production of scar tissue. This can lead to severe adhesions and cysts that serve to protect bacteria from immune system response.

Signs and Symptoms

Dull, diffuse abdominal pain is the most common sign of peritonitis. It can have a fast or insidious onset, depending on underlying causes. Anorexia and nausea are often present, along with fever and rapid heart rate.

Treatment

If the abdominal inflammation or infection can be treated without surgery, this is obviously the preferred course. Open or laparoscopic surgery may be required, however, to repair perforations or ruptures.

Medications

- Oral or intravenous antibiotics for bacterial infection

Massage?

RISKS	Acute peritonitis is a medical emergency, and contraindicates massage until the crisis is over.
BENEFITS	A client who has fully recovered from peritonitis can enjoy the same benefits from massage as the rest of the population.

Pityriasis Rosea

Definition: What Is It?

Pityriasis rosea is an idiopathic, self-limiting rash that usually affects teenagers and young adults. Its name derives from the Greek for "pink bran" because the lesions are round, pinkish, and slightly itchy.

Etiology: What Happens?

The etiology of pityriasis rosea is unclear, but it seems to have a strong link with a viral trigger: many cases erupt after a recent upper respiratory tract infection. It does not appear to be contagious however, so the rash may be a side effect of viral exposure rather than the result of direct damage to the tissues. It is rare for a person to have pityriasis rosea more than once.

Signs and Symptoms

Pityriasis rosea typically begins with a single, round, pinkish lesion on the trunk; this is called the "herald patch." This is followed within the next two weeks with many similar lesions, often in a symmetrical "Christmas tree" pattern on the body. The lesions, which are not intensely itchy, are usually confined to the back, chest, or abdomen. It is most common among people between 10 and 35 years old. The rash lasts two to eight weeks, and then spontaneously disappears, leaving little or no discoloration.

It is useful to get a professional diagnosis for pityriasis rosea because this noncontagious rash resembles both ringworm and secondary syphilis: both potentially communicable conditions that require treatment to eradicate.

Treatment

Often no treatment is prescribed for this benign, self-limiting condition. Home care may include avoiding harsh or drying soaps and using soothing lotion. Exposure to ultraviolet light may be recommended, as this appears to speed healing. When medication is prescribed, it is to deal with symptoms only.

Medications

- Corticosteroid cream for itching
- Antihistamines for itching

Massage?

RISKS	It is important to work with this condition only when a definitive diagnosis has been obtained, because pityriasis resembles other skin conditions that are potentially communicable. Massage may exacerbate itching, so this rash may be a local contraindication while it is present.
BENEFITS	Massage won't speed healing or otherwise directly improve pityriasis rosea, but if it can be conducted without making the itching worse, a client with this condition can enjoy the same benefits of bodywork as the rest of the population.

Pleurisy

Definition: What Is It?

Pleurisy refers to inflammation of the pleurae: the epithelial membranes that line the thoracic cavity. Pleuritis is a synonym.

Etiology: What Happens?

The outer surface of each lung is covered by an epithelial membrane called the visceral pleura; the inner surface of the thoracic cavity is lined with a similar membrane called the parietal pleura. In normal conditions, the visceral and parietal layers of the pleurae secrete a small amount of lubricating fluid that allows the two surfaces to slip and slide easily over each other with every breath. Pleurisy develops when the visceral and parietal layers develop inflammation. This causes the layers to stick together, making breathing painful. Further, prolonged inflammation can allow the pleural space to fill with fluid. This compresses the lungs and creates a risk of empyema: infection in the pleural space.

Causes of pleurisy include lung infection, chest trauma, the congestion that occurs with heart failure, inhaled chemicals or toxins, autoimmune diseases (specifically rheumatoid arthritis and lupus), cancers of the lung or pleurae, pulmonary embolism, and abdominal problems that can put pressure on the thoracic cavity, including pancreatitis, gallbladder disease, and cirrhosis.

Signs and Symptoms

Pleurisy typically involves stabbing chest pain with inhalation. The pain is usually unilateral and has a sudden onset in conjunction with a predisposing factor: a respiratory infection, a flare of autoimmune disease, a chest trauma, or something else. It is important to get a confirmed diagnosis of pleurisy: chest muscle strains or costochondritis look very similar, but require different treatment options.

Treatment

Pleurisy is treated according to underlying causes. Drugs can treat bacterial infections, autoimmune diseases, and emboli. Other causes may have to be treated with a combination of medication and surgical procedures.

Nonpharmacologic interventions for pleurisy start with external splinting of the chest wall, but may include thoracentesis (needle aspiration of the pleural space); decortication, a procedure to remove infectious material and scar tissue; or pleurodesis, which introduces an irritant to the pleural space that essentially "glues" the layers together in order to prevent future episodes of pleural effusion.

Medications

- Aspirin, ibuprofen, NSAIDs to control pain and inflammation
- Antibiotics for bacterial infections
- Anticoagulants for pulmonary embolism
- Immunosuppressants for autoimmune disease

Massage?

RISKS	Pleurisy is sometimes a sequence of serious underlying diseases that have implications for massage: these must be explored before safety is assured.
BENEFITS	A client whose pleurisy is identified and being treated may be a good candidate for any bodywork that he or she can tolerate, as long as infections are no longer communicable. Massage that focuses on breathing muscles and awareness may be welcomed. A client who has fully recovered from pleurisy can enjoy the same benefits of massage as the rest of the population.

Polymyalgia Rheumatica

Definition: What Is It?

The name polymyalgia rheumatica (PMR) describes "multiple muscle and joint pain," and this is an apt label for a condition that involves aching, stiff sore muscles and joints that persist for months or years and then spontaneously goes away. This idiopathic condition mostly affects women of Northern European ancestry between 50 and 80 years old.

Etiology: What Happens?

The etiology of PMR is poorly understood, but most experts agree that it involves a combination of it involves a combination of genetic predisposition, exposure to an environmental trigger, and abnormal monocyte activation, along with the presence of several proinflammatory cytokines. Signs of recent infection with a variety of common viruses are common with PMR, so some researchers theorize that these are the trigger.

An episode of PMR typically affects the neck, shoulders, hip, and proximal limbs. Joints muscles are painful, possibly because the fasciae, bursae, and synovial capsules are mildly inflamed. Fortunately, joint inflammation is nonerosive; that is, no permanent damage occurs.

Signs and Symptoms

Deep, aching pain of the neck, shoulders, and hips is the hallmark of PMR. The pain usually has a short onset, developing over a matter of a few days. It is worst after periods of inactivity, and morning stiffness persists for an hour or more every day. PMR may begin on one side, but it becomes bilateral. Proximal joints are the first site of pain, but the muscles of the upper arms and thighs are usually also stiff and painful. Range of motion becomes limited as well.

Some people experience low-grade fever, malaise, fatigue, and weight loss when PMR begins. Distal edema happens to some, with accompanying carpal tunnel syndrome if edema affects the wrists.

Types of Polymyalgia Rheumatica

- **Giant cell arteritis (GCA):** While GCA isn't exactly a subtype of PMR, the two conditions are frequently seen together, and experts agree that they are somehow linked. About 20% of people with PMR develop GCA, and about 60% of people with GCA had PMR first.

GCA is also called temporal arteritis or cranial arteritis. In this situation, the medium-sized blood vessels in the head and face become inflamed. The risk of permanent vision loss or stroke is significant. Symptoms of GCA include jaw and scalp pain, headache, and visual impairment. These are signals that a person must seek immediate medical help to decrease inflammation.

Treatment

PMR usually goes away by itself two to three years after it begins, but the quality of life for patients is severely impacted during the process. It responds to long-term, low-dose steroids, so this is the treatment of choice. Vitamin D and calcium supplements may be suggested to deal with the bone thinning that accompanies long-term steroid use. PMR patients are counseled to stay as active as possible: this condition puts no limitations on physical activity, as long as pain isn't exacerbated.

Medications

- Corticosteroids to control inflammation (low dose, for up to three years)
- High-dose corticosteroids for giant cell arteritis

Massage?

RISKS	Massage that is too vigorous may exacerbate pain for a client with PMR rather than relieve it. People with PMR are also likely to be taking long-term corticosteroids, which have some cautions for massage. Clients with symptoms of giant cell arteritis (which can include headache) must see a health care provider right away.
BENEFITS	Gentle massage that is soothing and nonchallenging may help decrease pain and stiffness in clients with PMR.

Rheumatic Heart Disease

Definition: What Is It?

Rheumatic heart disease is a complication of a bacterial infection, usually with *Streptococcus pyogenes*. The vast majority of people with rheumatic heart disease experience this in early childhood as "strep throat." For reasons that are not clear, about 0.3% to 3% of people who have strep throat develop a condition called rheumatic fever several weeks later. Rheumatic fever is a systemic condition that causes joint pain and inflammation, rash, and sometimes uncontrollable twitching called Sydenham chorea. Of the people who develop rheumatic fever, anywhere from 39% to 60% are at risk to develop rheumatic heart disease.

Thanks to effective antibiotics against strep throat and improved health care delivery systems, rheumatic heart disease is now rare in developed countries. However, this condition can cause extensive damage to the heart, and it is still the leading reason behind mitral valve replacement surgeries in the United States.

Etiology: What Happens?

Rheumatic heart disease does not mark a resurgence of a streptococcal infection. Rather, most experts believe that an immune system mistake causes B-cells and T-cells to misidentify normal tissues as outposts of bacteria. This makes rheumatic heart disease, for all intents and purposes, an autoimmune disorder.

These immune system attacks against healthy tissues are typically initiated by repeated exposure to *Streptococcus pyogenes*; that is, each repeated episode of strep throat raises the risk that the immune system will one day cause rheumatic fever and then rheumatic heart disease. The whole heart may be affected, but the worst outcomes occur when the endocardium that covers the mitral valve is attacked. This can lead to mitral valve stenosis, atrial fibrillation, a high risk of thromboembolism, stroke, congestive heart failure, and even death.

Signs and Symptoms

Signs and symptoms of rheumatic heart disease are similar to those for more typical versions of heart failure: shortness of breath, chest discomfort, edema, and cough. In addition, palpitations may develop, and abnormal heart sounds, including murmurs in a new pattern, may be heard through a stethoscope.

Treatment

The mainstay of treatment for rheumatic heart disease is bed rest and management of issues relating to congestive heart failure. Surgery to correct damaged valves may be recommended.

Medications

- Prophylactic antibiotics against recurring infection with *Streptococcus pyogenes*
- Salicylates for pain and inflammation
- In acute cases steroidal anti-inflammatories
- Diuretics for heart failure management

Massage?

RISKS	Rheumatic heart disease can lead to mitral valve stenosis, congestive heart failure, and death. These extremes are rare but not unheard of in the United States. Any massage that presents significant challenges to homeostasis may be too intense for a person with a compromised system to withstand.
BENEFITS	Massage for a person with a heart weakened by rheumatic heart disease can be restorative and beneficial as long as the client's limited ability to adapt is respected. Massage that presents challenges no greater than the client's typical daily activities is safe and appropriate.

Sarcoidosis

Definition: What Is It?

Sarcoidosis is an idiopathic disease in which abnormal immune system activity leads to the formation of tiny clumps of white blood cells and other matter called granulomas. These trigger an inflammatory response that can cause extensive tissue damage and scarring. Sarcoidosis can affect any organ system, but it is most often associated with lung and skin problems.

Etiology: What Happens?

The exact triggers that begin the process of sarcoidosis are not fully understood. Most experts suggest that a combination of genetic predisposition and environmental exposures to pathogens or irritating substances create a reaction that leads to granulomas, inflammation, scarring, and damage in a variety of tissues.

The majority of people diagnosed with sarcoidosis have it in their lungs, raising the theory that the trigger may be an inhaled pathogen or irritant. The granulomas can develop in virtually any tissues, however, including the skin, lymph nodes, kidneys, liver, bones, heart, and brain.

Unlike many autoimmune diseases, sarcoidosis does not appear to run in cycles of flare and remission. Rather, the majority of people diagnosed with this disease have it in a relatively mild or harmless form that runs through its course over several years and then spontaneously resolves with no permanent damage. Some people develop serious organ damage, however. Sarcoidosis is very rarely fatal.

Signs and Symptoms

Signs and symptoms of sarcoidosis vary according to severity and which tissues are affected. Many people have no specific symptoms, but evidence of the disease is found on a chest x-ray taken for some other reason. Some patients begin with fever, fatigue, weight loss, and malaise. Lung damage causes dyspnea and chest pain. If lymph nodes are affected they become enlarged; this is most consistent in the thorax. Eyes may become painful with tearing and light sensitivity. The risk of permanent damage to the eye is significant, and symptoms should be reported as quickly as possible. Skin lesions vary from discoloration to a rash on the lower leg to large nodules or ulcers that may appear on the face or hands.

Types of Sarcoidosis

- **Lofgren syndrome:** This form of sarcoidosis involves enlarged lymph nodes, especially in the thorax. Erythema nodosum is a rash of red or purplish bumps that appear over the ankles and shins. Joint pain, especially at the ankles, is common with this type. Lofgren syndrome is typically acute and short-lived, and is associated with a positive prognosis for the disease.
- **Lupus pernio:** This involves dramatic and potentially disfiguring plaques and nodules on the face, inside the nasal passages, and on the digits.
- **Subcutaneous nodular sarcoidosis:** Also called Darier-Rousy sarcoidosis, this involves small flesh-colored or purplish nodules on the extremities or trunk. The lesions are not painful. This form of sarcoidosis usually signals a mild course of the disease.

Complications

Complications of sarcoidosis happen in fewer than half of the people diagnosed with this disease, but they can be serious. Pulmonary fibrosis can permanently limit lung function and raise the risk of pneumonia. If this disease affects the eyes, then color sensitivity can be lost, while glaucoma, cataracts, light sensitivity, and even blindness can develop. Changes with how calcium is managed in the body can lead to kidney damage. It is rare, but sarcoidosis can affect the nervous system, affecting the pituitary and hypothalamus or causing damage to cranial nerve VII (this is a type of Bell palsy). In the heart, it interferes with the electrical conduction system.

Treatment

Many cases of sarcoidosis are subtle enough that they don't require intrusive treatment before they simply dissipate. Treatments are aimed at controlling symptoms and complications, preventing progression, and limiting lung damage.

Medications

- NSAIDs for Lofgren syndrome
- Bronchodilators for lung dysfunction
- Steroidal anti-inflammatories to suppress inflammation and immune system activity
- TNF-alpha inhibitors (infliximab) to suppress immune system activity
- Antirejection drugs to suppress immune system activity
- Antimalarial drugs to manage calcium processing and skin lesions

Massage?

RISKS	Sarcoidosis sometimes involves skin lesions that may be portals of entry for infection. Patients with lung damage may be uncomfortable lying flat for prolonged periods. Some patients may use immunosuppressant drugs to manage this disease, so they may be vulnerable to infection.
BENEFITS	Activity limitations for sarcoidosis patients are related only to lung involvement: it is safe for them to exercise within tolerance. This means that forms of bodywork that stay within those parameters are also likely to be safe. While massage is unlikely to alter the course of this condition, it can certainly add to a patient's quality of life. People who have a history of sarcoidosis that has resolved can enjoy the same benefits from massage as the rest of the population.

Thromboangiitis Obliterans

Definition: What Is It?

Also called Buerger disease, thromboangiitis obliterans (TAO) is a condition of small arteries and veins in the feet, hands, toes, and fingers. It is seen most often in people between 20 and 50 years old. It leads to painful ulcers on the fingers and toes, with a high risk of gangrene and amputation. Unlike other conditions that affect circulation, TAO is not related to atherosclerotic plaques, hypercoagulability, or diabetes.

Etiology: What Happens?

Thromboangiitis obliterans is a condition in which small arteries and veins in the extremities (almost exclusively the hands, feet, fingers, and toes) become inflamed and blocked by tiny blood clots. The result is nonhealing ulcers on the digits, a high risk for gangrene infection, and a need for amputation.

While the exact etiology of TAO is unknown, one unifying factor in all patients is tobacco use. Cigarettes are the most common form of use, but this disease has been seen in tobacco chewers and cigar smokers as well. Even the use of nicotine patches has been seen to stimulate progression of the disease. Experts theorize that some people have a genetic predisposition toward vascular inflammation and the development of tiny blood clots, and this tendency is triggered by nicotine exposure.

Signs and Symptoms

Signs and symptoms of TAO include intermittent claudication, resting pain, Raynaud phenomenon, parasthesia in the affected limbs, painful ulcers on the digits, and possible gangrene, which means amputation will probably be necessary. Most TAO patients have these signs in more than one extremity.

Treatment

Treatment for TAO begins and ends with the cessation of tobacco use. People with TAO are also counseled to be extremely careful about footwear, to treat infections on the feet or hands very aggressively, and to avoid vasoconstrictive drugs and extreme cold environments.

Surgical intervention to replace damaged blood vessels is sometimes attempted, but the success rate is relatively low. Sympathectomy to alter vasoconstriction and pain sensation may be recommended. This procedure has some short-term benefits, but long-term benefits have not been established.

Medications

Medical treatment for TAO has not had a great deal of success. Some options include the following:

- NSAIDs for inflammation and pain management
- Vasodilators
- Anticoagulants

Massage?

RISKS	TAO involves pain, poor circulation, and damaged skin at the hands and feet. Any massage or bodywork must be adapted to accommodate these complications.
BENEFITS	People with TAO have no limitations on exercise outside of their own tolerance. Their proximal limbs and trunk are likely to be healthy, and massage in these areas is probably safe and appropriate. In addition, TAO patients are probably dealing with smoking cessation. Any stress relief that massage provides during this difficult time can be welcome.

Uterine Prolapse

Definition: What Is It?

Uterine prolapse describes a situation in which the uterus protrudes into the vaginal canal. It can range from very mild to complete descent of the organ. It is almost exclusively seen in postmenopausal women who have vaginally delivered children, especially if any of those children were over 9 pounds at birth.

Etiology: What Happens?

The uterus is held in suspension in the pelvic cavity by a fascia, supporting ligaments and the tone and tightness of the muscles in the pelvic floor, which is determined by healthy nerve transmission to the muscles involved. If the fasciae, ligaments, muscles, and nerves are damaged, then the integrity of the pelvic floor can be compromised. A history of childbirth can weaken this important group of structures, but multiple other factors are often involved. Among these are neuropathy, pelvic tumors, general connective tissue weakness, and any condition that adds to intra-abdominal pressure, such as obesity, chronic obstructive pulmonary disease, or long-term constipation.

When the pelvic floor is seriously compromised and the ligaments that should stabilize the uterus are loose, the uterus can protrude into the vaginal space. This can occur on a continuum of severity, so minor cases cause no symptoms or problems, but major cases can cause the whole uterus to descend out of the pelvic cavity.

Signs and Symptoms

Mild cases of uterine prolapse cause no symptoms. More severe cases can involve a feeling of fullness and discomfort in the vagina, low back pain, problems with voiding the bladder or the rectum, and painful sexual intercourse. Vaginal spotting may be present if the cervix develops ulcerations.

Complications

Complications from uterine prolapse are mostly related to long-term severe cases that are not adequately treated. They can include a risk of urinary tract infection, permanent incontinence, ulcerations on the cervix, and prolapse of other pelvic organs, including the bladder (cystocele) and rectum (rectocele).

Treatment

If the extent of uterine prolapse is mild and no symptoms or complications have arisen, no treatment is recommended. A more serious situation calls for treatment, which often begins with the use of a pessary: this is a device that is inserted into the vagina to give mechanical support to the cervix and the rest of the uterus. It is removed for sexual activity and for frequent cleaning. Pessaries can be a temporary or permanent solution to uterine prolapse. If they are unsuccessful, surgery may be recommended.

Surgery for uterine prolapse ranges from reattaching loosened ligaments, to inserting a sling to support the uterus, to full hysterectomy. It can be conducted via the vagina, as open abdominal surgery, or laparoscopically.

Medications

- Estrogen replacement therapy (ERT) to improve muscle tone in the pelvic floor—if risks for ERT don't outweigh benefits
- Topical estrogen applied via pessary
- Postsurgical analgesics

Massage?

RISKS	Massage has few risks for a client with uterine prolapse, unless she has an extreme situation that has not been treated by a physician.
BENEFITS	While massage may not influence the process or prognosis of uterine prolapse, it can certainly add to the quality of life of a person undergoing this type of physical challenge. A person who has undergone surgery to repair a prolapsed uterus and has fully recovered can enjoy the same benefits from massage as the rest of the population.

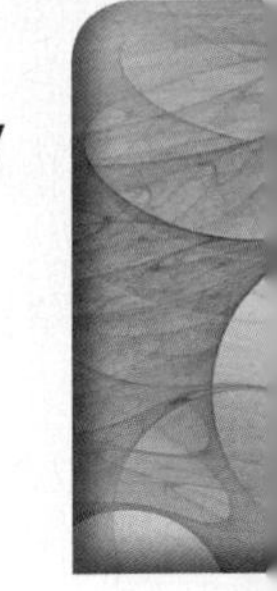

Bibliography

Chapter 1

1. Centers for Disease Control and Prevention. Guideline for Hand Hygiene in Health-Care Settings: Recommendations of the Healthcare Infection Control Practices Advisory Committee and the HICPAC/SHEA/APIC/IDSA Hand Hygiene Task Force. MMWR Morbidity and Mortality Weekly Report. 2002;51(No. RR-16). URL: http://www.cdc.gov/mmwr/PDF/rr/rr5116.pdf. Accessed winter 2010.
2. Dermal Absorption as an Exposure Route. Children's Environmental Health Project. ©2000 Canadian Association of Physicians for the Environment. URL: http://www.cape.ca/children/derm2.html. Accessed winter 2010.
3. Friedlander E. Inflammation and Repair. URL: http://www.pathguy.com/lectures/inflamma.htm. Accessed winter 2010.
4. Healthcare Wide Hazards. Occupational Safety & Health Administration. URL: http://www.osha.gov/SLTC/etools/hospital/hazards/univprec/univ.html. Accessed winter 2010.
5. Inflammation: What You Need To Know. ©1995–2009 The Cleveland Clinic Foundation. URL: http://my.clevelandclinic.org/symptoms/Inflammation/hic_Inflammation_What_You_Need_To_Know.aspx. Accessed winter 2010.
6. King M. Collagen. Indiana University School of Medicine. ©1996–2010 Michael W. King, PhD. URL: http://themedicalbiochemistrypage.org/extracellularmatrix.html. Accessed winter 2010.
7. Policy: Human Body Fluids Precautions. Sen. Doc. No. 90-028. © 2009 University of Massachusetts Amherst. URL: http://www.umass.edu/research/bodyfluid.html. Accessed winter 2010.
8. Ramachandran T. Prion-Related Diseases. © 1994–2009 by Medscape. URL: http://emedicine.medscape.com/article/1168941-overview. Accessed winter 2010.
9. Rudy S, Parham-Vetter P. Percutaneous absorption of topically applied medication. ©2009 CBS Interactive Inc. URL: http://findarticles.com/p/articles/mi_hb6366/is_2_15/ai_n29000203/?tag=content;col1. Accessed winter 2010.
10. Rutala W, Weber D; the Healthcare Infection Control Practices Advisory Committee (HICPAC). Guideline for Disinfection and Sterilization in Healthcare Facilities, 2008. URL: http://www.cdc.gov/ncidod/dhqp/pdf/guidelines/Disinfection_Nov_2008.pdf. Accessed winter 2010.
11. Siegel J, Rhinehart E, Jackson M, et al. 2007 Guideline for Isolation Precautions: Preventing Transmission of Infectious Agents in Healthcare Settings. URL: http://www.cdc.gov/ncidod/dhqp/pdf/isolation2007.pdf. Accessed winter 2010.
12. Siegel J, Rhinehart E, Jackson M, et al.; the Healthcare Infection Control Practices Advisory Committee. Management of Multidrug-Resistant Organisms in Healthcare Settings, 2006. URL: http://www.cdc.gov/ncidod/dhqp/pdf/ar/mdroguideline2006.pdf. Accessed winter 2010.
13. The Inflammatory Process. The American Dental Hygienists' Association. URL: http://www.adha.org/CE_courses/course13/inflammatory_process.htm. Accessed winter 2010.
14. Viruses. American Society of Microbiology. URL: http://www.microbeworld.org/index.php?option=com_content&view=category&layout=blog&id=77&Itemid=72. Accessed winter 2010.

Chapter 2

Acne Rosacea

1. Alai N. Rosacea. ©2009 MedicineNet, Inc. URL: http://www.medicinenet.com/rosacea/article.htm
2. Banasikowska A, Singh S. Rosacea. ©1994–2009 Medscape. URL: http://emedicine.medscape.com/article/1071429-overview. Accessed winter 2010.
3. Frequently Asked Questions. National Rosacea Society. ©1996–2009 National Rosacea Society. URL: http://www.rosacea.org/patients/faq.php. Accessed winter 2010.
4. Rosacea. http://www.dermnetnz.org/nzds.html. New Zealand Dermatological Society Incorporated. ©2009 New Zealand Dermatological Society Incorporated. URL: http://dermnetnz.org/acne/rosacea.html. Accessed winter 2010.
5. Rosacea. American Osteopathic College of Dermatology. ©2010 AOCD. URL: http://www.aocd.org/skin/dermatologic_diseases/rosacea.html. Accessed winter 2010.
6. Standard grading system for rosacea: Report of the National Rosacea Society Expert Committee on the Classification and Staging of Rosacea. Journal of the American Academy of Dermatology 2004;50:907–912. ©2004 American Academy of Dermatology. URL: http://www.rosacea.org/grading/gradingsystem.pdf. Accessed winter 2010.

Acne Vulgaris

1. Fulton J. Acne Vulgaris. ©1994–2009 Medscape. URL: http://emedicine.medscape.com/article/1069804-overview. Accessed winter 2010.
2. Guidelines of care for acne vulgaris management. American Academy of Dermatology. ©2007 American Academy of Dermatology, Inc. URL: http://www.aad.org/research/_doc/ClinicalResearch_Acne%20Vulgaris.pdf. Accessed winter 2010.
3. Keri J, Nijhawan R. Diet and Acne. ©2008 Expert Reviews Ltd. URL: http://www.medscape.com/viewarticle/579326. Accessed winter 2010.

4. Thielitz A, Gollnick H. Overview of New Therapeutic Developments for Acne. ©2009 Expert Reviews Ltd. URL: http://www.medscape.com/viewarticle/587306. Accessed winter 2010.
5. What is Acne. American Academy of Dermatology. ©2010 American Academy of Dermatology. URL: http://www.skincarephysicians.com/acnenet/acne.html. Accessed winter 2010.

Animal Parasites

1. Cordoro K, Wilson B, Kauffman C. Scabies. © 1994–2010 by Medscape. URL: http://emedicine.medscape.com/article/1109204-overview. Accessed winter 2010.
2. Flinders D, Schweinitz P. Pediculosis and Scabies. © 2004 American Academy of Family Physicians. URL: http://www.aafp.org/afp/20040115/341.html. Accessed winter 2010.
3. Guenther L, Maguiness S, Austin T. Pediculosis. © 1994–2010 by Medscape.URL: http://emedicine.medscape.com/article/225013-overview. Accessed winter 2010.
4. Lice. ©2010 WebMD, Inc. URL: http://www.emedicinehealth.com/lice/article_em.htm. Accessed winter 2010.
5. Perlstein D, Shiel W Jr. Head Lice Infestation (Pediculosis). ©1996–2010 MedicineNet. URL: http://www.medicinenet.com/head_lice/article.htm. Accessed winter 2010.
6. Pubic Lice (Crabs). MedicineNet. ©1996–2010 MedicineNet, Inc.URL: http://www.medicinenet.com/script/main/art.asp?articlekey=33588. Accessed winter 2010.
7. Rockoff A, Stoppler M. Scabies. MedicineNet. ©1996–2010 MedicineNet, Inc. URL: http://www.medicinenet.com/script/main/art.asp?articlekey=11922. Accessed winter 2010.
8. Scabies. Centers for Disease Control and Prevention. URL: http://www.cdc.gov/scabies/index.html. Accessed winter 2010.
9. What are body lice? Centers for Disease Control and Prevention. URL: http://www.cdc.gov/lice/body/factsheet.html. Accessed winter 2010.

Burns

1. Cox R. Burns, Chemical. ©1994–2010 Medscape. http://emedicine.medscape.com/article/769336-overview. Accessed winter 2010.
2. Goodis J, Schraga E. Burns, Thermal. ©1994–2010 Medscape. http://emedicine.medscape.com/article/769193-overview. Accessed winter 2010.
3. Melsaether C, Rosen C. Burns, Ocular. ©1994–2010 Medscape.URL: http://emedicine.medscape.com/article/798696-overview. Accessed winter 2010.
4. Morien A, Garrison D, Smith NK. Range of motion improves after massage in children with burns: a pilot study. Journal of Bodywork and Movement Therapies 2008;12(1):67–71. URL: http://www.ncbi.nlm.nih.gov/pubmed/19083657?itool=EntrezSystem2.PEntrez.Pubmed.Pubmed_ResultsPanel.Pubmed_RVDocSum&ordinalpos=4. Accessed winter 2010.
5. Roh YS, Cho H, Oh JO, et al. Effects of skin rehabilitation massage therapy on pruritus, skin status, and depression in burn survivors. Taehan Kanho Hakhoe Chi 2007;37(2):221–226. URL: http://www.ncbi.nlm.nih.gov/pubmed/17435407?itool=EntrezSystem2.PEntrez.Pubmed.Pubmed_ResultsPanel.Pubmed_RVDocSum&ordinalpos=8. Accessed winter 2010.

Decubitus Ulcers

1. Bedsores (pressure sores). Mayo Clinic. © 1998–2010 Mayo Foundation for Medical Education and Research (MFMER). URL: http://mayoclinic.com/health/bedsores/DS00570. Accessed winter 2010.
2. Duimel-Peeters IG, Hulsenboom MA, Berger MP, et al. Massage to prevent pressure ulcers: knowledge, beliefs and practice. A cross-sectional study among nurses in the Netherlands in 1991 and 2003. Journal of Clinical Nursing 2006;15(4):428–435.
3. Mawson A, Siddiqui F, Biundo J Jr. Enhancing host resistance to pressure ulcers: a new approach to prevention. Preventive Medicine 1993;22(3):433–450. URL: http://www.ncbi.nlm.nih.gov/pubmed/8327423?ordinalpos=1&itool=EntrezSystem2.PEntrez.Pubmed.Pubmed_ResultsPanel.Pubmed_SingleItemSupl.Pubmed_Discovery_RA&linkpos=5&log$=relatedreviews&logdbfrom=pubmed. Accessed winter 2010.
4. Revis D Jr. Decubitus Ulcers. © 1994–2010 Medscape. URL: http://emedicine.medscape.com/article/190115-overview. Accessed winter 2010.
5. Shahin ES, Dassen T, Halfens RJ. Pressure ulcer prevention in intensive care patients: guidelines and practice. Journal of Evaluation in Clinical Practice. 2009;15(2):370–374. URL: http://www.ncbi.nlm.nih.gov/pubmed/19335499?itool=EntrezSystem2.PEntrez.Pubmed.Pubmed_ResultsPanel.Pubmed_RVDocSum&ordinalpos=1. Accessed winter 2010.
6. URL: http://www.ncbi.nlm.nih.gov/pubmed/16553756?itool=EntrezSystem2.PEntrez.Pubmed.Pubmed_ResultsPanel.Pubmed_RVDocSum&ordinalpos=9. Accessed winter 2010.
7. Werdin F, Tennenhaus M, Schaller H, et al. Evidence-based Management Strategies for Treatment of Chronic Wounds. ePlasty 2009;9:e19. © 1994–2010 Medscape. URL: http://www.medscape.com/viewarticle/709000. Accessed winter 2010.

Dermatitis, Eczema

1. Allergic Contact Rashes. American Academy of Dermatology. © 2009 American Academy of Dermatology. URL: http://www.aad.org/public/publications/pamphlets/skin_allergic.html. Accessed winter 2010.
2. An Introduction to Probiotics. Department of Health and Human Services National Institutes of Health (NIH). URL: http://nccam.nih.gov/health/probiotics/. Accessed winter 2010.
3. Eczema/Atopic Dermatitis. American Academy of Dermatology. ©2009 American Academy of Dermatology. URL: http://www.aad.org/public/publications/pamphlets/skin_eczema.html. Accessed winter 2010.
4. Guidelines of care for atopic dermatitis. American Academy of Dermatology. © 2004 by the American Academy of Dermatology, Inc. URL: http://www.aad.org/research/_doc/ClinicalResearch_atopic%20Dermatitis%20Part%20I.pdf. Accessed winter 2010.

5. Hoffjan S, Stemmler S. Epidermal Differentiation Complex in Ichthyosis Vulgaris. The British Journal of Dermatology 2007;157(3):441–449. ©1994–2010 Medscape. URL: http://www.medscape.com/viewarticle/564078_4. Accessed winter 2010.
6. http://www.medscape.com/viewarticle/572227. Accessed winter 2010.
7. Kedrowski D. Hand Dermatitis: A Review of Clinical Features, Diagnosis, and Management. ©2008 Jannetti Publications, Inc.
8. Lam J, Friedlander S. Atopic Dermatitis: A Review of Recent Advances in the Field. ©2008 Future Medicine Ltd. URL: http://www.medscape.com/viewarticle/586561. Accessed winter 2010.
9. Norton A. Acupuncture May Ease the Itch of Eczema. ©2009 Reuters Health Information. URL: http://www.medscape.com/viewarticle/714235. Accessed winter 2010.
10. Perry A, Trafeli J. Hand Dermatitis: Review of Etiology, Diagnosis, and Treatment. Journal of the American Board of Family Medicine 2009;22(3):325–330. © 1994–2010 Medscape. URL: http://www.medscape.com/viewarticle/710375. Accessed winter 2010.
11. Poison Ivy, Oak & Sumac. American Academy of Dermatology. © 2009 American Academy of Dermatology. URL: http://www.aad.org/public/publications/pamphlets/skin_poison.html. Accessed winter 2010.
12. Seborrheic Dermatitis. American Academy of Dermatology Association. ©2009 American Academy of Dermatology Association. URL: http://www.aad.org/public/publications/pamphlets/common_seb_dermatitis.html. Accessed winter 2010.
13. Treadwell P. Eczema and Infection. ©2008 Lippincott Williams & Wilkins. URL: http://www.medscape.com/viewarticle/578781. Accessed winter 2010.

Fungal Infections of the Skin

1. Burkhart CG, Gottwald L, Burkhart CN. Tinea Versicolor. © 1994–2009 by Medscape. URL: http://emedicine.medscape.com/article/1091575-overview
2. Jock Itch. National Institutes of Health. URL: http://www.nlm.nih.gov/medlineplus/ency/article/000876.htm. Accessed winter 2010.
3. Kao G. Tinea Capitis. © 1994–2009 Medscape. URL: http://emedicine.medscape.com/article/1091351-overview. Accessed winter 2010.
4. Lesher J Jr. Tinea Corporis. © 1994–2009 by Medscape. URL: http://emedicine.medscape.com/articvle/1091473-overview. Accessed winter 2010.
5. Rashid R, Miller A, Silverberg M. Tinea. © 1994–2010 Medscape. URL: http://emedicine.medscape.com/article/787217-overview. Accessed winter 2010.
6. Robbins C, Elewski B. Tinea Pedis. © 1994–2009 by Medscape. URL: http://emedicine.medscape.com/article/1091684-overview. Accessed winter 2010.
7. Tinea capitis. National Institutes of Health. URL: http://www.nlm.nih.gov/medlineplus/ency/article/000878.htm. Accessed winter 2010.
8. Tinea versicolor. National Institutes of Health. URL: http://www.nlm.nih.gov/medlineplus/ency/article/001465.htm. Accessed winter 2010.
9. Tosti A. Onychomycosis. © 1994–2009 Medscape. URL: http://emedicine.medscape.com/article/1105828-overview. Accessed winter 2010.
10. Wiederkehr M, Schwartz R. Tinea Cruris. © 1994–2009 Medscape. URL: http://emedicine.medscape.com/article/1091806-overview. Accessed winter 2010.

Herpes Simplex

1. Genital Herpes. Centers for Disease Control and Prevention. URL: http://www.cdc.gov/std/Herpes/STDFact-Herpes.htm. Accessed winter 2010.
2. Herpes Simplex. American Academy of Dermatology Association. © 2009 American Academy of Dermatology. URL: http://www.aad.org/public/publications/pamphlets/viral_herpes_simplex.html. Accessed winter 2010.
3. Kramer A, Schwebke I, Kampf G. How long do nosocomial pathogens persist on inanimate surfaces? A systematic review. © 2006 Kramer et al. Licensee BioMed Central Ltd. URL: http://www.biomedcentral.com/1471-2334/6/130. Accessed winter 2010.
4. Omori M. Herpetic Whitlow. © 1994–2009 Medscape. http://emedicine.medscape.com/article/788056-overview. Accessed winter 2010.
5. Salvaggio M, Lutwick L, Seenivasan M, et al. Herpes Simplex. © 1994–2009 Medscape. URL: http://emedicine.medscape.com/article/218580-overview. Accessed winter 2010.
6. Torres G, Schinstine M, Krusinski P, et al. Herpes Simplex. © 1994–2009 by Medscape. URL: http://emedicine.medscape.com/article/1132351-overview. Accessed winter 2010.

Psoriasis

1. Alai N. Psoriasis. MedicineNet. ©1996–2010 MedicineNet, Inc. URL: http://www.medicinenet.com/script/main/art.asp?articlekey=459. Accessed winter 2010.
2. Azfar R, Gelfand J. Psoriasis and Metabolic Disease: Epidemiology and Pathophysiology. Current Opinion in Rheumatology 2008;20(4):416–422. Medscape. © 1994–2010 by WebMD LLC. URL: http://www.medscape.com/viewarticle/576496. Accessed winter 2010.
3. Hoffjan S, Stemmler S. On the Role of the Epidermal Differentiation Complex in Ichthyosis Vulgaris, Atopic Dermatitis and Psoriasis. The British Journal of Dermatology 2007;157(3):441–449. © 1994–2010 Medscape. http://www.medscape.com/viewarticle/564078. Accessed winter 2010.
4. Lui H, Mamelak A. Psoriasis, Plaque. Medscape. © 1994–2010 Medscape. URL: http://emedicine.medscape.com/article/1108072-overview. Accessed winter 2010.
5. Psoriasis Triggers. American Academy of Dermatology. ©2010 American Academy of Dermatology. URL: http://www.skincarephysicians.com/psoriasisnet/triggers.html. Accessed winter 2010.
6. Schmid-Ott G, Jaeger B, Boehm T, et al. Immunological Effects of Stress in Psoriasis. The British Journal of Dermatology 2009;160(4):782–785. Medscape. © 1994–2010 by WebMD LLC. URL: http://www.medscape.com/viewarticle/589969. Accessed winter 2010.

7. Steele T, Rogers C, Jacob S. Herbal Remedies for Psoriasis: What Are Our Patients Taking? Dermatology Nursing 2007;19(5):448–463. © 1994–2010 by WebMD LLC. URL: http://www.medscape.com/viewarticle/567028. Accessed winter 2010.
8. Types of psoriasis. National Psoriasis Foundation. ©2010 National Psoriasis Foundation/USA. URL: http://www.psoriasis.org/netcommunity/learn_types. Accessed winter 2010.
9. Types of psoriatic arthritis. National Psoriasis Foundation. ©2010 National Psoriasis Foundation/USA. URL: http://www.psoriasis.org/netcommunity/learn_psatypes. Accessed winter 2010.
10. What is Psoriasis? American Academy of Dermatology. © 2010 American Academy of Dermatology. URL: http://www.skincarephysicians.com/psoriasisnet/whatis.html. Accessed winter 2010.

Scar Tissue

1. Patiño O, Novick C, Merlo A, et al. Massage in hypertrophic scars. The Journal of Burn Care and Rehabilitation 1999;20(3):268–271; discussion 267. URL: http://www.ncbi.nlm.nih.gov/pubmed/10342484. Accessed winter 2010.
2. Scars. MedicineNet. ©1996–2010 MedicineNet, Inc. URL: http://www.medicinenet.com/script/main/art.asp?articlekey=43240. Accessed winter 2010.
3. What is a scar? American Academy of Dermatology. © 2010 American Academy of Dermatology. http://www.aad.org/public/publications/pamphlets/cosmetic_scar.html. Accessed winter 2010.
4. What is a scar? University of Virginia Health System. © 2010 by the Rector and Visitors of the University of Virginia. URL: http://www.healthsystem.virginia.edu/uvahealth/adult_derm/scars.cfm. Accessed winter 2010.
5. Wong T, Mcgrath J, Navsaria H. The Role of Fibroblasts in Tissue Engineering and Regeneration. The British Journal of Dermatology 2007;156(6):1149–1155. © 1994–2010 Medscape. URL: http://www.medscape.com/viewarticle/558003. Accessed winter 2010.

Seborrheic Keratosis

1. Balin A. Seborrheic Keratosis. Medscape. © 1994–2010 by Medscape. URL: http://emedicine.medscape.com/article/1059477-overview. Accessed winter 2010.
2. Seborrheic Keratoses. American Academy of Dermatology. © 2010 American Academy of Dermatology. http://www.aad.org/public/publications/pamphlets/common_seb_keratoses.html. Accessed winter 2010.
3. Seborrheic keratosis. Mayo Clinic. © 1998–2010 Mayo Foundation for Medical Education and Research. URL: http://www.mayoclinic.com/health/seborrheic-keratosis/DS00846. Accessed winter 2010.

Skin Cancer

1. Basal cell carcinoma. Mayo Clinic. © 1998–2010 Mayo Foundation for Medical Education and Research. URL: http://www.mayoclinic.com/health/basal-cell-carcinoma/DS00925. Accessed winter 2010.
2. Bowen's Disease. American Osteopathic College of Dermatology. © 2010 AOCD, URL: http://www.aocd.org/skin/dermatologic_diseases/bowens_disease.html. Accessed winter 2010.
3. Four Types of Melanoma. American Academy of Dermatology. © 2010 American Academy of Dermatology. URL: http://www.skincarephysicians.com/skincancernet/four_types.html. Accessed winter 2010.
4. Gandey A. Malignant Melanomas Often Look Noticeably Different From Other Moles. Medscape. © 1994–2010 Medscape. URL: http://www.medscape.com/viewarticle/569114. Accessed winter 2010.
5. How Is Melanoma Staged? American Cancer Society. ©2010 American Cancer Society. URL: http://www.cancer.org/docroot/CRI/content/CRI_2_4_3X_How_is_melanoma_staged_50.asp. Accessed winter 2010.
6. Intraocular (Eye) Melanoma Treatment. National Cancer Institute. URL: http://www.cancer.gov/cancertopics/pdq/treatment/intraocularmelanoma/healthprofessional/allpages. Accessed winter 2010.
7. Leukoplakia. Mayo Clinic. © 1998–2010 Mayo Foundation for Medical Education and Research (MFMER). URL: http://www.mayoclinic.com/health/leukoplakia/DS00458. Accessed winter 2010.
8. Lober B, Lober C. Actinic Keratosis is Squamous Cell Carcinoma. Southern Medical Journal 2000;93(7). © 1994–2010 by Medscape. URL: http://www.medscape.com/viewarticle/410575. Accessed winter 2010.
9. McIntyre W, Downs M, Bedwell S. Treatment Options for Actinic Keratoses. Journal of the American Academy of Family Physicians. © 2007 American Academy of Family Physicians. URL: http://www.aafp.org/afp/2007/0901/p667.html. Accessed winter 2010.
10. Skin Cancer Fact Sheet. American Academy of Dermatology. © 2010 American Academy of Dermatology. URL: http://www.aad.org/media/background/factsheets/fact_skincancer.html. Accessed winter 2010.
11. Skin Cancer Statistics. Centers for Disease Control and Prevention. URL: http://www.cdc.gov/cancer/skin/statistics/index.htm. Accessed winter 2010.
12. Skin Cancer: Basal Cell and Squamous Cell. American Cancer Society. ©2008 American Cancer Society. URL: http://documents.cancer.org/118.00/118.00.pdf. Accessed winter 2010.
13. Spencer J, Basile A. Actinic Keratosis. Medscape. © 1994–2010 Medscape. URL: http://emedicine.medscape.com/article/1099775-overview. Accessed winter 2010.
14. What You Need to Know About Skin Cancer. National Cancer Institute. URL: http://www.cancer.gov/cancertopics/wyntk/skin/allpages. Accessed winter 2010.
15. What you need to know: Melanoma. National Cancer Institute. URL: http://www.cancer.gov/cancertopics/wyntk/melanoma. Accessed winter 2010.

Staphylococcus Infections of the Skin

1. Boils and carbuncles. Mayo clinic. ©1998–2009 Mayo Foundation for Medical Education and Research. URL: http://mayoclinic.com/health/boils-and-carbuncles/DS00466. Accessed winter 2010.

2. Folliculitis. Mayo clinic. ©1998–2009 Mayo Foundation for Medical Education and Research. URL: http://mayoclinic.com/health/folliculitis/DS00512. Accessed winter 2010.
3. Jovanovic M, Kihiczak G, Schwartz R. Hidradenitis Suppurativa. ©1994–2009 Medscape. URL: http://emedicine.medscape.com/article/1073117-overview. Accessed winter 2010.
4. Lanigan M. Pilonidal Cyst and Sinus. ©1994–2009 Medscape. URL: http://emedicine.medscape.com/article/788127-overview. Accessed winter 2010.
5. Martinez J. MRSA Skin Infection in Athletes. ©1994–2009 Medscape. URL: http://emedicine.medscape.com/article/108972-overview. Accessed winter 2010.
6. MRSA. Mayo clinic. ©1998–2009 Mayo Foundation for Medical Education and Research. URL: http://mayoclinic.com/health/mrsa/DS00735. Accessed winter 2010.
7. Satter E. Folliculitis. ©1994–2009 Medscape. URL: http://emedicine.medscape.com/article/1070456-overview. Accessed winter 2010.
8. Tolan R, Baorto E, Baorto D. *Staphylococcus Aureus* Infection. ©1994–2009 Medscape. URL: http://emedicine.medscape.com/article/971358-overview. Accessed winter 2010.

Streptococcal Infections of the Skin

1. Davis L, Cole J, Benbenisty K. Erysipelas. ©1994–2009 Medscape. URL: http://emedicine.medscape.com/article/1052445-overview. Accessed winter 2010.
2. Humphrey I, Halsey E. Cellulitis. ©1994–2009 Medscape. URL: http://emedicine.medscape.com/article/214222-overview. Accessed winter 2010.
3. MRSA and the Workplace. The National Institute for Occupational Safety and Health (NIOSH). URL: http://www.cdc.gov/niosh/topics/mrsa/. Accessed winter 2010.
4. Nochimson G. Erysipelas. ©1994–2009 Medscape. http://emedicine.medscape.com/article/782452-overview. Accessed winter 2010.
5. Schwartz R, Kapila R. Necrotizing Fasciitis. ©1994–2009 Medscape. URL: http://emedicine.medscape.com/article/1054438-overview. Accessed winter 2010.

Warts

1. Common Warts. Mayo Clinic. © 1998–2010 Mayo Foundation for Medical Education and Research. URL: http://www.mayoclinic.com/health/common-warts/DS00370. Accessed winter 2010.
2. Crowe M. Molluscum Contagiosum. Medscape. © 1994–2010 by Medscape. URL: http://emedicine.medscape.com/article/910570-overview. Accessed winter 2010.
3. Duct Tape More Effective than Cryotherapy for Warts. Journal of the American Academy of Family Physicians. © 2003 by the American Academy of Family Physicians. URL: http://www.aafp.org/afp/2003/0201/p614.html. Accessed winter 2010.
4. Lipke M. An Armamentarium of Wart Treatments. Clinical Medicine & Research. ©2006 Marshfield Clinic. URL: http://www.clinmedres.org/cgi/content/full/4/4/273. Accessed winter 2010.
5. Plantar Warts. Mayo Clinic. © 1998–2010 Mayo Foundation for Medical Education and Research. URL: http://www.mayoclinic.com/health/plantar-warts/DS00509. Accessed winter 2010.
6. Shanley J. Papillomavirus. Medscape. © 1994–2010 Medscape. URL: http://emedicine.medscape.com/article/224516-overview. Accessed winter 2010.
7. Shenefelt P. Warts, Nongenital. Medscape. © 1994–2010 Medscape. URL: http://emedicine.medscape.com/article/1133317-overview. Accessed winter 2010.
8. Siegel R. Human Papillomavirus. Stanford University. URL: http://virus.stanford.edu/papova/HPV.html. Accessed winter 2010.
9. Warts. American Academy of Dermatology. © 2010 American Academy of Dermatology. URL: http://www.aad.org/public/publications/pamphlets/common_warts.html. Accessed winter 2010.

Chapter 3

Adhesive Capsulitis

1. Adhesive Capsulitis: A Patient's Guide to Adhesive Capsulitis. Copyright © 2009–2011 Medical Multimedia Group, L.L.C. URL: http://www.eorthopod.com/content/adhesive-capsulitis. Accessed winter 2011.
2. Cy H, et al. The effectiveness of manual therapy in the management of musculoskeletal disorders of the shoulder: a systematic review. Manual Therapy 2009;14(5):463–474. [Epub May 21, 2009.] URL: http://www.ncbi.nlm.nih.gov/pubmed/19467911. Accessed winter 2011.
3. Guler-Uysal F, et al. Comparison of the early response to two methods of rehabilitation in adhesive capsulitis. Swiss Medical Weekly 2004;134(23–24):353–358. URL: http://www.ncbi.nlm.nih.gov/pubmed/15318285. Accessed winter 2011.
4. Jewell DV, et al. Interventions associated with an increased or decreased likelihood of pain reduction and improved function in patients with adhesive capsulitis: a retrospective cohort study. Physical Therapy 2009;89(5):419–429. [Epub Mar 6, 2009.] URL: http://www.ncbi.nlm.nih.gov/pubmed/19270045. Accessed winter 2011.
5. Roy A, et al. Adhesive Capsulitis. © 1994–2011 by WebMD LLC. URL: http://emedicine.medscape.com/article/326828-overview. Accessed winter 2011.
6. Shiel W, et al. Frozen Shoulder (Adhesive Capsulitis). © 1996–2011 MedicineNet, Inc. URL: http://www.medicinenet.com/script/main/art.asp?articlekey=2023. Accessed winter 2011.
7. Sokk J, et al. Shoulder muscle strength and fatigability in patients with frozen shoulder syndrome: the effect of 4-week individualized rehabilitation. Electromyography and Clinical Neurophysiology 2007;47(4–5):205–213. URL: http://www.ncbi.nlm.nih.gov/pubmed/17711038. Accessed winter 2011.

Baker Cyst

1. Baker's Cyst/Popliteal Cysts. © 1996–2011 Data Trace Internet Publishing, LLC. URL: http://www.wheelessonline.com/ortho/bakers_cyst_popliteal_cysts. Accessed winter 2011.

2. Bui-Mansfield L, et al. Copyright © 1994–2011 by WebMD LLC. URL: http://emedicine.medscape.com/article/387399-overview. Accessed winter 2011.
3. Nordqvist C. What Is A Baker's Cyst (Popliteal Cyst)? What Causes A Baker's Cyst? April 07, 2010. © Medical News Today. URL: http://www.medicalnewstoday.com/articles/184714.php. Accessed winter 2011.
4. Popliteal Cysts: A Patient's Guide to Popliteal Cysts. Copyright © 2009–2011 Medical Multimedia Group, L.L.C. URL: http://www.eorthopod.com/content/popliteal-cysts. Accessed winter 2011.

Bunion

1. Bunions. Copyright ©1995–2011 by the American Academy of Orthopaedic Surgeons. URL: http://orthoinfo.aaos.org/topic.cfm?topic=a00155. Accessed winter 2011.
2. Bunions. © 1998–2011 Mayo Foundation for Medical Education and Research (MFMER). URL: http://www.mayoclinic.com/health/bunions/DS00309. Accessed winter 2011.
3. Laughlin R. Bunion. Copyright © 1994–2011 by WebMD LLC. URL: http://emedicine.medscape.com/article/1235796-overview. Accessed winter 2011.
4. Shiel W. Bunions. ©1996–2011 MedicineNet, Inc. URL: http://www.medicinenet.com/bunions/article.htm. Accessed winter 2011.
5. Torkki M, et al. Hallux Valgus: Wait and See, Orthosis, or Surgery? Copyright © 2002 by the American Academy of Family Physicians. URL: http://www.aafp.org/afp/2002/0101/p126.html. Accessed winter 2011.

Bursitis

1. Bursitis. © 1998–2011 Mayo Foundation for Medical Education and Research (MFMER). URL: http://www.mayoclinic.com/health/bursitis/DS00032. Accessed winter 2011.
2. Gonsalves A, et al. Bursitis. Copyright © 1994–2011 by WebMD LLC. URL: http://emedicine.medscape.com/article/1267823-overview. Accessed winter 2011.
3. Hip Bursitis. Copyright ©1995–2011 by the American Academy of Orthopaedic Surgeons. URL: http://orthoinfo.aaos.org/topic.cfm?topic=a00409. Accessed winter 2011.
4. Shiel W. ©1996–2011 MedicineNet, Inc. URL: http://www.medicinenet.com/bursitis/article.htm. Accessed winter 2011.

Carpal Tunnel Syndrome

1. Carpal Tunnel Syndrome Fact Sheet. National Institute of Neurological Disorders and Stroke. URL: http://www.ninds.nih.gov/disorders/carpal_tunnel/detail_carpal_tunnel.htm. Accessed winter 2011.
2. Fuller D. Carpal Tunnel Syndrome. Copyright © 1994–2011 by WebMD LLC. URL: http://emedicine.medscape.com/article/1243192-overview. Accessed winter 2011.
3. Lowe W. Suggested variations on standard carpal tunnel syndrome assessment tests. Journal of Bodywork Movement Therapies 2008;12(2):151–157. URL: http://www.ncbi.nlm.nih.gov/pubmed?term=whitney%20lowe. Accessed winter 2011.
4. Matullo K, et al. Characterization of a First Thoracic Rib Ligament: Anatomy and Possible Clinical Revelance. Copyright © 1994–2011 by WebMD LLCn. URL: http://www.medscape.com/viewarticle/732226. Accessed winter 2011.
5. Russell B. Carpal tunnel syndrome and the "double crush" hypothesis: a review and implications for chiropractic. Chiropractic & Osteopathy 2008;16:2. © 2008 Russell. URL: http://www.ncbi.nlm.nih.gov/pmc/articles/PMC2365954/?tool=pubmed. Accessed winter 2011.
6. Simpson RL, et al. Multiple compression neuropathies and the double-crush syndrome. The Orthopedic Clinics of North America 1996;27(2):381–388. URL: http://www.ncbi.nlm.nih.gov/pubmed/8614586. Accessed winter 2011.

Cervical Spondylosis

1. Al-Shatoury H, et al. Cervical Spondylosis. Copyright © 1994–2011 by WebMD LLC. URL: http://emedicine.medscape.com/article/306036-overview. Accessed winter 2011.
2. Cervical Spondylosis and Spondylotic Cervical Myelopathy. © 2010–2011 Merck Sharp & Dohme Corp., a subsidiary of Merck & Co., Inc.. URL: http://www.merckmanuals.com/professional/print/sec16/ch224/ch224d.html. Accessed winter 2011.
3. Vokshoor A. Spondylolisthesis, Spondylolysis, and Spondylosis. Copyright © 1994–2011 by WebMD LLC. URL: http://emedicine.medscape.com/article/1266860-overview. Accessed winter 2011.
4. Walker K. Alternative Treatments for Spondylosis. © 1999–2011 Vertical Health, LLC. URL: http://www.spineuniverse.com/conditions/spondylosis/drugs-medications-injections-spondylosis. Accessed winter 2011.
5. What Is Cervical Spondylosis (Cervical Osteoarthritis)? What Causes Cervical Spondylosis? © Medical News Today Nov 24, 2009. URL: http://www.medicalnewstoday.com/articles/172015.php. Accessed winter 2011.
6. Young W. Cervical Spondylotic Myelopathy: A Common Cause of Spinal Cord Dysfunction in Older Persons. Copyright © 2000 by the American Academy of Family Physicians. URL: http://www.aafp.org/afp/20000901/1064.html. Accessed winter 2011.

Compartment Syndrome

1. Burning Thigh Pain (Meralgia Paresthetica). Copyright ©1995–2011 by the American Academy of Orthopaedic Surgeons. URL: http://orthoinfo.aaos.org/topic.cfm?topic=A00340#Symptoms. Accessed winter 2011.
2. Chronic Compartment Syndrome. © American Academy of Podiatric Sports Medicine. URL: http://www.aapsm.org/chroniccompartment.html. Accessed winter 2011.
3. Chronic External Compartment syndrome. © 1998–2011 Mayo Foundation for Medical Education and Research. URL: http://www.mayoclinic.com/health/chronic-exertional-compartment-syndrome/DS00789. Accessed winter 2011.
4. Compartment Syndrome. Copyright ©1995–2011 by the American Academy of Orthopaedic Surgeons. URL: http://

orthoinfo.aaos.org/topic.cfm?topic=A00204. Accessed winter 2011.
5. Paula R. Compartment Syndrome, Extremity. Copyright © 1994–2011 by WebMD LLC. URL: http://emedicine.medscape.com/article/828456-overview. Accessed winter 2011.
6. Wedro B. Compartment Syndrome. ©1996–2011 MedicineNet, Inc. URL: http://www.medicinenet.com/script/main/art.asp?articlekey=117129. Accessed winter 2011.

Disc Disease

1. Baldwin N. Lumbar Disc Disease: The Natural History. Copyright © 1994–2011 by WebMD LLC. URL: http://www.medscape.com/viewarticle/442526. Accessed winter 2011.
2. Herniated Disk. © 1998–2011 Mayo Foundation for Medical Education and Research (MFMER). URL: http://www.mayoclinic.com/health/herniated-disk/DS00893. Accessed winter 2011.
3. Humphreys S, et al. Clinical Evaluation and Treatment Options for Herniated Lumbar Disc. Copyright © 1999 by the American Academy of Family Physicians. URL: http://www.aafp.org/afp/990201ap/575.html. Accessed winter 2011.
4. Kraft S. What Is A Herniated Disk (Ruptured Or Slipped Disk)? What Causes A Herniated Disk? © Medical News Today Jun 16, 2010. URL: http://www.medicalnewstoday.com/articles/191979.php. Accessed winter 2011.
5. Lumbar Degenerative Disc Disease: A Patient's Guide to Lumbar Degenerative Disc Disease. © Copyright 2009–2011 Medical Multimedia Group, L.L.C. URL: http://www.eorthopod.com/content/lumbar-degenerative-disc-disease. Accessed winter 2011.
6. Sahrakar K, et al. Lumbar Disc Disease. Copyright © 1994–2011 by WebMD LLC. URL: http://emedicine.medscape.com/article/249113-overview. Accessed winter 2011.
7. Windsor R, et al. Cervical Discogenic Pain Syndrome. Copyright © 1994–2011 by WebMD LLC. URL: http://emedicine.medscape.com/article/93761-overview. Accessed winter 2011.

Dupuytren Contracture

1. Barnes C, et al. Knuckle Pads. Copyright © 1994–2011 by WebMD LLC. URL: http://emedicine.medscape.com/article/1074379-overview. Accessed winter 2011.
2. Dupuytren's Contracture. Copyright ©1995–2011 by the American Academy of Orthopaedic Surgeons.URL: http://orthoinfo.aaos.org/topic.cfm?topic=A00008. Accessed winter 2011.
3. DuPuytren's Contracture. © 1998–2011 Mayo Foundation for Medical Education and Research. URL: http://www.mayoclinic.com/health/dupuytrens-contracture/DS00732. Accessed winter 2011.
4. Dupuytren's disease (Morbus Dupuytren or Dupuytren's contracture). International Dupuytren Society. URL: http://www.dupuytren-online.info/dupuytrens_contracture.html. Accessed winter 2011.
5. Mathew S, et al. Dupuytren Contracture. Copyright © 1994–2011 by WebMD LLC. URL: http://emedicine.medscape.com/article/329414-overview. Accessed winter 2011.

Ganglion Cysts

1. Genova R, et al. Ganglion Cyst. Copyright © 1994–2011 by WebMD LLC. URL: http://emedicine.medscape.com/article/1243454-overview. Accessed winter 2011.
2. Ganglion Cysts. © 2011 American Society for Surgery of the Hand. URL: http://www.assh.org/Public/HandConditions/Pages/GanglionCysts.aspx?PF=1. Accessed winter 2011.
3. Ganglion (Cyst) of the Wrist. Copyright ©1995–2011 by the American Academy of Orthopaedic Surgeons. URL: http://orthoinfo.aaos.org/topic.cfm?topic=A00006&return_link=0. Accessed winter 2011.
4. Ganglion cysts. © 1998–2011 Mayo Foundation for Medical Education and Research (MFMER). URL: http://www.mayoclinic.com/health/ganglion-cysts/DS00767. Accessed winter 2011.

Gout

1. Gout. National Institute of Arthritis and Musculoskeletal and Skin Diseases (NIAMS). URL: http://www.niams.nih.gov/Health_Info/Gout/default.asp. Accessed winter 2011.
2. Miller A, et al. Gout. Copyright © 1994–2011 by WebMD LLC. URL: http://emedicine.medscape.com/article/329958-overview. Accessed winter 2011.
3. Nordqvist C. What Is Gout? What Causes Gout? © Medical News Today Apr 02, 2009. URL: http://www.medicalnewstoday.com/articles/144827.php. Accessed winter 2011.

Hammertoe

1. Hammertoe and mallet toe. © 1998–2011 Mayo Foundation for Medical Education and Research (MFMER). URL: http://www.mayoclinic.com/health/hammertoe-and-mallet-toe/DS00480. Accessed winter 2011.
2. Hammertoe. Copyright © 2011 American College of Foot and Ankle Surgeons. URL: http://www.footphysicians.com/footankleinfo/hammertoes.htm. Accessed winter 2011.
3. Hammertoe. Connecticut Surgical Group. URL: http://www.ctsurgical.com/ed_podiatry_hammertoe.php. Accessed winter 2011.
4. Watson A. Hammertoe Deformity. Copyright © 1994–2011 by WebMD LLC. URL: http://emedicine.medscape.com/article/1235341-overview. Accessed winter 2011.

Hernia

1. Nicks B, et al. Hernias. Copyright © 1994–2011 by WebMD LLC. URL: http://emedicine.medscape.com/article/775630-overview. Accessed winter 2011.
2. Menon A, et al. Hernia Reduction. Copyright © 1994–2011 by WebMD LLCe. URL: http://emedicine.medscape.com/article/149608-overview. Accessed winter 2011.

3. Qureshi W. Hiatal Hernia. Copyright © 1994–2011 by WebMD LLC. URL: http://emedicine.medscape.com/article/178393-overview. Accessed winter 2011.
4. Hernia. © A.D.A.M., Inc. URL: http://www.ncbi.nlm.nih.gov/pubmedhealth/PMH0001956/. Accessed winter 2011.
5. Inguinal Hernia. National Institute of Diabetes and Digestive and Kidney Diseases. URL: http://digestive.niddk.nih.gov/ddiseases/pubs/inguinalhernia/index.htm. Accessed winter 2011.

Joint Disruptions

1. Banit D, et al. Atlantoaxial Instability. Copyright © 1994–2011 by WebMD LLC. URL: http://emedicine.medscape.com/article/1265682-overview. Accessed winter 2011.
2. Malanga G, et al. Patellar Injury and Dislocation. Copyright © 1994–2011 by WebMD LLC. URL: http://emedicine.medscape.com/article/90068-overview. Accessed winter 2011.
3. McCarthy J. Developmental Dysplasia of the Hip. Copyright © 1994–2011 by WebMD LLC. URL: http://emedicine.medscape.com/article/1248135-overview. Accessed winter 2011.
4. Polansky R, et al. Joint Reduction, Finger Dislocation. Copyright © 1994–2011 by WebMD LLC. URL: http://emedicine.medscape.com/article/109206-overview. Accessed winter 2011.
5. Tham E, et al. Dislocation, Hip. Copyright © 1994–2011 by WebMD LLC. URL: http://emedicine.medscape.com/article/823471-overview. Accessed winter 2011.

Joint Replacement Surgery

1. Arthritis. National Institute of Arthritis and Musculoskeletal and Skin Diseases (NIAMS). URL: http://www.niams.nih.gov/Health_Info/Joint_Replacement/default.asp. Accessed winter 2011.
2. Preparing for Joint Replacement Surgery. © 1995–2011 American Academy of Orthopaedic Surgeons. URL: http://orthoinfo.aaos.org/topic.cfm?topic=A00220. Accessed winter 2011.
3. Shiel W. Total Hip Replacement. ©1996–2011 MedicineNet, Inc. URL: http://www.medicinenet.com/script/main/art.asp?articlekey=497. Accessed winter 2011.
4. Shiel W. Total Knee Replacement. ©1996–2011 MedicineNet, Inc. URL: http://www.medicinenet.com/script/main/art.asp?articlekey=498. Accessed winter 2011.
5. Shoulder Joint Replacement. © 1995–2011 American Academy of Orthopaedic Surgeons. URL: http://orthoinfo.aaos.org/topic.cfm?topic=A00094. Accessed winter 2011.
6. Total Joint Replacement. © 1995–2011 American Academy of Orthopaedic Surgeons. URL: http://orthoinfo.aaos.org/topic.cfm?topic=A00233. Accessed winter 2011.

Lyme Disease

1. Lyme Disease Treatment and Prognosis. Centers for Disease Control and Prevention. URL: http://www.cdc.gov/ncidod/dvbid/lyme/ld_humandisease_treatment.htm. Accessed winter 2011.
2. Lyme Disease. © 2006 American Lyme Disease Foundation, Inc. URL: http://www.aldf.com/lyme.shtml. Accessed winter 2011.
3. Lyme Disease. © 1998–2011 Mayo Foundation for Medical Education and Research (MFMER). URL: http://www.mayoclinic.com/health/lyme-disease/DS00116. Accessed winter 2011.
4. Meyerhoff J. Lyme Disease. Copyright © 1994–2011 by WebMD LLC. URL: http://emedicine.medscape.com/article/330178-overview. Accessed winter 2011.
5. Other Tick-Borne Diseases. © 2006 American Lyme Disease Foundation, Inc. URL: http://www.aldf.com/majorTick.shtml. Accessed winter 2011.
6. Tick Removal. Centers for Disease Control and Prevention. URL: http://www.cdc.gov/ncidod/dvbid/lyme/ld_tickremoval.htm. Accessed winter 2011.

Muscular Dystrophy

1. Bushby K. Diagnosis and management of Duchenne muscular dystrophy part 1: diagnosis, and pharmacological and psychosocial management. The Lancet Neurology 2010;9(1):77–93. URL: http://www.thelancet.com/journals/lancet/article/PIIS1474-4422(09)70271-6/abstract. Accessed winter 2011.
2. Carter G. Rehabilitation Management of Neuromuscular Disease. Copyright © 1994–2011 by WebMD LLC. URL: http://emedicine.medscape.com/article/321397-overview. Accessed winter 2011.
3. Do T. Muscular Dystrophy. Copyright © 1994–2011 by WebMD LLC. URL: http://emedicine.medscape.com/article/1259041-overview. Accessed winter 2011.
4. Muscular Dystrophy: Hope Through Research. National Institute of Neurological Disorders and Stroke (NINDS). URL: http://www.ninds.nih.gov/disorders/md/detail_md.htm. Accessed winter 2011.
5. Muscular dystrophy. © 1998–2011 Mayo Foundation for Medical Education and Research (MFMER). URL: http://www.mayoclinic.com/health/muscular-dystrophy/DS00200. Accessed winter 2011.
6. Muscular dystrophy. © 2011 University of Maryland Medical Center (UMMC). URL: http://www.umm.edu/altmed/articles/muscular-dystrophy-000113.htm.Accessed winter 2011.

Myofascial Pain Syndrome

1. Acupuncture And Myofascial Trigger Therapy Treat Same Pain Areas. MediLexicon International Ltd. © 2004–2011. URL: http://www.medicalnewstoday.com/articles/107422.php. Accessed winter 2011.
2. Finley J. Myofascial Pain. Copyright © 1994–2011 by WebMD LLC. URL: http://emedicine.medscape.com/article/313007-overview. Accessed winter 2011.
3. Froese B. Cervical Myofascial Pain. Copyright © 1994–2011 by WebMD LLC. URL: http://emedicine.medscape.com/article/305937-overview. Accessed winter 2011.
4. Myofascial pain syndrome. © 1998–2011 Mayo Foundation for Medical Education and Research (MFMER). URL: http://www.mayoclinic.com/health/myofascial-pain-syndrome/DS01042. Accessed winter 2011.

5. Myofascial Pain Syndrome. © Copyright 1995–2009 The Cleveland Clinic Foundation. URL: http://my.clevelandclinic.org/disorders/chronic_pain/hic_myofascial_pain_syndrome.aspx. Accessed winter 2011.
6. Pain Management: Myofascial Pain Syndrome (Muscle Pain). ©2005–2011 WebMD, LLC. URL: http://www.webmd.com/pain-management/guide/myofascial-pain-syndrome. Accessed winter 2011.

Osgood-Schlatter Disease

1. Bhatia M, et al. Osgood-Schlatter Disease. Copyright © 1994–2011 by WebMD LLC. URL: http://emedicine.medscape.com/article/91249-overview. Accessed winter 2011.
2. McFarland E, et al. Patient Guide to Osgood-Schlatter Disease. Johns Hopkins Orthopaedic Surgery. URL: http://www.hopkinsortho.org/osgood-schlatter_html. Accessed winter 2011.
3. Osgood-Schlatter Disease (Knee Pain). © 1995–2011 American Academy of Orthopaedic Surgeons. URL: http://orthoinfo.aaos.org/topic.cfm?topic=a00411. Accessed winter 2011.
4. Osgood-Schlatter disease. © 1998–2011 Mayo Foundation for Medical Education and Research (MFMER). URL: http://www.mayoclinic.com/health/osgood-schlatter-disease/DS00392. Accessed winter 2011.

Osteoarthritis

1. Abramson S, et al. Development in the Scientific Understanding of Osteoarthritis. Copyright © 1994–2011 by WebMD LLC. URL: http://www.medscape.com/viewarticle/714866?src=mp&spon=17&uac=78486SY. Accessed winter 2011.
2. Lozada C, et al. Osteoarthritis. Copyright © 1994–2011 by WebMD LLC. URL: http://emedicine.medscape.com/article/330487-overview. Accessed winter 2011.
3. Osteoarthritis. © 2011 Arthritis Foundation. URL: http://www.arthritis.org/disease-center.php?disease_id=32&df=definition. Accessed winter 2011.
4. Osteoarthritis. National Institute of Arthritis and Musculoskeletal and Skin Diseases (NIAMS). URL: http://www.niams.nih.gov/Health_Info/Osteoarthritis/default.asp. Accessed winter 2011.
5. Perlman A, et al. Massage Therapy for Osteoarthritis of the Knee. Archives of Internal Medicine 2006;166:2533–2538. URL: http://archinte.ama-assn.org/cgi/content/full/166/22/2533. Accessed winter 2011.
6. Reginster J, et al. Current Role of Glucosamine in the Treatment of Osteoarthritis. Copyright © 1994–2011 by WebMD LLC. URL: http://www.medscape.com/viewarticle/557058. Accessed winter 2011.

Osteoporosis

1. Factors to Consider When Choosing a Treatment. © 2011 National Osteoporosis Foundation. URL: http://www.nof.org/aboutosteoporosis/managingandtreating/choosingtreatment. Accessed winter 2011.
2. Nalamachu S, et al. Osteoporosis (Primary). Copyright © 1994–2011 by WebMD LLC. URL: http://emedicine.medscape.com/article/311331-overview. Accessed winter 2011.
3. Osteoporosis Medicines: What You Need To Know. © 2011 National Osteoporosis Foundation. URL: http://www.nof.org/aboutosteoporosis/managingandtreating/medicinesneedtoknow. Accessed winter 2011.
4. Osteoporosis Overview. NIH Osteoporosis and Related Bone Diseases. National Resource Center. URL: http://www.niams.nih.gov/Health_Info/Bone/Osteoporosis/overview.asp. Accessed winter 2011.
5. Serota A, et al. Osteoporosis (Secondary). Copyright © 1994–2011 by WebMD LLC. http://emedicine.medscape.com/article/311449-overview. Accessed winter 2011.
6. Werner R. Osteoporosis and Hyperkyphosis: What Does Calcium Have to Do With It? © 2011 Associated Bodywork & Massage Professionals. URL: http://www.massagetherapy.com/articles/index.php/article_id/1260/Osteoporosis-and-Hyperkyphosis:-What-Does-Calcium-Have-to-Do-With-It. Accessed winter 2011.

Osteomyelitis

1. Eck J. Osteomyelitis (Bone Infection). ©1996–2011 MedicineNet, Inc. URL: http://www.medicinenet.com/osteomyelitis/article.htm. Accessed winter 2011.
2. King R, et al. Osteomyelitis. Copyright © 1994–2011 by WebMD LLC. URL: http://emedicine.medscape.com/article/785020-overview. Accessed winter 2011.
3. Osteomyelitis. © 1998–2011 Mayo Foundation for Medical Education and Research (MFMER). URL: http://www.mayoclinic.com/health/osteomyelitis/DS00759. Accessed winter 2011.
4. Osteomyelitis. © 1995–2011 The Cleveland Clinic Foundation. URL: http://my.clevelandclinic.org/disorders/osteomyelitis/hic_osteomyelitis.aspx. Accessed winter 2011.

Osteosarcoma

1. Bone Cancer. © 1998–2011 Mayo Foundation for Medical Education and Research (MFMER). URL: http://www.mayoclinic.com/health/bone-cancer/DS00520. Accessed winter 2011.
2. Bone Tumor. © 1995–2011 American Academy of Orthopaedic Surgeons. URL: http://orthoinfo.aaos.org/topic.cfm?topic=A00074. Accessed winter 2011.
3. Chansky H, et al. Metastatic Carcinoma. Copyright © 1994–2011 by WebMD LLC. URL: http://emedicine.medscape.com/article/1253331-overview. Accessed winter 2011.
4. Chordoma. © 1995–2011 American Academy of Orthopaedic Surgeons. URL: http://orthoinfo.aaos.org/topic.cfm?topic=A00084. Accessed winter 2011.
5. Enchondroma. © 1995–2011 American Academy of Orthopaedic Surgeons. URL: http://orthoinfo.aaos.org/topic.cfm?topic=A00085. Accessed winter 2011.
6. Ewing's Sarcoma. © 1995–2011 American Academy of Orthopaedic Surgeons. URL: http://orthoinfo.aaos.org/topic.cfm?topic=A00082. Accessed winter 2011.

7. Giant Cell Tumor of Bone. © 1995–2011 American Academy of Orthopaedic Surgeons. URL: http://orthoinfo.aaos.org/topic.cfm?topic=A00080. Accessed winter 2011.
8. Mehlman C, et al. Osteosarcoma. Copyright © 1994–2011 by WebMD LLC. URL: http://emedicine.medscape.com/article/1256857-overview. Accessed winter 2011.
9. Nelson R. SIR 2009: Novel Treatment Relieves Metastatic Bone Pain. Copyright © 1994–2011 by WebMD LLC. URL: http://www.medscape.com/viewarticle/589486. Accessed winter 2011.

Patellofemoral Syndrome

1. Juhn M. Patellofemoral Pain Syndrome: A Review and Guidelines for Treatment. Copyright © 1999 by the American Academy of Family Physicians. URL: http://www.aafp.org/afp/991101ap/2012.html. Accessed winter 2011.
2. Patellofemoral Pain Syndrome. © American Academy of Family Physicians. URL: http://familydoctor.org/online/famdocen/home/healthy/physical/injuries/479.html. Accessed winter 2011.
3. Patellofemoral Problems: A Patient's Guide to Patellofemoral Problems. © Medical Multimedia Group, L.L.C. URL: http://www.eorthopod.com/content/patellofemoral-problems. Accessed winter 2011.
4. Potter P, et al. Patellofemoral Syndrome. Copyright © 1994–2011 by WebMD LLC. URL: http://emedicine.medscape.com/article/308471-overview. Accessed winter 2011.
5. Servi J. Patellofemoral Joint Syndromes. Copyright © 1994–2011 by WebMD LLC. URL: http://emedicine.medscape.com/article/90286-overview. Accessed winter 2011.

Plantar Fasciitis

1. Glatter R. Plantar Fasciitis: Evidence-Based Management. Copyright © 1994–2011 by WebMD LLC. URL: http://www.medscape.com/viewarticle/562437. Accessed winter 2011.
2. Plantar Fasciitis and Bone Spurs. © 1995–2011 American Academy of Orthopaedic Surgeons. URL: http://orthoinfo.aaos.org/topic.cfm?topic=a00149. Accessed winter 2011.
3. Plantar Fasciitis, Heel Spurs, Heel Pain. © 1997–2011 Plantar Fasciitis Organization. URL: http://www.plantar-fasciitis.org/. Accessed winter 2011.
4. Young C, et al. Treatment of Plantar Fasciitis. Copyright © 2001 by the American Academy of Family Physicians. URL: http://www.aafp.org/afp/2001/0201/p467.html?ref=SevSevil.Com. Accessed winter 2011.
5. Young C. Plantar Fasciitis. Copyright © 1994–2011 by WebMD LLC. URL: http://emedicine.medscape.com/article/86143-overview. Accessed winter 2011.

Ples Planus, Pes Cavus

1. Buchanan M. Pes planus. Copyright © 1994–2011 by WebMD LLC. URL: http://emedicine.medscape.com/article/1236652-overview. Accessed winter 2011.
2. Pes planus—Overview. © 2011 University of Maryland Medical Center. URL: http://www.umm.edu/ency/article/001262all.htm. Accessed winter 2011.
3. Turner N. Pes Cavus. Copyright © 1994–2011 by WebMD LLC. URL: http://emedicine.medscape.com/article/1236538-overview. Accessed winter 2011.
4. Wheeless C. Pes Cavus. © 1996–2009 Data Trace Internet Publishing, LLC. URL: http://www.wheelessonline.com/ortho/pes_cavus. Accessed winter 2011.
5. Wheeless C. Pes Planus/Flat Foot. © 1996–2009 Data Trace Internet Publishing, LLC. URL: http://www.wheelessonline.com/ortho/pes_planus_flat_foot. Accessed winter 2011.

Scoliosis

1. Brauser D. Hyperkyphosis Associated With Increased Mortality in Older Women With Vertebral Fractures. Copyright © 1994–2011 by WebMD LLC. URL: http://www.medscape.com/viewarticle/703647. Accessed winter 2011.
2. Corenman D. Hyperkyphosis/Scheuermann's Disease. Neck and Back.com. URL: http://neckandback.com/conditions/hyperkyphosis-scheuermanns-disease. Accessed winter 2011.
3. Dalton E. Straight Talk: Symptomatic Scoliosis. © 2003 Associated Bodywork and Massage Professionals. URL: http://www.massageandbodywork.com/Articles/AprilMay2006/scoliosis.html. Accessed winter 2011.
4. Kyphosis. © 1998–2011 Mayo Foundation for Medical Education and Research (MFMER). URL: http://www.mayoclinic.com/health/kyphosis/DS00681/. Accessed winter 2011.
5. Mehlman C. Idiopathic Scoliosis. Copyright © 1994–2011 by WebMD LLC. URL: http://emedicine.medscape.com/article/1265794-overview. Accessed winter 2011.
6. Scoliosis. © 2011 University of Rochester Medical Center. URL: http://www.urmc.rochester.edu/ortho/patient/content.cfm?pageid=P08121. Accessed winter 2011.

Shin Splints

1. Massage for Anterior Shin Splints. © 2011 Natural Wellness®. URL: http://www.integrative-healthcare.org/mt/archives/2006/02/massage_for_ant.html. Accessed winter 2011.
2. Shin splints. © 1998–2011 Mayo Foundation for Medical Education and Research (MFMER). URL: http://www.mayoclinic.com/health/shin-splints/DS00271. Accessed winter 2011.
3. Shiel W. Shin Splints. ©1996–2011 MedicineNet, Inc. URL: http://www.medicinenet.com/script/main/art.asp?articlekey=2031. Accessed winter 2011.
4. Stickley C, et al. Crural Fascia and Muscle Origins Related to Medial Tibial Stress Syndrome Symptom Location. Copyright © 1994–2011 by WebMD LLC. URL: http://www.medscape.com/viewarticle/711305. Accessed winter 2011.
5. Shin Splints. © 2005–2011 WebMD, LLC. URL: http://www.webmd.com/fitness-exercise/shin-splints. Accessed winter 2011.
6. Walker B. Shin Splints and Shin Splints Treatment. Copyright (c)© 2011 The Stretching Institute. URL: http://www.thestretchinghandbook.com/archives/shin-splints.php. Accessed winter 2011.

7. Shin splints. © 1997–2011 A.D.A.M., Inc. URL: http://www.nlm.nih.gov/medlineplus/ency/article/003177.htm. Accessed winter 2011.

Spasms, Cramps

1. Albertin A, et al. The effect of manual therapy on masseter muscle pain and spasm. Electromyography and Clinical Neurophysiology 2010;50(2):107–112. URL: http://www.ncbi.nlm.nih.gov/pubmed/20405786. Accessed winter 2011.
2. Charley horse. © 1997–2011 A.D.A.M., Inc. URL: http://www.nlm.nih.gov/medlineplus/ency/article/002066.htm. Accessed winter 2011.
3. Wedro B. Muscle Spasms. © 1994–2011 MedicineNet, Inc. URL: http://www.medicinenet.com/muscle_spasms/article.htm. Accessed winter 2011.

Spondylolisthesis

1. Dawson E. Spondylolisthesis. © 1999–2011 Vertical Health, LLC. URL: http://www.spineuniverse.com/conditions/spondylolisthesis/spondylolisthesis. Accessed winter 2011.
2. Froese B. Lumbar Spondylolysis and Spondylolisthesis. Copyright © 1994–2011 by WebMD LLC. URL: http://emedicine.medscape.com/article/310235-overview. Accessed winter 2011.
3. Heary R. Spondylolisthesis: Introduction and Illustrative Cases. Copyright © 1994–2011 by WebMD LLC. URL: http://www.medscape.com/viewarticle/439164. Accessed winter 2011.
4. Herkowitz H, et al. The Diagnosis and Management of Degenerative Lumbar Spondylolisthesis. Copyright © 1994–2011 by WebMD LLC. URL: http://www.medscape.com/viewarticle/722299. Accessed winter 2011.
5. Irani Z, et al. Spondylolisthesis. Copyright © 1994–2011 by WebMD LLC. URL: http://emedicine.medscape.com/article/396016-overview. Accessed winter 2011.
6. Litao A, et al. Lumbosacral Spondylolysis. Copyright © 1994–2011 by WebMD LLC. URL: http://emedicine.medscape.com/article/95691-overview. Accessed winter 2011.
7. Meyerding H. Spondylolisthesis. © 2011 The Journal of Bone and Joint Surgery, Inc. URL: http://www.ejbjs.org/cgi/reprint/13/1/39. Accessed winter 2011.
8. Pearson A, et al. Degenerative Spondylolisthesis versus Spinal Stenosis: Does a Slip Matter? Comparison of Baseline Characteristics and Outcomes (SPORT). Copyright © 1994–2011 by WebMD LLC. URL: http://www.medscape.com/viewarticle/716556. Accessed winter 2011.

Sprains

1. Fong D, et al. Understanding acute ankle ligamentous sprain injury in sports. Sports Medicine, Arthroscopy, Rehabilitation Therapy and Technology 2009;1:14. © Fong et al; licensee BioMed Central Ltd. URL: http://www.ncbi.nlm.nih.gov/pmc/articles/PMC2724472/?tool=pubmed. Accessed winter 2011.
2. Hupperets M, et al. Effect of unsupervised home based proprioceptive training on recurrences of ankle sprain: randomised controlled trial. Copyright © 1994–2011 by WebMD LLC. URL: http://www.medscape.com/viewarticle/707073. Accessed winter 2011.
3. Sprains, Strains, and Other Soft-Tissue Injuries. © 1995–2011 American Academy of Orthopaedic Surgeons. URL: http://orthoinfo.aaos.org/topic.cfm?topic=A00304. Accessed winter 2011.
4. Three-Phase Rehab for High Ankle Sprains. © 2010–2011 Medical Multimedia Group, LLC. URL: http://nwos-spokane.com/orthopaedic-advisor.html?disp_type=news_detail&area=19&news_id=0cc8a06caa6f1c18b62260c14bf56a8fAccessed winter 2011.

Strain

1. Muscle Strain. © 1994–2011 WebMD, LLC. URL: http://www.emedicinehealth.com/muscle_strain/article_em.htm. Accessed winter 2011.
2. Muscle Strains in the Thigh. © 1995–2011 American Academy of Orthopaedic Surgeons. URL: http://orthoinfo.aaos.org/topic.cfm?topic=a00366. Accessed winter 2011.
3. Wasielewski N. Does Eccentric Exercise Reduce Pain and Improve Strength in Physically Active Adults With Symptomatic Lower Extremity Tendinosis? A Systematic Review. Journal of Athletic Training 2007;42(3):409–421. © National Athletic Trainers' Association, Inc. URL: http://www.ncbi.nlm.nih.gov/pmc/articles/PMC1978463/?tool=pubmed. Accessed winter 2011.

Temporomandibular Joint Syndrome

1. Peckham C. Prolotherapy: An Expert Interview with Paul H. Goodley MD. ©1994–2011 Medscape, LCC. http://www.medscape.com/viewarticle/707539. Accessed winter 2011.
2. TMJ disorders. © 1998–2011 Mayo Foundation for Medical Education and Research (MFMER). http://www.mayoclinic.com/health/tmj-disorders/DS00355. Accessed winter 2011.
3. TMJ Disorders. National Institute of Dental and Craniofacial Research. http://www.nidcr.nih.gov/OralHealth/Topics/TMJ/TMJDisorders.htm. Accessed winter 2011.
4. Tsai V, et al. Temporomandibular Joint Syndrome. Copyright © 1994–2011 by WebMD LLC. http://emedicine.medscape.com/article/809598-overview. Accessed winter 2011.

Tendonopathies

1. Hargrove R, et al. Achilles Tendon Pathology. Copyright © 1994–2011 by WebMD LLC. URL: http://emedicine.medscape.com/article/1235456-overview. Accessed winter 2011.
2. Gonzales P, et al. Biceps Tendinopathy. Copyright © 1994–2011 by WebMD LLC. URL: http://emedicine.medscape.com/article/327227-overview. Accessed winter 2011.
3. Meals R. De Quervain Tenosynovitis. Copyright © 1994–2011 by WebMD LLC. URL: http://emedicine.medscape.com/article/1243387-overview. Accessed winter 2011.
4. Hyman G, et al. Jumper's Knee. Copyright © 1994–2011 by WebMD LLC. URL: http://emedicine.medscape.com/article/89569-overview. Accessed winter 2011.
5. DeBerardino T, et al. Supraspinatus Tendonitis. Copyright © 1994–2011 by WebMD LLC. URL: http://emedicine.

medscape.com/article/93095-overview. Accessed winter 2011.

6. Steele M, et al. Tendonitis. Copyright © 1994–2011 by WebMD LLC. URL: http://emedicine.medscape.com/article/809692-overview. Accessed winter 2011.
7. Wasielewski N. Does Eccentric Exercise Reduce Pain and Improve Strength in Physically Active Adults with Symptomatic Lower Extremity Tendinosis? A Systematic Review. Journal of Athletic Training 2007;42(3):409–421. © National Athletic Trainers' Association, Inc. URL: http://www.ncbi.nlm.nih.gov/pmc/articles/PMC1978463/?tool=pubmed. Accessed winter 2011.
8. Shulman R. Tendinopathy—a complete guide. Sports Injury Bulletin. URL: http://www.sportsinjurybulletin.com/archive/tendinopathy. Accessed winter 2011.
9. Tendonitis and Tenosynovitis. © EMIS 2010. URL: http://www.patient.co.uk/health/Tenosynovitis.htm. Accessed winter 2011.
10. Norvell J, et al. Tenosynovitis. Copyright © 1994–2011 by WebMD LLC. URL: http://emedicine.medscape.com/article/809777-overview. Accessed winter 2011.

Thoracic Outlet Syndrome

1. Physical Therapy Corner: Thoracic Outlet Syndrome. © 2000–2011 by the Plone Foundation et al. URL: http://www.nismat.org/ptcor/thoracic_outlet. Accessed winter 2011.
2. Singh M, et al. Thoracic Outlet Syndrome. Copyright © 1994–2011 by WebMD LLC. URL: http://emedicine.medscape.com/article/1143532-overview. Accessed winter 2011.
3. Thoracic Outlet Syndrome. © 1995–2011 American Academy of Orthopaedic Surgeons. URL: http://orthoinfo.aaos.org/topic.cfm?topic=a00336#Cause. Accessed winter 2011.
4. Thoracic outlet syndrome. © 1998–2011 Mayo Foundation for Medical Education and Research (MFMER). URL: http://www.mayoclinic.com/health/thoracic-outlet-syndrome/DS00800. Accessed winter 2011.
5. What is Thoracic Outlet Syndrome? National Institute of Neurological Disorders and Stroke (NINDS). URL: http://www.ninds.nih.gov/disorders/thoracic/thoracic.htm. Accessed winter 2011.

Whiplash

1. Hunter O, et al. Cervical Sprain and Strain. Copyright © 1994–2011 by WebMD LLC. URL: http://emedicine.medscape.com/article/306176-overview. Accessed winter 2011.
2. Vernon H, et al. Chronic Mechanical Neck Pain in Adults Treated by Manual Therapy: A Systematic Review of Change Scores in Randomized Controlled Trials of a Single Session. Journal of Manual and Manipulative Therapy 2008;16(2):E42–E52. © 2008 Journal of Manual & Manipulative Therapy. URL: http://www.ncbi.nlm.nih.gov/pmc/articles/PMC2565115/?tool=pubmed. Accessed winter 2011.
3. Whiplash. © 1998–2011 Mayo Foundation for Medical Education and Research (MFMER). URL: http://www.mayoclinic.com/health/whiplash/DS01037. Accessed winter 2011.
4. Cobo E, et al. What Factors have Influence on Persistence of Neck Pain after a Whiplash? Copyright © 1994–2011 by WebMD LLC. URL: http://www.medscape.com/viewarticle/721609. Accessed winter 2011.
5. Kumar S, et al. Looking Away From Whiplash: Effect of Head Rotation in Rear Impacts. Copyright © 1994–2011 by WebMD LLC. URL: http://www.medscape.com/viewarticle/502445. Accessed winter 2011.
6. Whiplash and Whiplash-Associated Disorders. © 2006 North American Spine Society. URL: http://www.spine.org/Documents/whiplash_2006.pdf. Accessed winter 2011.

Chapter 4

Addiction

1. Black S, et al. Chair Massage for Treating Anxiety in Patients Withdrawing from Psychoactive Drugs. Journal of Alternative and Complementary Medicine 2010;16(9):979–987. URL: http://www.ncbi.nlm.nih.gov/pubmed/20799900. Accessed winter 2011.
2. Drug Addiction. © 1998–2011 Mayo Foundation for Medical Education and Research. URL: http://www.mayoclinic.com/health/drug-addiction/DS00183. Accessed winter 2011.
3. Drugs, Brains, and Behavior: The Science of Addiction. The National Institute on Drug Abuse (NIDA). URL: http://drugabuse.gov/pdf/tib/soa.pdf. Accessed winter 2011.
4. New Advances in Alcoholism Treatment. National Institute on Alcohol Abuse and Alcoholism. URL: http://pubs.niaaa.nih.gov/publications/aa49.htm. Accessed winter 2011.
5. NIDA InfoFacts: Understanding Drug Abuse and Addiction. The National Institute on Drug Abuse (NIDA). URL: http://www.nida.nih.gov/infofacts/understand.html. Accessed winter 2011.
6. Pill To Fight Alcoholism: Neurologists Find Topiramate Effective For Treatment Of Alcoholism. © 1995–2010 ScienceDaily LLC. URL: http://www.sciencedaily.com/videos/2008/1110-pill_to_fight_alcoholism.htm. Accessed winter 2011.
7. Principles of Drug Addiction Treatment: A Research-Based Guide. The National Institute on Drug Abuse (NIDA). URL: http://www.nida.nih.gov/PDF/PODAT/PODAT.pdf. Accessed winter 2011.
8. Tompson W, et al. Alcoholism. © 2011 Medscape. URL: http://emedicine.medscape.com/article/285913-overview. Accessed winter 2011.

Alzheimer Disease

1. Alzheimer Myths. © 2011 Alzheimer's Association. URL: http://www.alz.org/alzheimers_disease_myths_about_alzheimers.asp. Accessed winter 2011.
2. Alzheimer's Disease Facts and Figures. © 2011 Alzheimer's Association. URL: http://www.alz.org/documents_custom/report_alzfactsfigures2010.pdf. Accessed winter 2011.
3. Alzheimer's Disease Treatment. National Institute on Aging. URL: http://www.nia.nih.gov/Alzheimers/AlzheimersInformation/Treatment/. Accessed winter 2011.

4. Alzheimer's disease. © 1998–2011 Mayo Foundation for Medical Education and Research (MFMER). URL: http://www.mayoclinic.com/health/alzheimers-disease/DS00161. Accessed winter 2011.
5. Alzheimer's Disease. National Institute of Health. NIH Publication No. 08-6423. URL: http://www.nia.nih.gov/NR/rdonlyres/7DCA00DB-1362-4755-9E87-96DF669E-AE20/13991/ADFactSheetFINAL2510.pdf. Accessed winter 2011.
6. Anderson H. Alzheimer Disease. © 2011 Medscape. URL: http://emedicine.medscape.com/article/1134817-overview. Accessed winter 2011.
7. Know the 10 Signs. © 2011 Alzheimer's Association. URL: http://www.alz.org/alzheimers_disease_10_signs_of_alzheimers.asp. Accessed winter 2011.
8. Stages of Alzheimer's. © 2011 Alzheimer's Association. URL: http://www.alz.org/alzheimers_disease_stages_of_alzheimers.asp. Accessed winter 2011.
9. What is Alzheimer's. © 2011 Alzheimer's Association. URL: http://www.alz.org/alzheimers_disease_what_is_alzheimers.asp#. Accessed winter 2011.

Amyotrophic Lateral Sclerosis

1. ALS (Amyotrophic Lateral Sclerosis) Fact Sheet. National Institute of Neurological Disorders and Stroke (NINDS). URL: http://www.ninds.nih.gov/disorders/amyotrophiclateralsclerosis/detail_ALS.htm. Accessed winter 2011.
2. Amyotrophic Lateral Sclerosis (ALS). © 2011 American Speech-Language-Hearing Association. URL: http://www.asha.org/public/speech/disorders/ALS.htm. Accessed winter 2011.
3. Amyotrophic lateral sclerosis. ©2011 A.D.A.M., Inc. URL: http://www.ncbi.nlm.nih.gov/pubmedhealth/PMH0001708/. Accessed winter 2011.
4. Armon C. Amyotrophic Lateral Sclerosis. © 2011 Medscape. URL: http://emedicine.medscape.com/article/1170097-overview. Accessed winter 2011.
5. Blatzheim K. Interdisciplinary Palliative Care, Including Massage, in Treatment of Amyotrophic Lateral Sclerosis. Journal of Bodyworks and Movement Therapies 2009;13(4):328–335. [Epub Jul 10, 2008.] URL: http://www.ncbi.nlm.nih.gov/pubmed/19761955. Accessed winter 2011.

Anxiety Disorders

1. Anxiety Disorders. The National Institute of Mental Health (NIMH). URL: http://www.nimh.nih.gov/health/publications/anxiety-disorders/complete-index.shtml. Accessed winter 2011.
2. Bernstein B. Generalized Anxiety Disorder. © 2011 Medscape. http://emedicine.medscape.com/article/1356176-overview. Accessed winter 2011.
3. Cutshall SM, et al. Effect of massage therapy on pain, anxiety, and tension in cardiac surgical patients: a pilot study. © 1998–2011 Mayo Foundation for Medical Education and Research. URL: http://www.ncbi.nlm.nih.gov/pubmed/20347840. Accessed winter 2011.
4. Effective Treatments Available for Anxiety Disorder. © 1998–2011 Mayo Foundation for Medical Education and Research. URL: http://www.mayoclinic.org/news2009-mchi/5201.html. Accessed winter 2011.
5. Friedman S, et al. Anxiety Disorder, Specific Phobia. © 2011 Medscape. URL: http://emedicine.medscape.com/article/917056-overview. Accessed winter 2011.
6. Generalized anxiety disorder. © 1998–2011 Mayo Foundation for Medical Education and Research. URL: http://www.mayoclinic.com/health/generalized-anxiety-disorder/DS00502. Accessed winter 2011.
7. Hatayama T, et al. The Facial Massage Reduced Anxiety and Negative Mood Status, and Increased Sympathetic Nervous Activity. Biomedical Research 2008;29(6):317–320. National Center for Biotechnology Information. URL: http://www.ncbi.nlm.nih.gov/pubmed/19129675?ordinalpos=2&itool=Email.EmailReport.Pubmed_ReportSelector.Pubmed_RVDocSum. Accessed winter 2011.
8. Hatayama T, et al. The facial massage reduced anxiety and negative mood status, and increased sympathetic nervous activity. National Institute of Health (NIH). URL: http://www.ncbi.nlm.nih.gov/pubmed/19129675. Accessed winter 2011.
9. Morgan A, et al. Outcomes of Self-help Efforts in Anxiety Disorder. © 2011 Medscape. URL: http://www.medscape.com/viewarticle/711635. Accessed winter 2011.
10. Obsessive-compulsive disorder (OCD). © 1998–2011 Mayo Foundation for Medical Education and Research. URL: http://www.mayoclinic.com/health/obsessive-compulsive-disorder/DS00189. Accessed winter 2011.
11. Obsessive-Compulsive Disorder. National Institute of Mental Health (NIMH). URL: http://report.nih.gov/nihfactsheets/viewfactsheet.aspx?csid=54&key=o#o. Accessed winter 2011.
12. Price C. Body-oriented therapy in recovery from child sexual abuse: an efficacy study. Alternative Therapies in Health and Medicine 2005;11(5):46–57. URL: http://www.ncbi.nlm.nih.gov/pmc/articles/PMC1933482/?tool=pubmed. Accessed winter 2011.
13. Sherman KJ, et al. Effectiveness of Therapeutic Massage for Generalized Anxiety Disorder: A Randomized Controlled Trial. Depress Anxiety 2010;27(5):441–450. National Center for Biotechnology Information. URL: http://www.ncbi.nlm.nih.gov/pubmed/20186971?itool=Email.EmailReport.Pubmed_ReportSelector.Pubmed_RVDocSum&ordinalpos=1. Accessed winter 2011.
14. Social Anxiety Disorder (social phobia). © 1998–2011 Mayo Foundation for Medical Education and Research. URL: http://www.mayoclinic.com/health/social-anxiety-disorder/DS00595. Accessed winter 2011.
15. Tynan W. Anxiety Disorder, Obsessive-Compulsive Disorder. © 2011 Medscape. URL: http://emedicine.medscape.com/article/1826591-overview. Accessed winter 2011.
16. Yates W. Anxiety Disorders. © 2011 Medscape. URL: http://emedicine.medscape.com/article/286227-overview. Accessed winter 2011.

Attention Deficit Hyperactivity Disorder

1. Adult ADHD (attention-deficit/hyperactivity disorder). © 1998–2011 Mayo Foundation for Medical Education and

Research (MFMER). URL: http://www.mayoclinic.com/health/adult-adhd/DS01161. Accessed winter 2011.
2. Attention Deficit Hyperactivity Disorder (ADHD). National Institute of Mental Health. URL: http://www.nimh.nih.gov/health/publications/attention-deficit-hyperactivity-disorder/complete-index.shtml. Accessed winter 2011.
3. Brooks M. 'Meta-Cognitive' Therapy Effective for Adult ADHD. © 2011 Medscape. URL: http://www.medscape.com/viewarticle/718932. Accessed winter 2011.
4. Maddigan B. The Effects of Massage Therapy & Exercise Therapy on Children/Adolescents with Attention Deficit Hyperactivity Disorder. © 2011 Canadian Academy of Child and Adolescent Psychiatry. URL: http://www.ncbi.nlm.nih.gov/pmc/articles/PMC2538473/?tool=pubmed. Accessed winter 2011.
5. Scudder L. The Changing Epidemiology of ADHD: An Expert Interview with Susan Visser, MS. © 2011 Medscape. URL: http://www.medscape.com/viewarticle/735440. Accessed winter 2011.
6. Soreff S, et al. Psychiatric Manifestations of Attention Deficit Hyperactivity Disorder. © 2011 Medscape. URL: http://emedicine.medscape.com/article/289350-overview. Accessed winter 2011.

Autism Spectrum Disorder

1. Autism Overview: What We Know. URL: http://www.nichd.nih.gov/publications/pubs/upload/introduction_autism.pdf. Accessed winter 2011.
2. Autism Spectrum Disorders (ASDs). National Institute of Child Health & Development. URL: http://www.nichd.nih.gov/health/topics/asd.cfm. Accessed winter 2011.
3. Autism Spectrum Disorders (Pervasive Developmental Disorders). The National Institute of Mental Health (NIMH). URL: http://www.nimh.nih.gov/health/publications/autism/complete-index.shtml. Accessed winter 2011.
4. Bernstein B. Childhood Disintegration Disorder. © 2011 Medscape. URL: http://emedicine.medscape.com/article/916515-overview. Accessed winter 2011.
5. Brasic J, et al. Autism. © 2011 Medscape. URL: http://emedicine.medscape.com/article/912781-print. Accessed winter 2011.
6. Chiu S, et al. Pervasive Developmental Disorder. © 2011 Medscape. URL: http://emedicine.medscape.com/article/914683-overview. Accessed winter 2011.
7. Effective Treatments Available for Anxiety Disorder. ©1998–2011 Mayo Foundation for Medical Education and Research. URL: http://www.mayoclinic.org/news2009-mchi/5201.html. Accessed winter 2011.
8. Facts About ASDs. © 2011 Centers for Disease Control and Prevention. URL: http://www.cdc.gov/ncbddd/autism/facts.html. Accessed winter 2011.
9. Lee MS, et al. Massage therapy for children with autism spectrum disorders: a systematic review. © Physicians Postgraduate Press, Inc. URL: http://www.ncbi.nlm.nih.gov/pubmed/21208598. Accessed winter 2011.
10. What is Asperger Syndrome? National Institute of Health. URL: http://www.nichd.nih.gov/health/topics/asperger_syndrome.cfm. Accessed winter 2011.
11. What is Autism? © 2011 Autism Speaks Inc. URL: http://www.autismspeaks.org/whatisit/index.php. Accessed winter 2011.

Bell Palsy

1. Bell's Palsy Fact Sheet: What is Bell's Palsy? National Institute of Neurological Disorders and Stroke. URL: http://www.ninds.nih.gov/disorders/bells/detail_bells.htm. Accessed spring 2011.
2. Bell's palsy. © 1998–2011 Mayo Foundation for Medical Education and Research (MFMER). URL: http://www.mayoclinic.com/health/bells-palsy/DS00168. Accessed spring 2011.
3. Causes of Facial Palsy. © Bell's Palsy Information Site. URL: http://www.bellspalsy.ws/cause.htm. Accessed spring 2011.
4. Lindsay RW, et al. Comprehensive Facial Rehabilitation Improves Function in People with Facial Paralysis: A 5-year Experience at the Massachusetts Eye and Ear Infirmary. Physical Therapy 2010;90(3):391–397. [Epub Jan 21, 2010]. URL: http://www.ncbi.nlm.nih.gov/pubmed/20093325?itool=Email.EmailReport.Pubmed_ReportSelector.Pubmed_RVDocSum&ordinalpos=1. Accessed spring 2011.
5. Manikandan N. Effect of Facial Neuromuscular Re-education on Facial Symmetry in Patients with Bell's Palsy: A Randomized Controlled Trial. Clinical Rehabilitation 2007;21(4):338–343. URL: http://www.ncbi.nlm.nih.gov/pubmed/17613574. Accessed spring 2011.
6. Monnell K, et al. Bell Palsy. © 2011 Medscape. URL: http://emedicine.medscape.com/article/1146903-overview. Accessed spring 2011.

Cerebral Palsy

1. Cerebral Palsy: Hope Through Research. National Institute of Neurological Disorders and Stroke. URL: http://www.ninds.nih.gov/disorders/cerebral_palsy/detail_cerebral_palsy.htm. Accessed spring 2011.
2. Cerebral Palsy. Centers for Disease Control and Prevention. URL: http://www.cdc.gov/ncbddd/dd/cp2.htm. Accessed spring 2011.
3. Cerebral Palsy. © 1998–2011 Mayo Foundation for Medical Education and Research. URL: http://www.mayoclinic.com/health/cerebral-palsy/DS00302. Accessed spring 2011.
4. Deep Muscle Massage Helpful for Cerebral Palsy Patients. © 2011 Cerebral Palsy Source. URL: http://www.cerebralpalsysource.com/News_and_Articles/deep-massage/index.html. Accessed spring 2011.
5. Treatment of 140 Cerebral Palsied Children with a Combined Method Based on Traditional Chinese Medicine (TCM) and Western Medicine. Published online 2004 December 20. doi: 10.1631/jzus.2005.B0057. © Journal of Zhejiang University Science. URL: http://www.ncbi.nlm.nih.gov/pmc/articles/PMC1390761/?tool=pubmed. Accessed spring 2011.
6. Thorngood C, et al. Physical Medicine and Rehabilitation for Cerebral Palsy. © 2011 Medscape. URL: http://emedicine.medscape.com/article/310740-overview. Accessed spring 2011.

Charcot-Marie-Tooth Disorder

1. Charcot-Marie-Tooth Disease Fact Sheet. National Institute of Neurological Disorders and Stroke (NINDS). URL: http://www.ninds.nih.gov/disorders/charcot_marie_tooth/detail_charcot_marie_tooth.htm. Accessed winter 2011.
2. Charcot-Marie-Tooth disease. © 1998–2011 Mayo Foundation for Medical Education and Research. URL: http://www.mayoclinic.com/health/charcot-marie-tooth-disease/DS00557. Accessed winter 2011.
3. Charcot-Marie-Tooth Disorders. © 2011 Charcot-Marie-Tooth Association. URL: http://www.charcot-marie-tooth.org/about_cmt/overview.php. Accessed winter 2011.
4. Kedlaya D. Charcot-Marie-Tooth Disease. © 2011 Medscape. URL: http://emedicine.medscape.com/article/315260-overview. Accessed winter 2011.

Complex Regional Pain Syndrome

1. Complex regional pain syndrome. © 1998–2011 Mayo Foundation for Medical Education and Research. URL: http://www.mayoclinic.com/health/complex-regional-pain-syndrome/DS00265. Accessed spring 2011.
2. CRPS RSD Overview: CRPS Origins—When was It First Studied: The Origins of Complex Regional Pain Syndrome—CRPS. © 2011 American RSDHope. URL: http://www.rsdhope.org/Showpage.asp?PAGE_ID=3&PGCT_ID=546. Accessed spring 2011.
3. Four Stages of RSDS. © 2011 American RSDHope. URL: http://www.rsdhope.org/ShowPage.asp?PAGE_ID=5. Accessed spring 2011.
4. Groeneweg G, et al. Regulation of Peripheral Blood Flow in Complex Regional Pain Syndrome Clinical Implication for Symptomatic Relief and Pain Management. BMC Musculoskeletal Disorder 2009;10:116. National Center for Biotechnology Information. URL: http://www.ncbi.nlm.nih.gov/pubmed/19775468. Accessed spring 2011.
5. Lee J, et al. Early Aggressive Treatment Improves Prognosis in Complex Regional Pain Syndrome. Practitioner 2011;255(1736):23–26, 3. National Center for Biotechnology Information. URL: http://www.ncbi.nlm.nih.gov/pubmed?term=massage%20AND%20crps. Accessed spring 2011.
6. Reflex Sympathetic Dystrophy/ Complex Regional Pain Syndromes (CRPS): State-of-the-Science. National Institute of Neurological Disorders and Stroke. URL: http://www.ninds.nih.gov/news_and_events/proceedings/reflex_sympathetic_dystrophy_2001.htm. Accessed spring 2011.
7. RSD–CRPS Treatments: Drug Therapies for RSD/CRPS. © 2011 American RSDHope. URL: http://www.rsdhope.org/Showpage.asp?PAGE_ID=155&PGCT_ID=3822. Accessed spring 2011.
8. Wheeler A. Complex Regional Pain Syndromes. © 2011 Medscape. URL: http://emedicine.medscape.com/article/1145318-overview. Accessed spring 2011.

Depression

1. Bhalla R, et al. Depression. © 2011 WebMD LLC. URL: http://emedicine.medscape.com/article/286759-overview. Accessed winter 2011.
2. Bipolar Disorder. National Institute of Mental Health. URL: http://www.nimh.nih.gov/health/publications/bipolar-disorder/complete-index.shtml. Accessed winter 2011.
3. Depression. National Institute of Mental Health. URL: http://www.nimh.nih.gov/health/publications/depression/complete-index.shtml. Accessed winter 2011.
4. Field T, et al. Benefits of Combining Massage Therapy with Group Interpersonal Psychotherapy in Prenatally Depressed Women. Journal of Bodywork and Movement Therapies 2009;13(4):297–303. URL: http://www.ncbi.nlm.nih.gov/pmc/articles/PMC2785018/?tool=pubmed. Accessed winter 2011.
5. Hou WH, et al. Treatment Effects of Massage Therapy in Depressed People: A Meta-Analysis. The Journal of Clinical Psychiatry 2010;71(7):894–901. [Epub Mar 23, 2010.] URL: http://www.ncbi.nlm.nih.gov/pubmed/20361919. Accessed winter 2011.
6. Joy S. Postpartum Depression. © 2011 WebMD LLC. URL: http://emedicine.medscape.com/article/271662-overview. Accessed winter 2011.
7. Langenfeld S, et al. Dysthemic Disorder. © 2011 WebMD LLC. URL: http://emedicine.medscape.com/article/290686-overview. Accessed winter 2011.
8. Major depression. © 2011 A.D.A.M., Inc. URL: http://www.ncbi.nlm.nih.gov/pubmedhealth/PMH0001941/. Accessed winter 2011.
9. Massage Therapy for Depression. © 2011 Massachusetts General Hospital. URL: http://www.womensmentalhealth.org/posts/massage-therapy-for-depression/. Accessed winter 2011.
10. Vale S. Depressive Symptoms, Risk of Stroke and the Stress Response. © 2011 American Heart Association, Inc. URL: http://stroke.ahajournals.org/cgi/content/full/38/6/e34. Accessed winter 2011.

Dystonia

1. Classification of Dystonia. © 2011 WE MOVE. URL: http://www.mdvu.org/library/disease/dystonia/. Accessed winter 2011.
2. Dystonia. © 1998–2011 Mayo Foundation for Medical Education and Research (MFMER). URL: http://www.mayoclinic.com/health/dystonia/DS00684. Accessed winter 2011.
3. Dystonias Fact Sheet. National Institute of Neurological Disorder and Stroke. URL: http://www.ninds.nih.gov/disorders/dystonias/detail_dystonias.htm. Accessed winter 2011.
4. Moberg-Wolff E, et al. Dystonias. © 2011 Medscape. URL: http://emedicine.medscape.com/article/312648-overview. Accessed winter 2011.
5. Reynolds N, et al. Torticollis. © 2011 Medscape. URL: http://emedicine.medscape.com/article/1152543-overview. Accessed winter 2011.
6. What is Dystonia? © 2011 DMRF (Dystonia Medical Research Foundation). URL: http://www.dystonia-foundation.org/pages/what_is_dystonia_/26.php. Accessed winter 2011.

Eating Disorders

1. Anorexia Nervosa. Office on Women's Health. URL: http://www.womenshealth.gov/faq/anorexia-nervosa.pdf. Accessed winter 2011.
2. Binge Eating Disorder. Office on Women's Health. URL: http://www.womenshealth.gov/faq/binge-eating-disorder.pdf. Accessed winter 2011.
3. Body Image. The National Women's Health Information Center. URL: http://www.womenshealth.gov/bodyimage/eatingdisorders/. Accessed winter 2011.
4. Bulimia Nervosa. Office on Women's Health. URL: http://www.womenshealth.gov/faq/bulimia-nervosa.pdf. Accessed winter 2011.
5. Eating Disorders. National Institute of Mental Health (NIMH). URL: http://www.nimh.nih.gov/health/publications/eating-disorders/complete-index.shtml. Accessed winter 2011.
6. Treatment. © 2011 Academy for Eating Disorders. URL: http://www.aedweb.org/Treatment/1533.htm. Accessed winter 2011.

Encephalitis

1. Assis F, et al. Viral Encephalitis. © 2011 Medscape. URL: http://emedicine.medscape.com/article/1166498-overview. Accessed winter 2011.
2. Cunha B. West Nile Encephalitis. © 2011 Medscape. URL: http://emedicine.medscape.com/article/234009-overview. Accessed winter 2011.
3. Encephalitis. © 1998–2011 Mayo Foundation for Medical Education and Research (MFMER). URL: http://www.mayoclinic.com/health/encephalitis/DS00226. Accessed winter 2011.
4. Meningitis and Encephalitis Fact Sheet. National Institute of Neurological Disorders and Stroke. URL: http://www.ninds.nih.gov/disorders/encephalitis_meningitis/detail_encephalitis_meningitis.htm. Accessed winter 2011.
5. West Nile virus. © 1998–2011 Mayo Foundation for Medical Education and Research (MFMER). URL: http://www.mayoclinic.com/health/west-nile-virus/DS00438. Accessed winter 2011.

Fibromyalgia

1. Castro-Sanchez A, et al. Benefits of Massage-Myofascial Release Therapy on Pain, Anxiety, Quality of Sleep, Depression, and Quality of Life in Patients with Fibromyalgia. © 2011 Adelaida María Castro-Sánchez, et al. URL: http://www.ncbi.nlm.nih.gov/pmc/articles/PMC3018656/. Accessed spring 2011.
2. Chakrabarty S, et al. Fibromyalgia. American Family Physician 2007;76(2):247–254. © American Academy of Family Physicians. URL: http://www.aafp.org/afp/2007/0715/p247.html. Accessed spring 2011.
3. Ekici G, et al. Comparison of Manual Lymph Drainage Therapy and Connective Tissue Massage in Women with Fibromyalgia: A Randomized Controlled Trial. National Center for Biotechnology Information. URL: http://www.ncbi.nlm.nih.gov/pubmed/19243724. Accessed spring 2011.
4. Fibromyalgia: Summaries of Research. National Institute of Arthritis and Musculoskeletal and Skin Diseases. URL: http://www.niams.nih.gov/News_and_Events/Spotlight_on_Research/2004/fibro_sum.asp. Accessed spring 2011.
5. Harth M, et al. The Fibromyalgia Tender Points: Use Them or Lose Them? A Brief Review of the Controversy. © The Journal of Rheumatology Publishing Company Limited. URL: https://www.jrheum.com/subscribers/07/05/914.html. Accessed spring 2011.
6. Kalichman L. Massage Therapy for Fibromyalgia Symptoms. Rheumatology International 2010;30(9):1151–1157. [Epub Mar 20, 2010.] National Center for Biotechnology Information. URL: http://www.ncbi.nlm.nih.gov/pubmed/20306046. Accessed spring 2011.
7. Smith H, et al. Fibromyalgia: An Afferent Processing Disorder Leading to a Complex Pain Generalized Syndrome 2011;14;E217–E245. The Official Journal of the American Society of Interventional Pain Physicians. URL: http://www.painphysicianjournal.com/linkout_vw.php?issn=1533-3159&vol=14&page=E217. Accessed spring 2011.
8. Winfield J, et al. Fibromyalgia. © 2011 Medscape. URL: http://emedicine.medscape.com/article/329838-overview. Accessed spring 2011.

Headache

1. Chawla J, et al. Migraine Headache. © 2011 WebMD. URL: http://emedicine.medscape.com/article/1142556-overview#showall. Accessed spring 2011.
2. Cluster headache. © 1998–2011 Mayo Foundation for Medical Education and Research (MFMER). URL: http://www.mayoclinic.com/health/cluster-headache/DS00487. Accessed spring 2011.
3. Headache. National Institute of Neurological Disorders and Stroke (NINDS) URL: http://www.ninds.nih.gov/disorders/headache/detail_headache.htm. Accessed spring 2011.
4. Moraska A, et al. Changes in Psychological Parameters in Patients with Tension-type Headache Following Massage Therapy: A Pilot Study. The Journal of Manual & Manipulative Therapy 2009;17(2):86–94. © Journal of Manual & Manipulative Therapy. URL: http://www.ncbi.nlm.nih.gov/pmc/articles/PMC2700492/?tool=pubmed. Accessed spring 2011.
5. Rebound headaches. © 1998–2011 Mayo Foundation for Medical Education and Research (MFMERS). URL: http://www.mayoclinic.com/health/rebound-headaches/DS00613. Accessed spring 2011.
6. Sargeant L, et al. Headache, Cluster. © 2011 WebMD. URL: http://emedicine.medscape.com/article/792150-overview#showall. Accessed spring 2011.
7. Singh M. Muscle Contraction Tension Headache. © 2011 WebMD. URL: http://emedicine.medscape.com/article/1142908-overview. Accessed spring 2011.

Herpes Zoster

1. Anderson W. Varicella-Zoster Virus. © 2011 Medscape. URL: http://emedicine.medscape.com/article/231927-overview. Accessed winter 2011.

2. McElveen W, et al. Postherpetic Neuralgia. © 2011 Medscape. URL: http://emedicine.medscape.com/article/1143066-overview. Accessed winter 2011.
3. Shingles (Herpes Zoster). Centers for Disease Control and Prevention. URL: http://www.cdc.gov/shingles/hcp/clinical-overview.html. Accessed winter 2011.
4. Shingles. © 1998–2011 Mayo Foundation for Medical Education and Research (MFMER). URL: http://www.mayoclinic.com/health/shingles/DS00098. Accessed winter 2011.

Huntington Disease

1. Huntington's Disease: Hope Through Research. National Institute of Neurological Disorders and Stroke. URL: http://www.ninds.nih.gov/disorders/huntington/detail_huntington.htm. Accessed winter 2011.
2. Huntington's disease. © 1998–2011 Mayo Foundation for Medical Education and Research (MFMER). URL: http://www.mayoclinic.com/health/huntingtons-disease/DS00401. Accessed winter 2011.
3. Miller M. HD Research—Past and Future. © 2011 Huntington's Disease Society of America. URL: http://www.hdsa.org/research/past-and-future.html. Accessed winter 2011.
4. Overview of Huntington's Disease. © 2011 WE MOVE. URL: http://www.wemove.org/hd/hd.html. Accessed winter 2011.
5. Sharon I, et al. Huntington Disease Dementia. © 2011 Medscape. URL: http://emedicine.medscape.com/article/289706-overview. Accessed winter 2011.
6. What Is Huntington's Disease (HD)? © 2011 Huntington's Disease Society of America. URL: http://www.hdsa.org/about/our-mission/what-is-hd.html. Accessed winter 2011.

Meniere Disease

1. Meniere's Disease Start Page. © 2011 Meniere's Disease Information Center. URL: http://www.menieresinfo.com/start.html. Accessed spring 2011.
2. Meniere's disease. © 2011 A.D.A.M. URL: http://www.ncbi.nlm.nih.gov/pubmedhealth/PMH0001721/. Accessed spring 2011.
3. Meniere's disease. © 1998–2011 Mayo Foundation for Medical Education and Research (MFMER). URL: http://www.mayoclinic.com/health/menieres-disease/DS00535. Accessed spring 2011.
4. NIDCD Fact Sheet: Meniere's Disease. National Institute on Deafness and Other Communication Disorders. URL: http://www.nidcd.nih.gov/staticresources/health/hearing/MeineresFS.pdf. Accessed spring 2011.
5. Wilkerson R. Meniere Disease. © 2011 WebMD. URL: http://emedicine.medscape.com/article/792902-overview. Accessed spring 2011.

Meningitis

1. Meningitis and Encephalitis Fact Sheet. National Institute of Neurological Disorders and Stroke. URL: http://www.ninds.nih.gov/disorders/encephalitis_meningitis/detail_encephalitis_meningitis.htm. Accessed winter 2011.
2. Meningitis: Clinical Information for Healthcare Professionals. Centers for Disease Control and Prevention. URL: http://www.cdc.gov/meningitis/clinical-info.html. Accessed winter 2011.
3. Meningitis. © 1998–2011 Mayo Foundation for Medical Education and Research (MFMER). URL: http://www.mayoclinic.com/health/meningitis/DS00118. Accessed winter 2011.
4. Razonable R, et al. Meningitis. © 2011 Medscape. URL: http://emedicine.medscape.com/article/232915-overview. Accessed winter 2011.

Multiple System Atrophy

1. Diedrich A, et al. Multiple System Atrophy. © 2011 Medscape. URL: http://emedicine.medscape.com/article/1154583-overview. Accessed winter 2011.
2. Multiple system atrophy (MSA). © 1998–2011 Mayo Foundation for Medical Education and Research (MFMER). URL: http://www.mayoclinic.com/health/shy-drager-syndrome/DS00989. Accessed winter 2011.
3. Multiple System Atrophy Fact Sheet. National Institute of Neurological Disorders and Stroke (NINDS). URL: http://www.ninds.nih.gov/disorders/msa/detail_msa.htm. Accessed winter 2011.
4. Multiple System Atrophy. © 2011 National Dysautonomia Research Foundation (NDRF). URL: http://www.ndrf.org/MSA.htm. Accessed winter 2011.
5. Overview of Multiple System Atrophy. © 2011 WE MOVE. URL: http://www.wemove.org/msa/. Accessed winter 2011.

Parkinson Disease

1. Hauser R, et al. Parkinson Disease. © 2011 Medscape. URL: http://emedicine.medscape.com/article/1151267-overview. Accessed winter 2011.
2. Craig LH, et al. Controlled pilot study of the effects of neuromuscular therapy in patients with Parkinson's disease. © 2011 Movement Disorder Society. URL: http://www.ncbi.nlm.nih.gov/pubmed/17044088. Accessed winter 2011.
3. Ferry P, et al. Use of Complementary Therapies and Non-prescribed Medication in Patients with Parkinson's Disease. Postgraduate Medicinal Journal 2002;78:612–614. URL: http://www.ncbi.nlm.nih.gov/pmc/articles/PMC1742510/pdf/v078p00612.pdf. Accessed winter 2011.
4. Parkinson's Disease: Hope Through Research. National Institute of Neurological Disorders and Stroke. URL: http://www.ninds.nih.gov/disorders/parkinsons_disease/detail_parkinsons_disease.htm. Accessed winter 2011.
5. Parkinson's disease. © 1998–2011 Mayo Foundation for Medical Education and Research (MFMER). URL: http://www.mayoclinic.com/health/parkinsons-disease/DS00295. Accessed winter 2011.
6. Paterson C, et al. A Pilot Study of Therapeutic Massage for People with Parkinson's disease: the Added Value of User Involvement. Complementary Therapies in Clinical Practice 2005;11(3):161–171. URL: http://www.ncbi.nlm.nih.gov/pubmed/16005833. Accessed winter 2011.

7. Rao S, et al. Parkinson's Disease: Diagnosis and Treatment. American Family Physician 2006;74(12):2046–2054. URL: http://www.aafp.org/afp/2006/1215/p2046.html. Accessed winter 2011.

Peripheral Neuropathy

1. About Peripheral Neuralpathy. © The Neuropathy Association. URL: http://www.neuropathy.org/site/PageServer?pagename=About_Facts. Accessed winter 2011.
2. Peripheral Neuropathy Fact Sheet. National Institute of Neurological Disorders and Stroke. URL: http://www.ninds.nih.gov/disorders/peripheralneuropathy/detail_peripheralneuropathy.htm. Accessed winter 2011.
3. Peripheral neuropathy. © 1998–2011 Mayo Foundation for Medical Education and Research. URL: http://www.mayoclinic.com/health/peripheral-neuropathy/DS00131. Accessed winter 2011.
4. Poncelet A. An Algorithm for the Evaluation of Peripheral Neuropathy. © American Academy of Family Physicians. URL: http://www.aafp.org/afp/980215ap/poncelet.html. Accessed winter 2011.

Polio

1. Munis F, et al. Postpolio Syndrome. © 2011 Medscape. URL: http://emedicine.medscape.com/article/306920-overview. Accessed winter 2011.
2. Post-Polio Syndrome Fact Sheet. National Institute of Neurological Disorders and Stroke. URL: http://www.ninds.nih.gov/disorders/post_polio/detail_post_polio.htm. Accessed winter 2011.
3. Post-Polio Syndrome for Health Professionals. © Post-Polio Health International. URL: http://www.post-polio.org/edu/pabout3.html#hea. Accessed winter 2011.
4. Vidyadhara S, et al. Poliomyelitis. © 2011 Medscape. URL: http://emedicine.medscape.com/article/1259213-overview. Accessed winter 2011.

Seizure disorder

1. Cavazos J. Seizures and Epilepsy, Overview and Classification. © 2011 WebMD. URL: http://emedicine.medscape.com/article/1184846-overview#showall. Accessed spring 2011.
2. Epilepsy: Know the Facts. Epilepsy Foundation. URL: http://www.epilepsyfoundation.org/about/upload/EFA270.pdf. Accessed spring 2011.
3. Frequently Asked Questions. Centers for Disease Control and Prevention. URL: http://www.cdc.gov/epilepsy/basics/faqs.htm. Accessed spring 2011.
4. Seizures and Epilepsy: Hope Through Research. National Institute of Neurological Disorders and Stroke (NINDS). URL: http://www.ninds.nih.gov/disorders/epilepsy/detail_epilepsy.htm. Accessed spring 2011.

Sleep Disorders

1. Can't Sleep? What to Know About Insomnia. © National Sleep Foundation. URL: http://www.sleepfoundation.org/article/sleep-related-problems/insomnia-and-sleep. Accessed spring 2011.
2. Lubit R, et al. Sleep Disorders. © 2011 WebMD. URL: http://emedicine.medscape.com/article/287104-overview. Accessed spring 2011.
3. Narcolepsy and Sleep. © National Sleep Foundation. URL: http://www.sleepfoundation.org/article/sleep-related-problems/narcolepsy-and-sleep. Accessed spring 2011.
4. Periodic Limb Movements in Sleep. © National Sleep Foundation. URL: http://www.sleepfoundation.org/article/sleep-related-problems/periodic-limb-movements-sleep. Accessed spring 2011.
5. Restless Legs Syndrome and Sleep. © National Sleep Foundation. URL: http://www.sleepfoundation.org/article/sleep-related-problems/restless-legs-syndrome-rls-and-sleep. Accessed spring 2011.
6. Sleep Aids and Insomnia. © National Sleep Foundation. URL: http://www.sleepfoundation.org/article/sleep-related-problems/sleep-aids-and-insomnia. Accessed spring 2011.
7. Sleep Apnea. © 1998–2011 Mayo Foundation for Medical Education and Research (MFMER). URL: http://www.mayoclinic.com/health/sleep-apnea/DS00148. Accessed spring 2011.
8. What Is Insomnia. National Heart Lung and Blood Institute (NHLBI). URL: http://www.nhlbi.nih.gov/health/dci/Diseases/inso/inso_all.html. Accessed spring 2011.

Spina Bifida

1. Foster M. Spina Bifida. © 2011 Medscape. URL: http://emedicine.medscape.com/article/1266529-overview.
2. Kolaski K. Myelomeningocele. © 2011 Medscape. URL: http://emedicine.medscape.com/article/311113-overview. Accessed spring 2011.
3. Spina Befida. © 2011 March of Dimes Foundation. URL: http://www.marchofdimes.com/birthdefects_spinabifida.html. Accessed spring 2011.
4. Spina Bifida Fact Sheet. National Institute of Neurological Disorders and Stroke. URL: http://www.ninds.nih.gov/disorders/spina_bifida/detail_spina_bifida.htm. Accessed spring 2011.
5. Spina Bifida. Centers for Disease Control and Prevention. URL: http://www.cdc.gov/ncbddd/spinabifida/facts.html. Accessed spring 2011.
6. Tethering Spinal Cord. © Spina Bifida Association of America. URL: http://www.spinabifidaassociation.org/site/c.liKWL7PLLrF/b.2700295/k.6B9E/Tethering_Spinal_Cord.htm. Accessed spring 2011.

Spinal Cord Injury

1. Benzel E. Spinal Cord Injury (SCI): Damage Control and Treatment. © Vertical Health, LLC. URL: http://www.spineuniverse.com/conditions/spinal-cord-injury/spinal-cord-injury-sci-damage-control-treatment. Accessed spring 2011.
2. Campagnolo D. Autonomic Dysreflexia in Spinal Cord Injury. © 2011 Medscape. URL: http://emedicine.medscape.com/article/322809-overview. Accessed spring 2011.
3. Campagnolo D. Heterotopic Ossification in Spinal Cord Injury. © 2011 Medscape. URL: http://emedicine.medscape.com/article/322003-print. Accessed spring 2011.

4. Cardenas D, et al. Treatments for Chronic Pain in Persons with Spinal Cord Injury: A Survey Study. Journal of Spinal Cord Medicine 2006;29(2):109–117. © American Paraplegia Society. URL: http://www.ncbi.nlm.nih.gov/pmc/articles/PMC1864800/?tool=pubmed. Accessed spring 2011.
5. Heutink M, et al. Chronic Spinal Cord Injury Pain: Pharmacological and Non-pharmacological Treatments and Treatment Effectiveness. Disability and Rehabilitation 2011;33(5):433–440. [Epub Aug 9, 2010.] URL: http://www.ncbi.nlm.nih.gov/pubmed/20695788. Accessed spring 2011.
6. Manella C, et al. Gait Characteristics, Range of Motion, and Spasticity Changes in Response to Massage in a Person with Incomplete Spinal Cord Injury: Case Report. International Journal of Therapeutic Massage & Bodywork: Research, Education, & Practice 2011;4(1). © International Journal of Therapeutic Massage & Bodywork. http://www.ijtmb.org/index.php/ijtmb/article/view/108/157. Accessed spring 2011.
7. Saulino M et al. Rehabilitation of Persons with Spinal Cord Injuries. © 2011 Medscape. URL: http://emedicine.medscape.com/article/1265209-overview. Accessed spring 2011.
8. Spinal Cord Injury (SCI): Fact Sheet. Centers for Disease Control and Prevention. URL: http://www.cdc.gov/TraumaticBrainInjury/scifacts.html. Accessed spring 2011.
9. Spinal Cord Injury: Hope Through Research: A Short History of the Treatment of Spinal Cord Injury. National Institute of Neurological Disorders and Stroke. URL: http://www.ninds.nih.gov/disorders/sci/detail_sci.htm. Accessed spring 2011.
10. Spinasanta S. Drugs and Medications for Spinal Cord Injury. © Vertical Health, LCC. URL: http://www.spineuniverse.com/conditions/spinal-cord-injury/drugs-medications-spinal-cord-injury. Accessed spring 2011.

Stroke

1. Becker J, et al. Stroke, Ischemic. © 2011 Medscape. URL: http://emedicine.medscape.com/article/793904-overview. Accessed spring 2011.
2. Bruno-Petrina A. Motor Recovery in Stroke. © 2011 Medscape. URL: http://emedicine.medscape.com/article/324386-overview. Accessed spring 2011.
3. Culebras A. Sleep and Stroke. © 2011 Medscape. URL: http://www.medscape.com/viewarticle/713990?src=mp&spon=17&uac=78486SY. Accessed spring 2011.
4. Stroke Treatment. © National Stroke Foundation. URL: http://www.stroke.org/site/PageServer?pagename=treatment. Accessed spring 2011.
5. Stroke: Hope Through Research. National Institute of Neurological Disorders and Stroke. URL: http://www.ninds.nih.gov/disorders/stroke/detail_stroke.htm. Accessed spring 2011.
6. Stroke. © 1998–2011 Mayo Foundation for Medical Education and Research (MFMER). URL: http://www.mayoclinic.com/health/stroke/DS00150. Accessed spring 2011.

Traumatic Brain Injury

1. Concussion and Mild TBI. Centers for Disease Control and Prevention. URL: http://www.cdc.gov/concussion/index.html. Accessed spring 2011.
2. Dawodu S. Traumatic Brain Injury (TBI)—Definition, Epidemiology, Pathophysiology. © 2011 Medscape. URL: http://emedicine.medscape.com/article/326510-overview. Accessed spring 2011.
3. Krafft R. Trigeminal Neuralgia. American Family Physician 2008;77(9):1291–1296. © American Academy of Family Physicians. URL: http://www.aafp.org/afp/2008/0501/p1291.html. Accessed spring 2011.
4. Mild TBI/Concussion Overview. The Center of Excellence for Medical Multimedia. URL: http://www.traumaticbraininjuryatoz.org/Mild-TBI.aspx. Accessed spring 2011.
5. Moderate to Severe TBI Overview. The Center of Excellence for Medical Multimedia. URL: http://www.traumaticbraininjuryatoz.org/Moderate-to-Severe-TBI.aspx. Accessed spring 2011.
6. Pangilinan P, et al. Classification and Complications of Traumatic Brain Injury. © 2011 Medscape. URL: http://emedicine.medscape.com/article/326643-overview. Accessed spring 2011.
7. Singh M, et al. Trigeminal Neuralgia. © 2011 Medscape. URL: http://emedicine.medscape.com/article/1145144-overview. Accessed spring 2011.
8. Traumatic Brain Injury: Hope Through Research. National Institute of Neurological Disorders and Stroke. URL: http://www.ninds.nih.gov/disorders/tbi/detail_tbi.htm. Accessed spring 2011.

Tremor

1. Burke D, et al. Essential Tremor. © 2011 Medscape. http://emedicine.medscape.com/article/1150290-overview. Accessed winter 2011.
2. Chen J, et al. Essential Tremor: Diagnosis and Treatment. © 2011 Medscape. URL: http://www.medscape.com/viewarticle/461397. Accessed winter 2011.
3. Essential Tremor. © 1998–2011 Mayo Foundation for Medical Education and Research. URL: http://www.mayoclinic.com/health/essential-tremor/DS00367. Accessed winter 2011.
4. Kenney C, et al. Tourette's Syndrome. American Family Physician 2008;77(5):651–658. © American Academy of Family Physicians. URL: http://www.aafp.org/afp/2008/0301/p651.html. Accessed winter 2011.
5. Tremor Fact Sheet. National Institute of Neurological Disorders and Stroke. URL: http://www.ninds.nih.gov/disorders/tremor/detail_tremor.htm. Accessed winter 2011.

Trigeminal Neuralgia

1. Trigeminal Neuralgia Fact Sheet. National Institute of Neurological Disorders and Stroke. URL: http://www.ninds.nih.gov/disorders/trigeminal_neuralgia/detail_trigeminal_neuralgia.htm. Accessed spring 2011.
2. Trigeminal Neuralgia Treatment. © Department of Neurosurgery, University of Pittsburgh. URL: http://www.ninds.nih.gov/disorders/trigeminal_neuralgia/detail_trigeminal_neuralgia.htm
3. Trigeminal neuralgia. © 1998–2011 Mayo Foundation for Medical Research and Education. URL: http://www.ninds.nih.gov/disorders/trigeminal_neuralgia/detail_trigeminal_neuralgia.htm. Accessed spring 2011.

Vestibular Balance Disorders

1. Balance Disorders. National Institute on Deafness and Other Communication Disorders. URL: http://www.nidcd.nih.gov/health/balance/balance_disorders.asp. Accessed spring 2011.
2. Balance Procedures Manual. NHanes. URL: http://www.cdc.gov/nchs/data/nhanes/ba.pdf. Accessed spring 2011.
3. Boston M, et al. Inner Ear Labyrinthitis. © 2011 WebMD. URL: http://emedicine.medscape.com/article/856215-overview. Accessed spring 2011.
4. Li J, et al. Benign Paroxysmal Positional Vertigo. © 2011 WebMD. URL: http://emedicine.medscape.com/article/884261-overview. Accessed spring 2011.
5. Samy H, et al. Dizziness, Vertigo, and Imbalance. © 2011 WebMD. URL: http://emedicine.medscape.com/article/1159385-overview. Accessed spring 2011.

Chapter 5

Anemia

1. Abrahamian F, et al. Anemia, Chronic. © Medscape 1994–2011. URL: http://emedicine.medscape.com/article/780176-overview#showall. Accessed summer 2011.
2. Anemia. © 1994–2011 by WebMD. 2011. URL: http://www.emedicinehealth.com/anemia/article_em.htm. Accessed summer 2011.
3. Anemia. © Mayo Foundation for Medical Education and Research (MFMER) 1998–2011. URL: http://www.mayoclinic.com/health/anemia/DS00321. Accessed summer 2011.
4. Conrad M, et al. Anemia. © 1994–2011 by WebMD. URL: http://emedicine.medscape.com/article/198475-overview#showall. Accessed summer 2011.
5. Iron and Iron Deficiency. Centers for Disease Control and Prevention. URL: http://www.cdc.gov/nutrition/everyone/basics/vitamins/iron.html. Accessed summer 2011.
6. What is Anemia. National Heart Lung and Blood Institute. URL: http://www.nhlbi.nih.gov/health/dci/Diseases/anemia/anemia_all.html. Accessed summer 2011.
7. What is Aplastic Anemia. National Heart Lung and Blood Institute. URL: http://www.nhlbi.nih.gov/health/dci/Diseases/aplastic/aplastic_all.html. Accessed summer 2011.
8. What is Pernicious Anemia. National Heart Lung and Blood Institute. URL: http://www.nhlbi.nih.gov/health/dci/Diseases/prnanmia/prnanmia_all.html. Accessed summer 2011.

Aneurysm

1. Aneurysm. © A.D.A.M., Inc. 2011. URL: http://www.ncbi.nlm.nih.gov/pubmedhealth/PMH0002109/. Accessed summer 2011.
2. Cerebral Aneurysm Fact Sheet. National Institute of Neurological Disorders and Stroke. URL: http://www.ninds.nih.gov/disorders/cerebral_aneurysm/detail_cerebral_aneurysm.htm. Accessed summer 2011.
3. Nelson B, et al. Thoracic Aneurysm. © Medscape. URL: http://emedicine.medscape.com/article/761627-overview#showall. Accessed summer 2011.
4. O'Connor R, et al. Abdominal Aneurysm. © 1994–2011 by WebMD. URL: http://emedicine.medscape.com/article/756735-overview#showall. Accessed summer 2011.
5. What is an Aneurysm. National Heart Lung and Blood Institute. URL: http://www.nhlbi.nih.gov/health/dci/Diseases/arm/arm_all.html. Accessed summer 2011.

Atherosclerosis

1. Boudi B, et al. Noncoronary Atherosclerosis. © 1994–2011 WebMD. URL: http://emedicine.medscape.com/article/1950759-overview#showall. Accessed summer 2011.
2. Coronary Artery Disease. © 1996–2011 Texas Heart Institute. URL: http://www.texasheartinstitute.org/HIC/Topics/Cond/CoronaryArteryDisease.cfm. Accessed summer 2011.
3. Peripheral Arterial Diseases in the Legs. Centers for Disease Control and Prevention. URL: http://www.cdc.gov/DHDSP/data_statistics/fact_sheets/docs/fs_PAD.pdf. Accessed summer 2011.
4. Rimmerman C. Coronary Artery Disease. © 2000–2011 The Cleveland Clinic Foundation. URL: http://www.clevelandclinicmeded.com/medicalpubs/diseasemanagement/cardiology/coronary-artery-disease/. Accessed summer 2011.
5. Vascular Disease. © 1996–2011 Texas Heart Institute. URL: http://www.texasheartinstitute.org/HIC/Topics/Cond/pvd.cfm. Accessed summer 2011.
6. What is Atherosclerosis. National Heart Lung and Blood Institute. URL: http://www.nhlbi.nih.gov/health/dci/Diseases/Atherosclerosis/Atherosclerosis_All.html. Accessed summer 2011.
7. What is Carotid Artery Disease. National Heart Lung and Blood Institute. URL: http://www.nhlbi.nih.gov/health/dci/Diseases/catd/catd_all.html
8. What is Coronary Artery Disease. National Heart Lung and Blood Institute. URL: http://www.nhlbi.nih.gov/health/dci/Diseases/Cad/CAD_All.html. Accessed summer 2011.

Heart Attack

1. Heart Attack. Centers for Disease Control and Prevention. URL: http://www.cdc.gov/heartdisease/heart_attack.htm. Accessed summer 2011.
2. Heart Disease & Stroke Statistics: 2010 Update At-A-Glance. American Heart Association. URL: http://dbbs.wustl.edu/dbbs/website.nsf/forms/forms/$file/HeartStrokeUpdate2010.pdf. Accessed summer 2011.
3. Kondur A, et al. Complications of Myocardial Infarction. © 1994–2011 WebMD. URL: http://emedicine.medscape.com/article/164924-overview#showall. Accessed summer 2011.
4. What is A Heart Attack. American Heart Association. American Stroke Association. URL: http://www.heart.org/idc/groups/heart-public/@wcm/@hcm/documents/downloadable/ucm_304570.pdf. Accessed summer 2011.
5. WhatisAHeartAttack.NationalHeartLungandBloodInstitute. URL: http://www.nhlbi.nih.gov/health/dci/Diseases/HeartAttack/HeartAttack_All.html. Accessed summer 2011.

6. Zafari A, et al. Myocardial Infarction. © 1994–2011 WebMD. URL: http://emedicine.medscape.com/article/155919-overview#showall. Accessed summer 2011.

Heart Failure

1. Heart Failure. The Journal of the American Medical Association. URL: http://jama.ama-assn.org/content/297/22/2548.full.pdf. Accessed summer 2011.
2. Heart Failure. © 2010 Romeo, Ortiz, Miller, Ha, Cheesman, Kim, Rademacher, and Jaski. URL: http://www.heartfailure.org/eng_site/hf.asp. Accessed summer 2011.
3. Heart Failure and Your Neuroendocrine System. © 2010 Romeo, Ortiz, Miller, Ha, Cheesman, Kim, Rademacher, and Jaski. http://www.heartfailure.org/eng_site/hf_neuroendocrine.asp. Accessed summer 2011.
4. Heart Failure Medications. © American Heart Association, Inc. URL: https://www.amhrt.org/HEARTORG/Conditions/HeartFailure/PreventionTreatmentofHeartFailure/Medications-for-Heart-Failure_UCM_306342_Article.jsp. Accessed summer 2011.
5. Heart failure. © 2011 A.D.A.M., Inc. URL: http://www.ncbi.nlm.nih.gov/pubmedhealth/PMH0001211/. Accessed summer 2011.
6. What is Heart Failure? National Heart Lung and Blood Institute. URL: http://www.nhlbi.nih.gov/health/dci/Diseases/Hf/HF_All.html. Accessed summer 2011.

Hemophilia

1. Kessler C, et al. Acquired Hemophilia. © 1994–2011 by WebMD. URL: http://emedicine.medscape.com/article/211186-overview#showall. Accessed summer 2011.
2. Sawaf H, et al. Hemophilia A and B. © 1994–2011 by WebMD. URL: http://emedicine.medscape.com/article/955590-overview#showall. Accessed summer 2011.
3. Hemophilia A (Factor VIII Deficiency). © 2006 National Hemophilia Foundation. URL: http://www.hemophilia.org/NHFWeb/MainPgs/MainNHF.aspx?menuid=180&contentid=45&rptname=bleeding. Accessed summer 2011.
4. Hemophilia B (Factor IX). © 2006 National Hemophilia Foundation. URL: http://www.hemophilia.org/NHFWeb/MainPgs/MainNHF.aspx?menuid=181&contentid=46&rptname=bleeding. Accessed summer 2011.
5. Hemophilia. © 1995–2011 The Cleveland Clinic. URL: http://my.clevelandclinic.org/disorders/hemophilia/hic_what_is_hemophilia.aspx. Accessed summer 2011.
6. Hemophilia. © 1998–2011 Mayo Foundation for Medical Education and Research (MFMER). URL: http://www.mayoclinic.com/health/hemophilia/DS00218. Accessed summer 2011.
7. What is Hemophilia? National Heart Lung and Blood Institute. URL: http://www.nhlbi.nih.gov/health/dci/Diseases/hemophilia/hemophilia_all.html. Accessed summer 2011.
8. Mowen K. Turning Hurt into Relief. © 2002 Associated Bodywork & Massage Professionals. URL: http://www.massageandbodywork.com/Articles/OctNov1999/hemophilia.html. Accessed summer 2011.
9. Von Willebrand disease. © 2006 National Hemophilia Foundation. URL: http://www.hemophilia.org/NHFWeb/MainPgs/MainNHF.aspx?menuid=182&contentid=47&rptname=bleeding. Accessed summer 2011.
10. Von Willebrand. National Heart Lung and Blood Institute. URL: http://www.nhlbi.nih.gov/health/dci/Diseases/vWD/vWD_All.html

Hypertension

1. Olney C. The Effect of Therapeutic Back Massage in Hypertensive Persons: A Preliminary Study. © 2011 SAGE Publications. Biological Research for Nursing 2005;7(2):98–105. URL: http://brn.sagepub.com/content/7/2/98.abstract. Accessed summer 2011.
2. Morbidity and Mortality Weekly Report (MMWR). Centers for Disease Control and Prevention. URL: http://www.cdc.gov/mmwr/preview/mmwrhtml/mm6004a4.htm?s_cid=mm6004a4_w. Accessed summer 2011.
3. High Blood Pressure (Hypertension). © 1996–2011 Texas Heart Institute. URL: http://www.texasheartinstitute.org/HIC/Topics/Cond/hbp.cfm. Accessed summer 2011.
4. Riaz K, et al. Hypertension. © 1994–2011 WebMD. URL: http://emedicine.medscape.com/article/241381-overview. Accessed summer 2011.
5. Jefferson LL. Exploring Effects of Therapeutic Massage and Patient Teaching in the Practice of Diaphragmatic Breathing on Blood Pressure, Stress, and Anxiety in Hypertensive African-American Women: An Intervention Study. National Center for Biotechnology Information, U.S. National Library of Medicine. Journal of National Black Nurses Association 2010;21(1):17–24. URL: http://www.ncbi.nlm.nih.gov/pubmed/20857772. Accessed summer 2011.
6. Cambron JA, Dexheimer J, Coe P. Changes in Blood Pressure After Various Forms of Therapeutic Massage: A Preliminary Study. The Journal of Alternative and Complementary Medicine. 2006;12(1):65–70. doi:10.1089/acm.2006.12.65. URL: http://www.liebertonline.com/doi/abs/10.1089/acm.2006.12.65. Accessed summer 2011.
7. What is High Blood Pressure? National Heart Lung and Blood Institute. URL: http://www.nhlbi.nih.gov/health/dci/Diseases/Hbp/HBP_All.html Accessed summer 2011.

Leukemia

1. Acute Lymphoblastic Leukemia. © 2011 The Leukemia & Lymphoma Society. URL: http://www.lls.org/#/diseaseinformation/leukemia/acutelymphoblasticleukemia/. Accessed summer 2011.
2. Acute Myeloid Leukemia. © The Leukemia & Lymphoma Society. URL: http://www.lls.org/#/diseaseinformation/leukemia/acutemyeloidleukemia/. Accessed summer 2011.
3. Chronic Lymphocytic Leukemia. © 2011 The Leukemia and Lymphoma Societ. URL: http://www.lls.org/#/diseaseinformation/leukemia/chroniclymphocyticleukemia/. Accessed summer 2011.
4. Chronic Myeloid Leukemia. © 2011 The Leukemia and Lymphoma Society. URL: http://www.lls.org/#/diseaseinformation/leukemia/chronicmyeloidleukemia/. Accessed summer 2011.

5. Leukemia. National Institute on Aging. URL: http://nihseniorhealth.gov/leukemia/toc.html. Accessed summer 2011.
6. What is Leukemia? National Cancer Institute. URL: http://www.cancer.gov/cancertopics/wyntk/leukemia/AllPages. Accessed summer 2011.

Myeloma

1. Besa E. Multiple Myeloma. © 1994–2011 WebMD. URL: http://emedicine.medscape.com/article/204369-overview#showall. Accessed summer 2011.
2. Blood Cancers: Leukemia, Lymphoma, and Myeloma. Centers for Disease Control and Prevention. URL: http://www.cdc.gov/Features/HematologicCancers/. Accessed summer 2011.
3. Hu W, et al. Myeloma. © 2011 WebMD. URL: http://www.emedicinehealth.com/myeloma/article_em.htm. Accessed summer 2011.
4. Multiple myeloma. © 1998–2011 Mayo Foundation for Medical Education and Research (MFMER). URL: http://www.mayoclinic.com/health/multiple-myeloma/DS00415. Accessed summer 2011.
5. What You Need to Know About Multiple Myeloma. National Cancer Institute. URL: http://www.cancer.gov/cancertopics/wyntk/myeloma/AllPages. Accessed summer 2011.

Raynaud Syndrome

1. Denton C. Raynaud's. © 2010 Raynaud's & Scleroderma Association. URL: http://www.raynauds.org.uk/raynauds/raynauds. Accessed summer 2011.
2. Narayanan S, et al. Raynaud Phenomenon. © 1994–2011 WebMD. URL: http://emedicine.medscape.com/article/331197-overview. Accessed summer 2011.
3. Raynaud's Phenomenon. National Institute of Arthritis and Musculoskeletal and Skin Diseases. URL: http://www.niams.nih.gov/Health_Info/Raynauds_Phenomenon/default.asp. Accessed summer 2011.
4. Raynaud's phenomenon: what is it? © 2011 Arthritis Foundation. URL: http://www.arthritis.org/disease-center.php?disease_id=22&df=definition. Accessed summer 2011.
5. What is Raynaud's? National Heart Lung and Blood Institute. URL: http://www.nhlbi.nih.gov/health/dci/Diseases/raynaud/ray_all.html. Accessed summer 2011.

Sickle Cell Disease

1. Distenfeld A, et al. Sickle Cell Anemia. © 1994–2011 WebMD. URL: http://emedicine.medscape.com/article/205926-overview. Accessed summer 2011.
2. Lemanek KL, et al. A Randomized Controlled Trial of Massage Therapy in Children with Sickle Cell Disease. National Center for Biotechnology Information. Journal of Pediatric Psychology 2009;34(10):1091–1096. URL: http://www.ncbi.nlm.nih.gov/pubmed/19282374. Accessed summer 2011.
3. Oliver-Carpenter G, et al. Disease Management, Coping, and Functional Disability in Pediatric Sickle Cell Disease. National Center for Biotechnology Information. Journal of the National Medical Association 2011;103(2):131–137. URL: http://www.ncbi.nlm.nih.gov/pubmed/21443065. Accessed summer 2011.
4. Sickle Cell Disease (SCD). Centers for Disease Control and Prevention. URL: http://www.cdc.gov/NCBDDD/sicklecell/index.html. Accessed summer 2011.
5. Sickle Cell Disease. National Heart Lung and Blood Institute. URL: http://report.nih.gov/nihfactsheets/ViewFactSheet.aspx?csid=116&key=S. Accessed summer 2011.
6. What is Sickle Cell Anemia. National Heart Lung and Blood Institute. URL: http://www.nhlbi.nih.gov/health/dci/Diseases/Sca/SCA_All.html. Accessed summer 2011.

Thrombophlebitis, Deep Vein Thrombosis

1. Bareau D. Deep Vein Thrombosis and Pulmonary Embolism. Centers for Disease Control and Prevention. URL: http://wwwnc.cdc.gov/travel/yellowbook/2010/chapter-2/deep-vein-thrombosis-pulmonary-embolism.aspx. Accessed summer 2011.
2. Beckman M, et al. Venous Thromboembolism. © 2011 Elsevier. American Journal of Preventive Medicine 2010;38(4 Suppl):S495–S501. URL: http://www.ajpm-online.net/article/S0749–3797(09)00946–5/fulltext. Accessed summer 2011.
3. Deep Vein Thrombosis (DVT). © Society for Vascular Surgery. URL: https://www.vascularweb.org/vascularhealth/Pages/deep-vein-thrombosis-(-dvt-)-.aspx. Accessed summer 2011.
4. Deep Vein Thrombosis and Pulmonary Embolism. National Center on Birth Defects and Developmental Disabilities. URL: http://www.cdc.gov/ncbddd/blooddisorders/documents/BBV_PNV_C0_1159_Thrombosis_R1mtr.pdf. Accessed summer 2011.
5. Deep Vein Thrombosis Cause. © 1995–2011 American Academy of Orthopaedic Surgeons. URL: http://orthoinfo.aaos.org/topic.cfm?topic=A00219. Accessed summer 2011.
6. Deep Vein Thrombosis. © 2004–2011 American Academy of Family Physicians. URL: http://familydoctor.org/online/famdocen/home/common/heartdisease/basics/. Accessed summer 2011.
7. Gardiner E, et al. Arterial Thrombosis: Going, Gone. © The American Society of Hematology. URL: http://bloodjournal.hematologylibrary.org/content/116/13/2201.full. Accessed summer 2011.
8. Ouellette D, et al. Pulmonary Embolism. © 1994–2011 WebMD. URL: http://emedicine.medscape.com/article/300901-overview#showall. Accessed summer 2011.
9. Thrombophlebitis. © 1997–2011 A.D.A.M., Inc. URL: http://www.nlm.nih.gov/medlineplus/ency/article/001108.htm. Accessed summer 2011.
10. Thrombophlebitis. © 1998–2011 Mayo Foundation for Medical Education and Research. URL: http://www.mayoclinic.com/health/thrombophlebitis/DS00223. Accessed summer 2011.
11. Venous and Arterial Thrombosis: A Continuous Spectrum of the Same Disease. © The European Society of Cardiology 2004. URL: http://eurheartj.oxfordjournals.org/content/26/1/3.full. Accessed summer 2011.

12. What is Deep Vein Thrombosis. National Heart Lung and Blood Institute. URL: http://www.nhlbi.nih.gov/health/dci/Diseases/Dvt/DVT_All.html. Accessed summer 2011.

Varicose Veins

1. Alaiti S, et al. Sclerotherapy. © 1994–2011 WebMD. URL: http://emedicine.medscape.com/article/1271091-overview#showall. Accessed summer 2011.
2. Esophageal Varicose. © 1998–2011 Mayo Foundation for Medical Education and Research. URL: http://www.mayoclinic.com/health/esophageal-varices/DS00820. Accessed summer 2011.
3. Nabili S, et al. Varicose Veins & Spider Veins. © 2011 MedicineNet. URL: http://www.medicinenet.com/script/main/art.asp?articlekey=514. Accessed summer 2011.
4. Thornton S, et al. Hemorrhoids. © 1994–2011 WebMD. URL: http://emedicine.medscape.com/article/195401-overview. Accessed summer 2011.
5. Weiss R, et al. Varicose Veins and Spider Veins. © 1994–2011 WebMD. URL: http://emedicine.medscape.com/article/1085530-overview. Accessed summer 2011.
6. What are Hemorrhoids. © 2005–2011 WebMD. URL: http://www.webmd.com/a-to-z-guides/hemorrhoids-topic-overview. Accessed summer 2011.
7. What Are Varicose Veins. National Heart Lung and Blood Institute. URL: http://www.nhlbi.nih.gov/health/dci/Diseases/vv/vv_all.html. Accessed summer 2011.
8. White W, et al. Varicocele. © 1994–2011 WebMD. URL: http://emedicine.medscape.com/article/438591-overview#showall. Accessed summer 2011.

Chapter 6

Allergies

1. Ghaffar A. Immunology. © 2009 The Board of Trustees of the University of South Carolina. URL: http://pathmicro.med.sc.edu/ghaffar/hyper00.html. Accessed summer 2011.
2. Guy A, et al. Angioedema in Emergency Medicine. © 1994–2011 WebMD. URL: http://emedicine.medscape.com/article/756261-overview. Accessed summer 2011.
3. Johnson R, et al. Anaphylactic Shock: Pathophysiology, Recognition, and Treatment. Seminars in Respiratory and Critical Care Medicine 2004;25(6):695–703. © 2004 Thieme Medical Publishers. URL: http://www.medscape.com/viewarticle/497498_3. Accessed summer 2011.
4. Multiple Chemical Sensitivities. U.S. Department of Labor Occupational Safety & Health Administration. URL: http://www.osha.gov/SLTC/multiplechemicalsensitivities/index.html. Accessed summer 2011.
5. Multiple Chemical Sensitivity. © 1994–2011 WebMD. URL: http://www.webmd.com/allergies/multiple-chemical-sensitivity?print=true. Accessed summer 2011.
6. Tips to Remember. © American Academy of Allergy, Asthma & Immunology. URL: http://www.aaaai.org/patients/publicedmat/tips/whatisallergicreaction.stm. Accessed summer 2011.

Ankylosing Spondylitis

1. Ankylosing Spondylitis. © 1998–2011 Mayo Foundation for Medical Education and Research. URL: http://www.mayoclinic.com/health/ankylosing-spondylitis/DS00483. Accessed summer 2011.
2. Ankylosing Spondylitis. © Arthritis Foundation. URL: http://www.arthritis.org/disease-center.php?disease_id=2&df=definition. Accessed summer 2011.
3. Ankylosing Spondylitis. National Institute of Arthritis and Musculoskeletal and Skin Diseases. URL: http://www.niams.nih.gov/health_info/Ankylosing_Spondylitis/default.asp. Accessed summer 2011.
4. Brent L, et al. Ankylosing Spondylitis and Undifferentiated Spondyloarthropathy. © 1994–2011 WebMD. URL: http://emedicine.medscape.com/article/332945-overview#showall. Accessed summer 2011.
5. Chunco R. The Effects of Massage on Pain, Stiffness, and Fatigue Levels Associated with Ankylosing Spondylitis: A Case Study. International Journal of Therapeutic Massage and Bodywork. URL: http://www.ijtmb.org/index.php/ijtmb/article/view/118/155. Accessed summer 2011.

Chronic Fatigue Syndrome

1. Chronic Fatigue Syndrome (CFS). Centers for Disease Control and Prevention. URL: http://www.cdc.gov/cfs/general/symptoms/index.html. Accessed summer 2011.
2. Chronic Fatigue Syndrome (CFS). Centers for Disease Control and Prevention. URL: http://www.cdc.gov/cfs/general/causes/index.html. Accessed summer 2011.
3. Chronic Fatigue Syndrome: General Information Treatment for CFS. Centers for Disease Control and Prevention. URL: http://www.cdc.gov/cfs/general/treatment/index.html. Accessed summer 2011.
4. Chronic Fatigue Syndrome: General Information. Centers for Disease Control and Prevention. URL: http://www.cdc.gov/cfs/general/index.html. Accessed summer 2011.
5. Cunha B, et al. Chronic Fatigue Syndrome. © 1994–2011 WebMD. URL: http://emedicine.medscape.com/article/235980-overview#showall. Accessed summer 2011.
6. Fukuda K, et al. The Chronic Fatigue Syndrome: A Comprehensive Approach to its Definition and Study. © The CFIDS Association of America, Inc. URL: http://www.cfids.org/about-cfids/case-definition.asp. Accessed summer 2011.
7. Hitt E. Chronic Fatigue Syndrome Not Linked to XMRV. © 1994–2011 WebMD. URL: http://www.medscape.com/viewarticle/741121. Accessed summer 2011.
8. Shiel W. Chronic Fatigue Syndrome (CFS). © 1994–2011 WebMD. URL: http://www.emedicinehealth.com/chronic_fatigue_syndrome/article_em.htm. Accessed summer 2011.

Crohn Disease

1. About Crohn's Disease. © 2009 Crohn's & Colitis Foundation of America. URL: http://www.ccfa.org/info/about/crohns. Accessed summer 2011.
2. Achkar J. Inflammatory Bowel Disease. © 2011 American College of Gastroenterology. URL: http://www.acg.gi.org/patients/gihealth/ibd.asp. Accessed summer 2011.

3. Crohn's disease. © 1997–2011 A.D.A.M., Inc. URL: http://www.nlm.nih.gov/medlineplus/ency/article/000249.htm. Accessed summer 2011.
4. Crohn's disease. © 1998–2011 Mayo Foundation for Medical Education and Research. URL: http://www.mayoclinic.com/health/crohns-disease/DS00104. Accessed summer 2011.
5. Crohn's disease. National Institute of Diabetes and Digestive and Kidney Diseases. URL: http://digestive.niddk.nih.gov/ddiseases/pubs/crohns/. Accessed summer 2011.
6. Rowe W, et al. Inflammatory Bowel Disease. © 1994–2011 WebMD. URL: http://emedicine.medscape.com/article/179037-overview#showall. Accessed summer 2011.
7. Rowe W, et al. Inflammatory Bowel Disease. © 1994–2011 WebMD. URL: http://www.emedicinehealth.com/inflammatory_bowel_disease/article_em.htm. Accessed summer 2011.

Edema

1. Edema Overview. © 1994–2011 WebMD. URL: http://www.webmd.com/heart-disease/heart-failure/edema-overview. Accessed summer 2011.
2. Edema. © 1995–2009 The Cleveland Clinic Foundation. URL: http://my.clevelandclinic.org/disorders/edema/hic_edema.aspx. Accessed summer 2011.
3. Edema. © 1998–2011 Mayo Foundation for Medical Research and Education. URL: http://www.mayoclinic.com/health/edema/DS01035. Accessed summer 2011.

Fever

1. Dalal S, et al. Pathophysiology and Management of Fever. The Journal of Supportive Oncology. http://d.yimg.com/kq/groups/15854266/652670728/name/feb+neu+2.pdf. Accessed summer 2011.
2. Davis C. Fever in Adults. © 1994–2011 WebMD. URL: http://www.emedicinehealth.com/fever_in_adults/article_em.htm. Accessed summer 2011.
3. Fever. U.S. National Library of Medicine. URL: http://www.nlm.nih.gov/medlineplus/ency/article/003090.htm. Accessed summer 2011.

HIV AIDS

1. Biological Catch-22 Prevents Induction of Antibodies that Block HIV. Duke University Medical Center. URL: http://www.sciencedaily.com/releases/2009/12/091215102105.htm. Accessed summer 2011.
2. Estimates of New HIV Infections in the United States. Centers for Disease Control and Prevention. URL: http://www.cdc.gov/hiv/topics/surveillance/resources/factsheets/pdf/incidence.pdf. Accessed summer 2011.
3. HIV Drug Resistance. World Health Organization. URL: http://www.who.int/hiv/facts/WHD2011-HIVdr-fs-final.pdf. Accessed summer 2011.
4. Human immunodeficiency virus (HIV). © 1994–2011 Edward C. Klatt MD. URL: http://library.med.utah.edu/WebPath/TUTORIAL/AIDS/HIV.html. Accessed summer 2011.
5. Kennedy R. HIV AIDS. © 2011 The Doctors' Medical Library. URL: http://www.medical-library.net/hiv_aids.html. Accessed summer 2011.
6. Kennedy R. HIV AIDS. © 2011 The Doctors' Medical Library. URL: http://www.medical-library.net/hiv_aids.html. Accessed summer 2011.
7. Mohammed I, et al. The Pathophysiology and Clinical Manifestations of HIV/AIDS. AIDS in Nigeria. URL: http://www.apin.harvard.edu/Chapter6.pdf. Accessed summer 2011.
8. Tuberculosis and HIV. © WHO 2011. URL: http://www.who.int/hiv/topics/tb/en/index.html. Accessed summer 2011.

Lupus

1. Bartels C, et al. Systemic Lupus Erythematosus. © 1994–2011 WebMD. URL: http://emedicine.medscape.com/article/332244-overview#showall. Accessed summer 2011.
2. Hoffman R, et al. Mixed Connective-Tissue Disease. © 1994–2010 Medscape. URL: http://emedicine.medscape.com/article/335815-overview. Accessed summer 2011.
3. Lupus. National Institute of Arthritis and Musculoskeletal and Skin Diseases. URL: http://www.niams.nih.gov/Health_Info/Lupus/default.asp. Accessed summer 2011.
4. Mixed Connective Tissue Disease. © 1998–2010 Mayo Foundation for Medical Education and Research. URL: http://www.nlm.nih.gov/medlineplus/connectivetissuedisorders.html. Accessed summer 2011.
5. Schwartz R, et al. Mixed Connective Tissue Disease. © 1994–2010 Medscape. URL: http://emedicine.medscape.com/article/1066445-overview. Accessed summer 2011.
6. Systemic Lupus Erythematosus. © 2011 A.D.A.M. URL: http://www.ncbi.nlm.nih.gov/pubmedhealth/PMH0001471/. Accessed summer 2011.
7. Understanding Lupus. © 2011 Lupus Foundation of America, Inc. URL: http://www.lupus.org/webmodules/webarticlesnet/templates/new_learnunderstanding.aspx?articleid=2231&zoneid=523. Accessed summer 2011.

Lymphangitis

1. Erysipelas Cellulitis Lymphangitis. National Center for Emergency Medical Informatics. URL: http://www.ncemi.org/cse/cse1111.htm. Accessed summer 2011.
2. Lymphangitis. © 2011 A.D.A.M., Inc. URL: http://www.ncbi.nlm.nih.gov/pubmedhealth/PMH0004551/. Accessed summer 2011.
3. Pitetti R, et al. Lymphangitis. © 1994–2011 WebMD. URL: http://emedicine.medscape.com/article/966003-overview. Accessed summer 2011.

Lymphoma

1. Adult Hodgkin Lymphoma Treatment (PDQ®). National Cancer Institute. URL: http://www.cancer.gov/cancertopics/pdq/treatment/adulthodgkins/Patient/AllPages. Accessed summer 2011.
2. Balentine J, et al. Lymphoma. © 1994–2011 WebMD, LLC. URL: http://www.emedicinehealth.com/lymphoma/article_em.htm. Accessed summer 2011.

3. Burkitt Lymphoma. © 1997–2011 A.D.A.M., Inc. URL: URL of this page: http://www.nlm.nih.gov/medlineplus/ency/article/001308.htm. Accessed summer 2011.
4. Gajra A, et al. Lymphoma, B-Cell. © 1994–2011 WebMD. URL: http://emedicine.medscape.com/article/202677-overview. Accessed summer 2011.
5. Hodgkin Lymphoma. © 2010 Lymphoma Research Foundation. URL: http://www.lymphoma.org/site/pp.asp?c=chKOI6PEImE&b=1574105. Accessed summer 2011.
6. Integrative Medicine & Complementary and Alternative Therapies as Part of Blood Cancer Care. The Leukemia & Lymphoma Society. URL: http://www.lls.org/content/nationalcontent/resourcecenter/freeeducationmaterials/treatments/pdf/integrativemedicinecamtherapies.pdf. Accessed summer 2011.
7. What You Need To Know About Hodgkin Lymphoma. National Cancer Institute. URL: http://www.cancer.gov/cancertopics/wyntk/hodgkin/AllPages. Accessed summer 2011.
8. What You Need To Know About Non-Hodgkin Lymphoma. National Cancer Institute. URL: http://www.cancer.gov/cancertopics/wyntk/non-hodgkin-lymphoma/AllPages. Accessed summer 2011.

Mononucleosis

1. Cunha B, et al. Infectious Mononucleosis. © 1994–2011 WebMD. URL: http://emedicine.medscape.com/article/222040-overview#showall. Accessed summer 2011.
2. Doerr S, et al. Mononucleosis (Mono). © 1994–2011 WebMD. URL: http://www.emedicinehealth.com/script/main/art.asp?articlekey=58850&pf=3&page=1. Accessed summer 2011.
3. Epstein-Barr Virus and Infectious Mononucleosis. National Center for Infectious Diseases. URL: http://www.cdc.gov/ncidod/diseases/ebv.htm. Accessed summer 2011.
4. Mononucleosis. © 1995–2009 The Cleveland Clinic Foundation. URL: http://my.clevelandclinic.org/disorders/mononucleosis/hic_overview.aspx. Accessed summer 2011.
5. Mononucleosis. © 1998–2011 Mayo Foundation for Medical Education and Research. URL: http://www.mayoclinic.com/health/mononucleosis/DS00352. Accessed summer 2011.

Multiple Sclerosis

1. Goodin, et al. Disease Modifying Therapies in Multiple Sclerosis. Report of the Therapeutics and Technology Assessment Subcommittee of the American Academy of Neurology and the MS Council for Clinical Practice Guidelines. URL: http://advocacyforpatients.org/pdf/ms/ms_aan.pdf. Accessed summer 2011.
2. Luzzio C, et al. Multiple Sclerosis. © 1994–2011 WebMD. URL: http://emedicine.medscape.com/article/1146199-overview. Accessed summer 2011.
3. Multiple Sclerosis. © 2011 A.D.A.M., Inc. URL: http://www.ncbi.nlm.nih.gov/pubmedhealth/PMH0001747/. Accessed summer 2011.
4. Multiple Sclerosis: Hope Through Research. National Institute of Neurological Disorders and Stroke. URL: http://www.ninds.nih.gov/disorders/multiple_sclerosis/detail_multiple_sclerosis.htm. Accessed summer 2011.
5. Multiple Sclerosis: Just the Facts. © 2010 National MS Society. URL: www.nationalmssociety.org/download.aspx?id=22. Accessed summer 2011.
6. What is Multiple Sclerosis. © 2010 National Multiple Sclerosis Society. URL: http://www.nationalmssociety.org/about-multiple-sclerosis/index.aspx. Accessed summer 2011.

Myasthenia Gravis

1. Clinical Overview of MG. © 2010 Myasthenia Gravis Foundation of America, Inc. URL: http://www.myasthenia.org/HealthProfessionals/ClinicalOverviewofMG.aspx. Accessed summer 2011.
2. Congenital Myasthenia. © 2010 Myasthenia Gravis Foundation of America, Inc. URL: http://www.myasthenia.org/LinkClick.aspx?fileticket=7X4UXeybJH4%3d&tabid=84. Accessed summer 2011.
3. Facts About Autoimmune Myasthenia Gravis for Patients and Families. © 2010 Myasthenia Gravis Foundation of America, Inc. URL: http://www.myasthenia.org/LinkClick.aspx?fileticket=PNk_GqQc0Ws%3d&tabid=84. Accessed summer 2011.
4. Goldenberg W, et al. Myasthenia Gravis in Emergency Medicine. © 1994–2011 WebMD. URL: http://emedicine.medscape.com/article/793136-overview#showall. Accessed summer 2011.
5. Myasthenia Gravis Fact Sheet. National Institute of Neurological Disorders and Stroke. URL: http://www.ninds.nih.gov/disorders/myasthenia_gravis/detail_myasthenia_gravis.htm. Accessed summer 2011.
6. Myasthenia Gravis. © A.D.A.M., Inc. URL: http://www.ncbi.nlm.nih.gov/pubmedhealth/PMH0001731/. Accessed summer 2011.

Polymyalgia Rheumatica

1. Polymyalgia Rheumatica and Giant Cell Arthritis. National Institute of Arthritis and Musculoskeletal and Skin Diseases. URL: http://www.niams.nih.gov/Health_Info/Polymyalgia/default.asp. Accessed summer 2011.
2. Polymyalgia Rheumatica. © 1998–2010 Mayo Foundation for Medical Education and Research. URL: http://www.mayoclinic.com/health/polymyalgia-rheumatica/DS00441. Accessed summer 2011.
3. Saad E, et al. Polymyalgia Rheumatica. © 1994–2010 Medscape. URL: http://emedicine.medscape.com/article/330815-overview. Accessed summer 2011.

Rheumatoid Arthritis

1. Miller M, et al. Juvenile Rheumatoid Arthritis. © 1994–2011 WebMD, LLC. URL: http://www.emedicinehealth.com/juvenile_rheumatoid_arthritis/article_em.htm. Accessed summer 2011.
2. Rheumatoid Arthritis. © 2011 A.D.A.M., Inc. URL: http://www.ncbi.nlm.nih.gov/pubmedhealth/PMH0001467/. Accessed summer 2011.

3. Rheumatoid Arthritis. National Institute of Arthritis and Musculoskeletal and Skin Diseases. URL: http://www.niams.nih.gov/Health_Info/Rheumatic_Disease/default.asp
4. Shiel W, et al. Rheumatoid Arthritis. © 1994–2011 WebMD. URL: http://www.emedicinehealth.com/rheumatoid_arthritis/article_em.htm. Accessed summer 2011.
5. Temprano K, et al. Rheumatoid Arthritis. © 1994–2011 Mescape. URL: http://emedicine.medscape.com/article/331715-overview#showall. Accessed summer 2011.
6. What People With Rheumatoid Arthritis Need to Know About Osteoporosis. National Institute of Arthritis and Musculoskeletal and Skin Diseases. URL: http://www.niams.nih.gov/Health_Info/Bone/Osteoporosis/Conditions_Behaviors/osteoporosis_ra.asp. Accessed summer 2011.

Scleroderma

1. Jimenez S, et al. Scleroderma. © 1994–2011 WebMD LLC. URL: http://emedicine.medscape.com/article/331864-overview#showall. Accessed summer 2011.
2. Scleroderma. © A.D.A.M., Inc. URL: http://www.ncbi.nlm.nih.gov/pubmedhealth/PMH0001465/. Accessed summer 2011.
3. Scleroderma. National Institute of Arthritis and Musculoskeletal and Skin Diseases. URL: http://www.niams.nih.gov/Health_Info/Scleroderma/default.asp. Accessed summer 2011.
4. What is Scleroderma? Copyright © 2001–2011 Scleroderma Foundation URL: http://www.scleroderma.org/medical/overview.shtm. Accessed summer 2011.
5. Your Medications: A Guide to Better Understanding. Copyright © 2001–2011 Scleroderma Foundation. URL: http://www.scleroderma.org/medical/medication.shtm. Accessed summer 2011.

Ulcerative Colitis

1. About Ulcerative Colitis and Proctitis. © 2008 Crohn's and Colitis Foundation of America. URL: http://www.ccfa.org/info/about/ucp. Accessed summer 2011.
2. Achkar J. Inflammatory Bowel Disease. © 2011 American College of Gastroenterology. URL: http://www.acg.gi.org/patients/gihealth/ibd.asp. Accessed summer 2011.
3. Basson M, et al. Ulcerative Colitis. © 1994–2011 WebMD. URL: http://emedicine.medscape.com/article/183084-overview#showall. Accessed summer 2011.
4. Rowe W, et al. Inflammatory Bowel Disease. © 1994–2011 WebMD. URL: http://emedicine.medscape.com/article/179037-overview#showall. Accessed summer 2011.
5. Rowe W, et al. Inflammatory Bowel Disease. © 1994–2011 WebMD. URL: http://www.emedicinehealth.com/inflammatory_bowel_disease/article_em.htm. Accessed summer 2011.
6. Ulcerative Colitis. © 2008 American Society of Colon & Rectal Surgeons. URL: http://www.fascrs.org/patients/conditions/ulcerative_colitis/. Accessed summer 2011.
7. Ulcerative Colitis. National Institute of Diabetes and Digestive and Kidney Diseases. URL: http://digestive.niddk.nih.gov/ddiseases/pubs/colitis/. Accessed summer 2011.

Chapter 7

Acute Bronchitis

1. Acute Bronchitis. © 2001–2011 American Academy of Family Physicians. URL: http://www.nlm.nih.gov/medlineplus/acutebronchitis.html. Accessed summer 2011.
2. Bronchitis (Chest Cold). Centers for Disease Control and Prevention. URL: http://www.cdc.gov/getsmart/antibiotic-use/URI/bronchitis.html. Accessed summer 2011.
3. Bronchitis. Copyright © 2011, A.D.A.M., Inc. URL: http://www.ncbi.nlm.nih.gov/pubmedhealth/PMH0002078/. Accessed summer 2011.
4. Fayyaz J, et al. Bronchitis. © 1994–2011 WebMD LLC. URL: http://emedicine.medscape.com/article/297108-overview#showall. Accessed summer 2011.

Asthma

1. Asthma in Adults Fact Sheet. © 2011 American Lung Association. URL: http://www.lungusa.org/lung-disease/asthma/resources/facts-and-figures/asthma-in-adults.html. Accessed summer 2011.
2. Asthma. © The Ohio State University Medical Center. URL: http://medicalcenter.osu.edu/patientcare/healthcare_services/lung_diseases/lung/asthma/Pages/index.aspx. Accessed summer 2011.
3. Asthma. National Heart Lung and Blood Institute. URL: http://www.nhlbi.nih.gov/health/dci/Diseases/Asthma/Asthma_All.html. Accessed summer 2011.
4. Guill M. Asthma Update: Epidemiology and Pathophysiology. Pediatrics in Review 2004;25(9). URL: http://hsc.unm.edu/emermed/ped/physicians/residents/articles/Asthma%20Update%20Epidemiology%20and%20Pathophysiology.pdf. Accessed summer 2011.
5. Morris M, et al. Asthma. © 1994–2011 WebMD LLC. URL: http://emedicine.medscape.com/article/296301-overview#showall. Accessed summer 2011.
6. Pathophysiology of Asthma. © 2011 Cygnus Interactive. URL: http://www.emsworld.com/print/EMS-World/Pathophysiology-of-Asthma/1$2257. Accessed summer 2011.

Chronic Bronchitis

1. Chronic Bronchitis. © The Ohio State University Medical Center. URL: http://medicalcenter.osu.edu/patientcare/healthcare_services/lung_diseases/lung/bronchitis/Pages/index.aspx. Accessed summer 2011.
2. COPD. National Institutes of Health Senior Health. URL: http://nihseniorhealth.gov/copd/toc.html. Accessed summer 2011.
3. What is Chronic Bronchitis. © 2011 American Lung Association. URL: http://www.lungusa.org/lung-disease/bronchitis-chronic/understanding-chronic-bronchitis.html. Accessed summer 2011.

Common Cold

1. Common Cold and Runny Nose. Centers for Disease Control and Prevention. URL: http://www.cdc.gov/

getsmart/antibiotic-use/URI/colds.html. Accessed summer 2011.

2. Common Cold. © 1998–2011 Mayo Foundation for Medical Education and Research. URL: http://www.mayoclinic.com/health/common-cold/DS00056. Accessed summer 2011.
3. Common Cold. © The Ohio State University Medical Center. URL: http://medicalcenter.osu.edu/patientcare/healthcare_services/lung_diseases/cold/pages/index.aspx. Accessed summer 2011.
4. Common Cold. National Institute of Allergy and Infectious Diseases. URL: http://www.niaid.nih.gov/Pages/default.aspx. Accessed summer 2011.
5. What a Common Cold is. © 1999–2007 Commoncold, Inc. URL: http://www.commoncold.org/undrstn4.htm. Accessed summer 2011.

Cystic Fibrosis

1. Cystic Fibrosis. Genetics Home Reference, National Library of Medicine. URL: http://ghr.nlm.nih.gov/condition/cystic-fibrosis. Accessed summer 2011.
2. Frequently Asked Questions. © 2011 Cystic Fibrosis Foundation. URL: http://www.cff.org/AboutCF/Faqs/. Accessed summer 2011.
3. Sharma G. Cystic Fibrosis. © 1994–2011 WebMD LLC. URL: http://emedicine.medscape.com/article/1001602-overview#showall. Accessed summer 2011.
4. Understanding Cystic Fibrosis. © 2011 American Lung Association. URL: http://www.lungusa.org/lung-disease/cystic-fibrosis/. Accessed summer 2011.
5. What Is Cystic Fibrosis. National Heart Lung and Blood Institute. URL: http://www.nhlbi.nih.gov/health/dci/Diseases/cf/cf_all.html. Accessed summer 2011.

Emphysema

1. Chronic Obstructive Pulmonary Disease (COPD) Fact Sheet. © 2011 American Lung Association. URL: http://www.lungusa.org/lung-disease/copd/resources/in-depth-resources.html. Accessed summer 2011.
2. Chronic Obstructive Pulmonary Disease. © 2011 A.D.A.M., Inc. URL: http://www.ncbi.nlm.nih.gov/pubmedhealth/PMH0001153/. Accessed summer 2011.
3. Demirjian B, et al. Emphysema. © 2004–2011 WebMD LLC. URL: http://emedicine.medscape.com/article/298283-overview#showall. Accessed summer 2011.
4. Pulmonary Emphysema. © The Ohio State University Medical Center. URL: http://medicalcenter.osu.edu/patientcare/healthcare_services/lung_diseases/lung/emphysema/Pages/index.aspx. Accessed summer 2011.
5. What is COPD. National Heart Lung and Blood Institute. URL: http://www.nhlbi.nih.gov/health/dci/Diseases/Copd/Copd_All.html. Accessed summer 2011.

Influenza

1. 2009 H1N1 Flue ("Swine Flu") and You. Centers for Disease Control and Prevention. URL: http://www.cdc.gov/h1n1flu/qa.htm. Accessed summer 2011.
2. About the Flu. U.S. Department of Health & Human Services. URL: http://www.flu.gov/individualfamily/about/index.html. Accessed summer 2011.
3. Avian Influenza (Bird Flu). U.S. Department of Health & Human Services. URL: http://www.pandemicflu.gov/general/avian.html. Accessed summer 2011.
4. Key Facts about Influenza (Flue) & Flu Vaccine. Centers for Disease Control and Prevention. URL: http://www.cdc.gov/flu/keyfacts.htm. Accessed summer 2011.
5. Seasonal Influenza (Flu). Centers for Disease Control and Prevention. URL: http://www.cdc.gov/flu/about/disease/symptoms.htm. Accessed summer 2011.

Laryngeal Cancer

1. Fact Sheet: Laryngeal (Voice Box) Cancer. © 2010 American Academy of Otolaryngology—Head and Neck Surgery. URL: http://www.entnet.org/HealthInformation/laryngealCancer.cfm. Accessed summer 2011.
2. Johnson J, et al. Malignant Tumors of the Larynx. Copyright © 1994–2011 by WebMD LLC. URL: http://emedicine.medscape.com/article/848592-overview#showall. Accessed summer 2011.
3. Throat Cancer. © 1998–2010 Mayo Foundation for Medical Education and research. URL: http://www.mayoclinic.com/health/oral-and-throat-cancer/DS00349. Accessed summer 2011.
4. What You Need to Know About Cancer of the Larynx. National Cancer Institute. URL: http://www.cancer.gov/cancertopics/wyntk/larynx. Accessed summer 2011.

Lung Cancer

1. Lung Cancer 101: About Lung Cancer. © 2011 Cancer Care, Inc. URL: http://www.lungcancer.org/reading/. Accessed summer 2011.
2. Lung Cancer Fact Sheet. © 2011 American Lung Association. URL: http://www.lungusa.org/lung-disease/lung-cancer/resources/facts-figures/lung-cancer-fact-sheet.html. Accessed summer 2011.
3. Lung Cancer Statistics. Centers for Disease Control and Prevention. URL: http://www.cdc.gov/cancer/lung/statistics/index.htm. Accessed summer 2011.
4. Stevenson M, et al. Small Cell Lung Cancer Staging. Copyright © 1994–2011 by WebMD LLC. URL: http://emedicine.medscape.com/article/2006716-overview. Accessed summer 2011.
5. Stöppler M, et al. Lung Cancer. © 2011 WebMD LLC. URL: http://www.emedicinehealth.com/script/main/art.asp?articlekey=58829&pf=3&page=1. Accessed summer 2011.
6. What You Need To Know About Lung Cancer. National Cancer Institute. URL: http://www.cancer.gov/cancertopics/wyntk/lung. Accessed summer 2011.

Pleurisy

1. Pleurisy—Overview. © 1995–2010 Healthwise, Incorporated. URL: http://www.webmd.com/lung/tc/pleurisy-overview. Accessed summer 2011.
2. Pleurisy. © 2011 Mayo Foundation for Medical Education and Research. URL: http://www.mayoclinic.com/health/pleurisy/DS00244. Accessed summer 2011.

3. Schiffman G. Pleurisy (Pleuritis). © 2010 MedicineNet, Inc. URL: http://www.medicinenet.com/script/main/art.asp?articlekey=19782. Accessed summer 2011.

Pneumonia

1. Kamangar N. Bacterial Pneumonia. © 1994–2011 WebMD LLC. URL: http://emedicine.medscape.com/article/300157-overview. Accessed summer 2011.
2. Mosenifer Z. Viral Pneumonia. © 1994–2011 WebMD LLC. URL: http://emedicine.medscape.com/article/300455-overview. Accessed summer 2011.
3. Pneumonia Can Be Prevented—Vaccines Can Help. Centers for Disease Control and Prevention. URL: http://www.cdc.gov/Features/Pneumonia/. Accessed summer 2011.
4. Pneumonia. © 1995–2011 The Cleveland Clinic Foundation. URL: http://my.clevelandclinic.org/disorders/Pneumonia/hic_Pneumonia.aspx. Accessed summer 2011.
5. Understanding Pneumonia. © 2011 American Lung Association. URL: http://www.lungusa.org/lung-disease/pneumonia/. Accessed summer 2011.

Sinusitis

1. Becker D, et al. Allergic and Non-Allergic Sinusitis for the Primary Care Physician: Pathophysiology, Evaluation and Treatment. Copyright © 2110, Daniel G. Becker, MD and Samual S. Becker, MD. URL: http://www.noseandsinus.com/book10.pdf. Accessed summer 2011.
2. Pfaar O. et al. Pathophysiology of itching and sneezing in allergic rhinitis. Swiss Medical Weekly 2009;139(3–4):35–40. URL: http://www.smw.ch/docs/PdfContent/smw-12468.pdf. Accessed summer 2011.
3. Radojicic C. Sinusitis. © 2000–2011 The Cleveland Clinic Foundation. URL: http://www.clevelandclinicmeded.com/medicalpubs/diseasemanagement/allergy/rhino-sinusitis/. Accessed summer 2011.
4. Sinus Infection. © 2005–2007 WebMD Inc. URL: http://www.webmd.com/allergies/sinus-infection. Accessed summer 2011.
5. Sinusitis. © 2011 A.D.A.M., Inc. URL: http://www.ncbi.nlm.nih.gov/pubmedhealth/PMH0001670/. Accessed summer 2011.
6. Tips to Remember: Sinusitis. © 2010 American Academy of Allergy, Asthma & Immunology. URL: http://www.aaaai.org/patients/publicedmat/tips/sinusitis.stm. Accessed summer 2011.

Tuberculosis

1. Extensively Drug-Resistant Tuberculosis (XDR TB). Centers for Disease Control and Prevention. URL: http://www.cdc.gov/tb/publications/factsheets/drtb/xdrtb.pdf. Accessed summer 2011.
2. Multidrug-Resistant Tuberculosis (MDR TB). Centers for Disease Control and Prevention. URL: http://www.cdc.gov/tb/publications/factsheets/drtb/MDRTB.pdf. Accessed summer 2011.
3. Mycobacterium tuberculosis and Tuberculosis. © 2011 Todar K. URL: http://textbookofbacteriology.net/themicrobialworld/tuberculosis.html. Accessed summer 2011.
4. Questions and Answers About Tuberculosis 2009. U.S. Department of Health and Human Services, Centers for Disease Control and Prevention. URL: http://www.cdc.gov/tb/publications/faqs/pdfs/qa.pdf. Accessed summer 2011
5. Tuberculosis. © 2011 World Health Organization. URL: http://www.who.int/mediacentre/factsheets/fs104/en/. Accessed summer 2011.
6. Tuberculosis: General Information. Centers for Disease Control and Prevention. URL: http://www.cdc.gov/tb/publications/factsheets/general/tb.htm. Accessed summer 2011.

Chapter 8

Candidiasis

1. Candidiasis. Centers for Disease Control and Prevention. URL: http://www.cdc.gov/nczved/divisions/dfbmd/diseases/candidiasis/index.html. Accessed summer 2011.
2. Hidalgo J. Candidiasis. © 1994–2011 WebMD LLC. URL: http://emedicine.medscape.com/article/213853-overview#showall. Accessed summer 2011.
3. Kessel K, et al. Common Complementary and Alternative Therapies for Yeast Vaginitis and Bacterial Vaginosis: A Systematic Review. © 2003 Lippincott Williams & Wilkins, Inc.
4. Khan MS, et al. Anti-Candidal Activity of Essential Oils Alone and in Combination with Amphotericin B or Fluconazole Against Multi-Drug Resistant Isolates of *Candida albicans*. National Center for Biotechnology Information, U.S. National Library of Medicine. URL: http://www.ncbi.nlm.nih.gov/pubmed/21756200. Accessed summer 2011.
5. St. Ãppler M. Candidiasis (Yeast Infection). © 2011 WebMD, LLC. URL: http://www.emedicinehealth.com/script/main/art.asp?articlekey=58847&pf=3&page=1. Accessed summer 2011.

Celiac Disease

1. Brooks M. Celiac Disease Diagnosis Up 4-Fold Worldwide. © 2010 WebMD, LLC. URL: http://www.medscape.com/viewarticle/726127. Accessed summer 2011.
2. Celiac Disease–Sprue. © 2011 A.D.A.M., Inc. URL: http://www.ncbi.nlm.nih.gov/pubmedhealth/PMH0001280/. Accessed summer 2011.
3. Celiac Disease. © 1998–2011 Celiac Disease Foundation (CDF). URL: http://www.celiac.org/index.php?option=com_content&view=article&id=3&Itemid=9. Accessed summer 2011.
4. Celiac Disease. National Institute of Diabetes and Digestive and Kidney Diseases. URL: http://digestive.niddk.nih.gov/ddiseases/pubs/celiac/index.htm. Accessed summer 2011.

Cirrhosis

1. Cirrhosis. © 2002–2011 The Regents of The University of California. URL: http://www.ucsfhealth.org/conditions/cirrhosis/. Accessed summer 2011.

2. Cirrhosis. © 2011 American Liver Foundation. URL: http://www.liverfoundation.org/abouttheliver/info/cirrhosis/. Accessed summer 2011.
3. Cirrhosis. National Digestive Diseases Information Clearinghouse (NDDIC). URL: http://digestive.niddk.nih.gov/ddiseases/pubs/cirrhosis/. Accessed summer 2011.
4. NAFLD: Non-Alcoholic Fatty Liver Disease. © 2011 American Liver Foundation. URL: http://www.liverfoundation.org/abouttheliver/info/nafld/. Accessed summer 2011.
5. Niederau C. NAFLD and NASH. © Mauss (ed.) Hepatology 2010 (free textbook)URL: http://www.hepatologytextbook.com/hep_chapt25.pdf. Accessed summer 2011.
6. Wolf D. Cirrhosis. © 1994–2011 WebMD, LLC. URL: http://emedicine.medscape.com/article/185856-overview#showall. Accessed summer 2011.

Colorectal Cancer

1. Cagir B. Rectal Cancer. © 1994–2011 WebMD LLC. URL: http://emedicine.medscape.com/article/281237-overview#showall. Accessed summer 2011.
2. Colon and Rectum Cancer Staging. American Joint Committee on Cancer, American Cancer Society. URL: http://www.cancerstaging.org/staging/posters/colon8.5x11.pdf. Accessed summer 2011.
3. Colorectal Cancer Overview. © 2011 American Cancer Society. URL: http://www.cancer.org/acs/groups/cid/documents/webcontent/003047-pdf.pdf. Accessed summer 2011.
4. General Information About Colon Cancer. National Cancer Institute. URL: http://www.cancer.gov/cancertopics/pdq/treatment/colon/HealthProfessional. Accessed summer 2011.
5. What I need to know about Colon Polyps. National Digestive Diseases Information Clearinghouse (NDDIC). URL: http://digestive.niddk.nih.gov/ddiseases/pubs/colonpolyps_ez/. Accessed summer 2011.
6. What You Need To Know About Cancer of the Colon and Rectum. National Cancer Institute. URL: http://www.cancer.gov/cancertopics/wyntk/colon-and-rectal/AllPages. Accessed summer 2011.

Diverticular Disease

1. Diverticular Disease. © 2009 American Society of Colon and Rectal Surgeons. URL: http://www.fascrs.org/patients/conditions/diverticular_disease/. Accessed summer 2011.
2. Diverticular Disease. © 2010 WebMD, LLC. URL: http://www.webmd.com/digestive-disorders/diverticular-disease. Accessed summer 2011.
3. Diverticular Disease. © The Ohio State University Medical Center. URL: http://medicalcenter.osu.edu/patientcare/healthcare_services/digestive_disorders/diverticular_disease/pages/index.aspx. Accessed summer 2011.
4. Hobson K, et al. Etiology and Pathophysiology of Diverticular Disease. © Theme Medical Publishers. URL: http://www.ncbi.nlm.nih.gov/pmc/articles/PMC2780060/. Accessed summer 2011.
5. Nguyen M. Diverticulitis. © 1994–2011 WebMD LLC. URL: http://emedicine.medscape.com/article/173388-overview#showall. Accessed summer 2011.
6. What I Need To Know About Diverticular Disease. National Digestive Diseases Information Clearing House (NDDIC). URL: http://digestive.niddk.nih.gov/ddiseases/pubs/diverticular/. Accessed summer 2011.

Esophageal Cancer

1. Absi A, et al. Esophageal cancer. © 2000–2011 The Cleveland Clinic Foundation. URL: http://www.clevelandclinicmeded.com/medicalpubs/diseasemanagement/hematology-oncology/esophageal-cancer/. Accessed summer 2011.
2. Esophageal Cancer. © 2007 American Cancer Society, Inc. URL: http://www.cancer.org/acs/groups/content/@nho/documents/document/esophagealcancerpdf.pdf. Accessed summer 2011.
3. Herbella F. Esophageal Cancer. © 1994–2011 WebMD LLC. URL: http://emedicine.medscape.com/article/277930-overview#showall. Accessed summer 2011.
4. Rhodes T. Esophageal Cancer Staging. © 1994–2011 WebMD LLC. URL: http://emedicine.medscape.com/article/2003224-overview. Accessed summer 2011.
5. What You Need To Know About Cancer of the Esophagus. National Cancer Institute. URL: http://www.cancer.gov/cancertopics/wyntk/esophagus. Accessed summer 2011.

Gallstones

1. Dieting and Gallstones. Weight-control Information Network. URL: http://win.niddk.nih.gov/publications/gallstones.htm#safely. Accessed summer 2011.
2. Gallstones. © 2000–2011 American Academy of Family Physicians. URL: http://familydoctor.org/online/famdocen/home/common/digestive/disorders/555.printerview.html. Accessed summer 2011.
3. Gallstones. © 2011 A.D.A.M., Inc. URL: http://www.ncbi.nlm.nih.gov/pubmedhealth/PMH0001318/. Accessed summer 2011.
4. Heuman D. Cholelithiasis. © 1994–2011 WebMD LLC. URL: http://emedicine.medscape.com/article/175667-overview#showall. Accessed summer 2011.
5. Understanding Gallstones. © 2011 American Gastroenterological Association. URL: http://www.gastro.org/patient-center/digestive-conditions/gallstones. Accessed summer 2011.

Gastroenteritis

1. Diskin A. Gastroenteritis in Emergency Medicine. © 1994–2011 WebMD LLC. URL: http://emedicine.medscape.com/article/775277-overview#showall. Accessed summer 2011.
2. Viral Gastroenteritis. National Center for Immunization and Respiratory Diseases. URL: http://www.cdc.gov/ncidod/dvrd/revb/gastro/faq.htm. Accessed summer 2011.
3. Viral Gastroenteritis. National Institute of Diabetes and Digestive and Kidney Diseases. URL: http://digestive.niddk.nih.gov/ddiseases/pubs/viralgastroenteritis/. Accessed summer 2011.
4. Wedro B. Gastroenteritis (Stomach Flu). © 2011 WebMD LLC. URL: http://www.emedicinehealth.com/script/main/art.asp?articlekey=59278&pf=3&page=1#Prevention. Accessed summer 2011.

Gastroesophageal Reflux Disease

1. Azodo I, et al. Barrett's Esophagus. © 2011 American College of Gastroenterology. URL: http://www.acg.gi.org/patients/gihealth/barretts.asp. Accessed summer 2011.
2. Gastroesophageal Reflux Disease. © 2011 A.D.A.M., Inc. URL: http://www.ncbi.nlm.nih.gov/pubmedhealth/PMH0001311/. Accessed summer 2011.
3. Heartburn, Gastroesophageal Reflux (GER), and Gastroesophageal Reflux Disease (GERD). National Digestive Diseases Information Clearinghouse (NDDIC). URL: http://digestive.niddk.nih.gov/ddiseases/pubs/gerd/. Accessed summer 2011.
4. O'Malley P. Pathophysiology of GERD and Ulcer Disease. © 2003 Lippincott Williams & Wilkins. URL: http://www.medscape.com/viewarticle/465049_2. Accessed summer 2011.
5. Reflux or GERD. NIH Office of Communications. URL: http://newsinhealth.nih.gov/issue/apr2011/feature2. Accessed summer 2011.
6. Simic J, et al. Gastroesophageal Reflux Disease (GERD). © 2011 WebMD LLC. URL: http://www.emedicinehealth.com/reflux_disease_gerd/article_em.htm. Accessed summer 2011.
7. Treatment of GERD. © 1998–2011 International Foundation for Functional Gastrointestinal Disorders, Inc. URL: http://www.aboutgerd.org/site/about-gerd/treatment/. Accessed summer 2011.

Hepatitis

1. Lenz J. Hepatitis A—Epidemiology, Transmission, and Natural History. Hepatology—A clinical textbook. Hepatology 2010. URL: http://www.hepatologytextbook.com/hep_chapt01.pdf. Accessed summer 2011.
2. Hepatitis A FAQs for Health Professionals. Centers for Disease Control and Prevention. URL: http://www.cdc.gov/hepatitis/HAV/HAVfaq.htm. Accessed summer 2011.
3. Hepatitis A. © 2011 WHO. URL: http://www.who.int/mediacentre/factsheets/fs328/en/index.html. Accessed summer 2011.
4. Hepatitis B FAQs for Health Professionals. Centers for Disease Control and Prevention. URL: http://www.cdc.gov/hepatitis/HBV/HBVfaq.htm. Accessed summer 2011.
5. Hepatitis B. © 2011 WHO. URL: http://www.who.int/mediacentre/factsheets/fs204/en/index.html. Accessed summer 2011.
6. Hepatitis C FAQs for Health Professionals. Centers for Disease Control and Prevention. URL: http://www.cdc.gov/hepatitis/HCV/HCVfaq.htm. Accessed summer 2011.
7. Hepatitis C. © 2011 WHO. URL: http://www.who.int/mediacentre/factsheets/fs164/en/index.html. Accessed summer 2011.
8. Jhaveri R. What's New in the Alphabet Soup of Viral Hepatitis: An Update on Hepatitis A and B in Kids. © 2011 WebMD, LLC. URL: http://www.medscape.com/viewarticle/743651?src=mp&spon=17. Accessed summer 2011.
9. Wasmuth J. Hepatitis B—Epidemiology, Transmission and Natural History. Hepatology—A Clinical Textbook. URL: http://www.hepatologytextbook.com/hep_chapt02.pdf. Accessed summer 2011.
10. Wasmuth J. Hepatitis C—Epidemiology, Transmission and Natural History. Hepatology—A Clinical Textbook. URL: http://www.hepatologytextbook.com/hep_chapt03.pdf. Accessed summer 2011.

Irritable Bowel Syndrome.

1. Diagnosis, Pathophysiology, and Treatment of Irritable Bowel Syndrome. © 1994–2011 Medscape LLC. URL: http://www.medscape.org/viewarticle/463481. Accessed summer 2011.
2. Freeman K. Irritable Bowel Syndrome. © 2000–2011 The Cleveland Clinic Foundation. URL: http://www.clevelandclinicmeded.com/medicalpubs/diseasemanagement/gastroenterology/irritable-bowel-syndrome/. Accessed summer 2011.
3. Irritable Bowel Syndrome. © 2007 The Board of Trustees of the University of Illinois. URL: http://www.mckinley.illinois.edu/handouts/irritable_bowel_syndrome/irritable_bowel_syndrome.html. Accessed summer 2011.
4. Irritable Bowel Syndrome. National Digestive Diseases Information Clearinghouse (NDDIC) or National Institute of Diabetes and Digestive and Kidney Diseases (NIDDK). URL: http://digestive.niddk.nih.gov/ddiseases/pubs/ibs/. Accessed summer 2011.
5. Lehrer J. Irritable Bowel Syndrome. © 1994–2011 WebMD LLC. URL: http://emedicine.medscape.com/article/180389-overview#showall. Accessed summer 2011.
6. Shen Y, et al. Complementary and Alternative Medicine for Treatment of Irritable Bowel Syndrome. Canadian Family Physician. URL: http://www.ncbi.nlm.nih.gov/pmc/articles/PMC2642499/pdf/0550143.pdf. Accessed summer 2011.

Liver Cancer

1. Adult Primary Liver Cancer Treatment (PDQ®). National Cancer Institute. URL: http://www.cancer.gov/cancertopics/pdq/treatment/adult-primary-liver/Patient/AllPages. Accessed summer 2011.
2. Hepatocellular Carcinoma. © 1994–2011 WebMD LLC. URL: http://emedicine.medscape.com/article/197319-overview#showall. Accessed summer 2011.
3. What is Liver Cancer. © 2011 American Cancer Society. URL: http://www.cancer.org/Cancer/LiverCancer/OverviewGuide/index. Accessed summer 2011.
4. What You Need To Know About Liver Cancer. National Cancer Institute. URL: http://cancer.gov/cancertopics/wyntk/liver.pdf. Accessed summer 2011.

Pancreatic Cancer

1. Dragovich T. Pancreatic Cancer. © 1994–2011 WebMD LLC. URL: http://emedicine.medscape.com/article/280605-overview#showall. Accessed summer 2011.
2. Frequently Asked Questions. © 2000–2011 Pancreatica. URL: http://www.pancreatica.org/index.cfm/faqs.htm. Accessed summer 2011.
3. Gardner T. Acute Pancreatitis. © 1994–2011 WebMD LLC. URL: http://emedicine.medscape.com/article/181364-overview#showall. Accessed summer 2011.

4. How is Pancreatic Cancer Staged. © 2011 American Cancer Society. URL: http://www.cancer.org/cancer/pancreaticcancer/detailedguide/pancreatic-cancer-staging. Accessed summer 2011.
5. Obideen K. Chronic Pancreatitis. © 1994–2011 WebMD LLC. URL: http://emedicine.medscape.com/article/181554-overview#showall. Accessed summer 2011.
6. Pancreatitis. © 2011 University of Maryland Medical Center (UMMC). URL: http://www.umm.edu/altmed/articles/pancreatitis-000122.htm. Accessed summer 2011.
7. Pancreatitis. National Digestive Diseases Information Clearinghouse (NDDIC). URL: http://digestive.niddk.nih.gov/ddiseases/pubs/pancreatitis/. Accessed summer 2011.
8. Stevens T, et al. Acute Pancreatitis. © 2000–2011 The Cleveland Clinic Foundation. URL: http://www.clevelandclinicmeded.com/medicalpubs/diseasemanagement/gastroenterology/acute-pancreatitis/. Accessed summer 2011.
9. What You Need To Know About Cancer of the Pancreas. National Cancer Institute. URL: http://nci.nih.gov/cancertopics/wyntk/pancreas.pdf. Accessed summer 2011.

Peptic Ulcers

1. Anand BS. Peptic Ulcer Disease. © 1994–2011 WebMD LLC. URL: http://emedicine.medscape.com/article/181753-overview#showall. Accessed summer 2011.
2. *H. Pylori* and Peptic Ulcers. National Digestive Diseases Information Clearinghouse (NDDIC). URL: http://digestive.niddk.nih.gov/ddiseases/pubs/hpylori/index.aspx. Accessed summer 2011.
3. HR Mertz, et al. Peptic Ulcer Pathophysiology. The Medical Clinics of North America 1991;75(4): 799–814. URL: http://www.ncbi.nlm.nih.gov/pubmed/2072787. Accessed summer 2011.
4. NSAIDs and Peptic Ulcers. National Digestive Diseases Information Clearinghouse (NDDIC). URL: http://digestive.niddk.nih.gov/ddiseases/pubs/nsaids/index.aspx. Accessed summer 2011.
5. Ulcers: What You Can Do to Heal Your Ulcer. American Academy of Family Physicians. © 1996–2011 American Academy of Family Physicians. URL: http://familydoctor.org/online/famdocen/home/common/digestive/disorders/186.html. Accessed summer 2011.
6. What I Need To Know About Peptic Ulcers. National Digestive Diseases Information Clearinghouse (NDDIC). URL: http://digestive.niddk.nih.gov/ddiseases/pubs/pepticulcers_ez/. Accessed summer 2011.

Stomach Cancer

1. Cabebe E. Gastric Cancer. © 1994–2011 WebMD LLC. URL: http://emedicine.medscape.com/article/278744-overview#showall. Accessed summer 2011.
2. Stomach Cancer. © 1998–2011 American Academy of Family Physicians. URL: http://familydoctor.org/online/famdocen/home/common/cancer/types/817.html. Accessed summer 2011.
3. Stomach Cancer. © 2011 Cedars-Sinai. URL: http://www.cedars-sinai.edu/Patients/Health-Conditions/Stomach-Cancer.aspx. Accessed summer 2011.
4. Stomach Cancer. American Cancer Society. URL: http://www.cancer.org/acs/groups/cid/documents/webcontent/003141-pdf.pdf. Accessed summer 2011.
5. What You Need To Know About Stomach Cancer. National Cancer Institute. URL: http://www.cancer.gov/cancertopics/wyntk/stomach/AllPages. Accessed summer 2011.

Chapter 9

Diabetes Mellitus

1. 2011 National Diabetes Fact Sheet. Centers for Disease Control and Prevention. URL: http://www.cdc.gov/diabetes/pubs/general11.htm#what. Accessed summer 2011.
2. Adams L, et al. Nonalcoholic Fatty Liver Disease Increases Risk of Death among Patients with Diabetes: A Community-based Cohort Study. © 2010 Nature Publishing Group. URL: http://www.medscape.com/viewarticle/735152. Accessed summer 2011.
3. Castro-Sanchez A, et al. Connective Tissue Reflex Massage for Type 2 Diabetic Patients with Peripheral Arterial Disease: Randomized Controlled Trial. Evidence Based Complementary and Alternative Medicine 2009. URL: http://www.ncbi.nlm.nih.gov/pubmed/19933770. Accessed summer 2011.
4. Diabetes Overview. The National Diabetes Information Clearinghouse. URL: http://diabetes.niddk.nih.gov/dm/pubs/overview/index.aspx. Accessed summer 2011.
5. Diabetic Neuropathies: The Nerve Damage of Diabetes. The National Diabetes Information Clearinghouse. URL: http://diabetes.niddk.nih.gov/dm/pubs/neuropathies/index.aspx. Accessed summer 2011.
6. Hendrick B. CDC: 26 Million Americans Have Diabetes. © 1994–2011 WebMD Inc. URL: http://www.medscape.com/viewarticle/736400. Accessed summer 2011.
7. Khardori R. Type 1 Diabetes Mellitus. © 1994–2011 WebMD LLC. URL: http://emedicine.medscape.com/article/117739-overview#showall. Accessed summer 2011.
8. Khardori R. Type 2 Diabetes Mellitus. © 1994–2011 WebMD LLC. URL: http://emedicine.medscape.com/article/117853-overview#showall. Accessed summer 2011.
9. Kidney Disease of Diabetes. The National Kidney and Urologic Diseases Information Clearinghouse. URL: http://kidney.niddk.nih.gov/KUDiseases/pubs/kdd/index.aspx. Accessed summer 2011.
10. Marsh K, et al. Vegetarian Diets and Diabetes. © 2011 Sage Publications Inc. URL: http://www.medscape.com/viewarticle/739101. Accessed summer 2011.
11. National Diabetes Statistics, 2011. The National Diabetes Information Clearinghouse. URL: http://diabetes.niddk.nih.gov/dm/pubs/statistics/index.aspx. Accessed summer 2011.

Hyperthyroidism

1. Anderson P. Hyperthyroidism Increases Stroke Risk in Young Adults. © 1994–2011 by WebMD LLC. URL: http://www.medscape.com/viewarticle/719675. Accessed summer 2011.

2. Graves' Disease. The National Endocrine and Metabolic Diseases Information Service. URL: http://www.endocrine.niddk.nih.gov/pubs/graves/. Accessed summer 2011.
3. Hyperthyroidism. The National Endocrine and Metabolic Diseases Information Service. URL: http://www.endocrine.niddk.nih.gov/pubs/Hyperthyroidism/. Accessed summer 2011.
4. Lee S. Hyperthyroidism. © 1994–2011 WebMD LLC. URL: http://emedicine.medscape.com/article/121865-overview#showall. Accessed summer 2011.
5. NINDS Thyrotoxic Myotherapy Information Page. National Institute of Neurological Disorders and Stroke. URL: http://www.ninds.nih.gov/disorders/thyrotoxic_myopathy/thyrotoxic_myopathy.htm. Accessed summer 2011.
6. Schraga E. Hyperthyroidism, Thyroid Storm, and Graves Disease. © 1994–2011 WebMD LLC. URL: http://emedicine.medscape.com/article/767130-overview#showall. Accessed summer 2011.

Hypothyroidism

1. Bharaktiya S. Hypothyroidism. © 1994–2011 WebMD LLC. URL: http://emedicine.medscape.com/article/122393-overview#showall. Accessed summer 2011.
2. Gurnell M, et al. What Should be Done When Thyroid Function Tests Do Not Make Sense? © 2011 Blackwell Publishing. URL: http://www.medscape.com/viewarticle/743248?src=mp&spon=17. Accessed summer 2011.
3. Hypothyroidism. The National Endocrine and Metabolic Diseases Information Service. URL: http://www.endocrine.niddk.nih.gov/pubs/Hypothyroidism/. Accessed summer 2011.
4. Stabouli S, et al. Hypothyroidism and Hypertension. Copyright © 1994–2011 by WebMD LLC. URL: http://www.medscape.com/viewarticle/733788. Accessed summer 2011.
5. Yamada M, et al. Mechanisms Related to the Pathophysiology and Management of Central Hypothyroidism. © 2008 Nature Publishing Group. URL: http://www.medscape.com/viewarticle/584468. Accessed summer 2011.

Metabolic Syndrome

1. Cassels C. Meditation Improves Endothelial Function in Metabolic Syndrome. © 1994–2011 WebMD LLC. URL: http://www.medscape.com/viewarticle/739296. Accessed summer 2011.
2. Hughes S. Metabolic Syndrome Increases CV Risk by Twofold. © 2011 Medscape LLC. URL: http://www.medscape.com/viewarticle/729468. Accessed summer 2011.
3. Lam J, et al. Obstructive Sleep Apnea and the Metabolic Syndrome. © 2009 Expert Reviews Ltd. URL: http://www.medscape.com/viewarticle/706601. Accessed summer 2011.
4. Metabolic Syndrome Linked to Cognitive Decline in Older Adults. © 1994–2011 WebMD LLC. URL: http://www.medscape.com/viewarticle/736817. Accessed summer 2011.
5. Wang S. Metabolic Syndrome. © 1994–2011 WebMD LLC. URL: http://emedicine.medscape.com/article/165124-overview#showall. Accessed summer 2011.
6. What is Metabolic Syndrome. National Heart Lung and Blood Institute. URL: http://www.nhlbi.nih.gov/health/health-topics/topics/ms/. Accessed summer 2011.

Thyroid Cancer

1. Lentsch E. Thyroid Cancer Staging. © 1994–2011 WebMD LLC. URL: http://emedicine.medscape.com/article/2006643-overview. Accessed summer 2011.
2. Lentsch E. Thyroid Cancer Treatment Protocols. © 1994–2011 WebMD LLC. URL: http://emedicine.medscape.com/article/2007769-overview. Accessed summer 2011.
3. Sharma P. Thyroid Cancer. © 1994–2011 WebMD LLC. URL: http://emedicine.medscape.com/article/851968-overview#showall. Accessed summer 2011.
4. Spinasanta S. Incidence and Types of Thyroid Cancer. National Cancer Institute. URL: http://www.endocrineweb.com/guides/thyroid-cancer/thyroid-cancer-symptoms-possible-causes-risk-factors. Accessed summer 2011.
5. What You Need to Know About Thyroid Cancer. National Cancer Institute. URL: http://www.cancer.gov/cancertopics/wyntk/thyroid/AllPages. Accessed summer 2011.

Chapter 10

Bladder Cancer

1. Bladder Cancer. © 2011 A.D.A.M., Inc. URL: http://www.ncbi.nlm.nih.gov/pubmedhealth/PMH0001517/. Accessed fall 2011.
2. Bladder Cancer. © 2011 American Cancer Society, INC. URL: http://www.cancer.org/cancer/bladdercancer/detailedguide/bladder-cancer-staging. Accessed fall 2011.
3. Bladder Cancer. © 2011 American Urological Association Foundation. URL: http://www.urologyhealth.org/urology/index.cfm?article=100. Accessed fall 2011.
4. Bladder Cancer. © 2011 Memorial Sloan-Kettering Cancer Center. URL: http://www.mskcc.org/mskcc/html/280.cfm. Accessed fall 2011.
5. Bladder Cancer. © 2011 The University of Texas MD Anderson Cancer Center. URL: http://www.mdanderson.org/patient-and-cancer-information/cancer-information/cancer-types/bladder-cancer/index.html. Accessed fall 2011.
6. Steinberg D. Bladder Cancer. © 1994–2011 WebMD LLC. URL: http://emedicine.medscape.com/article/438262-overview#showall. Accessed fall 2011.
7. The Bladder. National Cancer Institute. URL: http://www.cancer.gov/cancertopics/wyntk/bladder/AllPages. Accessed fall 2011.

Interstitial Cystitis

1. IC Treatment Guidelines. © 2011 Interstitial Cystitis Association. URL: http://www.ichelp.org/Page.aspx?pid=429. Accessed fall 2011.
2. Interstitial Cystitis/Painful Bladder Syndrome. National Kidney and Urologic Diseases Information Clearinghouse. URL: http://kidney.niddk.nih.gov/kudiseases/pubs/interstitialcystitis/. Accessed fall 2011.

3. Metts J. Interstitial Cystitis: Urgency and Frequency Syndrome. American Family Physician. 2001;64(7):1199–1207. © 2001 American Academy of Family Physicians. URL: http://www.aafp.org/afp/2001/1001/p1199.html. Accessed fall 2011.
4. Rovner E. Interstitial Cystitis. © 1994–2011 WebMD LLC. URL: http://emedicine.medscape.com/article/441831-overview#showall. Accessed fall 2011.

Kidney Stones

1. Fathallah-Shaykh S. Uric Acid Stones. © 1994–2011 WebMD LLC. URL: http://emedicine.medscape.com/article/983759-overview#showall. Accessed fall 2011.
2. Kidney Stones in Adults. National Kidney & Urologic Diseases Information Clearinghouse. URL: http://kidney.niddk.nih.gov/kudiseases/pubs/stonesadults/. Accessed fall 2011.
3. Kidney Stones. © 1998–2011 Mayo Foundation for Medical Education and Research. URL: http://my.clevelandclinic.org/disorders/kidney_stones/np_overview.aspx. Accessed fall 2011.
4. Kidney Stones. © 2011 National Kidney Foundation, Inc. URL: http://www.kidney.org/atoz/content/kidneystones.cfm. Accessed fall 2011.
5. Wedro B. Kidney Stones. © 2011 WebMD LLC. URL: http://www.emedicinehealth.com/kidney_stones/article_em.htm. Accessed fall 2011.

Polycystic Kidney disease

1. General Information About Inheritance. © 2010 PKD Foundation. URL: http://www.pkdcure.org/tabid/1354/Default.aspx. Accessed fall 2011.
2. Polycystic Kidney Disease. © 1998–2010 Mayo Foundation for Medical Education and Research. URL: http://www.mayoclinic.com/health/polycystic-kidney-disease/DS00245. Accessed fall 2011.
3. Polycystic Kidney Disease. National Kidney and Urologic Diseases Information Clearinghouse. URL: http://kidney.niddk.nih.gov/kudiseases/pubs/polycystic/. Accessed fall 2011.
4. Torra R. Polycystic Kidney Disease. © 1990–2010 Medscape. URL: http://emedicine.medscape.com/article/244907-overview. Accessed fall 2011.
5. Verghese P, et al. Polycystic Kidney Disease. © 1994–2010 Medscape. URL: http://emedicine.medscape.com/article/983281-overview. Accessed fall 2011.

Pyelonephritis

1. Aronoff S. Pyelonephritis. Copyright © 1994–2011 by WebMD LLC. URL: http://emedicine.medscape.com/article/968028-overview#showall. Accessed fall 2011.
2. Pyelonephritis (Kidney Infection) in Adults. National Institute of Diabetes and Digestive and Kidney Diseases. URL: http://kidney.niddk.nih.gov/kudiseases/pubs/pyelonephritis/. Accessed fall 2011.
3. Pyelonephritis. © 2011 University of Maryland Medical Center. URL: http://www.umm.edu/ency/article/000522all.htm. Accessed fall 2011.
4. Ramakrishnan K, et al. Diagnosis and Management of Acute Pyelonephritis in Adults. © 2005 American Academy of Family Physicians. URL: http://www.aafp.org/afp/2005/0301/p933.html. Accessed fall 2011.

Renal Cancer

1. Kidney Cancer: Who's at Risk. National Cancer Institute. URL: http://www.cancer.gov/cancertopics/wyntk/kidney. Accessed fall 2011.
2. Quinn D. Multikinase Inhibitors and Renal Cell Cancer: How They Work and the Promise They Hold. Oncology Issues March/April 2007. URL: http://accc-cancer.org/oncology_issues/articles/marapr07/quinn.pdf. Accessed fall 2011.
3. Renal Cell Carcinoma (RCC). © 1998–2010 Healthcommunities.com, Inc. URL: http://www.urologychannel.com/kidney-cancer/index.shtml. Accessed fall 2011.
4. Sachdeva K, et al. Renal Cell Carcinoma. © 1994–2010 Medscape. URL: http://emedicine.medscape.com/article/281340-overview. Accessed fall 2011.
5. Wilms' Tumor. © 1998–2010 Mayo Foundation for Medical Education and Research. URL: http://www.mayoclinic.com/health/wilms-tumor/DS00436. Accessed fall 2011.

Renal Failure

1. Arora P. Chronic Renal Failure. © 1994–2011 WebMD LLC. URL: http://emedicine.medscape.com/article/238798-overview#showall. Accessed fall 2011.
2. Chronic Kidney Disease (CKD). © 2011 National Kidney Disease Foundation, Inc. URL: http://www.kidney.org/kidneydisease/ckd/index.cfm. Accessed fall 2011.
3. Kathuria P. Chronic Kidney Disease. © 2011 WebMD, LLC. URL: http://www.emedicinehealth.com/chronic_kidney_disease/article_em.htm. Accessed fall 2011.
4. Kidney and Urologic Diseases Statistics for the United States. National Institute of Diabetes and Digestive and Kidney Diseases. URL: http://kidney.niddk.nih.gov/kudiseases/pubs/kustats/. Accessed fall 2011.
5. Kidney Failure: Choosing a Treatment That's Right for You. National Institute of Diabetes and Digestive and Kidney Diseases. URL: http://kidney.niddk.nih.gov/kudiseases/pubs/choosingtreatment/index.aspx. Accessed fall 2011.
6. Workeneh B. Acute Renal Failure. © 1994–2011 WebMD LLC. URL: http://emedicine.medscape.com/article/243492-overview. Accessed fall 2011.

Urinary Tract Infection

1. Balentine J. Urinary Tract Infections (UTIs). © 2011 WebMD LLC. URL: http://www.emedicinehealth.com/urinary_tract_infections/article_em.htm. Accessed fall 2011.
2. Brusch J. Urinary Tract Infection in Females. © 1994–2011 WebMD LLC. URL: http://emedicine.medscape.com/article/233101-overview#showall. Accessed fall 2011.
3. Urinary Tract Infection—Treatment. © 2011 University of Maryland Medical Center. URL: http://www.umm.edu/patiented/articles/what_treatments_symptoms_of_urinary_tract_infections_000036_7.htm. Accessed fall 2011.

4. Urinary Tract Infection (UTI). U.S. Department of Health and Human Services, Office on Women's Health. URL: http://www.womenshealth.gov/publications/our-publications/fact-sheet/urinary-tract-infection.pdf. Accessed fall 2011.
5. Urinary Tract Infections in Adults. National Kidney and Urologic Diseases Information Clearinghouse. URL: http://kidney.niddk.nih.gov/kudiseases/pubs/utiadult/. Accessed fall 2011.

Chapter 11

Benign Prostatic Hyperplasia

1. Benign Prostatic Hyperplasia (BPH). © 2000–2011 American Academy of Family Physicians. URL: http://familydoctor.org/online/famdocen/home/men/prostate/148.html. Accessed fall 2011.
2. Deters L. Benign Prostatic Hyperplasia. Copyright © 1994–2011 by WebMD LLC. URL: http://emedicine.medscape.com/article/437359-overview. Accessed fall 2011.
3. Prostate Enlargement: Benign Prostatic Hyperplasia. National Kidney and Urologic Diseases Information Clearinghouse. URL: http://kidney.niddk.nih.gov/kudiseases/pubs/pdf/ProstateEnlargement.pdf. Accessed fall 2011.

Breast Cancer

1. Breast Cancer Overview. 2010 Copyright American Cancer Society. URL: http://www.cancer.org/acs/groups/cid/documents/webcontent/003037-pdf.pdf. Accessed fall 2011.
2. Breast Cancer Treatment (PDQ). National Cancer Institute. URL: http://www.cancer.gov/cancertopics/pdq/treatment/breast/healthprofessional/page3. Accessed fall 2011.
3. Breast Cysts. © 1998–2011 Mayo Foundation for Medical Education and Research (MFMER).URL: http://www.mayoclinic.com/health/breast-cysts/DS01071. Accessed fall 2011.
4. General Information About Breast Cancer. National Cancer Institute. URL: http://www.cancer.gov/cancertopics/pdq/treatment/breast/Patient/page1. Accessed fall 2011.
5. Ivins M. Who Needs Breasts, Anyway? TIME Magazine Feb. 18, 2002. Copyright © 2011 Time Inc. URL: http://www.time.com/time/magazine/article/0,9171,1001832,00.html. Accessed fall 2011.
6. Mayer M, et al. Breast Disorders and Breast Cancer Screening. Copyright © 2000–2011 The Cleveland Clinic Foundation. URL: http://www.clevelandclinicmeded.com/medicalpubs/diseasemanagement/womens-health/breast-disorders-and-cancer-screening/. Accessed fall 2011.
7. Stages of Breast Cancer. National Cancer Institute. URL: http://www.cancer.gov/cancertopics/pdq/treatment/breast/Patient/page2. Accessed fall 2011.
8. Swart R. Breast Cancer. Copyright © 1994–2011 by WebMD LLC. URL: http://emedicine.medscape.com/article/1947145-overview#showall. Accessed fall 2011.
9. What You Need To Know About Breast Cancer. National Cancer Institute. URL: http://www.cancer.gov/cancertopics/wyntk/breast/WYNTK_breast.pdf. Accessed fall 2011.

Cervical Cancer

1. Boardman C. Cervical Cancer Staging. Copyright © 1994–2011 by WebMD LLC. URL: http://emedicine.medscape.com/article/2006486-overview. Accessed fall 2011.
2. Cervical Cancer Screening Guidelines. Centers for Disease Control and Prevention. URL: http://www.cdc.gov/cancer/cervical/pdf/guidelines.pdf. Accessed fall 2011.
3. Cervical Cancer Treatment (PDQ). National Cancer Institute. URL: http://www.cancer.gov/cancertopics/pdq/treatment/cervical/Patient/AllPages. Accessed fall 2011.
4. Cervical Cancer. 2010 Copyright American Cancer Society. URL: http://www.cancer.org/acs/groups/cid/documents/webcontent/003094-pdf.pdf. Accessed fall 2011.
5. Cervical Cancer. Centers for Disease Control and Prevention. URL: http://www.cdc.gov/cancer/cervical/pdf/Cervical_FS_0510.pdf. Accessed fall 2011.
6. Fact Sheet: Human Papilloma Viruses and Cancer. U.S. Department of Health and Human Services, National Institutes of Health. URL: http://www.cancer.gov/cancertopics/factsheet/Risk/Fs3_20.pdf. Accessed fall 2011.
7. Rich W. Cancer of the Cervix. © 2003 GYNCANCER.COM. URL: http://www.gyncancer.com/cervix.html. Accessed fall 2011.
8. What You Need to Know About Cervical Cancer. National Cancer Institute. URL: http://www.cancer.gov/cancertopics/wyntk/cervix/AllPages. Accessed fall 2011.

Dysmenorrhea

1. Dysmenorrhea. © Copyright 1995–2009 The Cleveland Clinic Foundation. URL: http://my.clevelandclinic.org/disorders/dysmenorrhea/hic_dysmenorrhea.aspx. Accessed fall 2011.
2. French L. Dysmenorrhea. Copyright © 2005 by the American Academy of Family Physicians. URL: http://www.aafp.org/afp/2005/0115/p285.html. Accessed fall 2011.
3. Holder A. Dysmenorrhea in Emergency Medicine. Copyright © 1994–2011 by WebMD LLC. URL: http://emedicine.medscape.com/article/795677-overview#showall. Accessed fall 2011.
4. Menstrual Cramps (Dysmenorrhea). © The Board of Trustees of the University of Illinois, 2008. URL: http://www.mckinley.illinois.edu/handouts/menstrual_cramps.html. Accessed fall 2011.
5. Painful menstrual periods. Copyright 1997–2011, A.D.A.M. URL: http://www.nlm.nih.gov/medlineplus/ency/article/003150.htm. Accessed fall 2011.
6. Premenstrual dysphoric disorder. Copyright © 2011, A.D.A.M., Inc. URL: http://www.ncbi.nlm.nih.gov/pubmedhealth/PMH0004461/. Accessed fall 2011.
7. Primary Dysmenorrhea Consensus Guideline. SOGC Clinical Practice Guideline No 169, December 2005, 1117–1130. URL: http://www.sogc.org/guidelines/public/169E-CPG-December2005.pdf. Accessed fall 2011.

Endometriosis

1. About endometriosis. © 2005–2011 endometriosis.org. URL: http://endometriosis.org/endometriosis/. Accessed fall 2011.

2. Damewood M. Pathophysiology and management of endometriosis. © 2010 CBS Interactive. URL: http://findarticles.com/p/articles/mi_m0689/is_n1_v37/ai_13218685/. Accessed fall 2011.
3. Endometriosis Overview. Womens Surgery Group 2009. URL: http://www.womenssurgerygroup.com/conditions/Endometriosis/overview.asp. Accessed fall 2011.
4. Facts About Endometriosis. World Endometriosis Society and the World Endometriosis Research Foundation May 2011. URL: http://www.endometriosis.ca/facts-about-endometriosis.pdf. Accessed fall 2011.
5. Stoppler M. Endometriosis. © 2011 WebMD, LLC. URL: http://www.emedicinehealth.com/endometriosis/article_em.htm. Accessed fall 2011.
6. Valiani M. The effects of massage therapy on dysmenorrhea caused by endometriosis. Iranian Journal of Nursing and Midwifery Research 2010 Autumn;15(4):167–171. © Iranian Journal of Nursing and Midwifery Research. URL: http://www.ncbi.nlm.nih.gov/pmc/articles/PMC3093183/?tool=pubmed. Accessed fall 2011.

Fibroid Tumors

1. Evans P. Uterine Fibroid Tumors: Diagnosis and Treatment. American Family Physician 2007;75(10):1503–1508. URL: http://www.aafp.org/afp/2007/0515/p1503.html. Accessed fall 2011.
2. Uterine fibroids. © BMJ Publishing Group Limited 2011. URL: http://bestpractice.bmj.com/best-practice/monograph/567/basics/pathophysiology.html. Accessed fall 2011.
3. Uterine Fibroids. National Women's Health Information Center, U.S. Department of Health and Human Services, Office on Women's Health. URL: http://www.womenshealth.gov/publications/our-publications/fact-sheet/uterine-fibroids.pdf. Accessed fall 2011.
4. Uterine Fibroids. Copyright March 2009 by the American College of Obstetricians and Gynecologists. URL: http://www.acog.org/publications/patient_education/bp074.cfm. Accessed fall 2011.

Menopause

1. Breast Cancer after Use of Estrogen plus Progestin in Postmenopausal Women. WHI Clinical Coordinating Center. URL: http://www.whi.org/findings/ht/eplusp_bc2.php. Accessed fall 2011.
2. Kovacs P. What Influences the Timing of Menopause? American Journal of Obstetrics & Gynecology. 2011;205:34.e1–e13. URL: http://www.medscape.com/viewarticle/747499. Accessed fall 2011.
3. Medical Encyclopedia: Hormone replacement therapy (HRT). Copyright 2002 A.D.A.M., Inc. URL: http://www.nlm.nih.gov/medlineplus/ency/article/007111.htm. Accessed fall 2011.
4. Menopause Overview. Copyright © 1994–2011 by WebMD LLC. URL: http://emedicine.medscape.com/article/264088-overview#showall. Accessed fall 2011.
5. Menopause: What to Expect When Your Body is Changing. Copyright © 1996–2011 American Academy of Family Physicians. URL: http://familydoctor.org/online/famdocen/home/women/reproductive/menopause/125.html. Accessed fall 2011.
6. Risks and Benefits of Estrogen Plus Progestin in Healthy Postmenopausal Women. JAMA 2002;288:321–333. © 2002 American Medical Association. URL: http://jama.ama-assn.org/cgi/content/abstract/288/3/321. Accessed fall 2011.
7. Rossouw J. Release of the Results of the Estrogen Plus Progestin Trial of the Women's Health Initiative: Findings and Implications. Women's Health Initiative, National Heart, Lung, and Blood Institute July 9, 2002. URL: http://www.whi.org/findings/ht/eplusp_press_rossouw.php. Accessed fall 2011.
8. Shoupe D. Individualizing Hormone Therapy to Minimize Risk. Women's Health. 2011;7(4):475–485. © 2011 Future Medicine Ltd. URL: http://www.medscape.com/viewarticle/747269. Accessed fall 2011.
9. The Hormone Therapy Story. Contents © 2011 The North American Menopause Society. URL: http://www.menopause.org/MG4.pdf. Accessed fall 2011.
10. WHI Study Data Confirm Short-Term Heart Disease Risks of Combination Hormone Therapy for Postmenopausal Women. National Heart, Lung, and Blood Institute. URL: http://www.nih.gov/news/health/feb2010/nhlbi-15.htm. Accessed fall 2011.

Ovarian Cancer

1. Cancer of the ovary. Copyright © 2000–2011 The Cleveland Clinic Foundation. URL: http://www.clevelandclinicmeded.com/medicalpubs/diseasemanagement/womens-health/gynecologic-malignancies/. Accessed fall 2011.
2. Green A. Ovarian Cancer. Copyright © 1994–2011 by WebMD LLC. URL: http://emedicine.medscape.com/article/255771-overview#showall. Accessed fall 2011.
3. Ovarian Cancer Overview. 2010 Copyright American Cancer Society. URL: http://www.cancer.org/acs/groups/cid/documents/webcontent/003070-pdf.pdf. Accessed fall 2011.
4. Ovarian Cancer Staging System, FIGO System & TNM System. © 1998–2010 HealthCommunities.com, Inc. All Rights Reserved. URL: http://www.healthcommunities.com/ovarian-cancer/figo-system-tnm-system.shtml. Accessed fall 2011.
5. What every woman should know. © 2000–2011 Johns Hopkins University. URL: http://pathology2.jhu.edu/ovca/menu_understanding.cfm. Accessed fall 2011.
6. What You Need To Know About Ovarian Cancer. National Cancer Institute. URL: http://www.cancer.gov/cancertopics/wyntk/ovary/wyntk_ovarian.pdf. Accessed fall 2011.

Ovarian Cysts

1. Helm W. Ovarian Cysts. Copyright © 1994–2011 by WebMD LLC URL: http://emedicine.medscape.com/article/255865-overview#showall. Accessed fall 2011.
2. Ovarian Cysts and Tumors. © 2010 WebMD, LLC. URL: http://women.webmd.com/ovarian-cysts. Accessed fall 2011.
3. Ovarian Cysts. © Copyright 1995–2009 The Cleveland Clinic Foundation. URL: http://my.clevelandclinic.org/disorders/ovarian_cysts/hic_ovarian_cysts.aspx. Accessed fall 2011.
4. Ovarian cysts. Copyright October 2009 by the American College of Obstetricians and Gynecologists. URL: http://

www.acog.org/publications/patient_education/bp075.cfm. Accessed fall 2011.

5. Ovarian Cysts. U.S. Department of Health and Human Services, Office on Women's Health. URL: http://www.womenshealth.gov/publications/our-publications/fact-sheet/ovarian-cysts.pdf. Accessed fall 2011.
6. Polycystic Ovaries and PCOS. Copyright © 2011 PCOSandFibroids.com. URL: http://www.pcosandfibroids.com/. Accessed fall 2011.
7. Polycystic ovary syndrome. Copyright © 2011, A.D.A.M., Inc. URL: http://www.ncbi.nlm.nih.gov/pubmedhealth/PMH0001408/. Accessed fall 2011.

Pregnancy

1. Goodier R. Managing Asthma During Pregnancy Can Reduce Perinatal Risks. Reuters Health Information © 2011. URL: http://www.medscape.com/viewarticle/748304. Accessed fall 2011.
2. HELLP Syndrome and Your Pregnancy. Copyright © 2000–2011 American Academy of Family Physicians. URL: http://familydoctor.org/online/famdocen/home/women/pregnancy/complications/456.html. Accessed fall 2011.
3. Pregnancy complications: Asthma. © 2010 March of Dimes Foundation. URL: http://www.marchofdimes.com/printableArticles/complications_asthma.html. Accessed fall 2011.
4. Pregnancy complications: Depression. © 2010 March of Dimes Foundation. URL: http://www.marchofdimes.com/printableArticles/complications_depression.html. Accessed fall 2011.
5. Pregnancy-Induced Hypertension. Copyright © 2000–2011 American Academy of Family Physicians. URL: http://familydoctor.org/online/famdocen/home/women/pregnancy/complications/064.html. Accessed fall 2011.
6. Prenatal Massage: Massage During Pregnancy. © 2000–2011 American Pregnancy Association. URL: http://www.americanpregnancy.org/pregnancyhealth/prenatalmassage.html. Accessed fall 2011.
7. Sepilian V. Ectopic Pregnancy. Copyright © 1994–2011 by WebMD LLC. URL: http://emedicine.medscape.com/article/2041923-overview#showall. Accessed fall 2011.
8. Trupin S. Common Pregnancy Complaints and Questions. Copyright © 1994–2011 by WebMD LLC. URL: http://emedicine.medscape.com/article/259724-overview#showall. Accessed fall 2011.

Premenstrual Syndrome

1. Moreno M. Premenstrual Syndrome. © 1994–2011 by WebMD LLC. URL: http://emedicine.medscape.com/article/953696-overview#showall. Accessed fall 2011.
2. Premenstrual Dysphoric Disorder (PMDD). Copyright © 2003–2011 American Academy of Family Physicians. URL: http://familydoctor.org/online/famdocen/home/women/mental/752.html. Accessed fall 2011.
3. Premenstrual Syndrome. Copyright © March 2010 by the American College of Obstetricians and Gynecologists. URL: http://www.acog.org/publications/patient_education/bp057.cfm. Accessed fall 2011.
4. Premenstrual Syndrome. National Women's Health Information Center, U.S. Department of Health and Human Services, Office on Women's Health. URL: http://www.womenshealth.gov/publications/our-publications/fact-sheet/premenstrual-syndrome.pdf. Accessed fall 2011.

Prostate Cancer

1. About the Prostate. © 2011 Prostate Cancer Foundation. URL: http://www.pcf.org/site/c.leJRIROrEpH/b.5699537/k.BEF4/Home.htm. Accessed fall 2011.
2. Prostate Cancer Treatment Options. Copyright © 2003–2011 American Academy of Family Physicians. URL: http://familydoctor.org/online/famdocen/home/common/cancer/treatment/264.html. Accessed fall 2011.
3. Prostate Cancer. 2010 Copyright American Cancer Society. URL: http://www.cancer.org/acs/groups/cid/documents/webcontent/003134-pdf.pdf. Accessed fall 2011.
4. Prostate Cancer. Copyright © 1999–2011 American Academy of Family Physicians. URL: http://familydoctor.org/online/famdocen/home/common/cancer/types/361.html. Accessed fall 2011.
5. Prostate-Specific Antigen (PSA) Test. National Cancer Institute. URL: http://www.cancer.gov/cancertopics/fact-sheet/detection/PSA. Accessed fall 2011.
6. PSA. ©2001–2011 by American Association for Clinical Chemistry. URL: http://labtestsonline.org/understanding/analytes/psa/tab/test. Accessed fall 2011.
7. SEER Stat Fact Sheets: Prostate Cancer. National Cancer Institute. URL: http://seer.cancer.gov/statfacts/html/prost.html. Accessed fall 2011.
8. What You Need To Know About Prostate Cancer. National Cancer Institute. URL: http://www.cancer.gov/cancertopics/wyntk/prostate.pdf. Accessed fall 2011.

Prostatitis

1. Prostatitis. © 1998–2011 Mayo Foundation for Medical Education and Research (MFMER). URL: http://www.mayoclinic.com/health/prostatitis/DS00341. Accessed fall 2011.
2. Prostatitis. Copyright © 2000–2011 American Academy of Family Physicians. URL: http://familydoctor.org/online/famdocen/home/men/prostate/581.html. Accessed fall 2011.
3. Prostatitis: Disorders of the Prostate. National Kidney and Urologic Diseases Information Clearinghouse. URL: http://kidney.niddk.nih.gov/kudiseases/pubs/pdf/Prostatitis.pdf. Accessed fall 2011.
4. Turek P. Prostatitis. Copyright © 1994–2011 by WebMD LLC. URL: http://emedicine.medscape.com/article/785418-overview#showall. Accessed fall 2011.
5. Watson R. Chronic Pelvic Pain Syndrome and Prostatodynia. Copyright © 1994–2011 by WebMD LLC. URL: http://emedicine.medscape.com/article/437745-overview#showall. Accessed fall 2011.

Sexually Transmitted Infections

1. Bacterial Vaginosis—CDC Fact Sheet. Centers for Disease Control and Prevention. URL: http://www.cdc.gov/STD/bv/STDFact-Bacterial-Vaginosis.htm. Accessed fall 2011.

2. Chlamydia—CDC Fact Sheet. Centers for Disease Control and Prevention. URL: http://www.cdc.gov/std/chlamydia/chlamydia-fact-sheet-press-August-2011.pdf. Accessed fall 2011.
3. Chlamydia. © 2000–2011 American Academy of Family Physicians. URL: http://familydoctor.org/online/famdocen/home/common/sexinfections/sti/204.html. Accessed fall 2011.
4. Fact Sheet: Genital HPV. Centers for Disease Control and Prevention. URL: http://www.cdc.gov/std/hpv/hpv-fact-sheet.pdf. Accessed fall 2011.
5. Gonorrhea—CDC Fact Sheet. Centers for Disease Control and Prevention. URL: http://www.cdc.gov/std/gonorrhea/gonorrhea-fact-sheet-April-2011.pdf. Accessed fall 2011.
6. Molluscum contagiosum. Copyright © 2011, A.D.A.M., Inc. URL: http://www.ncbi.nlm.nih.gov/pubmedhealth/PMH0001829/. Accessed fall 2011.
7. Nongonococcal Urethritis (NGU) in Men. The Cleveland Clinic © 1995–2011. URL: http://my.clevelandclinic.org/disorders/nongonococcal_urethritis/hic_nongonococcal__urethritis_ngu_in_men.aspx. Accessed fall 2011.
8. Sexually Transmitted Infections: Overview. U.S. Department of Health and Human Services, Office on Women's Health. URL: http://www.womenshealth.gov/publications/our-publications/fact-sheet/sexually-transmitted-infections.pdf. Accessed fall 2011.
9. STI Detection and Prevention. Copyright © 2000–2011 American Academy of Family Physicians. URL: http://familydoctor.org/online/famdocen/home/common/sexinfections/sti/165.html. Accessed fall 2011.
10. Syphilis—CDC Fact Sheet. for Disease Control and Prevention. URL: http://www.cdc.gov/std/syphilis/syphilis-Fact-Sheet.pdf. Accessed fall 2011.
11. Syphilis. Copyright © 1999–2011 American Academy of Family Physicians. URL: http://familydoctor.org/online/famdocen/home/common/sexinfections/sti/380.html. Accessed fall 2011.
12. Trichomoniasis—CDC Fact Sheet. for Disease Control and Prevention. URL: http://www.cdc.gov/std/Trichomonas/Trichomoniasis-Fact-Sheet.pdf. Accessed fall 2011.

Testicular Cancer

1. Brown C. Testicular Cancer: An Overview. Urologic Nursing 2004;24(2). © 2004 Society of Urologic Nurses and Associates. URL: http://www.medscape.com/viewarticle/473629. Accessed fall 2011.
2. Testicular Cancer Info: Staging. Copyright © 2001–2007 The Testicular Cancer Resource Center. URL: http://tcrc.acor.org/staging.html. Accessed fall 2011.
3. Testicular Cancer. ©2011 American Cancer Society. URL: http://www.cancer.org/Cancer/TesticularCancer/DetailedGuide/index. Accessed fall 2011.
4. Testicular Cancer. Copyright © 2010 testicular-cancer.us. URL: http://testicular-cancer.us/. Accessed fall 2011.
5. Testicular Cancer: Questions and Answers. National Cancer Institute. URL: http://www.cancer.gov/cancertopics/factsheet/Sites-Types/Fs6_34.pdf. Accessed fall 2011.
6. The Testicular Cancer Hall of Fame! Copyright © 1997–2009 The Testicular Cancer Resource Center. URL: http://tcrc.acor.org/celeb.html. Accessed fall 2011.

Uterine Cancer

1. Chiang JW. Uterine Cancer. Copyright © 1994–2011 by WebMD LLC. URL: http://emedicine.medscape.com/article/258148-overview. Accessed fall 2011.
2. Endometrial (Uterine) Cancer. Copyright © 2011 American Cancer Society. URL: http://www.cancer.org/acs/groups/cid/documents/webcontent/003097-pdf.pdf. Accessed fall 2011.
3. Endometrial Cancer Treatment (PDQ). National Cancer Institute. URL: http://www.cancer.gov/cancertopics/pdq/treatment/endometrial/Patient/AllPages. Accessed fall 2011.
4. Rich W. Cancer of the Uterus. © 2003 GYNCANCER.COM. URL: http://www.gyncancer.com/uterus.html. Accessed fall 2011.
5. Uterine Cancer Overview. Copyright © 2011 NexCura, Inc. URL: http://www.cancerfacts.com/GeneralContent/Uterine/gen_overview.asp?CB=11. Accessed fall 2011.
6. Uterine Cancer. Centers for Disease Control and Prevention. URL: http://www.cdc.gov/cancer/uterine/pdf/Uterine_FS_0510.pdf. Accessed fall 2011.
7. What You Need To Know About Cancer of the Uterus. National Cancer Institute. URL: http://www.cancer.gov/cancertopics/wyntk/uterus.pdf. Accessed fall 2011.

Chapter 12

Cancer

1. Are the number of cancer cases increasing or decreasing in the world? ©WHO 2011. URL: http://www.who.int/features/qa/15/en/index.html. Accessed fall 2011.
2. Berrettoni BA, Carter JR. Mechanisms of cancer metastasis to bone. Journal of Bone and Joint Surgery America 1986;68:308–312. URL: http://jbjs.org/article.aspx?articleid=19693. Accessed fall 2011.
3. Cancer Fact sheet No. 297. © WHO 2011. URL: http://www.who.int/mediacentre/factsheets/fs297/en/index.html. Accessed fall 2011.
4. Cancer Prevention Overview (PDQ) Health Professional Version. National Cancer Institute. URL: http://www.cancer.gov/cancertopics/pdq/prevention/overview/HealthProfessional#Section_132. Accessed fall 2011.
5. Cancer Vaccines. National Cancer Institute Fact Sheet. URL: http://www.cancer.gov/cancertopics/factsheet/Therapy/cancer-vaccines. Accessed fall 2011.
6. Chronological History of ACS Recommendations for the Early Detection of Cancer in Asymptomatic People. © 2011 American Cancer Society, Inc. URL: http://www.cancer.org/Healthy/FindCancerEarly/CancerScreeningGuidelines/chronological-history-of-acs-recommendations. Accessed fall 2011.
7. Emanuel L, et al. Combating Compassion Fatigue and Burnout in Cancer Care. Medscape Nurses © 2011 WebMD,

LLC. URL: http://www.medscape.com/viewarticle/742941?src=mp&spon=17. Accessed fall 2011.

8. Known and Probable Human Carcinogens. © 2011 American Cancer Society, Inc. URL: http://www.cancer.org/Cancer/CancerCauses/OtherCarcinogens/GeneralInformationaboutCarcinogens/known-and-probable-human-carcinogens. Accessed fall 2011.
9. Metastatic Cancer. National Cancer Institute Fact Sheet. URL: http://www.cancer.gov/cancertopics/factsheet/Sites-Types/metastatic. Accessed fall 2011.
10. Screening for various cancers. ©WHO 2011. URL: http://www.who.int/cancer/detection/variouscancer/en/index.html. Accessed fall 2011.
11. SEER Stat Fact Sheets: All Sites. National Cancer Institute. URL: http://seer.cancer.gov/statfacts/html/all.html. Accessed fall 2011.
12. The World Health Organization's Fight Against Cancer: Strategies that prevent, cure and care. © World Health Organization 2007. URL: http://www.who.int/cancer/publicat/WHOCancerBrochure2007.FINALweb.pdf. Accessed fall 2011.
13. What is Cancer Cell and Gene Therapy? ©2011–2012 Alliance for Cancer Gene Therapy. URL: http://www.acgt-foundation.org/cgt.html. Accessed fall 2011.

Extra Conditions At a Glance

Abortion, Spontaneous and Elective

1. Medical Abortion. © 1998–2010 Mayo Foundation for Medical Education and Research (MFMER). URL: http://www.mayoclinic.com/health/medical-abortion/MY00819. Accessed fall 2011.
2. Puscheck E. Early Pregnancy Loss. Copyright © 1994–2011 by WebMD LLC. URL: http://emedicine.medscape.com/article/266317-overview. Accessed fall 2011.
3. Trupin S, et al. Elective Abortion. Copyright © 1994–2011 by WebMD LLC.
4. URL: http://emedicine.medscape.com/article/252560-overview. Accessed fall 2011.

Acromegaly

1. Acromegaly. National Institute of Diabetes and Digestive and Kidney Diseases (NIDDK). URL: http://www.endocrine.niddk.nih.gov/pubs/acro/acro.aspx. Accessed summer 2011.
2. Khandwala H. Acromegaly. © 1994–2011 WebMD LLC. URL: http://emedicine.medscape.com/article/116366-overview. Accessed summer 2011.

Addison Disease

1. Addison's Disease. © 1998–2010 Mayo Foundation for Medical Education and Research. URL: http://www.mayoclinic.com/health/addisons-disease/DS00361. Accessed summer 2011.
2. Adrenal Insufficiency and Addison's Disease. The National Endocrine and Metabolic Diseases Information Service. URL: http://www.endocrine.niddk.nih.gov/pubs/addison/addison.htm. Accessed summer 2011.
3. Griffing G, et al. Addison Disease. © 1994–2011 Medscape. URL: http://emedicine.medscape.com/article/116467-overview. Accessed summer 2011.

Avascular Necrosis

1. Avascular Necrosis of the Hip: A Patient's Guide to Avascular Necrosis of the Hip. © Medical Multimedia Group, L.L.C. URL: http://www.eorthopod.com/content/avascular-necrosis-hip. Accessed winter 2011.
2. Avascular Necrosis. © Mayo Clinic. URL: http://www.mayoclinic.com/health/avascular-necrosis/DS00650. Accessed winter 2011.
3. Harris George. Legg-Calve-Perthes Disease. © Medscape. URL: http://emedicine.medscape.com/article/1248267-overview. Accessed winter 2011.
4. Legg-Calve-Perthes Disease. © Mayo Clinic. URL: http://www.mayoclinic.com/health/legg-calve-perthes-disease/DS00654. Accessed winter 2011.
5. Legg-Calve-Pethes Disease Increases Cardiovascular Risk. © Reuters Health Information. URL: http://www.medscape.com/viewarticle/721403. Accessed winter 2011.
6. Legg-Calve'-Perthes Disease: The National Osteonecrosis Foundation. © National Osteonecrosis Foundation. URL: http://www.nonf.org/perthesbrochure/perthes-brochure.htm. Accessed winter 2011.
7. Osteonecrosis. Niams. 2009. URL: http://www.niams.nih.gov/Health_Info/Osteonecrosis/#nidcr. Accessed winter 2011.
8. Tofferi J, et al. Avascular Necrosis. © Medscape. URL: http://emedicine.medscape.com/article/333364-overview. Accessed winter 2011.

Bronchiectasis

1. Bronchiectasis. © 2011 National Jewish Health. URL: http://www.nationaljewish.org/healthinfo/conditions/bronchiectasis/index.aspx. Accessed summer 2011.
2. Bronchiectasis. National Heart Lung and Blood Institute. URL: http://www.nhlbi.nih.gov/health/dci/Diseases/brn/brn_all.html. Accessed summer 2011.
3. Emmons E. Bronchiectasis. © 1994–2010 Medscape. URL: http://emedicine.medscape.com/article/296961-overview. Accessed summer 2011.

Carditis

1. Carditis. © 1996–2010 Neal Chamberlain. URL: http://www.atsu.edu/faculty/chamberlain/Website/lectures/tritzid/carditis.htm. Accessed summer 2011.

2. Kulick D, et al. Endocarditis. © 2010 MedicineNet, Inc. URL: http://www.medicinenet.com/script/main/art.asp?articlekey=1949. Accessed summer 2011.
3. Kulick D, et al. Myocarditis. © 2010 MedicineNet, Inc. URL: http://www.medicinenet.com/script/main/art.asp?articlekey=6474. Accessed summer 2011.
4. Wedro B, et al. Pericarditis. © MedicineNet, Inc. URL: http://www.medicinenet.com/script/main/art.asp?articlekey=444. Accessed summer 2011.

Charcot-Marie-Tooth Syndrome

1. Charcot-Marie-Tooth Disease Fact Sheet. National Institute of Neurological Disorders and Stroke. URL: http://www.ninds.nih.gov/disorders/charcot_marie_tooth/detail_charcot_marie_tooth.htm. Accessed spring 2011.
2. Charcot-Marie-Tooth disease. Copyright © 2011, A.D.A.M., Inc. URL: http://www.ncbi.nlm.nih.gov/pubmedhealth/PMH0001741/. Accessed spring 2011.
3. I have CMT. © 2006—2011 Charcot-Marie-Tooth Association. URL: http://www.cmtausa.org/index.php?option=com_content&view=category&layout=blog&id=3&Itemid=28. Accessed spring 2011.

Cushing Syndrome

1. Adler G. Cushing Syndrome. © 1994–2010 Medscape. URL: http://emedicine.medscape.com/article/117365-overview. Accessed summer 2011.
2. Cushing Syndrome. © 1997–2010 A.D.A.M., Inc. URL: http://www.nlm.nih.gov/medlineplus/ency/article/000410.htm. Accessed summer 2011.
3. Cushing's Syndrome. © 1998–2010 Mayo Foundation for Medical Education and Research. URL: http://www.mayoclinic.com/health/cushings-syndrome/DS00470. Accessed summer 2011.
4. Cushing's Syndrome. The National Endocrine and Metabolic Diseases Information Service. URL: http://endocrine.niddk.nih.gov/pubs/cushings/cushings.aspx. Accessed summer 2011.
5. Margulies P. Cushing's Syndrome. National Adrenal Diseases Foundation. URL: http://www.nadf.us/docs/nadf_cushings.pdf. Accessed summer 2011.
6. NINDS Cushing's Syndrome Information Page. National Institute of Neurological Disorders and Stroke. URL: http://www.ninds.nih.gov/disorders/cushings/cushings.htm?css=print. Accessed summer 2011.

Diabetes Insipidus

1. Cooperman M. Diabetes Insipidus. © 1994–2011 WebMD LLC. URL: http://emedicine.medscape.com/article/117648-overview. Accessed summer 2011.
2. Diabetes Insipidus. © 1998–2010 Mayo foundation for Medical Education and Research. URL: http://www.mayoclinic.com/health/diabetes-insipidus/DS00799. Accessed summer 2011.
3. Diabetes Insipidus. National Kidney & Urologic Diseases Information Clearinghouse (NKUDIC). URL: http://kidney.niddk.nih.gov/KUDiseases/pubs/insipidus/index.aspx. Accessed summer 2011.

Ehlers-Danlos Syndrome

1. Ceccolini E, et al. Ehlers-Danlos Syndrome. © Medscape. URL: http://emedicine.medscape.com/article/1114004-overview. Accessed winter 2011.
2. Ehlers-Danlos Syndrome. Genetics Home Reference. URL: http://ghr.nlm.nih.gov/condition/ehlers-danlos-syndrome. Accessed winter 2011.
3. Ehlers-Danlos Syndrome. © 1998–2011 Mayo Foundation for Medical Education and Research (MFMER). URL: http://www.mayoclinic.com/health/ehlers-danlos-syndrome/DS00706. Accessed winter 2011.
4. What Are The Types of EDS? © TerranTribune Inc. URL: http://www.ednf.org/index.php?option=com_content&task=view&id=1348&Itemid=88888969. Accessed winter 2011.

Fractures

1. Bennell K, et al. Effects of an Exercise and Manual Therapy Program on Physical Impairments, Function and Quality-of-life in People with Osteoporotic Vertebral Fracture: A Randomised, Single-blind Controlled Pilot Trial. © Medscape. URL: http://www.medscape.com/viewarticle/717981. Accessed winter 2011.
2. Bone Fracture Repair. © A.D.A.M., Inc. URL: http://www.nlm.nih.gov/medlineplus/ency/article/002966.htm. Accessed winter 2011.
3. Fractures: An Overview. © American Academy of Orthopaedic Surgeons. URL: http://orthoinfo.aaos.org/topic.cfm?topic=a00139. Accessed winter 2011.
4. Stress Fractures. © American Academy of Orthopaedic Surgeons. URL: http://orthoinfo.aaos.org/topic.cfm?topic=A00112. Accessed winter 2011.
5. Wedro B. Fracture. © MedicineNet, Inc. URL: http://www.medicinenet.com/script/main/art.asp?articlekey=2035. Accessed winter 2011.

Glomerulonephritis

1. Glomerulonephritis. © 1996–2011 Aetna InteliHealth Inc. URL: http://www.intelihealth.com/IH/ihtIH/c/9339/31198.html. Accessed fall 2011.
2. Glomerulonephritis. © 1998–2010 Mayo Foundation for Medical Education and Research. URL: http://www.mayoclinic.com/health/glomerulonephritis/DS00503. Accessed fall 2011.
3. Glomerulonephritis. © 1997–2011, A.D.A.M., Inc. URL: http://www.nlm.nih.gov/medlineplus/ency/article/000484.htm. Accessed fall 2011.

Guillain-Barre Syndrome

1. Davids H, et al. Guillain-Barre Syndrome. © 2011 Medscape. URL: http://emedicine.medscape.com/article/315632-overview. Accessed winter 2011.
2. Guillain-Barre Syndrome Fact Sheet. National Institute of Neurological Disorders and Stroke. URL: http://www.ninds.nih.gov/disorders/gbs/detail_gbs.htm. Accessed winter 2011.
3. Guillain-Barre Syndrome. ©1998–2011 Mayo Foundation for Medical Education and Research (MFMER). URL: http://

www.mayoclinic.com/health/guillain-barre-syndrome/DS00413. Accessed winter 2011.

Heterotopic Ossification

1. Moore D, et al. Heterotopic Ossification. © Medscape. URL: http://emedicine.medscape.com/article/390416-overview. Accessed winter 2011.
2. Myositis Ossificans. © PhysioAdvisor. URL: http://www.physioadvisor.com.au/10635850/myositis-ossificans-physioadvisor.htm. Accessed winter 2011.
3. Soft Tissue Calcifications. © UW Radiology. URL: http://www.rad.washington.edu/academics/academic-sections/msk/teaching-materials/online-musculoskeletal-radiology-book/soft-tissue-calcifications/?searchterm=heterotopicossification. Accessed winter 2011.

Hyperparathyroidism

1. Hyperparathyroidism. © 1998–2011 Mayo Foundation for Medical Education and Research. URL: http://www.mayoclinic.com/health/hyperparathyroidism/DS00396. Accessed summer 2011.
2. Hyperparathyroidism. National Endocrine and Metabolic Diseases Information Service. URL: http://www.endocrine.niddk.nih.gov/pubs/hyper/hyper.htm. Accessed summer 2011.
3. Kim L, et al. Hyperparathyroidism. © 1994–2011 Medscape. URL: http://emedicine.medscape.com/article/127351-overview. Accessed summer 2011.

Hypoparathyroidism

1. Definition of Hypoparathyroidism and Related Disorders. Copyright © 1999–2011, Hypoparathyroidism Association, Inc. URL: http://www.hpth.org/about-hpth/definition.html. Accessed summer 2011
2. Gonzalez-Campoy J. Hypoparathyroidism. © 1994–2010 Medscape. URL: http://emedicine.medscape.com/article/122207-overview. Accessed summer 2011.
3. Hypoparathyroidism. © 1998–2011 Mayo Foundation for Medical Education and Research. URL: http://www.mayoclinic.com/health/hypoparathyroidism/DS00952. Accessed summer 2011.
4. Hypoparathyroidism. National Institute of Child Health & Human Development. URL: http://www.nichd.nih.gov/health/topics/hypoparathyroidism.cfm. Accessed summer 2011.

Ichthyosis

1. DiGiovanna J, Robinson-Bostom L. Ichthyosis: Etiology, Diagnosis, and Management. American Journal of Clinical Dermatology 2003;4(2):81–95. ©2003 Adis Data Information BV. URL: http://adisonline.com/dermatology/pages/articleviewer.aspx?year=2003&issue=04020&article=00002&type=abstract. Accessed winter 2010.
2. Hoffjan S, Stemmler S. On the Role of the Epidermal Differentiation Complex in Ichthyosis Vulgaris, Atopic Dermatitis and Psoriasis. The British Journal of Dermatology 2007;157(3):441–449. © 1994–2010 Medscape http://www.medscape.com/viewarticle/564078. Accessed winter 2010.
3. Ichthyosis vulgaris. Mayo Clinic. © 1998–2010 Mayo Foundation for Medical Education and Research (MFMER). URL: http://mayoclinic.com/health/ichthyosis-vulgaris/DS00734. Accessed winter 2010.
4. Schwartz R, Okulicz J. Ichthyosis Vulgaris, Hereditary and Acquired. © 1994–2010 by Medscape. URL: http://emedicine.medscape.com/article/1112753-overview. Accessed winter 2010.
5. Types of Ichthyosis. Foundation for Ichthyosis and Related Skin Type's. (F.I.R.S.T.). © 2010 F. I. R. S. T. URL: http://www.scalyskin.org/column.cfm?ColumnID=14. Accessed winter 2010.
6. What is Ichthyosis? Lamellar.org. © 2004 Lamellar.org. URL: http://lamellar.org/Etiology%20of%20the%20Disease.htm. Accessed winter 2010.

Impetigo

1. Amini S, Burdick A. Impetigo. Medscape. © 1994–2010 by Medscape. URL: http://emedicine.medscape.com/article/1052709-overview. Accessed winter 2010.
2. Davis L. Ecthyma. Medscape. © 1994–2010 by Medscape. URL: http://emedicine.medscape.com/article/1052279-overview. Accessed winter 2010.
3. Impetigo. Mayo Clinic. © 1998–2010 Mayo Foundation for Medical Education and Research URL: http://mayoclinic.com/health/impetigo/DS00464. Accessed winter 2010.
4. Rashid R, Miller A, Silverberg M. Impetigo. Medscape. © 1994–2010 by Medscape. URL: http://emedicine.medscape.com/article/783562-overview. Accessed winter 2010.
5. Rockoff A. Impetigo (Impetigo Contagiosa). MedicineNet. ©1996–2010MedicineNet,Inc.URL:http://www.medicinenet.com/script/main/art.asp?articlekey=11919. Accessed winter 2010.

Jaundice

1. Marks J. Jaundice. © 2010 MedicineNet, Inc. URL: http://www.medicinenet.com/script/main/art.asp?articlekey=1899. Accessed summer 2011.

Lichen planus

1. Chuang T, Stitle L. Lichen Planus. Medscape. © 1994–2010 by Medscape. URL: http://emedicine.medscape.com/article/1123213-overview. Accessed winter 2010.
2. Lichen Planus. Mayo Clinic. © 1998–2010 Mayo Foundation for Medical Education and Research. URL: http://www.mayoclinic.com/health/lichen-planus/DS00782. Accessed winter 2010.
3. Lichen Planus. American Academy of Dermatology. © 2010 American Academy of Dermatology. URL: http://www.aad.org/public/publications/pamphlets/common_lichen.html. Accessed winter 2010.
4. Lichen Planus. American Osteopathic College of Dermatology. ©2010 American Osteopathic College of Dermatology, URL: http://www.aocd.org/skin/dermatologic_diseases/lichen_planus.html. Accessed winter 2010.

Malaria

1. Malaria. © Mayo Foundation for Medical Education and Research. URL: http://www.mayoclinic.com/health/malaria/DS00475. Accessed summer 2011.
2. Malaria. National Institute of Allergy and Infectious Diseases. URL: http://www.niaid.nih.gov/topics/malaria/documents/malaria.pdf. Accessed summer 2011.
3. Perez-Jorge E, et al. Malaria. © 1994–2011 Medscape. URL: http://emedicine.medscape.com/article/221134-overview. Accessed summer 2011.

Marfan Syndrome

1. Channell K, et al. Marfan Syndrome. © Medscape. URL: http://emedicine.medscape.com/article/1258926-overview. Accessed winter 2011.
2. Marfan Syndrome. © American Heart Association, Inc. URL: http://www.americanheart.org/presenter.jhtml?identifier=4672. Accessed winter 2011.
3. Marfan Syndrome. National Institute of Arthritis and Musculoskeletal and Skin Disease (NIAMS). URL: http://www.niams.nih.gov/Health_Info/Marfan_Syndrome/default.asp. Accessed winter 2011.

Myasthenia Gravis

1. Goldenberg W, et al. Myasthenia Gravis. © Medscape. URL: http://emedicine.medscape.com/article/793136-overview. Accessed winter 2011.
2. Myasthenia Gravis Fact Sheet. National Institute of Neurological Disorders and Stroke (NINDS). URL: http://www.ninds.nih.gov/disorders/myasthenia_gravis/detail_myasthenia_gravis.htm. Accessed winter 2011.
3. What is Myasthenia Gravis (MG)? © Myasthenia Gravis Foundation of America and James F. Howard Jr, MD. URL: http://www.myasthenia.org/hp_clinicaloverview.cfm. Accessed winter 2011.

Osteogenesis Imperfecta

1. Exercise and Activity: Key Elements in the Management of OI. National Institute of Arthritis and Musculoskeletal and Skin Diseases (NIAMS). URL: http://www.niams.nih.gov/Health_Info/Bone/Osteogenesis_Imperfecta/exercise_activity.asp. Accessed winter 2011.
2. Facts about Osteogenesis Imperfecta. © OI Foundation URL: http://www.oif.org/site/PageServer?pagename=AOI_Facts. Accessed winter 2011.
3. Osteogenesis Imperfecta: A Guide for Nurses. National Institute of Arthritis and Musculoskeletal and Skin Diseases (NIAMS). URL: http://www.niams.nih.gov/Health_Info/Bone/Osteogenesis_Imperfecta/nurses_guide.asp. Accessed winter 2011.
4. Plotkin H. Osteogenesis Imperfecta. © Medscape. URL: http://emedicine.medscape.com/article/947588-overview. Accessed winter 2011.

Osteomalacia

1. Osteomalacia. © 1998–2011 Mayo Foundation for Medical Education and Research (MFMER). URL: http://www.mayoclinic.com/health/osteomalacia/DS00935. Accessed winter 2011.
2. Osteomalacia. © Susan Ott, MD. URL: http://courses.washington.edu/bonephys/hypercalU/opmal2.html. Accessed winter 2011.
3. Osteomalacia. © The Cleveland Clinic Foundation. URL: http://my.clevelandclinic.org/disorders/osteomalacia/hic_osteomalacia.aspx. Accessed winter 2011.
4. Wheeless C. Osteomalacia. © Data Trace Internet Publishing, LLC. URL: http://www.wheelessonline.com/ortho/osteomalacia. Accessed winter 2011.

Osteomyelitis

1. Eck J. Osteomyelitis (Bone Infection). © MedicineNet, Inc. URL: http://www.medicinenet.com/osteomyelitis/article.htm. Accessed winter 2011.
2. King R, et al. Osteomyelitis. © Medscape. URL: http://emedicine.medscape.com/article/785020-overview. Accessed winter 2011.
3. Osteomyelitis. © 1998–2011 Mayo Foundation for Medical Education and Research (MFMER). URL: http://www.mayoclinic.com/health/osteomyelitis/DS00759. Accessed winter 2011.
4. Osteomyelitis. © The Cleveland Clinic Foundation. URL: http://my.clevelandclinic.org/disorders/osteomyelitis/hic_osteomyelitis.aspx. Accessed winter 2011.

Paget Disease

1. Carbone L, et al. Paget Disease. © Medscape. URL: http://emedicine.medscape.com/article/334607-overview. Accessed winter 2011.
2. Matthews B, et al. Paget's Disease of Bone. © Medscape. URL: http://www.medscape.com/viewarticle/713989. Accessed winter 2011.
3. Paget's Disease of Bone. © American Academy of Orthopaedic Surgeons. URL: http://orthoinfo.aaos.org/topic.cfm?topic=A00076. Accessed winter 2011.
4. Paget's disease of bone. © 1998–2011 Mayo Foundation for Medical Education and Research (MFMER). URL: http://www.mayoclinic.com/health/pagets-disease-of-bone/DS00485. Accessed winter 2011.

Pelvic Inflammatory Disease

1. Haggerty C. Diagnosis and Treatment of Pelvic Inflammatory Disease. Women's Health. 2008;4(4):383–397. © Future Medicine Ltd. URL: http://www.medscape.com/viewarticle/576815. Accessed fall 2011.
2. Jaiyeoba O. Recommendations and Rationale for the Treatment of Pelvic Inflammatory Disease. Expert Reviews Anti-Infective Therapy 2011;9(1):61–70. © Expert Reviews Ltd. URL: http://www.medscape.com/viewarticle/738853. Accessed fall 2011.
3. Pelvic Inflammatory Disease (PID)—CDC Fact Sheet. Centers for Disease Control and Prevention. URL: http://www.cdc.gov/std/pid/stdfact-pid.htm. Accessed fall 2011.
4. Pelvic Inflammatory Disease (PID). © 2011 Planned Parenthood Federation of America Inc. URL: http://www.plannedparenthood.org/health-topics/stds-hiv-safer-sex/

pelvic-inflammatory-disease-pid-4278.htm. Accessed fall 2011.

5. Pelvic Inflammatory Disease (PID). Copyright © 2000–2011 American Academy of Family Physicians. URL: http://familydoctor.org/online/famdocen/home/women/reproductive/sti/213.html. Accessed fall 2011.
6. Pelvic Inflammatory Disease. Copyright © April 2010 by the American College of Obstetricians and Gynecologists. URL: http://www.acog.org/publications/patient_education/bp077.cfm. Accessed fall 2011.

Peritonitis

1. Appendicitis. © 1998–2011 Mayo Foundation for Medical Education and Research. URL: http://www.mayoclinic.com/health/appendicitis/DS00274. Accessed summer 2011.
2. Peralta R, et al. Peritonitis and Abdominal Sepsis. © 1994–2011 Medscape. URL: http://emedicine.medscape.com/article/192329-overview. Accessed summer 2011.
3. Peritonitis—Secondary. © 1997–2011 A.D.A.M., Inc. URL: http://www.nlm.nih.gov/medlineplus/ency/article/000651.htm. Accessed summer 2011.
4. Peritonitis—Spontaneous. © 1997–2011 A.D.A.M., Inc. URL: http://www.nlm.nih.gov/medlineplus/ency/article/000648.htm. Accessed summer 2011.
5. Peritonitis. © 1998–2011 Mayo Foundation for Medical Education and Research. URL: http://www.mayoclinic.com/health/peritonitis/DS00990. Accessed summer 2011.
6. Peritonitis. © 2006 University of Maryland Medical Center (UMMC). URL: http://www.umm.edu/altmed/articles/peritonitis-000127.htm. Accessed summer 2011.

Polymyalgia Rheumatica

1. Polymyalgia rheumatica. © 1998–2011 Mayo Foundation for Medical Education and Research. URL: http://www.mayoclinic.com/health/polymyalgia-rheumatica/DS00441. Accessed spring 2011.
2. Polymyalgia rheumatica. © 2010 American College of Rheumatology URL: http://www.rheumatology.org/practice/clinical/patients/diseases_and_conditions/polymyalgiarheumatica.asp. Accessed spring 2011.
3. Polymyalgia rheumatica. Copyright © 2011, A.D.A.M., Inc. URL: http://www.ncbi.nlm.nih.gov/pubmedhealth/PMH0001452/. Accessed spring 2011.

Rheumatic Heart Disease

1. Chin T, et al. Rheumatic Heart Disease. © 1994–2011 Medscape. URL: http://emedicine.medscape.com/article/891897-overview. Accessed summer 2011.
2. Perlstein D, et al. Rheumatic Fever (Acute Rheumatic Fever or ARF). © 2010 MedicineNet. URL: http://www.medicinenet.com/script/main/art.asp?articlekey=104259. Accessed summer 2011.
3. Rheumatic fever. © 1998–2010 Mayo Foundation for Medical Education and Research. URL: http://www.mayoclinic.com/health/rheumatic-fever/DS00250. Accessed summer 2011.
4. Rheumatic Heart Disease/Rheumatic Fever. © 2010 American Heart Association. URL: http://www.americanheart.org/presenter.jhtml?identifier=4709. Accessed summer 2011.
5. Wallace M, et al. Rheumatic Fever. © 1994–2010 Medscape. URL: http://emedicine.medscape.com/article/236582-overview. Accessed summer 2011.

Sarcoidosis

1. Gould K, et al. Sarcoidosis. © 1994–2010 Medscape. URL: http://emedicine.medscape.com/article/1123970-overview. Accessed summer 2011.
2. Sarcoidosis. © 1998–2010 Mayo Foundation for Medical Education and Research. URL: http://www.mayoclinic.com/health/sarcoidosis/DS00251. Accessed summer 2011.
3. Understanding Sarcoidosis. © 2010 American Lung Association. URL: http://www.lungusa.org/lung-disease/sarcoidosis/understanding-sarcoidosis.html. Accessed summer 2011.
4. What is Sarcoidosis. National Heart Lung and Blood Institute. URL: http://www.nhlbi.nih.gov/health/dci/Diseases/sarc/sarc_all.html. Accessed summer 2011.

Thromboangiitis Obliterans

1. Arkkila P. Thromboangiitis Obliterates (Buerger's disease). © 2006 Arkkila. Orphanet J Rare Dis 2006; 1:14. URL: http://www.ncbi.nlm.nih.gov/pubmed/16722538. Accessed summer 2011.
2. Buerger's Disease. © 1998–2010 Mayo Foundation for Medical Education and Research. URL: http://www.mayoclinic.com/health/buergers-disease/DS00807. Accessed summer 2011.
3. DisHanly E, et al. Buerger Disease (Thromboangiitis Obliterans). © 1994–2011 WebMD. URL: http://emedicine.medscape.com/article/460027-overview. Accessed summer 2011.
4. Published online 2006 April 27. doi: 10.1186/1750–1172–1–14. URL: http://www.ncbi.nlm.nih.gov/pmc/articles/PMC1523324/.
5. Thromboangiitis Obliterans. © 1997–2010 A.D.A.M. URL: http://www.nlm.nih.gov/medlineplus/ency/article/000172.htm. Accessed summer 2011.

Uterine Prolapse

1. Lazarou G. Uterine Prolapse. Copyright © 1994–2011 by WebMD LLC. URL: http://emedicine.medscape.com/article/264231-overview. Accessed fall 2011.
2. Uterine Prolapse. © 1998–2010 Mayo Foundation for Medical Education and Research (MFMER). URL: http://www.mayoclinic.com/health/uterine-prolapse/DS00700. Accessed fall 2011.
3. Uterine Prolapse. Copyright © 1995–2010 The Cleveland Clinic Foundation. URL: http://my.clevelandclinic.org/disorders/uterine_prolapse/hic_uterine_prolapse.aspx. Accessed fall 2011.

Glossary

Note: This glossary contains brief definitions of many terms found in *A Massage Therapist's Guide to Pathology*. Many entries also contain a reference to a particular condition where that term may be found: this is intended to direct readers to the body of the text. Thus, the definition of acne fulminans concludes with "See *acne vulgaris*" to indicate where this term is used in context.

Ablate (ah-BLATE) To remove or destroy function.

Abrasion (ah-BRA-zhun) A scrape involving injury to the epithelial layer of the skin or mucous membranes.

Absence seizure (AB-sens SE-zhur) A type of seizure characterized by lack of activity with occasional clonic movements.

Acanthosis nigricans (ak-an-THO-sis nig-rih-KANZ) An eruption of velvet warty benign growths and hyperpigmentation occurring in the skin of the axillae, neck, anogenital area, and groins; may be associated with endocrine disorders. See *metabolic syndrome*.

Acetaminophen (ah-set-ah-MIN-o-fen) A drug with antifever and analgesic effects similar to aspirin but with limited anti-inflammatory action.

Acetylcholine (ah-set-il-KO-lene) The neurotransmitter at cholinergic synapses. It causes cardiac inhibition, vasodilation, gastrointestinal peristalsis, and other parasympathetic effects.

Acinar (AS-ih-ner) Describing a cell that is grape shaped and produces a secretion released through a small lumen.

Acne fulminans (AK-ne FUL-mih-nanz) Severe scarring acne with fever and joint pain; seen most often in teenage boys. See *acne vulgaris*.

Acral lentiginous melanoma (AK-ral len-TIH-jih-nus mel-ah-NO-mah) Pigmented lesions usually on the nail bed, fingers, palms, soles, or between toes. See *skin cancer*.

Acromegaly (ak-ro-MEG-ah-le) A disorder marked by progressive enlargement of peripheral parts of the body, linked to excessive secretion of growth hormone.

Acromioclavicular joint sprain (ah-KRO-me-o-klah-VIK-yu-lar joynt sprane) An injury to the ligaments that support the acromioclavicular joint.

Acropachy (AK-ro-pak-e, ah-KROP-ak-e) The swelling and clubbing of fingers associated with severe forms of hyperthyroidism.

Actinic cheilitis (ak-TIN-ik ki-LI-tis) Actinic keratosis lesions that appear on the lip. See *skin cancer*.

Actinic keratosis (ak-TIN-ik ker-ah-TO-sis) A premalignant warty lesion occurring on the sun-exposed skin of the face or hands in aged light-skinned persons. See *skin cancer*.

Acute (ah-KUTE) A stage of injury or infection that is short-term and severe.

Acute exertional compartment syndrome (ah-KUTE eg-ZER-shun-al kom-PART-ment SIN-drome) A serious injury involving excessive swelling of leg muscles that may dangerously compress blood vessels and peripheral nerves. See *shin splints*.

Acute granulocytic leukemia (ah-KUTE gran-yu-lo-SIT-ik lu-KE-me-ah) Synonym for acute myelogenous leukemia. See *leukemia*.

Acute idiopathic polyneuritis (ah-KUTE ih-de-o-PATH-ik pol-e-nu-RI-tis) Synonym for Guillain-Barré syndrome.

Acute inflammatory demyelinating polyneuropathy (AIDP) (ah-KUTE in-FLAM-ah-tor-e de-MI-el-ih-na-ting pol-e-nu-ROP-ath-e) A form of Guillain-Barré syndrome.

Acute lymphoblastic leukemia (ah-KUTE lim-fo-BLAS-tik lu-KE-me-ah) Synonym for acute lymphocytic leukemia. See *leukemia*.

Acute lymphoid leukemia (ah-KUTE LIM-foid lu-KE-me-ah) Synonym for acute lymphocytic leukemia. See *leukemia*.

Acute myelocytic leukemia (ah-KUTE mi-el-o-SIT-ik lu-KE-me-ah) Synonym for acute myelogenous leukemia. See *leukemia*.

Acute myelogenous leukemia (ah-KUTE mi-el-OJ-en-us lu-KE-me-ah) Aggressive cancer of the myeloid class of blood cells. See *leukemia*.

Acute vestibular neuronitis (ah-KUTE ves-TIB-yu-lar nu-ro-NI-tis) Inflammation of the vestibular portion of cranial nerve VIII; a type of vestibular balance disorder.

Acyclovir (a-SI-klo-vir) An antiviral agent often used in the treatment of herpes simplex.

Adenocarcinoma (ah-den-o-kar-sih-NO-mah) A malignant neoplasm of epithelial cells in glandular or glandlike pattern.

Adenoma (ad-en-O-mah) A benign neoplasm, usually occurring in epithelial tissue. See *colorectal cancer*.

Adhesion (ad-HE-zhun) The joining or uniting of two surfaces. Layers of connective tissue may adhere, which limits movement and increases the risk of injury.

Adhesive capsulitis (ad-HE-siv kap-su-LI-tis) A condition involving inflammatory thickening of a joint capsule, usually at the shoulder, leading to loss of range of motion. Also known as frozen shoulder.

Adipocyte (AD-ih-po-site) Fat cell; a connective tissue cell distended with one or more fat globules.

Adjunctive therapy (ad-JUNC-tiv THER-a-pe) Any accessory treatment used in combination to enhance a primary treatment.

Adjuvant (AD-ju-vent) A substance added to a medication that affects the action of the drug in a predictable way.

Adson test (AD-sun test) A test for thoracic outlet syndrome. The patient is seated with the head extended and rotated toward the affected side. With deep inspiration there is a diminution or total loss of radial pulse on that side.

Adventitia (ad-ven-TIH-shah) The outermost connective tissue layer that covers organs and vessels.

Aerobic metabolism (a-RO-bik meh-TAB-o-lizm) Metabolism that occurs in the presence of adequate oxygen, which reduces the overall production of toxic waste products.

Aflatoxin (AF-lah-tok-sin) B1 A toxin produced by some strains of *Aspergillus flavus* that causes cancer in some animals. See *liver cancer*.

Agglutination (ah-glu-tin-A-shun) The process by which suspended red blood cells or other particles are caused to adhere and form clumps. See *chemical dependency*.

Agoraphobia (ah-gor-ah-FO-be-ah) A mental disorder characterized by an irrational fear of leaving the familiar setting of home or venturing into the open; often associated with panic attacks. See *anxiety disorders*.

Albumin (al-BYU-min) Any of several naturally occurring blood proteins, some of which contribute to blood clotting capacity.

Alcoholism (AL-ko-hol-izm) Chronic alcohol abuse, dependence, or addiction; chronic excessive drinking of alcoholic beverages resulting in impairment of health and/or social or occupational functioning and increasing adaptation to the effects of alcohol, requiring increasing doses to achieve and sustain a desired effect. See *chemical dependency*.

Aldosterone (al-DOS-ter-one) A hormone manufactured in the adrenal cortex. It helps to maintain appropriate fluid balance by influencing sodium reabsorption in the kidneys; the principal mineralocorticoid.

Alkaline phosphatase (AL-kah-lin FOS-fah-tase) A phosphatase with an optimum pH above 7.0, present in many tissues; low levels of this enzyme are seen in cases of hypophosphatasia. See *Paget disease, osteoporosis*.

Allergen (AL-er-jen) A substance that elicits an allergic reaction.

Allergic rhinitis (ah-LER-jik ri-NI-tis) Synonym for hay fever. See *sinusitis*.

Allodynia (al-o-DIN-e-ah) Condition in which a normally painless stimulus causes pain.

Allogenic transplant (al-o-JEN-ik TRANZ-plant) A graft transplanted between genetically different individuals of the same species.

Alpha-1-antitrypsin (AL-fah 1 an-te-TRIP-sin) A protein that protects the inner lining of alveoli. See *emphysema*.

Alpha-blockers (AL-fah BLOK-erz) A class of medications employed to help control hypertension.

Alpha-fetoprotein (AL-fah FE-to-pro-tene) An antigen present in the fetus, associated with neural tube defects. See *spina bifida*.

Alveolus, alveoli (al-VE-o-lus, al-VE-o-li) A small cavity or socket; specifically, the terminal epithelial structures in the lungs where gaseous exchange takes place.

Alzheimer disease (ALZ-hi-mer dih-ZEZE) Progressive mental deterioration manifested by losses of memory, ability to calculate, and visual-spatial orientation; confusion; disorientation.

Amantadine (ah-MAN-tah-dene) An antiviral agent sometimes used to treat influenza.

Ambulatory (AM-bu-lah-tor-e) Able to walk; not confined to bed or a wheelchair.

Amebiasis (am-e-BI-ah-sis) Protozoan infection, usually with *Entamoeba histolytica*.

Amenorrhea (ah-men-or-E-ah) Absence or abnormal cessation of menses.

Amine (AM-ene) A positively charged ion found only in association with negatively charged ions; amines combine with acids to form salts.

Amino acid (ah-ME-no AS-id) An organic acid in which one of the hydrogen atoms on a carbon atom has been replaced by NH_2, a type of ammonia. A building block of proteins.

Amniocentesis (am-ne-o-sen-TE-sis) Transabdominal aspiration of fluid from the amniotic sac for diagnostic purposes.

Amphiarthrosis, amphiarthroses (am-fe-arth-RO-sis) A joint in which the two bones are joined by fibrocartilage.

Amyloidosis (am-ih-loyd-O-sis) A disease characterized by extracellular accumulation of amyloid proteins in various organs and tissues. See *myeloma*.

Amyotrophic lateral sclerosis (am-e-o-TRO-fik LAT-er-al skler-O-sis) A disease of the motor tracts of the lateral columns and anterior horns of the spinal cord, causing progressive muscular atrophy, increased reflexes, fibrillary twitching, and spastic irritability of muscles. Also called Lou Gehrig disease.

Anaerobic metabolism (an-ah-RO-bik meh-TAB-o-lizm) Metabolism that takes place without adequate supplies of oxygen. It may result in excessive buildup of toxic waste products.

Anaphylaxis (an-ah-fil-AK-sis) An immediate, transient allergic reaction characterized by contraction of smooth muscle and dilation of capillaries.

Androgen (AN-dro-jen) A hormone that stimulates activity of sex organs.

Anergy (AN-er-je) Lack of ability to generate a sensitivity reaction to substances expected to be antigenic, immunogenic, or allergenic in that individual. See *HIV/AIDS*.

Aneurysm (AN-yur-izm) Circumscribed dilation of an artery or a cardiac chamber, in direct communication with the lumen, usually due to an acquired or congenital weakness of the wall of the artery or chamber.

Angina (an-JI-nah) A severe, often constricting pain. Usually refers to angina pectoris.

Angioedema (an-je-o-eh-DE-mah) Recurrent large circumscribed areas of subcutaneous edema of sudden onset, usually disappearing within 24 hours, frequently seen as an allergic reaction to foods or drugs. See *allergic reactions*.

Angiogenesis (an-je-o-JEN-eh-sis) Development of new blood vessels.

Angiogram (AN-je-o-gram) Radiograph of blood vessels after injection of contrast material.

Angioneurotic edema (an-je-o-nu-ROT-ik eh-DE-mah) Hives on the face and neck and swelling to the point that breathing becomes difficult.

Angioplasty (AN-je-o-plas-te) Recanalization of a blood vessel, usually by means of balloon dilation and/or the placement of a stent.

Angular cheilitis (ANG-u-ler ki-LI-tis) Inflammation of the lips and production of fissures that radiate from the angles of the mouth.

Ankle-brachial index (ANG-kel BRA-ke-al IN-dex) A comparison of blood pressure between the ankle and the arm, used to identify risk of peripheral artery disease. See *atherosclerosis*.

Ankylosing spondylitis (ANG-kih-lo-sing spon-dih-LI-tis) Arthritis of the spine; more common in the male, often with the rheumatoid factor absent and the human leukocyte antigen present. The strong familial aggregation suggests an important genetic factor.

Anoxia (an-OX-e-ah) Absence of oxygen.

Anterior knee pain syndrome (an-TE-re-or ne PANE SIN-drome) Synonym for patellofemoral syndrome.

Antibody (AN-ti-bod-e) An immunoglobulin molecule produced by B cells and designed to react with specific antigens.

Anticholinergic (an-te-kol-ih-NER-jik) Antagonistic to the action of parasympathetic or other cholinergic nerve fibers, for example, atropine.

Anticoagulant (an-te-co-AG-yu-lent) An agent that prevents or inhibits clotting of the blood.

Antidiuretic hormone (an-ti-di-ur-EH-tik HOR-mone) Also called vasopressin, a hormone that suppresses the output of urine.

Antigen (AN-tih-jen) Any substance that elicits an immune response on contact with sensitive cells.

Antigenic shift (an-tih-JEN-ik shift) The merging of genetic material that may occur when two subtypes of pathogens simultaneously coinfect a single host. See *influenza*.

Antinuclear antibody (an-ti-NU-kle-ar AN-ti-bod-e) An antibody showing an affinity for cell nuclei, demonstrated by exposing a cell substrate to the serum to be tested, followed by exposure to an anti–human globulin serum; found in the serum of a high proportion of patients with systemic lupus erythematosus, rheumatoid arthritis, and certain collagen diseases, in some of their healthy relatives, and in about 1% of normal individuals.

Antrectomy (an-TREK-to-me) Removal of the antrum (distal half) of the stomach in treatment of peptic ulcer.

Anular (AN-yu-lar) Ring shaped.

Anulus fibrosis (AN-u-lus fi-BRO-sis) Fibrous ring of tissue in an intervertebral disc.

Aphasia (ah-FA-zha) Impaired or absent comprehension or production of, or communication by, speech, writing, or signs; due to an acquired lesion of the dominant cerebral hemisphere. See *stroke*.

Aphtha, aphthae (AF-thah, AF-the) Small ulcer on a mucous membrane, usually in the mouth.

Aplastic (a-PLAS-tik) Referring to conditions characterized by defective regeneration,for example, varieties of cancer.

Apnea (AP-ne-ah) Absence of breathing.

Aponeurosis (ap-o-nu-RO-sis) A fibrous sheet or flat expanded tendon giving attachment to muscular fibers and serving as the means of origin or insertion of a flat muscle; it sometimes serves as a fascia for other muscles.

Apophysitis (ah-pof-ih-SI-tis) Inflammation of a bony process or outgrowth.

Apoptosis (ap-op-TO-sis) Programmed cell death.

Arachinodonic acid (ah-rak-ih-DON-ik AS-id) An essential fatty acid associated with hypersensitivity reactions on the skin.

Arachnoid (ah-RAK-noyd) A delicate membrane of spider web–like filaments that lies between the dura mater and the pia mater.

Arbovirus (AR-buh-vi-rus) A large group of RNA viruses, often spread by arthropod vectors such as mosquitoes, ticks, sand flies, and midges.

Arrhythmia (ah-RITH-me-ah) Irregularity of the heartbeat.

Arteriogram (ar-TE-re-o-gram) Radiographic image of an artery after injection of a contrast medium.

Arteriole (ar-TE-re-ole) A minute artery continuous with a capillary network.

Arteriosclerosis (ar-TE-re-o-skler-O-sis) Hardening of the arteries; types generally recognized are atherosclerosis, Mönckeberg arteriosclerosis, and arteriolosclerosis.

Arteriovenous malformation (ar-ter-i-o-VE-nus mal-for-MA-shun) An abnormal connection between veins and arteries, usually found in the cranium.

Arthrochalasia EDS (arth-ro-kah-LA-zha EDS) A type of Ehlers-Danlos syndrome involving easily dislocating hip joints.

Arthroplasty (AR-thro-plas-te) Joint replacement surgery.

Ascites (ah-SI-teze) The accumulation of serous fluid in the peritoneal cavity. See *cirrhosis, liver cancer*.

Aspergillosis (as-per-gil-O-sis) The presence of *Aspergillus*, a genus of fungi, in the tissues or on a mucous surface of humans and animals, and the symptoms produced thereby.

Asphyxia (as-FIX-e-ah) Impaired or absent exchange of carbon dioxide and oxygen in the respiratory system.

Astrocyte (AS-tro-site) Star-shaped glial cells in the central nervous system; they help provide the blood-brain barrier.

Ataxic (ah-TAX-ik) Unable to coordinate muscle activity for smooth movement.

Atelectasis (at-el-EK-tah-sis) Absence of gas from a part or whole of the lung; pulmonary collapse.

Atherosclerosis (ath-er-o-skler-O-sis) Hardening of the arteries characterized by the formation of lipid deposits in the intima of large arteries. Deposits lead to fibrosis, calcification, and a narrowing of the lumen.

Athetoid (ATH-eh-toyd) Referring to slow, writhing, involuntary movement of fingers and hands, sometimes of toes and feet.

Atopic (a-TOP-ic) Relating to an allergic reaction.

ATP energy crisis Describing the vicious circle of involuntary muscle cell contraction that leads to an increased need for fuel, and a decreased supply of blood due to local ischemia.

Atrial fibrillation (A-tre-al fib-rih-LA-shun) Fibrillation in which the normal rhythmical contractions of the cardiac atria are replaced by rapid irregular twitchings of the muscular wall. See *embolism*.

Atrium, atria (A-tre-um, A-tre-ah) A chamber or cavity connected to other cavities; specifically the superior chambers of the heart.

Atrophic (a-TRO-fik) Denoting tissue or organ wasting.

Atrophic gastritis (a-TRO-fik gas-TRI-tis) A condition in which long-term inflammation interferes with acid-producing cells in the stomach; a risk factor for stomach cancer.

Atrophy (AT-ro-fe) A wasting of tissues from a number of causes, including diminished cellular proliferation, ischemia, malnutrition, and death.

Auscultation (aw-skul-TA-shun) Listening to sounds made by various body parts as a diagnostic tool.

Autoantibody (aw-to-AN-ti-bod-e) Antibody occurring in response to antigenic constituents of the host's tissue; reacts with the inciting tissue component.

Autodigestion (aw-to-di-JES-chun) Enzymatic digestion of cells (especially dead or degenerate) by enzymes present within them. See *pancreatitis*.

Autogenic transplant (aw-to-JEN-ic TRANZ-plant) The transplant of a substance that originated within the patient's body, as in bone marrow cells. Also called autologous transplant.

Autoimmune (AW-to-ih-MUNE) Arising from and directed against the individual's tissues.

Autoimmune polyglandular syndrome (au-to-ih-MUNE pol-e GLAN-du-lar SIN-drome) A group term for conditions that frequently appear together or within families, including Graves disease, type I diabetes, systemic lupus erythematosus, and others.

Autologous transplant (aw-TOL-o-gus TRANZ-plant) Synonym for autogenic transplant.

Autologous Describing a transplant of tissue in which one person serves as both the donor and recipient.

Autonomic dysreflexia (aw-to-NOM-ik dis-re-FLEX-e-ah) A syndrome occurring in some persons with spinal cord lesions and resulting from functional impairment of the autonomic nervous system. Symptoms include hypertension, bradycardia, severe headaches, pallor below and flushing above the cord lesion, and convulsions.

Avascular (a-VAS-ku-lar) Without blood or lymphatic vessels.

Avulsion (ah-VUL-zhun) A tearing away or forcible separation.

Axon (AK-son) The process of a nerve cell that conducts impulses away from the cell body.

Babesiosis (bah-be-ze-O-sis) An infection with a species of protozoan parasites, transferred to humans by tick bites.

Babinski sign (bah-BIN-ske sine) Extension of the great toe and abduction of the other toes instead of the normal flexion reflex to plantar stimulation, considered indicative of central nervous system injury.

Bacteremia (bak-te-RE-me-ah) The presence of viable bacteria in circulating blood.

Balloon sinusotomy (bah-LOON si-nus-OT-o-me) Procedure involving the use of tiny balloons on catheters to correct nasal sinus structural anomalies.

Barotrauma (BA-ro-traw-mah) Scuba diving injury involving a rapid change in pressure that can damage the inner ear. See *vestubular balance disorders*.

Barrel chest (BA-rel chest) An occasional symptom of emphysema, in which the intercostal muscles hold the rib cage out as wide as possible.

Barrett esophagus (BA-ret e-SOF-ah-gus) Chronic ulceration of the lower esophagus, often associated with gastroesophageal reflux disorder; sometimes a precursor to adenocarcinoma of the esophagus.

Basal ganglia (BA-sal GANG-le-ah) Large masses of gray matter at the base of the cerebral hemispheres.

Basal layer (BA-sal LA-er) Also called the stratum basale; the deepest layer of the epidermis.

Basophil (BA-so-fil) A phagocytic leukocyte.

Bell law The ventral spinal roots are motor, while the dorsal spinal roots are sensory.

Bence Jones proteins Protein fragments found in association with multiple myeloma.

Benign (be-NINE) Denoting the mild character of an illness or nonmalignant character of a neoplasm.

Benign paroxysmal positional vertigo (be-NINE pah-rok-SIZ-mal po-SIH-shun-al VER-tih-go) A recurrent form of vertigo caused by otoliths outside of the vestibule. See *vestibular balance disorders*.

Benign prostate hypertrophy (be-NINE PROS-tate hy-PER-tro-fe) A nodular hyperplasia of the prostate; the gland thickens in a way that may obstruct the urethra.

Benzene (BEN-zene) A highly toxic hydrocarbon from light coal tar oil, used as a solvent.

Benzodiazapine (ben-zo-di-AH-zah-pene) Any of a group of psychotropic drugs with sedative action; used as antianxiety drugs or sleeping aids. See *anxiety disorders*.

Beta amyloid (BA-tah AM-ih-loyd) A type of protein associated with formation of plaque in the brain. See *Alzheimer disease*.

Beta-blocker (BA-tah BLOK-er) A type of drug that limits sympathetic reactions, specifically as they relate to the cardiovascular system.

Beta cell (BA-tah sel) Cell in the pancreas that secretes insulin.

Bile Yellowish-brown or green fluid produced in the liver, stored in the gallbladder, and released into the duodenum to aid in the digestion of fats.

Biliary colic (BIL-e-a-re KOL-ik) Intense spasmodic pain in the right upper quadrant of the abdomen from impaction of a gallstone in the cystic duct.

Bilirubin (BIL-ih-ru-bin) A dark bile pigment formed from the hemoglobin of dead erythrocytes.

Biological response modifiers (bi-o-LOJ-ik-ul re-SPONS MOD-ih-fi-erz) Substances that alter the interaction between the body's immune defenses and cancer cells to boost, direct, or restore the body's ability to fight the disease.

Biophosphates (bi-o-FOS-fates) A group of medications that inhibit reabsorption of bone; often recommended in the treatment of osteoporosis.

Biopsy (BI-op-se) Process of removing tissue from patients for diagnostic examination.

Bipolar disease (bi-PO-lar dih-ZEZE) Synonym for manic-depressive psychosis.

Bismuth (BIZ-muth) A metallic element used in several medicines, specifically in those designed to affect stomach acidity.

Bisphosphonate (bis-FOS-fo-nate) A class of drugs used to treat osteoporosis; they encourage osteoclasts to undergo apoptosis.

Blastomycosis (blast-o-mi-KO-sis) A type of fungal infection that usually begins in the respiratory system. See *pneumonia*.

Blepharospasm (BLEF-ah-ro-spazm) Involuntary spasmodic contraction of the orbicularis oculi muscles. See *dystonia*.

Blood-brain barrier (blud-brane BA-re-er) A selective filter in a continuous layer of endothelial cells connected by tight junctions; prevents or inhibits the passage of ions or large compounds from the blood to the brain tissue.

Bolus (BO-lus) A masticated morsel of food or other substance ready to be swallowed.

Bone scan A diagnostic test to look for bone cancer or infections, to evaluate unexplained pain, or to diagnose fractures.

Borrelia burgdorferi (bo-RE-le-ah burg-DOR-fer-i) A species of bacteria that causes Lyme disease; transferred to humans through tick bites.

Botulinum (BOT-yu-lin-um) A potent neurotoxin from *Clostridium botulinum*.

Bouchard nodes (boo-SHAR nodez) Enlargement of the proximal interphalangeal joints due to bone spurs associated with osteoarthritis.

Bovine spongiform encephalopathy (BO-vine SPUN-jih-form en-sef-ah-LOP-ath-e) A disease of cattle first reported in 1986 in Great Britain; characterized clinically by apprehensive behavior, hyperesthesia, and ataxia and histologically by spongiform changes in the gray matter of the brainstem; caused by a prion, like spongiform encephalopathies of other animals, for example, scrapie in cattle and Creutzfeldt-Jakob disease in human beings. See *Alzheimer disease*.

Bowen disease (BO-wen dih-ZEZE) A form of intraepidermal carcinoma characterized by the development of slowly enlarging pinkish or brownish papules or eroded plaques covered with a thickened horny layer. See *skin cancer*.

Bowman capsule (BO-man KAP-sule) The beginning of a nephron that surrounds the glomerulus.

Brachytherapy (BRAK-e-THER-ah-pe) Radiotherapy in which the source of the radiation is implanted into the tissues to be treated.

Bradykinesia (brad-e-kin-E-se-a) A decrease in the spontaneity of movement.

Bronchiectasis (bronk-e-ek-TA-sis) Chronic dilation of the bronchi or bronchioles, often as a consequence of inflammatory disease or obstruction.

Bruxism (BRUK-sizm) Jaw clenching that results in rubbing and grinding of teeth, especially during sleep.

Buerger disease (BUR-ger diz-EZE) Inflammation of the intima of a blood vessel with thrombosis. See *Raynaud syndrome*.

Bulbar (BUL-bar) Bulb-shaped, referring to a problem involving the medulla oblongata.

Bulla, bullae (BUL-ah, BUL-ee) A bubblelike structure, specifically the air-filled blisters on the lung formed by fused alveoli in emphysema.

Burkitt lymphoma (BUR-kit lym-FO-mah) A form of malignant lymphoma frequently involving the jaw and abdominal lymph nodes. Geographic distribution of Burkitt lymphoma suggests that it is found in areas with endemic malaria. It is primarily a B-cell neoplasm and is believed to be caused by Epstein-Barr virus, a member of the family *Herpesviridae*.

Bursectomy (bur-SEK-to-me) Surgical removal of a bursa.

Calcitonin (kal-sih-TO-nin) A hormone that increases the deposition of calcium and phosphate in bone.

Calcium channel blockers (KAL-se-um CHAN-el BLOK-erz) A class of medications that prevents the passage of calcium through membranes; used to treat hypertension, angina pectoris, and arrhythmia.

Calcium oxalate (KAL-se-um OK-sah-late) A sediment in urine and renal calculi. See *kidney stones*.

Calcium phosphate (KAL-se-um FOS-fate) Calcium salts of phosphoric acid.

Calcium pyrophosphate dihydrate (KAL-se-um pi-ro-FOS-fate di-HI-drate) Substance deposited in pseudogout, leading to acute attacks of joint inflammation. See *gout*.

Callus (KAL-us) A thickening of the keratin layer of the epidermis as a result of repeated friction or intermittent pressure.

Campylobacter jejuni (KAM-pih-lo-bak-ter jeh-JU-ni) A species that causes acute gastroenteritis of sudden onset with constitutional symptoms (malaise, myalgia, arthralgia, and headache) and cramping abdominal pain.

Campylobacter pylori (KAM-pih-lo-bak-ter pi-LOR-i) Synonym for *Helicobacter pylori*. See *ulcers*.

Candida albicans (KAN-di-dah AL-bih-kanz) A genus of yeastlike fungi.

Capsaicin (kap-SA-zin) Red pepper, hot pepper.

Capsid (KAP-sid) A complete virus particle that is structurally intact and infectious.

Carbuncle (KAR-bunk-el) A group of local infections of hair follicles with connecting sinuses; a group of boils.

Carcinoma (kar-sih-NO-mah) Any of a variety of malignant neoplasms deriving from epithelial tissue.

Cardia of stomach (KAR-de-ah ov STUM-ak) Proximal end of the stomach.

Cardiac tamponade (KAR-de-ak TAM-po-nade) Pathological compression of the heart, related to increased volume of the pericardium.

Cardiomyopathy (kar-de-o-mi-OP-ath-e) Disease of the myocardium; a primary disease of heart muscle in the absence of a known underlying etiology.

Cataplexy (KAT-ah-plex-e) A transient attack of extreme generalized muscular weakness, often precipitated by an emotional state such as laughing, surprise, fear, or anger. See *sleep disorders*.

Catheter atherectomy (KATH-eh-ter ath-er-EK-to-me) Removal of atherosclerotic plaque through a catheter; usually applied to carotid arteries.

Cauda equina (KAW-dah e-KWI-nah) Bundle of spinal nerve roots that runs through the lumbar cistern; it comprises the roots of all the spinal nerves below L_1. From Latin: *horse tail*. See *ankylosing spondylitis, disc disease*.

Causalgia (kaw-ZAL-je-ah) Persistent severe burning sensation, usually following partial injury of a peripheral nerve, accompanied by trophic changes including thinning of skin and loss of sweat glands and hair follicles. See *complex regional pain syndrome*.

Celiac sprue (SE-le-ak spru) Chronic inflammation and atrophy of the mucosa of the small intestine, related to an allergy to gluten. See *celiac sprue*.

Cellular immunity (SEL-u-lar ih-MU-nih-te) Also called cell-mediated immunity. Immune responses that are initiated by T cells and mediated by T cells, macrophages, or both.

Cervical dystonia (SER-vih-kul dis-TO-ne-ah) A state of abnormal tendency in skeletal muscles that affect the neck.

Cervical rib (SER-vih-kal rib) An abnormally wide transverse process of a cervical vertebra or a supernumerary rib that articulates with a cervical vertebra but does not articulate with the sternum. C7 is the vertebra most often affected.

Cervical spondylitic myelopathy (SER-vih-kal spon-dih-LIH-tik mi-el-OP-ath-e) Damage to the spinal cord due to osteophytic pressure. See *spondylosis*.

Chancre (KAN-ker) The primary lesion of syphilis, which begins at the site of infection after an interval of 10 to 30 days as a papule or area of infiltration, of dull red color, hard, and insensitive; the center usually becomes eroded or breaks down into an ulcer that heals slowly after 4 to 6 weeks. See *sexually transmitted diseases*.

Chemonucleolysis (ke-mo-nu-kle-OL-ih-sis) Injection of chymopapain into the nucleus pulposus of a herniated disc.

Chemotherapy (ke-mo-THER-ah-pe) The treatment of disease by chemical means, that is, drugs.

Chiari II formation (ke-AR-e for-MA-shun) A malformation of the brain, involving a downward displacement of the cerebellum through the foramen magnum.

Childhood disintegrative disorder (child-hood dis-IN-teh-gra-tiv dis-OR-der) A type of autism spectrum disorder involving a dramatic loss of vocabulary, motor, and communication skills.

Chimeric (ki-MER-ik) Any macromolecule fusion formed by two or more macromolecules from different species or from different genes. See *scleroderma*.

Chlamydia (klah-MIH-de-ah) A genus of bacteria that is a causative factor for pelvic inflammatory disease and other infections; the chief agent of bacterial sexually transmitted diseases in the United States.

Chlamydia trachomatis (klah-MIH-de-ah trak-o-MAH-tis) Spherical organism that causes a variety of infections, including conjunctivitis, pelvic inflammatory disease, and others.

Cholangitis (ko-lan-JI-tis) Inflammation of the bile duct or biliary tree.

Cholecyst (KO-leh-sist) Synonym for gallbladder.

Choledocholithiasis (ko-led-o-ko-lih-THI-ah-sis) Presence of a gallstone in the common bile duct.

Cholelithiasis (ko-leh-lih-THI-ah-sis) Presence of stones in the gallbladder or bile ducts.

Cholinesterase inhibitors (ko-lin-ES-ter-ase in-HIB-ih-torz) Class of drugs that improve myoneural function; used for myasthenia gravis, Alzheimer disease.

Chondrocyte (KON-dro-site) A nondividing cartilage cell.

Chondroitin sulfate (kon-DROY-tin SUL-fate) One of the substances in the extracellular matrix of connective tissue.

Chondromalacia patellae (kon-dro-mah-LA-she-a pah-TEL-a) Degenerative condition in the articular cartilage of the kneecap caused by abnormal compression or shearing forces at the knee joint; may cause patellalgia (knee pain).

Choriocarcinoma (KOR-e-o-kar-sih-NO-mah) A highly malignant neoplasm. Hemorrhagic metastases are found in the lungs, liver, brain, and vagina; choriocarcinoma may follow any type of pregnancy, especially hydatidiform mole, and occasionally originates in teratoid neoplasms of the ovaries or testes. See *testicular cancer*.

Christmas disease (KRIS-mas dih-ZEZE) Synonym for hemophilia B, involving a deficiency in clotting factor IX.

Chronic (KRON-ik) Having low intensity, lasting a long time; refers to a disease or disorder.

Chronic exertional compartment syndrome (KRON-ik eg-ZER-shun-al kom-PART-ment SIN-drome) The accumulation of fluid pressure in one or more of the tough fascial compartments of the lower leg. See *shin splints*.

Chronic granulocytic leukemia (KRON-ik gran-u-lo-SIT-ik lu-KE-me-ah) Synonym for chronic myelogenous leukemia. See *leukemia*.

Chronic myeloid leukemia (KRON-ik MI-eh-loyd lu-KE-me-ah) Synonym for chronic myelogenous leukemia. See *leukemia*.

Chronic venous insufficiency (KRON-ik VE-nus in-suh-FISH-en-se) A condition resulting from valve damage in veins that leads to permanent edema, skin discoloration or ulcers, and very slow healing in the affected area.

Chyme (kime) Semifluid mass of partly digested food in the stomach or small intestine.

Cilium, cilia (sil-e-um, sil-e-ah) Hairlike motile extension of the surface of certain epithelial cells.

Circadian rhythm (sir-KA-de-an RITH-em) Relating to biological variations or rhythms that last approximately 24 hours. From Latin *circa* (*about*) and *dies* (*day*).

Cirrhosis (sir-O-sis) Progressive disease of the liver characterized by damage to hepatocytes and accumulation of scar tissue.

Clonic spasm (KLON-ik spazm) Alternating involuntary contraction and relaxation of a muscle.

Coagulability (ko-ag-yu-lah-BIL-ih-te) Ability to clot.

Cobalamin (ko-BAL-ah-mene) General term for compounds containing the nucleus of vitamin B_{12}.

Coccidioidomycosis (kok-sid-e-OY-do-mi-KO-sis) A potentially fatal fungal disease, usually of the respiratory tract.

Coelomic metaplasia (se-LO-mik) A theory for the etiology of endometriosis based on the fact that coelomic epithelium is the common ancestor of endometrial and peritoneal cells, and may undergo metaplasia, or a change in formation, later in life.

Cognitive-behavioral therapy (KOG-nih-tiv be-HA-vyor-al THER-ah-pe) A technique in psychotherapy that uses guided self-discovery, imaging, self-instruction, and other elicited cognitions as the principal mode of treatment.

Colchicine (KOL-chih-sene) An alkaloid obtained from autumn crocus used for the treatment of gout.

Colic (KOL-ik) An abnormal contraction of smooth muscle, particularly in the digestive tract.

Collagen (KOL-ah-jen) A major protein forming the white fibers of connective tissue.

Collagenase (ko-LAJ-eh-nase) A proteolytic dissolving enzyme that acts on one or more of the collagens.

Colonoscopy (kol-o-NOS-ko-pe) A visual examination of the internal surface of the colon by means of a long fiberoptic endoscope.

Colostomy (ko-LOS-to-me) An artificial opening from the skin to the colon.

Colposcopy (kol-POS-ko-pe) Examination of the vagina and cervix by means of an endoscope.

Comedo (ko-ME-do) A dilated hair follicle filled with bacteria; the principal lesion of acne vulgaris. Plural— comedos, comedones.

Comedome (KO-meh-dome) A dilated hair follicle filled with bacteria and other substances; an acne lesion.

Comminuted (KOM-ih-nu-ted) Broken into several pieces; denoting especially a fractured bone.

Comorbidity (ko-mor-BID-ih-te) Condition of having multiple pathologies simultaneously.

Complement (KOM-pleh-ment) A combination of many serum proteins that react with each other in various ways to disable antigens and assist immune system response.

Complex regional pain syndrome (KOM-plex RE-jun-al PAIN SIN-drome) A chronic pain syndrome; sometimes called *complex regional pain syndrome*.

Compression (kum-PRESH-un) Squeezing together; a decrease in the dimension of a structure because of forces exerted from outside.

Concentric (kun-SEN-trik) Describing a muscle contraction that pulls attachments closer together, that is, toward the center.

Concussion (kun-KUSH-un) An injury of the brain resulting from a blow or violent shaking; may lead to partial or complete loss of function.

Condyle (KON-dile) A rounded articular surface at the extremity of a bone.

Condyloma acuminatum (kon-dih-LO-mah-tah ah-ku-min-AH-tum) A warty growth on the external genitals or at the anus, consisting of fibrous overgrowths covered by thickened epithelium showing koilocytosis, due to sexually transmitted infection with human papillomavirus; malignant change is associated with particular types of the virus. Also known as genital warts. See *sexually transmitted diseases*.

Congenital (kon-JEN-ih-tal) Referring to mental or physical traits that exist at birth.

Congenital nevus (kon-JEN-ih-tal NE-vus) A benign local overgrowth of melanin-forming cells of the skin present at birth or appearing early in life.

Consolidation (kon-sol-ih-DA-shun) Solidification into a firm, dense mass, specifically with cellular exudate in the lungs during pneumonia.

Constriction (kon-STRIK-shun) A narrowed portion of a luminal structure.

Contact inhibition (KON-takt in-hih-BIH-shun) The tendency of basal cells involved in healing to stop reproducing when they encounter cells from the other side of the wound.

Contracture (kun-TRAK-chur) Muscle shortening due to spasm or fibrosis, loss of balance between antagonists, or loss of motion of the adjacent joint.

Contralateral (kon-trah-LAT-er-al) Relating to the opposite side, as when pain is felt or paralysis occurs on the side opposite to that of the lesion.

Contusion (kun-TU-zhun) Any mechanical injury resulting in hemorrhage beneath unbroken skin.

Cor pulmonale (kor pul-mo-NAL) Right-sided ventricular hypertrophy, often arising from disease of the lungs.

Corpus callosum (KOR-pus kal-LOS-um) The plate of nerve fibers interconnecting the cortical hemispheres.

Corpus luteum (KOR-pus LU-te-um) The site of egg release on follicles of the ovaries immediately after ovulation.

Corticosteroid injection (kor-tih-ko-STER-oyd in-JEK-shun) An injection of a specific steroid into an injured area for its anti-inflammatory and/or connective tissue–dissolving properties.

Cortisol (KOR-tih-sol) A glucocorticoid secreted by the adrenal cortex. It acts on carbohydrate metabolism and influences the growth and nutrition of connective tissue.

Cortisone (KOR-tih-sone) A form of cortisol that may be injected into specific areas to act as an anti-inflammatory or to help dissolve connective tissue.

Counter-irritant (kown-tur-IR-ih-tent) An agent that causes irritation or mild inflammation of the skin to relieve symptoms of a deeper inflammatory process.

Coup de sabre (koo deh SAHB) Linear scleroderma over the forehead.

Coup-contrecoup (koo-KON-treh-koo) Pattern of brain injury involving a primary impact on one side of the skull and a secondary impact as the brain bounces to the opposite side of the cranium. See *traumatic brain injury*.

COX-2 inhibitors A class of nonsteroidal anti-inflammatory drugs that work by blocking COX (cyclooxygenase) 2 enzyme, which is involved in the inflammation pathway.

Coxsackie virus (kok-SAK-e VI-rus) A group of viruses first isolated in Coxsackie, New York. They may be responsible for several human diseases, including meningitis and juvenile diabetes.

C-reactive protein A beta-globulin found in the serum of various persons with certain inflammatory, degenerative, and neoplastic diseases. See *heart attack*, *atherosclerosis*.

Creatine kinase (KREE-ah-tene) An enzyme used in muscle contraction that allows transformation of adenosine diphosphate into adenosine triphosphate and creatine; levels of creatine kinase are sometimes elevated following a heart attack. See *muscular dystrophy*.

Crepitus (KREP-ih-tus) A crackling sound resembling the noise heard on rubbing hair between the fingers.

CREST syndrome *C*alcinosis, *R*aynaud phenomenon, *e*sophageal motility disorders, *s*clerodactyly, and *t*elangiectasia. See *scleroderma*.

Crisis (KRI-sis) A sudden change, usually for the better, in the course of an acute disease.

Cruciate ligament sprain (KROO-she-ate LIG-ah-ment spranez) Major ligaments that crisscross the knee in the anteroposterior direction, providing stability in that plane.

Crust (krust) A hard outer covering; a scab.

Cryomyolysis (kri-o-mi-OL-ih-sis) A procedure using liquid nitrogen to freeze uterine fibroid tumors.

Cryptococcus neoformans (KRIP-to-kok-us ne-o-FOR-manz) A species of yeastlike fungi that reproduce by budding. See *HIV/AIDS*.

Cryptorchism, cryptorchidism (krip-TOR-kizm) Failure of one or both of the testes to descend. See *testicular cancer*.

Cryptosporidium (krip-to-spor-IH-de-um) A genus of sporozoans that are common parasites of humans with impaired immunity. See *gastroenteritis*.

Cyanosis (si-ah-NO-sis) A bluish or purplish coloration of the skin and mucous membranes due to deficient oxygenation of the blood. See *Raynaud syndrome*, *anemia*.

Cyclooxygenase-1 pathway (si-klo-OX-ih-jen-ase-1 PATH-way) The sequence of events that leads to an inflammatory process: this is interrupted by anti-inflammatories.

Cyclooxygenase-2 (si-klo-OX-ih-jen-ase) See *COX-2 inhibitors*.

Cystadenoma (sist-ah-den-O-ma) A benign neoplasm derived from glandular epithelium. See *ovarian cysts*.

Cystine (SIS-tene) A type of acid that can form deposits of crystals in the urine or in the kidneys.

Cystocele (SIS-to-sele) Hernia of the bladder, often into the vagina.

Cystoscope (SIS-to-skope) A lighted tubular endoscope for examining the interior of the bladder.

Cytokine (SI-to-kine) Hormonelike proteins secreted by many cells and involved in cell-to-cell communication.

Cytomegalovirus (si-to-MEG-ah-lo-vi-rus) A group of viruses in the Herpesviridae family infecting humans and animals. Mononucleosis.

Cytotoxic drug (si-to-TOX-ik drug) A drug that is detrimental or destructive to certain cells.

Dactylitis (dak-tih-LI-tis) Inflammation of the fingers.

de Quervain tenosynovitis (deh kare-VA ten-o-sin-o-VI-tis) Inflammation of the tendons of the first dorsal compartment of the wrist, which includes the extensor pollicis brevis and the abductor pollicis longus.

Debridement (da-brede-MONH) Excision of dead tissue and foreign matter from a wound.

Decortication (de-kor-tih-KA-shun) Removal of the cortex, or external layer, of any organ or structure.

Decubitus ulcer (de-KU-bih-tus UL-ser) Focal ischemic necrosis of skin and underlying tissues at sites of constant pressure or recurring friction in persons confined to bed or immobilized by illness.

Degeneration (de-jen-er-A-shun) A retrogressive pathological change in tissues, in consequence of which their functions may be impaired or destroyed.

Degenerative joint disease (de-JEN-er-ah-tiv JOYNT dih-ZEZE) Synonym for osteoarthritis.

Dementia (de-MEN-sha) The loss, usually progressive, of cognitive and intellectual functions without impairment of perception or consciousness.

Dendrite (DEN-drite) The process of a nerve cell that carries impulses toward the cell body.

Dermabrasion (der-mah-BRA-zhun) Procedure to remove acne scars or pits from the skin using sandpaper, rotating wire brushes, or other abrasive materials.

Dermatitis herpetiformis (der-mah-TI-tis her-pet-ih-FOR-mis) A chronic disease of the skin marked by a symmetrical itching eruption of vesicles and papules that occur in groups; relapses are common; associated with gluten-sensitive enteropathy. See *celiac sprue*.

Dermatome (DER-mah-tome) The area of skin supplied by cutaneous branches from a single spinal nerve.

Dermatophyte (der-MAT-o-fite) A fungus that causes superficial infections of the skin, hair, and nails.

Dermatophytosis (der-mat-o-fi-TO-sis) An infection of the hair, skin, or nails caused by any one of the dermatophytes. The lesions are characterized by erythema, small papular vesicles, fissures, and scaling. See *fungal infections*.

Dermatosparaxis EDS (der-mat-o-spah-RAK-sis) A type of Ehlers-Danlos syndrome involving loose, sagging skin even in young children, and ligament laxity.

Dermographia (der-mo-GRAF-e-ah) A form of urticaria in which wheals develop where the skin has been stroked.

Dermoid cyst (DER-moyd SIST) A tumor consisting of displaced ectodermal structures along lines of embryonic fusion, the wall being formed of epithelium-lined connective tissue, including skin appendages and containing keratin, sebum, and hair. See *testicular cancer, ovarian cysts*.

DEXA Dual-energy x-ray absorptiometry. Use of low-dose x-radiation of two different energies to measure bone mineral content at different anatomic sites.

Dextroamphetamine (dex-tro-am-FET-ah-mene) A medication for central nervous system stimulation.

Diabetes insipidus (di-ah-BE-teze in-SIP-ih-dus) Chronic excretion of very large amounts of pale urine of low specific gravity, causing dehydration and extreme thirst; ordinarily results from inadequate output of pituitary antidiuretic hormone.

Diaphoresis (di-ah-for-E-sis) Perspiration.

Diaphysis (di-AH-fih-sis) The shaft of a long bone.

Diarthrosis, diarthroses (di-arth-RO-sis, di-arth-RO-seze) Also called synovial joint. A joint in which articulating surfaces are covered by articular cartilage and held together by a capsular ligament, which is lined with a synovial membrane. Some degree of freedom of movement is possible with diarthrotic joints.

Diastole (DI-ah-stole) Normal postsystolic dilation of the heart cavities, during which they fill with blood.

Diethylstilbesterol (di-eth-il-stil-BES-ter-ol) An estrogenic compound that used to be used to prevent miscarriage; it is associated with a risk of cervical cancer in the daughters of women who took it.

Diffuse axonal injury (dih-FUSE AK-so-nal IN-jur-e) Injury to white matter in the central nervous system that is frequently associated with a persistent vegetative state. See *traumatic brain injury*.

Diffuse idiopathic skeletal hyperostosis (DISH) (dih-FUSE id-e-o-PATH-ik SKEL-eh-tal hi-per-os-TO-sis) A common condition involving the deposition of calcium deposits along the anterior longitudinal ligament of the spine.

Diffuse large cell lymphoma (dih-FUSE larj sell lim-FO-mah) A type of intermediate-grade lymphoma.

Diffuse mixed cell lymphoma (dih-FUSE mixt sell lim-FO-mah) A type of intermediate-grade lymphoma.

Diffuse scleroderma (dih-FUSE skler-o-DER-mah) A form of systemic scleroderma characterized by sudden onset and early involvement of internal organs.

Diffusion (dih-FU-zhun) Random movement of small particles in solution to a uniform distribution within a closed space.

Dihydrotestosterone (DHT) (di-hi-dro-tes-TOS-ter-one) An androgenic hormone with the same uses and actions as testosterone. Elevated levels are associated with an increased risk of benign prostatic hyperplasia.

Dilation (di-LA-shun) The enlargement of a hollow structure or opening.

Dilation and curettage (di-LA-shun and ku-reh-TAHJH) Dilation of the cervix and scraping of the endometrium to remove growths or other abnormal tissues or to obtain material for tissue diagnosis.

Dimethyl sulfoxide (DMSO)(di-METH-il sul-FOX-ide) A penetrating solvent-enhancing absorption of therapeutic agents through the skin.

Dioxin (di-OX-in) A contaminate in some herbicides; associated with toxicity, some forms of cancer, and birth defects.

Diphtheria (dif-THE-re-ah) A highly infectious bacterial disease that begins in the nose and throat; can resemble mononucleosis.

Diplegia (di-PLE-je-ah) Paralysis of corresponding parts on both sides of the body.

Discoid lupus erythematosus (DIS-koid LU-pus eh-rih-them-ah-TO-sis) Autoimmune disease involving lesions on the skin. See *lupus*.

Diskectomy (dis-KEK-to-me) Excision of part or all of an intervertebral disk. See *disc disease*.

Diuretic (di-u-REH-tik) A chemical agent that increases urine output.

Diverticulum, diverticula (div-er-TIK-u-lum, div-er-TIK-u-lah) A pouch or sac opening from a tubular or saccular organ, for example, the colon or urinary bladder.

DMARDs Disease-modifying antirheumatic drugs. Agents that apparently alter the course and progression of rheumatoid arthritis; more rapidly acting other substances (not DMARDs) suppress inflammation and decrease pain, but do not prevent cartilage or bone erosion or progressive disability.

DOMS Delayed-onset muscle soreness.

Dopamine (DO-pah-mene) A neurotransmitter in the basal ganglia.

Double crush syndrome (DUB-el KRUSH SIN-drome) Irritation of peripheral nerves at multiple sites, leading to confusing signs and symptoms. See *carpal tunnel syndrome.*

Double depression (DUB-ul de-PRESH-un) Comorbidity of dysthymia with an episode of major depressive disorder.

Ductal ectasia (DUK-tal ek-TA-zha) Inflammation of the ducts of the breast. See *breast cancer.*

Dupuytren contracture (du-pwe-TRAH kon-TRAK-cher) A disease of the palmar fascia resulting in thickening and shortening of fibrous bands on the palmar surface of the hand and fingers resulting in a characteristic flexion deformity of the fourth and fifth digits.

Dura mater (DU-rah MA-ter) A tough, fibrous membrane forming the outer covering of the central nervous system.

Dural ectasia (DUR-al ek-TA-zha) Stretching and weakening of the dura mater with age; associated with Marfan syndrome.

Dysarthria (dis-ARTH-re-ah) Disturbance of speech related to paralysis or spasticity. See *stroke.*

Dyshidrosis (dis-hi-DRO-sis) A skin eruption with blisters and itching that usually appears on the volar surface of the hands or feet.

Dysmobility (dis-mo-BIL-ih-te) Inefficient or uncoordinated peristalsis in the gastrointestinal tract. See *scleroderma.*

Dyspepsia (dis-PEP-se-ah) Upset stomach: pain, burning, nausea, and gas.

Dysphagia (dis-FA-je-a) Difficulty in swallowing.

Dysplasia, dysplastic (dis-PLA-zha, dis-PLAS-tik) Abnormal tissue development.

Dysplastic nevus (dis-PLAS-tik NE-vus) Atypical mole associated with an increased risk of developing into malignant melanoma. See *skin cancer.*

Dyspnea (disp-NE-ah) Shortness of breath.

Dysreflexia (dis-re-FLEX-e-ah) A condition of disordered or inappropriate responses to stimuli.

Dyssomnia (dis-SOM-ne-a) Inability to achieve or maintain sleep.

Dysthymia (dis-THI-me-ah) Chronic mood disorder involving long-term, low-grade depression.

Dystonia (dis-TO-ne-ah) A state of abnormal (too much or too little) muscle tone.

Dystrophic (dis-TRO-fik) Relating to progressive changes that may result from defective nutrition of a tissue or organ.

Dystrophin (dis-TRO-fin) A protein found in the sarcolemma of normal muscle tissue; it is missing in individuals with some forms of muscular dystrophy.

Escherichia coli (E-KO-li, esh-er-IK-e-ah KO-li) A species of bacteria linked with infections of the gastrointestinal or urinary tracts.

EAST Elevated arm stress test. See *thoracic outlet syndrome.*

Eccentric contraction (ek-SEN-trik kun-TRAK-shun) A lengthening action in which a muscle's attachments are drawn away from each other while the muscle is activated.

Ecchymosis (ek-ih-MO-sis) A purplish patch caused by blood leaking into the skin; a bruise.

Echocardiogram (ek-o-KAR-de-o-gram) The record obtained by the use of ultrasound in the investigation of the heart and great vessels and diagnosis of cardiovascular lesions.

Eclampsia (e-KLAMP-se-ah) One or more convulsions not attributable to other cerebral conditions. In this case, related to pregnancy-induced hypertension.

Ecthyma (ek-THI-mah) A form of streptococcal infection of the skin. See *impetigo.*

Eczema (EG-zeh-mah) Generic term for inflammatory conditions of the skin, particularly with blistering in the acute stage, often accompanied by sensations of itching and burning.

Edema (eh-DE-mah) An accumulation of an excessive amount of watery fluid in cells, tissues, or serous membranes.

Ehrlichiosis (er-lik-e-O-sis) A tickborne bacterial infection of humans and dogs. See *Lyme disease*.

Elastin (e-LAS-tin) A yellow, elastic fibrous protein that contributes to the connective tissue of elastic structures.

Electrocauterization (e-lek-tro-kaw-ter-i-ZA-shun) Cauterization by passage of high-frequency current through tissue or by metal that has been electrically heated.

Electroencephalogram (EEG) (e-lek-tro-en-SEF-ah-lo-gram) A recording of electrical potentials of the brain, derived from electrodes attached to the scalp.

Electrolyte (e-LEK-tro-lite) Any compound that in solution conducts electricity and is decomposed by it.

Electromyography (EMG) (e-lek-tro-mi-OG-raf-e) A recording of electrical activity in muscle tissue.

Electronystagmogram (e-lek-tro-nis-TAG-mo-gram) A test to measure the extent of horizontal or vertical nystagmus. See *vestibular balance disorders*.

ELISA Enzyme-linked immunosorbent assay. In vitro binding assay in which an enzyme and its substrate (rather than a radioactive substance) serve as the indicator system; in positive results, the two yield a colored or other easily recognizable substance. See *HIV/AIDS*.

Embolization (em-bo-li-ZA-shun) Therapeutic introduction of various substances into the circulation to occlude vessels, either to arrest or prevent hemorrhaging or to devitalize a structure or organ by occluding its blood supply.

Embryonic carcinoma (em-bre-ON-ik kar-sih-NO-mah) A type of testicular cancer.

Emery-Dreifuss muscular dystrophy (EM-er-e DRI-fus MUS-ku-lar DIS-tro-fe) A generally benign type of muscular dystrophy that typically begins in the shoulder girdle and then spreads distally; an X-linked inherited disorder.

Emollient (e-MOL-i-ent) An agent that softens or soothes the skin.

Empyema (em-pi-E-mah) Pus in a body cavity; usually refers to the thorax. See *pneumonia*.

Encephalitis (en-sef-ah-LI-tis) Inflammation of the brain.

Endarterectomy (en-dar-ter-EK-to-me) Excision of the diseased layers of an artery along with atherosclerotic plaques.

Endemic (en-DEM-ik) Present in a community or among a group of people; said of a disease prevailing continually in a region.

Endo- (EN-do) A prefix indicating within, inner, absorbing, or containing.

Endocarditis (en-do-kar-DI-tis) Inflammation of the the innermost tunic of the heart.

Endogenous (en-DOJ-en-us) Originating or produced within the organism or one of its parts.

Endolymph (EN-do-limf) The fluid in the membranous labyrinth of the inner ear.

Endometrioma (en-do-me-tre-O-mah) Mass of abnormal tissue in the endometrium. See *ovarian cysts*.

Endometritis (en-do-meh-TRI-tis) Inflammation of the endometrium.

Endometrium (en-do-ME-tre-um) The inner layers of the uterine wall.

Endomysium (en-do-MI-ze-um) The connective tissue sheath surrounding muscle fibers.

Endoscopic retrograde cholangiopancreatography (ERCP) (en-do-SKOP-ik RET-ro-grade ko-lan-je-o-pan-kre-ah-TOG-raf-e) A diagnostic procedure to detect problems in the liver, gallbladder, bile ducts, or pancreas. See *gallstones*.

Endoscopy (en-DOS-ko-pe) Examination of the interior of a hollow area by means of a special instrument, an endoscope.

Endosteum (en-DOS-te-um) A layer of cells lining the inner surface of bone in the central medullary cavity of long bones.

Endovascular (en-do-VAS-kyu-lar) Referring to procedures conducted within blood vessels.

Enterovirus (EN-ter-o-vi-rus) Any of a diverse group of viruses that attack the intestines.

Enzyme (EN-zime) A protein that acts as a catalyst to induce chemical changes in other substances while remaining unchanged itself.

Eosinophil (e-o-SIN-o-fil) A class of phagocytic white blood cells with antiparasitic functions.

Ephelis, ephelides (eh-FElis, eh-FE-lih-deze) Freckles.

Epi- (EP-e) Prefix indicating upon, following, or subsequent to.

Epicondylitis (ep-ih-kon-dih-LI-tis) Infection or inflammation of an epicondyle.

Epidermis (ep-ih-DER-mis) The superficial epithelial portion of the skin.

Epidermodysplasia verruciformis (ep-ih-dur-mo-dis-PLA-ze-ah veh-ru-sih-FOR-mis) A rare genetic skin disorder characterized by abnormal susceptibility to human papillomaviruses, causing widespread warts.

Epidermophyton (ep-ih-der-MOF-ih-ton, ep-ih-der-mo-FI-ton) A genus of fungi whose macroconidia are clavate and smooth walled. The only species, *Epidermophyton floccosum*, is a common cause of tinea pedis and tinea cruris. See *fungal infections*.

Epididymis (ep-ih-DIH-dih-mus) A tube on the posterior aspect of the testes in which sperm mature.

Epimysium (ep-ih-MIS-e-um) The connective tissue membrane surrounding a skeletal muscle.

Epinephrine (ep-ih-NEF-rin) The chief hormone of the adrenal medulla; a potent stimulant of the sympathetic response.

Epistaxis (ep-ih-STAK-sis) Profuse bleeding from the nose.

Epitenon (e-PIT-en-on) Sheath that wraps around tendons; also a synonym for tenosynovial sheath.

Epithelium (ep-ih-THE-le-um) A purely cellular avascular layer covering all free surfaces including skin, mucous, and serous glands.

Epstein-Barr virus (EP-stine BAR VI-rus) A herpesvirus that causes infectious mononucleosis and is implicated in Burkitt lymphoma.

Ergot (ER-got) The resistant, overwintering stage of the parasitic ascomycetous fungus *Claviceps purpurea*. Ergot induces uterine contractions, controls bleeding, and alleviates certain localized vascular disorders, such as migraine headaches.

Ernest syndrome (ER-nest SIN-drome) A condition involving a weakened and irritated stylomandibular ligament; frequently mistaken for temporomandibular joint disorder. See *temporomandibular joint disorder*.

Erysipelas (er-ih-SIP-eh-lus) A specific acute, cutaneous inflammatory disease caused by beta-hemolytic streptococci and characterized by hot, red, edematous, brawny, and sharply defined eruptions; usually accompanied by severe constitutional symptoms. See *cellulitis*.

Erythema (er-i-THE-mah) Redness of the skin due to capillary dilation.

Erythema migrans (er-i-THE-mah MI-granz) A type of rash, usually seen as an early symptom of Lyme disease.

Erythrocyte (e-RITH-ro-site) A mature red blood cell.

Erythrodermic psoriasis (e-rith-ro-DER-mik so-RI-ah-sis) A generalized form of psoriasis that can cover 85% or more of the body.

Erythropoietin (EPO)(e-rith-ro-POY-eh-tin) A hormone secreted by the kidneys and possibly other tissues that stimulates the formation of red blood cells.

Essential (e-SEN-shal) Of unknown etiology, specifically in reference to hypertension.

Estradiol (es-tra-DI-ol) The most potent naturally occurring estrogen in mammals.

Estriol (ES-tre-ol) Estrogenic metabolite of estradiol; usually the predominant estrogenic metabolite found in urine, especially during pregnancy.

Estrogen (ES-tro-jen) A group of hormones secreted by the ovaries, placenta, testes, and possibly other tissues. Estrogens influence secondary sexual characteristics and the menstrual cycle.

Estrogen dominance (ES-tro-jen DOM-ih-nens) A metabolic state in which endogenous and exogenous forms of estrogen overbalance progesterone levels.

Estrogen replacement therapy (ERT) (ES-tro-jen re-PLASE-ment THER-ah-pe) A treatment for the prevention or slowing of osteoporosis by replacing some of the hormones that are lost or diminished with the onset of menopause.

Estrone (ES-trone) A metabolite of estradiol.

Excitotoxicity (ek-si-to-tox-IH-sih-te) A pathologic state in which nerve cells are damaged by excessive exposure to excitatory neurotransmitters, especially glutamate.

Exenteration (ek-sen-ter-A-shun) Removal of internal organs and tissues, usually to ablate cancer.

Exogenous (eg-ZOJ-en-us) Originating or produced outside the organism.

Exophthalmus (ex-of-THAL-mus) Protrusion of one or both eyeballs.

External scar tissue (ex-TER-nal SKAR TISH-u) Scar tissue that develops outside of the injured structure, often binding that structure to other nearby structures in adhesions.

Extracorporeal shockwave lithotripsy (ex-trah-kor-POR-e-al SHOK-wave LITH-o-trip-se) Breaking up of renal or ureteral calculi by focused ultrasound energy.

Extramedullary plastocytoma (ex-trah-MED-u-la-re plas-to-si-TO-mah) Growth of myeloma tumors outside of bone tissue.

Exudate (EK-su-date) Any fluid that has seeped out of a tissue or its capillaries because of inflammation or injury.

Facioscapulohumeral dystrophy (FASH-e-o-SKAP-u-lo-HU-mer-al DIS-tro-fe) A relatively benign, slowly progressive type of muscular dystrophy involving the muscles of the face, shoulders, and arms.

Familial adenomatous polyposis (fah-MIL-e-al ad-en-O-mah-tus pol-e-PO-sis) An inherited trait characterized by formation of epithelial polyps in the colon; may be associated with an increased risk of colorectal cancer.

Fascicle, fasciculi (FASH-i-kel, fah-SHIK-u-li) A band or bundle of fibers, specifically muscle fibers.

Fasciculation (fash-ik-u-LA-shun) Involuntary contractions or twitchings of fasciculi.

Fasciotomy (fash-e-OT-o-me) A surgical procedure to cut fascia in order to relieve internal pressure and avoid permanent damage.

Fat necrosis (fat nek-RO-sis) The death of fat cells, often in the breast.

Fecalith (FE-kah-lith) A hard mass composed of solidified or petrified feces. See *diverticular disease*.

Festinating gait (FES-tin-a-ting GATE) Gait in which the trunk is flexed, legs are stiff but flexed at the knees and hips, and the steps are short and progressively more rapid.

Fetal alcohol syndrome (fe-tal AL-ko-hol SIN-drome) A specific pattern of fetal malformation and health problems among offspring of mothers who are chronic alcoholics.

Fibrillation (fib-ril-A-shun) Exceedingly rapid contractions or twitching of muscular fibrils.

Fibrillin (FIB-ril-in) A protein of connective tissue. See *Marfan syndrome*.

Fibrin (FI-brin) An elastic filamentous protein that aids in coagulation of the blood.

Fibrinogen (fi-BRIN-o-jen) A globulin of the blood plasma that is converted into fibrin by the action of thrombin in the presence of ionized calcium to produce coagulation of the blood.

Fibroadenoma (fi-bro-ad-en-O-mah) A benign neoplasm of glandular epithelium, in which fibroblasts and other connective tissue proliferate. See *breast cancer*.

Fibroblast (FI-bro-blast) A cell capable of forming collagen fibers.

Filtration (fil-TRA-shun) The process of passing a liquid or gas through a filter.

Fimbria, fimbriae (FIM-bre-ah, FIM-bre-a) Any fringelike structure. Ovarian fimbriae extend over the ovaries.

Fistula, fistulae (FIS-tu-lah, FIS-tu-le) An abnormal passage from one epithelial surface to another.

Fixation (fik-SA-shun) The condition of being firmly attached or set. In regard to the spine, being excessively limited in movement between individual vertebrae.

Flaccid paralysis (FLAK-sid pah-RAL-ih-sis, FLAS-id pah-RAL-ih-sis) Paralysis with a loss of muscle tone, although sensation is present.

Focal dystonia (FO-kal dis-TO-ne-ah) A movement disorder that affects only one region of the body.

Focal epithelial hyperplasia (Heck disease) (FO-kul ep-ih-THE-le-ul hi-pur-PLA-ze-a) A skin condition characterized by white and pink papules in the mouth.

Folate (FO-late) A form of folic acid.

Folic acid (FO-lik AS-id) Member of the vitamin B complex necessary for the normal formation of red blood cells.

Follicular cleaved cell lymphoma (fo-LIK-u-lar kleved sell lim-FO-mah) A type of low-grade lymphoma.

Follicular large cell lymphoma (fo-LIK-u-lar larj sell lim-FO-mah) A type of intermediate-grade lymphoma.

Follicular mixed cell lymphoma (fo-LIK-u-lar mixt sell lim-FO-mah) A type of low-grade lymphoma.

Folliculitis (fo-lik-u-LI-tis) Inflammatory reaction in hair follicles leading to papules or pustules.

Fomite (FO-mite) An object such as a sheet, a tool, or clothing that can harbor and transmit an infectious agent.

Fragile X syndrome (FRAJ-il X SIN-drome) Genetic anomaly associated with developmental disability and autism spectrum disorder.

Frozen shoulder (FRO-zen SHOL-der) See *adhesive capsulitis*.

Fulminant (FUL-mi-nant) Occurring suddenly, with great intensity or severity.

Fulminant colitis (FUL-mi-nant ko-LI-tis) Sudden and extreme onset of colon inflammation seen with ulcerative colitis.

Fundoplication (fun-do-plih-KA-shun) Suture of the fundus of the stomach around the esophagus to prevent reflux with hiatal hernia.

Furuncle (FYU-runk-el) A local bacterial infection in a hair shaft. A boil.

Gamma globulin (GAM-ah GLOB-u-lin) A preparation of proteins of human plasma containing the antibodies of normal adults.

Gamma-aminobutyric acid (GABA) (GAM-ah ah-me-no-bu-TIR-ik AS-id) A principal inhibitory neurotransmitter.

Gardner syndrome (GARD-ner SIN-drome) A type of familial adenomatous polyposis; a genetic risk factor for colorectal cancer.

Gastritis (gas-TRI-tis) Inflammation, especially mucosal, of the stomach.

Gastrostomy (gas-TROS-to-me) Establishment of a new opening into the stomach.

Geniculate ganglion (jen-IK-u-late GANG-le-on) A ganglion of the fibers conveyed by the facial nerve, located within the facial canal, containing the sensory neurons innervating the taste buds on the anterior two-thirds of the tongue and a small area on the external ear. Bell palsy.

Geste antagoniste (jhest an-tag-o-NEEST) The habit of repeatedly touching an area affected with dystonia to reduce the severity of local contractions.

Giardia (je-AR-de-ah) A genus of parasitic flagellates that colonize the gastrointestinal tract of many mammals.

Gigantism (JI-gan-tizm) A condition of abnormal size or overgrowth of the entire body or of any of its parts. See *acromegaly*.

Gliadin (GLI-ah-din) A class of protein, separable from wheat and rye glutens. See *celiac sprue*.

Globus pallidus (GLO-bus PAL-id-us) The inner and lighter gray portion of the lentiform nucleus. See *Parkinson disease*.

Glomerular filtrate (glo-MARE-yu-lar FIL-trate) The liquid pushed from the glomerulus into the Bowman capsule.

Glomerular filtration rate (glo-MARE-yu-lar fil-TRA-shun RATE) The amount of fluid that passes from the glomeruli to the nephron within a given amount of time.

Glomerulations (glo-mare-yu-LA-shunz) Pinpoint hemorrhages of the bladder wall, seen with some cases of interstitial cystitis.

Glomerulonephritis (glo-MARE-yu-lar nef-RI-tis) Inflammation of the glomerulus and Bowman capsule.

Glomerulus (glo-MARE-yu-lus) A tuft of capillary loops surrounded by the Bowman capsule at the beginning of each nephric tubule in the kidney.

Glucagon (GLU-kah-gon) A hormone secreted by the pancreas; elevates blood sugar concentration.

Glucocorticoid (glu-ko-KOR-ti-koyd) Any steroidlike compound capable of influencing metabolism; also exerts an anti-inflammatory effect. Cortisol is the most potent of the naturally occurring glucocorticoids.

Glucosamine sulfate (glu-KO-sah-mene SUL-fate) An amino sugar used to support cartilaginous repair in osteoarthritis.

Glutamate (GLU-tah-mate) A salt or ester of glutamic acid, an amino acid that occurs in proteins; the sodium salt is monosodium glutamate. See *amyotrophic lateral sclerosis*.

Gluten (GLU-ten) The insoluble protein constituent of wheat and other grains.

Gluten-sensitive enteropathy (GLU-ten SEN-sih-tiv en-ter-OP-ath-e) Synonym for celiac sprue.

Glycogen (GLI-ko-jen) A substance found primarily in the liver and muscles that is easily converted into glucose.

Goiter (GOY-ter) Chronic enlargement of the thyroid gland not due to a neoplasm. May be related to both hyperthyroidism and hypothyroidism.

Golfer's elbow (GOL-ferz EL-bo) Synonym for medial epicondylitis.

Golgi tendon organ (GOL-je TEN-don OR-gan) A proprioceptive sensory nerve ending embedded in tendon fibers. It is activated by changes in tendon tension.

Grand mal seizure (grand MAL SE-zhur) Also called generalized tonic clonic seizure. Characterized by a sudden onset of tonic contraction of the muscles, giving way to clonic convulsive movements.

Granulation tissue (gran-u-LA-shun TISH-u) Vascular connective tissue that forms on the surface of a healing wound.

Granulocyte (GRAN-u-lo-site) A mature granular leukocyte.

Granuloma (gran-u-LO-mah) A nodular inflammatory lesion, usually composed of epithelial cells, but may contain specialized leukocytes as well. See *inflammation*.

Granulomatosis enteritis (gran-u-lo-mah-TO-sis en-ter-I-tis) A term that was once used to refer to Crohn disease.

Graves disease (graves dih-ZEZE) An organ-specific autoimmune disease of the thyroid gland. See *hyperthyroidism*.

Graves ophthalmopathy (graves of-thal-MOP-ath-e) Exophthalmos caused by increased water content of retroocular orbital tissues; associated with thyroid disease, usually hyperthyroidism.

Greater omentum (GRA-ter o-MEN-tum) A fold of peritoneum holding fat cells that hangs like an apron in front of the intestines.

Growth hormone (GH) (growth HOR-mone) See *somatotrophin*.

Guaifenesin (gwi-FEN-ih-sen) An expectorant that reduces the viscosity of sputum; sometimes recommended in the treatment of fibromyalgia syndrome.

Guillain-Barré syndrome (ge-YAH bar-RA SIN-drome) A self-limiting demyelinating syndrome related to autoimmune dysfunction, surgical complication, some vaccines, Hodgkin disease, and some types of drug reactions. Motor and/or sensory dysfunction begins in the extremities and moves proximally, sometimes leading to respiratory failure, before function is restored within weeks or months.

Guttate psoriasis (GUT-ate so-RI-ah-sis) A type of psoriasis that appears in round small patches, often following streptococcal infections.

HAART Highly active antiretroviral therapy. *See HIV/AIDS*

Haemophilus influenzae (he-MOF-ih-lus in-flu-EN-za) A species in the respiratory tract that causes acute respiratory infections including pneumonia, acute conjunctivitis, bacterial meningitis, and purulent meningitis in children, rarely in adults.

Hallux valgus (HAL-lux VAL-gus) A deviation of the great toe toward the lateral side of the foot; bunion.

Hand-foot syndrome A possible complication of chemotherapy in which the skin on the palms and soles becomes red, swollen, numb, and flaky. It usually resolves within a few weeks of finishing a chemotherapy treatment.

Hashimoto thyroiditis (hah-shih-MO-to thi-royd-I-tis) Diffuse infiltration of the thyroid gland with lymphocytes, resulting in diffuse goiter, progressive destruction of the parenchyma, and hypothyroidism. See *hypothyroidism*.

Haustrum, haustra (HAW-strum, HAW-strah) One of a series of sacs or pouches, as seen in the colon.

Heberden nodes (HE-ber-den nodez) Small bone spurs that form on the distal phalanges of the hands in association with osteoarthritis.

Helicobacter pylori (hel-ik-o-BAK-ter pi-LOR-i) Species of bacteria associated with peptic ulcers.

HELLP A mnemonic for *h*emolysis, *e*levated *l*iver enzymes, *l*ow *p*latelet count; associated with pregnancy-induced hypertension.

Hemagglutinin (hem-ah-GLU-tih-nin) A type of protein found in the outer coating of influenza and other antigens; it causes the agglutination of red blood cells.

Hematologic (he-mah-to-LOJ-ik) Relating to the blood.

Hematoma (he-mah-TO-mah) A localized mass of extravasated blood that is relatively or completely confined within an organ or tissue, a space, or a potential space; the blood is usually clotted, and depending on how long it has been there, may manifest various degrees of organization and decolorization.

Hematuria (he-mah-TYU-re-ah) Any condition in which the urine contains blood or red blood cells.

Heme (heme) The oxygen-carrying, color-bearing group of hemoglobin.

Hemiplegia (hem-ih-PLE-je-ah) Paralysis of one side of the body.

Hemo- (HE-mo) A prefix denoting blood.

Hemochromatosis (he-mo-kro-mah-TO-sis) A genetic disorder characterized by the absorption of too much iron in the blood; sometimes associated with liver cancer.

Hemodialysis (he-mo-di-AL-ih-sis) Dialysis of soluble substances and water from the blood by diffusion through a semipermeable membrane.

Hemoglobin (HE-mo-glo-bin) Red protein of erythrocytes which binds to oxygen.

Hemoglobin A1c test A test of blood glucose that reflects trends over a 3-month period. See *diabetes*.

Hemolysis (he-MOL-ih-sis) Destruction of blood cells.

Hemolytic (he-mo-LIH-tik) Destructive to blood cells.

Hemolytic uremic syndrome (he-mo-LIH-tik u-RE-mik SIN-drome) Hemolytic anemia and thrombocytopenia with acute renal failure.

Hemophilia (he-mo-FELE-e-ah) An inherited disorder of blood coagulation characterized by a permanent tendency to hemorrhages, spontaneous or traumatic, due to a defect in the blood coagulating mechanism.

Hemophilic arthritis (he-mo-FIL-ik arth-RI-tis) Joint damage and inflammation associated with bleeding into joint cavities seen with hemophilia.

Hemoptysis (he-MOP-tis-is) Expectoration of blood derived from the lungs or bronchi as a result of pulmonary or bronchial hemorrhage.

Hemorrhage (HEM-or-aj) An escape of blood through ruptured vessels.

Hemorrhoid (HEM-or-oyd) A varicose condition of the external or internal rectal veins causing painful swellings at the anus.

Hepatocellular carcinoma (hep-at-o-SEL-u-lar kar-sih-NO-mah) A carcinoma derived from parenchymal cells of the liver. See *liver cancer*.

Hepatocyte (hep-AT-o-site) An active liver cell.

Hepatorenal syndrome (hep-AT-o-RE-nal SIN-drome) Occurrence of acute renal failure in patients with disease of the liver or biliary tract, apparently due to decreased renal blood flow.

Hereditary nonpolyposis colorectal cancer syndrome (her-ED-ih-ta-re non-pol-ih-PO-sis KO-lo-rek-tal KAN-ser SIN-drome) A genetic condition that predisposes some people toward the development of colorectal and other cancers.

Herniated disc (HER-ne-a-ted DISK) Protrusion of a degenerated or fragmented intervertebral disk into the intervertebral foramen with potential compression of a nerve root or into the spinal canal with potential compression of the cauda equina in the lumbar region or the spinal cord at higher levels. See *disc disease*.

Herpetic keratitis (hur-PET-ik ker-ah-TI-tis) Inflammation of the cornea and possibly conjunctiva due to infection with herpes simplex virus.

Heterophile (HET-er-o-file) A neutrophilic leukocyte. See *mononucleosis*.

Heterotopic ossification (het-er-o-TOP-ik os-if-ih-KA-shun) The formation of calcium deposits in soft tissues, particularly seen with spinal cord injury patients. See *myositis ossificans, spinal cord injury*.

Hidradenitis suppurativa (hi-drad-en-I-tis SUP-per-a-tee-va) Chronic suppurative folliculitis of apocrine sweat gland–bearing skin, producing abscesses with scarring. See *boils*.

High-density lipoprotein (HDL) (hi-DEN-sih-te LI-po-pro-tene) A compound in plasma containing both lipids and proteins; HDLs are associated with a reduced risk of cardiovascular disease.

Hip dysplasia (hip dis-PLA-zhah) A type of hip dislocation.

Hippocampus (HIP-o-KAMP-us) A structure in the brain located deep within the temporal lobe. It is part of the limbic system, and it is involved in the consolidation of information from short-term memory to long-term memory.

Hirsutism (HIR-zu-tizm) Presence of excessive bodily and facial terminal hair in a male pattern, especially in women; may develop in children or adults as the result of androgen (male hormone) excess due to tumors, drugs, or medications. See *ovarian cysts.*

Histamine (HIS-tah-mene) A secretion of some cells that is a powerful stimulant of gastric secretion, a constrictor of bronchial smooth muscle, and a vasodilator.

Histoplasmosis (his-to-plaz-MO-sis) An infectious disease caused by *Histoplasma capsulatum*, usually acquired by inhalation of fungal spores, and manifested by a primary lung infection.

Hobnail liver (HOB-naled LIV-er) Characteristically knobby, bumpy appearance of a liver with advanced cirrhosis.

Homans sign (HO-manz sine) A pain at the back of the knee or calf when the ankle is slowly dorsiflexed with the knee bent. This test indicates incipient or established thrombosis in the veins of the leg.

Homeostasis (ho-me-o-STA-sis) A state of equilibrium in the body with respect to various functions and the chemical compositions of fluids and tissues.

Hürthle cell carcinoma (HUR-tel sel kar-sih-NO-mah) A type of thyroid tumor; may be benign or malignant.

Human herpesvirus 6 (HU-man HER-pez-vi-rus) A herpesvirus found in certain lymphoproliferative disorders. See *mononucleosis.*

Human papillomavirus (HPV) (HU-man pap-il-O-mah vi-rus) Class of DNA viruses that cause genital and cutaneous warts.

Human T-cell lymphotropic virus (HU-man T-sell lim-fo-TRO-fik VI-rus) A group of viruses (subfamily Oncovirinae, family Retroviridae) that are lymphotropic with a selective affinity for the helper/inducer cell subset of T lymphocytes and that are associated with adult T-cell leukemia and lymphoma.

Humoral immunity (HU-mor-al ih-MU-nih-te) Immunity associated with circulating antibodies, as opposed to cellular immunity.

Hunner ulcer (HUN-er UL-ser) A focal and often multiple star-shaped lesion involving all layers of the bladder wall; a sign of interstitial cystitis.

Hyaluronic acid (hi-al-yur-ON-ik AS-id) A gelatinous material in tissue spaces that acts as a lubricant and shock absorbant.

Hydrocephalus (hi-dro-SEF-ah-lus) A condition marked by an excessive accumulation of cerebrospinal fluid resulting in dilation of the cerebral ventricles and raised intracranial pressure; may also result in enlargement of the cranium and atrophy of the brain. See *cerebral palsy.*

Hyper- (HI-per) A prefix denoting excessive, above normal.

Hyperacusis (hi-per-ah-KU-sis) Abnormal acuteness of hearing due to irritability of sensory nerves. See *Bell palsy.*

Hyperalgesia (hi-per-al-JE-ze-ah) Extreme sensitivity to painful stimuli. See *peripheral neuropathy.*

Hyperglycemia (hi-per-gli-SE-me-ah) An abnormally high concentration of glucose in the circulating blood.

Hyperkinesia (hi-per-kin-E-ze-ah) Excessive muscular activity.

Hyperkyphosis (hi-per-ki-FO-sis) A deformity of the spine characterized by extensive flexion. See *postural deviations.*

Hyperlordosis (hi-per-lor-DO-sis) A deformity of the spine characterized by excessive extension. See *postural deviations.*

Hyperosmolality (hi-per-oz-mo-LAL-ih-te) Increased concentration of a solution expressed as osmoles of solute per kilogram of serum water. See *diabetes.*

Hyperplasia (hi-per-PLA-zha) An increase in the number of cells in a tissue or organ, outside of tumor formation.

Hyperreflexia (hi-per-re-FLEX-e-ah) A condition in which the deep tendon reflexes are exaggerated.

Hypersensitivity (hi-per-sen-sih-TIV-ih-te) An exaggerated response to the stimulus of a foreign agent.

Hyperthermia (hi-per-THER-me-ah) High body temperature; fever.

Hypertonic (hi-per-TON-ik) Having an increased degree of tension.

Hypertrophic scar (hi-per-TRO-fik SKAR) An elevated scar resembling a keloid but that does not spread into surrounding tissues.

Hypertrophy (hy-PER-tro-fe) General increase in bulk of a part or organ, due to increase in size but not in number of the individual tissue elements.

Hyperuricemia (hi-per-ur-ih-SE-me-ah) Enhanced blood concentrations of uric acid.

Hypnagogic hallucination (hip-nah-GOJ-ik hah-lu-sih-NA-shun) Vivid hallucination that occurs on waking from sleep; occurs with narcolepsy. See *sleep disorders*.

Hypnic myoclonia (HIP-nik mi-o-KLO-ne-ah) The startling sensation that a person is about to fall; it often occurs while nearly asleep.

Hypo- (HI-po) A prefix denoting deficient, below normal.

Hypoglycemia (hi-po-gli-SE-me-ah) An abnormally low concentration of glucose in circulating blood.

Hypokinesia (hi-po-kih-NE-zha) Diminished or slowed movement.

Hypothermia (hi-po-THER-me-ah) In humans, a body temperature significantly below 98.6°F (37°C).

Hypotonic (hi-po-TON-ik) Having a reduced degree of tension.

Hypoxia (hi-POX-e-ah) Below-normal levels of oxygen in the body.

Iatrogenic (e-at-ro-GEN-ik) A response to medical or surgical treatment, usually unfavorable.

Ichthyosis (ik-the-O-sis) Congenital disorders of keratinization characterized by noninflammatory dryness and scaling of the skin, often associated with other defects and with abnormalities of lipid metabolism.

Icterus (IK-ter-us) Synonym for jaundice, a yellowish staining of the skin, sclerae, and mucous membranes that occurs with cirrhosis and other liver diseases.

IDDM Insulin-dependent diabetes mellitus. Obsolete term for type I diabetes mellitus.

Idiopathic (id-e-o-PATH-ik) Denoting a disease of unknown cause.

Idiopathic endolymphatic hydrops (id-e-o-PATH-ik en-do-lim-FAT-ik HI-drops) Synonym for Ménière disease.

Idiopathic environmental intolerance (id-e-o-PATH-ik en-vi-ron-MEN-tal in-TOL-er-ans) Synonym for multiple chemical sensitivity syndrome. See *allergic reactions*.

Imatinib (im-ah-TIN-ib) Drug used to suppress cellular replication for one type of leukemia.

Immunoblastic lymphoma (im-u-no-BLAS-tik lim-FO-mah) A type of high-grade lymphoma.

Impetigo (im-peh-TI-go) A contagious superficial pyoderma caused by *Staphylococcus aureus* or group A streptococci; begins with a superficial flaccid vesicle that ruptures and forms a thick yellowish crust, most commonly on the face of children.

In situ (in SI-tu) At the site only; refers to early stages of cancer development.

Incarceration (in-kar-ser-A-shun) The entrapment of a hernia that cannot be repaired without surgery.

Incision (in-SIH-zhun) A cut or surgical wound.

Indomethacin (in-do-METH-ah-sin) A nonsteroidal analgesic agent used in the treatment of various types of arthritis.

Induction (in-DUK-shun) The introduction of chemotherapeutic drugs into the central nervous system.

Infantile paralysis (IN-fan-tile pah-RAL-ih-sis) Synonym for polio.

Infarction (in-FARK-shun) Sudden insufficiency of arterial or venous blood supply due to emboli, thrombi, vascular torsion, or necrosis.

Inflammatory bowel disease (in-FLAM-mah-tor-e BOW-el dih-ZEZE) Umbrella term for Crohn disease and ulcerative colitis.

Infundibulum (in-fun-DIB-u-lum) Funnel-shaped structure or passage; the link between the pituitary gland and the hypothalamus.

Inguinal orchiectomy (ING-wih-nal or-ke-EK-to-me) Removal of one or both testes through the abdominal cavity. See *testicular cancer.*

Insulin (IN-su-lin) A hormone secreted by beta cells in the pancreas that promotes the utilization of glucose in tissue cells.

Integumentary (in-teg-u-MEN-tar-e) Relating to the skin.

Interferon (in-ter-FE-ron) A class of proteins with antiviral properties.

Interleukin-1 (IN-ter-lu-kin) A cytokine that enhances the proliferation of T helper cells and the growth and differentiation of B cells.

Intermittent claudication (in-ter-MIT-ent klaw-dih-KA-shun) Condition caused by transient ischemia, usually of calf muscles, brought on by walking.

Internal scar tissue (in-TER-nal SKAR TISH-u) Scar tissue that accumulates within the injured structure, for example, tendon, muscle, or ligament.

Interpersonal therapy (in-ter-PER-so-nul THER-ah-pe) Type of psychotherapy focusing on interpersonal relationships and skills.

Interstitial (in-ter-STIH-shal) Relating to spaces within a tissue or organ but excluding such spaces as body cavities or potential space.

Intertrigo (in-ter-TRI-go) A cutaneous yeast infection that grows in skin folds around the groin, axilla, and under the breasts.

Intrathecal pump (in-tra-THE-kal pump) Device for introducing drugs directly into the central nervous system. See *complex regional pain syndrome.*

Intravenous pyelography (in-trah-VE-nus pi-el-O-grah-fe) Radiological study of the kidney, ureters, and usually the bladder, performed with the aid of a contrast agent injected intravenously.

Intrinsic factor (in-TRIN-zik FAK-tor) A mucoprotein in the stomach necessary for the absorption of vitamin B_{12}.

Inverse psoriasis (IN-verse so-RI-ah-sis) Psoriasis in which lesions are red, thickened, and clustered around skin folds.

Iritis (i-RI-tis) Inflammation of the iris of the eye.

Ischemia (is-KE-me-ah) Local anemia due to a mechanical obstruction of the blood supply.

Ischemic penumbra The area surrounding an ischemic stroke.

Isometric (i-so-MET-rik) Describing a muscle contraction in which the muscle does not change its length.

Isotonic (i-so-TON-ik) Describing a muscle contraction in which the muscle does not change its tone.

Itch-scratch cycle The vicious circle in which a skin problem causes itching, the person scratches it, the damage causes more itching, and so on.

IUD Intrauterine device. A plastic or metal device to be inserted into the uterus for contraception.

Ixodes (ik-SO-dez) A genus of hard ticks, many of which are parasitic to humans and which may be the vector for the spread of some diseases. See *Lyme disease.*

Joint mice Freely floating bits of cartilage inside joint capsules, usually at the knee or talotibial joints.

Jumper's knee Synonym for patellofemoral syndrome.

Kaposi sarcoma (kah-PO-seze sar-KO-mah) A malignant neoplasm occurring in the skin and sometimes in lymph nodes or viscera; clinically manifested by cutaneous lesions consisting of reddish-purple to dark-blue macules, plaques, or nodules; Seen most commonly in men over 60 years of age and in AIDS patients.

Keloid scar (KE-loyd skar) A nodular mass of scar tissue that may occur after surgery, a burn, or cutaneous diseases.

Keratin (KER-ah-tin) A substance present in cuticular structures, for example, hair, nails, and horns.

Keratinocyte (ker-AT-in-o-site) A cell of the epidermis that produces keratin.

Kerion (KE-re-on) A secondary bacterial infection of tinea capitis, leading to a raised boggy lesion.

Ketoacidosis (ke-to-as-id-O-sis) Acidosis caused by enhanced production of ketonic acids.

Ketogenic (ke-to-JEN-ik) Giving rise to ketones in metabolism.

Ketone (KE-tone) A potentially toxic product of metabolism; the most widely recognized ketone is acetone.

Kinin (KI-nin) Any of a variety of chemicals with physiological effects on cell activity, including visceral muscle contraction along with vascular muscle relaxation, which leads to vasodilation.

Klebsiella (kleb-se-EL-ah) A genus of bacteria that may or may not be pathogenic, depending on the individual type.

Koebner phenomenon (KOBE-ner fen-OM-en-on) Heightened susceptibility to the effects of trauma and chemical exposure; sometimes seen in people with psoriasis and lichen planus.

Kupffer cells (KUP-fer selz) Phagocytic cells found in the liver.

Labyrinthitis (lab-ih-rin-THI-tis) Inflammation of the labyrinth of the inner ear; may be associated with vertigo and/or hearing loss. See *vestibular balance disorders*.

Laceration (las-er-A-shun) A torn or jagged wound.

Lactobacillus (lak-to-bah-SIL-us) A genus of bacteria that are part of the normal flora of the mouth, intestinal tract, and vagina.

Lamivudine (lah-MIH-vu-dene) A reverse transcriptase inhibitor used to treat HIV and hepatitis B.

Lanugo (lah-NU-go) Fine, soft, lightly pigmented hair, associated with fetal development and advanced anorexia nervosa.

Laparoscopy (lap-ah-ROS-ko-pe) Examination of the abdominal contents with a scope passed through the abdominal wall.

Laparotomy (lap-ah-ROH-to-me) Incision into the abdominal wall.

Lavage (lah-VAJH) The washing out of a hollow cavity by repeated injections and rejections of fluid.

Ledderhose disease (LED-er-hoze dih-ZEZE) A condition similar to Dupuytren contracture that develops on the plantar surface of the foot. Also called *plantar fibromatosis*.

Legg-Calve-Perthes disease (leg KAHL-va PER-tez) Epiphysial necrosis of the upper end of the femur. See *avascular necrosis*.

Leiomyoma (li-o-mi-O-mah) A benign neoplasm derived from smooth muscle tissue. See *fibroid tumors*.

Lentigo (len-TI-go) A brown macule or spot resembling a freckle.

Leprosy (LEP-ro-se) A chronic bacterial infection caused by *Mycobacterium leprae* affecting the cooler body parts, especially the skin, peripheral nerves, and testes. Leprosy is classified into two main types, lepromatous and tuberculoid, representing extremes of immunological response. Also called Hansen disease.

Lesion (LE-zhun) A wound or injury; a pathogenic change in tissues.

Lesser-Trelat sign (LA-za-tra-LAH sine) The sudden onset of multiple seborrheic keratoses, often with an inflammatory base. This may be a sign of internal malignancy.

Letrozole (LET-ro-zole) A medication used to reduce the risk of recurrent breast cancer.

Leukocyte (LU-ko-site) A type of blood cell formed in several types of tissues, involved in immune reactions. A white blood cell.

Leukoplakia (lu-ko-PLA-ke-ah) A white patch of oral mucous membrane that cannot be wiped off and cannot be diagnosed clinically; biopsy may show malignant or premalignant changes. See *skin cancer*.

Levodopa (lev-o-DO-pah) The biologically active form of dopa; a precursor of dopamine.

Levulose (LEV-yu-lose) Fructose; fruit sugar.

Lewy body disease (LU-we BOD-e dih-ZEZE) A degenerative cerebral disorder of elderly people characterized by progressive dementia or psychosis; can resemble Alzheimer disease and Parkinson disease.

Leydig cell tumor (LI-dig sel TU-mor) A type of testicular cancer.

Lhermitte sign (ler-METE sine) Sudden electric-like shocks extending down the spine on flexion of the head. See *muscular dystrophy, multiple sclerosis*.

Lichenification (li-ken-ih-fih-KA-shun) Leathery hardening and thickening of the skin; can be caused by scratching in areas of eczema and contact dermatitis.

Ligamenta flava (lig-ah-MEN-tah FLAH-vah) A pair of yellow elastic fibrous structures that bind the laminae of adjoining vertebrae.

Ligamentum flava, flavum (lig-uh-MEN-tum FLA-va, FLA-vum) Ligaments that connect the lamina of the vertebrae from inside the vertebral canal.

Limb-girdle dystrophy (lim GIR-del DIS-tro-fe) One of the less well defined types of muscular dystrophy; characterized by weakness and wasting, usually symmetrical, of the pelvic girdle muscles, the shoulder girdle muscles, or both, but not the facial muscles.

Limbic system (LIM-bik SIS-tem) A group of brain structures and their connections that exert important influence on the endocrine and autonomic nervous systems. The limbic system is associated with motivational and mood states.

Limited systemic scleroderma (LIM-ih-ted sis-TEM-ik skler-o-DERM-ah) A form of scleroderma that carries a relatively low risk of internal organ involvement.

Linea alba (LIN-e-ah AL-bah) Fibrous band that runs vertically from the xiphoid process to the pubis; site of attachment for abdominal muscles.

Lipoprotein (lip-o-PRO-tene) Complexes or compounds containing lipid and protein. Plasma lipoproteins are characterized as very low density lipoprotein (VLDL), intermediate density lipoprotein (IDL), low density lipoprotein (LDL), high density lipoprotein (HDL), and very high density lipoprotein (VHDL). Levels of lipoproteins are important in assessing the risk of cardiovascular disease.

Lithium (LITH-e-um) An element of the alkali metal group used to treat depression and other mood disorders.

Lithotripsy (LITH-o-trip-se) The crushing of a stone in the renal pelvis, ureter, or bladder by mechanical force or sound waves.

Low-density lipoprotein (LDL) (lo-DEN-sih-te lip-o-PRO-tene) A compound in plasma containing both lipids and proteins; associated with an increased risk of cardiovascular disease.

Lumen (LU-men) The space in the interior of a tubular structure.

Lymphadenitis (lim-FAD-en-I-tis) Inflammation of a lymph node or nodes.

Lymphadenoma (lim-FAD-en-O-mah) Enlarged lymph node; may be associated with cancer.

Lymphangion (lim-FAN-je-on) A lymphatic vessel.

Lymphedema (lim-feh-DE-mah) Swelling as a result of obstruction or damage to lymph nodes.

Lymphoblastic lymphoma (lim-fo-BLAST-ik lim-FO-mah) A type of high-grade lymphoma.

Lymphocyte (LIM-fo-site) A white blood cell formed in lymphatic tissues.

Lymphocytic lymphoma (lim-fo-SIT-ik lim-FO-mah) A type of low-grade lymphoma.

Lymphokines (LIM-fo-kinez) A group of hormonelike substances that mediate immune responses; released by lymphocytes.

Lynch syndrome (LINCH SIN-drome) A synonym for hereditary nonpolyposis colorectal cancer syndrome, a genetic risk factor for colorectal cancer.

Macrophage (MAK-ro-fahj) A type of phagocytic white blood cell.

Macrosomia (mak-ro-SO-me-ah) Condition in which a fetus grows abnormally large as a consequence of gestational diabetes.

Magnetic resonance imaging (MRI) (mag-NET-ik REZ-o-nans IM-ah-jing) A diagnostic modality in which the magnetic nuclei of a patient are aligned in a strong, uniform magnetic field. The signals they emit are converted into images that permit three-dimensional reference to soft tissues.

Malaise (mah-LAZE) A feeling of general discomfort or uneasiness.

Malar rash (MA-lar rash) A rash of the cheeks or cheek bones, often associated with lupus or erysipelas.

Malignant (mah-LIG-nant) Having the property of locally invasive and destructive growth and metastasis.

Malignant hypertension (mah-LIG-nant hi-per-TEN-shun) Severe hypertension that runs a rapid course, causing necrosis of arteriolar walls in kidney and retina, hemorrhages, and death most frequently due to uremia or rupture of a cerebral vessel.

Malocclusion (mal-o-KLU-zhun) Any deviation from a physiologically acceptable contact of opposing dentitions.

Mast cell A white blood cell found in connective tissue that contains heparin and histamine.

Mastitis (mas-TI-tis) Infection of the breast.

Matrix (MA-trix) The intercellular substance of a tissue.

Medial tibial stress syndrome (ME-de-al TIB-e-al STRES SIN-drome) Pain at the posteromedial border of the tibia that occurs in conjunction with exercise. See *shin splints*.

Meige syndrome (MEZH-eh SIN-drome) A type of dystonia that combines blepharospasm and oromandibular dystonia.

Melanin (MEL-ah-nin) Dark brown to black pigment formed in the skin and some other tissues.

Melanocyte (mel-AN-o-site) A pigment-producing cell in the basal layer of the epidermis.

Melatonin (MEL-ah-to-nin) A substance secreted by the pineal gland that suppresses some glandular function; associated with circadian rhythm.

Menarche (men-AR-ke) A woman's first menstrual period.

Meningitis (men-in-JI-tis) Inflammation of the membranes of the brain or spinal cord.

Meniscus (men-IS-kus) A crescent-shaped fibrocartilaginous structure of the knee, the acromioclavicular and sternoclavicular, and the temporomandibular joints.

Menses (MEN-seze) Periodic hemorrhage from the uterine mucosa; usually preceded by ovulation but not by fertilization.

Meralgia parasthetica (mer-AL-je-ah pare-as-THET-ik-ah) Paresthesia at the lateral aspect of the distal thigh, in the distribution of the lateral femoral cutaneous nerve.

Mesangial glomerulonephritis (mes-AN-je-al glo-MARE-yu-lo-nef-RI-tis) A type of glomerulonephritis associated with immune system abnormalities and the loss of erythrocytes into the urine.

Mesentery (MES-en-ter-e) A double layer of peritoneum attached to the abdominal wall and enclosing a portion of the abdominal viscera.

Mesothelioma (mes-o-the-le-O-mah) A malignant neoplasm derived from cells of the pleura or peritoneum.

Metabolite (meh-TAB-o-lite) Any product of metabolism, especially catabolism.

Metaplasia (met-ah-PLA-zhia) Abnormal transformation of adult, fully differentiated tissue into another type of tissue. See *endometriosis*.

Metastasis (met-AS-tah-sis) The spread of a disease process from one part of the body to another, as with the spread of cancer.

Methicillin-resistant Staphylococcus aureus (MRSA)(METH-ih-sil-in re-ZIS-tant staf-ih-lo-KOK-us OR-e-us) Common infective bacterium that does not respond to the methicillin family of antibiotics.

Methylphenidate (meth-il-FEN-ih-date) A central nervous system stimulant often used to treat attention deficit hyperactivity disorder.

Microaerophilic (mi-kro-air-o-FIL-ik) Referring to a type of bacteria that requires oxygen, although less than is available in the air.

Microbe (MI-krobe) Any very minute organism.

Micrographia (mi-kro-GRAF-e-ah) Handwriting that grows progressively smaller and more cramped. See *Parkinson disease*.

Microsporum (mi-kro-SPOR-um) A genus of pathogenic fungi causing dermatophytosis. See *fungal infections*.

Mineralocorticoid (min-er-al-o-KOR-tih-koyd) One of the steroids from the adrenal cortex that influence salt metabolism.

Mitochondrion (mi-to-KON-dre-on) An organelle of the cell cytoplasm; the principal energy source of the cell.

Mittelschmerz (MIT-el-shmertz) Abdominal pain occurring at the time of ovulation.

Molluscum contagiosum (mo-LUS-kum kon-ta-je-O-sum) A contagious disease of the skin caused by proliferation of a virus of the family Poxviridae and characterized by the appearance of small, pearly epidermal growths. In adults, it typically occurs on or near the genitals and is sexually transmitted. See *sexually transmitted diseases, warts*.

Monoamine oxidase inhibitor (MAOI) (MON-o-ah-mene OX-ih-dase in-HIB-ih-tor) A class of antidepressants that inhibit the breakdown of certain neurotransmitters.

Monoclonal immunoglobulins (MON-o-klo-nal im-u-no-GLOB-u-linz) A type of antibodies produced by B cells affected by myeloma. Also called M proteins.

Monocyte (MON-o-site) A relatively large leukocyte; normally comprises 3% to 7% of the leukocytes in circulating blood.

Mononeuropathy (mon-o-nur-OP-ath-e) Disorder involving a single nerve.

Mononucleosis (mon-o-nu-kle-O-sis) Presence of abnormally large numbers of mononuclear leukocytes in the circulating blood, especially with reference to forms that are not normal.

Mosaic warts (mo-ZA-ik warts) Numerous closely formed plantar warts forming a mosaic appearance.

Motility (mo-TIL-ih-te) The power of spontaneous movement.

Movie-goer's knee Synonym for *patellofemoral syndrome*.

MRSA See *methicillin-resistant* Staphylococcus aureus.

Mucolytic (myu-ko-LIT-ik) Capable of dissolving, digesting, or liquefying mucus.

Mucopolysaccharide (myu-ko-pol-e-SAK-ah-ride) Protein-polysaccharide complex, obtained from proteoglycans. See *hyperthyroidism*.

Mucormycosis (myu-kor-mi-KO-sis) A fungal infection associated with genera of the class Zygomycetes. Also called zygomycosis. See *diabetes*.

Mucormycosis (myu-ker-mi-KO-sis) A fungal infection caused by fungi in the order Mucorales. It frequently involves the sinuses, brain, or lungs.

Mucosal-associated lymphoid-type lymphoma (myu-KO-sal ah-SO-se-a-ted LIM-foyd tipe lim-FO-mah) A type of cancer usually associated with *Helicobacter pylori*. See *ulcers*.

Mucous cyst (MYU-kus SIST) A type of ganglion cyst most often seen on the distal interphalangeal joint of older people.

Multiple crush syndrome A phenomenon of nerve entrapment and irritation at multiple sites; it can be exacerbated by the fact that a single nerve irritation can cause the entire nerve swell, making it more vulnerable in other areas

Multiple system atrophy (MUL-tih-pel SIS-tem AT-ro-fe) A central nervous system disorder leading to stiffness, rigidity, loss of balance, poor coordination, and other symptoms. See *tremor*.

Muscle spindle (MUH-sel SPIN-del) Proprioceptor that wraps around specialized muscle fibers to relay information about the relative length of the muscle fibers.

Myalgic encephalomyelitis (mi-AL-jik en-sef-ah-lo-mi-el-I-tis) Inflammation of the brain and spinal cord characterized by muscle pain. See *chronic fatigue syndrome*.

Myasthenia gravis (mi-as-THE-ne-ah GRAV-is) Immunological disorder of neuromuscular transmission, marked by fluctuating weakness, especially of the oculofacial muscles and the proximal limb muscles.

Mycobacterium (mi-ko-bak-TE-re-um) Genus of bacteria that causes tuberculosis in humans.

Mycoplasma (mi-ko-PLAZ-mah) A specialized type of bacteria that do not possess a true cell wall but are bound by a three-layered membrane.

Mycosis (mi-KO-sis) Any disease caused by a fungus.

Myelin (MI-eh-lin) A membrane composed of fat and protein molecules that surrounds nerve fibers.

Myelodysplastic anemia (mi-el-o-dis-PLAS-tik ah-NE-me-ah) A primary neoplastic stem cell disorder characterized by peripheral blood cytopenias and prominent maturation abnormalities in the bone marrow; evolves progressively and may transform into leukemia.

Myeloid cell (MI-el-oyd sel) Any cell that develops into a granulocyte of blood; also refers to any bone marrow cell.

Myocardial infarction (mi-o-KAR-de-al in-FARK-shun) Synonym for *heart attack*.

Myoclonic (mi-o-KLON-ik) Related to one or a series of shocklike contractions of a group of muscles; of variable regularity, synchrony, and symmetry, generally due to a central nervous system lesion.

Myofibril (mi-o-FI-bril) One of the fine longitudinal fibrils in skeletal or cardiac muscle fiber.

Myofibroblast (mi-o-FI-bro-blast) A contractile connective tissue cell with properties of both smooth muscle cells and fibroblasts.

Myopia (mi-O-pe-ah) Optical condition in which only rays from a finite distance from the eye focus on the retina; nearsightedness. See *Marfan syndrome*.

Myositis ossificans (mi-o-SI-tis OS-ih-fih-kanz) Ossification of inflammatory tissue within a muscle, usually at the site of a hematoma due to blunt trauma.

Myotonia (mi-o-TO-ne-ah) Delayed relaxation of a muscle after a strong contraction.

Myrmecia (mir-ME-she-ah) Synonym for deep palmar plantar warts.

Myrmecia (mur-ME-she-ah) A form of wart in which the lesion has a domed surface.

Myxedema coma (mik-seh-DE-mah KO-mah A state of profound unconsciousness related to extreme hypothyroidism.

NAFLD Nonalcoholic fatty liver disease. See *cirrhosis*.

Nailfold capillaroscopy (nale fold kap-il-ah-ROS-ko-pe) A diagnostic test to look for signs of arteriole distortion seen with Raynaud syndrome.

Narcolepsy (NAR-ko-lep-se) A sleep disorder characterized by recurring episodes of sleep during the day and interrupted sleep at night.

Necrosis (nek-RO-sis) Pathological death of one or more cells or of a portion of tissue or organ.

Necrotizing fasciitis (NEK-ro-ti-zing fah-SHI-tis) Also called "flesh-eating bacteria," this is an infection of deep layers of the skin. Causative agents can include Group A streptococcus, *Staphylococcus aureus*, and others.

Needle aponeurotomy (NE-del ap-o-nur-OT-o-me) A procedure to treat Dupuytren contracture with tiny punctures to release the palmar aponeurosis.

Negative feedback loop A metabolic process in which the output of a system opposes changes to the input of a system, so stability is achieved.

Neisseria gonorrhoeae (ni-SE-re-a gon-o-RE-a) A species that causes gonorrhea and other infections in humans; the type species of the genus *Neisseria*.

Neisseria meningitidis (ni-SE-re-a men-in-JIH-tih-dis) A bacterial species found in the nasopharynx; the causative agent of meningococcal meningitis.

Neoadjuvant therapy (ne-o-AD-ju-vent THER-ah-pe) Chemotherapy or radiation given before cancer surgery or other intervention to increase the chance of success.

Neoplasm (NE-o-plazm) An abnormal tissue that grows by cellular proliferation more rapidly than normal and continues to grow after the stimuli that initiated the new growth cease.

Nephrolithiasis (nef-ro-lih-THI-ah-sis) Presence of renal calculi.

Nephron (NEF-ron) A long convoluted tubular structure; the functional unit of the kidney.

Nerve growth factor A protein that helps to control the development of sympathetic neurons and other nerve tissue; associated with heightened pain sensitivity.

Neuralgia-inducing cavitational osteonecrosis (NICO) (nur-AL-je-a in-DU-sing kav-ih-TA-shun-al os-te-o-nek-RO-sis) Tissue death at the site of extracted teeth that causes pain in the face. Also called *osteomyelitis*.

Neuraminidase (nur-am-IN-ih-daze) One of a group of proteins found in the external surface of influenza viruses.

Neurilemma (nur-ih-LEM-mah) A cell that enfolds one or more axons of the peripheral nervous system.

Neuroendocrine (nur-o-EN-do-krin) Descriptive of cells that release hormones in response to a neural stimulus. See *pancreatic cancer*.

Neurofibrillary tangle (nur-o-FIB-rih-la-re TANG-el) Intraneural accumulations of filaments with twisted, contorted patterns; associated with Alzheimer disease.

Neurogenic bladder (NUR-o-jen-ik BLAD-er) Bladder dysfunction that originates with nervous system damage.

Neuroma (nur-O-mah) General term for any neoplasm derived from cells of the nervous system, especially Morton neuroma. See *pes planus, pes cavus*.

Neuron (NUR-on) The functional unit of the nervous system; consists of the nerve cell body, the dendrites, and the axon.

Neuropeptide (nur-o-PEP-tide) Any of a variety of peptides found in neural tissue; for example, endorphins, enkephalins.

Neuroplasticity (nur-o-plas-TIS-ih-te) Describes the ability of the central nervous system to change functionally and structurally as a result of injury or damage.

Neutrophil (NU-tro-fil) A type of mature white blood cell formed in the bone marrow.

Neutrophilic (nu-tro-FIL-ik) Characterized by the presence of neutrophils.

Nevus, nevi (NE-vus, NE-vi) A malformation of the skin colored by hyperpigmentation or increased vascularity.

NIDDM Non–insulin-dependent diabetes mellitus. Obsolete term for type II diabetes mellitus.

Nit The ovum of a head or body louse.

Nociceptor (no-si-SEP-tor) A peripheral nerve organ or mechanism for the reception and transmission of painful or injurious stimuli.

Nocturia (nok-TUR-e-ah) Urinating at night.

Nodular (NOD-u-lar) Having nodes or knotlike swellings.

Nonalcoholic steatohepatitis (NASH) (non-al-ko-HOL-ik ste-AT-o-hep-ah-TI-tis) Inflammation of fatty tissue in the liver not associated with alcohol abuse.

Non-Burkitt lymphoma (non-BUR-kit lim-FO-mah) A type of high-grade lymphoma.

Nongonococcal urethritis (non-gon-o-KOK-al u-re-THRI-tis) Urethritis not from gonococcal infection; *Chlamydia trachomatis* is the most common agent. See *sexually transmitted diseases*.

Nonseminoma (non-sem-ih-NO-mah) A type of testicular cancer.

Nonsteroidal anti-inflammatory drug (NSAID) (non-ster-OYD-al AN-te-in-FLAM-ah-tor-e drug) Any collection of anti-inflammatory drugs that do not include steroidal compounds. Examples include aspirin, acetaminophen, ibuprofen, and naproxen.

Nontropical sprue Synonym for celiac sprue.

Noradrenaline (nor-ah-DREN-ah-lin) See *norepinephrine*.

Norepinephrine (nor-ep-ih-NEF-rin) A hormone produced in the adrenal medulla; secreted in response to hypotension and physical stress.

Norovirus (NOR-o-vi-rus) Genus name for the group of viruses provisionally described as Norwalk-like viruses.

Nosocomial (no-so-KO-me-al) Of a disease acquired while being treated in a hospital; specifically applied to some varieties of pneumonia.

Noxious (NOK-shus) Injurious, harmful.

Nucleus pulposus (NU-kle-us pul-PO-sus) The soft fibrocartilage central portion of an intervertebral disk.

Numb-likeness A condition characterized by reduced sensation but not total numbness.

Nummular eczema (NUM-u-lar (EG-zeh-mah) Discrete coin-shaped patches of eczema.

Obturator hernia (OB-tur-a-tur HER-ne-ah) Tissue that bulges through a hole in fascia covering the obturator foramen.

Occult (o-KULT) Hidden; concealed; not manifest.

Oculopharyngeal muscular dystrophy (ok-u-lo-fah-RIN-je-al MUS-ku-lar DIS-tro-fe) An inherited progressive form of muscular dystrophy that often involves ptosis and problems with swallowing.

Oligodendrocyte (ol-ih-go-DEN-dro-site) One of the three types of glial cells, the other two being astrocytes and microglia, that together with nerve cells compose the tissue of the central nervous system.

Olivopontocerebellar atrophy (OL-ih-vo-PON-to-ser-ah-BEL-ar AT-ro-fe) A central nervous system movement disorder that is part of multiple system atrophy. See *tremor*.

Oncogene (ONK-o-jene) Any of a family of genes which, under normal circumstances, code for proteins related to cell growth, but which foster malignant processes if mutated or activated by contact with specific viruses.

Onycholysis (on-ih-KOL ih-sis) Loosening of the nails, beginning at the free border and usually incomplete. See *psoriasis, fungal infections*

Onychomycosis (on-ih-ko-mi-KO-sis) Fungal infection of the nails.

Oocyte (o-o-site) The female sex cell.

Oophorectomy (o-o-for-EK-to-me) Surgical removal of the ovaries.

Oophoritis (o-o-for-I-tis) Inflammation of an ovary.

Orchiectomy (or-ke-EK-to-me) Removal of one or both testes.

Orchitis (or-KI-tis) Inflammation of the testes.

Orthotics (or-THOT-iks) The science of making and fitting of orthopedic appliances. Also used to refer to orthopedic appliances that are made to adjust the alignment and weight-bearing stress in the feet.

Os coxae (oz KOK-se) The fused unit containing the ilium, ischium, and pubis.

Oscillation (os-il-A-shun) A to-and-fro movement. See *tremor*.

Osgood-Schlatter disease (OZ-good SHLAT-er dih-ZEZE) Inflammation or partial avulsion of the tibial tuberosity due to traction forces.

Osteitis deformans (os-te-I-tis de-FOR-manz) Synonym for *Paget disease*.

Osteoblast (OS-te-o-blast) A bone-forming cell.

Osteoclast (OS-te-o-klast) A cell functioning in the absorption and removal of osseus tissue.

Osteocyte (OS-te-o-site) A cell of osseous tissue that occupies a lacuna and has cytoplasmic processes that extend to contact other osteocytes.

Osteomalacia (os-te-o-mah-LA-shah) A disease characterized by progressive softening and bending of the bones.

Osteomyelitis (os-te-o-mi-el-I-tis) Inflammation of the bone marrow and adjacent bone tissue.

Osteonecrosis (os-te-o-nek-RO-sis) The death of bone en mass, as distinguished from caries ("molecular death") or relatively small foci of necrosis in bone.

Osteopenia (os-te-o-PE-ne-ah) Pathological thinning of bones; may be a precursor to osteoporosis.

Osteophyte (OS-te-o-fite) A bony outgrowth or protuberance.

Osteotomy (os-te-OT-o-me) The cutting of bone, usually using a saw or chisel.

Ostomy (OS-to-me) Artificial opening (stoma) into the trachea, urinary tract, or gastrointestinal tract.

Otolith (O-to-lith) Tiny ear stone of hardened material found in the vestibule of the inner ear.

Overuse syndrome (O-ver use SIN-drome) Synonym for patellofemoral syndrome.

Oxygen free radical (OX-ih-jen fre RAD-ih-kal) An atom or atom group carrying an unpaired electron and no charge. They may promote heart disease, cancer, Alzheimer disease, and other progressive disorders.

Pain-spasm-pain cycle Self-perpetuating cycle of pain, which causes spasm, which increases pain, ad infinitum.

Palliative (PAL-le-ah-tiv) Denoting alleviation of symptoms without curing the underlying disease.

Palmar fasciitis (PAL-mar fash-I-tis) Synonym for Dupuytren contracture.

Palpable (PAL-pah-bel) Perceptible to touch.

Palpitation (pal-pih-TA-shun) Forcible or irregular pulsation of the heart perceptible to the patient, usually with an increase in frequency or force, with or without an irregularity in rhythm.

Pancolitis (pan-ko-LI-tis) Inflammation of the entire colon. See *ulcerative colitis*.

Pap test Microscopic examination of cells scraped usually from the uterine cervix and stained with Papanicolaou stain to look for signs of cancer.

Papain (puh-PA-in) An enzyme derived from papayas that is used to tenderize meat or dissolve connective tissue.

Paraplegia (pare-ah-PLE-je-ah) Paralysis of both lower extremities and generally the lower trunk.

Parasomnia (pare-ah-SOM-ne-ah) Disruption of the sleep state.

Parathyroid hormone (PTH) (pare-ah-THI-royd HOR-mone) A hormone secreted by the parathyroid glands that raises serum calcium levels by causing bone resorption.

Parenchyma (pare-en-KI-mah) The distinguishing or specific cells of a gland or organ, contained within a connective tissue framework stroma.

Paresis (pah-RE-sis) Partial or incomplete paralysis.

Paresthesia (pare-es-THE-zha) An abnormal sensation, such as burning, prickling, tickling, or tingling.

Parkinsonism (PAR-kin-son-izm) A neurological syndrome that has signs and symptoms of Parkinson disease.

Pars interarticularis (pars in-ter-ar-tik-yu-LARE-is) The region between the superior and inferior articulating facets of a vertebra; may be fractured with spondylolisthesis.

Patellar tendinitis (pah-TEL-ar ten-din-I-tis) Injury to the insertion of the quadriceps group.

Patellofemoral syndrome (pa-TELL-o-fem-o-ral SIN-drome) Anterior knee pain as a result of a structural or functional malfunction between the patella and distal femur.

Patent foramen ovale (PAT-ent FOR-ah-men o-VAH-le) A condition in which the valve in the atrial septum does not fully close postnatally.

Pathogen (PATH-o-jen) Any virus, microorganism, or substance causing disease.

Pediculosis (ped-ik-yu-LO-sis) The state of being infested with lice.

Pediculus (ped-IK-yu-lus) A genus of parasitic lice that live in the hair and feed periodically on blood. Important species include *Pediculus humanus* var. *capitis*, the head louse of man; *Pediculus humanus* var. *corporis*, also called *Pediculus corporis*, the body louse or clothes louse, which lives and lays nits in clothing and feeds on the human body.

Pedunculate (peh-DUNK-u-late) Having a pedicle; suspended by a stalk.

Peptide (PEP-tide) A compound of two or more amino acids.

Percutaneous nephrolithotomy (per-ku-TA-ne-us nef-ro-lith-OT-o-me) Incision through the skin directly to the kidney for the removal of a renal calculus.

Percutaneous transluminal coronary angioplasty (PCTA) (per-kyu-TA-ne-us trans-LU-min-al KOR-o-na-re AN-je-o-plast-e) A surgical procedure for enlarging a narrowed coronary vessel by inflating and withdrawing through the narrowed region a balloon on the tip of a catheter.

Perforation (per-for-A-shun) Abnormal opening in a hollow organ.

Perfusion (per-FU-zhun) The forcing of fluid to flow through the vascular bed of a tissue or through the lumen of a hollow structure.

Perfusion pressure (per-FYU-zhun PRESH-ur) The gradient between arterial blood pressure and venous pressure in a comparable location.

Peri- (PER-ih) Prefix denoting *around*, *about*, or *near*.

Pericarditis (per-ih-kar-DI-tis) Inflammation of the pericardium.

Perilymph fistula (PER-ih-limf FIS-tu-lah) An abnormal portal that allows fluid to move between the inner ear and the middle ear. See *vestibular balance disorders*.

Perimenopause (per-ih-MEN-o-pawz) The 3- to 5-year period before the final cessation of the menstrual cycle, during which estrogen levels begin to drop.

Perimysium (per-ih-MI-se-um) The fibrous sheath enveloping each of the primary bundles of skeletal muscle fibers.

Periodic limb movement disorder (PLMD) A disorder characterized by periodic episodes of repetitive and highly stereotyped limb movements that occur during sleep. See *sleep disorders*.

Periosteum (per-e-OS-te-um) The thick fibrous membrane covering every surface of a bone except the articular cartilage.

Periostitis (per-e-os-TI-tis) Inflammation of the periosteum. See *shin splints*.

Peripheral vascular disease (per-IF-er-al VAS-ku-lar dih-ZEZE) Condition related to the consequences of atherosclerosis in the extremities, especially the legs; can include blood clots, stasis dermatitis, skin ulcers, and infections.

Pervasive development disorders Synonym for autism spectrum disorders.

Pes cavus Condition characterized by increased height of the foot's medial longitudinal arch.

Pes planus A condition in which the longitudinal arch is broken down, the entire sole touching the ground. Flatfoot.

PET scan Positron emission tomography; use of nuclear medicine and digital imaging to observe chemical and electrical activity in living tissue.

Petit mal (peh-TE MAL) A brief seizure characterized by arrest of activity and occasional clonic movements.

Peyronie disease (pa-ro-NE) A condition in which the skin on the shaft of the penis becomes thickened and scarred. Can be associated with Dupuytren contracture.

Phalen maneuver (FA-len mah-NU-ver) Maneuver in which the wrist is maintained in flexion for 60 seconds or more; the sensation of paresthesia or other symptoms may indicate carpal tunnel syndrome.

Pheochromocytoma (fe-o-kro-mo-si-TO-mah) Benign adrenal tumor that can cause increased secretion of epinephrine. Associated with a form of thyroid cancer.

Phlebectomy (fleb-EK-to-me) Excision of a segment of a vein, especially to treat varicose veins.

Phlegm (flem) Abnormal amounts of mucus, especially as expectorated from the mouth.

Photodynamic therapy (fo-to-di-NAM-ik THER-ah-pe) A treatment option that destroys some types of cancer cells through the use of a fixed-frequency laser light in combination with a photosensitizing agent.

Photosensitivity (fo-to-sen-sih-TIV-ih-te) Abnormal sensitivity to light, especially of the eyes.

Phyllodes tumor (FIL-odez TU-mor) A low-grade, rarely metastasizing form of breast neoplasm. See *breast cancer*.

Phyto- (FI-to) Having to do with plants.

Phytoestrogen (fi-to-ES-trah-jen) Plant-based chemical with an estrogenic effect on the body.

Pia mater (PI-ah MA-ter, PE-ah MA-ter) A delicate fibrous membrane firmly adherent to the brain and spinal cord.

Pilonidal cyst (pi-lo-NI-dal sist) An abscess in the sacral region containing hair, which may act as a foreign body leading to chronic inflammation.

Pinna (PIN-na) A feather, wing, or fin—used to describe the ear.

Pitting edema (PIT-ing eh-DE-mah) Edema that retains for a time the indentation produced by pressure.

Placenta abruptio (plah-SEN-tah ab-RUP-te-o) Premature separation of the placenta.

Plantar fibromatosis (PLAN-tar fi-bro-mah-TO-sis) A condition similar to Dupuytren contracture, appearing on the foot. Also called Ledderhose disease.

Plaque (plak) A small differentiated area on a surface; atheromatous plaques form well-defined yellow areas or swellings on the intimal surface of an artery.

Plasmapheresis (plaz-mah-fer-E-sis) Removal of whole blood from the body, separation of its cellular elements, and reinfusion of them suspended in saline or another plasma substitute.

Plastocytoma (plas-to-si-TO-mah) A collection of proliferating cancerous immature B cells found outside bone tissue. See *myeloma*.

Platelet (PLATE-let) An irregularly shaped fragment of a megakaryocyte that aids in blood clotting.

Pleurisy (PLU-rih-se) Inflammation of the pleurae.

Plexus (PLEK-sus) A network or interjoining of nerves, blood vessels, or lymphatic vessels.

Pneumococcus (nu-mo-KOK-us) Synonym for *Streptococcus pneumoniae*.

Pneumocystis carinii pneumonia Former name for *Pneumocystis jiroveci* pneumonia.

Pneumocystis jiroveci pneumonia Pneumonia resulting from infection with *Pneumocystis carinii*, frequently seen in the immunologically compromised, such as persons with AIDS, or steroid-treated individuals, the elderly, or premature or debilitated babies. A protozoan infection of the lungs associated with impaired immunity. Formerly called *Pneumocystis carinii* pneumonia.

Pneumothorax (nu-mo-THOR-ax) The presence of air or gas in the pleural cavity.

Podagra (po-DAG-rah) Severe foot pain, usually associated with acute gouty arthritis at the metatarsal-phalangeal joint of the great toe.

Poliomyelitis (pol-e-o-mi-el-I-tis) An inflammatory process involving the gray matter of the spinal cord.

Poly- (POL-e) Many; multiplicity.

Polyarteritis nodosa (pol-e-ar-ter-I-tis no-DO-sah) A disease involving segmental inflammation and necrosis of medium-size and small arteries.

Polycythemia (pol-e-si-THE-me-ah) An increase above normal in the number of red cells in the blood.

Polydipsia (pol-e-DIP-se-ah) Excessive thirst that is relatively prolonged. See *diabetes*.

Polyendocrine deficiency syndrome (pol-e-EN-do-krin de-FISH-en-se SIN-drome) An autoimmune condition associated with Addison disease in which the adrenal glands, along with other endocrine structures, are impaired.

Polyneuropathy (pol-e nu-ROP-ath-e) A disease process involving a number of peripheral nerves.

Polyp (POH-lip) Any mass of tissue that bulges outward or upward from a normal surface level so that it is easily visible.

Polyphagia (pol-e-FA-je-ah) Excessive eating. See *diabetes*.

Polysomnography (pol-e-som-NOG-raf-e) Continuous monitoring of normal and abnormal physiological functioning during sleep.

Polyuria (pol-e-U-re-ah) Excessive excretion of urine. See *diabetes*.

Popliteal cyst (pop-LIT-e-al sist, pop-lit-E-al sist) Synonym for Baker cyst.

Popliteal fossa (pop-LIT-e-al fos-ah, pop-lit-E-al fos-ah) The diamond-shaped space posterior to the knee bounded superficially by the diverging biceps femoris and semimembranosus muscles above and inferiorly by the two heads of the gastrocnemius muscle.

Portal hypertension (POR-tal hi-per-TEN-shun) Elevation of pressure in the hepatic portal circulation due to cirrhosis or other fibrotic change in liver tissue.

Postherpetic neuralgia (post-her-PET-ik nu-RAL-je-ah) A pain that lasts after the lesions related to herpes zoster have healed.

Postmastectomy pain syndrome (post-mas-TEK-to-me pane SIN-drome) A chronic pain syndrome that occurs after breast surgery; pain is often located in the axilla, shoulder, arm, and chest wall.

Postpartum psychosis (post-PAR-tum si-KO-sis) A group of mental illnesses following the childbirth with a sudden onset of psychotic symptoms; may be linked to bipolar disorder in some patients.

Posturography (pos-tur-OG-raf-e) A measurement of postural stability under varying visual and proprioceptive inputs. See *vestibular balance disorders*.

Prednisone (PRED-nih-zone) An analog of cortisol; used as a steroidal anti-inflammatory.

Preeclampsia (pre-e-KLAMP-se-ah) Development of hypertension with proteinuria or edema, or both, due to pregnancy.

Premenstrual dysphoric disorder (PMDD) (pre-MEN-stru-al dis-FOR-ik dis-OR-der) A pervasive pattern occurring during the last week of the luteal phase in most menstrual cycles for at least a year and remitting within a few days of the onset of the follicular phase; the symptoms are comparable in severity to those seen in a major depressive episode, distinguishing this disorder from the far more common premenstrual syndrome.

Pretibial myxedema (pre-TIB-e-al mik-seh-DE-mah) A rash that occurs in the tibial region, specifically associated with hyperthyroidism.

Priapism (PRI-ah-pizm) Persistent erection of the penis, accompanied by pain and tenderness.

Prion (PRI-on) Small infectious proteinaceous particle on nonnucleic acid; the causative agent for bovine spongiform encephalopathy, Creutzfeldt-Jakob disease, kuru, and others.

Prodromic (pro-DRO-mik) Relating to the early or premonitory symptom of a disease, especially herpes simplex.

Progestin (pro-JEST-in) A hormone of the corpus luteum.

Proliferants (pro-LIF-er-ants) Injected substances that are designed to stimulate the growth of new collagen fibers, which with appropriate stretching and exercise, lie down in alignment with the original fibers.

Proliferative inflammatory atrophy (pro-LIF-er-ah-tiv in-FLAM-ah-tor-e A-tro-fe) Condition of the prostate and other tissues involving chronic inflammation, which leads to cellular proliferation and an increased risk of cancer.

Prophylaxis (pro-fil-AK-sis) Prevention of a disease or of a process that can lead to a disease.

Proprioceptor (pro-pre-o-SEP-tor) Sensory end organs that relay information about position and muscle tension.

Proptosis (prop-TO-sis) Protruding eyes; exophthalmos. See *hyperthyroidism*.

Prostadynia (pros-tah-DIN-e-ah) Synonym for chronic pelvic pain syndrome; associated with prostate pain.

Prostaglandins (PROS-tah-glan-din) Substances in many tissues with effects such as vasodilation, vasoconstriction, and stimulation of smooth muscle tissue.

Prostate-specific antigen (PSA) (PROS-tate speh-SIF-ik AN-tih-jen) A glycoprotein found in normal seminal fluid and produced in prostate epithelial cells. Elevated levels of PSA are associated with prostatic enlargement and an increased risk of prostate cancer.

Prostatic intrathelial neoplasia (pros-TAT-ik in-tra-THE-le-al ne-o-PLA-zhah) Microscopic lesion in the prostate that may be a precursor to prostate cancer.

Prosthesis, prostheses (pros-THE-sis, pros-THE-seze) Fabricated substitute for a diseased or mission part of the body.

Protease inhibitor (PRO-te-aze) A group of AIDS drugs that work to interrupt the maturing phase of the virus.

Proteoglycan (pro-te-o-GLI-kan) A large protein molecule made of chains of linear carbohydrate polymers that are negatively charged.

Pruritis (pru-RI-tis) Itchiness.

Pseudogout (SU-do-gowt) Acute episodes of synovitis caused by calcium pyrophosphate crystals as opposed to urate crystals, as in true gout.

Pseudohypertrophy (SU-do- hy-PER-tro-fe) Increase in size of an organ or a part, due not to increase in size or number of the specific functional elements but to that of some other tissue, fatty or fibrous. See *muscular dystrophy*

Pseudomembranous colitis (su-do-MEM-brah-nus ko-LI-tis) Intestinal inflammation due to infection with *Clostridium difficile*; often related to prolonged antibiotic therapy.

Pseudomonas aeruginosa (su-do-MO-nah ah-ru-jin-O-sah) Species of aerobic bacteria that sometimes infect humans, especially when the host is otherwise compromised. See *cystic fibrosis*.

Psoralen (SOR-ah-len) A phototoxic drug used in the treatment of psoriasis.

Psoriasis (sor-I-ah-sis) A common inherited condition characterized by the eruption of reddish, silvery-scaled maculopapules, predominantly on the elbows, knees, scalp, and trunk.

Psychodynamic therapy (si-ko-di-NAM-ik THER-ah-pe) Therapy based on the psychological forces that underlie human behavior.

Psychoneuroimmunology (si-ko-nur-o-ih-myu-NOL-o-je) Study of emotional or other psychological states that affect the immune system, rendering an individual susceptible to a disease or the course of a disease.

Psychosis (si-KO-sis) A mental and behavioral disorder affecting a person's capacity to recognize reality, communicate, and relate to others.

Pthirus pubis (THI-rus PU-bis) A species of pubic or crab lice.

Ptosis (TO-sis) A sinking down or prolapse of an organ, specifically the eyelid. See *myasthenia gravis*.

Pugilistic parkinsonism (pu-jih-LIS-tik PAR-kin-son-izm) A disorder of professional boxers who receive multiple blows to the head and in whom symptoms progress even after they stop fighting. See *Parkinson disease*.

Purine (pyur-EEN) An organic compound that contains nitrogen; found in high concentration in meat and organs, and seafood.

Pustular psoriasis (PUS-tyu-lar so-RI-ah-sus) Psoriasis with pustule formation in the normal and psoriatic skin.

Pustule (PUS-tyule) A small, circumscribed elevation of the skin containing purulent material.

PUVA Oral administration of *p*soralen and subsequent exposure to long-wavelength *u*ltra*v*iolet-*A* light; used to treat psoriasis.

Pyelogram (PI-el-o-gram) A radiograph of the kidneys and ureters following the injection of a contrast medium.

Pyelography (pi-el-OG-rah-fe) Radiological study of the kidneys, ureters, and bladder.

Pyrogen (PI-ro-jen) A fever-inducing agent.

Q-angle The angle formed by the line of traction of the quadriceps tendon on the patella and the line of traction of the patellar tendon on the tibial tubercle. See *patellofemoral syndrome*.

Quadriplegia (kwoh-drih-PLE-je-ah) Paralysis of all four limbs. Also called tetraplegia.

Quercetin (KWER-seh-tin) A bioflavonoid with antihistamine and anti-inflammatory properties. See *prostatitis*.

Radiation (ra-de-A-shun) The sending forth of light, short radio waves, ultraviolet or x-rays, or any other waves for treatment, diagnosis, or other purpose.

Radicular pain (rah-DIK-u-lar pane) Pain felt along the pathway of a spinal nerve.

Radiculopathy (rah-dik-u-LOP-ath-e) Any disorder of the spinal nerve roots.

Radioimmunotherapy (ra-de-o-ih-my-no-THER-ah-pe) The use of radiation with medication to target specific tumor cells.

Radioisotope (ra-de-o-I-so-tope) An isotope that changes to a more stable state by emitting radiation.

Rales (RALE-ez) Term for an extra sound heard on auscultation of breath sounds.

Ramsay Hunt syndrome type 1 Facial paralysis, ear pain, and herpes zoster resulting from viral infection of the seventh cranial nerve and geniculate ganglion.

RANK ligand inhibitors A class of drugs used to treat osteoporosis that interferes with bone resorption.

Raynaud syndrome (ra-NO SIN-drome) Idiopathic bilateral cyanosis of the digits due to arterial and arteriolar contraction.

Rectocele (REK-to-sele) Prolapse or herniation of the rectum; also called proctocele.

Reduction (re-DUK-shun) The restoration, by surgical or manipulative procedures, of a part to its normal anatomic relation.

Reed-Sternberg cells Large transformed lymphocytes, indicative of Hodgkin disease.

Regional enteritis (RE-joh-nal en-tur-I-is) Synonym for Crohn disease.

Reiter syndrome (RI-tur sin-drome) A combination of symptoms, including urethritis, cutaneous lesions, arthritis, and diarrhea. One or more of these symptoms may recur at intervals, but the arthritis may be persistent.

Relaxin (re-LAK-sin) A hormone secreted during pregnancy that allows the softening and lengthening of the pubis symphysis, along with other connective tissues.

Renal calculus (RE-nal KAL-kyu-lus) A stone or pebble formed in the kidney collection system. See *kidney stones*.

Renal colic (RE-nal KOH-lik) Severe pain caused by the impaction or passage of a calculus in the ureter or renal pelvis.

Renin (REN-in) An enzyme produced by the kidneys that is involved in vasoconstriction and hypertension.

Repetitive stress injury (re-PET-ih-tiv STRESS IN-jur-e) Any injury related to wear and tear brought about by repeated, especially percussive, movements. See *carpal tunnel syndrome*.

Restenosis (re-sten-O-sis) Recurrence of stenosis after corrective surgery on the heart valve; narrowing of a structure, usually a coronary artery, following the removal or reduction of a previous narrowing.

Restless leg syndrome A sense of uneasiness, twitching, or restlessness that occurs in the legs after going to bed. See *sleep disorders*.

Reticulocyte (reh-TIK-u-lo-site) An immature red blood cell.

Retinoin (RET-ih-no-in) A class of keratolytic drugs derived from retinoic acid and used for treatment of severe acne and psoriasis.

Retinopathy (ret-ih-NOH-path-e) Noninflammatory degenerative disease of the retina.

Retrovirus (RET-ro-vi-rus) A virus in the family Retroviridae. They possess RNA, which serves as a template for synthesis of DNA in the host cell.

Rett syndrome A progressive and severe form of autism found mainly in girls.

Rheumatic (ru-MAT-ik) Characterized by muscle or joint pain.

Rheumatoid spondylitis (RU-mah-toid spon-dih-LI-is) See *ankylosing spondylitis*.

Rhinitis (ri-NI-tis) Inflammation of the nasal mucous membrane.

Rhinophyma (ri-no-FI-mah) Hypertrophy of the nose with follicular dilation, resulting from hyperplasia of sebaceous glands with fibrosis and increased vascularity. See *acne rosacea*.

Rhupus (RU-pus) Term for a common comorbidity of lupus and rheumatoid arthritis.

Rickettsia rickettsii (rih-KET-se-ah rih-KET-se-i) The agent of Rocky Mountain spotted fever and its geographic variants; transmitted by infected ixodid ticks, especially *Dermacentor andersoni* and *Dermacentor variabilis*. See *Lyme disease*.

Rimantadine (ri-MAN-tah-dene) An antiviral agent that closely resembles amantadine but is often better tolerated.

Ringworm A fungal infection of the keratin component of hair, skin, or nails. Tinea.

Rodent ulcer (RO-dent UL-ser) A slowly enlarging ulcerated basal cell carcinoma, usually on the face. See *skin cancer*.

Rotavirus (RO-tah-vi-rus) A group of RNA viruses, some of which cause human gastroenteritis. These viruses are major causes of infant diarrhea throughout the world.

Rotoscoliosis (ro-to-sko-li-O-sis) Combined lateral and rotational deviation of the vertebral column.

Rubella (ru-BEL-ah) An acute exanthematous disease caused by the rubella virus *Rubivirus*, with enlargement of lymph nodes but usually with little fever or constitutional reaction; a high incidence of birth defects in children results from maternal infection during the first several months of fetal life (congenital rubella syndrome). See *mononucleosis*.

S-adenosyl-methionine (SAM) (S-ah-DEN-o-sil meh-THI-o-nine) An amino acid associated with mood improvement. See *depression*.

Salmonella (sal-mo-NEL-ah) A group of bacteria associated with gastrointestinal tract infections and food poisoning.

Salpingitis (sal-pin-JI-tis) Inflammation of the fallopian (uterine) tube.

Sarcoidosis (sar-koyd-O-sis) A systemic granulomatous disease of unknown cause, especially involving the lungs with fibrosis.

Sarcolemma (sar-ko-LEM-ah) The plasma membrane of a muscle fiber.

Sarcoma (sar-KO-mah) A neoplasm of connective tissue.

Sarcomere (SAR-ko-mere) The segment of a myofibril between Z lines; the functioning contractile unit of striated muscle.

Sarcoptes scabiei (sar-KOP-teze SKA-be-i) The itch mite, varieties of which are distributed worldwide and affect humans and many animals. The mite burrows into the skin and lays eggs within the burrow; intense itching and rash develop near the burrow in about a month.

Savant (sah-VAHNT) A condition in which people with developmental disorders have one or more areas of expertise or ability.

Scheuermann disease (SHOY-er-mahn dih-ZEZE) Epiphysial osteonecrosis of adjacent vertebral bodies in the thoracic spine. See *postural deviations*.

Schistosoma haematobium (skis-to-SO-ma he-mah-TO-be-um) The vesical blood fluke, a species that occurs as a parasite in the portal system and mesenteric veins of the bladder, causing human schistosomiasis haematobium, and rectum; found throughout Africa and the Middle East; See *bladder cancer*.

Schwann cells (shwahn selz) Cells forming a continuous envelope around each fiber of peripheral nerves.

Sclerodactyly (skler-o-DAK-tih-le) Stiffness and tightness of the skin of the fingers, with atrophy of the soft tissue and osteoporosis of the distal phalanges of the hands and feet; a limited form of progressive systemic sclerosis. See *scleroderma*.

Scleroderma (skler-o-DER-mah) Thickening and induration of the skin caused by new collagen formation; either a manifestation of progressive systemic sclerosis or localized morphea.

Scoliosis (sko-le-O-sis) Abnormal lateral curve of the vertebral column.

Seasonal affective disorder (SAD) (SE-zon-al ah-FEK-tiv dis-OR-der) A depressive disorder that is exacerbated by short days and that subsides in spring and summer.

Sebaceous gland (seh-BA-shus gland) Gland in the dermis that usually opens into hair follicles and secretes an oily semifluid; sebum.

Seborrheic (seb-o-RE-ik) Relating to overactivity of the sebaceous glands resulting in an excessive amount of sebum. See *eczema*.

Seborrheic keratosis (seb-o-RE-ik ker-ah-TO-sis) Superficial benign skin lesions of proliferating epithelial cells.

Sebum (SE-bum) The secretion produced by sebaceous glands.

Second impact syndrome Exacerbation of a head injury by another before the first has fully healed.

Selective estrogen receptor modulators (SERMs) (seh-LEK-tiv ES-tro-jen re-SEP-tur MOD-u-la-terz) A group of medications developed to reduce the risk of some recurrent cancers; can also be used for osteoporosis.

Selective serotonin reuptake inhibitors (SSRIs) (seh-LEK-tiv SER-o-to-nin re-UP-take in-HIB-ih-torz) A class of drugs used in the treatment of depression that selectively prevent the reuptake of serotonin in the brain.

Self-limited disease A disease that resolves spontaneously with or without treatment.

Seminiferous tubules (sem-ih-NIF-er-us TU-byulez) The glandular part of testicles that contain the sperm-producing cells.

Seminoma (sem-ih-NO-mah) A type of germ cell tumor. See *testicular cancer.*

Sentinel lymph node (SEN-tih-nal LIMF node) The first lymph node to receive lymph drainage from a malignant tumor; if it is found clear of metastasis, all of the other nearby nodes are clear also.

Septicemia (sep-tih-SE-me-ah) Systemic disease caused by the spread of microorganisms and their toxins in the circulating blood. See *cellulitis, lymphangitis.*

Seronegative (ser-o-NEG-ah-tiv) Denoting the absence of specific antibodies in serum.

Serotonin (ser-o-TO-nin) A chemical found in many tissues. In the brain it is a neurotransmitter associated with mood disorders; in the body it can be a vasoconstrictor, can stimulate smooth muscle contraction, and can inhibit gastric secretion.

Sertoli cell tumor (ser-TO-le sel TU-mor) A testicular tumor containing Sertoli cells, which may cause feminization. See *testicular cancer.*

Severe acute respiratory syndrome (SARS) A highly contagious respiratory illness caused by a type of coronavirus.

Shigella (shih-GEL-ah) A genus of bacteria associated with gastrointestinal infection.

Shoulder-hand syndrome Synonym for complex regional pain syndrome.

Shy-Drager syndrome (SHI-DRA-ger SIN-drome) A progressive central nervous system disorder involving tremor, muscle wasting, hypotension, and other symptoms. See *tremor.*

Sigmoidoscopy (sig-moid-OS-ko-pe) Endoscopic inspection of the sigmoid flexure of the colon.

Sine scleroderma An unusual form of systemic scleroderma with significant organ involvement and minimal affect on the skin.

Sinoatrial node (si-no-A-tre-al node) The mass of specialized cardiac fibers that act as the pacemaker for the heart.

Sinusotomy (si-nu-OT-o-me) A surgical procedure involving making an incision into a sinus.

Sitz bath Immersion of only the perineum and buttocks, with the legs being outside the tub.

Sjögren syndrome (SHOR-gren SIN-drome) An autoimmune disorder with a collection of signs and symptoms, including conjunctivitis, dryness of mucous membranes, and bilateral enlargement of the parotid glands. See *rheumatoid arthritis, lupus, scleroderma.*

Sleep paralysis (slepe pah-RAL-ih-sis) Brief episodic loss of voluntary movement that occurs when falling asleep (hypnagogic sleep paralysis) or when awakening (hypnopompic sleep paralysis). See *sleep disorders.*

Sodium urate (SO-de-um YUR-ate) Uric acid.

Somatomedin C (so-mat-o-ME-din C) A peptide that stimulates growth in bone and cartilage. See *acromegaly.*

Somatotropin (so-mat-o-TRO-pin) A hormone produced in the anterior pituitary that promotes body growth, fat mobilization, and inhibition of glucose utilization.

Sonogram (SON-o-gram) A diagnostic technique that uses ultrasound waves to create a computer image.

Spastic paralysis (SPAS-tik pah-RAL-ih-sis) Central nervous system damage resulting in permanent muscle contraction; combines aspects of hypertonia, hypokinesia, and dysreflexia.

Spasticity (spas-TIS-ih-te) A state of increased muscle tone with exaggerated muscle tendon reflexes. See *cerebral palsy, spinal cord injury, amyotrophic lateral sclerosis*

Specific immunity (speh-SIF-ik ih-MYU-nih-te) The immune state in which an altered reactivity is directed solely against the antigens that stimulated it.

Specific muscle weakness Degeneration and weakening of muscles supplied by specifically damaged motor neurons, as opposed to general muscle weakness, which may not be related to nerve damage.

Sphincter (sfink-tur) A muscle that encircles a duct, tube, or orifice.

Sphygmomanometer (sfig-mo-man-OM-eh-ter) Blood pressure cuff.

Spigelian hernia (spih-GALE-e-an HER-ne-ah) A hernia through the spigelian fascia, which is the layer on the lateral aspect of the rectus abdominus.

Spina bifida meningocele (SPI-nah BIF-ih-dah men-ING-go-sele) Protrusion of the membranes of the brain or spinal cord through a defect in the skull or vertebral column.

Spina bifida myelomeningocele (SPI-nah BIF-ih-dah mi-el-o-men-ING-go-sele) Protrusion of the spinal cord and its membranes through a defect in the vertebral column.

Spina bifida occulta (SPI-nah BIF-ih-dah o-KUL-tah) Spina bifida in which there is a spinal defect but no protrusion of the cord or its membrane, although there is often some abnormality in their development.

Spirochete (SPI-ro-kete) A type of bacteria shaped like undulating spiral rods. See *ulcers, Lyme disease, syphilis*.

Spirometry (spi-ROM-et-re) A test to measure respiratory gases using a spirometer.

Splenomegaly (splen-o-MEG-ah-le) Enlargement of the spleen. See *mononucleosis, anemia*.

Spondyloarthropathy (spon-dih-lo-arth-ROH-path-e) Group name for dysfunction or disease at spinal joints.

Spondylolisthesis (spon-dih-lo-lis-THE-sis) Forward movement of the body of one of the lumbar vertebrae on the vertebra below it or on the sacrum.

Spondylolysis (spon-dih-lo-LI-sis) Degeneration of the articulating part of the vertebra.

Spondylosis (spon-dih-LO-sis) Stiffening of the vertebra; often applied nonspecifically to any lesion of the spine of a degenerative nature.

Sporadic (spor-AD-ik) Occurring irregularly, haphazardly.

Sputum (SPYU-tum) Expectorated matter, especially mucus or mucopurulent matter expectorated in diseases of the air passages.

Squamous (SKWA-mus) Relating to or covered with scales.

St. Anthony's fire Any of several inflammatory infections of the skin, especially erysipelas. See *cellulitis*.

Staghorn calculus (STAG-horn KAL-kyu-lus) A calculus occurring in the renal pelvis, with branches extending into the calices. See *kidney stones*.

Staging (STA-jing) The classification of distinct phases or periods in the course of a disease.

Stapedius (stah-PE-de-us) Muscle that connects the eardrum (tympanum) to the stapes.

Staphylococcus (staf-ih-lo-KOK-us) A type of bacteria formed of spherical cells that divide to make irregular clusters.

Starling equilibrium (star-lingz ek-wih-LIB-re-um) Also called Starling hypothesis (hi-POTH-eh-sis) The principle that the amount of fluid squeezed out of circulatory capillaries should be almost equal to the amount being drawn into lymphatic capillaries.

Status epilepticus (STAT-us ep-ih-LEP-tih-kus) Repeated seizure or a seizure prolonged for at least 30 minutes; may be convulsive tonic-clonic, nonconvulsive absence, complex partial, partial epilepsia partialis continuans, or subclinical electrographic status epilepticus. See *seizure disorders*.

Steatorrhea (ste-at-o-RE-ah) Passage of large amounts of feces due to failure to digest and absorb nutrients, especially fats. Often linked to absence of bile salts in the gastrointestinal tract.

Stein-Leventhal syndrome (stine LEV-en-thal SIN-drome) Synonym for polycystic ovary disease. See *ovarian cysts*.

Stenosis (sten-O-sis) A stricture or narrowing of any canal.

Stent A device to hold tissue in place or provide support.

Steroids (STER-oydz) A large group of chemical compounds including some hormones and drugs of a particular molecular composition. Some steroids include gonadal and adrenal hormones.

Stereotactic radiotherapy (ster-e-o-TAK-tik ra-de-o-THER-ah-pe) Three-dimensional approach to radiation therapy.

Stoma (STO-mah) An artificial opening between two cavities or between a hollow area and the surface of the body.

Stomatitis (sto-mah-TI-tis) Inflammation of the mucous membrane of the mouth.

Strabismus (strah-BIS-mus) A lack of parallelism in the visual axes of the eyes. See *cerebral palsy*.

Stratum basale (STRAT-um bah-SAL) The deepest layer of the epidermis, composed of dividing stem cells and anchoring cells.

Streptococcus (strep-to-KOK-us) A type of bacteria formed of spherical cells that occur in pairs or in long or short chains.

Streptococcus pneumoniae (strep-to-KOK-us nu-MO-ne-a) A species of diplococci frequently occurring in pairs or chains. Normal inhabitants of the respiratory tract and the cause of lobar pneumonia, otitis media, meningitis, sinusitis, and other infections.

Striatonigral degeneration (stro-at-o-NIH-gral de-jen-ur-A-shun) A movement disorder that may appear with Shy-Drager syndrome and olivopontocerebellar atrophy in a condition called multiple system atrophy. See *tremor*.

Stricture (STRIK-cher) A narrowing or stenosis of a tube, duct, or hollow structure.

Stroma (STRO-mah) The framework, usually made of connective tissue, of an organ, gland, or other tissue.

Stromal cell tumor (STRO-mal sel TU-mur) A tumor that arises from connective tissue stroma rather than epithelium. See *breast cancer*.

Struvite (STRU-vite) A compound of magnesium ammonium phosphate found in some renal calculi. See *kidney stones*.

Sty A pus-forming infection of a gland or hair follicle; inflammation of the sebaceous gland of the eyelash.

Subacute (sub-ah-KYUTE) Between acute and chronic, denoting medium duration or relatively mild severity.

Subacute cutaneous lupus (sub-ah-KYUTE kyu-TA-ne-us) A group of skin disorders related to lupus erythematosus; may progress to systemic lupus.

Subcutaneous (sub-kyu-TA-ne-us) Beneath the skin.

Subluxation (sub-luk-SA-shun) An incomplete dislocation; although a relationship is altered, contact between joint surfaces remains.

Substance P A neurotransmitter that is primarily involved in pain transmission and is one of the most potent compounds affecting smooth muscle tissue. See *fibromyalgia*.

Substantia nigra (sub-STAN-te-ah NIG-rah) A large mass composed of pigmented cells in the brainstem. The site of dopamine synthesis.

Sudeck atrophy (SU-dek AT-ro-fe) Synonym for *complex regional pain syndrome*.

Sulcus, sulci (SUL-kus, SUL-si) One of the grooves or furrows on the surface of the brain.

Superficial fascia (su-per-FISH-al FASH-a) A loose fibrous envelope of connective tissue under the skin containing fat, blood vessels, and nerves.

Superior vena cava syndrome (su-PE-re-or VE-na KA-va SIN-drome) Obstruction of the superior vena cava by benign or malignant lesions that cause engorgement of the blood vessels of the face, neck, and arms. See *lung cancer*.

Symbiosis (sim-be-O-sis) The biological association of two or more species to their mutual benefit.

Sympathectomy (sim-pa-THEK-to-me) Excision of a section of a sympathetic nerve or one or more of the sympathetic ganglia. See *complex regional pain syndrome*.

Synarthrosis, synarthroses (sin-ar-THRO-sis, sin-ar-THRO-sez) A fibrous joint, sometimes said to be immovable.

Syncytial (sin-SIH-shal) Relating to a mass formed by the secondary union of originally separated cells.

Syndesmophyte (sin-DEZ-mo-fite) A bone spur attached to a ligament.

Syndrome X A synonym for *metabolic syndrome*.

Synkinesis (sin-kin-E-sis) Involuntary movement that follows a voluntary one. See *Bell palsy*.

Synovectomy (sin-o-VEK-to-me) The excision of part or all of the synovial membrane of a joint.

Synovial joint (sin-O-ve-al joynt) A diarthrosis, or freely movable joint.

Systemic lupus erythematosus (sis-TEM-ik LU-pus eh-rih-the-mah-TO-sus) An inflammatory connective tissue disease with variable features including fever, weakness and fatigability, joint pains or arthritis resembling rheumatoid arthritis, and diffuse erythematous skin lesions on the face, neck, or upper extremities.

Systole (SIS-tole) The contraction of the heart, specifically of the ventricles.

Tachycardia (tak-e-KAR-de-a) Rapid heartbeat, usually applied to rates greater than 100 beats per minute.

Tamoxifen (tah-MOX-ih-fen) An antiestrogen agent used in the treatment of breast cancer.

Tau (tow) A protein that helps to maintain the structure of the cytoskeleton; found in the plaques of persons with Alzheimer disease.

Telangiectasia (tel-an-je-ek-TA-ze-ah) Dilation of previously existing small vessels, most commonly in the skin. Also called *spider veins*. See *scleroderma*, *varicose veins*, *acne rosacea*.

Tender point One of many predictable bilateral pairs of points that produce a painful response with a minimum of pressure 4 kg; used to help diagnose fibromyalgia.

Tendinosis (ten-din-O-sis) The condition of chronic tendon injury without inflammation. See *tendinopathies*.

Tennis elbow (TEH-nis EL-bo) A synonym for *lateral epicondylitis*.

Tenosynovitis (ten-o-sin-o-VI-tis) Inflammation of a tendon and its enveloping sheath.

TENS, transcutaneous electrical nerve stimulation A device to control pain with electrical stimulation applied through the skin to the nerves.

Teratoma (ter-ah-TO-mah) A neoplasm that contains tissues not normally found in the tissue in which it arises; usually found as benign ovarian cysts in women and malignant testicular growths in men. See *testicular cancer, ovarian cysts*.

Terminal ileitis (TER-min-al il-e-I-tis) Synonym for *Crohn disease*.

Testosterone (tes-TOS-teh-rone) A naturally occurring androgen found in testes and other tissues.

Tethered cord (TETH-erd CORD) A group of malformations that all involve restricting the free movement of the spinal cord within the spinal canal.

Tetraplegia (tet-rah-PLE-je-a) Quadriplegia.

Thalassemia (thal-ah-SE-me-ah) Any of a group of inherited disorders of hemoglobin metabolism.

Thenar (THE-nar) Referring to the fleshy mass on the lateral side of the palm; the ball of the thumb.

Thermal capsulorraphy (THER-mal kap-su-LOR-ah-fe) The use of heat to shrink and repair a joint capsule, specifically at the shoulder, to prevent future dislocations.

Thermography (ther-MOG-raf-e) The making of a regional temperature map of the body, obtained by using an infrared sensing device.

Thrombocyte (THROM-bo-site) Platelet.

Thrombocytopenia (throm-bo-si-to-PE-ne-ah) Decreased number of thrombocytes.

Thromboembolism (throm-bo-EM-bo-lism) An embolism (traveling clot) that originated from a thrombus (lodged clot).

Thrombosis (throm-BO-sis) Formation or presence of a clot.

Thrush Infection of the oral tissues with *Candida albicans*; often an opportunistic infection in persons with AIDS or other conditions that depress the immune system. See *HIV/AIDS, Candida*.

Thymoma (thi-MO-ma) A neoplasm originating in the thymus; usually benign. See *myasthenia gravis*.

Thymosin (THI-mo-sin) A hormone that restores thymus function.

Thyrotoxic myopathy (thi-ro-TOX-ik mi-OP-ath-e) A neuromuscular disorder connected to hyperthyroidism that involves weakness, the breakdown of muscle tissue, and intolerance to heat.

Thyrotoxicosis (thi-ro-tox-ih-KO-sis) Describing the presence of excessive levels of endogenous or exogenous thyroid hormone.

Thyroxin (thi-ROK-sin) Tetraiodothyronine (T_4); a secretion of the thyroid gland.

Tibial tuberosity apophysitis (TIB-e-al tu-ber-OS-ih-te ap-of-ih-SI-tis) Inflammation of the tibial tuberosity; synonym for Osgood-Schlatter disease.

Tic douloureux (tik doo-lo-ROO) A synonym for *trigeminal neuralgia*.

Tinea (TIN-e-ah) A fungal infection of the keratin component of hairs, skin, or nails.

Tinea barbae (TIN-e-ah BAR-ba) Tinea of the beard, occurring as a follicular infection or as a granulomatous lesion; the primary lesions are papules and pustules. See *fungal infections*.

Tinea capitis (TIN-e-ah KAP-ih-tus) A common fungus infection of the scalp caused by various species of *Microsporum* and *Trichophyton* on or within hair shafts. See *fungal infections*.

Tinea corporis (TIN-e-ah KOR-por-is) A well-defined, scaling, macular eruption of dermatophytosis that frequently forms annular lesions and may appear on any part of the body. See *fungal infections*.

Tinea cruris (TIN-e-ah KRU-ris) A form of tinea imbricata occurring in the genitocrural region, including the inner side of the thighs, the perineal region, and the groin. See *fungal infections*.

Tinea manus (TIN-e-ah MAN-us) Ringworm of the hand, usually referring to infections of the palmar surface. See *fungal infections*.

Tinea pedis (TIN-e-ah PED-is) Dermatophytosis of the feet, especially of the skin between the toes, caused by one of the dermatophytes, usually a species of *Trichophyton* or *Epidermophyton;* the disease consists of small vesicles, fissures, scaling, maceration, and eroded areas between the toes and on the plantar surface of the foot; See *fungal infections*.

Tinea unguium (TIN-e-ah UNG-we-um) Ringworm of the nails due to a dermatophyte. See *fungal infections*.

Tinea versicolor (TIN-e-ah VER-sih-koh-lor) An eruption of tan or brown branny patches on the skin of the trunk, often appearing white, in contrast with hyperpigmented skin after exposure to the summer sun; caused by growth of *Malassezia furfur* in the stratum corneum with minimal inflammatory reaction. See *fungal infections*.

Tinel sign (te-NEL sine) Distally radiating pain or tingling caused by tapping over the site of a superficial nerve, indicating inflammation or entrapment of that nerve; a test used to help identify carpal tunnel syndrome.

Tinnitus (TIN-ih-tus, tin-I-tus) A sensation of noises ringing, whistling, or booming in the ears.

Tissue plasminogen activator (tPA) (TISH-u plaz-MIN-o-jen AK-tiv-a-tor) A genetically engineered protein that acts as a powerful thrombolytic clot-busting agent.

Titer (TI-ter) The standard of strength of a volumetric test solution; the assay value of an unknown measure by volumetric means.

Tonic spasm (TON-ik SPAZ-em) Continuous involuntary spasm of skeletal muscle.

Tonic-clonic seizure (TON-ik KLON-ik SE-zher) The sudden onset of tonic contraction of muscles, giving way to clonic convulsive movements. Grand mal seizure.

Tonometer (to-NOM-eh-ter) An instrument for determining pressure or tension.

Tophus, tophi (TO-fus, TO-fi) Deposits of uric acid and urates in tissue around joints and other areas; seen with gout.

Topical immunomodulators (TINs) (TOP-ih-kal im-u-no-MOD-u-la-torz) A class of anti-inflammatory ointments used as an alternative to steroidal applications in the treatment of atopic dermatitis. See *eczema*.

Torsion (TOR-shun) A twisting of a structure along its long axis.

Torticollis (tor-tih-KOL-is) A contraction, often spasmodic, of the muscles of the neck, chiefly those supplied by the spinal accessory nerve; the head is drawn to one side and usually rotated so that the chin points to the other side.

Toxic megacolon (TOK-sik MEG-ah-ko-lon) Acute nonobstructive dilation of the colon.

Toxoplasma gondii (TOX-o-plaz-mah GON-de-i) A widespread parasitic species of sporozoan; may cause mononucleosis.

Transcriptase (tran-SKRIP-tase) An enzyme that converts RNA to DNA in the AIDS virus.

Transcutaneous (tranz-kyu-TA-ne-us) Denoting the passage of substances through unbroken skin.

Treponema pallidum (trep-o-NE-mah PAL-ih-dum) A species of spirochetal bacteria that causes syphilis in humans.

Trichomoniasis (trik-o-mo-NI-ah-sis) Disease caused by infection with a protozoan of the genus *Trichomonas*.

Trichophyton (trih-KOF-ih-ton) A genus of pathogenic fungi that cause dermatophytosis in humans and animals. See *fungal infections*.

Tricyclic antidepressants (tri-SIK-lik an-te-de-PRES-ants) A chemical group of drugs that share a three-ringed nucleus, for example, amitriptyline, imipramine.

Trigger point A small area in which muscle fibers have been injured and not healed normally. Pressure on a trigger point elicits moderate to severe pain in specific referring patterns.

Triiodothyronine (tri-I-o-do-THI-ro-nene) T_3, a secretion of the thyroid gland. See *hypothyroidism*.

Trophic (TRO-fik) Relating to or dependent on nutrition; resulting from interruption of nerve supply.

Trophic ulcer (TRO-fik UL-ser) Ulcer resulting from cutaneous sensory denervation.

Tubercle (TU-ber-kel) A nodule or bump; may refer to bony prominences, elevations on the skin or other tissues, or to the lesions caused by infection with *Mycobacterium tuberculosis*.

Tuberous sclerosis (TU-bur-us skler-O-sis) A rare multisystem genetic disease that causes nonmalignant tumors to grow in the brain and other vital organs. Can be connected to developmental delay and other neurological problems, including autism spectrum disease.

Tumor (TU-mor) Any swelling, usually denoting a neoplasm.

Tumor necrosis factor (TU-mur nek-RO-sis fak-tor) A polypeptide hormone produced by activated macrophages; can initiate fever.

Tumor suppressor gene (TU-mur suh-PRES-ur jene) A gene with the function of suppressing cellular proliferation; loss of this gene leads to a heightened susceptibility to cancer.

Tunica intima (TU-nih-kah IN-tih-mah) The innermost coat of a blood or lymphatic vessel.

Tunica media (TU-nih-kah ME-de-ah) The middle, usually muscular coat of a blood vessel or lymphatic vessel.

Turcot syndrome (tur-KO SIN-drome) A subgroup of a genetic predisposition to colorectal cancer; part of familial adenomatous polyposis.

Tyrosine (TI-ro-zene) An amino acid present in most proteins.

Umbilicus (um-BIL-ih-kus) The pit in the center of the abdominal wall marking the site where the umbilical cord entered the fetus.

Unilateral (u-nih-LAT-er-al) Confined to one side only.

Ureaplasma urealyticum (u-re-ah-PLAZ-mah u-re-ah-LIH-tih-kum) A species of bacteria that cause infections in the genitourinary tract. See *sexually transmitted diseases*.

Uremia (yu-RE-me-a) An excess of urea and other nitrogenous waste in the blood.

Ureterolithiasis (u-re-ter-o-lith-I-ah-sis) A kidney stone lodged in the ureter.

Ureteroscopic stone removal (u-re-ter-o-SKOP-ik STONE re-mu-val) Removal of a calculus in the mid to lower ureters with a ureteroscope.

Urogram (YUR-o-gram) Radiographic record of any part of the urinary tract.

Urticaria (ur-tih-KA-re-ah) An eruption of itching wheals; synonym for hives.

Uveitis (yu-ve-I-tis) Inflammation of the uveal tract iris, ciliary body, and choroid of the eye. See *ulcerative colitis*.

Vagotomy (va-GOT-o-me) Division of the vagus nerve.

Valgus (VAL-gus) Laterally deviated.

Vapocoolant (VA-po-koo-lant) A topical anesthetic aerosol spray used for pain relief and stretching of muscles affected by trigger points. See *myofascial pain syndrome*.

Varicocele (VAR-ih-ko-sele) A condition manifested by abnormal dilation of the veins of the spermatic cord, caused by incompetent valves in the internal spermatic vein and resulting in impaired drainage of blood into the spermatic cord veins when the patient assumes the upright position.

Varix, varices (VAR-ix, VAR-ih-sez) A dilated vein.

Varus (VAR-us) Medially deviated.

Vas deferens (vas DEF-er-enz) The secretory duct of the testicle, running from the epididymis to the prostatic urethra, where it terminates as the ejaculatory duct.

Vasculitis (vas-ku-LI-tis) Inflammation of a blood or lymphatic vessel.

Venography (ve-NOG-rah-fe) A radiographic demonstration of a vein after the injection of a contrast medium.

Ventricle (VEN-trih-kul) A normal cavity, specifically in the brain or heart.

Venule (VEN-yule, VE-nyule) A venous branch continuous with a capillary.

Verruca (veh-RU-ka) A wart composed of a thickened keratin layer of the epidermis.

Vesicle (VES-ih-kul) A small, circumscribed fluid-filled elevation of the skin; a blister.

Vesicouretal reflux (VES-ih-co-u-RE-tul RE-flux) Backward flow of urine from bladder into ureter.

Villus, villi (VIL-us, VIL-i) A projection from the surface, especially of a mucous membrane.

Virchow triad (FERE-kow TRI-ad) A description of precipitating factors for clot formation; injury to endothelium, hypercoagulability, and venous stasis.

Viremia (vih-RE-me-ah) The presence of a virus in the bloodstream.

Virion (VI-re-on) The complete virus particle that is intact and infectious.

Virulent (VIR-u-lent) Extremely toxic, denoting a markedly pathogenic microorganism.

Von Willebrand disease (fon vil-eh-BRAHNT) A disease characterized by the tendency to bleed primarily from the mucous membranes and prolonged bleeding time.

von Willebrand factor A blood glycoprotein that helps platelets to adhere to wound sites.

Wernicke-Korsakoff syndrome (VER-nih-ke KOR-sah-kof SIN-drome) A combination of conditions related to prolonged alcohol abuse and thiamin deficiency, including tremor, psychosis, confusion, memory loss, and delirium tremens.

Wheal (wele) A reddened, itchy, changeable edematous area of the skin that is caused by exposure to an allergenic substance in a susceptible individual.

Wolff law (volf law) A law stating that every change in the form and/or function of a bone is followed by changes in internal and external architecture of the bone.

Wright test (rite test) A thoracic outlet syndrome test in which the hand is placed over the head and the head is turned toward the affected side. If this exacerbates symptoms or reduces the strength of the pulse of the affected side, impingement to the axillary artery and lower brachial plexus nerves is suspected.

Xeroderma (ze-ro-DER-mah) Excessively dry skin; a mild form of ichthyosis.

Xeroderma pigmentosum (ze-ro-DER-mah pig-men-TO-sum) A genetic disorder that impedes the ability to heal from overexposure to ultraviolet radiation.

Yolk sac tumor Malignant neoplasm occurring in the gonads. See *testicular cancer*.

Yuppie flu Vernacular for a set of signs and symptoms that may be diagnosed as chronic fatigue syndrome.

Zygapophysial joint (zi-gah-po-FIZ-e-al) Relating to a zygapophysis or articular process of a vertebra.

Illustration Credits

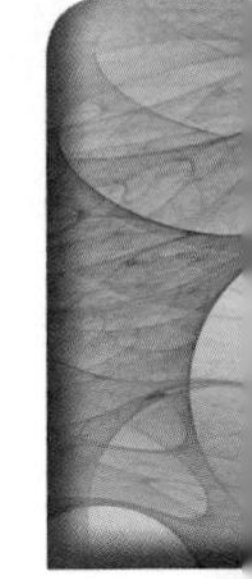

Chapter 1

1.1 Public Images Library, Centers for Disease Control and Prevention.
1.2 McClatchey KD. Clinical Laboratory Medicine, 2nd ed. Philadelphia: Lippincott Williams & Wilkins, 2002.
1.3 McClatchey KD. Clinical Laboratory Medicine, 2nd ed. Philadelphia: Lippincott Williams & Wilkins, 2002.
1.4 Koneman EW, Allen SD, Janda WM, Schreckenberger PC, Winn WC. Color Atlas and Textbook of Diagnostic Microbiology, 5th ed. Philadelphia: Lippincott Williams & Wilkins, 1997.
1.5 Sun T. Parasitic Disorders: Pathology, Diagnosis, and Management, 2nd ed. Philadelphia: Lippincott Williams & Wilkins, 1999.
1.6 Public Images Library, Centers for Disease Control and Prevention.
1.7 Koneman EW, Allen SD, Janda WM, Schreckenberger PC, Winn WC. Color Atlas and Textbook of Diagnostic Microbiology, 5th ed. Philadelphia: Lippincott Williams & Wilkins, 1997.

Chapter 2

2.2 Goodheart HP. Goodheart's Photoguide of Common Skin Disorders, 2nd ed. Philadelphia: Lippincott Williams & Wilkins, 2003.
2.3 Goodheart HP. Goodheart's Photoguide of Common Skin Disorders, 2nd ed. Philadelphia: Lippincott Williams & Wilkins, 2003.
2.4 Koneman EW, Allen SD, Janda WM, Schreckenberger PC, Winn WC. Color Atlas and Textbook of Diagnostic Microbiology, 5th ed. Philadelphia: Lippincott Williams & Wilkins, 1997.
2.5 Goodheart HP. Goodheart's Photoguide of Common Skin Disorders, 2nd ed. Philadelphia: Lippincott Williams & Wilkins, 2003.
2.6 Koneman EW, Allen SD, Janda WM, Schreckenberger PC, Winn WC. Color Atlas and Textbook of Diagnostic Microbiology, 5th ed. Philadelphia: Lippincott Williams & Wilkins, 1997.
2.7 Goodheart HP. Goodheart's Photoguide of Common Skin Disorders, 2nd ed. Philadelphia: Lippincott Williams & Wilkins, 2003.
2.8 McClatchey KD. Clinical Laboratory Medicine, 2nd ed. Philadelphia: Lippincott Williams & Wilkins, 2002.
2.9 Goodheart HP. Goodheart's Photoguide of Common Skin Disorders, 2nd ed. Philadelphia: Lippincott Williams & Wilkins, 2003.
2.10 Goodheart HP. Goodheart's Photoguide of Common Skin Disorders, 2nd ed. Philadelphia: Lippincott Williams & Wilkins, 2003.
2.11 Sutton DA, Fothergill AW, Rinaldi MG. Guide to Clinically Significant Fungi. Baltimore: Williams & Wilkins, 1998.
2.12 Goodheart HP. Goodheart's Photoguide of Common Skin Disorders, 2nd ed. Philadelphia: Lippincott Williams & Wilkins, 2003.
2.13 Goodheart HP. Goodheart's Photoguide of Common Skin Disorders, 2nd ed. Philadelphia: Lippincott Williams & Wilkins, 2003.
2.14 Image provided by Stedmans. (Dr Barankin Dermatology Collection 2)
2.15 Goodheart HP. Goodheart's Photoguide of Common Skin Disorders, 2nd ed. Philadelphia: Lippincott Williams & Wilkins, 2003.
2.16 Public Images Library, Centers for Disease Control and Prevention.
2.17 Goodheart HP. Goodheart's Photoguide of Common Skin Disorders, 2nd ed. Philadelphia: Lippincott Williams & Wilkins, 2003.
2.18 Goodheart HP. Goodheart's Photoguide of Common Skin Disorders, 2nd ed. Philadelphia: Lippincott Williams & Wilkins, 2003.
2.19 Image provided by Stedmans. (Dr Barankin Dermatology Collection)
2.20 Goodheart HP. Goodheart's Photoguide of Common Skin Disorders, 2nd ed. Philadelphia: Lippincott Williams & Wilkins, 2003.
2.21 Goodheart HP. Goodheart's Photoguide of Common Skin Disorders, 2nd ed. Philadelphia: Lippincott Williams & Wilkins, 2003.
2.22 Rubin E, Gorstein F, Schwarting R, Strayer DS. Rubin's Pathology: Clinicopathologic Foundations of Medicine, 4th ed. Philadelphia: Lippincott Williams & Wilkins, 2005.
2.23 Image provided by Stedmans. (Dr Barankin Dermatology Collection)
2.24 Rassner G. Atlas of Dermatology, 3rd ed. Philadelphia: Lea & Febiger, 1994.
2.25 Goodheart HP. Goodheart's Photoguide of Common Skin Disorders, 2nd ed. Philadelphia: Lippincott Williams & Wilkins, 2003.
2.26 Goodheart HP. Goodheart's Photoguide of Common Skin Disorders, 2nd ed. Philadelphia: Lippincott Williams & Wilkins, 2003.
2.27 Goodheart HP. Goodheart's Photoguide of Common Skin Disorders, 2nd ed. Philadelphia: Lippincott Williams & Wilkins, 2003.

2.28 Sauer GC, Hall JC. Manual of Skin Diseases, 7th ed. Philadelphia: Lippincott Raven, 1966.
2.29 Goodheart HP. Goodheart's Photoguide of Common Skin Disorders, 2nd ed. Philadelphia: Lippincott Williams & Wilkins, 2003.
2.30 Goodheart HP. Goodheart's Photoguide of Common Skin Disorders, 2nd ed. Philadelphia: Lippincott Williams & Wilkins, 2003.
2.31 Goodheart HP. Goodheart's Photoguide of Common Skin Disorders, 2nd ed. Philadelphia: Lippincott Williams & Wilkins, 2003.
2.32 Goodheart HP. Goodheart's Photoguide of Common Skin Disorders, 2nd ed. Philadelphia: Lippincott Williams & Wilkins, 2003.
2.33 Image provided by Stedmans. (Dr Barankin Dermatology Collection)
2.34 Goodheart HP. Goodheart's Photoguide of Common Skin Disorders, 2nd ed. Philadelphia: Lippincott Williams & Wilkins, 2003.
2.35 Stedman's Medical Dictionary.
2.36 Courtesy of the American Cancer Society, Atlanta, GA.
2.37 Image provided by Stedmans. (Dr Barankin Dermatology Collection)
2.38 Tasman W, Jaeger E. the Wills Eye Hospital Atlas of Clinical Ophthalmology, 2nd ed. Philadelphia: Lippincott Williams & Wilkins, 2003.
2.39 Goodheart HP. Goodheart's Photoguide of Common Skin Disorders, 2nd ed. Philadelphia: Lippincott Williams & Wilkins, 2003.
2.40 Goodheart HP. Goodheart's Photoguide of Common Skin Disorders, 2nd ed. Philadelphia: Lippincott Williams & Wilkins, 2003.
2.41 Image provided by Stedmans. (Dr Barankin Dermatology Collection)
2.42 Smeltzer SC, Bare BG. Brunner & Suddarth's Textbook of Medical-Surgical Nursing, 9th ed. Philadelphia: Lippincott Williams & Wilkins, 2000.
2.43 Rubin E, Farber JL. Pathology, 3rd ed. Philadelphia: Lippincott Williams & Wilkins, 1999.
2.44 Goodheart HP. Goodheart's Photoguide of Common Skin Disorders, 2nd ed. Philadelphia: Lippincott Williams & Wilkins, 2003.
2.45 Rubin E, Gorstein F, Schwarting R, Strayer DS. Rubin's Pathology: Clinicopathologic Foundations of Medicine, 4th ed. Philadelphia: Lippincott Williams & Wilkins, 2005.
2.46 Goodheart HP. Goodheart's Photoguide of Common Skin Disorders, 2nd ed. Philadelphia: Lippincott Williams & Wilkins, 2003.
2.47 Asset provided by Anatomical Chart Co.
2.48 Image provided by Stedmans. (Dr Barankin Dermatology Collection)
2.49 Image provided by Stedmans. (Dr Barankin Dermatology Collection)
2.50 Fleisher GR, Ludwig S, Baskin MN. Atlas of Pediatric Emergency Medicine. Philadelphia: Lippincott Williams & Wilkins, 2005.
2.51 Willis MC. Medical Terminology: The Language of Health Care. Baltimore: Williams & Wilkins, 1996.
2.52 Rubin E, Gorstein F, Schwarting R, Strayer DS. Rubin's Pathology: Clinicopathologic Foundations of Medicine, 4th ed. Philadelphia: Lippincott Williams & Wilkins, 2005.

Chapter 3

3.2 Asset provided by Anatomical Chart Co.
3.5 Asset provided by Anatomical Chart Co.
3.6 Berg D, Worzala K. Atlas of Adult Physical Diagnosis. Philadelphia: Lippincott Williams & Wilkins, 2006.
3.7 Roentgen EJ. Diagnosis of Diseases of Bone, 3rd ed. Baltimore: Williams & Wilkins, 1981.
3.8 Asset provided by Anatomical Chart Co.
3.9 Rubin E, Gorstein F, Schwarting R, Strayer DS. Rubin's Pathology: Clinicopathologic Foundations of Medicine, 4th ed. Philadelphia: Lippincott Williams & Wilkins, 2005.
3.12 Barker LR, Burton JR, Zieve PD. Principles of Ambulatory Medicine, 4th ed. Baltimore: Williams & Wilkins, 1995.
3.13 Rubin E, Gorstein F, Schwarting R, Strayer DS. Rubin's Pathology: Clinicopathologic Foundations of Medicine, 4th ed. Philadelphia: Lippincott Williams & Wilkins, 2005.
3.14 Berg D, Worzala K. Atlas of Adult Physical Diagnosis. Philadelphia: Lippincott Williams & Wilkins, 2006.
3.15 Asset provided by Anatomical Chart Co.
3.16 Fleisher GR, Ludwig S, Baskin MN. Atlas of Pediatric Emergency Medicine. Philadelphia: Lippincott Williams & Wilkins, 2004.
3.17 Baker CL. The Hughston Clinic Sports Medicine Book. Baltimore: Williams & Wilkins, 1995.
3.18 Asset provided by Anatomical Chart Co.
3.19 Asset provided by Anatomical Chart Co.
3.20 Koneman EW, Allen SD, Janda WM, Schreckenberger PC, Winn WC. Color Atlas and Textbook of Diagnostic Microbiology, 5th ed. Philadelphia: Lippincott Williams & Wilkins, 1997.
3.21 Sanders CV, Nesbitt LT. The Skin and Infection: A Color Atlas and Text. Baltimore: Williams & Wilkins, 1995.
3.22 Asset provided by Anatomical Chart Co.
3.23 Asset provided by Anatomical Chart Co.
3.25 MacNab I, McCulloch J. Neck Ache and Shoulder Pain. Baltimore: Williams & Wilkins, 1994.
3.26 MacNab I, McCulloch J. Neck Ache and Shoulder Pain. Baltimore: Williams & Wilkins, 1994.
3.27 Asset provided by Anatomical Chart Co.
3.29 Asset provided by Anatomical Chart Co.
3.31 Moore KL, Dalley AF. Clinically Orietned Anatomy, 4th ed. Baltimore: Lippincott Williams & Wilkins, 1999.
3.34 Asset provided by Anatomical Chart Co.
3.35 Asset provided by Anatomical Chart Co.
3.37 Berg D, Worzala K. Atlas of Adult Physical Diagnosis. Philadelphia: Lippincott Williams & Wilkins, 2006.
3.39 Asset provided by Anatomical Chart Co.
3.43 Frymoyer JW, Wiesel SW, etal. The Adult and Pediatric Spine. Philadelphia: Lippincott Williams & Wilkins, 2004.
3.44 Premkumar K. The Massage Connection, Anatomy and Physiology, 2nd ed. Baltimore: Lippincott Williams and Wilkins, 2004.

3.46 Bucci C. Condition-Specific Massage Therapy. Philadelphia: Lippincott Williams and Wilkins, 2011.
3.49 Asset provided by Anatomical Chart Co.
3.52 Asset provided by Anatomical Chart Co.
3.54 Asset provided by Anatomical Chart Co.

Chapter 4

4.3 Rubin E, Strayer DS. Rubin's Pathology: Clinicopathologic Foundations of medicine, 5th ed. Philadelphia: Lippincott Williams & Wilkins, 2008.
4.4 Asset provided by Anatomical Chart Co.
4.6 Fleisher GR, Ludwig W, Baskin MN. Atlas of Pediatric Emergency Medicine. Philadelphia: Lippincott Williams & Wilkins, 2004.
4.8 Asset provided by Anatomical Chart Co.
4.12 Courtesy of Robert Schwarzmann, MD, Philadelphia, PA.
4.13 Yochum TR, Rowe LJ. Essentials of Skeletal Radiology, 2nd ed. Baltimore: Williams & Wilkins, 1996.
4.15 Anatomical Chart Co.
4.23 Adapted from Smeltzer SC, Bare BG. Brunner & Suddarth's Textbook of Medical-Surgical Nursing, 9th ed. Philadelphia: Lippincott Williams & Wilkins, 2000.

Chapter 5

5.2 Cohen BJ, Wood DL. Memmler's The Human Body in Health and Disease, 9th ed. Philadelphia: Lippincott Williams & Wilkins, 2000.
5.3 Asset provided by Anatomical Chart Co.
5.8 Asset provided by Anatomical Chart Co.
5.9 Asset provided by Anatomical Chart Co.
5.11 Rubin E, Farber J. Pathology, 3rd ed. Philadelphia: Lippincott Williams & Wilkins, 1999.
5.13 Harwood-Nuss A, Wolfson AB, et al. The Clinical Practice of Emergency Medicine, 3rd ed. Philadelphia: Lippincott Williams & Wilkins, 2001.
5.14 Asset provided by Anatomical Chart Co.
5.16 Courtesy of International Scleroderma Network, www.sclero.org.
5.18 Moore KL, Dalley AF. Clinically Orietned Anatomy, 4th ed. Baltimore: Lippincott Williams & Wilkins, 1999.

Chapter 6

6.2 Rubin E, Gorstein F, Schwarting R, Strayer DS. Rubin's Pathology: Clinicopathologic Foundations of Medicine, 4th ed. Philadelphia: Lippincott Williams & Wilkins, 2005.
6.3 Reprinted with permission from Fitzpatrick J, Aeling J. Dermatology Secrets in Color, 2nd ed. Philadelphia: Hanley & Belfus, 2000.
6.4 Bickley LS. Bates' Guide to Physical Examination and History Taking, 7th ed. Philadelphia: Lippincott Williams & Wilkins, 1999.
6.5 Neville B, et al. Color Atlas of Clinical Oral Pathology. Philadelphia: Lea & Febiger, 1991.
6.6 Asset provided by Anatomical Chart Co.
6.7 DeVita VT, Hellamen S, Rosenberg S, et al. AIDS: Etiology, Diagnosis, Treatment, and Prevention, 4th ed. Philadelphia: Lippincott Williams & Wilkins, 1997.
6.8 Asset provided by Anatomical Chart Co.
6.9 Koopman WJ, Moreland LW. Arthritis and Allied Conditions: A Textbook of Rheumatology, 15th ed. Philadelphia: Lippincott Williams & Wilkins, 2005.
6.11 Goodheart HP. Goodheart's Photoguide of Common Skin Disorders, 2nd ed. Philadelphia: Lippincott Williams & Wilkins, 2003.
6.12 Porth CM. Essentials of Pathophysiology: Concepts of Altered Health States, 2nd ed. Philadelphia: Lippincott Williams & Wilkins, 2007.
6.14 Asset provided by Anatomical Chart Co.
6.16 Rubin E, Gorstein F, Schwarting R, Strayer DS. Rubin's Pathology: Clinicopathologic Foundations of Medicine, 4th ed. Philadelphia: Lippincott Williams & Wilkins, 2005.
6.17 Goodheart HP. Goodheart's Photoguide of Common Skin Disorders, 2nd ed. Philadelphia: Lippincott Williams & Wilkins, 2003.
6.18 Goodheart HP. Goodheart's Photoguide of Common Skin Disorders, 2nd ed. Philadelphia: Lippincott Williams & Wilkins, 2003.
6.19 Rubin E, Farber JL. Pathology. 3rd ed. Philadelphia: Lippincott Williams & Wilkins, 1999.
6.20 Goodheart HP. Goodheart's Photoguide of Common Skin Disorders, 2nd ed. Philadelphia: Lippincott Williams & Wilkins, 2003.
6.21 Goodheart HP. Goodheart's Photoguide of Common Skin Disorders, 2nd ed. Philadelphia: Lippincott Williams & Wilkins, 2003.
6.22 Adapted from ACC.

Chapter 7

7.1 Asset provided by Anatomical Chart Co.
7.3 Asset provided by Anatomical Chart Co.
7.5 Rubin E, Farber JL. Pathology. 3rd ed. Philadelphia: Lippincott Williams & Wilkins, 1999.
7.6 Asset provided by Anatomical Chart Co.
7.7 Asset provided by Anatomical Chart Co.
7.8 Asset provided by Anatomical Chart Co.
7.9 Rubin E, Farber JL. Pathology. 3rd ed. Philadelphia: Lippincott Williams & Wilkins, 1999.
7.10 Asset provided by Anatomical Chart Co.
7.11 Moore KL, Dalley AF. Clinically Oriented Anatomy, 4th ed. Baltimore: Lippincott Williams & Wilkins, 1999.

Chapter 8

8.2 Asset provided by Anatomical Chart Co.
8.4 Asset provided by Anatomical Chart Co.

8.5 Asset provided by Anatomical Chart Co.
8.6 Asset provided by Anatomical Chart Co.
8.7 Rubin E, Farber JL. Pathology. 3rd ed. Philadelphia: Lippincott Williams & Wilkins, 1999.
8.9 Asset provided by Anatomical Chart Co.
8.10 LifeArt image.
8.11 Asset provided by Anatomical Chart Co.
8.12 Sun T. Parasitic Disorders: Pathology, Diagnosis, and Management, 2nd ed. Philadelphia: Lippincott Williams & Wilkins, 1999.
8.13 Rubin E, Farber JL. Pathology. 3rd ed. Philadelphia: Lippincott Williams & Wilkins, 1999.
8.15 Rubin E, Farber JL. Pathology. 3rd ed. Philadelphia: Lippincott Williams & Wilkins, 1999.
8.16 Asset provided by Anatomical Chart Co.
8.17 LWW's Organism Central.

Chapter 9

9.1 Smeltzer SC, Bare BG. Brunner & Suddarth's Textbook of Medical-Surgical Nursing, 9th ed. Philadelphia: Lippincott Williams & Wilkins, 2000.
9.3 Weber J, Kelley J. Health Assessment in Nursing, 2nd ed. Philadelphia: Lippincott Williams & Wilkins, 2003.

Chapter 10

10.1 Asset provided by Anatomical Chart Co.
10.3 Rubin E, Gorstein F, Schwarting R, Strayer DS. Rubin's Pathology: Clinicopathologic Foundations of Medicine, 4th ed. Philadelphia: Lippincott Williams & Wilkins, 2005.
10.4 Asset provided by Anatomical Chart Co.
10.5 McConnell TH. The Nature Of Disease: Pathology for the Health Professions, Philadelphia: Lippincott Williams & Wilkins, 2007.
10.6 Asset provided by Anatomical Chart Co.

Chapter 11

11.3 Asset provided by Anatomical Chart Co.
11.4 Asset provided by Anatomical Chart Co.
11.5 Asset provided by Anatomical Chart Co.
11.6 Asset provided by Anatomical Chart Co.
11.7 Adapted from asset provided by Anatomical Chart Co.
11.8 Mitchell GW. The Female Breast and its Disorders. Baltimore: Williams & Wilkins, 1990.
11.9 Asset provided by Anatomical Chart Co.
11.11 Rubin E, Gorstein F, Schwarting R, Strayer DS. Rubin's Pathology: Clinicopathologic Foundations of Medicine, 4th ed. Philadelphia: Lippincott Williams & Wilkins, 2005.

Chapter 12

12.1 Gold DH, Weingeist TA. Color Atlas of the Eye in Systemic Disease. Philadelphia: Lippincott Williams & Wilkins, 2001.
12.2 Rubin E, Gorstein F, Schwarting R, Strayer DS. Rubin's Pathology: Clinicopathologic Foundations of Medicine, 4th ed. Philadelphia: Lippincott Williams & Wilkins, 2005.

Index

Note: Page numbers followed by f denote figures; those followed by t indicate tables.

B

D

H

M

N

O

Q

R

S

U